Fractures in Sport

Greg A. J. Robertson • Nicola Maffulli
Editors

Fractures in Sport

Springer

Editors
Greg A. J. Robertson
Edinburgh Orthopaedic Trauma Unit
Royal Infirmary of Edinburgh
Edinburgh
UK

Nicola Maffulli
Centre for Sports and Exercise Medicine
Queen Mary University of London
London
UK

ISBN 978-3-030-72035-3   ISBN 978-3-030-72036-0 (eBook)
https://doi.org/10.1007/978-3-030-72036-0

This Springer imprint is published by the registered company Springer Nature Switzerland AG
The registered company address is: Gewerbestrasse 11, 6330 Cham, Switzerland

Preface

David Beckham, Chris Froome, Henrik Larsson, Paula Radcliffe and Alex Smith, to name a few, have two things in common: they are all high-profile athletes, and they all suffered a fracture while playing their sport. We vividly remember the trauma of the event, yet these injuries had not just a physical effect. It is easy to overlook the anguish of the athlete at being unable to continue playing, the anxiety of the athlete and the team about whether and when they can return, and the onus on the treating physician to provide the optimal treatment possible to facilitate this. More specifically, those privileged surgeons and physicians may not necessarily have the luxury of keeping such patients in plaster on crutches for several weeks, as they gradually settle back into their sedentary jobs, with occasional light sessions in the gym and the pool. These elite professional patients are itching to return to weightbearing, training and sport, as soon as feasible—not only for their own personal achievement and mental well-being, but also for their own and their team's financial requirements. So, with an insight into the complexities of managing fractures in sport, the editors realised the need to provide high-quality, athlete-focussed fracture care for this population.

Fractures in Sport provides clinicians with a practically applicable sport-centred guide to fracture management for athletes. The focus is to provide the optimal management of fracture care for athletic patients and to facilitate the most expedient return to sport possible, with the lowest side effect.

The principles of fracture management have been extensively developed over the last century. However, the focus of most fracture-based research has been to optimise fracture care within the general population, particularly for the commonly encountered 'osteoporotic' fractures. When athletes do experience a fracture, however, we enter a completely different 'ball game', with major differences in mechanism of injury, common fracture locations, common fracture patterns, the physiological status of the patient, their pre-fracture functional level, the physiological response to fracture care and the functional expectations in post-fracture care. As such, while certain key factors from generic fracture care can be translated into the management of fractures in the athlete, the principles and practice of sport-related fracture care require specific defining, to provide optimal treatment and outcomes for these patients.

Until now, such principles were poorly defined, and most athletes have been managed using the standard principles of fracture care for the general population. This text attempts to provide an athlete-centred approach to fracture care. *Fractures in Sport* should be a valuable guide for practising and trainee orthopaedic surgeons, sports medicine physicians, family physicians, allied health professionals in orthopaedics and sports medicine, and medical students.

Fractures in Sport is divided into seven sections. The first section presents information relevant to the epidemiology and basic science principles of fracture management in athletes. The next three sections detail site-specific acute fracture assessment and management in athletes, covering the upper limb, the lower limb and the axial skeleton, respectively. The last three sections detail site-specific stress fracture assessment and management in athletes, covering the upper limb, the lower limb and the axial skeleton, respectively. Throughout, we aimed to enable readers to develop a deep understanding of the ideal management principles available to manage fractures in these high-functioning, and at times demanding, patients.

The editors have had a clear interest in fracture care of athletes for several years. Both have published leading research studies on this topic and have a robust knowledge of the current evidence-based recommendations that guide optimal practice in this field. The individual chapter authors are experts in each of the relevant fields of interest, based on their previous research and publications. Together, this text then provides the combined guidance of a group of internationally recognised experts in the fields of orthopaedic trauma, sports trauma, sports medicine and rehabilitation.

We thank all of the authors who have contributed to *Fractures in Sport*. Without their combined hard work and dedication, this project would not have been possible. Additionally, we would like to acknowledge the advice and support from the staff at the Edinburgh Orthopaedic Trauma Unit, who have been helpful in shaping the concept of the text, and the support and input of the Academic Department of the Faculty of Medicine, Surgery and Dentistry of the University of Salerno, together with the expertise of the Centre for Sport and Exercise Medicine, Barts and The Royal London School of Medicine, Queen Mary University of London. Last but not least, both the editors thank their families for their ever present support and understanding: to them, we remain deeply thankful.

The editors wish the reader every success in translating the knowledge from this book, to provide optimal care for the injured athletes who will come under their care.

Edinburgh, UK Greg A. J. Robertson
London, UK Nicola Maffulli

The original version of this book was revised. The correction to this book can be found at https://doi.org/10.1007/978-3-030-72036-0_30

Contents

Part I

Epidemiology and Basic Sciences

The Epidemiology of Acute Fractures in Sport

1

Charles M. Court-Brown

Learning Objectives

- To understand the epidemiology of sports related fractures
- To understand which sports are associated with the highest prevalence of fractures.
- To understand which fractures are most commonly seen in sports injuries.
- To appreciate the changing epidemiology of sports fractures.

There has been very little scientific work on the epidemiology of sports related fractures. Many studies have focused on different sports, where different body areas have been examined to determine the prevalence of sports injuries. However, it is often impossible to determine the prevalence of fractures as opposed to soft tissue injuries. The injuries are not infrequently combined into body areas such as upper and lower limbs or hand, foot and ankle and, in real terms, there is little information regarding the types of fractures caused by sport. In addition, good epidemiological data can only be obtained from well documented information about all the fractures in a defined population. This is usually impossible, as most large cities have several hospitals managing trauma, and it is difficult to collate information from all hospitals. In addition, most developed countries have a private medical system in addition and in parallel to a state system. The private system will deal with many of the less severe injuries, and to obtain good information all private surgeons would need to be successfully consulted. This is not realistic.

In Edinburgh, Scotland, up to about 2015, all minor and major trauma was treated in one hospital and there were no private acute trauma units. Thus, all fractures were reviewed and treated in one single hospital, The Royal Infirmary of Edinburgh. Scotland also has a good postcode system, and we have been able to reliably assess the epidemiology of all fractures by restricting the analysis of fractures to those from the City of Edinburgh, Midlothian and East Lothian. The Royal Infirmary is the only hospital treating orthopaedic trauma in these areas. The adult population (≥16 years) was 558,220 in 2010.

Another advantage of collecting epidemiological information in Edinburgh is that in three 1-year periods between 2000 and 2011 all fracture data were collected and analysed by experienced orthopaedic trauma surgeons. In the literature the implication is that all data, particularly 'Big Data', are accurate and correct: this is simply not the case. A study of fracture diagnosis by Emergency Department staff in the Royal Infirmary of Edinburgh in 2007/2008 showed that 25% of the fractures were incorrectly diagnosed, mainly by inexperienced staff [1]. This is important, as there have been many studies of large databases where it is highly likely that the initial diagnosis has been made by inexperienced medical staff. A number of studies of all in-patient and out-patient fractures during a year, where the diagnosis has been made by an experienced surgeon, have been undertaken. The information about sports fractures in this chapter comes from a prospective study undertaken between September 2010 and August 2011 [2]. All patients aged 16 years and above were included in the study. This study will be used to provide much of the data for this chapter. Where necessary, it will be compared with data from an equivalent study in 2000 [3].

The other difficulty in analysing sports related fractures is the long standing argument of what constitutes a sport. The definition of a sport often states that it is an activity that requires skill and physical fitness, and is played according to codified rules. Nevertheless, some authorities accept bridge, draughts and chess as sports [4]: the four dance fractures reported in this chapter may well have required greater physical fitness than fractures related to golf, bowling and curling!

There are about 8000 different sports in the world [5]. Many of these are played in a particular area by a small num-

C. M. Court-Brown (✉)
Professor of Orthopaedic Trauma, University of Edinburgh, Royal Infirmary of Edinburgh, Edinburgh, UK
e-mail: ccb@courtbrown.com

G. A. J. Robertson, N. Maffulli (eds.), *Fractures in Sport*, https://doi.org/10.1007/978-3-030-72036-0_1

ber of participants, and may well be very similar to other sports. For example, there are over 70 types of football and rugby, over 30 equestrian sports, and over 20 types of hockey [5]. Clearly it is impossible to determine the epidemiology of fractures caused by all sports, and the best than one can do is to determine the epidemiology of sports related fractures in the more popular sports. Even this is difficult because while soccer, or association football, tennis and basketball are global sports, cricket is mainly played in the United Kingdom and the British Commonwealth, and baseball is mainly played in the United States, Caribbean and Japan. This chapter will attempt to analyse the epidemiology of sports related fractures in a large UK City where all fractures were seen by an orthopaedic surgeon experienced in trauma. The literature will be examined, where possible, to determine the epidemiology of other sports. The sports that have been analysed will be divided into different types to allow comparison with sports that did not present in the study year or are played in other parts of the world. Fractures will be classified using the AO/OTA classification [6], and open fractures will be classified using the Gustilo classification [7, 8].

1.1 Overall Epidemiology

During the study year, 6996 fractures in adults ≥16 years of age were treated [2]. The overall incidence of adult fractures was 1351.7/10^5/year, and the average age was 53.2 years. Patients ≥65 years suffered 34.0% of the fractures, and 17.3% occurred in patients aged ≥80 years. There were six major causes of fracture these being sports injuries, falls from a standing height, falls from a low height (<6 ft) or down stairs, falls from a greater height, direct blows or assaults, and road traffic accidents. In addition, 0.9% of fractures were pathological, stress or spontaneous fractures or their cause was unknown. Table 1.1 shows the basic epidemiological characteristics of the different causes of fracture.

Table 1.1 shows that sport was the third commonest cause of fractures, accounting for 772 (11.1%) of all the fractures in the study year. In males, sport caused 19.4% of all fractures, whereas in females, sport only accounted for 3.8% of fractures. The high prevalence of sports fractures emphasizes the importance of investigating their epidemiology. Table 1.1 also indicates that sport fractures tend to be less severe than fractures from other causes. Only 0.6% of sports fractures were open, and only 2.2% of people with sports fractures presented with multiple fractures.

The age related distribution of sports fractures in 2010/2011 is shown in Fig. 1.1. In males, there is a gradual decline in the incidence of fractures with increasing age from

Table 1.1 The comparative epidemiology of all fractures treated in a 1 year period in 2010/2011. The different modes of injury are shown as is the prevalence of the different fracture types

	Sport	Fall	Low fall	Fall height	Direct blow	RTA	Other
Average age (years)	30.8	61.8	51.1	35.5	32.8	35.5	53.8
	%						
All fractures	11.1	62.5	4.3	2.3	13.6	5.2	0.9
Males	19.4	40.1	4.6	4.3	21.9	8.7	0.8
Females	3.8	82.4	3.9	0.5	6.3	2.1	0.8
Open fractures	0.6	0.5	3.1	10.6	5.8	6.4	0
Multiple fractures	2.2	3.9	6.7	32.6	5.7	16.0	0
Upper limb	%						
Clavicle	25.3	40.5	5.8	1.2	4.7	22.2	0.4
Scapula	8.1	40.5	13.5	10.8	0	27.0	0
Proximal humerus	4.2	85.4	5.4	0.2	1.5	2.5	0.8
Humeral diaphysis	8.6	71.4	4.3	0	11.4	1.4	2.9
Distal humerus	6.2	72.9	2.1	4.2	4.2	10.4	0
Proximal forearm	13.0	64.0	6.9	2.1	2.9	10.8	0.3
Forearm diaphyses	27.3	49.1	3.6	1.8	9.1	7.3	1.8
Distal radius/ulna	9.5	79.9	3.8	0.9	2.2	3.5	0.1
Carpus	18.6	58.8	4.1	1.5	9.8	6.7	0.5
Metacarpus	10.9	23.8	1.3	0.8	58.1	4.5	0.6
Finger phalanges	23.8	29.5	2.1	0.6	39.2	4.1	0.8
Total	13.3	56.3	3.8	1.0	19.2	5.9	0.5
Lower limb							
Proximal femur	0.8	93.4	2.7	0.4	0.1	0.9	1.7
Femoral diaphysis	1.2	70.4	3.7	4.9	0	9.9	9.9
Distal femur	2.8	86.1	5.6	2.8	0	2.8	0
Patella	2.0	75.5	4.1	2.0	4.1	10.2	2.0
Proximal tibia	25.4	33.9	15.3	3.4	8.5	13.6	0
Tibial diaphysis	26.1	44.9	5.8	2.9	4.3	15.9	0
Fibula	23.8	45.2	2.4	4.8	11.9	11.9	0
Distal tibia	7.1	38.1	7.1	33.3	2.4	11.9	0
Ankle	11.2	79.8	4.3	0.7	1.8	1.7	0.4
Hindfoot	7.8	15.6	14.3	53.2	5.2	2.6	1.3
Fibula	22.0	46.3	2.4	4.9	12.2	12.2	0
Midfoot	17.9	32.1	14.3	25.0	7.1	14.3	3.6
Metatarsus	8.8	71.6	4.1	1.1	8.6	3.9	1.9
Toe phalanges	15.7	16.7	2.0	0	61.8	2.9	1.0
Total	8.1	73.7	4.4	3.5	5.5	3.4	1.1
Axial skeleton							
Spine	8.7	23.1	22.1	26.9	1.0	16.3	1.9
Pelvis	3.4	82.4	3.4	2.5	0	9.2	0
Total	5.8	54.7	12.1	13.9	0.4	12.1	0.9

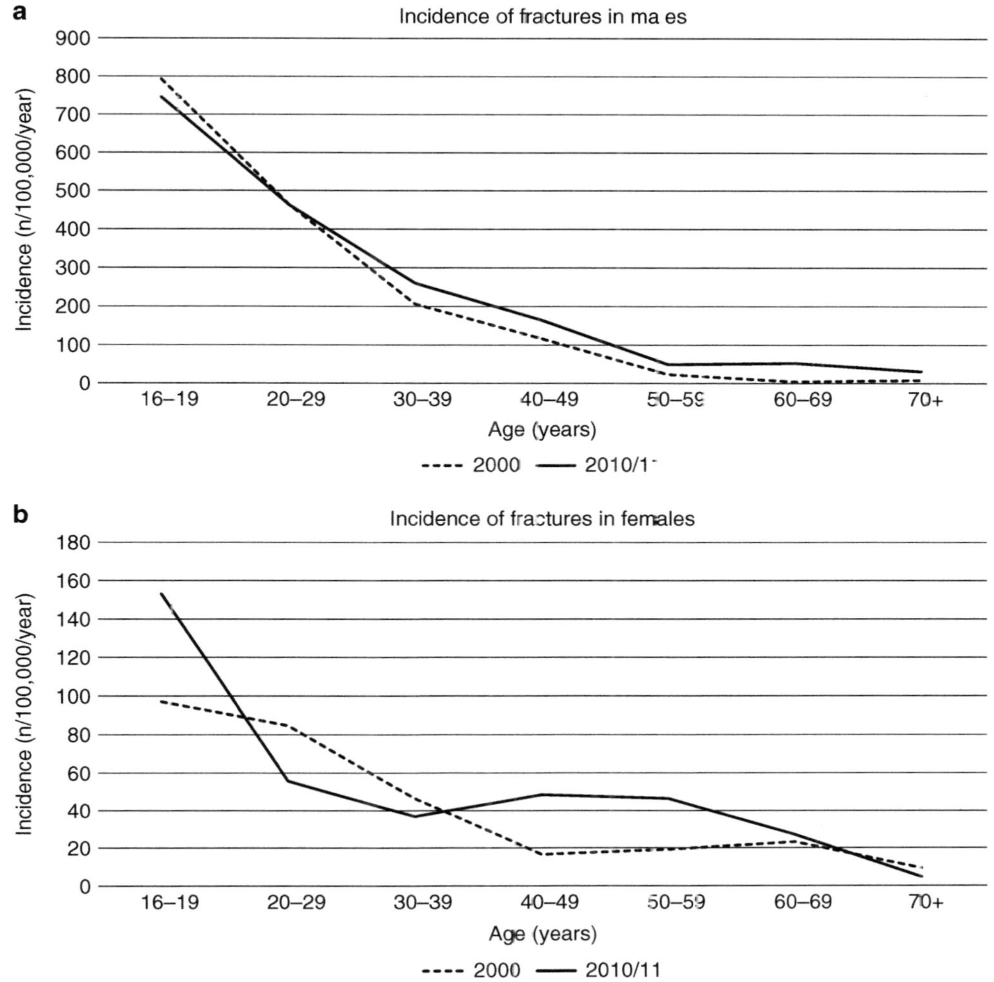

Fig. 1.1 (**a**) The changing incidence of sports fractures in males between 2000 and 2010/2011. (**b**) The changing incidence of sports fractures in females between 2000 and 2010/2011

745.7/10^5/year in 16–19 year old males to 30.5/10^5/year in males of 70+ years (Fig. 1.1a). In females, a similar decline in incidence, from 153/10^5/year to 4.3/10^5/year, is seen with increasing age, although Fig. 1.1b shows a slight increase in incidence in middle age.

Table 1.1 also shows the percentage of specific fractures caused by the different mechanisms of injury. Given the very high prevalence of fractures in older females following a fall from standing height, it is not surprising that there is no fracture where sports injuries cause the highest prevalence of fractures. However, it should be noted that sports injuries are the second commonest cause of fractures of the clavicle, proximal forearm, forearm diaphyses, distal radius and ulna and carpus in the upper limb, and of proximal tibial, tibial diaphysis, fibula, ankle and metatarsal fractures in the lower limb. Sports injuries cause a considerable number of fractures of the hand and wrist and foot and ankle: an overall analysis shows that sports injuries cause 13.8% of fractures of the hand and wrist, and 10.7% of fractures of the foot and ankle. In both areas, falls from a standing height are responsible for the highest prevalence of these fractures, causing 51.5% of hand and wrist fractures, and 67.9% of foot and ankle fractures.

Table 1.2 lists the fractures caused by sports injuries, and shows the prevalence of the different fractures. Overall, 72.0% of sports fractures are upper limb fractures, 26.3% are lower limb fractures, and only 1.7% are fractures of the axial skeleton. All areas have a similar male/female ratio, with about 80% of sports fractures occurring in males. Given the age distribution shown in Fig. 1.1, it is not surprising that the average age of people with sports fractures is 30.8 years, with a similar average age in upper limb and lower limb fractures, and a slightly higher average age in fractures of the axial skeleton. The average age of females with sports fractures is about 5 years more than in males.

Table 1.2 The numbers and percentages of the different sports fractures treated during the study year. The gender ratios, average ages and prevalence of open and multiple fractures are shown

Fractures	n	%	M/F (%)	Age (years) All	Male	Female	Open (%)	Multiple (%)
Upper limb								
Clavicle	65	8.4	91/9	28.0	27.2	36.3	0	1.5
Scapula	3	0.4	100/0	46.7	46.7	----	0	66.7
Proximal humerus	20	2.6	65/35	45.4	43.6	48.7	0	0
Humeral diaphysis	6	0.8	83/17	31.2	31.6	29.0	0	0
Distal humerus	3	0.4	100/0	43.3	43.3	----	0	0
Proximal forearm	49	6.3	78/22	31.6	31.2	32.9	0	8.2
Forearm diaphysis	15	1.9	93/7	32.2	31.6	44.0	0	0
Distal radius/ulna	116	15.0	80/20	32.3	30.7	38.7	0.9	1.7
Carpus	36	4.7	92/8	25.8	23.9	47.0	0	2.7
Metacarpus	85	11.0	89/11	28.0	27.7	30.4	0	6.2
Finger phalanges	158	20.5	82/18	29.1	29.3	28.2	1.3	1.9
Total	556	72.0	84/16	30.4	29.5	34.7	0.5	2.2
Lower limb								
Proximal femur	6	0.8	83/17	51.2	41.3	59.0	0	0
Femoral diaphysis	1	0.1	0/100	48.0	----	48.0	0	0
Distal femur	1	0.1	100/0	16.0	16.0	----	0	0
Patella	1	0.1	100/0	18.0	18.0	----	0	0
Proximal tibia	15	1.9	80/20	43.1	39.7	56.7	0	6.7
Tibial diaphysis	18	2.3	83/17	29.3	29.0	31.0	11.1	0
Fibula	9	1.2	100/0	32.8	32.8	----	0	0
Distal tibia	3	0.4	100/0	30.3	30.3	----	0	0
Ankle	80	10.4	77/23	32.0	30.8	36.1	0	2.5
Hindfoot	6	0.8	50/50	33.2	32.7	33.7	0	16.7
Midfoot	5	0.6	60/40	32.2	22.0	47.5	0	0
Metatarsus	41	5.3	73/27	26.9	26.7	27.4	0	2.6
Toe phalanges	16	2.1	94/6	25.2	25.1	27.0	0	0
Total	203	26.3	79/21	31.6	30.4	35.9	1.0	2.0
Axial skeleton								
Spine	9	1.2	44/56	34.7	40.2	30.2	0	28.6
Pelvis	4	0.5	50/50	37.5	34.5	40.5	0	0
Total	13	1.7	46/54	35.5	38.3	33.1	0	18.2
Overall total	772	100	82/18	30.8	29.8	35.0	0.6	2.2

There are a number of fractures where the average age is higher. This is true of fractures which normally present in older patients, such as proximal humeral, proximal femoral, femoral diaphyseal and spinal fractures, but fractures of the scapula, distal humerus, proximal tibia and midfoot also present at a slightly higher average age, particularly in females. This may represent a changing distribution of sports fractures, with an increased interest in sports by middle aged females, as suggested in Fig. 1.1.

Sports fractures are associated with a low prevalence of open fractures and multiple fractures compared with other causes of fracture (Table 1.1). Table 1.2 shows that tibial diaphyseal fractures are associated with the highest prevalence of open fractures and scapula fractures, hindfoot fractures and spinal fractures with the highest prevalence of multiple fractures. Open and multiple fractures will be discussed later in the chapter.

Table 1.3 shows the incidence of different sports fractures in different age groups in both males and females. The use of fracture incidence ($\times/10^5$/year) as opposed to simply using prevalence (%) is important, as the population numbers vary with age, and one can thus calculate the numbers of sports fractures seen in each group. One can also calculate the numbers of sports fractures that can be expected to occur in other geographical areas with similar sporting activities. Figure 1.1 shows that the incidence of sports fractures decreases with increasing age, but Table 1.3 allows us to calculate that males aged 50+ will present with 9.8% of the number of fractures that will occur in 16–35 year old males. The equivalent figure for females is 32.7%, which is probably higher than most orthopaedic surgeons would expect. The equivalent figures for upper and lower limb fractures in males are 7.8% and 15.4% in males, and 28.0% and 41.4% in females. In older females, one would expect a high number of fractures fol-

Table 1.3 The incidences of the sports fractures treated during the study year. The overall incidence of fractures in males and females and at three different age groups are shown

	Male incidence (×/10^5/year)				Female incidence (×/10^5/year)			
Fractures	All	16–35	36–49	50+	All	16–35	36–49	50+
Upper limb								
Clavicle	22.2	48.4	10.9	2.0	2.1	2.8	2.9	0.8
Scapula	1.1	0	4.7	0	0	0	0	0
Proximal humerus	4.9	3.9	7.8	4.1	2.4	1.9	2.9	2.5
Humeral diaphysis	1.9	2.9	3.1	0	0.3	0.9	0	0
Distal humerus	1.1	1.9	0	1.0	0	0	0	0
Proximal forearm	14.9	26.2	12.4	3.0	3.8	5.7	4.4	1.7
Forearm diaphysis	5.2	10.7	3.1	1.0	0.3	0	1.4	0
Distal radius/ulna	35.0	62.0	35.8	6.1	7.8	8.5	11.7	5.1
Carpus	12.4	30.0	3.1	0	1.0	0.9	1.5	0.8
Metacarpus	28.6	58.1	20.2	3.0	3.1	6.6	1.5	0.8
Finger phalanges	48.5	93.0	42.0	6.1	9.9	20.8	7.3	1.7
Total	175.2	337.1	143.0	26.4	30.8	48.2	33.7	13.5
Lower limb								
Proximal femur	1.9	1.0	1.6	3.0	0.3	0	0	0.8
Femoral diaphysis	0	0	0	0	0.3	0	1.5	0
Distal femur	0.4	1.0	0	0	0	0	0	0
Patella	0.4	1.0	0	0	0	0	0	0
Proximal tibia	4.5	5.8	4.7	3.0	1.0	0	0	2.5
Tibial diaphysis	5.6	11.6	3.1	1.0	1.0	1.9	1.5	0
Fibula	3.8	6.8	3.1	1.0	0	0	0	0
Distal tibia	1.1	1.9	1.6	0	0	0	0	0
Ankle	23.3	44.6	10.9	9.1	6.2	10.4	2.9	4.2
Hindfoot	1.1	2.9	0	0	1.0	1.9	0	0.8
Midfoot	1.1	2.9	0	0	0.7	0.9	0	0.8
Metatarsus	11.3	26.2	3.1	1.0	3.8	8.5	1.5	0.8
Toe phalanges	5.6	12.6	3.1	0	0.3	0.9	0	0
Total	60.2	118.2	31.1	18.3	14.7	24.6	7.3	10.2
Axial skeleton								
Spine	1.5	1.0	4.7	0	1.7	3.8	0	0.8
Pelvis	0.8	1.0	1.6	0	0.7	0.9	0	0.8
Total	2.3	2.0	6.2	0	2.4	4.7	0	1.7
Overall total	237.6	457.3	180.3	44.7	47.9	77.6	41.0	25.4

lowing a fall, but it is apparent that they have a relatively high prevalence of sports fractures.

If one extrapolates the data in Table 1.3, in the United Kingdom it is likely that there will be about 125,000 sports fractures each year in people aged ≥16 years. If one applies the data to the United States, it would seem that about 800,000 adults will present with sports fractures each year. This highlights the workload imposed by sports fractures.

Table 1.4 lists the 42 different sports that resulted in fractures during the study year. The numbers and prevalence of the fractures caused by each sport are given together with the gender ratio, average ages and the prevalence of open and multiple fractures. Although 11.1% of all fractures resulted from sports injuries, only 13 sports caused more than 10 fractures in the study year. The remaining 29 sports together only caused 12.2% of all the fractures, less than the fractures resulting from soccer or rugby, and about the same as those associated with cycling. These three sports caused 64.8% of all the sports fractures. Analysis of the gender ratio shows that, while the overall male/female ratio was 82/18, in 6 sports fractures were more commonly seen in females. These were ice skating, horse-riding, sledging, trampolining, badminton, and dancing. In addition, in skiing, snowboarding, roller skating, athletics and bowling the percentage of females presenting with a fracture was higher than average. In several sports the age of patients with fractures was notably higher than average. A number of these were in sports frequently played by older people, such as bowling, fishing and curling and golf, but in other sports such as cycling, skiing, horse-riding, ice skating, athletics, badminton, gymnastics and tennis the age was greater than the overall average, particularly in females.

There were only four sports that resulted in open fractures. This may be one of the few orthopaedic complications of cricket, but skate boarding, rugby and cycling were also associated with open fractures. Only eight sports were associated with multiple fractures.

One must be careful when interpreting Table 1.4. It is tempting to assume that soccer, rugby and cycling are the most dangerous sports, but it is impossible to know how many participants there are in each sport. Clearly this will affect the number of fractures. However, the table does show the spectrum of sports fractures which will present to a busy UK hospital in 1 year.

Table 1.5 lists the incidences of the fractures caused by different sports. The incidence of soccer fractures in 50+ year males is 6.5% that of fractures in 16–35 year males, with the equivalent figures for rugby and cycling being 1.3% and 25.1%, suggesting that few older males play rugby but that cycling is popular. In females the incidence of fractures in 50+ year ladies was higher than in 16–35 year ladies in skiing, ice skating and badminton. Extrapolation of the data in Table 1.5 indicates that in the United Kingdom we can expect to have about 30,000 soccer related fractures each year in males in addition to 8500 fractures from rugby, 7500 from cycling and about 2000 from skiing and basketball. In females, the equivalent figures are about 1100 soccer fractures and 1200 for rugby, cycling, skiing and basketball fractures combined.

Table 1.4 The basic descriptors of the fractures in the different sports treated in the study year. The numbers, percentages, average patient age, gender ratio and prevalence of open and multiple fractures for each sport are shown

			M/F	Age (years)			Open	Multiple
Sports	n	%	(%)	All	Male	Female	(%)	(%)
Soccer	306	39.6	96/4	28.6	28.8	21.7	0	1.7
Rugby	102	13.2	87/13	24.8	24.7	25.5	1.0	0
Cycling	92	11.9	86/14	36.3	35.3	42.4	1.1	4.5
Skiing	33	4.3	61/39	37.6	34.1	42.9	0	0
Basketball	25	3.2	80/20	26.6	24.9	33.4	0	0
Horse riding	23	3.0	13/87	39.8	37.0	40.2	0	4.5
Snowboarding	17	2.2	76/24	23.2	23.2	23.2	0	0
Ice skating	14	1.8	29/71	43.8	37.2	46.4	0	7.7
Martial arts	14	1.8	93/7	25.1	23.6	44.0	0	0
Cricket	13	1.7	100/0	33.5	33.5	---	15.4	0
Hockey	13	1.7	77/23	28.1	31.2	18.0	0	0
Skateboarding	13	1.7	85/15	27.7	28.0	26.0	7.7	0
Sledging	13	1.7	23/77	28.2	32.0	27.1	0	18.2
Roller skating	8	1.0	62/38	23.4	23.0	24.0	0	0
Boxing	7	0.9	86/14	28.4	25.8	44.0	0	0
Motor sports	7	0.9	100/0	19.9	19.9	---	0	16.7
Golf	7	0.9	100/0	61.7	61.7	---	0	0
Trampolining	7	0.9	14/86	26.0	47.0	22.5	0	0
Athletics	6	0.8	50/50	34.2	25.7	42.7	0	0
Badminton	5	0.6	20/80	56.0	44.0	59.0	0	25.0
Gymnastics	5	0.6	80/20	35.2	32.0	48.0	0	0
Arm wrestling	4	0.5	100/0	40.5	40.5	---	0	0
Dancing	4	0.5	0/100	42.7	---	42.7	0	0
Tennis	4	0.5	50/50	46.2	46.5	46.0	0	0
Bowling	3	0.4	67/33	74.7	74.5	75.0	0	0
Mountaineering	3	0.4	100/0	41.3	41.3	---	0	0
Netball	3	0.4	0/100	20.0	---	20.0	0	0
Diving	2	0.3	100/0	41.0	41.0	---	0	50.0
Fishing	2	0.3	100/0	60.0	60.0	---	0	0
Gaelic football	2	0.3	100/0	24.0	24.0	---	0	0
Softball	2	0.3	0/100	32.0	---	32.0	0	0
Squash	2	0.3	100/0	36.5	36.5	---	0	0
Weightlifting	2	0.3	100/0	33.5	33.5	---	0	0
American football	1	0.1	100/0	20.0	20.0	---	0	0
Cross ball	1	0.1	0/100	22.0	---	22.0	0	0
Curling	1	0.1	0/100	59.0	---	59.0	0	0
Curve ball	1	0.1	0/100	22.0	---	22.0	0	0
Lacrosse	1	0.1	100/0	35.0	35.0	---	0	0
Swimming	1	0.1	100/0	19.0	19.0	---	0	0
Volleyball	1	0.1	100/0	25.0	25.0	---	0	0
Water polo	1	0.1	0/100	19.0	---	19.0	0	0
Wrestling	1	0.1	100/0	28.0	28.0	---	0	0
Total	772	100	82/18	30.8	29.8	35.0	0.6	2.2

Table 1.5 The incidences of the fractures caused by each sport. The overall incidence and the incidences in three different age groups are shown

	Male incidence (×/10^5/year)				Female incidence (×/10^5/year)			
Sport	All	16–35	36–49	50+	All	16–35	36–49	50+
Soccer	115.1	235.4	74.6	15.2	4.1	11.4	0	0
Rugby	33.5	79.4	9.3	1.0	4.4	11.4	2.9	0
Cycling	29.7	40.7	42.0	10.2	4.4	4.7	7.3	3.4
Skiing	7.5	10.7	9.3	3.0	4.4	3.8	5.9	4.2
Basketball	7.5	18.4	0	1.0	1.7	3.8	2.9	0
Horse riding	1.1	1.0	3.1	0	6.8	7.6	8.8	5.1
Snowboarding	4.9	11.6	1.6	0	1.4	3.8	0	0
Ice skating	1.5	2.9	0	1.0	3.4	1.9	7.3	3.4
Martial arts	4.9	11.6	1.6	0	0.3	0	1.5	0
Cricket	4.9	7.7	7.8	0	0	0	0	0
Hockey	3.8	6.8	4.7	0	1.0	2.8	0	0
Skateboarding	4.1	7.7	4.7	0	0.7	1.9	1.5	0
Sledging	1.1	1.9	1.6	0	3.4	7.6	1.5	0.8
Roller skating	1.9	4.8	0	0	1.0	2.8	0	0
Boxing	2.3	4.8	1.6	0	0.3	0	1.5	0
Motor sports	2.6	6.8	0	0	0	0	0	0
Golf	2.6	0	0	7.1	0	0	0	0
Trampolining	0.4	0	1.6	0	2.1	5.7	0	0
Athletics	1.1	1.9	1.6	0	1.0	0.9	1.5	0.8
Badminton	0.4	0	1.6	0	1.4	0	0	3.4
Gymnastics	1.5	1.9	3.1	0	0.3	0	1.5	0
Arm wrestling	1.5	1.9	1.6	1.0	0	0	0	0
Dancing	0	0	0	0	1.4	1.9	0	1.7
Tennis	0.8	1.0	0	1.0	0.7	0	1.5	0.8
Bowling	0.8	0	0	2.0	0.3	0	0	0.8
Mountaineering	1.1	1.0	3.1	0	0	0	0	0
Netball	0	0	0	0	1.0	2.8	0	0
Diving	0.8	0	3.1	0	0	0	0	0
Fishing	0.8	0	1.6	1.0	0	0	0	0
Gaelic football	0.8	1.9	0	0	0	0	0	0
Softball	0	0	0	0	0.7	0.9	1.5	0
Squash	0.8	1.0	0	1.0	0	0	0	0
Weightlifting	0.8	1.0	1.6	0	0	0	0	0
American football	0.4	1.0	0	0	0	0	0	0
Cross ball	0	0	0	0	0.3	0.9	0	0
Curling	0	0	0	0	0.3	0	0	0.8
Curve ball	0	0	0	0	0.3	0.9	0	0
Lacrosse	0.4	1.0	0	0	0	0	0	0
Swimming	0.4	1.0	0	0	0	0	0	0
Volleyball	0.4	1.0	0	0	0	0	0	0
Water polo	0	0	0	0	0.3	0.9	0	0
Wrestling	0.4	1.0	0	0	0	0	0	0
Total	237.6	457.3	180.3	44.7	47.9	77.6	46.8	25.4

1.2 Types of Sport

Table 1.6 shows the epidemiology of fractures in different types of sport. The sports shown in Table 1.4 have been divided into ball sports and sports where a ball is not used. They have then been subdivided into sports where there is no physical contact and sports where there is physical contact between players. A fifth type of sport was added because of the potential difference in fracture epidemiology. This type includes sports undertaken at speeds faster than running or at a height. Table 1.6 shows that soccer has been considered separately from other non-contact ball sports. This was done because it is the most popular sport in the world but also because, while it may theoretically be a non-contact sport, few people believe that! Non-contact ball sports include sports such as basketball, cricket, golf, field hockey and tennis. Contact ball sports include rugby, American football and Gaelic football, and contact non-ball sports include martial arts, boxing and arm wrestling. Non-contact sports played without a ball include athletics, gymnastics, fishing and weightlifting. Sports which are undertaken at speed, or at a height, include cycling, skiing, skateboarding, motor sports, horse riding and trampolining. These subdivisions have been used to analyse the effect of different types of sport on fracture epidemiology, and to suggest what range of fractures might be seen in other sports if one knows how they are played.

Table 1.6 shows that non-contact sports, excluding soccer, caused relatively few fractures in the study year. This is also true of non-contact non-ball sports. Non-contact ball sports resulted in a higher prevalence of upper and lower limb fractures than non-contact non-ball sports, but the main difference was the higher prevalence of metacarpal and finger phalangeal fractures. The prevalence of fractures associated with physical contact non-ball sports is also low. There were three such sports, namely martial arts, boxing and arm wrestling. Table 1.6 shows that the highest prevalence of fractures occurred in soccer and in sports involving speed or a fall from a height. It is perhaps surprising that there was a higher prevalence of fractures in soccer, but soccer is by far the most popular sport, and Table 1.6 shows that 96% of the fractures occurred in males, many of whom were young.

One might reasonably assume that higher-energy fractures associated with speed or height might have a higher prevalence, but Table 1.6 shows that they tend to occur in older patients and 35% occurred in females. However, all

Table 1.6 The sports have been divided into six different types. See text for details. The prevalence of all fractures in the six different types of sport are shown together with gender ratios, average age and prevalence of open and multiple fractures

	Ball sports			Other sports		
	Non-contact		Physical contact	Non-contact	Physical contact	Speed/height
	Soccer	Other				
Fractures (%)	39.6	10.5	13.6	2.8	3.4	30.1
Average age (year)	28.6	35.6	24.5	38.1	28.5	34.2
Gender ratio (%)	96/4 %	73/27	88/12	54/46	92/8	65/35
Upper limb						
Clavicle	32.3	4.6	15.4	0	1.5	46.1
Scapula	0	0	0	0	0	100
Proximal humerus	10.0	15.0	5.0	0	0	70.0
Humeral diaphysis	16.7	0	0	16.7	16.7	50.0
Distal humerus	66.7	33.3	0	0	0	0
Proximal forearm	30.6	4.1	0	4.1	4.1	57.1
Forearm diaphysis	66.7	0	20.0	0	13.3	0
Distal radius/ulna	58.6	4.3	4.3	0.8	1.7	30.2
Carpus	41.7	11.1	8.3	0	5.6	33.3
Metacarpus	29.4	11.8	23.5	1.2	9.4	24.7
Finger phalanges	34.8	20.3	25.9	2.5	1.9	14.6
Total	38.5	10.8	14.9	1.6	3.8	30.4
Lower limb						
Proximal femur	0	16.6	0	16.6	0	66.7
Femoral diaphysis	0	0	50.0	0	0	50.0
Distal femur	100	0	0	0	0	0
Patella	100	0	0	0	0	0
Proximal tibia	33.3	0	0	13.3	0	53.3
Tibial diaphysis	50.0	5.6	16.7	0	0	27.8
Fibula	30.0	10.0	30.0	0	10.0	20.0
Distal tibia	33.3	0	33.3	0	0	33.3
Ankle	46.2	15.0	13.7	3.7	2.5	18.7
Hindfoot	16.7	0	0	16.7	0	66.7
Midfoot	40.0	20.0	20.0	20.0	0	0
Metatarsus	51.2	7.3	4.9	12.2	2.4	22.0
Toe phalanges	68.7	12.5	6.2	0	6.2	6.2
Total	45.3	10.3	10.8	6.4	2.5	24.6
Axial skeleton						
Spine	0	0	0	0	0	100
Pelvis	0	0	0	0	0	100
Total	0	0	0	0	0	100
Open fractures	0	2.5	1.0	0	0	0.9
Multiple fractures	1.7	1.2	0	0	0	4.5

fractures of the axial skeleton occurred in speed/height sports, with 46.1% occurring in winter sports and 23.1% in horse riding.

Table 1.2 shows that fractures of the hand and wrist account for 71.0% of all sports related upper limb fractures, and fractures of the foot and ankle account for 72.9% of all lower limb fractures. Table 1.7 shows the distribution of sports related fractures of the hand and wrist and foot and ankle in the different types of sports. There were relatively few fractures in either location in the non-ball non-contact or contact sports. Most hand and wrist fractures occurred as a result of soccer injuries, although physical contact sports, such as rugby, caused a number of phalangeal and metacarpal fractures, with speed/height sports mainly causing metacarpal, carpal and distal radial fractures.

The location of finger phalangeal fractures was similar in all types of sport. Most fractures occur in the ring and little fingers, but there was a high prevalence of thumb fractures in speed/height sports. A similar distribution is seen in metacarpal fractures the only difference being a higher prevalence of fractures in the thumb in non-contact ball sports. These occurred in hockey, lacrosse and cricket, where a bat or stick

Table 1.7 The prevalence of finger phalangeal, metacarpal, carpal, distal radial, ankle hindfoot and midfoot, metatarsal and toe fractures in each different of sport. Each fracture type has been subdivided into different locations or types and the prevalence of each location or type is given

	Ball sports			Other sports		
	No contact		Physical contact	No contact	Physical contact	Speed/height
	Soccer	Other sports				
	%					
Fractures						
Phalanges	34.8	20.3	25.9	2.5	1.9	14.6
Thumb	12.7	18.7	9.8	12.5	25.0	34.8
Index	7.3	12.5	7.3	0	0	4.3
Middle	10.9	9.4	17.1	12.5	0	13.0
Ring	34.5	25.0	31.7	25.0	25.0	30.4
Little	34.5	18.7	34.1	50.0	50.0	17.4
Metacarpus	29.4	11.8	23.5	1.2	9.4	24.7
Thumb	4.0	30.0	5.0	0	0	9.5
Index	20.0	20.0	20.0	0	25.0	14.3
Middle	16.0	0	20.0	0	0	19.0
Ring	8.0	30.0	40.0	0	12.5	19.0
Little	52.0	20.0	15.0	100	62.5	38.1
Carpus	41.7	11.1	8.3	0	5.6	33.3
Scaphoid	80.0	75.0	100	0	100	75.0
Triquetrum	20.0	25.0	0	0	0	25.0
Distal radius	58.6	4.3	4.3	0.8	1.7	30.2
Type A	64.7	40.0	80.0	100	100	57.1
Type B	23.5	40.0	20.0	0	0	22.9
Type C	11.8	20.0	0	0	0	20.0
Ankle	46.2	15.0	13.7	3.7	2.5	18.7
Type A	31.6	33.3	27.3	33.3	0	26.7
Type B	50.0	50.0	45.4	66.6	50.0	60.0
Type C	18.4	16.7	27.3	0	50.0	13.3
Hindfoot/midfoot	27.2	9.1	9.1	18.2	0	36.4
Metatarsus	51.2	7.3	4.9	12.2	2.4	22.0
Hallux	9.5	0	0	0	100	11.1
2nd toe	9.5	33.3	0	0	0	11.1
3rd toe	4.8	33.3	0	0	0	11.1
4th toe	4.8	0	0	0	0	11.1
5th toe	71.4	33.3	100.0	100	0	55.6
Toes	68.7	12.5	6.2	0	6.2	6.2

is used, and the fractures probably resulted from a direct blow. Further analysis showed that 33.5% of phalangeal fractures occurred in the distal phalanx, 39.9% in the middle phalanx, or proximal phalanx of the thumb, and 26.6% in the proximal phalanx of the other fingers. There were very few phalangeal fractures in non-ball non-contact and contact sports, but in these types of sport the fracture distribution in the phalanges was very similar to the overall distribution.

Carpal fractures most commonly occur in soccer or speed/height sports, and about 80% involve the scaphoid. Distal radial fractures show a similar distribution, with 88.8% of them occurring as a result of soccer or a speed/height injury, presumably mainly as a result of a fall while running in soccer, and a relatively high-energy injury in speed/height injuries. Most distal radial fractures are Type A, although 20% of fractures following speed/height injuries were Type C in severity. The 20% prevalence of Type C fractures in non-contact ball sports resulted from only one fracture in basketball.

With regard to lower limb injuries, almost half of the ankle fractures occurred as a result of soccer, presumably as a result of a fall while running. Most ankle fractures were Type B fractures. Hindfoot and midfoot fractures are unusual in sport. There were only two sports calcaneal fractures: one occurred as a result of a fall from a height while horse riding, and the other from a fall while running. There were four talar fractures as a result of soccer, skiing, trampolining and rock climbing, and five midfoot fractures with two soccer injuries, the others being caused by dancing, rugby and badminton. Table 1.7 also shows that the distribution of metatarsal fractures is not dissimilar to that of metacarpal fractures. Most occurred as a result of soccer or were speed/height injuries, mostly of the fifth metatarsal. Most toe fractures resulted from soccer injuries.

1.3 Open Fractures

Tables 1.2 and 1.4 indicate that open fractures are uncommon in sports. This is not surprising given that most sports injuries are relatively low energy injuries. In the study year only 5 (0.6%) of fractures were open. There were two open tibia and fibula diaphyseal fractures from skateboarding and rugby, two open finger fractures from cricket, and one open distal radial fracture from mountain biking. Four were Gustilo Type I fractures, and the distal radial fracture was a Type IIIA fracture.

The rarity of open sports fractures means that analysis of the open fractures in 1 year gives little information. A review of all the open sports fractures presenting to the Royal Infirmary of Edinburgh between 1988 and 2010 shows that there were 114 open fractures in the 23 year period, an average of 5 per year. An analysis of these fractures is shown in Table 1.8. This shows the prevalence of open fractures in sports that resulted in at least two open fractures as well as the commonest three open fracture types in each sport. The percentage of Gustilo Type III fractures is also listed.

Overall, 54.4% of open fractures were upper limb fractures, 43.8% were lower limb fractures, and there were two open pelvic fractures from mountain biking. Table 1.8 shows that the overall distribution of open fractures was not dissimilar to that seen in the study year, with the most common open sports fractures being open tibia and fibula and finger fractures, which accounted for 63.1% of the open fractures in the 23 year period. Soccer, cycling and rugby caused 51.7% of the open fractures. Table 1.8 also shows that Gustilo Type III fractures are relatively uncommon, accounting for 14% of the open sports fractures. As a group, sport-related open fractures tend to be 'lower energy' open fracture injuries, with 53% of this cohort being Gustilo Type I injuries, and 33% being Gustilo Type II injuries. The epidemiology of open sports fractures has not changed much in the last 25–30 years. However, it is probable that, with increased participation in sports, fractures have become more common, but, with improved safety measures in many sports, open fractures have not increased in frequency.

Table 1.8 The epidemiology of open sports fractures between 1988 and 2010/2011. See text for details

	Open fractures		
Sports	(%)	Fracture type	Gustilo III (%)
Soccer	29.8	Tibia and fibula 55.9%, finger 11.8%, forearm diaphyses 11.8%	20.6
Cycling	11.4	Tibia and fibula 23.1%, proximal forearm 23.1%, finger 15.4%	15.4
Rugby	10.5	Finger 33.3%, tibia and fibula 25.0%, ankle 25.0%,	8.3
Winter sports	7.9	Finger 22.2%, proximal forearm 22.2%, humerus 11.1%	0
Hockey	7.0	Finger 100%	0
Horseriding	6.1	Tibia and fibula 28.6%, talus 14.3%, distal radius 14.3%	14.3
Basketball	3.5	Finger 66.7%, forearm diaphyses 33.3%	0
Shinty	2.6	Finger 100%	0
All sports		Finger 33.3%, tibia and fibula 29.8%, forearm diaphyses 7.9%	14.0

1.4 Multiple Fractures

Sixteen patients (2.2%) presented with multiple sports fractures. There were six patients with multiple finger and/or metacarpal fractures as a result of soccer, motorsports, sledging and cycling. Two patients presented with two thoracic spine fractures following injuries while sledging or diving. The remaining eight multiple fractures occurred as a result of soccer (talus/ankle, distal radius/proximal forearm), horse riding (proximal tibia/proximal forearm), cycling (scapula/clavicle, scapula/proximal forearm), ice skating (distal radius/carpus) and badminton (proximal forearm/ankle). Unsurprisingly, 15 (93.7%) patients were participating in soccer or speed/height sports when they sustained multiple fractures.

1.5 The Changing Epidemiology of Sports Fractures

With an expanding population and an increasing number of older people in the population, there will be more older people participating in different sports and, as a consequence, presenting with sports fractures. The epidemiology of all fractures in adults ≥16 years was initially examined in Edinburgh in 2000. Figure 1.1 shows the age-related incidence of sports fractures in the two 1-year periods in 2000 and 2010/2011. The overall incidence of sports fractures in 2000 was $119.7/10^5$/year. In 2010/2011 it was $138.3/10^5$/year, an increase of 15.5% in sports fractures in a decade. The incidence in males was $208.5/10^5$/year in 2000 and $237.6/10^5$/year in 2010/2011, an increase of 14.0%. In females, the equivalent figures were $39.4/10^5$/year and $47.9/10^5$/year, an increase of 21.6% in sports fractures.

Figure 1.1a suggests there was an increased incidence in males >20 years of age in 2010/2011 compared with 2000, and in females (Fig. 1.1b) there was greater increase in incidence between the ages of 30 and 60 years of age. Analysis of the incidence of fractures in the 30–60 year age groups in

Table 1.9 The epidemiology of sports fractures in patients aged ≥50 years. The number, percentage and gender ratio for each fracture and for each sport are given

Patients ≥ 50 years							
Sports	No	%	M/F	Fractures	No	%	M/F
Soccer	15	20.3	100/0	**Upper limb**	42	56.8	62/38
Cycling	14	18.9	71/29	Clavicle	3	4.1	67/33
Skiing	8	10.8	37/63	Proximal humerus	7	9.5	57/43
Golf	7	9.5	100/0	Distal humerus	1	1.4	100/0
Horse riding	6	8.1	0/100	Proximal forearm	5	6.8	60/40
Ice skating	5	6.8	20/80	Forearm diaphyses	1	1.4	100/0
Badminton	4	5.4	0/100	Distal radius	12	16.2	50/50
Bowling	3	4.1	67/33	Carpus	1	1.4	0/100
Tennis	2	2.7	50/50	Metacarpus	4	5.4	75/25
Dancing	2	2.7	0/100	Finger phalanges	8	10.8	75/25
Basketball	1	1.4	100/0	**Lower limb**	30	40.5	60/40
Athletics	1	1.4	0/100	Proximal femur	4	5.4	75/25
Arm wrestling	1	1.4	100/0	Proximal tibia	6	8.1	50/50
Curling	1	1.4	0/100	Tibial diaphysis	1	1.4	100/0
Fishing	1	1.4	100/0	Fibula	1	1.4	100/0
Rugby	1	1.4	100/0	Ankle	14	18.9	64/36
Sledging	1	1.4	0/100	Hindfoot	1	1.4	0/100
Squash	1	1.4	100/0	Midfoot	1	1.4	0/100
				Metatarsus	2	2.7	50/50
				Axial skeleton	2	2.7	0/100
Open fractures		0		Spine	1	1.4	0/100
Multiple fractures		5.7		Pelvis	1	1.4	0/100
				Total	74		59/41

males and females shows a 32.4% increase in sports fractures in males and a 53.1% increase in females. The incidence of sports fractures in older adults is increasing, particularly in females. This is borne out by examining the average age of some of the patients with sports fractures listed in Table 1.4 and the male/female ratio of fractures in the 50+ year patients who sustained their fractures in 2010/2011 shown in Table 1.9. This ratio must reflect an increasing incidence of sports fractures in older people, and the increasing importance of females in society.

1.6 Sports Fractures in the Older Population

When investigating fractures in the older population, it is usual to look at patients aged ≥65 years. However, while it is clear that older people are presenting with more sports fractures only 23 patients in this age group presented with fractures, giving an incidence of $22.9/10^5$/year. A review of male and female patients aged ≥50 years who presented with sports fractures showed an incidence of $34.2/10^5$/year, and this group has been examined to analyse the differences in the sports that fractures in older patients and the location of the fractures.

Table 1.9 shows that 18 different sports caused fractures in the ≥50 year patients in the study year. The sports that caused most fractures in the older group were not dissimilar to the sports that resulted in fractures in the overall group (Table 1.4). Soccer, cycling and skiing caused 50% of the fractures in the ≥50 year patients, having been responsible for 57.1% of the fracture in the overall group (Table 1.4). Rugby is clearly not played by many older adults! In 11 sports, more than 20% of the fractures occurred in patients aged ≥50 years. These were skiing, golf, horse riding, ice skating, badminton, bowling, tennis, dancing, arm wrestling, curling, fishing and squash. The male/female ratio of these sports is 39/61. Some sports have a high number of older participants. Examples are golf, bowling, dancing, curling and fishing. However, there is also a relatively high number of older people participating in sports such as horse riding, most winter sports and racquet sports such as tennis, badminton and squash.

A review of the fractures that the older population present with (Table 1.9) shows a lower prevalence of upper limb fractures and a higher prevalence of lower limb fractures in the older population. However, there is a higher prevalence of proximal humeral and distal radial fractures in the older population, the fractures expected to be seen in older patients. There is a lower prevalence of finger and metacarpal fractures in the older patients, although 75% of these still occur in soccer or speed/height injuries.

The higher prevalence of lower limb fractures in the older group is largely down to the numbers of ankle, proximal femoral and proximal tibial fractures in this group. Ankle fractures are the commonest fracture in ≥50 year patients, and are usually caused by a twist or fall with falls during sport, and are usually at a higher velocity than from a standing height. Two of the proximal femoral fractures occurred as a result of a cycling accident, and the other two as a result of falls during curling and tennis in patients aged 59 and 63 years. Cycling proximal femoral fractures will be discussed in the section on cycling fractures.

There is a high prevalence of proximal tibial fractures in older patients, with 40% occurring in the ≥50 year age group. Five of the six fractures occurred in soccer or speed/height sports such as cycling, skiing and horse riding, with one following a fall while fishing in a 72 year old man.

1.7 Sports Fractures

Tables 1.10 and 1.11 show the fracture prevalence in all sports that resulted in at least five fractures during the study year. The sports that resulted in ten or more fractures are shown in Table 1.10, and the sports that resulted

Table 1.10 The prevalence of each fracture type for the sports which caused ten fractures or more in the study year

	Prevalence of fractures in different sports (%)												
Fractures	Soccer	Rugby	Cycling	Skiing	Basketball	Horse riding	Snow-boarding	Ice skating	Martial arts	Cricket	Hockey	Skate boarding	Sledging
Scapula	---	---	3.3	---	---	---	---	---	---	---	---	---	---
Clavicle	6.9	8.8	17.4	3.0	---	---	35.3	---	7.1	7.7	7.7	23.1	15.4
Proximal humerus	0.7	1.0	6.5	12.1	---	8.7	---	7.1	---	---	---	---	---
Humeral diaphysis	0.7	---	---	3.0	---	8.7	---	---	---	---	---	---	---
Distal humerus	0.7	---	---	---	---	---	---	---	---	---	---	---	---
Proximal forearm	4.9	---	18.5	6.1	---	8.7	---	7.1	7.1	---	7.7	15.4	----
Forearm diaphysis	3.0	2.9	0	---	---	---	---	---	7.1	---	---	---	---
Distal radius/ulna	22.3	4.9	13.0	12.1	16.0	13.0	17.6	57.1	7.1	7.7	---	7.7	---
Carpus	4.9	2.9	4.3	3.0	8.0	4.3	17.6	7.1	7.1	---	7.7	7.7	---
Metacarpus	8.2	19.6	10.9	9.1	16.0	8.7	11.8	---	28.6	7.7	15.4	7.7	7.7
Finger phalanges	18.0	38.2	9.8	24.2	44.0	4.3	11.8	7.1	7.1	69.2	53.8	---	7.7
Proximal femur	---	---	4.3	---	---	---	---	---	---	---	---	---	---
Femoral diaphysis	---	---	---	---	---	4.3	---	---	---	---	---	---	---
Distal femur	0.3	---	---	---	---	---	---	---	---	---	---	---	---
Patella	0.3	---	---	---	---	---	---	---	---	---	---	---	---
Proximal tibia	1.6	---	3.3	6.1	---	8.7	---	---	---	---	---	7.7	---
Tibial diaphysis	2.6	2.9	---	3.0	---	---	---	7.1	---	---	---	15.4	7.7
Fibula	1.0	2.9							7.1	---	---	7.7	---
Distal tibia	0.3	1.0	---	---	---	---	---	---	---	---	---	---	---
Ankle	12.1	10.8	2.2	12.1	12.0	13.0	---	7.1	7.1	---	---	---	---
Hindfoot	0.3	---	---	3.0	---	4.3	---	---	---	---	---	---	---
Midfoot	0.7	1.0	---	---	---	---	---	---	---	---	---	---	---
Metatarsus	6.9	2.0	5.4	---	4.0	---	---	---	7.1	---	---	---	23.0
Toe phalanges	3.6	1.0	---	---	---	---	5.9	---	7.1	7.7	7.7	7.7	---
Pelvis	---	---	1.1	3.0	---	4.3	---	---	---	---	---	---	---
Spine	---	---	---	---	---	8.7	---	---	---	---	---	---	38.5

Table 1.11 The prevalence of each fracture type for the sports which caused 5–9 fractures in the study year

	Prevalence of fractures in different sports (%)							
Fractures	Roller skating	Boxing	Motor sports	Golf	Trampolining	Athletics	Badminton	Gymnastics
Clavicle	---	---	14.3	---	14.3	---	---	---
Proximal humerus	---	---	---	---	14.3	---	---	---
Humeral diaphysis	---	---	---	---	---	---	---	20.0
Proximal forearm	12.5	---	28.6	---	14.3	---	20.0	---
Forearm diaphysis	---	14.3	---	---	---	---	---	---
Distal radius/ulna	12.5	---	---	---	28.7	---	---	---
Carpus	12.5	14.3	---	---	---	---	20.0	---
Metacarpus	---	57.1	28.6	---	---	---	---	---
Finger phalanges	---	---	---	---	---	33.3	---	20.0
Tibial diaphysis	---	---	---	14.3	---	---	---	---
Fibula	12.5	---	---	14.3	---	---	---	---
Distal tibia	12.5	---	---	---	---	---	---	---
Ankle	37.5	14.3	14.3	71.4	---	33.3	40.0	20.0
Hindfoot	---	---	---	---	14.3	16.7	---	---
Midfoot	---	---	---	---	---	---	20.0	---
Metatarsus	---	---	---	---	14.3	16.7	---	40.0
Pelvis	---	---	14.3	---	---	---	---	---

in 5–9 fractures are shown in Table 1.11. The sports listed in Tables 1.10 and 1.11 caused 94.6% of the sports fractures in the study year. Tables 1.10 and 1.11 reconfirm the frequency with which upper limb fractures occur in sports. Table 1.2 shows that 72% of sports fractures occur in the upper limb, and Tables 1.10 and 1.11 show that, with the exception of ankle and metatarsal fractures, lower limb fractures are relatively unusual sports injuries. Table 1.1 shows that only fractures following a direct blow or assault have a lower prevalence of fractures of the axial skeleton than sports injuries.

1.8 Soccer

Soccer, the most popular sport in the world, is played globally. It is likely that the epidemiology of the soccer related fractures detailed in this chapter will be similar in other countries. As with all sports, it is impossible to know how many people actually play soccer, but it would seem reasonable to believe that its popularity is still growing. There is evidence of increased participation in soccer by young males [9] and comparison of the study year in 2010/2011 with the previous study year in 2000 shows that the overall incidence of soccer fractures increased slightly from $50.9/10^5$/year in 2000 to $55.5/10^5$/year in 2010/2011. However, as with all sports, we do not know whether this simply represents increased participation or more injuries, or both.

1.8.1 Upper Limb Fractures

Table 1.10 shows that soccer is associated with a high prevalence of hand and wrist fractures. Analysis of the study year showed an incidence of hand and wrist fractures of $29.2/10^5$/year, which compares with $27.3/10^5$/year in 2000. Further analysis shows that 34.1% of all sports hand fractures occur in soccer, usually as a result of catching a ball, a fall or a direct blow, and that 58.6% of all sports distal radial fractures occur as a result of a soccer injury, usually from a fall on an outstretched hand, particularly on synthetic turf [10]. In the study year there were more distal radial fractures from soccer than from road traffic accidents, direct blows, low fall falls from a height. The prevalence of hand and distal radial fractures from soccer are similar to other published reports [11, 12].

The distribution of hand fractures in soccer is shown in Table 1.7: about 70% of finger fractures and 60% of metacarpal fractures occur in the little and ring fingers. Further analysis shows that 73.7% of little finger fractures and 84.2% of ring finger fractures occur in the proximal phalanx. Analysis of the distal radial fractures shows that 64.7% were Type A fractures but 11.8% were Type C fractures.

The other upper limb fractures which occurred fairly frequently were fractures of the proximal forearm and clavicle fractures. Analysis of the proximal forearm fractures showed that 13 of 15 (86.7%) involved the proximal radius, and only 2 (13.3%) involved the proximal ulna. There were 21 clavicle fractures from soccer during the study year, 14 (66.7%) of which were diaphyseal and the remaining 7 (33.3%) were

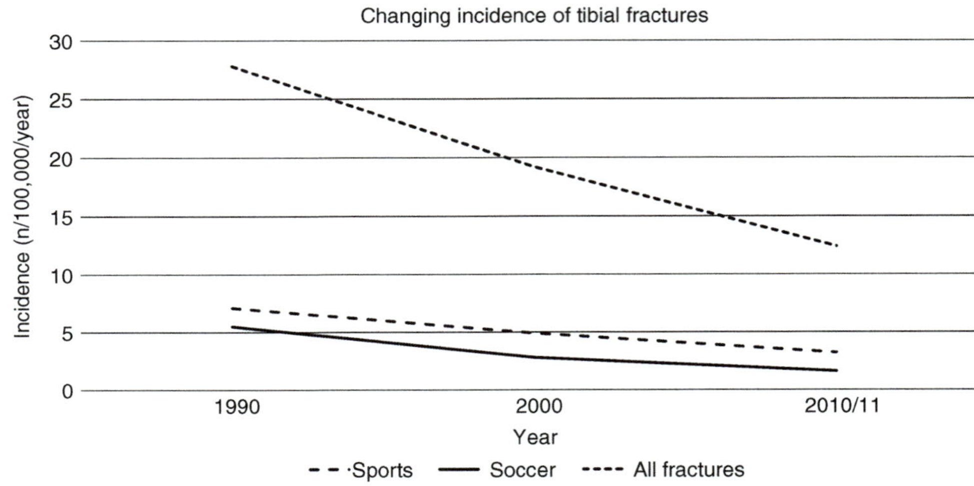

Fig. 1.2 The changing incidence of tibial diaphyseal fractures between 1990 and 2010/2011. See text for details

distal. There were no open soccer upper limb fractures, but four soccer players presented with multiple fractures, two with multiple metacarpal fractures, and one with multiple phalangeal fractures. The remaining patient presented with distal radial and radial head fractures.

1.8.2 Lower Limb Fractures

Table 1.10 shows that the commonest lower limb soccer fractures are those of the ankle and metatarsals. Table 1.7 shows that soccer is the commonest cause of both ankle and metatarsal sports fractures, accounting for almost half of the sports ankle fractures and more than half of the sports metatarsal fractures. Of the 21 metatarsal fractures, 15 (71.4%) involved the fifth metatarsal. There were no open or multiple metatarsal fractures. This was also the case for toe fractures.

Ankle fractures are the commonest soccer related lower limb fracture. The AO/OTA Types are listed in Table 1.7, and further analysis showed that 24 (64.9%) of the 37 ankle fractures were lateral malleolar fractures, 7 (18.9%) were medial malleolar fractures, 3 (8.1%) were bimalleolar, and 3 (8.1%) were trimalleolar fractures. Ankle fractures, unlike hand and wrist fractures, did show an increased incidence between 2000 and 2010/2011. The incidence in 2000 was $6.9/10^5$/year, but it rose to $14.3/10^5$/year in 2010/2011. It is difficult to know why this has occurred but, as with distal radial fractures, it may relate to the increased use of synthetic turf or possibly altered footwear.

Table 1.10 shows that only 2.6% of all soccer related fractures involved the tibial diaphysis. It has long been assumed that tibial diaphyseal fractures are a significant problem in soccer because of the illegal practice of stamping on an opponent's leg during a tackle. However, the incidence of tibial fractures is declining. To assess the changing incidence of tibial fractures, the equivalent populations of Edinburgh and the surrounding areas in 1990, 2000 and the study year of 2010/2011 were analysed. The changing incidence of tibial fractures in the overall population, the sports population and the soccer population is shown in Fig. 1.2. In 20 years, the overall incidence of tibial fractures decreased from $27.8/10^5$/year to $12.4/10^5$/year. In sports, it decreased from $7.1/10^5$/year to $3.2/10^5$/year, and in soccer from $5.5/10^5$/year to $1.6/10^5$/year. The overall incidence has decreased mainly as a result of improved road safety and work legislation, but it is likely that the decrease in soccer fractures is mainly associated with the increased use of shin guards. This has been pointed out in a study from the Netherlands [13] and a recent study from Nigeria has highlighted the problems of not wearing shin guards [14]. The improved situation regarding tibial fractures is also demonstrated by the fact that, in 1990, 9.4% of the soccer tibial fractures were open, but there were no open tibial fractures in 2000 and 2010/2011. There were also no patients with multiple fractures.

1.9 Rugby

A list of the prevalence of the different fractures caused by rugby is shown in Table 1.10. As with soccer, it is difficult to know how many people play rugby, but there was a slight increase in the incidence in rugby fractures between 2000 and 2010/2011. In 2000, the incidence was $16.1/10^5$/year, and in 2010/2011 it was $18.3/10^5$/year. During this period, the numbers of people playing rugby likely increased, with increased professionalism in rugby during this decade. However, as with soccer, there have been improved safety rules which have presumably have resulted in fewer fractures.

Rugby accounted for 13.2% of the sports fractures in the study year. Table 1.10 shows that the distribution of the fractures was fairly similar to that of soccer with one major difference. In rugby, there was a much higher prevalence of hand fractures and a much lower prevalence of distal radial fractures. In the lower limb, the distribution of fractures was very similar to soccer, with fewer metatarsal fractures.

1.9.1 Upper Limb Fractures

Analysis of the hand fractures in rugby shows that 57.8% of all rugby fractures were metacarpal or finger phalangeal fractures. A predominance of hand fractures in rugby was also noted by Elzinga and Chung [11]: back row forwards, centres and scrum halves were particularly susceptible to hand fractures. The incidence of rugby hand fractures does not seem to have increased significantly between 2000 and 2010/2011. In 2000, it was $9.2/10^5$/year and it 2010/2011 it was $11.1/10^5$/year.

The distribution of hand fractures is shown in Table 1.7. In the ball sports, physical contact column 102 of the 105 fractures were caused by rugby and the hand fracture prevalence is almost identical to that of rugby. As in soccer, about 45% of the finger phalangeal fractures and 50% of the metacarpal fractures occur in the ring and little fingers, with 69.2% of the little finger fractures and 75% of the ring finger fractures being in the proximal phalanx. The prevalence of distal radial fractures in rugby is only 4.9% (Table 1.10) this being very similar to non-soccer, non-contact ball sports (Table 1.7). Presumably, this is mainly because rugby players fall less frequently with their hands on the ground and more often on other players. The more benign nature of rugby distal radial fractures is emphasised by the fact that there were no Type C fractures. Of the 9 clavicle fractures, 7 (77.8%) were diaphyseal with the rest all being lateral in location. As in soccer, there were no open upper limb fractures and there were also no multiple fractures.

1.9.2 Lower Limb Fractures

The only lower limb fracture which is commonly seen in rugby injuries is the ankle fracture. There were 11 fractures, and all were lateral malleolar fractures. There were 3 (27.3%) Type A fractures, 5 (45.4%) Type B fractures, and 3 (27.3%) Type C fractures. Unlike soccer, tibial diaphyseal fractures are uncommon in rugby. Figure 1.2 shows the incidences in soccer between 1990 and 2010/2011. In rugby, the incidence in 2000 was $0.8/10^5$/year and in 2010/2011 it was $0.5/10^5$/year. However, one of the tibial fractures in the study year was open. There were no other open lower limb fractures, and there were no multiple fractures.

1.9.3 Axial Skeleton Fractures

There were no rugby spinal or pelvic fractures in the study year, but Morrissey et al. have documented two acetabular fractures in young males which were sustained while playing rugby [15].

1.10 Cycling

The complete epidemiology of cycling fractures involves the analysis of fractures caused by sport and fractures caused by road traffic accidents. Cycling has become much more popular in the last 20 years or so. It is estimated that in the United Kingdom two million adults cycle on a weekly basis [16], and there is good evidence of increasing injury. In a New Zealand study it was shown that hospital admissions following cycling injuries increased by 16.8% per year between 2012 and 2016 [17]. A study from the United States showed that the incidence of cycling injuries increased from $701/10^5$/year in 1997 to $1164/10^5$/year in 2013. The highest incidence of injuries was in younger cyclists, but there was a considerable increase in the number of older cyclists [18].

A review of the increasing incidence of cycle fractures shows that in 2000 sports cycling fractures had a incidence of $5.9/10^5$/year, and road accident cycling fractures had an incidence of $21/10^5$/year. In 2010/2011, the equivalent figures were $16.5/10^5$/year and $30.6/10^5$/year respectively. Thus, the incidence of cycle fractures has risen considerably, and will presumably continue to rise. In this chapter, the fractures related to sports cycling will be analysed, but, if information is required about road cycling fractures in 2010/2011, it is contained in the study by Court-Brown et al. [19]. Sport cycling can be divided into road cycling and mountain biking. There are differences between them, but the two disciplines will be combined in this chapter. Information about the epidemiology of fractures in both types of cycling is in the study by Court-Brown et al. [19]. Cycling caused 11.9% of the sports fractures treated during the study year. Table 1.10 gives the prevalence of the different fractures, and Table 1.4 shows that the average age of female cyclists was about 9 years older than males.

1.10.1 Upper Limb Fractures

Table 1.10 shows that 83.7% of sports cycling fractures were upper limb fractures, but unlike soccer and rugby, only 25% were hand fractures. In previous studies, clavicle fractures are the commonest cycling fracture [20, 21], and Table 1.10 shows that 27.2% of all sports cycling fractures occurred around the shoulder. There were 16 clavicle fractures, 6 proximal humeral fractures, and 3 scapular fractures. There were no scapular fractures in any other sport, and cycling accounted for 24.6% of all clavicle fractures and 30% of all proximal humeral fractures. The high prevalence of proximal humeral fractures is interesting, as this is classically a fracture of older females. All cycling proximal humeral fractures occurred in males, but 50% occurred in males aged 43–48 years. Four (66.7%) of the proximal humeral fractures were Type A fractures, the remainder being Type C. Of the clavicle fractures, 50% were diaphyseal and 50% were lateral.

All three scapular fractures occurred when the bicycle fell on one side, and the cyclist landed on his shoulder. All occurred in males, and the average age was 46.7 years. Two were scapular body fractures and one was a glenoid fracture. The severity of these fractures is highlighted by the fact that two patients had multiple fractures, one presenting with scapula and clavicle fractures, and the other with scapula and proximal forearm fractures.

The other relatively unusual sports upper limb fracture is the proximal forearm fracture. In cycling, this usually occurs when the bicycle falls to one side. There were 17 proximal forearm cycling fractures, being 34.7% of all the proximal forearm fractures in the study year. The male/female ratio was 76/24, and 7 (41.2%) of the cyclists were at least 40 years of age. Thirteen (76.5%) were proximal radial fractures, 3 (17.6%) were proximal ulna fractures, and 1(5.9%) was a proximal radius and ulna fracture.

Hand fractures are less prevalent than in other sports. Analysis shows that 55.5% were fractures of the little and ring fingers all of these being proximal phalangeal fractures. The distribution of metacarpal fractures was similar, with 50% involving the ring and little finger metacarpals. All of the carpal fractures were scaphoid waist fractures. There were 12 distal radial fractures, of which 5 (41.7%) were Type A, 5 (41.7%) were Type B, and 2 (16.7%) were Type C fractures. One of the Type C fractures was a Gustilo Type IIIa open fracture. There were no other open upper limb fractures in the study year. However, 4 (5.5%) of the cyclists with upper limb fractures presented with multiple fractures. The two scapular fractures have been detailed, and there were two patients with multiple metacarpal fractures.

1.10.2 Lower Limb Fractures

Lower limb fractures are relatively unusual in cycling. There were two ankle fractures and three proximal tibial fractures. Tables 1.10 and 1.11 show that proximal tibial fractures are uncommon in sport, and in cycling the three fractures were in males, two of whom were at least 50 years of age. The most unusual lower limb fracture is the proximal femoral fracture which occurred in four male cyclists. It is usually a fracture of osteoporotic elderly ladies and occurs as a result of a fall from a standing height. There were two intertrochanteric fractures in men in their thirties and two femoral neck fractures in two men aged 55 and 57 years. Femoral neck fractures occur in cyclists because the cyclists' shoes are clipped to the pedals, and when the bicycle falls to one side the cyclist lands on his or her hip [22]. There were no open lower limb cycling fractures, and no cyclist with a lower limb fracture presented with multiple fractures.

1.10.3 Axial Skeleton Fractures

There was one pelvic fracture in the study year in a 45 year old man who fell off a mountain bike. However, cycling is a speed/height sport and one can expect serious injuries. Table 1.6 shows that all axial skeletal fractures in the study year occurred in this type of sport. In a study from the National Centre for Pelvic and Acetabular surgery in Ireland, Fenelon et al. [23] showed that cycling injury referrals increased by 90% between 2016 and 2017, and there were more cycling referrals than motorbike injury referrals. The mean age of the patients was 51.7 years. Some referrals would have been as a result of road traffic accidents, but it does seem likely that, with the increasing interest in cycling, there will be more pelvic fractures.

There were no spinal fractures as a result of sports cycling in the study year, but a review of sports cervical spine injuries in the United States showed that the incidence of cycling cervical fractures increased between 2000 and 2015. In males, cycling was the commonest cause of cervical fractures; in females, it was the second commonest cause after horse riding [24].

Cycling has a very different spectrum of fractures from most other sports. Not only are there a number of higher energy fractures, but one sees fractures that are more commonly seen in older patients as a result of low energy injuries. Examples are fractures of the proximal humerus, proximal forearm proximal femur, and pelvis. With the increasing popularity of cycling in the older population, this is likely to continue.

1.11 Skiing and Snowboarding

Skiing and snowboarding will be considered together, as the sports have a number of obvious similarities and much of the recent literature has compared fractures in these sports. The epidemiology of skiing fractures in Edinburgh, shown in Table 1.10, is probably not representative of the overall epidemiology of skiing fractures. Scotland has reasonable skiing facilities, but they are not on a par with those of Central Europe or North America. The other difficulty is that many skiers in Edinburgh use a local artificial ski slope, and the spectrum of fractures from artificial ski slopes is different from that from snow slopes: artificial ski slopes result in more upper limb injuries compared with snow slopes [25].

In the study year, skiing accounted for 4.3% and snowboarding for 2.2% of sports fractures. Fractures in females were more commonly seen than in many other sports (Table 1.4), and almost 40% of skiing fractures occurred in females. In skiing, the average age was 14 years older than in snowboarding, and the average age in female skiers was about 9 years older than males. Snowboarding fractures occur in young males and females.

1.11.1 Upper Limb Fractures

Table 1.10 shows that 72.6% of skiing fractures and 94.1% of snowboarding fractures were upper limb fractures. In skiers, lower limb fractures are more common than upper limb fractures [26], and the higher prevalence of upper limb fractures in Table 1.10 probably relates to the use of the local artificial ski slope [27]. Snowboarders do not use the artificial ski slope, and upper limb fractures are more common than lower limb fractures in snowboarders [26]. Also, shoulder injuries are relatively common in skiers and snowboarders [26], and Table 1.10 confirms this.

A review of humeral fractures in skiers and snowboarders [28] identified a higher prevalence of proximal humeral fractures in skiers, and of diaphyseal and distal fractures in snowboarders. Table 1.10 shows that 12.1% of ski fractures were proximal humeral fractures, the second highest prevalence of proximal humeral fractures in all the sports shown in Tables 1.10 and 1.11. There were however no snowboarding humeral fractures in the study year. The four skiing proximal humeral fractures were not very severe. All were greater tuberosity fractures, with 2 Type A fractures and 2 Type B fractures. As with cycling, the average age was relatively high at 57 years. There was one skiing diaphyseal clavicle fracture, but Table 1.10 shows a high prevalence of snowboarding clavicle fractures. Of the six fractures, three were diaphyseal and three were lateral. Unlike the proximal humeral fractures, the average age of the patients with clavicle fractures was 27.0 years.

There was a similar prevalence of distal radial fractures in both sports, but a higher prevalence of carpal fractures in snowboarding, all being scaphoid fractures. Table 1.10 shows a higher prevalence of finger fractures in skiing: unlike soccer, rugby and cycling, there were few little and ring finger fractures, and 62.5% of the fractures were in the thumb. This probably results from having to grip a ski pole during a fall or falling onto an artificial ski slope. Thumb injuries are common on artificial ski slopes because of the shape of the matting, and tears of the thumb metacarpophalangeal ulnar collateral ligament are common [27]. There were no skiing upper limb open or multiple fractures in the study year.

1.11.2 Lower Limb Fractures

There were relatively few lower limb fractures in the study year. There was only one snowboarding toe fracture but there were a number of skiing fractures. Hindfoot fractures are unusual sports injuries, but there was one talar neck fracture (Table 1.10). Talar fractures are actually more common in snowboarding [26], and fractures of the lateral process of the talus might well be called a 'Snowboarders fracture' [29]. These fractures can mimic an ankle sprain, and may be missed. The four ankle skiing fractures were three lateral malleolar fractures and one trimalleolar fracture. Two of the ankle fractures were in skiers aged ≥50 years. There were no lower limb open or multiple fractures.

The spectrum of fractures from skiing on major snow slopes is actually very different from that shown in Table 1.10. This is particularly true of lower limb fractures. There are very few studies of skiing fracture epidemiology, but a study from the US in 2011/2012 used the National Trauma Data Base to examine 6055 injured skiers and snowboarders [26]. They noted a 0.3% mortality in both sports. Snowboarding had a higher prevalence of head injuries and abdominal organ injury than skiing, but the prevalence of chest injury and spinal injury was similar in both sports. Overall, 61% of the skiers and snowboarders had fractures, and the distribution of the fractures in both sports is shown in Table 1.12. Skiers had more lower limb fractures, and snowboarders had more upper limb fractures. The commonest upper limb frac-

Table 1.12 The prevalence of skiing and snowboarding fractures in a large US study. The statistical significance is shown. The study was carried out by Basques et al. [26]

	Fracture prevalence (%)		
	Skiing	Snowboarding	Significance
Upper limb			
Scapula	1.7	0.5	<0.001
Clavicle	3.7	3.5	ns
Proximal humerus	4.0	2.1	<0.001
Humeral diaphysis	1.1	2.1	ns
Distal humerus	1.1	3.3	<0.001
Proximal forearm	0.7	0.9	ns
Forearm diaphysis	0.8	2.7	<0.001
Distal radius/ulna	2.7	10.5	<0.001
Hand	2.1	2.1	ns
Lower limb			
Proximal femur	7.1	1.7	<0.001
Femoral diaphysis	5.6	3.6	<0.001
Distal femur	1.5	1.0	ns
Patella	0.5	0.3	ns
Proximal tibia	10.9	1.2	<0.001
Tibial diaphysis	12.3	3.2	<0.001
Ankle	2.5	1.7	<0.001
Foot	0.8	0.6	ns
Axial skeleton			
Pelvis	6.5	3.7	<0.001

ture in skiers was the proximal humeral fracture, with distal radial fractures being the commonest fracture in snowboarders.

Although there were few lower limb skiing fractures in the study year, 37.5% of the fractures were either proximal tibial or tibial diaphyseal fractures. These two fractures have always been associated with skiing, and Table 1.12 clearly shows that it is still the case. An analysis of snowboarding and skiing tibial fractures in Finland between 2006 and 2012 showed that tibial diaphyseal fractures were more common in skiers, and proximal tibial fractures were more common in snowboarders [30]. Snowboarders had more Type C fractures than skiers, and 17% of the snowboarders tibial fractures were open compared with 11% in skiers. In skiers, the commonest mode of injury was a fall, whereas snowboarders were more likely to sustain a tibial fracture by losing control while jumping. Clearly, both sports are potentially very dangerous and can cause more serious fractures than those shown in Table 1.10.

1.11.3 Axial Skeleton Fractures

There was one skiing pelvic fracture in the study year, but Table 1.12 shows that in major ski resorts pelvic fractures are not uncommon, particularly in skiers. An analysis of snowboarding pelvic fractures in Japan between 1998 and 2007 [31] showed that pelvic fractures accounted for 2% of snowboarding fractures, and that 20.8% of the patients had other injuries. The analysis showed that 85.5% of the fractures were stable, and 46.9% were pubic or ischial fractures. There was a higher prevalence of pelvic fractures in females (52.4%).

There were no spinal fractures in the study year, but they do occur. In an analysis of 114 thoracic and lumbar fractures, which were not transverse process or spinous process fractures, 71% of the fractures were compression fractures, 23% were burst fractures, 4.4% were distraction fractures, and 0.9% were rotational fractures. Snowboarders only incurred compression or burst fractures, and the distraction and rotational fractures occurred in skiers [32]. There were no neurological deficits in the study, but a review of spinal injuries in winter sports did quantify the prevalence of neurological deficits as well as discussing cervical fractures [33].

1.12 Basketball

Basketball caused 3.2% of the sports fractures in the study year. Table 1.4 shows that 20% of the fractures occurred in females and, as with cycling and skiing, the average age of the females was 9 years older than the males. As with many sports, there is very little published information about the epidemiology of basketball fractures, with most studies detailing lower limb soft tissue injuries. An Australian study examined basketball fractures that required hospitalisation: they were fractures of the forearm, hand and wrist, and the leg and ankle [34]. This is similar to the distribution of fractures shown in Table 1.10. There is another fracture which has been linked with basketball, ice hockey, baseball and golf: a fracture of the hook of the hamate [35, 36]. This is a stress fracture associated with prolonged gripping or prolonged ball shooting, as in basketball, although it can be caused by a direct blow.

1.12.1 Upper Limb Fractures

Table 1.10 shows that 84.0% of the basketball fractures in the study year were hand and wrist fractures, and 12.0% were ankle fractures. This is logical, as most basketball fractures will be caused by contact with the ball or an opponent or by a fall with the hand landing on a hard floor. As with soccer and rugby, most finger fractures were in the little and ring fingers (72.7%), and 84.6% of the finger fractures were located in the proximal phalanx. The distribution of metacarpal fractures was similar, with 75.0% being in the little and ring finger metacarpal. There was one scaphoid fracture and one triquetral fracture, and analysis of the distal radial fractures showed one Type A fracture, two Type B fractures and one Type C fracture. There were no upper limb open or multiple fractures.

1.12.2 Lower Limb Fractures

Analysis of the three ankle fractures showed that they were rotational injuries with two medial malleolar fractures and one lateral malleolar fracture. There were no lower limb open or multiple fractures.

1.13 Horse Riding

Horse riding, or equestrian activities, accounted for 3.0% of sports fractures in the study year. Horse riding is unusual, in that 87% of all equestrian fractures occurred in females with an average age of 40.2 years. In fact, females aged ≥40 years accounted for 52.2% of all equestrian fractures. The literature indicates that horse riding can be very dangerous [37–40], and Table 1.10 shows that it is associated with a broad spectrum of fractures. Horse riding was the only sport in the study year to cause both pelvic and spinal fractures and a femoral diaphyseal fracture.

1.13.1 Upper Limb Fractures

Analysis shows that 56.5% of equestrian fractures were upper limb fractures. Hand fractures were not as prevalent as in many sports. There was only one proximal phalangeal fracture in a ring finger and two metacarpal fractures in the index and little finger metacarpals. The carpal fracture was a triquetral fracture. There were three Type A distal radial fractures. However, Table 1.10 shows that humeral fractures are relatively unusual in sports injuries, and horse riding accounted for 33.3% of the humeral diaphyseal fractures and 10% of the proximal humeral fractures in the study year. There were two Type A3.2 humeral diaphyseal fractures, one Type A2.2 proximal humeral fracture, and one Type B1.1 proximal humeral fracture. Both proximal forearm fractures were radial head fracture in females, with an average age of 52.0 years. There were no open upper limb fractures, but one patient (8.3%) had a combination of a radial head fracture and a proximal tibial fracture.

1.13.2 Lower Limb Fractures

Lower limb fractures comprised 30.4% of the equestrian fractures. They were more unusual than the upper limb fractures, with a periprosthetic femoral diaphyseal fracture in a 51 year old female. The two proximal tibial fractures were Type B fractures, and the three ankle fractures were lateral malleolar fractures. There were no open lower limb fractures, and the only multiple fracture combination has been described.

1.13.3 Axial Skeleton Fractures

Tables 1.10 and 1.11 show that only sledging was associated with a higher prevalence of spinal fractures, and motor racing with a higher prevalence of pelvic fractures. There were no spinal cord injuries in the study year, but an analysis of sports related spinal cord injuries in 9 countries has shown that 11.4% are caused by horse riding [37]. The pelvic fracture was a fracture of the pubic rami and the spinal fractures were in the 12th thoracic and first lumbar vertebrae.

Equestrian activities can be dangerous. A study from Sweden analysing equestrian activities between 1997 and 2013 showed that 0.3% of equestrian injuries were fatal, and that under the age of 39 years all the fatalities were in females. Fractures were the most frequent type of injury resulting from equestrian activities [38]. A study of 1430 equestrian fractures in the United States gave the prevalence of fracture in different body areas including the shoulder (11.8%), humerus (6.9%), elbow (3.4%), forearm (15.3%), wrist (10.4%), hand (2.9%), finger (5.0%), femur (1.8%), knee (0.6%), leg (6.2%), ankle (4.1%), foot (2.1%), lumbar spine and pelvis (11.9%) and neck and cervical spine (0.6%). Only 0.8% of the fractures were open [39]. Another systematic review of articles analysing equestrian fractures indicated that 50.7% of fractures were upper limb fractures, 22.9% were lower limb fractures, 9.4% were spinal fractures, 4.7% were pelvic fractures and 11.6% were chest and torso fractures [40]. These figures are not dissimilar to those shown in Table 1.10.

Horse riding is a dangerous sport which can result in fractures that are often seen as a result of other modes of injury. There is a high prevalence of fractures in middle aged females, and with increasing longevity it seems likely that surgeons will have to treat a greater number of equestrian fractures in the future.

1.14 Ice Skating

Ice skating accounted for 1.8% of the sports fractures in the study year. Table 1.4 shows that, as with horse riding, sledging and trampolining, ice skating fractures are much more common in females, and the average age of the females was 9 years greater than in males. Ice skating fractures usually occur because of a fall on a very hard surface, and one would therefore expect a high prevalence of wrist fractures. Table 1.10 shows that this is indeed the case, with 57.1% of skating fractures being distal radial fractures. This is the highest prevalence of distal radial fractures in all sports. There were six Type A fractures and two Type C fractures. There was one triquetral fracture and one proximal phalangeal fracture in a ring finger. There was one radial head fracture, and one proximal humeral fracture which, as with proximal humeral fractures in skiing and cycling, occurred in a female aged 60 years.

A review of ice skating lower limb fractures showed that there was one lateral malleolar ankle fracture and a spiral tibial diaphyseal fracture. Both had occurred as a result of a fall. There were no open skating fractures, and the 7.7% prevalence of multiple fractures (Table 1.1) was a combination of a triquetral and distal radial fracture. An analysis of ice skating fractures in Cambridge, UK showed a similar distribution of fractures with 71.4% of the fractures being distal radial fractures [41]. Only 2.1% of the fractures were in the lower limb. Analysing children and adults, a bimodal fracture distribution was evident, with peaks between 0–16 years and 41–50 years of age.

1.15 Martial Arts

Martial arts caused 1.8% of the sports fractures seen in the study year. The sports that were involved were judo, karate, jujitsu, taekwondo and kick boxing. Table 1.1 shows that 93% of the fractures were in males, and the only female to sustain a fracture was 44 years of age. Analysis shows that 71.4% of the fractures were upper limb fractures and 28.6% were metacarpal fractures, all in the fifth metacarpal. Tables 1.10 and 1.11 show that martial arts and boxing have the highest prevalence of metacarpal fractures, presumably for the same reason. There was one diaphyseal clavicle fracture, one radial head fracture, one ulnar diaphyseal fracture, one scaphoid fracture, and one Type A distal radial fracture. The martial arts and boxing data confirms that distal radial fractures are generally not caused by punching. There were four lower limb fractures, with the lateral malleolar ankle fracture and the isolated fibular fracture being caused by a twist and fall, and the metatarsal and hallux fractures by a kick. There were no open or multiple fractures.

There is very little literature dealing with mixed martial arts fractures. In a study from Korea of all types of injury caused by martial arts, it was shown that 53.4% of the injuries were upper limb and 10.2% were lower limb. Overall 6.2% of the injuries were fractures [42].

1.16 Cricket

Cricket caused 1.7% of the sports fractures in the study year. All fractures occurred in males, with an average age of 33.5 years. Analysis showed that 30.8% of patients were ≥40 years of age. Table 1.10 shows that, not unexpectedly, 84.6% of the fractures were in the hand and wrist, and 69.2% were finger fractures. Cricket had the highest prevalence of finger fractures of all sports in the study year. A review of the finger fractures showed that 3 (33.3%) were in the little finger, 2 (22.2%) in the ring finger, 3 (33.3%) in the middle finger, and 1 (11.1%) in the thumb. Proximal phalangeal fractures were most commonly seen (36.4%), but in cricket 33.3% were distal fractures caused by catching a small hard ball. There was only one metacarpal fracture, one distal ulnar fracture and one diaphyseal clavicle fracture. In the lower limb, there was one hallux fracture following a fall while running. Table 1.4 shows that cricket had the highest prevalence of open fractures, these being two Gustilo Type I open finger fractures. No cricketers presented with multiple fractures.

Most cricket fractures are finger fractures, given the speed with which a hard ball is struck, and the fact that only wicket keepers wear gloves. Most finger fractures occur while fielding. Most lower limb injuries in cricket are soft tissue injuries, and head injuries and craniofacial injuries are not uncommon. Fast bowlers have a high incidence of lumbar spine injuries [43].

1.17 Hockey

Hockey, or field hockey, accounted for 1.7% of the sports fractures in the study year. The gender ratio was male/female ratio was 77/23 and 30% of the fractures occurred in males ≥40 years of age. Analysis shows that 92.3% of the fractures were upper limb fractures, and only cricket had a higher prevalence of finger phalangeal fractures, presumably because the hands of a hockey player are struck by the ball, hockey stick, or an opponent. A review of the finger fractures showed an even distribution with 1 (14.3%) little finger fracture, 2 (28.6%) thumb fractures, 3 (42.8%) ring finger fractures and 1 index finger fracture. There were three proximal, three distal and one middle phalangeal fracture. The two metacarpal fractures were in the thumb and index finger metacarpals. There was one scaphoid, one radial neck fracture and one lateral clavicle fracture. There was only one lower limb fracture, which was a lateral malleolar ankle fracture following a twist and fall while running. There were no open or multiple fractures.

1.18 Skateboarding

Skateboarding accounted for 1.7% of the fractures in the study year. The male/female ratio was 85/15, and both males and females had a low average age (Table 1.4). Skateboarding is acknowledged to be a dangerous sport [44], and Table 1.10 confirms a slightly unusual spectrum of fractures. Skateboarding had the second highest prevalence of clavicle and proximal forearm fractures of all the sports. It also had the highest prevalence of tibial diaphyseal fractures.

Analysis shows that 61.5% of skateboarding fractures were upper limb fractures. There were three diaphyseal clavicle fractures, one olecranon and one radial head fracture. Skateboarding hand fractures are unusual compared with most of the other sports in Tables 1.10 and 1.11. There were no finger fractures, and only one fifth metacarpal fracture. There was one scaphoid fracture and one Type A distal radial fracture. None of the upper limb fractures required surgery. There were no upper limb open or multiple fractures. Of the five lower limb fractures, there was a Type B ankle fracture, an isolated fibular diaphyseal fracture, and a Type B proximal tibial fracture. In addition, a patient presented with a closed Type A tibial diaphyseal fracture, and another with an open Type A tibial diaphyseal fracture. There were no lower limb multiple fractures.

Skateboarding is a very popular sport in young individuals, but, like cycling, skiing, snowboarding or horse riding, it can be dangerous. A study of 2270 people of all ages who were injured skateboarding in the United States showed that the severity of injury was worse if the skateboarders were >16 years of age [44]. In this age group, the mortality was 2.6% and 6.6% had an Injury Severity Score of ≥25. Analysis of the fractures in the >16 year group showed that 0.7% had humeral fractures, 10.4% had radius and ulnar fractures, 6.0% had femoral fractures, and 19.8% had tibia and fibula fractures. With the exception of the femoral fracture, these figures are not too dissimilar from Table 1.10.

1.19 Sledging

Sledging, or tobogganing, caused 1.7% of the sports fractures in the study year. Table 1.10 shows that it is associated with a very unusual spectrum of fractures, with 38.5% of sledging fractures being spinal fractures. This is much higher than any other sport. The literature confirms the high prevalence of spinal fractures from sledging [33]. In the study year, three of the five spinal fractures were thoracic, with one patient having T6 and T11 fractures and a second patient having a T12 fracture. The two patients with lumbar fractures had L1 and L2 fractures. These fractures indicate that most sledging spinal fractures are in the thoracolumbar area. This is in keeping with a previous Edinburgh study [45].

In the upper limb, there was one proximal phalangeal fracture of a ring finger and one little finger metacarpal fracture. There were two clavicle fractures, one being diaphyseal and the other lateral. In the lower limb, there were three metatarsal fractures and a Type A tibial diaphyseal fracture.

The relationship between sledging and spinal fractures is well known. They are likely to be caused by high speed collisions [33], but it has been suggested that sitting on a sledge with a flexed spine increases the risk of fracture [45]. The literature indicates that neurological compromise is unusual [33].

1.20 Roller Skating

Roller skating accounted for 1% of the fractures in the study year. There were more females with roller skating fractures, but the average ages of males and females were very similar, and indicates that roller skating is a sport for young people. Table 1.10 shows that lower limb injuries were more common than upper limb injuries, with three lateral malleolar ankle fractures, one isolated fibula fracture and a distal tibial fracture. A review of the upper limb fractures showed there was one triquetral fracture, a radial head fracture and a Type A distal radial fracture. There were no open or multiple fractures. A study from Hong Kong showed that 74.1% of roller skating fractures were upper limb fractures, with the commonest fractures being distal radial fractures (28.4%), ankle fractures (16%) and radius and ulnar fractures (14.8%) [46].

1.21 Boxing

Boxing accounted for 0.9% of the sports fractures in the study year. Seven of the eight fractures were in males, but there was a radial diaphyseal fracture in a 44 year old female. As one might expect, the other fractures were mostly hand fractures. There were no finger fractures, but boxing carries the highest prevalence of metacarpal fractures of all sports. However, only one metacarpal fracture was in the little finger metacarpal, this being the classic boxer's fracture. Two were in the index finger metacarpal and one in the ring finger metacarpal. There was one lower limb fracture, this being a lateral malleolar fracture following a twist and fall.

1.22 Motor Sports

Motor sports resulted in 0.9% of the fractures in the study year. All the fractures occurred in males aged between 17 and 24 years. There are a number of different motor sports, but the two sports that resulted in fracture in the study year were motocross and go karting. Analysis shows that 71.4% of the fractures were upper limb fractures with one diaphyseal clavicle fracture, two proximal ulna fractures, with one olecranon and one coronoid process fracture, and two metacarpal fractures in the middle and ring fingers. In the lower limb, there was one trimalleolar ankle fracture and there was also a pubic ramus fracture. There were no open fractures, but the two metacarpal fractures occurred in the same patient.

1.23 Golf

Golf accounted for 0.9% of the fractures in the study year. All occurred in males with an average age of 61.7 years. All were lower limb fractures, with 5 (71.4%) being ankle fractures. There was one isolated fibular diaphyseal fracture and one Type A tibial diaphyseal fracture. Of the five ankle fractures, three were lateral malleolar fractures and two were trimalleolar fractures. It is likely that the fact that all the golf fractures were lower limb fractures in males, is coincidental. A review of the three golf fractures that occurred in 2000 showed that two were distal radial fractures in females with an average age of 51.0 years. As golf courses can be wet and have an uneven terrain, it is probable that all the fractures followed a fall, with the fracture type simply depending on the type of fall. In recent years, there has been discussion about the hook of hamate fracture [35, 36], which has been diagnosed in golfers as well as in baseball, basketball and ice hockey players. In golfers, it is thought to be caused by prolonged gripping of golf clubs.

1.24 Trampolining

Trampolining accounted for 0.9% of the sports fractures in the study year. The male/female ratio was 14/86, and the only injured male was 47 years old. Obviously, most trampolining fractures are caused by falls from a height. Analysis shows that 71.4% of the fractures were upper limb fractures. There were two distal radial fractures, one being a Type A fracture and the other a Type B fracture. There was also a radial head fracture, a Type A proximal humeral fracture and a lateral clavicle fracture. In the lower limb there was a lateral process talus fracture and a fifth metatarsal fracture.

One might have expected more serious fractures from trampolining. In an Australian study between 2007 and 2013, 50 patients were reviewed and the results were very different from those in Table 1.11. Lower limb fractures were more common, and 26% of patients had tibial diaphyseal fractures, 24% had ankle fractures, and 14% cervical spine injuries. The complications included death, spinal cord injury, compartment syndrome and open fractures [47].

1.25 Athletics

Athletics caused 0.8% of the sports fractures in the study year. The male/female ratio was 50/50, but the average age of the females was 17 years greater than the males. Clearly, athletics takes many forms, but all the fractures were sustained while running. The only upper limb fractures were two little finger fractures sustained in falls. One was a proximal phalangeal fracture and the other a middle phalangeal fracture. In the lower limb, there were two lateral malleolar ankle fractures, a calcaneal fracture and a fifth metatarsal fracture. There were no open or multiple fractures.

1.26 Badminton, Tennis and Squash

Badminton, tennis and squash will be considered together. Badminton accounted for 0.6% of the sports fractures in the study year. Table 1.1 shows that it seems to be a sport of older females, as 80% of the fractures occurred in females with an average age of 59 years. There were two upper limb fractures, namely a scaphoid fracture and a proximal radius and ulna fracture. In the lower limb, there were two ankle fractures, one being lateral malleolar and the other medial malleolar. There was also a midfoot cuboid fracture. There were no open fractures, but one patient presented with the proximal radius and ulna fracture and the lateral malleolar fracture.

Tennis caused 0.5% of the fractures in the study year. As with badminton, the fractures were seen in older males and females. There were two fractures typical of older people. These were a Type B proximal humeral fracture in a 56 year old female, and a proximal femoral sub-capital fracture in a 63 year old male. As in badminton, most tennis fractures are caused by a fall. The other two fractures were a proximal phalangeal fracture of a thumb and a fifth metatarsal fracture. There were no open or multiple fractures. A study in the United States between 1990 and 2011 showed that soft tissue strains and sprains were the cause of most tennis injuries, but 14.6% of tennis injuries were fractures which were most commonly seen in older males [48].

Squash only resulted in 0.2% of the fractures in the study year. Both fractures were in the lower limb, one being a lateral malleolar fracture in a 52 year old man, and the other a third metatarsal fracture. Both were caused by a fall. There were no open or multiple fractures in tennis or squash.

1.27 Gymnastics

Gymnastics caused 0.6% of the fractures in the study year. The male/female ratio was 80/20, but the injured female was 16 years older than the average age of the males. Gymnastics covers a variety of different activities and exercises. A humeral diaphyseal fracture was sustained doing a bench press and the other fractures were simply the result of exercises which caused a fall. The 46 year old female sustained a proximal thumb fracture while doing a cartwheel. Two of the other males sustained fifth metatarsal fractures, with the other male sustaining a lateral malleolar ankle fracture. There were no open or multiple fractures.

1.28 Other Fractures

Table 1.13 contains details of the sports that resulted in less than five fractures during the study year. It is obvious that most sportsmen and women can have a fracture as a result of a fall or physical contact. Table 1.13 shows that 11 of the sports resulted in a metacarpal or finger phalangeal fracture, and 8 of these were ball sports. Table 1.7 shows that finger and metacarpal fractures commonly occur in ball sports. Arm wrestling predictably resulted in upper limb fractures, and diving caused two thoracic spine fractures in a 41 year old man. The association between diving and spinal fractures is well documented [24, 37].

Table 1.13 The fractures and number of fractures for the sports which caused less than five fractures in the study year

Sport	Fractures
Arm wrestling	Humeral diaphysis (1), distal radius/ulna (2), finger phalanx (2)
Dancing	Distal radius/ulna (1), metacarpal (1), cuboid (1), metatarsal (1)
Bowling	Proximal humerus (2), distal humerus (1)
Mountaineering	Finger phalanx (1), distal radius/ulna (1), talus (1)
Netball	Finger phalanx (3)
Diving	Spine (2)
Fishing	Proximal tibia (2)
Gaelic football	Clavicle (1), finger phalanx (1)
Softball	Clavicle (1), metacarpal (1)
Weightlifting	Olecranon (2)
American football	Finger phalanx (1)
Cross ball	Finger phalanx (1)
Curling	Proximal femur (1)
Curve ball	Finger phalanx (1)
Lacrosse	Metacarpal (1)
Swimming	Metatarsal (1)
Volleyball	Hallux (1)
Water polo	Metacarpal (1)
Wrestling	Radial neck (1)

Bowling, curling and fishing are usually favoured by older people, and again they are associated with fractures that one might expect to see in older people after a lower energy injury. Two proximal humeral fractures occurred in bowling, two proximal tibial fractures in fishing, and a proximal femoral fractures in a curler.

1.29 American Football

American football is a popular sport, but it is not played much in the United Kingdom and there was only one ring finger proximal phalangeal fracture in the study year. American football is not dissimilar to rugby in many ways, and one might well expect to see a spectrum of fractures similar to that of rugby shown in Table 1.10. In the upper limb, the dominant fractures are liable to be finger phalangeal, metacarpal and clavicle fractures, with the ankle fracture being common in the lower limb. This is supported by examining a study from the United States, of 986 fractures [49]. The study reported that 4.4% of all injuries in American football were fractures, and 39.9% of the fractures affected the hand and fingers, with 5.7% of the fractures being clavicle fractures. In the lower limb 19.9% of the fractures were fibular or ankle fractures, and 8.8% were metatarsal fractures. However, the authors reported that 20.8% of the metatarsal fractures were recurrent. The figures are not dissimilar to the data for rugby fractures shown in Table 1.10. However, in the US study, 1.8% of American football fractures were spinal and 0.4% were pelvic fractures.

1.30 Baseball

Baseball is a popular international sport, but it is not played much in the United Kingdom. It is highly likely that the fractures caused by baseball are very similar to those caused by cricket as both sports rely mainly on catching a hard ball thrown at speed. Table 1.10 shows that most cricket fractures are metacarpal or finger phalangeal fractures, and an analysis of the literature suggests that this is the case in baseball. The literature regarding baseball fractures is poor, but a study from the United States of 6226 baseball injuries, affecting the wrist and hand, showed that 10.6% of the injuries were fractures [50]. They showed that 32.2% of the fractures were metacarpal fractures, and 25.8% were finger phalangeal fractures. What was surprising was that 32% of the fractures were carpal fractures, with 87.7% of these being hook of hamate fractures. The literature is very deficient when it comes to lower limb baseball fractures, and what is available strongly suggests that, like cricket, most fractures are hand fractures, although a femoral diaphyseal fracture has been reported [51]. The hook of hamate fracture has been described in a number of sports such as baseball, ice hockey, basketball and golf [35, 36], and is thought mainly to arise from prolonged gripping. This fracture may be becoming increasingly recognised because of improved scanning.

1.31 Ice Hockey

As with many sports, there is little information about the epidemiology of ice hockey fractures. Ice hockey is a high velocity sport with contact between the player and a fast moving puck, hockey sticks, the ice, and the periphery of the ice rink. Fractures must be fairly common, and logically the distribution of fractures will be similar to that shown in Table 1.6 for the speed/height sports, although there is also a high prevalence of cervical spine injuries [52]. The literature indicates that clavicle and metacarpal fractures are relatively common [52], and a study of 50 major injuries in ice hockey showed that 10% were wrist fractures, 8% were metacarpal or phalangeal fractures, 4% were leg fractures, 12% were ankle fractures and 2% were foot fractures [53]. The literature also has a number of reports of other fractures, and two of four sports-related femoral diaphyseal fractures were reported as being from ice hockey [51]. The published scientific information suggests that the speed/height column in Table 1.6 is a reasonable approximation.

Review

Questions

1. What are the commonest sports related fractures seen in males and females?
2. What are the commonest sports that cause fractures?

Answers

1. These are shown in Tables 1.1, 1.2, 1.3, 1.10 and 1.11.
2. These are shown in Tables 1.4, 1.5, 1.10 and 1.11.

References

1. Aitken SA, Rodrigues MA, Duckworth AD, Clement ND, McQueen MM, Court-Brown CM. Determining the incidence of adult fractures: how accurate are emergency department data? Epidemiol Res Int. 2012;2012:Article ID 837928.
2. Court-Brown CM, Clement ND. The epidemiology of musculoskeletal injury. In: Tornetta P, Ricci WM, Ostrum RF, McQueen MM, McKee MD, editors. Rockwood and Green's fractures in adults. 9th ed. Philadelphia, PA: Wolters Kluwer; 2020. p. 123–87.
3. Court-Brown CM, Caesar B. Epidemiology of adult fractures: a review. Injury. 2006;37(8):691–7.
4. en.wikipedia.org/wiki/Sport.
5. en.Wikipedia.org/wiki/List_of_sports.
6. Fracture and dislocation compendium. Orthopaedic Trauma Association Committee for Coding and Classification. J Orthop Trauma. 1996;10(Suppl 1:v-ix):1–154.
7. Gustilo RB, Anderson JT. Prevention of infection in the treatment of one thousand and twenty-five open fractures of long bones: retrospective and prospective analyses. J Bone Joint Surg Am. 1976;58(4):453–8.
8. Gustilo RB, Mendoza RM, Williams DN. Problems in the management of type III (severe) open fractures: a new classification of type III open fractures. J Trauma. 1984;24(8):742–6.
9. De Putter CE, van Beeck EF, Burdorf A, Borsboom GJJM, Toet H, Hovius SER, Selles RW. Increase in upper extremity fractures in young male soccer players in the Netherlands, 1998-2009. Scand J Med Sci Sports. 2015;25(4):462–6.
10. Lawson GM, Hajducka C, McQueen MM. Sports fractures of the distal radius—epidemiology and outcome. Injury. 1995;26:33–6.
11. Elzinga KE, Chung KC. Finger injuries in football and rugby. Hand Clin. 2017;33(1):149–60.
12. Kuczinski A, Newman JM, Piuzzi NS, Sodhi N, Mont MA. Trends and epidemiologic factors contributing to soccer-related fractures that presented to emergency departments in the United States. Sports Health. 2019;11(1):27–31.
13. Vriend I, Valkenberg H, Schoots W, Goudswaard GJ, van der Meulen WJ, Backx FJG. Shinguards effective in preventing lower leg injuries in football: population-based trend analyses over 25 years. J Sci Med Sport. 2015;18(5):518–22.
14. Nwosa C. Tibial fractures following participation in recreational football: incidence and outcome. Niger J Clin Pract. 2019;22(4):492–5.
15. Morrissey DI, Good D, Leonard M. Acetabular fractures in skeletally immature rugby players. BMJ Case Rep. 2016;2016. pii: bcr2015211637. https://doi.org/10.1136/bcr-2015-2.
16. cyclinguk.org/statistics.
17. Singh N, Joe N, Amey J, Smith A, Christey G. Cycling-related injuries and cycling promotion: a trauma service perspective. NZ Med J. 2019;132(1494):41–8.
18. Fergus KB, Sanford T, Vargo J, Breyer BN. Trends in bicycle-related injuries, hospital admissions, and deaths in the USA 1997-2013. Traffic Inj Prev. 2019;20(5):550–5.
19. Court-Brown CM, Allan M, Davidson E, McQueen MM. The epidemiology of cycling fractures in adults. Emerg Med. 2013;3:2. https://doi.org/10.4172/2165-7548.1000139.
20. De Bernardo N, Barrios C, Vera P, Laiz C, Hadala M. Incidence and risk for traumatic and overuse injuries in top-level road cyclists. J Sports Sci. 2012;30(10):1047–53.
21. Haeberle HS, Navarro SM, Power EJ, Schickendantz MS, Farrow LD, Ramkumar PN. Prevalence and epidemiology of injuries among elite cyclists in the Tour de France. Orthop J Sports Med. 2018;6(9):2325967118793392. eCollection 2018.
22. Slootmans FC, Biert J, de Waard JW, de Waal Malefijt MC, Schoots FJ. Femoral neck fractures in bicyclists due to clipless pedals. Ned Tijdschr Geneeskd. 1995;139:1141–3.
23. Fenelon C, Murphy EP, Downey C, O'Daly BJ, Leonard M. A growing problem: cycling referrals to the National Centre for pelvic and acetabular fracture management in Ireland. Ir J Med Sci. 2019;188(3):855–9.
24. DePasse JM, Durand W, Palumbo MA, Daniels AH. Sex- and sport-specific epidemiology of cervical spine injuries sustained during sporting activities. World Neurosurg. 2019;122:e540–5.
25. Steedman DJ. Artificial ski slope injuries: a 1-year prospective study. Injury. 1986;17(3):208–12.
26. Basques BA, Gardner EC, Samuel AM, Webb ML, Lukasiewicz AM, Bohl DD, Grauer JN. Injury patterns and risk factors for orthopaedic trauma from snowboarding and skiing: a national perspective. Knee Surg Sports Traumatol Arthrosc. 2018;26(7):1916–26.
27. Keramidas E, Miller G. Adult hand injuries on artificial ski slopes. Ann Plast Surg. 2005;55(4):357–8.
28. Bissell BT, Johnson RJ, Shafritz AB, Chase DC, Ettlinger CF. Epidemiology and risk factors of humerus fractures among skiers and snowboarders. Am J Sports Med. 2008;36(10):1880–8.
29. Nicholas R, Hadley J, Paul C, James P. Snowboarder's fracture'; fracture of the lateral process of the talus. J Am Board Fam Pract. 1994;7(2):130–3.
30. Stenroos A, Pakarinen H, Jalkanen J, Mälkiä T, Handolin L. Tibial fractures in alpine skiing and snowboarding in Finland: a retrospective study on fracture types and injury mechanisms in 363 patients. Scand J Surg. 2015;104(2):127–31.
31. Ogawa H, Sumi H, Sumi Y, Shimizu K. Pelvic fractures resulting from snowboarding. Am J Sports Med. 2010;38(3):538–42.
32. Gertzbein SD, Khoury D, Bullington A, St John TA, Larson AI. Thoracic and lumbar fractures associated with skiing and snowboarding injuries according to the AO comprehensive classification. Am J Sports Med. 2012;40(8):1750–4.
33. Bigdon SF, Gewiess J, Hoppe S, Exadaktylos AK, Benneker LM, Fairhurst PG, Albers CE. Spinal injury in alpine winter sports: a review. Scand J Trauma Resusc Emerg Med. 2019;27(1):69. https://doi.org/10.1186/s13049-019-0645-z.
34. Flood L, Harrison JE. Epidemiology of basketball and netball injuries that resulted in hospital admission in Australia, 2000-2004. Med J Aust. 2009;3(4):87–90.
35. Husband JB. Hook of hamate and pisiform fractures in basketball and hockey players. Hand Clin. 2012;28:303.
36. Bansal A, Carlan D, Moley J, Goodson H, Goldfarb CA. Return to play and complications after hook of hamate fracture. J Hand Surg Am. 2017;42(10):803–9.
37. Chan CWL, Eng JJ, Tator CH, Krassioukov A. Epidemiology of sport-related spinal cord injuries: a systematic review. J Spinal Cord Med. 2016;39(3):255–64.

38. Meredith L, Thomson R, Ekman R, Kovaceva J, Ekbrand H. Equestrian-related injuries, predictors of fatalities and the impact on the public health system in Sweden. Public Health. 2019;168:67–75.
39. Loder R. The demographics of equestrian-related injuries in the United States: injury patterns, orthopaedic specific injuries, and avenues for injury prevention. J Trauma. 2008;65:447–60.
40. Young JD, Gelbs JC, Zhu DS, Gallacher SE, Sutton KM, Blaine TA. Orthopaedic injuries in equestrian sports. A current concepts review. Orthop J Sports Med. 2015;3(9):2325967115603924. https://doi.org/10.1177/2325967115603924.
41. Barr LV, Imam S, Crawford JR, Owen PJ. Skating on thin ice: a study of the injuries sustained at a temporary ice skating rink. Int Orthop. 2010;34(5):743–6.
42. Ji M. Analysis of injury types from mixed martial arts. J Phys Ther Sci. 2016;28(5):1544–6.
43. Pardiwala DN, Rao NN, Varshney AV. Injuries in cricket. Sports Health. 2018;10(3):217–22.
44. Lustenberger T, Talving P, Barmparas G, Schüriger B, Lam L, Inaba K, Demetriades D. Skateboard-related injuries: not to be taken lightly. A National Trauma Databank analysis. J Trauma. 2010;69:924–7.
45. Kelly M, Robinson CM. Fractures of the thoracolumbar vertebrae from sledging: a recurrent British winter problem. Injury. 2003;34(12):940–1.
46. Tse PYT, Shen WY, Chan KM, Leung PC. Roller skating—is it a dangerous sport? Br J Sports Med. 1987;21(3):125–6.
47. Arora V, Kimmel LA, Yu K, Gabbe BJ, Liew SM, Kamali Moaveni A. Trampoline related injuries in adults. Injury. 2016;47(1):192–6.
48. Gaw CE, Chounthirath T, Smith GA. Tennis-related injuries treated in United States emergency departments, 1990–2011. Clin J Sport Med. 2014;24(3):226–32.
49. Cairns MA, Hasty EK, Herzog MM, Ostrum RF, Kerr ZY. Incidence, severity, and time loss associated with collegiate football fractures, 2004-2005 to 2013-2014. Am J Sports Med. 2018;46(4):987–94.
50. Rhee P, Camp CL, D'Angelo J, Desai VS, Shin SS, Sheridan D, Conte S. Epidemiology and impact of hand and wrist injuries in minor and major league basebakk. Hand (NY). 2019. https://doi.org/10.1177/1558944719864450.
51. Sikka R, Fetzer G, Hunkele T, Sugarman E, Boyd J. Femur fractures in professional athletes: a case series. J Athl Train. 2015;50(4):442–8.
52. Mosenthal W, Kim M, Holzshu R, Hanypsiak B, Athiviraham A. Common ice hockey injuries and treatment: a current concepts review. Curr Sports Med Rep. 2017;16(5):357–62.
53. Mölsä J, Kujala U, Näsman O, Lehtipuu T-P, Airaksinen O. Injury profile in ice hockey from the 1970s through the 1990s in Finland. Am J Sports Med. 2000;28(3):322–7.

The Epidemiology of Stress Fractures in Sport

2

David N. Wasserstein and Falko Dahm

Abbreviations

BMI	Body mass index
MRI	Magnetic resonance imaging
SF	Stress fracture
WNBA	Women's National Basketball Association

Learning Objectives

- To determine the key features of stress fracture epidemiology, and to define the challenges of establishing valid incidence rates.
- To identify the key risk factors for developing stress fractures, and to illustrate the interplay between exposure and incidence.

2.1 Stress Fracture Epidemiology

Stress fractures affect thousands of athletes every year, and can occur in nearly every bone in the body. They are serious injuries, and if left untreated, can be career ending in professional athletes. Stress fractures are mostly described in active populations, and are expressed in units of exposure (e.g., number of stress fractures per athlete-years or per athlete-exposures). From the epidemiologic perspective, it is important to accurately determine the athletic exposures when defining the incidence. For retrospectively designed studies, the identification of patients through chart records or physician visits can be performed relatively easily; however, in such cases, the acquisition of accurate training or activity data leading to the stress fracture diagnosis, is almost impossible.

A second complicating factor in interpreting the literature, which defines the incidence of stress fractures in athletes, is the heterogeneity of the method of diagnosis used. Older studies relied on clinical diagnosis, either in isolation, or combined with basic imaging modalities such as x-ray, which have poor sensitivity [1, 2]. Even CT scans, which are more readily available than MRI scans in most countries, offer a limited sensitivity (42%) but a high specificity (100%) [3]. Many newer studies have utilized MRI techniques, which offers greater sensitivity (88%) and specificity (100%), and will identify stress fractures at an earlier stage [3]. MRI is sensitive enough to detect stress reactions, a precursor to stress fractures: thus, studies utilizing this method of detection will record a greater incidence of stress fracture injuries, but will be reporting on a broader spectrum of clinical disorder. In clinical practice, MRI scanning may not always be available: this is more commonly reserved for cases which are refractory to treatment or those with a more chronic duration [4].

This heterogeneity in diagnosis, study design, and accuracy of exposure preclude the pooling of data to formulate accurate incidence rates by sport or activity, at the current time. Therefore, this chapter will focus on a descriptive review of the literature, the most robust of which originates from military populations. Studies from various sports will also be reviewed and interpreted. A preference is given towards studies with a higher level of evidence, and those published within the last 15 years.

2.1.1 Stress Fractures: Military

Research performed on military personnel, especially on recruits, offers excellent opportunities to examine the epidemiology of stress injury and fracture. Patient activity, exposure and follow-up can be well controlled and documented, and large numbers of patients can be recruited, which allows

D. N. Wasserstein (✉) · F. Dahm
Sunnybrook Health Sciences Centre, Toronto, ON, Canada

University of Toronto, Toronto, ON, Canada
e-mail: david.wasserstein@utoronto.ca;
david.wasserstein@sunnybrook.ca; falko.dahm@mail.utoronto.ca

G. A. J. Robertson, N. Maffulli (eds.), *Fractures in Sport*, https://doi.org/10.1007/978-3-030-72036-0_2

for more homogeneous comparisons and higher level of evidence designs, such as prospective cohorts. The lack of validation to accurately extrapolate and apply this data to general or non-military populations, is the largest limiting factor of this research.

Most importantly, however, is that military personnel appear to have a higher incidence of stress fractures than the general population, due to the rapidly increased and high-volume exercise, associated with training. Accordingly, military studies on stress fractures have been performed all over the world, including the United States [1, 5–8], Finland [9], India [10] and Israel [11, 12].

Several of these studies found a higher incidence rate of stress fractures among females compared to males [5, 7, 13]. In the largest study of US Army recruits, the incidence of stress fractures was 79.9/1000 for female recruits, and 19.3/1000 for male recruits [7]. This pattern holds true internationally. An Israeli military study identified a similar discrepancy (ratio 2.1) of 'bone scan positive' stress fractures in females (23.9%) to males (11.2%) [12]. A Finnish study, reviewing 152,095 conscripts, also found a ratio of female to male bone stress injuries on MRI of 9:2 [9]. The overall incidence rate of stress fractures in this population was 311/100,000 person-years (95% confidence interval: 277–345).

There also appears to be a difference in the distribution of stress fracture location between male and female military personnel. Compared to males, females have higher reported rates of stress fractures of the pelvis [9, 12], sacrum [9], and tibia [9, 12].

Further subgroup analysis of the literature reveals additional risk factors, especially for female recruits.

Shaffer et al. identified a stress fracture rate of 5.1% in a cohort (n = 2962) of female US marine recruits [6]. All stress fractures occurred in the lower extremity, most commonly in the tibia, followed by the metatarsal bones, pelvis and femur. In regression analysis, the odds of developing a stress fracture, among recruits who were amenorrhoeic during the prior year, was more than five times higher than the baseline rate (odds ratio 5.64, 95% confidence interval 2.8–25.8). Lower aerobic performance, as determined by a timed run, also increased the odds of developing stress fractures in the pelvis and femur. Further studies identified a diagnosis of attention deficit hyperactivity disorder (ADHD) and a diagnosis of anemia to be independent risk factors for the development of stress fractures [11, 14].

Overall, the most common anatomic locations, where stress fractures develop, in military populations are the tibia and the metatarsals [5, 8, 11]. Stress fractures of the calcaneus were detected less frequently.

Sormaala et al. identified calcaneal stress fractures from MRI scans in recruits who had undergone an ankle MRI scan, for exercise induced heel or ankle pain [1]. The incidence rate of stress fractures among all recruits, during the study period, was 2.6/10,000 person-years (95% confidence interval 1.6–3.4). Most calcaneal stress fractures in this population were found in the posterior aspect of the bone, and 22/34 (65%) were associated with stress fractures in other tarsal bones. Interestingly, only 15% of these lesions could be detected on plain radiographs, which again, illustrates the higher sensitivity and improved ability of MRI scans to detect stress-related bone changes, at an earlier stage.

Several military studies also revealed that most stress fractures occurred within the first 3–4 months after enrollment [10, 15]. Pre-enrollment fitness training was found to be protective against developing stress injury in both male and female recruits [15, 16]. Screening for the most vulnerable personnel and the implementation of prevention programs, by adapting training loads during the high risk phases, have been suggested as prophylactic interventions to reduce the burden of disease [13, 15, 17].

2.1.2 Stress Fractures: Running

Runners are at higher risk of developing stress fractures, especially when training is conducted on rigid surfaces or on hills [18]. A training increase beyond distances of 32 km (20 miles) per week has also been associated with these injuries, as has a change of footwear [19]. The available data on the relationship of running volume to stress fracture development is limited in the current literature, so it remains difficult to provide prescriptive advice on this topic. Many of these athletes may also be competing in multiple sports, and establishing a direct causality to the running exposure can be challenging. Among runners, female long distance runners were found to be at the highest risk of developing stress fractures [20]. A prospective cohort study among 748 competitive high school cross-country and track and field runners found a 5.4% and 4.5% rate of stress fractures, in girls and boys respectively. Again, the most vulnerable anatomic regions were found to be the tibia and the metatarsal bones. In a multivariate model analysis, late menarche, low BMI and a prior history of stress fractures were identified to be significant risk factors to develop a new-onset stress fracture [21]. In a second, smaller cohort study of competitive high school runners, followed for 3 years, stress fractures were identified in 21/230 (9.1%) athletes, representing an incidence of 0.06 stress fractures per athlete exposure [22].

2.1.3 Stress Fractures: Tennis

Tennis players have a different injury risk pattern than runners. They are at risk of developing stress fractures especially in their racket arm and the lower extremities. In a study among 139 elite tennis players, the most common sites of stress fracture development were the navicular (5/18), pars interarticularis (3/18), metatarsals (2/18), tibia (2/18) and the lunate (2/18). In this cohort, stress fractures were more common among junior tennis players (20.3%) compared to professional tennis players (7.5%) [23]. Abrams et al. found that less frequent stress fracture locations, in tennis players, included the ischium, the first rib, the humerus, the sacrum, the patella, the hook of hamate, the ulna and the distal radius [24]. Unfortunately, none of these studies provided a metric for exposure, to calculate an incidence rate.

2.1.4 Stress Fractures: Basketball

Basketball players, similar to other sports mentioned above, mainly suffer from stress fractures to the lower extremity [25]. Basketball is a sport with a fast pace and high-impact exposure.

A study conducted on National Basketball Association professional basketball athletes reported on 76 bone stress injuries in 75 players [26], with a preponderance for the lower extremity. The distribution of injury location included the foot (55%), the ankle or fibula (21%), the tibia (17%), and the knee (7%). The most common stress fracture recorded was that of the fifth metatarsal. Half of the injuries occurred within the first 6 weeks of the season, which is in line with other studies, showing that stress fractures mainly occur secondary to an increase in skeletal loading. Bone stress injury is less common in basketball players [25, 26] compared to other sports, but are important, as they can lead to decreased player performance, and can even be career ending.

2.1.5 Stress Fracture: Pediatric and Adolescent Athletes

Pediatric and adolescent athletes are a special sub-population to examine, due to their physiology of hormonal changes and open physes. In a national survey study among 6831 adolescent girls aged 9–15, 267 (3.9%) of the cohort developed a stress fracture [27]. Multivariate modeling analysis demonstrated that running, basketball, cheerleading and gymnastics were all significant predictors for developing stress fracture. In a different retrospective case series by Niemeyer et al. [28], 19 children with 21 stress fractures were followed over a mean of 4.8 years. Most fractures occurred in the lower extremity, and the mean age at diagnosis was 14 years. They noted that tibial stress fractures were more likely to occur in sports which involved sudden 'stopping' manoeuvres, and that these injuries were the most difficult to treat, with the longest course of recovery.

2.1.6 Stress Fractures: Other Sports and Sites

Individual case reports and case series have been published, documenting the occurrence and incidence of stress fractures in various sports. Rib stress fractures not only occur in tennis players, as described above, but are also found in pitchers, weightlifters, competitive rowers, golfers and ballet dancers [19]. The ribs are also the most common site for stress fractures in golfers, specifically occurring on the lead-side of the athlete: however, in general, golfers do not experience frequent stress injuries [29]. Stress fractures of the metatarsals are most commonly seen in dancers, with the typical site being the base of the second metatarsal [30]. Other typical sites for stress fractures in dancers are the fibula, the tibia, the spine, and the hip [30]. Some sport specific case reports and case series are summarized in Table 2.1.

Table 2.1 Stress fracture epidemiology in various sports

Reference	Sport	Study design	N	Incidence	Notes
Ekegren et al. [31]	Ballet	Prospective cohort study	266	–	SF had the longest return to participation
McCarthy et al. [32]	Basketball (women)	Case series	37/506 (7.3%)	–	Injury reports of WNBA players at draft
Khan et al. [26]	Basketball (professional players)	Case series	76	–	55% foot (mainly fifth metatarsal), 21% ankle or fibula
Frost et al. [33]	Cricket	Prospective cohort study	248	–	Professional cohort; SF of the low back had the longest return to play
Ekstrand et al. [34]	Football	Prospective cohort study	51/2379 (2.1%)	0.04/1000 h	78% fifth metatarsal; 29% re-injury; 3–5 months absence
Pearce et al. [35]	Rugby	Prospective cohort study	12/899 (1.3%)	–	Navicular SF associated with the longest time off sport
Tenforde et al. [21]	Runners (adolescent)	Prospective cohort study	34/748 (4.5%)	–	n = 23 (5.4%) girls, n = 11 (4.0%) boys; Most common SF locations—tibia and metatarsal
Maquirriain et al. [23]	Tennis	Retrospective cohort study	18/139 (12.9%)	–	Follow up 2 years; imaging modality MRI

2.2 Conclusion

The reported incidence and occurrence of stress fractures in the literature is variable. The most robust data, originating from the military, suggests that new or intensified activity and female gender are the major risk factors for development of a stress injury. The most vulnerable phase for sustaining a stress fractures was found to be the first 3–4 months of increased exposure. Among athletes, the pattern of injury and the incidence and occurrence varies by sport and level of competition, with the strongest tendency in runners and high-volume running sports.

Clinical Pearls

- Stress fractures mainly occur in the lower extremity, especially in the tibia and the metatarsals.
- Female athletes are more susceptible to stress fractures, and thus consideration should be given to increasing their training loads and training intensity more gradually.
- Stress fractures often occur in a sport-specific pattern. Their diagnosis should always represent an alarm signal that prompts an interdisciplinary patient work up.

Review

Questions

1. *What group of people is at the highest risk of developing a stress fracture?*
   (a) Female Military Recruits
   (b) Male Tennis Players
   (c) Male Skiers
   (d) Female Racing Car Drivers
2. *What subpopulation has been studied closely to determine epidemiologic risk factors for stress fractures?*
   (a) Rugby Players
   (b) Military Personnel
   (c) Tennis Players
   (d) Swimmers
3. *Is it possible to develop stress fractures of the ribs?*
   (a) Rib stress fractures can occur in any sport with intensified respiratory activity.
   (b) Rib stress fractures have not been reported due to the elasticity of the thorax.
   (c) Rib stress fractures have been reported in pitchers, weightlifters, competitive rowers, golfers but can occur in other sports as well.
   (d) Rib stress fractures have been mostly reported in aquatic sports such as swimming and high diving.
4. *Which of the following patients in your clinic is at the highest risk to develop a stress fracture?*
   (a) 19-year-old male military recruit after 6 months of his basic training
   (b) 33-year-old professional basketball player during off-season
   (c) 19-year-old female long-distance runner, recovering from a training interruption due to hypermenorrhea.
   (d) 36-year-old female military officer during a winter skiing trip.

Answers

1. a.
2. b.
3. c
4. c.

References

1. Sormaala MJ, Niva MH, Kiuru MJ, Mattila VM, Pihlajamaki HK. Stress injuries of the calcaneus detected with magnetic resonance imaging in military recruits. J Bone Joint Surg Am. 2006;88(10):2237–42.
2. Shapiro M, Zubkov K, Landau R. Diagnosis of stress fractures in military trainees: A large-scale cohort. BMJ Mil Health. 2020;1–4.
3. Gaeta M, Minutoli F, Scribano E, et al. CT and MR imaging findings in athletes with early tibial stress injuries: comparison with bone scintigraphy findings and emphasis on cortical abnormalities. Radiology. 2005;235(2):553–61.
4. Wall J, Feller JF. Imaging of stress fractures in runners. Clin Sports Med. 2006;25(4):781–802.
5. Cosman F, Ruffing J, Zion M, et al. Determinants of stress fracture risk in United States Military Academy cadets. Bone. 2013;55(2):359–66.
6. Shaffer RA, Rauh MJ, Brodine SK, Trone DW, Macera CA. Predictors of stress fracture susceptibility in young female recruits. Am J Sports Med. 2006;34(1):108–15.
7. Knapik J, Montain SJ, McGraw S, Grier T, Ely M, Jones BH. Stress fracture risk factors in basic combat training. Int J Sports Med. 2012;33(11):940–6.
8. Lee D, Armed Forces Health Surveillance C. Stress fractures, active component, U.S. Armed Forces, 2004-2010. MSMR. 2011;18(5):8–11.
9. Mattila VM, Niva M, Kiuru M, Pihlajamaki H. Risk factors for bone stress injuries: a follow-up study of 102,515 person-years. Med Sci Sports Exerc. 2007;39(7):1061–6.
10. Takkar P, Prabhakar R. Stress fractures in military recruits: a prospective study for evaluation of incidence, patterns of injury and invalidments out of service. Med J Armed Forces India. 2019;75(3):330–4.
11. Ben-Ami IS, Ankory R, Kadar A, Rotman D, Snir N, Schermann H. The effect of previous methylphenidate use on incidence of stress fractures in military recruits: a retrospective cohort. J Bone Joint Surg Am. 2018;100(11):930–5.
12. Gam A, Goldstein L, Karmon Y, et al. Comparison of stress fractures of male and female recruits during basic training in the Israeli anti-aircraft forces. Mil Med. 2005;170(8):710–2.

13. Waterman BR, Gun B, Bader JO, Orr JD, Belmont PJ Jr. Epidemiology of lower extremity stress fractures in the United States Military. Mil Med. 2016;181(10):1308–13.
14. Yanovich R, Merkel D, Israeli E, Evans RK, Erlich T, Moran DS. Anemia, iron deficiency, and stress fractures in female combatants during 16 months. J Strength Cond Res. 2011; 25(12):3412–21.
15. Pihlajamaki H, Parviainen M, Kyrolainen H, Kautiainen H, Kiviranta I. Regular physical exercise before entering military service may protect young adult men from fatigue fractures. BMC Musculoskelet Disord. 2019;20(1):126.
16. Krauss MR, Garvin NU, Boivin MR, Cowan DN. Excess stress fractures, musculoskeletal injuries, and health care utilization among unfit and overweight female army trainees. Am J Sports Med. 2017;45(2):311–6.
17. Sanchez-Santos MT, Davey T, Leyland KM, et al. Development of a prediction model for stress fracture during an intensive physical training program: the Royal Marines Commandos. Orthop J Sports Med. 2017;5(7):2325967117716381.
18. Johanson MA. Contributing factors in microtrauma injuries of the lower extremity. J Back Musculoskelet Rehabil. 1992;2(4):12–25.
19. Kiel J, Kaiser K. Stress reaction and fractures. In: StatPearls. Treasure Island, FL: StatPearls; 2020.
20. Brunet ME, Cook SD, Brinker MR, Dickinson JA. A survey of running injuries in 1505 competitive and recreational runners. J Sports Med Phys Fitness. 1990;30(3):307–15.
21. Tenforde AS, Sayres LC, McCurdy ML, Collado H, Sainani KL, Fredericson M. Overuse Injuries in High School Runners: Lifetime Prevalence and Prevention Strategies. PM R. 2011;3:125–31.
22. Yagi S, Muneta T, Sekiya I. Incidence and risk factors for medial tibial stress syndrome and tibial stress fracture in high school runners. Knee Surg Sports Traumatol Arthrosc. 2013;21(3):556–63.
23. Maquirriain J, Ghisi JP. The incidence and distribution of stress fractures in elite tennis players. Br J Sports Med. 2006;40(5):454–9; discussion 459.
24. Abrams GD, Renstrom PA, Safran MR. Epidemiology of musculoskeletal injury in the tennis player. Br J Sports Med. 2012;46(7):492–8.
25. Drakos MC, Domb B, Starkey C, Callahan L, Allen AA. Injury in the national basketball association: a 17-year overview. Sports Health. 2010;2(4):284–90.
26. Khan M, Madden K, Burrus MT, et al. Epidemiology and impact on performance of lower extremity stress injuries in professional basketball players. Sports Health. 2018;10(2):169–74.
27. Field AE, Gordon CM, Pierce LM, Ramappa A, Kocher MS. Prospective study of physical activity and risk of developing a stress fracture among preadolescent and adolescent girls. Arch Pediatr Adolesc Med. 2011;165(8):723–8.
28. Niemeyer P, Weinberg A, Schmitt H, Kreuz PC, Ewerbeck V, Kasten P. Stress fractures in adolescent competitive athletes with open physis. Knee Surg Sports Traumatol Arthrosc. 2006;14(8):771–7.
29. Lee AD. Golf-related stress fractures: a structured review of the literature. J Can Chiropr Assoc. 2009;53(4):290–9.
30. Kadel N. Foot and ankle problems in dancers. Phys Med Rehabil Clin N Am. 2014;25(4):829–44.
31. Ekegren CL, Quested R, Brodrick A. Journal of Science and Medicine in Sport Injuries in pre-professional ballet dancers: Incidence, characteristics and consequences. J Sci Med Sport. 2014;17:271–75.
32. McCarthy MM, Voos JE, Nguyen JT, Callahan L, Hannafin JA. Injury profile in elite female basketball athletes at the Women's National Basketball Association combine. Am J Sports Med. 2013;41(3):645–51.
33. Frost WL, Chalmers DJ. Injury in elite New Zealand cricketers 2002-2008: descriptive epidemiology. Br J Sports Med. 2014;48(12):1002–7.
34. Ekstrand J, Torstveit MK. Stress fractures in elite male football players. Scand J Med Sci Sports. 2012;22(3):341–6.
35. Pearce CJ, Brooks JH, Kemp SP, Calder JD. The epidemiology of foot injuries in professional rugby union players. Foot Ankle Surg. 2011;17(3):113–8.

Acute Fracture Injuries in Sport

3

Greg A. J. Robertson, Alexander M. Wood,
Raju S. Ahluwalia, and Gary F. Keenan

Learning Objectives

- To develop an understanding of the basic science principles relevant to acute fractures in sport.
- To understand the role of fracture healing in facilitating an early return to sport.
- To determine the common injury patterns for acute fractures in sport, and to understand the associated biomechanical principles.
- To establish the optimal treatment methods for acute fractures in the athlete, and to understand the associated biomechanical principles.
- To understand the basic science principles of injury prevention for acute fractures in sport.

3.1 Introduction

Acute fractures in sport represent a unique set injuries, comprising a cohort of fractures that occur in a high-functioning, highly-motivated, athletic population, in which the goal is to return to sport as soon as possible [1–10]. The basic science principles, relevant to fracture healing and management of sport-related fractures, are largely similar to the basic science principles of fracture care in the general population [1, 11–22].

However, certain key factors differentiate this group from the general population, and so the relevant basic science principles need to be reconsidered, when approaching fracture care in the athlete [1–10]. These key factors comprise:

- Sport-related fractures predominantly occur in young, healthy, highly active individuals, in which bone metabolism is at its optimum, with potential for accelerated fracture healing times [1–10, 23, 24].
- These patients are highly-motivated to return to sport as early as possible, with the lowest morbidity possible, both for functional and financial reasons [1]. Thus treatment principles should be selected, with this in consideration [1, 6–10].
- In addition to the 'standard' principles of anatomical reduction, stable fixation, and timely rehabilitation, further treatment principles for these injuries include: surgical stabilisation of undisplaced unstable injuries [1, 6, 8]; promotion of 'internal' fixation methods (e.g. plate fixation instead of k-wire fixation) [1, 25]; and identification of stable injury patterns to avoid unnecessary surgery [1, 5, 10].
- Injury prevention plays a key role in this patient group, given the effect such fractures can have on an athlete's career [26]. Thus an in-depth as assessment of injury epidemiology [27–29], surveillance [26, 30–35] and biomechanics [11, 14, 17, 19–21] is necessary, to facilitate protective measures and reduce injury incidence.

With a view towards this 'accelerated' fracture care model for the athletic patient, this chapter will address the key basic principles in fracture treatment.

As an overview of the topics to be covered, these include:

- An assessment of fracture healing in the young athletic patient, in order to understand the interplay between fracture healing, fracture treatment and athlete rehabilitation.
- An improved understanding of the common injury patterns for fractures in sport, the causative biomechanics,

G. A. J. Robertson (✉)
Edinburgh Orthopaedic Trauma Unit, Royal Infirmary of Edinburgh, Edinburgh, UK

A. M. Wood
Oxford Trauma Unit, John Radcliffe Hospital, Oxford University Hospitals NHS Trust, Oxford, UK

R. S. Ahluwalia
Kings College Hospital, London NHS Trust & Kings Diabetic Foot Unit, London, UK
e-mail: r.ahluwalia1@nhs.net

G. F. Keenan
Edinburgh Orthopaedic Trauma Unit, Edinburgh, UK

G. A. J. Robertson, N. Maffulli (eds.), *Fractures in Sport*, https://doi.org/10.1007/978-3-030-72036-0_3

and the resultant fracture patterns. This allows the determination of fracture stability, a key factor in deciding treatment. This also facilitates the development of methods and equipment to aid fracture prevention. As an overview, in the athlete, a stable fracture is one with which full-weightbearing can occur, without a risk of displacement [1]. Conversely, an unstable fracture is one with which non-weightbearing or restrictive immobilisation is required, to prevent further fracture displacement [1].
- An assessment of the relevant basic sciences relating to management. This will provide a clear understanding, regarding the selection of the optimal treatment methods for common fracture types. The individual treatment methods, both conservative and surgical, will be reviewed to provide guidance on which of the techniques can facilitate the optimal return to sport.
- A review of injury prevention of fractures in sport, assessing the science of injury surveillance, and the biomechanical principles of injury prevention, and the evidence-based recommendations for protective equipment and adaptive practices in sport.

3.2 Fracture Healing

Fracture healing is the process by which traumatic osseous defects repair [12, 16, 19]. This can be divided into primary fracture healing and secondary fracture healing [12, 16, 19].

3.2.1 Primary Fracture Healing

Primary fracture healing is a process of direct bone healing [12, 16, 19]. It occurs through direct Haversian remodelling, with contact healing and gap healing [12, 16, 19]. Osteoblasts differentiate from mesenchymal stem cells and produce osteoid matrix at the fracture site, which is subsequently calcified [12, 16, 19]. Lamellar bone is formed directly when the fracture ends are in contact (i.e. <0.01 mm), during contact healing: while woven bone is formed provisionally to bridge fracture gaps, when present and of bridgeable size (i.e. <0.05 mm), during gap healing [12, 16, 19].

Remodelling of the fracture site occurs once osseous bridging has been achieved [12, 16, 19]. This occurs through the 'cutting cone' dynamic, with a front of osteoclasts removing the formed bone, followed by osteoblasts, which lay down organised osteoid matrix around a central advancing blood vessel to form an osteon [12, 16, 19]. In comparison to osteoblasts, osteoclasts differentiate from haematopoetic stem cells, with fusion of monocyte progenitors to form irregular multinucleated giant cells [12, 16, 19]. Osteoclasts function to resorb bone, while osteoblasts function to form bone, with both playing a key role in the bone remodelling unit [12, 16, 19].

Primary bone healing requires the fractures ends to be held with absolute stability, in direct contact to each other [12, 16, 19]. Absolute stability is defined by a fracture-site strain (i.e. the potential change in 'fracture gap' relative to the original length of the 'fracture gap' (%)) of less than 2% [12, 16, 19].

This method of fracture healing is observed with direct compression fracture fixation methods (i.e. lag screw and neutralisation, or compression plating) (Fig. 3.1) [12, 16, 17, 19].

The duration till fracture site healing is more prolonged with primary healing than with secondary healing [12, 16, 17, 19]. Due to the accompanying metalwork, and limited callus formation, it is also often difficult to accurately confirm radiographic healing with primary fracture healing [12, 16, 17, 19]. Stable fracture alignment with serial radiographic imaging is commonly used to guide progression of weight bearing and rehabilitation with this healing method [12, 16, 17, 19].

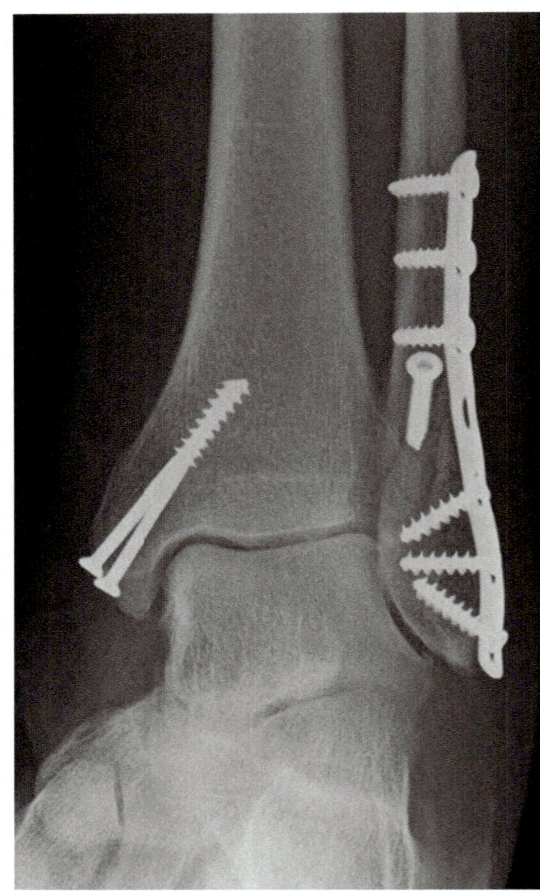

Fig. 3.1 Primary bone healing—an antero-posterior ankle radiograph of a supination external rotation type 4 ankle fracture treated with lag screw and neutralisation plate fixation (lateral malleolus), and partially threaded cancellous lag screw fixation (medial malleolus)

3.2.2 Secondary Fracture Healing

Secondary fracture healing is a process of indirect bone healing [12, 16, 19]. This involves both endochondral and intramembranous ossification [12, 16, 19]. Endochondral ossification follows a standard four stage fracture 'injury' model (Table 3.1) [12, 16, 19]:

1. haematoma formation, inflammatory cell invasion and granulation tissue formation (day 0–7);
2. 'soft' callus formation, comprising cartilage and fibrous tissue (day 7–28);
3. 'hard' callus formation, comprising osteoid and woven bone (day 28–120);
4. remodelling to form lamellar bone (day 120 onwards).

Endochondral ossification predominates within the intramedullary region of the fracture site, while intramembranous ossification occurs within the surrounding periosteal layer [12, 16, 19]. Fracture site micro-motion is required to promote callus formation [12, 16, 19]. This fracture repair mechanism occurs when fracture site strain is between 2 and 10%, with sufficient apposition of the fracture ends [12, 16, 19].

Within clinical practice, secondary fracture healing is observed with conservative treatment of adequately immobilised fractures (Figs. 3.2 and 3.3), and with surgical methods which provide relative fracture site stability (i.e. intra-medullary nailing, bridge plating) (Fig. 3.4) [12, 16, 17, 19].

Stability of secondary fracture healing is determined by both clinical and radiographic union [12, 17, 19, 36]. The definitions of these can vary, however, clinical union is com-

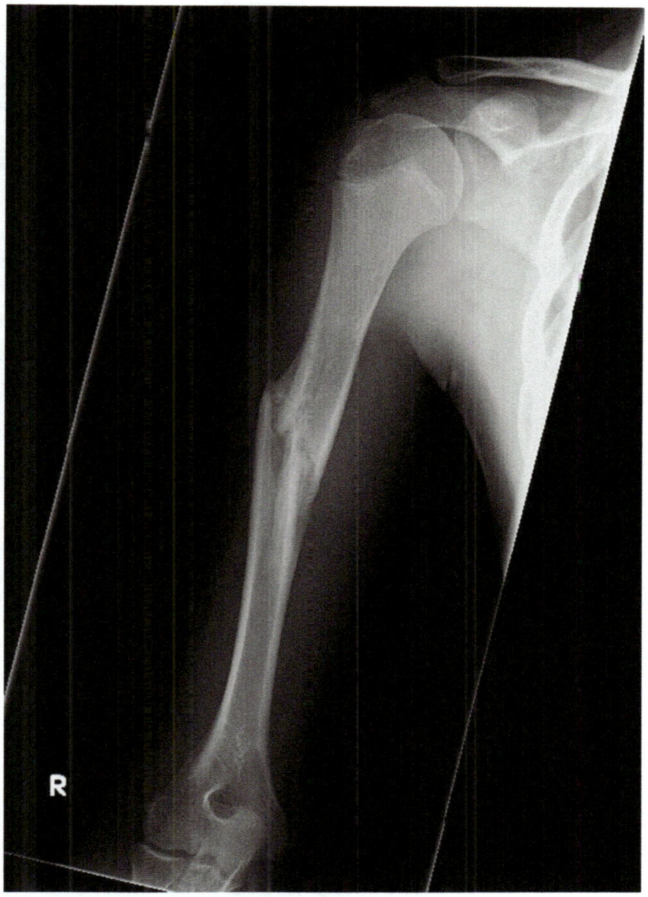

Fig. 3.2 Secondary bone healing—an oblique humeral radiograph of a humeral diaphyseal fracture treated with humeral brace immobilisation

Table 3.1 The stages of endochondral fracture healing

Stage	Time	Action	Cell types	Stability	Rehabilitation
Haematoma formation	At time of injury	Fracture haematoma develops from torn blood vessels, with subsequent fibrin clot formation. Pro-inflammatory mediators are then released from injured tissue and platelets.	Erythrocytes, platelets	Unstable	Rest and protect
Inflammation	0–7 days	Inflammatory cells migrate to the fracture site. Angiogenesis, phagocytosis and granulation tissue formation occur, with early recruitment of callus forming cells. Mediated by growth factors and cytokines.	Neutrophils, macrophages, fibroblasts, mesenchymal cells, osteoprogenitor cells, osteoclasts	Unstable	Rest and protect
Cartilaginous callus	7–28 days	Production of cartilaginous callus, comprising fibrous tissue and cartilage, through endochondral ossification at fracture site, with subsequent calcification. Production of bridging osseous callous in periosteum through intramembranous ossification.	Chondroblasts, fibroblasts, periosteal osteoblasts	Unstable	Non weight-bearing rehabilitation
Osseous callus	28–120 days	Replacement of cartilaginous callus with osteoid callus, followed by mineralisation, to form hard mineralised osteoid callus.	Chondroblasts, osteoblasts	Stable	Progressive weight-bearing rehabilitation
Remodelling	120 days+	Remodelling of the hard mineralised osteoid callus, from woven bone to organised lamellar bone, with re-establishment of the medullary canal. Involves the cutting cone process that occurs with primary bone healing.	Osteoclasts, osteoblasts	Stable	Return to sport as able

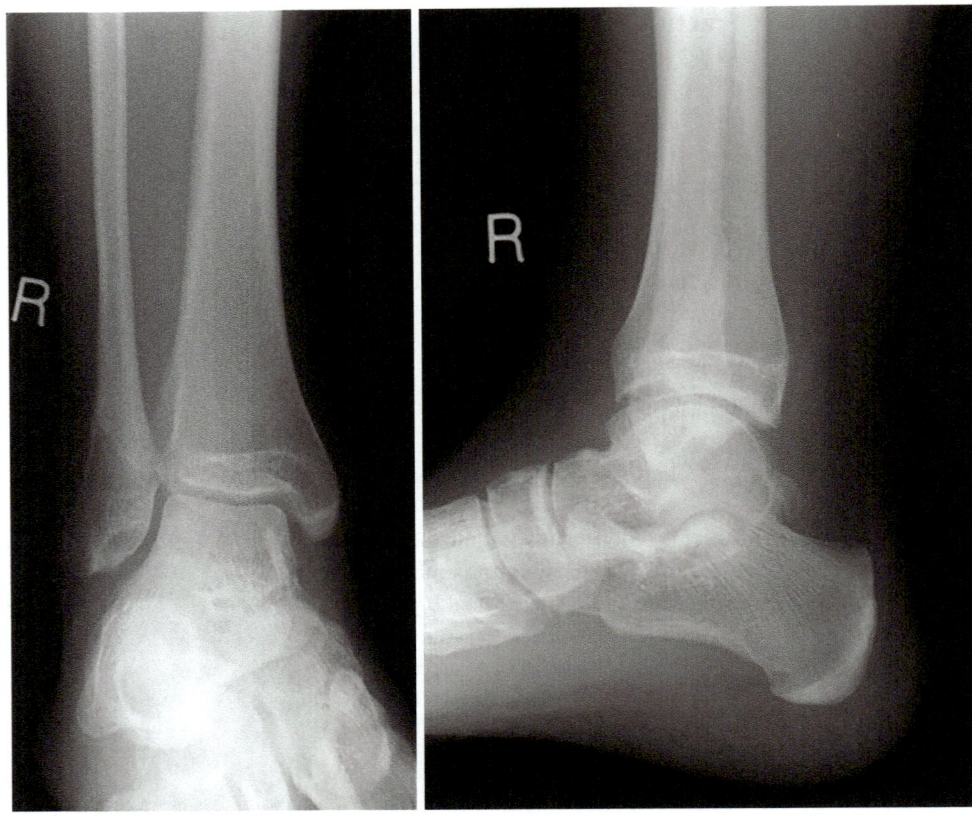

Fig. 3.3 Secondary bone healing—an antero-posterior ankle radiograph of a supination external rotation type 2 ankle fracture treated with 'moonboot' orthotic immobilisation

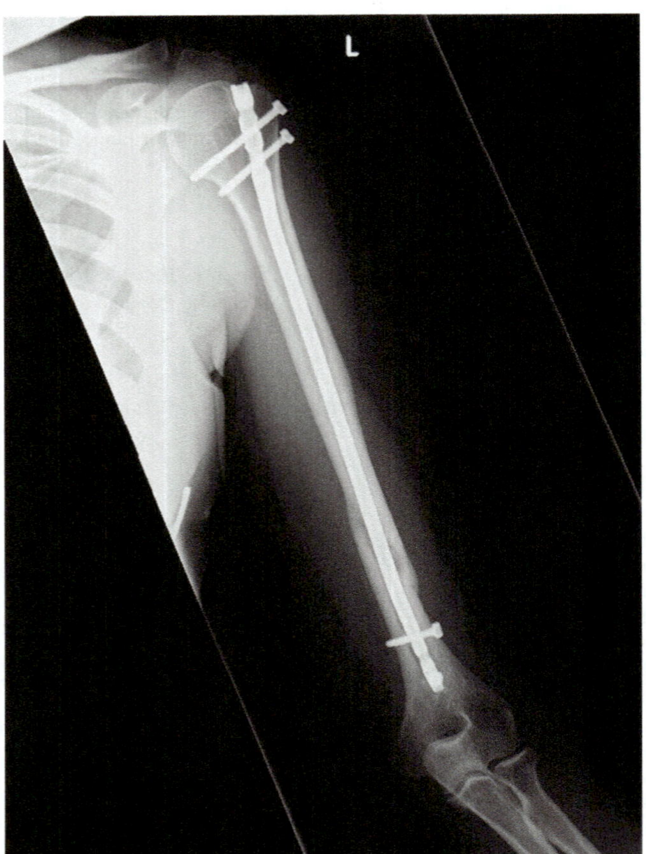

Fig. 3.4 Secondary bone healing—an oblique humeral radiograph of a humeral diaphyseal fracture treated with intra-medullary nailing

monly confirmed when there is no pain on physiological loading of the fracture site (e.g. with weightbearing) [12, 17, 19, 36]. Radiographic union is commonly confirmed when there is bridging callus noted across three of the four fracture cortices, on AP and lateral radiographs [12, 17, 19, 36]. The duration till fracture union varies depending on the location and nature of the fracture [12, 17, 19, 36]. Following establishment of fracture union, progressive weight-bearing and rehabilitation can be commenced [12, 17, 19, 36].

When fracture site strain exceeds 10%, there is insufficient fracture stability to facilitate bone formation, and this can lead to the development of a non-union [12, 16, 17, 19, 36].

3.2.3 Fracture Healing and Treatment

The type of fracture healing, which predominates within each of the main treatment modalities, is recorded in Table 3.2 [11–17].

The ability to determine whether a fracture pattern is suitable for conservative management, with secondary fracture healing, is dependent on accurate establishment of the stability of the injury [11–17].

The key factors for determining fracture stability are site-specific: however, as a generic rule, these include [11–17]:

1. Static fracture fragment displacement of less than 2 mm
2. Fracture fragment displacement of less than 2 mm on dynamic stress testing

Table 3.2 Fracture healing types by treatment modality

Treatment method	Type of bone healing	Process of bone healing
Conservative		
Cast	Secondary	Endochondral ossification (with periosteal bridging callus)
Surgical		
Compression plating	Primary	Haversian remodelling (contact healing and gap healing)
Lag screw and neutralisation plating	Primary	Haversian remodelling (contact healing and gap healing)
Bridge plating	Secondary	Endochondral ossification (with periosteal bridging callus)
Intra-medullary nailing	Secondary	Endochondral ossification (with periosteal bridging callus)
External fixation (rigid)	Primary	Haversian remodelling (contact healing and gap healing)
External fixation (dynamic)	Secondary	Endochondral ossification (with periosteal bridging callus)
K-wire fixation	Secondary	Endochondral ossification (with periosteal bridging callus)

3. A trial of full weight-bearing with subsequent fracture fragment displacement of less than 2 mm
4. The absence of angulation of the fracture fragments
5. The absence of comminution of the fracture fragments.

The mean safe time to return to sport for each fracture type is dependent on the location of the fracture, the configuration of the fracture, the treatment method selected, the type of fracture healing involved, and the activities involved [1]. As a rule, both clinical and radiological union are recommended prior to returning to sport [1]. This however is at the discretion of the treating physician and the athlete, with some patients wishing to return to sport prior to achieving complete union [1].

With specific relevance to the athletic patient, union times are theoretically faster in younger healthy patients, compared to the general population [1, 23, 24]. Laboratory based studies have confirmed that key components and promoters of the fracture healing process are present in higher quantities at a younger age [23, 24]. This should facilitate the young healthy athlete to be able to return to sport at the earliest possible stage, given the likelihood of expedient achievement of union [1, 11–17]. However, clinical testing has not been confirmed in this area, so each case should be directed by clinical and radiological evidence, along with surgeon experience [1, 23, 24].

There is a growing interest in the use of Orthobiologic Therapies to supplement fracture healing [37–40]. This topic is detailed in Sect. 6.1.

3.2.4 Non-union

Despite careful fracture management in the athletic population, fracture non-union remains a potential risk, with reported rate ranging from 1 to 2% [2–5]. Non-unions can be classified as: hypertrophic, atrophic, oligotrophic, septic or pseudo-arthrosis, based on clinical, radiological, histological and microbiological findings [17, 19, 22, 36]. Various definitions exist for non-union, which include:

(a) no evidence of fracture healing by 9 months post-injury, with no progression in fracture healing over the preceding 3months;
(b) no evidence of fracture healing beyond 6 months post-injury;
(c) failure of fracture healing within the expected timeframe for a specific fracture;
(d) no potential for fracture healing without further intervention [17, 19, 22, 36].

Fractures that fail to completely unite by 6 months post-injury should be considered delayed unions [17, 19, 22, 36].

In post-surgical cases, infection should always be considered as a cause for non-union, and investigated accordingly [17, 19, 22, 36]. Hypertrophic non-unions occur secondary to mechanical instability, with peripheral callus visible on the radiograph, though no bridging callus across the fracture site [17, 19, 22, 36]. Atrophic non-unions occur secondary to impaired biological conditions, with no evidence of callus on radiographs [17, 19, 22, 36]. Oligotrophic non-unions occur secondary to rigidly surgically-stabilised fractures with a significant gap between fracture ends, preventing bridging callus from forming [17, 19, 22, 36]. Given that athletes are predominantly young healthy patients, with a predilection to return to sport too early, hypertrophic non-union is more commonly observed in this patient cohort [2–5].

Infection, if present, requires identification and treatment as the first line of management [17, 19, 22, 36]. Following this, the management of hypertrophic non-unions comprises re-stabilisation of the fracture site (+/− the addition of an orthobiologic stimulus, often autologous bone graft) [17, 19, 22, 36]. The management of atrophic non-unions comprises debridement of the fracture ends to a healthy bleeding base, re-stabilisation and compression of the fracture ends, with the addition of an orthobiologic stimulus, often autologous bone graft [17, 19, 22, 36]. One must also consider and manage patient factors (e.g. systematic illness, such as diabetes) and iatrogenic factors (e.g. NSAIDs), that can lead to delayed union or non-union [17, 19, 22, 36].

3.3 Injury Patterns

3.3.1 Epidemiology and Classification

Fractures in the athlete often occur in set locations, with set injury patterns, according to the sport played, and the position played [1–10, 27–29, 41–48]. An understanding of these mechanisms of injury enable sports teams, sports physicians and orthopaedic surgeons to establish the common expected fracture patterns, and so develop optimal treatment plans [1].

Classification systems serve as a method of describing the location and nature of the fracture, which can guide treatment, allow for more accurate communication among clinicians, and facilitate the stratification of fracture types for research [49]. The majority of fracture classifications for acute fractures are site-specific, and each of the commonly used classifications are discussed in the relevant chapters [49]. As an overview, the AO/OTA (Arbeitsgemeinschaft für Osteosynthesefragen/Orthopaedic Trauma Association) classification provides a generic classification system that can be applied to all fracture types throughout the skeleton [49, 50]. Its predecessor (the AO Classification) has proved highly effective in coordinating recent epidemiological research on acute sport–related fractures, and both should be recommended [2–5, 27, 28, 41, 44, 51]. Regarding acute open sport-related fractures, the Gustilo classification has also proved highly effective in coordinating recent epidemiological research on this topic, and this should similarly be recommended (Table 3.3) [51, 52].

Acute sport-related fractures often differ significantly in location from the more common osteoporotic fractures seen in the aging general population [27, 28, 53]. For instance, the three commonest locations for osteoporotic fractures are the vertebrae, the distal radius and the proximal femur [53]. In comparison, the three commonest locations for sport-related fractures are finger phalanx, distal radius and metacarpals [27, 41]. Thus the cohort of acute sport-related fractures represents a unique entity [27, 41].

In terms of demographics, within the general population, three-quarters of all sport-related fractures occur in the upper limb, and one quarter in the lower limb [27, 28]. Similar ratios have been found in cohorts of amateur soccer players, rugby players and field hockey players [2–4]. Interestingly, however fracture locations and patterns can vary between amateur and professional sporting populations, with three quarters of all fractures in professional soccer players found to occur in the lower limb, and one quarter in the upper limb [29]. Variations in these ratios are also observed with sport-related open fracture, where three-fifths of such fractures occur in the upper limb, and two-fifths in the lower limb [51]. Fractures of the axial skeleton (pelvis and spine) are rare in sporting populations, and so analyses of their epidemiology and causative patterns are limited [27, 28].

To understand the common injury patterns, it is necessary to define the common causative sports for fractures. In the UK and Europe, the common causative sport for acute fractures comprise: soccer, rugby, snow-sports (skiing and snowboarding), cycling and horse-riding [27, 28]. In North America, the common causative sports comprise: American Football, soccer, basketball, wrestling and baseball [42, 43]. In Asia, the common causative sports comprise: soccer, basketball, high jump, rugby and martial arts [54].

3.3.2 Injury Patterns

Injury patterns can be analysed in a variety of ways [2–5, 27, 28]. A review of such patterns by individual playing positions can prove clinically useful: however, given the numerous potential positions and respective sports, such an analysis can be overly complex [2–5]. Thus, the authors choose to assess the common injury patterns by anatomic location, with segregation of these by each of the common sports [2–5].

Data from this research has provided a detailed insight into the mechanisms of injury for fractures sustained during soccer, rugby and field hockey (Table 3.4) [2–4]. This provides data on a 'lower limb' 'non-contact' sport (soccer), an 'upper limb' full-contact sport (rugby) and a 'stick and ball' sport (field hockey) [2–4]. The data from these three categories of sport can then be generalised to similar sports in other geographical regions [42, 43, 54].

In Table 3.4, data is presented on the commonest fracture patterns observed at each anatomic location [2–4].

This data shows that the majority of fractures, in the three sports, result from non-contact, low-energy mechanisms [2–4]. As a consequence, the common recorded fractures types are low-energy fracture patterns, such are oblique and spiral (Fig. 3.5) [2–4, 11, 19]. The exception to this is the transverse fracture pattern, which is commonly observed with tibial diaphyseal fracture: this is a high-energy fracture pattern (Fig. 3.6) [2–4, 11, 19]. Excluding this, it can be appreciated that the majority of sport-related fractures are low-energy injuries, within the spectrum of fracture injuries [2–4, 11, 19].

The high proportion of upper limb fractures is likely a reflection of the predominance of low-energy, non-contact mechanisms of injury, such as 'fall' and 'ball collision' [2–4]. Lower limb fractures often require a high-energy, 'contact' injury mechanism, and such mechanisms would appear to be less frequent within amateur athletes [2–4, 11, 19]. However, when comparing this data, with cohorts of profes-

Table 3.3 Sport-related open fractures—management principles by Gustilo classification

Gustilo grade	Wound size (cm)	Periosteal stripping	Contamination	Soft tissue coverage possible	Vascular injury requiring repair	Antibiotics	Soft tissue management	Fracture stabilisation
1	≤1	No	Minimal	Yes	No	1st generation cephalosporin	Direct closure	Site specific
2	1–10	No	Moderate	Yes	No	1st generation cephalosporin	Direct closure	Site specific
3a	>10	Yes	Severe	Yes	No	1st generation cephalosporin + aminoglycoside	Direct closure	Site specific +/− temporising Ex-Fix
3b	>10	Yes	Severe	No	No	1st generation cephalosporin + aminoglycoside	Rotational or free flap required	Site specific +/− temporising Ex-Fix
3c	>10	Dependent on injury severity	Severe	Dependent on injury severity	Yes	1st generation cephalosporin + aminoglycoside	Dependent on severity of soft tissue injury	Site specific +/− temporising Ex-Fix
Notes	High-risk environments include farmyards and marine environments. Add high-dose penicillin for farmyard injuries and heavily contaminated injuries. Add a fluoroquinolone or a 3rd/4th generation cephalosporin for freshwater injuries. Add doxycycline with a fluoroquinolone or a 3rd/4th generation cephalosporin for saltwater injuries. Tetanus management depends on injury contamination, timing of presentation and immunisation status.							

Ex-Fix external fixator

Table 3.4 Mechanisms of injury and fracture patterns

Fracture location	MMOI soccer[2]	MMOI rugby[3]	MMOI field hockey[4]	Most recorded fracture pattern
Upper limb				
Clavicle	Fall	Tackle	Ball strike	Mid-diaphyseal/non-comminuted
Proximal humerus	Fall	Tackle	–	Two-part involving greater tuberosity
Humeral diaphysis	–	Tackle	–	Spiral/non-comminuted
Olecranon	Fall	–	–	Articular/stable/non-comminuted
Radial head	Fall	Fall	–	Non-displaced/minimally displaced
Radius and ulna	Fall	Lineout	–	Non-comminuted
Radial diaphysis	Goals	Ruck	–	Non-comminuted
Ulna diaphysis	Goals	–	–	Non-comminuted
Distal radius	Fall	Fall	–	Extra-articular/non-comminuted
Distal ulna	–	Fall	Stick strike	Extra-articular/non-comminuted
Scaphoid	Fall	Fall	–	Waist/non-comminuted
Metacarpal	Goals	Tackle	Stick strike	Diaphyseal/oblique/non-comminuted
Finger phalanx	Goals	Tackle	Stick strike	Proximal/unicondylar
		Lower limb		
Proximal femur	–	–	–	Undisplaced trans-cervical
Femoral diaphysis	–	–	–	Spiral/non-comminuted
Distal femur				Partial-articular/frontal (Hoffa)
Proximal tibia	Twist	–	–	Tibial spine avulsion
Tibial plateau	Tackle	–	–	Lateral split (Schzakter I)
Patella	Fall	–	Ball strike	Transverse
Tibia	Tackle	Tackle	–	Diaphyseal/transverse
Fibula	Tackle	Twist	–	Spiral
Ankle	Tackle	Tackle	Inversion	Supination external rotation type 2 (isolated Weber B lateral malleolus)
Talus	Twist	Tackle	–	Lateral process fracture
Navicular	Tackle	–	–	Dorsal/transverse
Metatarsal	Tackle	Ruck	–	Diaphyseal/non-comminuted
Toe Phalanx	Tackle	–	–	Proximal/unicondylar
Pelvis	Fall	–	–	Stable public rami fracture (LC1)
Acetabulum	–	–	–	Post hemi-transverse and anterior column
Cervical spine				Lateral mass fracture of C1

MMOI most reported mechanism of injury, *LC1* lateral compression type 1 fracture

sional athletes, it is noticeable that professional sportspeople, particularly soccer players, record a significantly greater proportion of lower limb fractures [29]. This is likely a reflection of the higher energy injuries (often contact-related), sustained by professional athletes [11, 19, 29]. This also reflects the better conditioning of professional athletes, having a lower propensity to fall and sustain 'low-energy, non-contact' upper limb fractures [29].

This discrepancy between low-energy and high-energy fracture injuries, affecting the upper limb and the lower limb respectively, is particularly apparent when reviewing the incidence of open fractures in sport [51]. Open fractures are generally considered a higher energy injury, by the nature of the force required to break the overlying skin [11, 22, 51, 55]. Thus, it is unsurprising to note there is a significantly higher proportion of lower limb fractures in sport-related open fracture cohorts, compared to sport-related fracture cohorts as a whole [27, 28, 51].

Variations in injury patterns are also representative of the dynamics of the sport [27, 28, 41]. For instance, with field hockey, hand fractures predominate, secondary to contact with the ball or the stick [4, 41, 47, 48, 56]. As such, protective hand-gear may have a future role in reducing the fracture incidence within this sport [47]. This is a clear example of how a comprehensive overview of the expected injury patterns and their causative factors can facilitate injury prevention programmes for these fractures [57].

3.4 The Biomechanics of Fracture Injury

3.4.1 Force of Injury

Biomechanics forms a major part of fracture science [11, 13–15, 19]. The initial role of biomechanics in the field of 'fractures in sport' is to provide a clear understanding of the

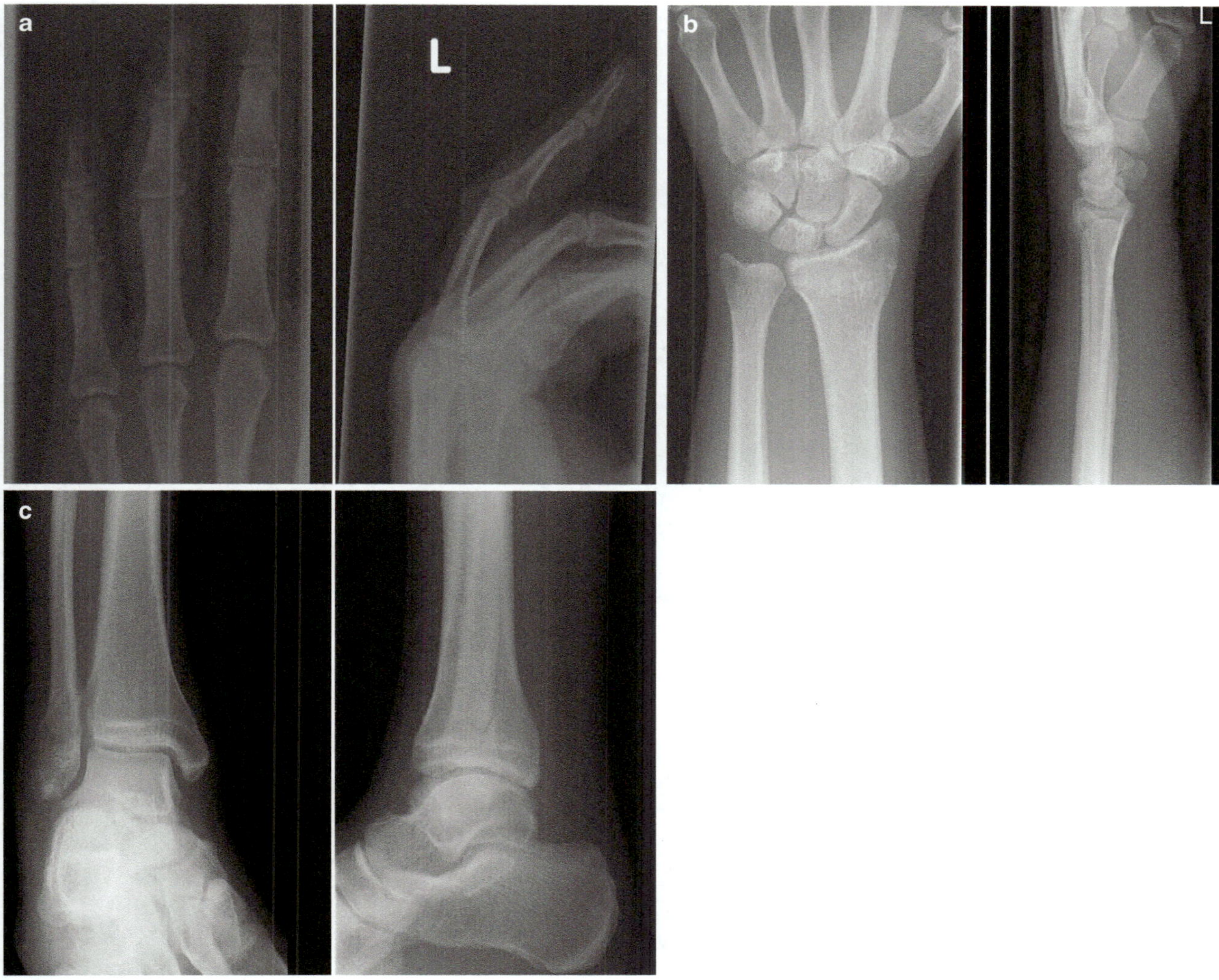

Fig. 3.5 The standard low-energy fracture patterns observed with sport-related fractures. (**a**) A minimally-displaced, non-comminuted, oblique fracture of the middle phalanx of a left little finger. (**b**) A minimally-displaced, non-comminuted, oblique fracture of a left distal radius. (**c**) A minimally-displaced, stable, non-comminuted, spiral, supination external rotation type 2 fracture of a right lateral malleolus

causative forces associated with each fracture [11, 13–15, 19]. The common causative mechanisms have been discussed above [2–4]. It is the resultant force imparted on the bone that determines the sustained fracture pattern [11, 19]. This then directs the mode of treatment [11, 13–15, 17, 19].

The main fracture loading mechanisms are: compression, tension, sheer, bending and torsion (Fig. 3.7) [11, 19]. These resultant fracture patterns are: spiral (secondary to torsion forces); oblique (secondary to compression forces or uneven bending forces); transverse (secondary to tension forces or pure bending forces); and butterfly (secondary to 'bending and compression' forces or 'torsion and compression' forces) [11, 19].

Among the common fracture patterns, such mechanisms of loading, and subsequent injury patterns, can be seen most obviously at the ankle and the tibia diaphysis [5, 11, 19, 58]. In the ankle, the Lauge-Hansen Classification clearly demonstrates the interplay between injury mechanism and fracture pattern [5, 11, 59]. While within tibial diaphysis, there is a logical, transparent link between the loading mechanism and the resultant fracture configuration [11, 19, 58]. Such fracture locations give a clear understanding of the causative injury mechanics, and so allow consideration to playing surface adjustments, footwear modifications, and targeted neuromuscular training to reduce the occurrence of these injuries [5, 11, 19, 58].

3.4.2 Bone Resistance

To understand the propensity of bone to fracture, it is necessary to view the stress-strain curve for bone (Fig. 3.8a) [11,

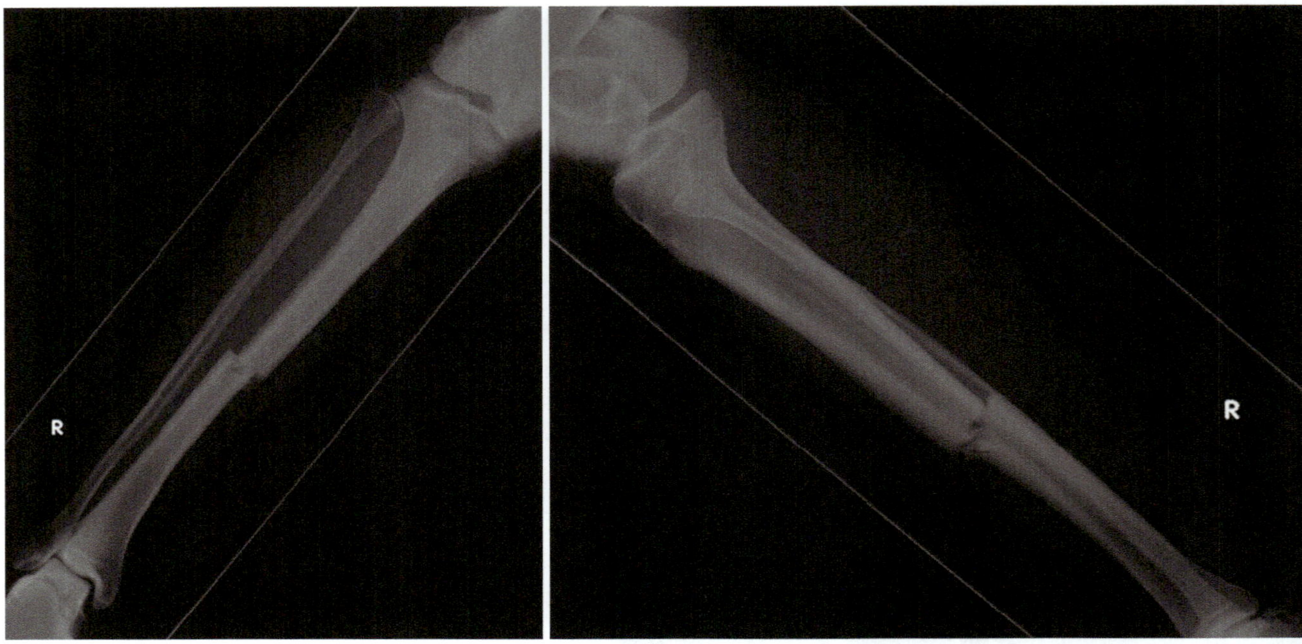

Fig. 3.6 A high-energy sport-related fracture pattern—a transverse fracture of the tibial diaphysis

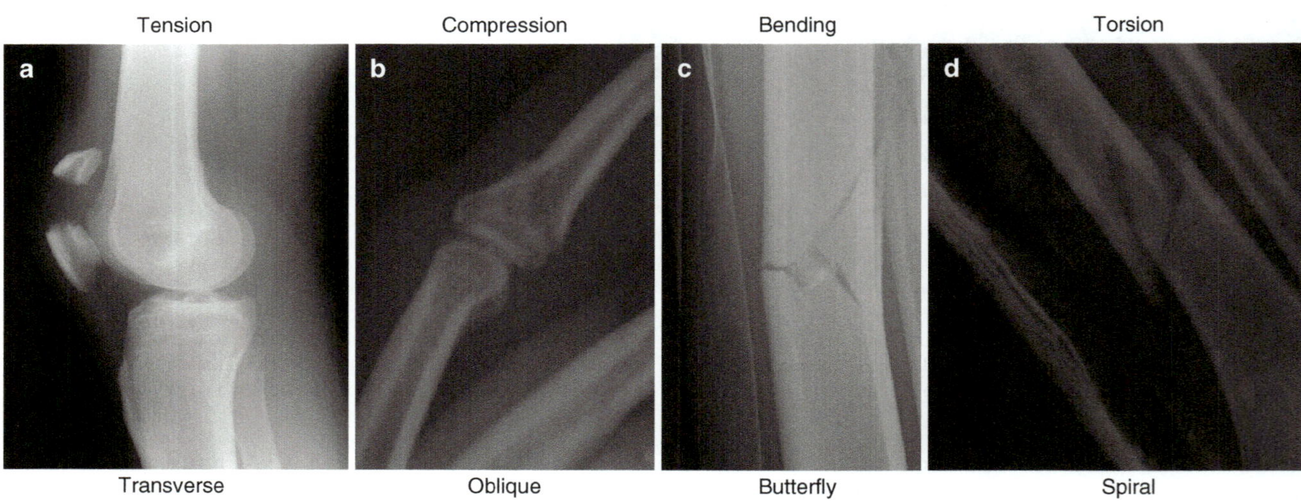

Fig. 3.7 Fracture patterns by mechanism of loading. (**a**) A transverse fracture pattern, secondary to 'tension' loading. (**b**) An oblique fracture pattern, secondary to 'compression' loading. (**c**) A 'butterfly' fracture pattern, secondary to 'bending' loading. (**d**) A spiral fracture pattern, secondary to 'torsional' loading

20, 22]. There are separate curves for both cortical bone and cancellous bone (Fig. 3.8b) [11, 20, 22]. Given bone's anisotropic nature, these curves also vary depending on the loading mechanism, acting on the bone (Fig. 3.8c) [11, 20, 22].

The key areas of each curve are the elastic region (the area of elastic deformation), the plastic region (the area of plastic deformation), the ultimate stress point and the fracture point [11, 20, 22]. Young's modulus of elasticity of bone is calculated from the gradient of the graph in the elastic zone (stress/strain) [11, 20, 22]. This provides a measure of resistance to deformity of the bone (i.e. stiffness) [11, 20, 22]. For cortical bone, Young's modulus is 10–30 GPa (GigaPascal) [11, 20, 22]. For cancellous bone, Young's modulus is 0.5–1.5 GPa [11, 20, 22]. By comparison, the Young's modulus of stainless steel is 190 GPa, and that of titanium is 110 GPa [11, 20, 22]. For cortical bone, the ultimate stress at failure in compression is approximately 200 N/m^2 (Newton per metre squared), while that in tension is approximately 150 N/m^2, and that in sheer approximately 80 N/m^2 [11, 20, 22].

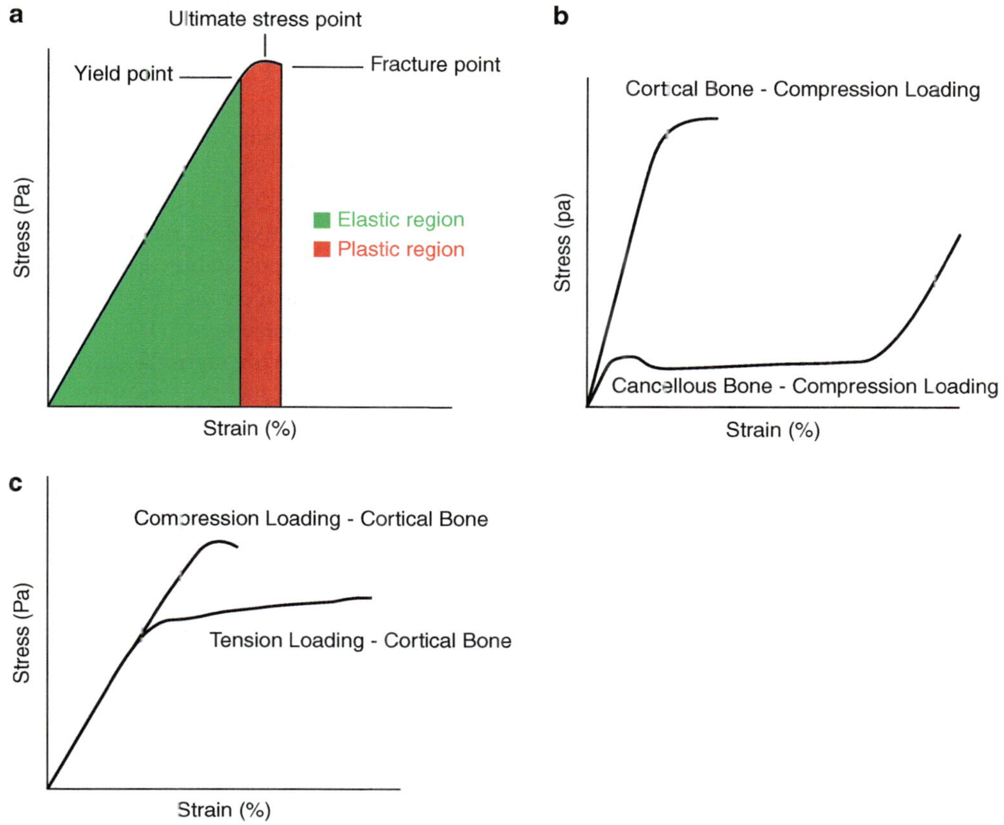

Fig. 3.8 The stress-strain curve of bone. (**a**) The stress –strain curve of cortical bone in compression loading. (**b**) The stress-strain curve of bone in compression loading—cortical vs. cancellous bone. (**c**) The stress-strain curve of cortical bone—compression loading vs. tension loading

Considering a bone, the resistance to bending, and subsequent fracture, is determined by the spatial distribution of the material, as well as the composition of the material [11, 20, 22]. The spatial distribution of an object is represented by the second moment area (SMA), which is proportional to the bending stress that an object can tolerate [11, 20, 22]. For cylindrically shaped bones, the SMA is proportional to the radius of the bone to the power 4 [11, 20, 22]. Thus, a cylindrical bone of double the radius, has 16 times the resistance to bending [11, 20, 22]. Similarly, for rectangular bones, the SMA is proportional to the thickness (perpendicular distance away from the neutral axis) of the bone to the power 3 [11, 20, 22]. Thus, a rectangular bone of double the thickness, has eight times the resistance to bending [11, 20, 22]. To note, for cortical bone, the required strain to cause a fracture is 2%, while that for cancellous bone is 75% [11, 19, 20, 22].

The concept of SMA is particularly relevant in callus formation during endochondral (secondary) fracture healing, where the increased radius and thickness of a bone can impart a significant increase in the bending rigidity of the healing fracture [11, 12, 19, 20, 22]. This concept is also relevant when considering the dimensions and material properties of fracture fixation materials, as discussed below [14, 15, 17].

Regarding the timescale of restoration of stability, studies have found that fracture healing restores normal osseous stiffness by around 4 weeks post-injury: however, other factors, such as the location and the structure of the bone, also influence time to fracture stability [12, 16, 19, 22]. With young athletic patients, fracture healing is often more rapid compared to the general population, allowing for reduced times to stability [23, 24]. An awareness of such dynamics can facilitate an accelerated return to weightbearing and rehabilitation for the athlete [1].

Over the course of an athlete's lifetime, there are variations in injury pattern observed at peri-articular sites: these variations comprise age-related presentations of avulsion injuries, soft tissue (ligament and tendon) injuries and fractures [11, 12, 19]. The resultant injury pattern is dependent on the nature and direction of the force [11, 12, 19]. However, with musculoskeletal injury, it is often the weakest structure that fails [11, 12, 19]. Thus in the skeletally immature patient, bones are weaker than ligaments, so avulsion injuries occur [11, 12, 19]. In the young adult, bones are stronger than ligaments, so ligament injuries predominate [11, 12, 19]. Then in the elderly skeleton, bones are weaker than ligaments, so fractures predominate [11, 12, 19].

3.4.3 Injury Stability

Determining the stability of a fracture pattern is key to establishing the optimal treatment modality [11, 19, 22]. Stable fracture patterns allow for early weight bearing with limited immobilisation, and so are suitable for conservative management [11, 13, 19]. However, non-operative management of unstable, undisplaced fracture patterns would require prolonged non-weightbearing with immobilisation, until fracture callus has stabilised the fracture: such fractures would thus benefit from surgical stabilisation, to facilitate early mobilisation and rehabilitation [11, 14, 19]. Biomechanical assessment of injury stability is often difficult in clinical practice, particularly due to associated pain limiting physical examination [11, 19, 22]. Markers of fracture instability are site-specific: however the generic instability markers are listed in Sect. 3.2 [11, 19, 22].

3.5 General Treatment Principles

3.5.1 Sport-Specific Principles

Fracture management in the athlete concords to the same principles as fracture management in the general population (Fig. 3.9a–i) [1]. These comprise anatomical reduction, stable fixation and early rehabilitation [1]. As such, undisplaced stable fractures are suitable for non-operative management. Displaced unstable fractures require operative management [1].

With undisplaced, potentially unstable, fractures, however, there is a growing divide in the treatment of such injuries in the athlete, compared to the general population [1, 6, 8, 60]. In the athlete, it is beneficial to convert an unstable fracture into a stabilised fracture, thus allowing early weight bearing and rehabilitation, facilitating an early return to sport

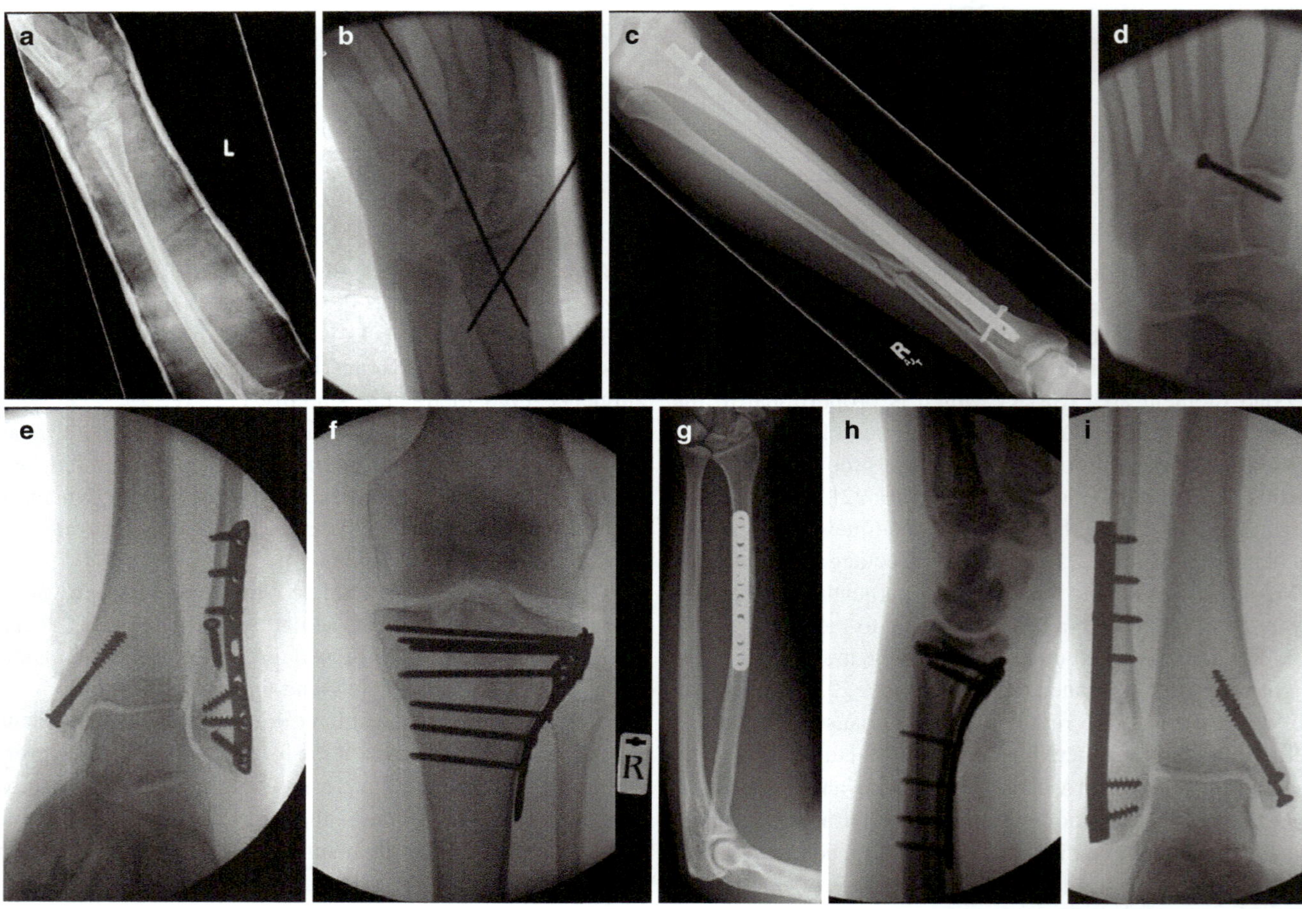

Fig. 3.9 Modes of treatment for sport-related fractures: (**a**) cast immobilisation. (**b**) K-wire fixation. (**c**) Intra-medullary nailing. (**d**) Screw fixation. (**e**) Lag screw and neutralisation plate fixation (lateral malleolus), with partially threaded cancellous lag screw fixation (medial malleolus). (**f**) Buttress plate fixation. (**g**) Compression plate fixation. (**h**) Locking plate fixation. (**i**) Bridge plate fixation (lateral malleolus), with partially threaded cancellous lag screw fixation (medial malleolus)

[1, 6, 8, 60]. Conservative management, which is often used in the general population to avoid the risks of surgery, would require a prolonged period of non-weightbearing, which would result in muscle wasting and deconditioning [1, 6, 8, 60]. As such, the benefits of surgical treatment in the athlete will likely out weight the risk of complications [1, 6, 8, 60]. Examples of such fractures include undisplaced tibial diaphyseal fractures (Fig. 3.10), undisplaced scaphoid waist fractures (Fig. 3.11) and undisplaced fifth metatarsal proximal metaphyseal-diaphyseal (Jones) fractures [1, 6, 8, 60].

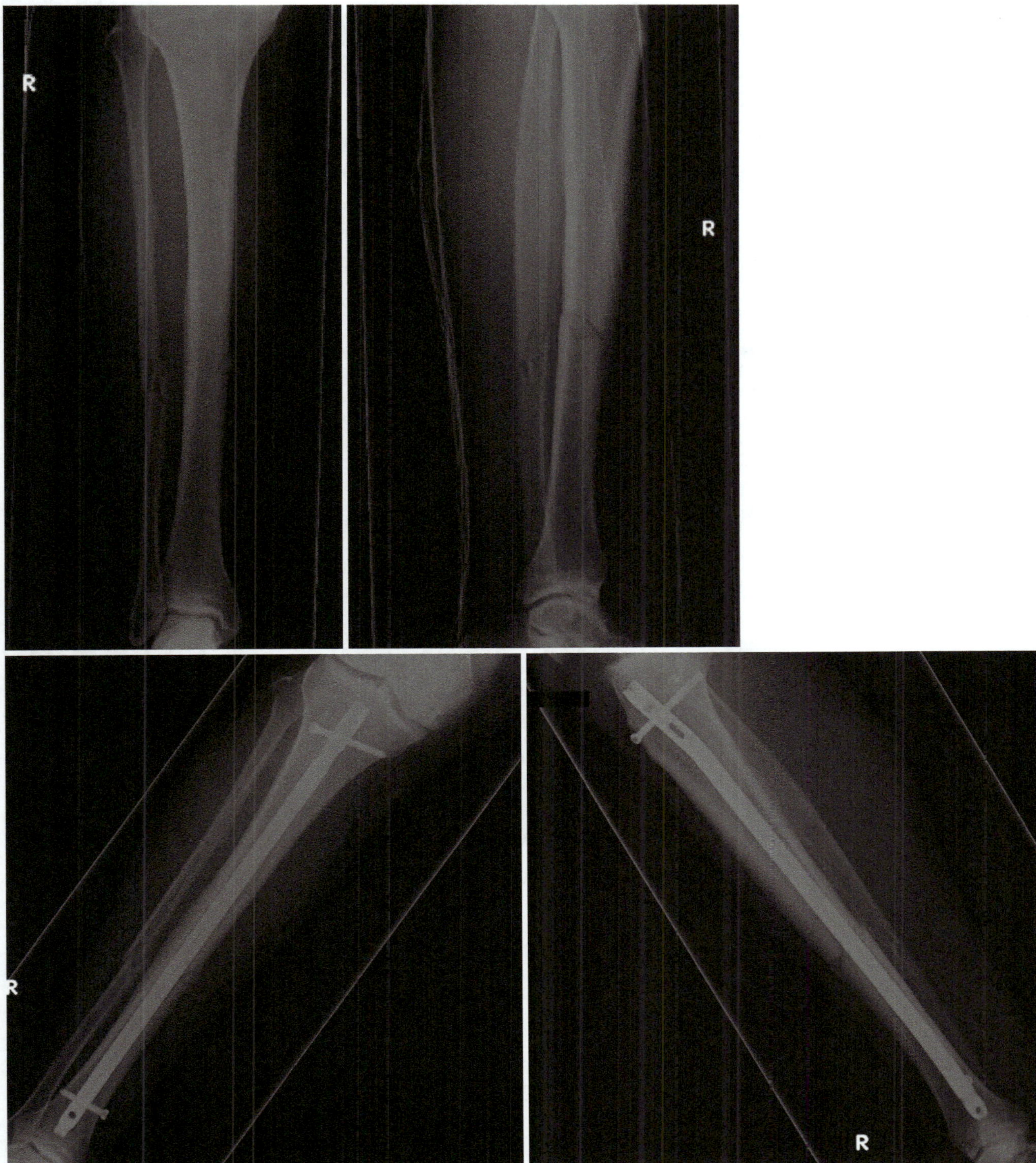

Fig. 3.10 Evidence-based management for sport-related fractures: intra-medullary nailing of a minimally displaced tibial diaphyseal fracture

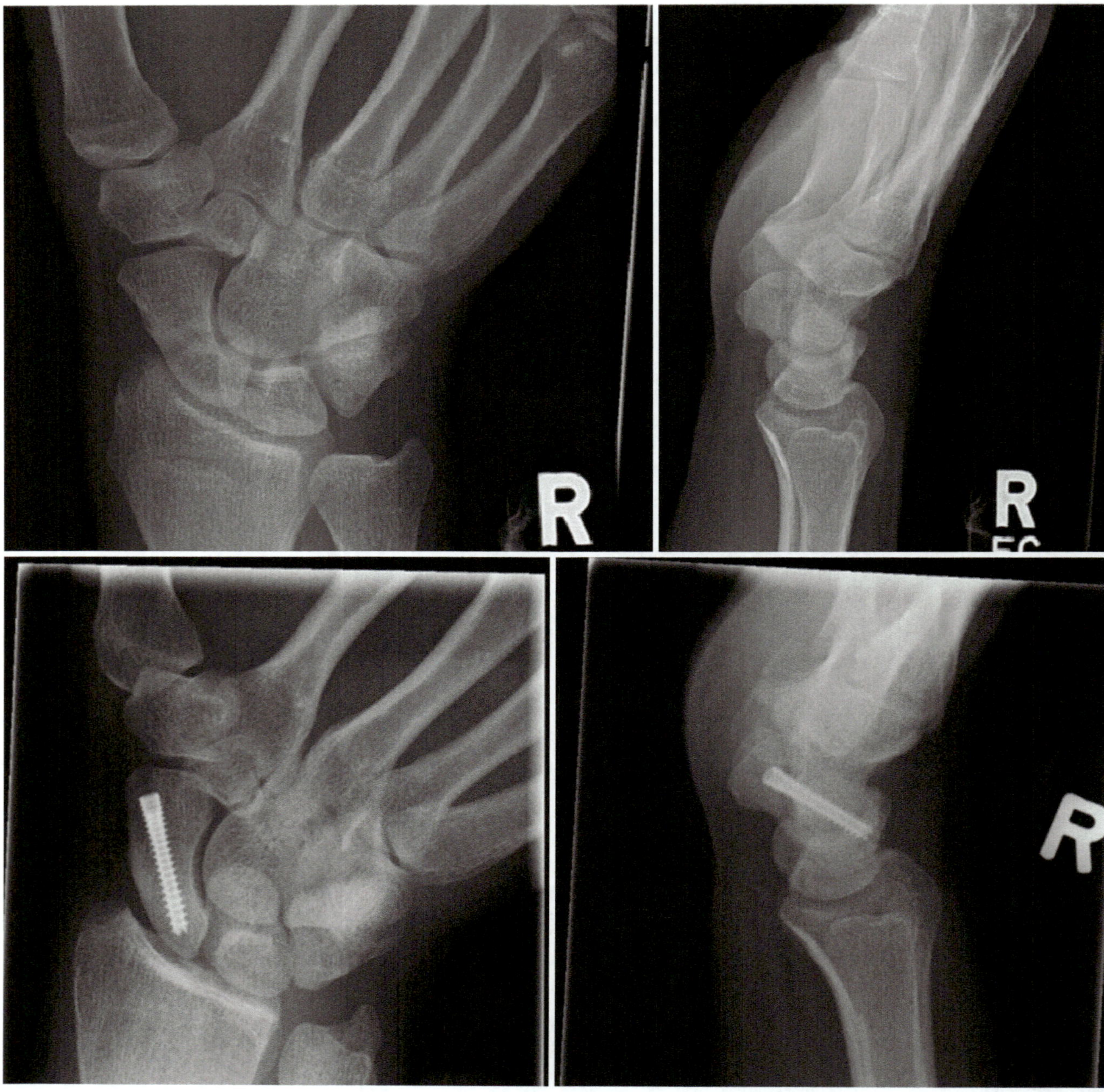

Fig. 3.11 Evidence-based management for sport-related fractures: percutaneous screw fixation of an undisplaced scaphoid waist fracture

The exception to this are the undisplaced proximal femoral and neck of femur fractures, which are routinely fixed in both athletes and the general population, to avoid the requirement for prolonged bed rest and to allow for early mobilisation [22].

To note, there are examples of displaced stable fractures, that are often treated conservatively in the general population, with satisfactory results [61, 62]. These include displaced middle-third clavicle fractures (Fig. 3.12) [61, 62]. However, given the high level of function required in the athlete, as well as the prolonged time to healing observed with these fractures, it is becoming increasingly accepted that surgical management of these injuries offers an accelerated return to sport, with an acceptable risk profile [7, 63]. Some displaced stable fractures can have minimal impact on overall function (displaced fifth metacarpal neck fracture), and the optimal treatment of these remains equivocal [22, 25, 64].

Lastly, it should be noted that it is important to be able to clearly define stable undisplaced fractures patterns from unstable undisplaced fracture patterns [1]. The stability (or instability) of the fracture pattern has often been assumed from established radiographic parameters (e.g. bimalleolar ankle fractures) [1, 5]. However, there is increasing evidence that a range of undisplaced fractures patterns, once thought to be unstable, are in fact stable: these injuries have been shown to achieve superior outcomes, including return rates and return times to sport, with conservative management over surgical management [1, 5, 10]. Examples include undisplaced bimalleolar ankle fractures, and undisplaced lisfranc injuries [1, 5, 10]. This is due to the avoidance of surgery, thus preventing scarring, and subsequent post-operative symptoms [1, 5, 10]. Stress testing should be used as an aid to determine the stability of such injuries, with regular radiographic follow-up performed, to confirm their stability [1, 5, 10].

The management of sport-related fractures can be divided into conservative and surgical techniques [1]. The exact choice of management is specific to the anatomic location of the fracture, and the configuration of the fracture [1]: however, a unifying set of management principles is provided in Table 3.5.

3.5.2 Conservative Management

To allow conservative management of an undisplaced fracture, appropriate immobilisation must be performed [13]. The choice of immobilisation is site and fracture-specific [13]. This is most commonly performed with cast or orthotic immobilisation [13]. These provide either three-point stabilisation or hydrostatic pressure stabilisation across the fracture site, preventing fracture movement, and allowing fracture healing in a stable environment [13]. Removable immobilisation should be favoured where possible, to facilitate early physiotherapy and mobilisation [1, 13]. There are however situations where formal immobilisation is not required, which include: when the fracture is anatomically positioned, such that cast immobilisation provides limited benefit over restricted movement (collar and cuff treatment of middle third clavicle fractures and proximal humeral fractures); and when the fracture is felt to be intrinsically stable due to the surrounding ligamentous attachments (e.g. buddy strapping of metacarpal fractures) [13, 22].

The design of the cast or the orthotic, and the duration of use of the immobilisation device is based on the location of the fracture [1, 13]. All such treatment regimens are flexible, and can be varied according to the perceived stability of the individual fracture pattern, the clinician's preference and experience, the centre's availability of resources, and relevant information from the patient's injury history (e.g. pre-treatment weight-bearing on an undisplaced lower limb fracture suggests it will be stable on further stressing) [1, 13].

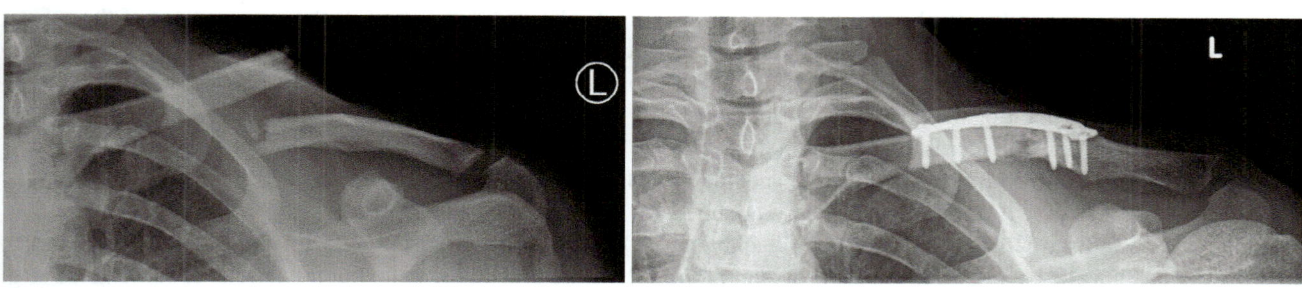

Fig. 3.12 Evidence-based management for sport-related fractures: open reduction and plate fixation of a displaced mid-diaphyseal clavicle fracture

Table 3.5 Sport-related fracture management recommendations by fracture stability and displacement

Stability	Displacement	Example	Treatment	Rational for treatment choice
Stable	Undisplaced[a]	– Undisplaced 'supination-external rotation' type 2 ankle #	Conservative	Avoid adverse post-surgical symptom profile.
Stable	Displaced	– Displaced middle third clavicle #	Consider surgical[b]	Restore function quicker. Reduce time to union. Accelerate rehabilitation.
Unstable	Undisplaced[a]	– Undisplaced tibial diaphyseal # – Undisplaced waist of scaphoid #	Surgical[b]	Achieve fracture stability to accelerate rehabilitation.
Unstable	Displaced	– Displaced radial diaphysis # – Displaced 'supination-external rotation' type 4 ankle #	Surgical[b]	Requirement for anatomical reduction and stable fixation.

[a]'Undisplaced' or 'minimally displaced'—i.e. displacement <2 mm
[b]'Internal' surgical fixation methods (e.g. plate fixation, intra-medullary nailing) recommended over 'external' surgical fixation methods (e.g. K-wire fixation), to accelerate rehabilitation
[#]Fracture

3.5.3 Surgical Management

The commonly used surgical techniques in fracture management include: open reduction internal fixation, percutaneous screw fixation, intra-medullary nail fixation, Kirschner Wire fixation and external frame fixation.

Open reduction and internal fixation involves re-alignment of the fracture by exploration of the site, followed by fixation with the use of plates and screws [14, 17, 22]. This is most commonly used for displaced intra-articular fractures, which require accurate joint surface reduction and stable fixation [14, 17, 22]. Other fracture patterns indicated for this treatment method include displaced fractures of the metaphyseal region of long bones (e.g. distal radius), and displaced fractures of small bones (e.g. metacarpal) that are not suitable for less invasive methods of surgical fixation [14, 17, 22, 65, 66]. Various modes of plating exist which include: neutralisation plating (used in conjunction with lag screw fixation), compression plating, buttress plating, anti-glide plating, locked plating, bridge plating and tension-band plating [14, 17, 22]. The biomechanical properties and indications for the different plating techniques are described below [14, 17, 22].

Percutaneous reduction and screw fixation involves re-alignment of a fracture by closed or minimal-access manipulation, followed by internal fixation with appropriate screw placement, using minimal-access skin incisions [14, 17, 22]. This is suitable for minimally displaced fractures which can be realigned by closed manipulation, and held by limited screw fixation (e.g. minimally displaced Lisfranc injuries, minimally displaced fifth metatarsal proximal diaphyseal-metaphyseal (Jones) fractures) [10, 14, 17, 22, 60].

Intra-medullary nail fixation involves re-alignment of a fracture by closed or minimal-access manipulation, followed by insertion of an intra-medullary nail into the medullary canal of the bone [14, 17, 22]. A reamed or an unreamed technique can be utilised [14, 17, 22]. A reamed technique allows a thicker nail to be inserted, which provides more rigid stability to the fracture [14, 17, 22]. Intra-medullary nailing is suitable for displaced fractures of the diaphysis of long bones (e.g. tibia), with acceptable degrees of comminution, which can be realigned by closed or open manipulation, and held appropriately with intra-medullary fixation [6, 14, 17, 22]. This technique can also be considered for appropriately positioned metaphyseal-diaphyseal junction fractures of long bones (e.g. distal tibia) [14, 17, 22].

Manipulation under Anaesthetic and Kirschner Wiring involves re-aligning a fracture under adequate anaesthesia, then stabilising the fracture, using two or three K-Wires, to provide intra-osseous three-point fixation of the fracture [14, 17, 22]. This is suitable for extra-articular, displaced, non-communited fractures (e.g. distal radius), and most commonly performed for fractures in the metaphyseal and diaphyseal regions of the hand and wrist [14, 17, 22, 66, 67].

External Frame Fixation involves the insertion of Steinman pins or K-Wires intra-osseously, on both sides of the fracture site, with assembly of an external frame that incorporates these attachments, to achieve stable anatomical alignment of the fracture [15, 22]. Less commonly used in the athletic patient, indications include: very distal intra-articular fractures, which are not amenable to internal fixation, and require joint-bridging for stability (e.g. distal, intra-articular distal radial fractures); or as a temporary fixation method, prior to proceeding with delayed definitive surgery (e.g. distal tibia) [15, 22, 65].

The choice of surgical method can be varied in accordance with the fracture pattern and the clinician's choice [14, 22]. With the athletic patient, there is a current focus to encourage stable 'internal' fixation methods over 'external' fixation methods (e.g. plate fixation instead of k-wire fixation), as this can facilitate the most accelerated post-operative mobilisation and rehabilitation possible (Fig. 3.13) [1, 6, 25, 64–67].

Post-operative immobilisation and rehabilitation varies on the method of surgical fixation used, the location of the fracture and the stability of fixation achieved [14, 22]. This can range from: full weightbearing post-operatively with minimal restrictions; to non-weightbearing with post-operative immobilisation, followed by a progressive weightbearing and mobilisation programme [14, 22].

As discussed in Sect. 6.1, the management of these fractures can be supplemented by Orthobiologic therapies to optimise fracture healing [37–40].

3.5.4 Open Fractures

Open fractures represent a significant high-energy injury in the athlete, with the potential for serious complications (e.g. osteomyelitis), if not treated appropriately [22, 51, 68]. Such sport-related injuries should thus be managed in accordance with the standard evidence-based treatment guidelines for the general population (Table 3.3) [22, 51, 52, 68].

With particular relevance to the athlete, clinicians managing these fractures should always determine the environment within which the injury was sustained [22, 51, 68]. Specifically, those sports played in farmyard terrain (e.g. quad biking), or in freshwater and saltwater environments (e.g. surfing), can result in severe wound-site contamination for the athlete [22, 51, 68]. These cases require immediate identification by the treating clinicians, to ensure the appropriate antibiotics are administered and urgent surgical debridement is performed (Table 3.3) [22, 51, 68].

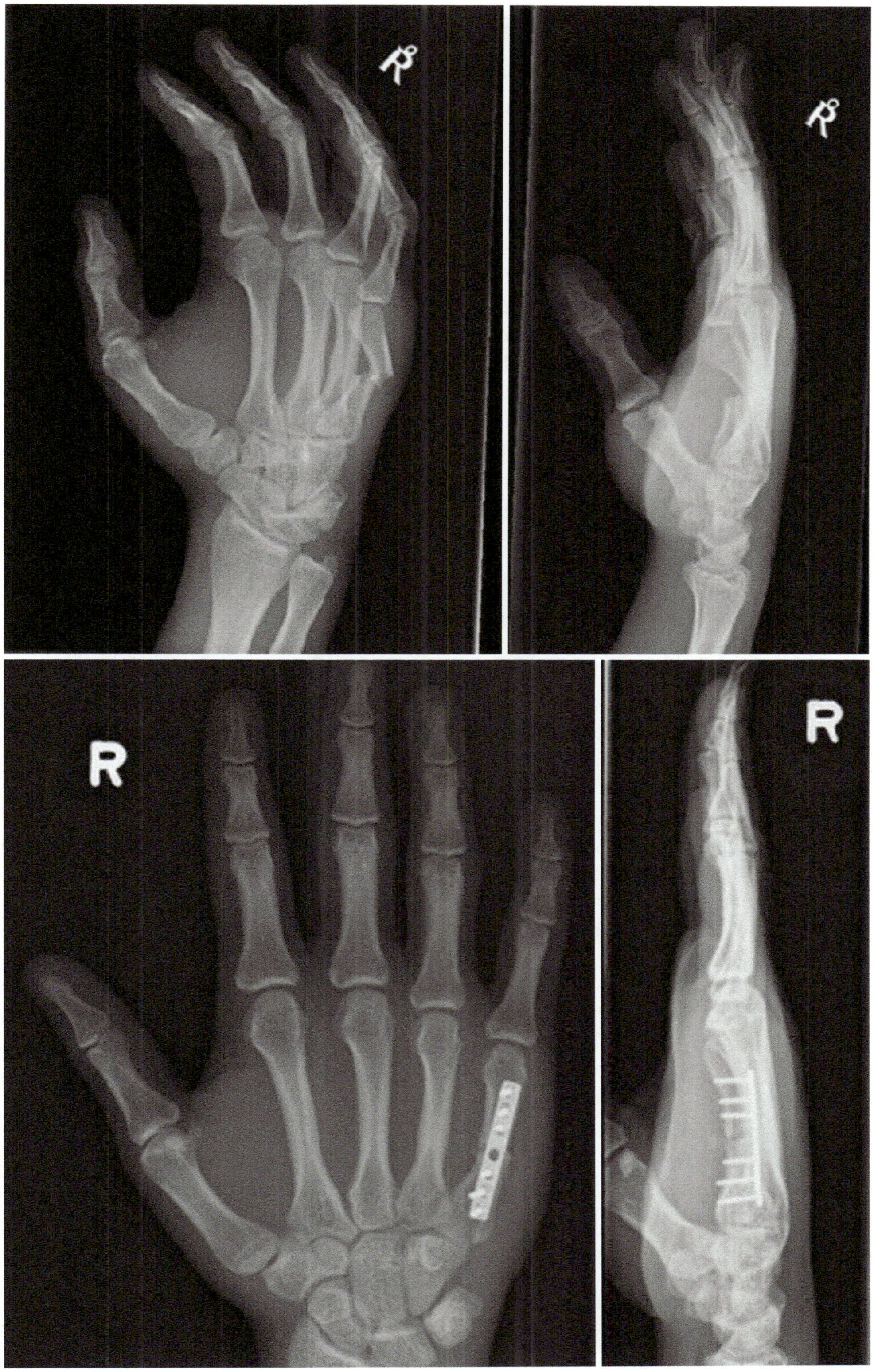

Fig. 3.13 Evidence-based management for sport-related fractures: open reduction and plate fixation of a displaced metacarpal diaphyseal fracture

3.6 The Biomechanics of Fracture Fixation

An understanding of the biomechanics of the treatment methods used for fracture stabilisation, provides the clinician a better ability to choose the optimal method [11, 17, 22].

3.6.1 Conservative Treatment Methods

Conservative management, with either plaster or orthotic immobilisation, utilises the principles of three-point fixation or hydrostatic pressure stabilisation about the fracture site, to maintain the fracture sufficiently stable, to allow secondary fracture healing to occur [13, 22]. This requires fracture site strain to be between 2 and 10%: often the internal stability of the fracture site accounts for a significant proportion of this [13, 19, 22]. Orthotic immobilisation is often preferred over cast immobilisation in the athletic population, as this allows for frequent removal and refitting, facilitating early mobilisation, to maintain joint range of motion, muscle bulk and proprioception, thus promoting an accelerated recovery [1, 13].

3.6.2 Surgical Treatment Methods

Regarding surgical fixation, 'internal' fixation provides the optimal treatment modality for the athlete, as this limits the need for post-operative immobilisation, facilitating an accelerated return to sport [1, 6, 25, 64–67]. Plate and screw fixation, screw fixation and intra-medullary nail fixation form the majority of the recommended fixation methods [1, 6, 14, 22, 25, 64–67].

3.6.3 Plate Fixation

Plate fixation is based on the principles of stable anatomic reduction with robust internal fixation [14, 17, 22]. It comprises application of a strip of metal, with holes in (i.e. a plate), across a fracture, which is then held in place by intraosseous screws [14, 17, 22]. The various modes of plate fixation are discussed above, and the methods of fracture healing observed with these are listed in Table 3.1 [14, 17, 22]. Plates are either made from stainless steel or titanium [14, 17, 22, 69].

Traditional 'non-locked' plates provide stability across a fracture, by the compression force that the screws exert on the plate, as they engage and hold in the bone [14, 17, 22]. 'Locked plating' is a relatively new technology, which provides a more robust method of fracture stabilisation, with the screws locking into the plate, providing a rigid fixed-angle construct [14, 17, 22]. Due this construct, locking plates can be considered as 'internal' external fixators [14, 17, 22].

Given the rigidity of the screw-plate interface in locking plates, reduction of the fracture prior to plate application is essential, and this can be facilitated by initial non-locked or lag screw insertion through the plate, in a mixed screw-type construct [14, 17, 22]. In comparison to conventional plating, locking plates, with the screw-plate interface contained within the locking system, have the additional benefit of avoiding compression of the periosteum, thus preserving periosteal blood flow [14, 17, 22]. 'Locked plating' is particularly useful for fractures located in metaphyseal regions, as well as those in osteoporotic bone [14, 17, 22].

Occasionally, bridge plating is utilised for comminuted fractures, where compression or lagging techniques cannot be achieved [14, 17, 19, 22]. These fractures heal by secondary (endochondral) fracture healing [14, 17, 19, 22]. The reduced rigidity and stability of the construct often requires restricted postoperative mobilisation to protect fracture healing, and this can be problematic for an athlete's rehabilitation [1, 14, 17, 22].

The resistance to bending of a plate is determined, by its bending rigidity [14, 20]. This is the product of the SMA and the Young's Modulus of the plate material [14, 20]. Considering Young's Modulus, a stainless steel plate has around twice the bending rigidity of that of an identically sized titanium plate [14, 20]. Similarly, considering the SMA, doubling the thickness of a plate results in an eightfold increase in the rigidity of the plate [14, 20, 23]. An overly-rigid fixation device should however be avoided, to prevent excessive stress shielding of the affected area, and to avoid the creation of stress risers proximal and distal to the plate [14, 20]. Of note, the rigidity of the plate and screw construct is also determined by the screw configuration [14, 17, 20]. The working length of the plate is determined by the distance between the two screws adjacent to the fracture site—the greater the distance, the longer the working length, and the less rigid the fixation construct [14, 17, 20]. For this reason, many surgeons use the near-far principle of screw placement [14, 17, 20].

Key factors to consider when using plate fixation in the athlete include: avoidance of an overly bulky plate, which can be too prominent and irritate the surrounding soft tissue structures (e.g. tendons); and utilisation of minimally-invasive plate insertion techniques, where possible, to preserve muscle function, minimise scarring and provide optimal function [1, 14, 17, 20, 22].

3.6.4 Screw Fixation

Screw fixation, in isolation, can be considered if the fracture pattern can be held sufficiently stable with this construct [14,

17, 22]. Screw design is pivotal in determining its biomechanical properties and resistance to pull-out [14, 17, 22]. The key dimensions are pitch, core diameter and thread diameter: variations in these are observed between cortical and cancellous screws, to optimise their function within each bone type [14, 17, 22]. Screws can exert compression at fracture sites through either variable pitch designs or use of lag techniques: in such instances, the screw should be orientated perpendicular to the fracture line [14, 17, 22].

Due to its cylindrical configuration, doubling the radius of the core diameter of a screw will result in a 16-fold increase in the bending rigidity of the screw [14, 20]. Regarding screw purchase in bone, doubling the radius of the thread diameter of a screw will result in a fourfold increase in the pull-out strength of the screw [14, 17, 22]. Reducing the screw pitch (i.e. a finer screw pitch) will also increase a screw's pull-out strength [14, 17, 22].

3.6.5 Intra-medullary Nail Fixation

Intra-medullary nailing imparts relative stability to the fracture site, and so secondary (endochondral) fracture healing occurs with this technique [14, 17, 22]. This allows preservation of periosteal blood supply, whilst restoring length and rotation [14, 17, 22]. Two-part fracture patterns can allow for compression at the fracture site: comminuted fractures, however, are bridged for stability, with static locking both proximally and distally [14, 17, 22]. Axially stable fracture patterns can be held with dynamically locked nails, to facilitate compression at fracture site, while axially unstable fracture are held with statically locked nails, to prevent fracture collapse [14, 17, 22].

Reaming allows for the maximal diameter nail possible, whilst also resulting in a uniform fit of the nail in the medullary canal, reducing its working length [14, 17, 22]. Both these factors serve to maximise the bending rigidity of the nail, and so provide maximum stability to the fracture site [14, 17, 22]. The bending rigidity of the nail is proportional to the radius of the nail to the power 4 (SMA), thus doubling the nail diameter will increase the bending rigidity 16-fold [14, 20]. The working length of the nail is the distance between the closest proximal contact point and the closet distal contact point to the fracture site: the shorter the working length, the more rigid the fixation construct [14, 17, 22]. Regarding the reaming process, while endosteal blood supply is initially disrupted by this, the periosteal blood supply rapidly expands to compensate, and so fracture site perfusion remains optimal [14, 17, 22].

Regarding athletes, intra-medullary nail fixation of a fracture provides a relatively minimally invasive method of fracture stabilisation, allowing almost immediate weight bearing, and early rehabilitation, with theoretical preservation of muscle bulk and function [1, 6, 14, 17, 22].

3.6.6 K-Wire Fixation

K-wire fixation aims to provide three-point stabilisation of the fracture, preventing fracture displacement, and allowing the fracture to heal by endochondral ossification [14, 17, 22]. However, the limited contact area achieved by the K-wires within the bone, can often result in limited stability compared to plate fixation [14, 17, 22]. Fracture reduction, with K-wire fixation, is almost always achieved indirectly, through manipulation and ligamentotaxis: such a method is often insufficiently accurate when performing reduction of intra-articular fractures [14, 17, 22]. However, this technique can be useful in the adolescent athlete, as it limits damage to the physis (growth plate), and so reduces the possibility of post-treatment growth disturbance [14, 17, 22, 44].

Similar to an intra-medullary nail, the rigidity of the each K-wire is proportional to the radius of the K-wire to the power 4 [14, 20]. However, as the radius of a K-wire is between six to ten times smaller than that of an intra-medullary nail, the stabilising effect of an individual K-wire is limited [14, 17, 22].

K-wires often remain protruding through the skin for 4–6 weeks post-operatively, protected by cast immobilisation [14, 17, 22]. Thus, rehabilitation and return to sport can be delayed with this fixation method, limiting its recommendation for elite athletes [1, 14, 22, 25, 64–67].

3.7 Fracture Prevention

Injury prevention is key to reduce the incidence of fracture injuries in the future [26, 33, 34, 57, 70]. Given the significant morbidity of such injuries in the athlete, it forms one of the most important areas in the treatment of these fractures [26, 33, 34, 57, 70].

3.7.1 Injury Surveillance

In order to instigate injury prevention measures, injury surveillance is required to qualify and quantify the extent of the problem, so appropriate measures and resources can be directed towards this [26, 33, 34, 57, 70].

Injury surveillance in sport is the process of ongoing and systematic collection of sports injury data, with its associated analysis, interpretation, dissemination and subsequent public health response [26, 33, 34, 70]. It aims to: detect trends in incidence; identify risk factors and causes; develop preventive and control measures, and evaluate the impact of the prevention measures [26, 33, 34, 70]. Such systems can capture data from all active players within their targeted population or can record injury data from a convenience sample or random stratified sample of their target population [26].

Injury surveillance in sport is often performed in the sports environment, with only a proportion of athletes requiring formal hospital assessment and treatment for their injury [26, 33, 34, 70]. As such, the definition of what constitutes an injury in the sporting environment is a key factor in this process, in order to consistently record the appropriate key events [26, 33, 34, 70]. Some surveillance systems employ injury definitions relating to time loss from participation in sport; other systems use medical-attention injury definitions, where a reportable injury must require some form of medical attention; and some systems use both definitions [26, 33, 34, 70]. Other systems include all injuries present [26, 33, 34, 70].

Similarly, the personnel who detect and confirm these injuries is another key factor in this process, as their training, medical knowledge and experience can vary, often influencing the diagnoses [26, 33, 34, 70]. Some systems utilise team doctors and physiotherapists to record injury data, while other systems use certified athletic trainers or non-medically trained technical personnel [26, 33, 34, 70].

These issues have been addressed by consensus statements to specify the recommended methods and modalities to collect injury surveillance data [34, 70].

There are 15 active injury surveillance systems in sport [26]. Eleven of these record data on elite or professional athletes, and four record data on non-professional athletes [26]. The recorded sports comprise: soccer (n = 3); rugby (n = 1); American Football (n = 1); Australian Football (n = 1); baseball (n = 1); skiing and snowboarding (n = 1); cricket (n = 1); and multiple sports (n = 6) [26].

All types of sports injury are included in these systems, ranging from muscle sprains to head injury [26, 30, 31, 42, 43, 45, 46, 48, 71–74]. Fracture data is often provided as a sub-cohort of injuries [30, 31, 42, 43, 45, 46, 48, 71–74]. While fracture injuries often have a more definite method of diagnosis (radiological imaging), many of these programmes combine acute and stress fractures within cohorts, as well as fractures from all body regions (i.e. facial fractures with limb fractures) [29–31, 42, 43, 45, 46, 48, 71–74]. Thus, analysis of the acute appendicular skeletal fracture data can be difficult [29–31, 42, 43, 45, 46, 48, 71–74].

Injury surveillance data allows clinicians to assess the injury patterns by mode of injury and playing position, within each sport, in order to determine potential injury prevention strategies for these fractures [26, 29–31, 33, 34, 70]. In recent years, surveillance type observational data has noted a decrease in the incidence of soccer-related tibial diaphyseal fractures, paralleled by the introduction of shin guards [58, 75, 76]. Similarly, surveillance data has also noted a decrease in the incidence of lacrosse-related finger fractures, paralleled by the introduction of protective hand-gear [47]. Both surveillance trends suggest the effectiveness of these protective equipment [47, 76]. However, more robust surveillance data and observational research is required to confirm these associations [47, 76].

However, despite such observations, injury surveillance currently plays a limited role in the prevention of sport-related fractures [26, 29, 30, 34]. This is due to a lack of formal targeted surveillance in this area [26, 29, 30, 34]. The future of injury surveillance for fractures in sport should focus on identifying 'high risk' groups for specific fracture types [2–5, 26, 29, 30, 34, 47, 48, 77]. When identified, the main mechanisms of injury and risk factors can then be identified, with considerations made of potential protective equipment [2–5, 26, 29, 30, 34, 47, 48, 77]. This equipment can then be introduced into these 'high risk' cohorts, and further surveillance data can then reveal the true effectiveness of these interventions [2–5, 26, 29, 30, 34, 47, 48, 77]. Identification of risk factors (e.g. playing terrain) can similarly allow modifications of practice (e.g. change of playing terrain), with the effect again formally assessed through ongoing surveillance [2–5, 26, 29, 30, 34, 47, 48, 77].

3.7.2 Protective Practice

Protective practice against fractures can be defined in two categories:

1. Protective Equipment
2. Modification of Technique and Practice

3.7.3 Protective Equipment

Regarding protective equipment, this is often specific to the anatomic location affected, and so these can be grouped by upper limb, lower limb and axial skeleton [47, 76–80].

Within the upper limb, the currently available protective equipment include shoulder pads and protective hand-gear [47, 77, 78].

Shoulder pads are a key area for injury prevention in contact sports (e.g. rugby, American Football, Ice Hockey), with an aim to reduce the incidence of clavicle and proximal humeral fractures [78]. However, despite their theoretical benefits, these have not been found to significantly reduce such injuries in rugby union [78]. The most comprehensive study to-date found no difference in the incidence of shoulder injuries in professional rugby union players between wearers and non-wearers of shoulder pads [78]. Thus, further research is required to define their value in contact sports [78].

Protective hand-gear is a key area for injury prevention in the stick and ball sports (e.g. hockey, lacrosse, shinty, ice hockey), with an aim to reduce the incidence of hand–related fractures [47]. While the use of such hand-gear is not routinely recommended in field hockey, it has been shown to be protective against hand fractures in lacrosse and ice hockey, where this is routinely used, with limited adverse effects on player dexterity [47].

To note goal-keeping gloves have been recommended by FIFA (The Fédération Internationale de Football Association), as a form of protective equipment for soccer goal-keepers [77]. However, there is no formal evidence, to confirm that their use reduces the incidence of hand fractures [77]. Further research in this area is required [77].

Within the lower limb, the currently available protective equipment include shin guards (Fig. 3.14) [76, 81, 82].

Formally recommended by FIFA, shin guards are a key area for injury prevention in soccer against tibial diaphsyeal fractures [77]. This is particularly relevant given that soccer accounts for 25% of all tibial diaphyseal fractures, with 83% of all soccer-related tibial fractures occurring due to tackle-related injuries [58, 83]. Biomechanical studies have found shin-guards to reduce tackle impact forces by up to 17% and strain forces by up to 51%, compared with the unguarded leg [84]. The material of the shin guard plays a significant role in its injury-prevention capacity, with carbon-fibre shin guards demonstrating superior protective abilities compared to polypropylene shin guards [85]. Other factors, which have been found to positively influence guard effectiveness, include increased thickness of material, increased compliance of material and even distribution of impact across the guard [84]. It has been hypothesised that the introduction of shin guards, and their subsequent design improvements, may explain the decreasing incidence of soccer-related tibial fractures seen in the available literature (soccer-related tibial fractures accounted for 25% of all tibial fractures in 1988–1990 [58]; 18% of all tibial fractures in 1990–1994 [75]; and 10% of all tibial fractures in 1997–2001 [76]). Given such findings, it would appear that the use of shin guards in soccer activities should be recommended [77].

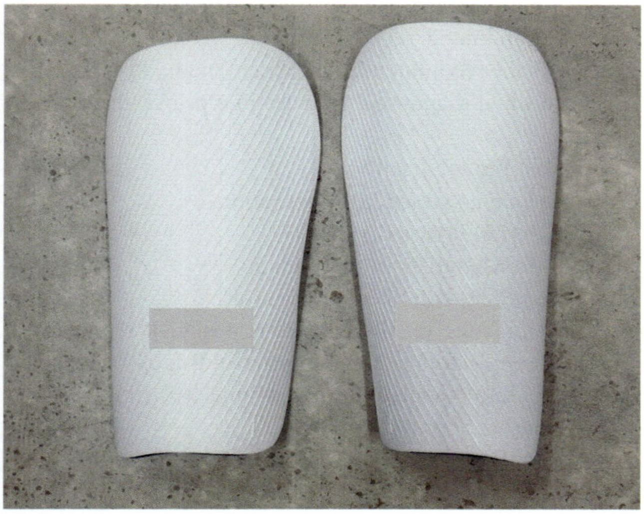

Fig. 3.14 A pair of commercially available polypropylene shin guards

Within the axial skeleton, the currently available protective equipment include head and neck support devices and thoraco-lumbar spine protectors [79, 80].

Laboratory-based evidence suggests that head and neck support devices, used in motor sports, can result in an 80% reduction in the flexion-distraction force produced by the head and neck [79]. However, the clinical evidence to support their use remains limited [79].

The use of thoraco-lumbar spine protectors remains controversial, and is currently not supported by evidence [80]. While these devices may protect the thoracolumbar spine, there are theoretical concerns that their rigidity may predispose the cervical spine to injury [80]. Further investigation into the benefits of such protectors is required before making formal recommendations [80].

3.7.4 Modification of Technique

Modification of technique can include modification of playing surface, modification of playing equipment or modification of playing technique [77, 86–90].

Data from Lawson et al. has found that an increased proportion of soccer-related distal radius fractures are sustained on synthetic grass pitches (54%), compared to grass pitches (28%) [86]. Logically, surfaces without adequate grip can precipitate slides and falls, while surfaces with uneven ground (e.g. poorly kept pitches with 'potholes') can also precipitate falls [86]. Given that 79% of soccer-related distal radial fractures occur secondary to a fall, it would appear that playing surface can have a significant influence on the risk of sustaining a sport-related distal radial fracture [86].

Theoretically, this should hold true for a number of sport-related fractures, particularly those of the upper limb, given that fall is a common mechanism of injury for the majority of these fractures [2, 3, 77, 86]. Thus, future research to establish the playing surfaces which precipitate the most falls, with appropriate modification or avoidance of these, should facilitate a reduction in the incidence of fractures within sporting populations [2, 3, 77, 86].

Similar to this, variations in footwear, particularly stud type and boot design, should have an influence, both on fall rates and injuries secondary to stud trapping, such as twisting and inversion [2, 3, 5, 77]. Stud trapping during sports can cause significant torsional forces to be transferred to the ankle and lower limb, providing an increased risk of fracture [2, 3, 5, 77]. As such, choice of footwear is likely to have a notable influence on rates of both upper limb and lower limb fractures [2, 3, 5, 77]. Thus, future research, which determines the types of footwear that have the highest risk of such injuries, with appropriate modification or avoidance, should also reduce the incidence of sport-related fractures [2, 3, 5, 77].

Lastly, a key factor to consider in injury prevention is the modification of high-risk sporting techniques, to reduce the incidence of certain mechanism-specific fracture types [87–90]. This area has the highest rate of clinical validation, with studies from American football and rugby demonstrating clear evidence of fracture reduction following legislation-based changes to players' technique [87–90]. This is most notable for cervical spinal injuries [87–90].

Within American football, the banning of spear tackling (tackling another player using the top of the head) in 1976 by the National Collegiate Athletic Association Football Rules Committee resulted in a reduction in the incidence of catastrophic cervical spinal injuries of 80% [87–89]. Similarly, within rugby union, the implementation of non-impact scrum laws by the French Rugby Union in 2010, resulted in a decrease in catastrophic cervical spine injuries of approximately 44% [90]. Such data clearly demonstrates that alteration of risk-associated behaviour can significantly reduce the incidence of sport-related traumatic injuries [87–90]. Further research, to accurately determine the modifiable sport-specific injury risks for each fracture type, is thus likely to have a significant influence on the incidence of sport-related fractures in the future [87–90].

3.8 Summary

This chapter provides an overview of the basic science principles relevant to the assessment and management of acute fractures in sport. A clear understanding of the process of fracture healing in the athlete, allows the clinician to determine the optimal treatment and rehabilitation for the patient. An appreciation of the common mechanisms of injury and the associated biomechanical principles allows for injury prediction and subsequent prevention. A robust knowledge of the treatment methods available, along with the guiding principles for application to sport-related fractures, enables athletes to be provided with the best possibility to return to sport, as early as possible. Fracture prevention is a multifaceted process, which forms a key component in minimising the adverse effects of these injuries in the future.

Clinical Pearls

- The basic science principles (i.e. fracture healing, injury biomechanics, treatment materials, injury surveillance) relevant to fracture care in the athlete, largely mirror those seen with standard fracture care. However, certain differences do exist.
- Injury stability is key to determine the optimal management of sport-related fractures. Unstable undisplaced fracture patterns should be surgically stabilised to avoid delays with conservative treatment. Stable undisplaced and minimally-displaced fracture patterns should be managed conservatively, to avoid the adverse symptom profile associated with surgical intervention.
- 'Internal' fixation methods (e.g. plate and screw fixation, screw fixation, intra-medullary nailing) should be favoured over 'external' fixation methods (e.g. K-wiring, external fixators) in the athlete, to facilitate an earlier return to training and sport.
- Protective equipment (e.g. shin guards for tibial diaphyseal fractures), alterations in playing technique (e.g. non-impact scrums to prevent neck injuries in rugby), and alterations in playing surfaces (e.g. playing on grass pitches instead of synthetic grass pitches to reduce the incidence of distal radial fractures) can all play a significant role in fracture prevention in the athlete.

Review

Questions

1. Which treatment method demonstrates primary fracture healing?
   (a) Intra-Medullary Nailing
   (b) K-Wire Fixation
   (c) Bridge Plate Fixation
   (d) Cast Immobilisation
   (e) Lag Screw and Neutralisation Plate Fixation
2. Which fracture pattern results from a tension force?
   (a) Transverse
   (b) Oblique
   (c) Spiral
   (d) Simple Wedge
   (e) Comminuted
3. What is the recommended treatment method for an undisplaced tibial diaphyseal fracture in a professional soccer player?
   (a) Cast Immobilisation
   (b) Sarmiento Brace Immobilisation
   (c) External Frame Fixation
   (d) Intra-Medullary Nail Fixation
   (e) Bed Rest with Skeletal Traction
4. Which practice results in the greatest risk reduction of catastrophic cervical spine injuries in Rugby Union?
   (a) The Implementation of Non-Impact Scrum Laws
   (b) Routine Scrum Cap Usage
   (c) Regular Lower Limb Proprioception Training
   (d) Routine Shoulder Pad Usage
   (e) Playing on Grass Surface Pitches

Answers

1. (e)—All the other treatment methods demonstrate secondary fracture healing (i.e. endochondral ossification with periosteal bridging callus).
2. (a)—Tension forces result in transverse fracture patterns (e.g. at the patella, olecranon and medial malleolus). Pure bending forces can also result in transverse fracture patterns (e.g. at the tibia diaphysis). None of the other listed fracture patterns result from tension forces.
3. (d)—An undisplaced tibial diaphyseal fracture is an unstable fracture pattern. In a professional soccer player, this should undergo 'internal' surgical stabilisation i.e. Intra-Medullary Nail Fixation. The other options either provide conservative management or 'external' surgical stabilisation – these would result in a delayed rehabilitation and a prolonged return to sport.
4. (a)—The implementation of non-impact scrum laws, in rugby union, has been found to result in a 44% reduction in catastrophic cervical spine injuries. None of the other injury prevention measures have been proven to reduce catastrophic cervical spine injuries.

References

1. Robertson GA, Wood AM. Fractures in sport: optimising their management and outcome. World J Orthop. 2015;6(11):850–63.
2. Robertson GA, Wood AM, Bakker-Dyos J, Aitken SA, Keenan AC, Court-Brown CM. The epidemiology, morbidity, and outcome of soccer-related fractures in a standard population. Am J Sports Med. 2012;40(8):1851–7.
3. Robertson GA, Wood AM, Heil K, Aitken SA, Court-Brown CM. The epidemiology, morbidity and outcome of fractures in rugby union from a standard population. Injury. 2014;45(4):677–83.
4. Robertson GA, Wood AM, Aitken SA, Court Brown CM. The epidemiology, management and outcome of field hockey related fractures in a standard population. Arch Trauma Res. 2017;6(4):76–81.
5. Robertson GA, Wood AM, Aitken SA, Court BC. Epidemiology, management, and outcome of sport-related ankle fractures in a standard UK population. Foot Ankle Int. 2014;35(11):1143–52.
6. Robertson GA, Wood AM. Return to sport after tibial shaft fractures: a systematic review. Sports Health. 2016;8(4):324–30.
7. Robertson GA, Wood AM. Return to sport following clavicle fractures: a systematic review. Br Med Bull. 2016;119(1):111–28.
8. Goffin JS, Liao Q, Robertson GA. Return to sport following scaphoid fractures: a systematic review and meta-analysis. World J Orthop. 2019;10(2):101–14.
9. Robertson GAJ, Wong SJ, Wood AM. Return to sport following tibial plateau fractures: a systematic review. World J Orthop. 2017;8(7):574–87.
10. Robertson GAJ, Ang KK, Maffulli N, Keenan G, Wood AM. Return to sport following Lisfranc injuries: a systematic review and meta-analysis. Foot Ankle Surg. 2019;25(5):654–64.
11. Bottlang M, Fitzpatrick DC, Claes L, Anderson DD. Biomechanics of fractures and fracture fixation. In: Tornetta III P, Ricci W, Ostrum RF, McQueen MM, McKee MD, Court Brown CM, editors. Rockwood and Green's fractures in adults. 9th ed. Philadelphia: Wolters Kluwer; 2019. p. 1–42.
12. Lopas LA, Mencias C, Kim HT, Hankenson KD, Ahn J. Bone, cartilage and tendon healing. In: Tornetta III P, Ricci W, Ostrum RF, McQueen MM, McKee MD, Court Brown CM, editors. Rockwood and Green's fractures in adults. 9th ed. Philadelphia: Wolters Kluwer; 2019. p. 43–60.
13. Court Brown CM, Davidson EK. Principles of nonoperative management of fractures. In: Tornetta III P, Ricci W, Ostrum RF, McQueen MM, McKee MD, Court Brown CM, editors. Rockwood and Green's fractures in adults. 9th ed. Philadelphia: Wolters Kluwer; 2019. p. 248–95.
14. Bishop JA, Behn AW, Gardner MJ. Principles and biomechanics of internal fixation. In: Tornetta III P, Ricci W, Ostrum RF, McQueen MM, McKee MD, Court Brown CM, editors. Rockwood and Green's fractures in adults. 9th ed. Philadelphia: Wolters Kluwer; 2019. p. 362–90.
15. Watson JT. Principles of external fixation. In: Tornetta III P, Ricci W, Ostrum RF, McQueen MM, McKee MD, Court Brown CM, editors. Rockwood and Green's fractures in adults. 9th ed. Philadelphia: Wolters Kluwer. 2019. p. 296–361.
16. Schmitz MR, DeHart MM, Qazi Z, Shuler FD. Orthopaedic biology. In: Miller MD, Thompson SR, editors. Miller's review of orthopaedics. 7th ed. Philadelphia, PA: Elsevier; 2015. p. 83–104.
17. Hak DJ, Mauffrey C. Trauma: biomechanics of fracture healing & biomechanics of open reduction and internal fixation. In: Miller MD, Thompson SR, editors. Miller's review of orthopaedics. 7th ed. Philadelphia, PA: Elsevier; 2015. p. 775–8.
18. Bates P, Moller-Madsen B, Noorani A, Ramachandran M. The basics of bone. In: Ramachandran M, editor. Basic orthopaedic sciences. 2nd ed. Boca Raton: CRC Press; 2017. p. 193–204.
19. Bates P, Yeo A, Ramachandran M. Bone injury, healing and grafting. In: Ramachandran M, editor. Basic orthopaedic sciences. 2nd ed. Boca Raton: CRC Press; 2017. p. 205–22.
20. Chatterjee S, Baring T, Blunn G. Biomaterial behaviour. In: Ramachandran M, editor. Basic orthopaedic sciences. 2nd ed. Boca Raton: CRC Press; 2017. p. 257–66.
21. Ramachandran M, Lee P. Basic concepts in biomechanics. In: Ramachandran M, editor. Basic orthopaedic sciences. 2nd ed. Boca Raton: CRC Press; 2017. p. 233–44.
22. Court Brown C, McQueen MM, Tornetta P III. Nonunions and bone defects. In: Tornetta III P, Einhorn T, editors. Trauma. Philadelphia: Lippincott Williams & Wilkins; 2006.
23. Clark D, Nakamura M, Miclau T, Marcucio R. Effects of aging on fracture healing. Curr Osteoporos Rep. 2017;15(6):601–8.
24. Gibon E, Lu L, Goodman SB. Aging, inflammation, stem cells, and bone healing. Stem Cell Res Ther. 2016;7:44.
25. Rettig AC, Ryan R, Shelbourne KD, McCarroll JR, Johnson F Jr, Ahlfeld SK. Metacarpal fractures in the athlete. Am J Sports Med. 1989;17(4):567–72.
26. Ekegren CL, Gabbe BJ, Finch CF. Sports injury surveillance systems: a review of methods and data quality. Sports Med. 2016;46(1):49–65.
27. Court-Brown CM, Wood AM, Aitken S. The epidemiology of acute sports-related fractures in adults. Injury. 2008;39(12):1365–72.
28. Aitken SA, Watson BS, Wood AM, Court-Brown CM. Sports-related fractures in South East Scotland: an analysis of 990 fractures. J Orthop Surg (Hong Kong). 2014;22(3):313–7.
29. Larsson D, Ekstrand J, Karlsson MK. Fracture epidemiology in male elite football players from 2001 to 2013: 'How long will this fracture keep me out?'. Br J Sports Med. 2016;50(12):759–63.
30. Junge A, Dvorak J. Injury surveillance in the World Football Tournaments 1998-2012. Br J Sports Med. 2013;47(12):782–8.
31. Junge A, Dvorak J. Football injuries during the 2014 FIFA World Cup. Br J Sports Med. 2015;49(9):599–602.
32. Dvorak J, Junge A, Grimm K, Kirkendall D. Medical report from the 2006 FIFA World Cup Germany. Br J Sports Med. 2007;41(9):578–81; discussion 81.

33. Junge A, Dvorak J, Graf-Baumann T, Peterson L. Football injuries during FIFA tournaments and the Olympic Games, 1998-2001: development and implementation of an injury-reporting system. Am J Sports Med. 2004;32(1 Suppl):80S–9S.
34. Junge A, Engebretsen L, Alonso JM, Renstrom P, Mountjoy M, Aubry M, et al. Injury surveillance in multi-sport events: the International Olympic Committee approach. Br J Sports Med. 2008;42(6):413–21.
35. Best JP, McIntosh AS, Savage TN. Rugby World Cup 2003 injury surveillance project. Br J Sports Med. 2005;39(11):812–7.
36. Ricci W. Principles of nonunion and bone defect treatment. In: Tornetta III P, Ricci W, Ostrum RF, McQueen MM, Mckee MD, Court Brown CM, editors. Rockwood and Green's fractures in adults. 9th ed. Philadelphia: Wolters Kluwer; 2019. p. 835–83.
37. Calcei JG, Rodeo SA. Orthobiologics for bone healing. Clin Sports Med. 2019;38(1):79–95.
38. Bray CC, Walker CM, Spence DD. Orthobiologics in pediatric sports medicine. Orthop Clin North Am. 2017;48(3):333–42.
39. Roberts TT, Rosenbaum AJ. Bone grafts, bone substitutes and orthobiologics: the bridge between basic science and clinical advancements in fracture healing. Organogenesis. 2012;8(4):114–24.
40. Toogood PA, Bahney C, Marcucio R, Miclau T. Biologic and biophysical technologies for the enhancement of fracture repair. In: Tornetta III P, Ricci WM, Ostrum RF, McQueen MM, MD MK, Court-Brown C, editors. Rockwood and Green's fractures in adults. 9th ed. Philadelphia: Wolters Kluwer Health; 2019. p. 61–79.
41. Aitken S, Court-Brown CM. The epidemiology of sports-related fractures of the hand. Injury. 2008;39(12):1377–83.
42. Swenson DM, Henke NM, Collins CL, Fields SK, Comstock RD. Epidemiology of United States high school sports-related fractures, 2008-09 to 2010-11. Am J Sports Med. 2012;40(9):2078–84.
43. Swenson DM, Yard EE, Collins CL, Fields SK, Comstock RD. Epidemiology of US high school sports-related fractures, 2005-2009. Clin J Sport Med. 2010;20(4):293–9.
44. Wood AM, Robertson GA, Rennie L, Caesar BC, Court-Brown CM. The epidemiology of sports-related fractures in adolescents. Injury. 2010;41(8):834–8.
45. Brooks JH, Fuller CW, Kemp SP, Reddin DB. Epidemiology of injuries in English professional rugby union: part 1 match injuries. Br J Sports Med. 2005;39(10):757–66.
46. Brooks JH, Fuller CW, Kemp SP, Reddin DB. Epidemiology of injuries in English professional rugby union: part 2 training injuries. Br J Sports Med. 2005;39(10):767–75.
47. Bowers AL, Baldwin KD, Sennett BJ. Athletic hand injuries in intercollegiate field hockey players. Med Sci Sports Exerc. 2008;40(12):2022–6.
48. Dick R, Hootman JM, Agel J, Vela L, Marshall SW, Messina R. Descriptive epidemiology of collegiate women's field hockey injuries: National Collegiate Athletic Association Injury Surveillance System, 1988-1989 through 2002-2003. J Athl Train. 2007;42(2):211–20.
49. Karam MD, Marsh JL. Classification of fractures. In: Tornetta III P, Ricci W, Ostrum RF, McQueen MM, McKee MD, Court Brown CM, editors. Rockwood and Green's fractures in adults. 9th ed. Philadelphia: Wolters Kluwer; 2019. p. 104–22.
50. Meinberg EG, Agel J, Roberts CS, Karam MD, Kellam JF. Fracture and dislocation classification compendium-2018. J Orthop Trauma. 2018;32(Suppl 1):S1–S170.
51. Wood AM, Robertson GAJ, MacLeod K, Porter A, Court-Brown CM. Epidemiology of open fractures in sport: one centre's 15-year retrospective study. World J Orthop. 2017;8(7):545–52.
52. Gustilo RB, Anderson JT. Prevention of infection in the treatment of one thousand and twenty-five open fractures of long bones: retrospective and prospective analyses. J Bone Joint Surg Am. 1976;58(4):453–8.
53. Court-Brown CM, Caesar B. Epidemiology of adult fractures: a review. Injury. 2006;37(8):691–7.
54. Hon WH, Kock SH. Sports related fractures: a review of 113 cases. J Orthop Surg (Hong Kong). 2001;9(1):35–8.
55. Court-Brown CM, Bugler KE, Clement ND, Duckworth AD, McQueen MM. The epidemiology of open fractures in adults. A 15-year review. Injury. 2012;43(6):891–7.
56. Murtaugh K. Injury patterns among female field hockey players. Med Sci Sports Exerc. 2001;33(2):201–7.
57. Parkkari J, Kujala UM, Kannus P. Is it possible to prevent sports injuries? Review of controlled clinical trials and recommendations for future work. Sports Med. 2001;31(14):985–95.
58. Shaw AD, Gustilo T, Court-Brown CM. Epidemiology and outcome of tibial diaphyseal fractures in footballers. Injury. 1997;28(5–6):365–7.
59. Lauge-Hansen N. Fractures of the ankle. II. Combined experimental-surgical and experimental-roentgenologic investigations. Arch Surg. 1950;60(5):957–85.
60. Roche AJ, Calder JD. Treatment and return to sport following a Jones fracture of the fifth metatarsal: a systematic review. Knee Surg Sports Traumatol Arthrosc. 2013;21(6):1307–15.
61. Robinson CM, Goudie EB, Murray IR, Jenkins PJ, Ahktar MA, Read EO, et al. Open reduction and plate fixation versus nonoperative treatment for displaced midshaft clavicular fractures: a multicenter, randomized, controlled trial. J Bone Joint Surg Am. 2013;95(17):1576–84.
62. Goudie EB, Clement ND, Murray IR, Lawrence CR, Wilson M, Brooksbank AJ, et al. The influence of shortening on clinical outcome in healed displaced midshaft clavicular fractures after nonoperative treatment. J Bone Joint Surg Am. 2017;99(14):1166–72.
63. Robertson GA, Wood AM, Oliver CW. Displaced middle-third clavicle fracture management in sport: still a challenge in 2018. Should you call the surgeon to speed return to play? Br J Sports Med. 2018;52(6):348–9.
64. Shaftel ND, Capo JT. Fractures of the digits and metacarpals: when to splint and when to repair? Sports Med Arthrosc Rev. 2014;22(1):2–11.
65. Henn CM, Wolfe SW. Distal radius fractures in athletes: approaches and treatment considerations. Sports Med Arthrosc. 2014;22(1):29–38.
66. Geissler WB. Operative fixation of metacarpal and phalangeal fractures in athletes. Hand Clin. 2009;25(3):409–21.
67. Gaston RG, Chadderdon C. Phalangeal fractures: displaced/nondisplaced. Hand Clin. 2012;28(3):395–401, x.
68. Rajasekaran S, Devendra A, Ramesh P, Dheenadhayalan J, Kamal CA. Initial management of open fractures. In: Tornetta III P, Ricci W, Ostrum RF, McQueen MM, McKee MD, Court Brown CM, editors. Rockwood and Green's fractures in adults. 9th ed. Philadelphia: Wolters Kluwer; 2019. p. 484–530.
69. Chatterjee S, Stammers J, Blunn G. Biomaterials. In: Ramachandran M, editor. Basic orthopaedic sciences. 2nd ed. Boca Raton: CRC Press; 2017. p. 257–66.
70. Hagglund M, Walden M, Bahr R, Ekstrand J. Methods for epidemiological study of injuries to professional football players: developing the UEFA model. Br J Sports Med. 2005;39(6):340–6.
71. Ekstrand J, Hagglund M, Walden M. Injury incidence and injury patterns in professional football: the UEFA injury study. Br J Sports Med. 2011;45(7):553–8.
72. Junge A, Langevoort G, Pipe A, Peytavin A, Wong F, Mountjoy M, et al. Injuries in team sport tournaments during the 2004 Olympic Games. Am J Sports Med. 2006;34(4):565–76.
73. Yard EE, Collins CL, Comstock RD. A comparison of high school sports injury surveillance data reporting by certified athletic trainers and coaches. J Athl Train. 2009;44(6):645–52.

74. Kerr ZY, Dompier TP, Snook EM, Marshall SW, Klossner D, Hainline B, et al. National collegiate athletic association injury surveillance system: review of methods for 2004-2005 through 2013-2014 data collection. J Athl Train. 2014;49(4):552–60.
75. Templeton PA, Farrar MJ, Williams HR, Bruguera J, Smith RM. Complications of tibial shaft soccer fractures. Injury. 2000;31(6):415–9.
76. Chang WR, Kapasi Z, Daisley S, Leach WJ. Tibial shaft fractures in football players. J Orthop Surg Res. 2007;2:11.
77. FIFA TFIdFA. F-MARC: football medicine manual. 2nd ed; 2016.
78. Headey J, Brooks JH, Kemp SP. The epidemiology of shoulder injuries in English professional rugby union. Am J Sports Med. 2007;35(9):1537–43.
79. Kaul A, Abbas A, Smith G, Manjila S, Pace J, Steinmetz M. A revolution in preventing fatal craniovertebral junction injuries: lessons learned from the head and neck support device in professional auto racing. J Neurosurg Spine. 2016;25(6):756–61.
80. Bigdon SF, Gewiess J, Hoppe S, Exadaktylos AK, Benneker LM, Fairhurst PG, et al. Spinal injury in alpine winter sports: a review. Scand J Trauma Resusc Emerg Med. 2019;27(1):69.
81. Giza E, Micheli LJ. Soccer injuries. Med Sport Sci. 2005;49:140–69.
82. Wong P, Hong Y. Soccer injury in the lower extremities. Br J Sports Med. 2005;39(8):473–82.
83. Court-Brown CM, McBirnie J. The epidemiology of tibial fractures. J Bone Joint Surg Br. 1995;77(3):417–21.
84. Francisco AC, Nightingale RW, Guilak F, Glisson RR, Garrett WE Jr. Comparison of soccer shin guards in preventing tibia fracture. Am J Sports Med. 2000;28(2):227–33.
85. Tatar Y, Ramazanoglu N, Camliguney AF, Saygi EK, Cotuk HB. The effectiveness of shin guards used by football players. J Sports Sci Med. 2014;13(1):120–7.
86. Lawson GM, Hajducka C, McQueen MM. Sports fractures of the distal radius-epidemiology and outcome. Injury. 1995;26(1):33–6.
87. Banerjee R, Palumbo MA, Fadale PD. Catastrophic cervical spine injuries in the collision sport athlete, part 1: epidemiology, functional anatomy, and diagnosis. Am J Sports Med. 2004;32(4):1077–87.
88. Boden BP, Jarvis CG. Spinal injuries in sports. Phys Med Rehabil Clin N Am. 2009;20(1):55–68, vii.
89. Torg JS, Guille JT, Jaffe S. Injuries to the cervical spine in American football players. J Bone Joint Surg Am. 2002;84(1):112–22.
90. Reboursiere E, Bohu Y, Retiere D, Sesboue B, Pineau V, Colonna JP, et al. Impact of the national prevention policy and scrum law changes on the incidence of rugby-related catastrophic cervical spine injuries in French Rugby Union. Br J Sports Med. 2018;52(10):674–7.

Stress Fracture Injuries in Sport

4

Timothy L. Miller and Christopher C. Kaeding

Learning Objectives

- The readers will be able to categorize bony stress injuries by severity and risk of fracture progression.
- The readers will be able to effectively communicate the site, severity, and risk level of bony stress fractures with colleagues in the field of Sports Medicine.
- The readers will be able to describe the biologic treatment options available to stimulate bone healing in athletes.
- The readers will be able to describe the surgical procedures available for stabilization and healing of high risk stress fractures as well as their indications, risks, and benefits.
- The readers will be able to describe the risks of continued participation despite severe, chronic, or recurrent stress fractures in elite athletes

4.1 Introduction

Stress fractures of bone, also known as fatigue fractures or march fractures, are common and troublesome injuries in athletes and military personnel. A multitude of biological and mechanical factors influence the body's ability to remodel bone and impact an individual's risk to develope a bony stress injury. These factors include sex, age, race, hormonal status, nutrition, neuromuscular function, and genetic factors. Other predisposing factors to consider include abnormal bony alignment, improper technique/biomechanics, poor running form, inadequate blood supply to specific bones, improper or worn-out footwear, and hard training surfaces. Understanding the classification and grade of stress fractures and their implications is the key to providing optimal care to patients with stress fractures, especially those with an injury at a high-risk site.

T. L. Miller (✉)
Orthopaedic Surgery and Sports Medicine at The Ohio State University Wexner Medical Center Jameson Crane Sports Medicine Institute, Ohio State University Athletics, Ohio State University Wexner Medical Center Endurance Medicine Team, Columbus, OH, USA
e-mail: Timothy.miller@osumc.edu

C. C. Kaeding
The Ohio State University Wexner Medical Center Sports Medicine, Department of Orthopaedics, Jameson Crane Sports Medicine Institute, Department of Athletics at The Ohio State University, Columbus, OH, USA
e-mail: christopher.kaeding@osumc.edu

4.2 The Holistic Approach to Stress Fractures

Stress fractures result from the loss of the normal balance between the production and repair of microcracks in bone. The principles of management include taking a holistic and systemic approach to individuals presenting with this injury. To decrease the production of microcracks, health care professionals must evaluate the patient's training regimen, biomechanics, and equipment. Maximizing the patient's biologic capacity to repair microcracks requires an assessment of the athlete's general health. This includes nutritional status, hormonal status, emotional status, and medication use.

Stress fractures are not a single consistent entity: they occur along a continuum of severity which can impact management and prognosis [1–4]. Not only does the extent of these injuries vary, but their clinical behavior varies according to their location and causative activity [5, 6]. No two stress fractures behave in exactly the same manner. Management protocols should be individualized to the patient, the causative activity, the anatomical site, and the severity of the fracture. The key principles for treating stress fractures in athletes are summarized in Table 4.1, and a treatment algorithm successfully employed by the authors is shown in Fig. 4.1.

Management of bony injuries aims to decrease the repetitive stress at the fracture site enough and for long enough to allow the body to restore the dynamic balance between damage and repair. This may include decreasing volume

G. A. J. Robertson, N. Maffulli (eds.), *Fractures in Sport*, https://doi.org/10.1007/978-3-030-72036-0_4

Table 4.1 Key treatment principles for a holistic approach to bony stress injuries

• Biomechanical and technique modification
• Pre-conditioning training
• Alternative training including training surfaces
• Nutritional optimization
• Hormonal balance
• Mental and emotional fitness and coping skills
• Surgical stabilization

and intensity of activity, equipment changes, technique changes, or cross training. One benefit to such a strategy is that the individual typically does not endure a substantial loss of conditioning while still allowing his or her body to repair the bony damage. If pain intensifies and activity modification alone is inadequate for healing, treatment should be escalated to include complete rest, immobilisation, or surgery.

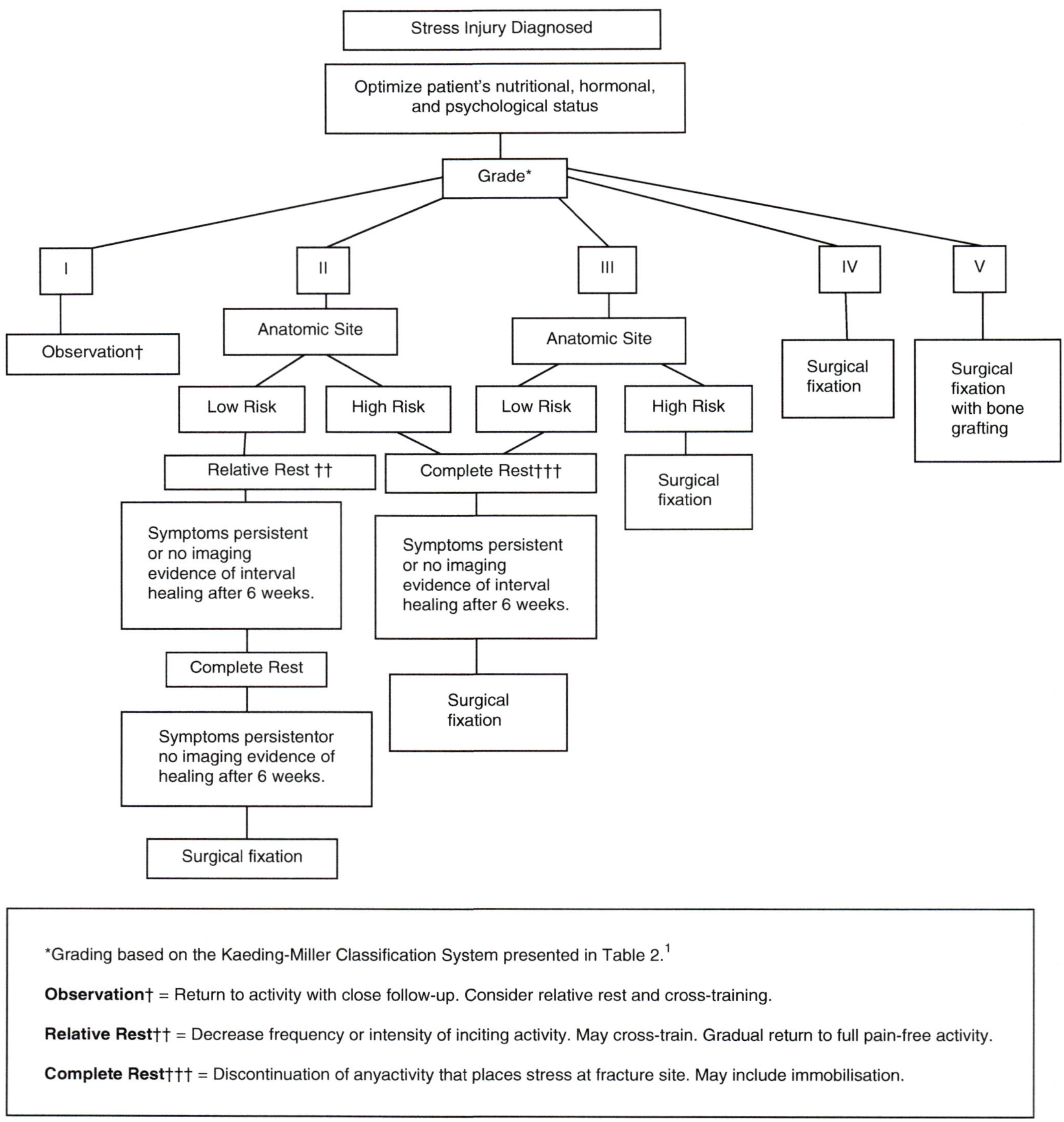

Fig. 4.1 Recommended treatment algorithm for stress injuries of bone

4.3 Athletes at Risk for Stress Fractures

4.3.1 Vitamin D Insufficiency

Most athletes should receive at least 800–1000 international units (and up to 5000 IU) of vitamin D_3 daily. This level of supplementation is safe and has a high therapeutic index. Serum 25(OH) D3 level is the investigation of choice to identify Vitamin D deficiency [7]. In those individuals with low vitamin D or low bone mineral density, the therapeutic goal for supplementation should range from at least 50 nmol/L (20 ng/mL) to as high as 90–100 nmol/L (36–40 ng/mL) based on the Food and Nutrition Board recommendations [7]. In general, the ideal serum level for athletes is 40–50 ng/mL. To achieve this goal as much 50,000 IU per may be prescribed for individuals with severe hypovitaminosis D. Although higher dietary intake of Vitamin D_3 may provide some protective effect against fractures, the exact role of Vitamin D in fracture prevention is still debated.

Recent studies have evaluated the association between serum Vitamin D_3 levels and stress fractures. A prospective study of Finnish military recruits found that the average serum vitamin D_3 concentration was significantly lower in the recruits who had sustained a stress fracture [8]. A randomized, double-blind, placebo-controlled study examined whether calcium and Vitamin D_3 intervention could reduce the incidence of stress fractures in female recruits during basic training [8]. This level 1 study suggested that calcium and Vitamin D_3 supplementation may have prevented a significant percentage of their recruits from sustaining a stress fracture and led to a significant decrease in morbidity and financial burden [8].

4.3.2 The Female Athlete Triad and Caloric Insufficiency

Inadequate caloric intake may play a role in amenorrhea, which has been linked to an increased incidence of stress fractures [9, 10]. Dietary intake and disordered eating patterns have been linked to amenorrhea in several studies. A concept that has been developed supporting the link between dietary intake and amenorrhea is the so-called "energy drain hypothesis". If caloric intake is too low, production of hormones such as estrogen and progesterone are moved lower on the body's list of priorities. These hormones may not be produced in amounts high enough to allow menstruation to occur [11]. Oligomenorrheic or amenorrheic female athletes are at increased risk secondary to decreased estrogen levels and increased osteoclastic activity [12].

Endocrine conditions and malabsorption can impair the delicate balance between bone formation and resorption, thus predisposing athletes to bony stress injuries. Stress fractures are associated with lower fat intake, lower calorie intake, eating disorders, and body weight of less than 75% of ideal body weight. The female athlete triad (menstrual irregularity, inadequate caloric intake, and decreased bone mineral density) has been associated with increased susceptibility to stress fractures. This increased risk is most commonly seen among female distance runners and military recruits, and is increased compared with males performing the same activities [13]. High-intensity training may suppress menses, which may exacerbate these risk factors [10].

Muscle fatigue can be a collaborative culprit in the development of stress fractures in overtrained athletes. Since the late twentieth century, it has been widely accepted that neuromuscular conditioning plays a significant role in enhancing the shock absorbing and energy dissipating function of muscles to the ground reaction forces occurring during impact loading. This neuromuscular tone is able to decrease the amount of energy directly absorbed by the bones and joints [14]. Thus, as they fatigue, muscles are less able to dissipate the applied external forces, allowing for more rapid accumulation of microtrauma to the bone [3]. A recent study of female track and field/cross-country runners indicated an increased risk of developing stress fractures if body mass index (BMI) was less than 19. In this case series female athletes with BMI of 19 or lower took significantly longer to return to unrestricted training and competition than those with a BMI above 19 [15, 16]. Decreased muscle mass was suggested as a risk factor for stress injuries and poor healing [15, 16].

4.3.3 The Male Endurance Athlete Tetrad

Male runners may also be predisposed to decreased bone mineral density [10], especially in the lumbar spine and radius. The cause of this decreased density is most likely multifactorial. Inadequate caloric intake, decreased testosterone levels, and a genetic predilection are suspected to be the main culprits. Decreased energy availability may be the key factor for low bone mineral density, and decreased testosterone levels are present in males endurance athletes. To prevent severe or irreversible effects of low bone mineral density, it is necessary to assess the nutritional behaviors of male endurance athletes as well as their female counterparts.

4.4 Pathophysiology

Healthy bone is constantly in balanced homeostasis between microcrack production and repair. The key modifiable risk factors in the development of overuse injuries of bone relate to the pre-participation condition of the bone and the frequency, duration and intensity of the causative activity [17].

Without pre-conditioning and acclimation to a particular activity, athletes are at significantly increased risk for the development of overuse and fatigue-related injuries of bone [18, 19]. Repeated episodes of bone strain can result in the accumulation of enough microdamage to become a clinically symptomatic stress reaction or stress fracture [2–4]. Fatigue failure of bone has three stages: crack initiation, crack propagation, and complete fracture.

Crack initiation typically occurs at sites of stress concentration during bone loading [3]. Stress concentration occurs at sites of differential bone consistency such as the lacunae or canuliculi [3]. Initiation of the microcrack alone is not sufficient to cause a symptomatic fracture. It is however the first step in bone remodeling, and may serve to increase bone density and strength. Crack propagation occurs if loading continues at a frequency or intensity above the level at which new bone can be laid down and microcracks repaired. Propagation, or extension of a microcrack, typically occurs along the cement lines of the bone, and is considered pathological. Continued loading and crack propagation allows for multiple cracks to coalesce to the point of becoming a clinically symptomatic stress fracture [3]. If the loading episodes are not modified or the reparative response is not increased, crack propagation can continue until a complete fracture occurs [3, 20].

4.5 Clinical Presentation

Pain that is initially present only during activity is common in patients presenting with a stress fracture. Symptom onset is usually insidious, and typically patients cannot recall a specific injury or trauma to the affected area. If activity level is not decreased or modified, symptoms persist or worsen. Those who continue to train without modification of their activities may develop pain with normal daily activity, and potentially sustain a complete fracture [4].

Physical examination reveals reproducible point tenderness with direct palpation of the affected bone site. There may or may not be swelling or a palpable soft tissue or bone reaction. Physical examination tests commonly used for assessing for stress fractures include the fulcrum test for long bones (Fig. 4.2a, b), where a 3-point bending moment is applied to a long bone, and the single leg stance and hop tests (Fig. 4.3) to evaluate pelvic and lower extremity stress injuries [7, 21]. The tuning fork test to identify sites of bone stress fractures has not been shown to be adequately sensitive or specific [7, 22].

4.6 Imaging Evaluation

4.6.1 Radiographs

Radiographs are most often negative early in the course of a stress fracture, especially in the first 2–3 weeks [23, 24]. As healing progresses, radiographic findings may be subtle and easily overlooked if the images are not thoroughly evaluated. Two-thirds of radiographs are initially normal, but about half ultimately provide evidence of a bony stress injury as healing progresses (Fig. 4.4a) [25]. This makes plain radiographs specific but not sensitive to identify and categorise stress fractures.

4.6.2 Bone Scintigraphy

Bone scintigraphy is nearly 100% sensitive for bony stress injuries, although it has a lower specificity than MRI [26]. It is especially useful to identify rib, pelvic, femoral, pelvic,

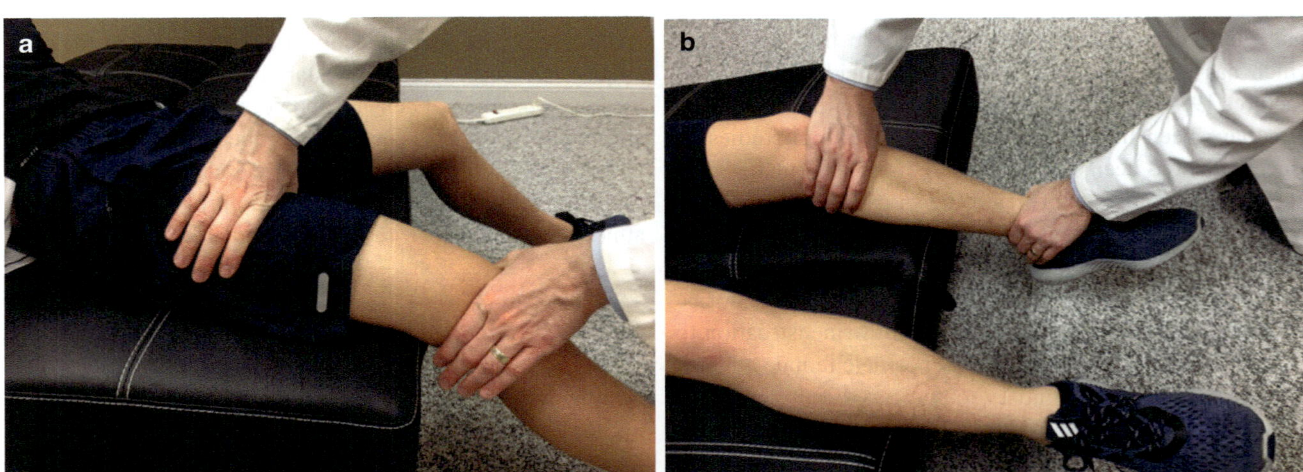

Fig. 4.2 Fulcrum test of the long bones. (**a**) Femoral shaft fulcrum test. (**b**) Tibial shaft fulcrum test.

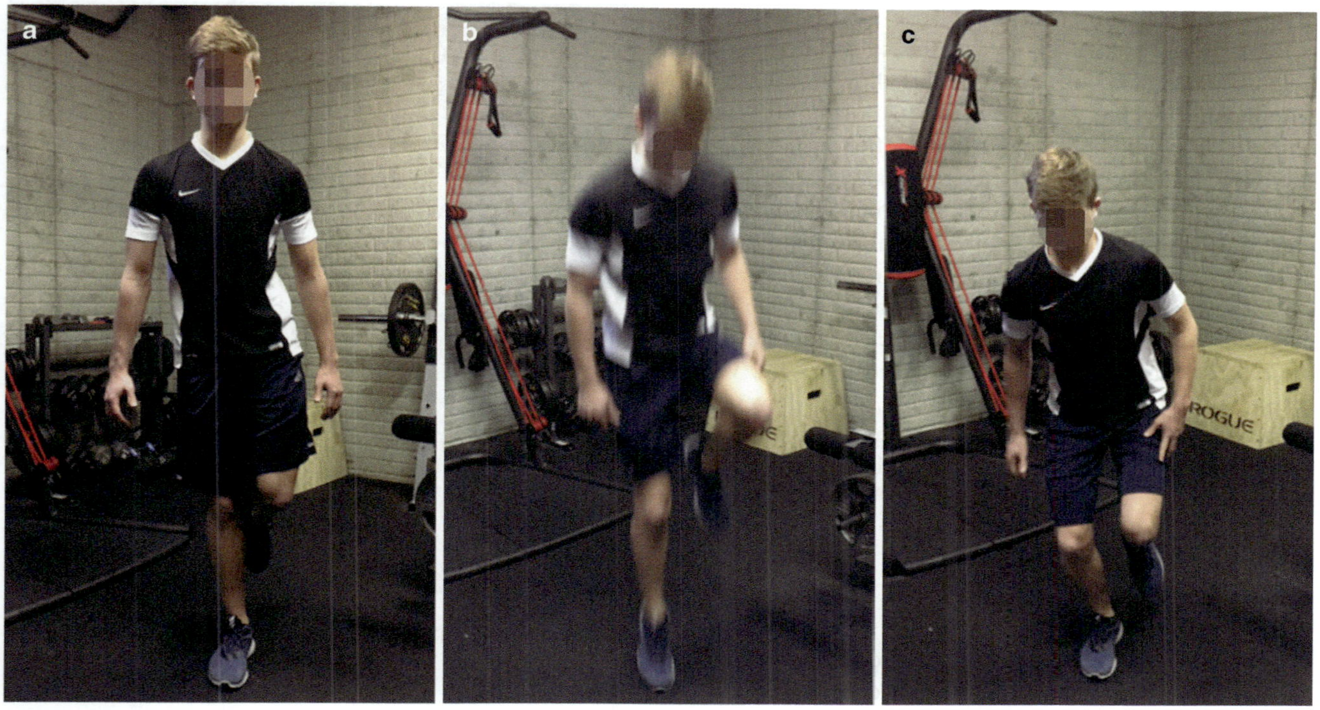

Fig. 4.3 (**a–c**) Soccer goalie demonstrates single leg stance and hop tests

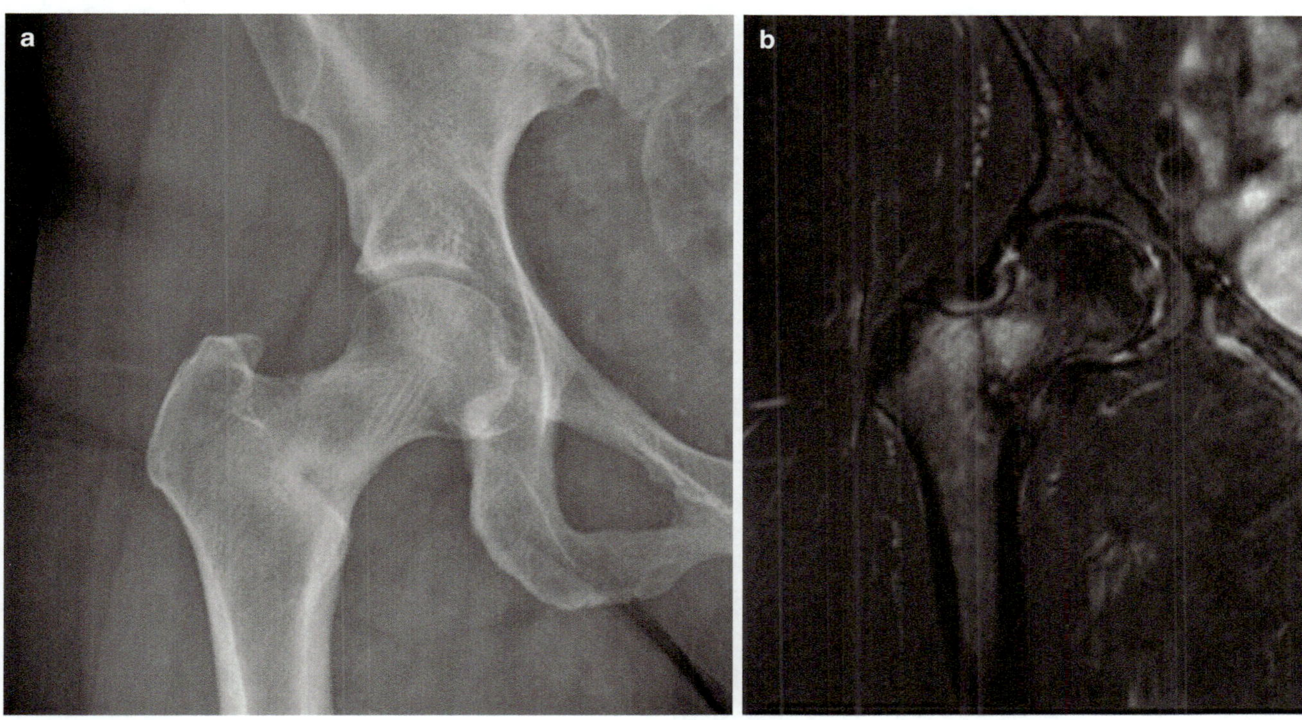

Fig. 4.4 (**a**) Anteroposterior radiograph of the hip in a 47 year-old female marathon runner with tension side femoral neck stress fracture with early callus formation. (**b**) T2 coronal MRI demonstrating nondisplaced transcervical femoral neck stress fracture in a 47 year-old female marathon runner

tibial, and tarsal stress fractures. Bone scans are typically positive in all phases of a triple-phase technetium scan (angiogram, blood pool, delayed). This allows for easier differentiation of stress fractures from periostitis, or medial tibial stress syndrome, as periostitis is often negative in the angiogram and blood pool phases and positive in the delayed image phase. Medial tibial stress syndrome also presents a more diffuse distribution along the medial border of the tibia as opposed to a focal "hotspot" indicating a stress fracture [27]. The greatest value of bone scintigraphy is its ability to diagnose multiple stress injuries. Bone scans will often demonstrate increased uptake in the affected bone 1–2 weeks before radiographic changes occur (Fig. 4.5). However, as the uptake on bone scan requires 12–18 months to normalize, bone scintigraphy is less helpful for guiding return to sports participation [26].

4.6.3 Computed Tomography (CT Scan)

In the setting of a chronic stress fracture computed tomography scan is beneficial for demonstrating evidence of healing by clearly showing the presence or absence of a nonunion [28, 29]. CT scan delineates bone well and is very useful to determine whether the fracture is complete or incomplete [28, 29]. It is of particular use in the case of tarsal navicular stress fractures (Fig. 4.6) and for stress injuries of the pars interarticularis [30].

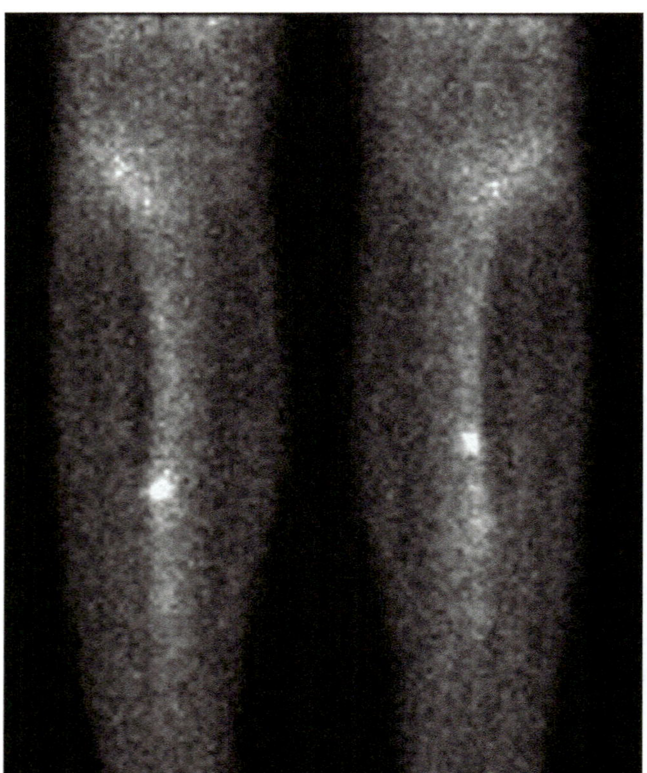

Fig. 4.5 Bone scan of bilateral tibias of a 19 year-old female college basketball player with multiple stress fractures of the bilateral anterior tibial diaphyses

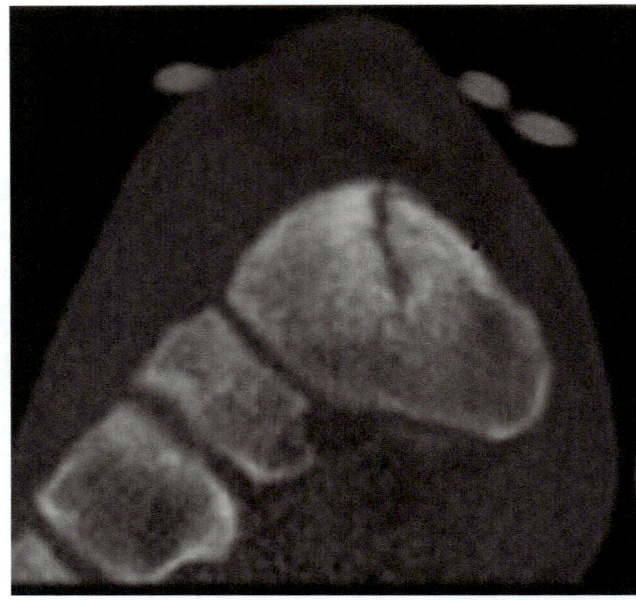

Fig. 4.6 Coronal CT scan demonstrating sagittal dorsal navicular stress fracture

4.6.4 Magnetic Resonance Imaging (MRI)

Currently, magnetic resonance imaging is the gold standard for diagnosing and classifying bony stress injuries. It has demonstrated superior sensitivity and specificity to bone scan and CT for associated soft tissue abnormalities, and may delineate injury earlier than bone scan [26]. Typical MRI findings on T2 sequences include a band of low signal corresponding to the fracture line, surrounded by diffuse high signal intensity representing marrow edema (Fig. 4.4b) [31]. Its sensitivity is similar to that of a bone scan, and it is much more precise in delineating the anatomic location, acuity, and extent of a bony injury [26]. MRI has additionally shown prognostic ability regarding time to healing a stress fracture and time to return to sport [15, 16].

4.6.5 Ultrasound

The use of ultrasound to diagnose a stress fracture has been advocated. In one study the authors validated the efficacy of ultrasound as a primary evaluation tool for bone stress injuries using MRI imaging as a standard. Though this option is not available in all sports medicine clinics and is dependent on the experience and skill of the operator, ultrasound is an inexpensive and increasingly available options for identifying stress injuries of bone [32].

4.6.6 Classification/Grading

Stress fractures are classified in a variety of ways [33]. They are most commonly categorized by the size of the fracture line, the anatomic site of injury, the biological healing potential of the injury location, the natural history of the particular fracture, or a combination of these features [1–7, 31]. Multiple authors have advocated classifying stress fractures as either "high-risk" or "low-risk" [3–6]. High-risk sites have at least one of the following characteristics: relative avascularity with or without retrograde blood supply and high tensile forces [7, 33]. These characteristics increase the risk of delayed or non-union, refracture, and significant long term consequences if a complete fracture occurs including avascular necrosis.

In addition to determining the risk level of a stress fracture, the extent of the fatigue failure or "grade" of the injury is necessary to describe and treat it [1, 4, 31]. A combined clinical and radiographic classification system developed by the authors is shown in Table 4.2 [1]. This system has shown high inter- and intra-observer reliability among sports medicine and orthopaedic clinicians [1]. Additionally, this system has high prognostic ability for time to healing and return to sports participation [3, 4, 15, 16]. The recommended treatment algorithm included in this chapter is based on the Kaeding-Miller classification system for stress fractures.

4.7 Risk Assessment

4.7.1 High Risk, Intermediate Risk, and Low Risk Stress Fractures

Low-risk stress fractures include the distal femur, the medial tibia, the ribs, the ulnar shaft, and the first through fourth metatarsals, all of which have a consistent blood supply and favorable natural history. These sites tend to be on the compression side of the bone, and respond well to activity modification. Low-risk stress fractures are less likely to recur, develop nonunion, or have a significant complication should they progress to complete fracture [5].

Intermediate risk stress fractures are those that occur near a high risk site, but have a favorable healing potential and biomechanical forces acting on them. Anatomic sites included in this group are the inferior surface of the femoral neck, the proximal femoral shaft, the inferior pubic ramus, and the pars intra-articularis. Rarely do these sites require surgical stabilization to allow healing, but, given their biomechanical features and proximity to high risk sites, they have an increased potential to extend into a high risk site if the fracture propagates.

Table 4.3 presents a list of anatomic locations considered high-risk for stress fracture propagation along with their recommended treatment strategies. A delay in treatment for a high-risk site may prolong the patient's period of complete rest, and potentially alter the treatment strategy to include surgical fixation with or without bone grafting. Given their location on the tension side of their respective bones, these fractures possess biomechanical properties that predispose them to propagation of the fracture line. In comparison to low-risk stress fractures, high-risk injuries are not likely to heal without complete rest and surgical stabilization. With less aggressive treatment, high-risk stress fractures tend to progress to nonunion or complete fracture, require operative management, and recur in the same location [3, 4, 6].

4.7.2 Management of High-Risk Stress Fractures

Treatment decision-making for high-risk stress fractures should be based on radiographic findings with less consideration given to symptom severity. The immediate goal of treatment of a high-risk stress fracture is to avoid propagation of the fracture. Typically, this requires either limited resistance, protected weightbearing, or surgical stabilization.

Table 4.2 Kaeding-Miller Stress Fracture Classification System. Shown is a combined clinical and radiographic classification system for stress fractures that has shown high intra- and inter-observer reliability and prognostic ability for healing

Grade	Pain	Radiographic findings (CT, MRI, Bone scan or X-ray)
I	–	Imaging evidence of stress FX No fracture line
II	+	Imaging evidence of stress FX No fracture line
III	+	Non-displaced fracture line
IV	+	Displaced fracture (>2 mm)
V	+	Nonunion

Table 4.3 Anatomic sites for high-risk stress fractures [6]

- Olecranon
- Scaphoid
- Femoral neck (tension side)
- Patella (tension side)
- Anterior tibial cortex
- Medial malleolus
- Talar neck
- Dorsal tarsal navicular cortex
- Fifth metatarsal proximal metaphysis
- Sesamoids of great toe

Ideally, while the fracture is healing a balance is maintained between the athlete maintaining fitness and minimizing the risk of fracture progression. While over-treatment of a low-risk stress fracture may result in unnecessary deconditioning and loss of playing time, under-treatment of a high-risk injury puts the athlete at risk of significant long-term complications.

The presence of a visible fracture line on a plain radiograph in a high-risk stress fracture should prompt serious consideration for surgical stabilization. Depending on injury severity, patients with stress injuries in high-risk locations may require immediate immobilisation and/or restriction from weight-bearing activities with close monitoring. If an incomplete fracture is present on plain radiographs with evidence of fracture on MRI or CT in a high-risk location, immobilisation and strict non-weight bearing is indicated. Worsening symptoms or radiographic evidence of fracture progression despite non-operative treatment is an indication for operative treatment. All complete fractures at high-risk sites should receive serious consideration for surgical treatment. In general, a low threshold for surgical fixation should be maintained for high risk stress fractures for several reasons. These include expediting healing, allowing earlier return to activity, and minimizing the risk of delayed union and re-fracture. In the case of a tension-side femoral neck stress fracture (Fig. 4.4a, b), urgent surgical fixation may be necessary to prevent a catastrophic fracture (Fig. 4.7) [6, 7, 21].

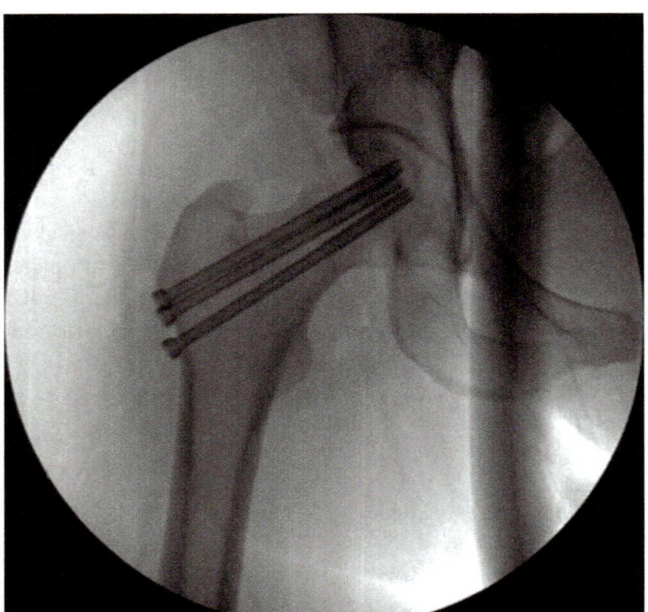

Fig. 4.7 Fluoroscopic radiographic image of the right hip following closed reduction and percutaneous screw fixation of a femoral neck stress fracture.

4.7.3 Management of Low Risk Stress Fractures

Low-risk stress fractures may be managed most often with relative rest and activity modification. Decision-making should be based in part on symptom severity. Athletes who experience enough pain to limit function should be treated with relative, if not complete, rest. The decision to continue activity despite the presence of a low-risk stress fracture and titrate the volume of activity to a low but functional pain level can be made after discussion with the athlete. A key point in this discussion is the possibility of progression to a complete fracture with this approach. If the goal is not to continue activity but to completely heal the fracture, then rest to a pain free level is required before return to athletic participation. Unless otherwise contraindicated, a patient may be permitted to maintain fitness by cross-training during this time with low impact alternatives such as cycling, swimming, elliptical training, stepping on a stepping machine, anti-gravity treadmill, or aquatic running.

4.7.4 Insufficiency Fractures

A distinction should be made between stress fractures and insufficiency fractures, although they are not mutually exclusive. Both are the result of the loss of balance between the production and repair of microdamage in bone. A stress fracture is the result of high loads placed on relatively normal bone, whereas an insufficiency fracture is the result of normal loads placed on bone with decreased osseous density or impaired healing capacity [34]. Insufficiency fractures occur most commonly in elderly females, but may occur in athletes with malabsorption conditions. An example of a subchondral insufficiency fracture of the medial femoral condyle is shown along with an intraoperative fluoroscopic image post treatment with intraosseous bioplasty procedure (Fig. 4.8a, b)

4.8 Return to Sports Participation

For most athletes, return to sport should only be allowed after proper treatment and complete healing of a stress fracture. Given the heterogeneity of these injuries, however, the time to return is difficult to predict. The Kaeding-Miller classification system presented in Table 4.2 is able to predict the expected time to return to athletic activity with the average to time to return to competitive running being 11–14 weeks with female athletes requiring greater time to return to sports [15, 16, 18].

Most early stress reactions at high-risk sites heal with non-operative management [6]. The key difference between a low-grade stress fracture at a high-risk location versus a

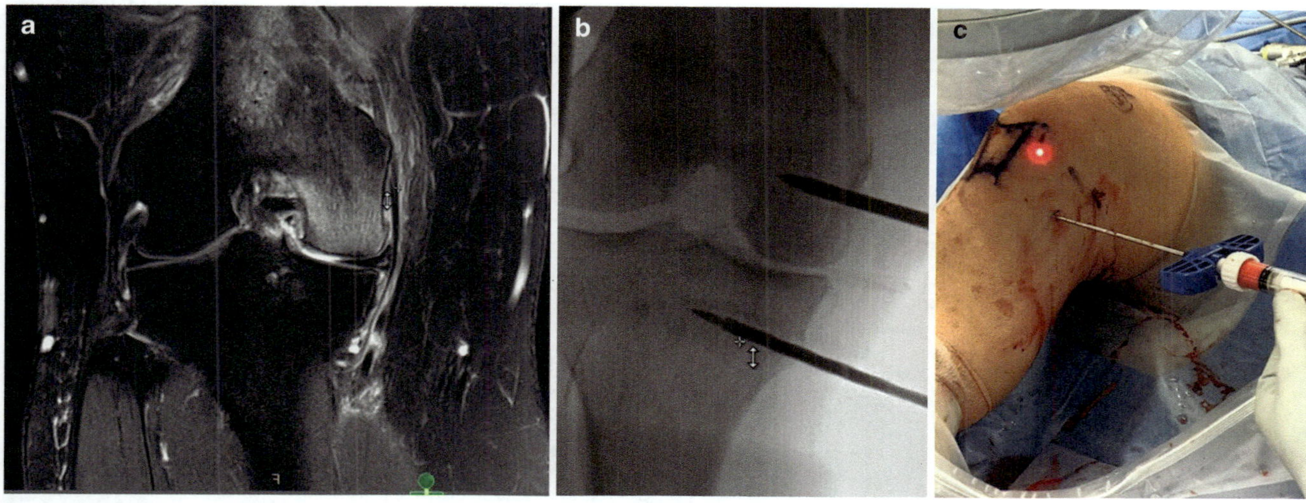

Fig. 4.8 (**a**) T2 coronal MRI demonstrating subchondral insufficiency fracture of the medial femoral condyle. (**b**) Intraoperative fluoroscopic radiograph during intraosseous bioplasty of the medial femoral condyle and medial tibial plateau. (**c**) Intraosseous bioplasty performed at the medial proximal tibia. Mixture of demineralized bone matrix and concentrated bone marrow aspirate are injected after core decompression has been completed

low-risk location is that with the low-risk site the athlete may be allowed to continue to train, whereas the high-risk injury requires complete heal prior to return to unrestricted activity. Regardless of the grade and location, the risk of continued participation should be discussed with each athlete, and the management of each fracture should be individualized. Cross-training while resting from the inciting activity allows maintenance of cardiovascular fitness while decreasing tensile, bending, and rotational forces at the healing fracture site [3, 7, 21, 35]. Return to participation should be a joint decision between the physician, athletic trainer, coach, and athlete.

4.9 Prevention of Stress Injuries to Bone

Prevention is the ideal treatment of stress injuries of bone and most other overuse injuries. An assessment of the athlete's risk should be made at pre-participation evaluations, especially in those with a history of previous stress fractures, and women with light or absent menses [2, 12, 21]. Correction of amenorrhea in females and calcium and Vitamin D_3 supplementation is recommended in addition to general nutritional optimization. If biomechanical abnormalities are encountered, the use of appropriately designed orthotic devices should be considered as an initial corrective measure. However, running gait analysis (Fig. 4.9) and appropriate running form or technique changes may be necessary to prevent future injuries. Unfit or unconditioned athletes including military recruits, particularly female athletes with menstrual irregularities, are at peak risk for stress injuries to bone and increased utilization of health care resources [18].

4.10 Biologic Healing Enhancement

4.10.1 Electrical Osseous Stimulation

Recent technological developments have given rise to the use of biologic treatment modalities for stress injuries to bone. These include the use of electronic bone stimulators, pulsed parathyroid hormone (Teriparatide), subchondroplasty, and concentrated bone marrow aspirate. Pulsed Electromagnetic Fields (PEMF) and Low Intensity Pulsed Ultrasound (LIPU) are FDA approved, non-invasive tools which increase the production of regulatory mediators required for physiological bone healing [36]. PEMF creates a magnetic field and a secondary electric impulse activating a series of enzyme reactions that up-regulate growth factors such as Bone Morphogenic Proteins, Transforming Growth Factor-β and Calmodulin leading to bone cell proliferation and fracture healing. LIPU appears to have a direct effect on ion channels for stimulating bone cell activity via mechanoreceptors [37]. Bone stimulators have been shown to be the most effective for delayed unions of the tibial shaft and fifth metatarsal shaft [38]. Additionally, evidence has demonstrated the value of therapeutic ultrasound specifically in tarsal navicular stress injuries [39].

4.10.2 Parathyroid Hormone Stimulation

The effect of Teriparatide on fracture healing has been evaluated with mixed results. Teriparatide achieves the primary endpoint of accelerated healing with improved early fracture callus formation compared to placebo [40]. Preclinical stud-

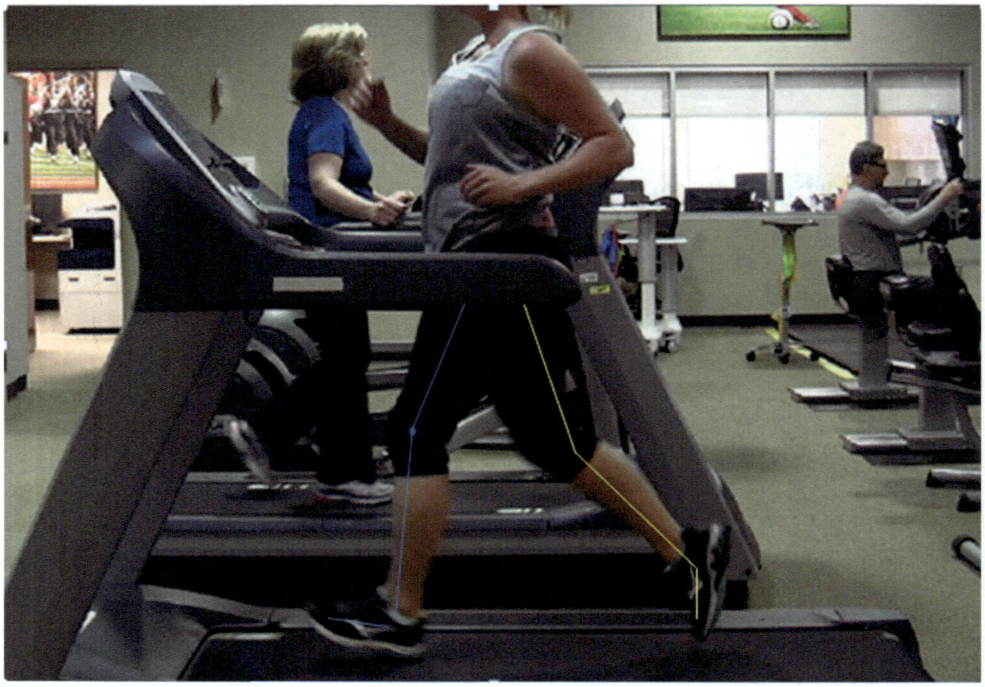

Fig. 4.9 Video running gait analysis performed on a 29 year-old female runner with recurrent tibial stress fractures

ies on rat models have shown that supra-physiologic doses of parathyroid hormone have demonstrated increased fracture site strength and callus quantity, with greater mineralization at the fracture site [40, 41].

4.10.3 Subchondroplasty and Intraosseous Bioplasty

Subchondroplasty is a recently developed procedure to increase the density and structural integrity of subchondral bone. This surgical technique is performed by drilling into subchondral bone with a cannulated guide pin. Under fluoroscopy, engineered calcium phosphate paste is injected into subchondral bony defects forming a macroporous scaffold for bone. Its application includes the treatment of subchondral insufficiency fractures most commonly of the distal femur and proximal tibia (Fig. 4.8b) [42]. Initial short term results have shown that subchondroplasty provides significant improvement in pain and functional capacity over the first 24 weeks following surgery [43]. Intraosseous bioplasty involves percutaneously performing a core decompression of the affected metaphyseal bone site and injecting a mixture of bone marrow concentrate, calcium chloride clot, and demineralized bone matrix (Fig. 4.8c). The long-term results of these treatment options are currently being investigated.

4.10.4 Bone Marrow Aspirate Concentrate (BMAC)

Bone Marrow Aspirate Concentrate is a biologic treatment employing an individual's own stem cells to stimulate bony healing. Osteoblastic progenitor cells are available in the bone marrow aspirate of the iliac crest, proximal aspect of the tibia, and calcaneus. The iliac crest provides the highest yield of osteoblastic progenitor cells, though BMAC can be extracted from other sites, including the proximal tibial metaphysis (Fig. 4.10) [44]. Percutaneous screw fixation of proximal fifth metatarsal fractures augmented with bone marrow aspirate concentrate provides predictable healing results while permitting athletes a return to sport at their previous levels of competition with few complications [45]. Autologous BMAC combined with PRP injection has been shown to improve bone healing in distraction osteogenesis of the tibia [46]. The local application of BMAC in the management of delayed healing is a promising alternative

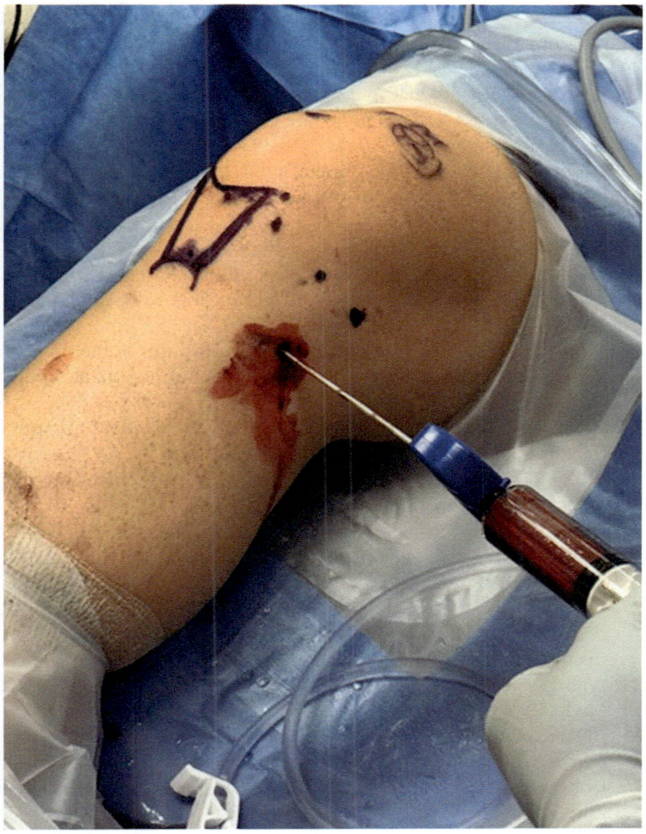

Fig. 4.10 Aspiration of bone marrow concentrate from the medial proximal tibial metaphysis

to autogenous bone grafting, and may help to reduce donor site morbidity [47, 48].

4.11 Summary

Stress fractures are common, particularly in endurance athletes and military recruits. The diagnosis can be made if a high index of suspicion is maintained and the proper imaging studies are obtained. The Kaeding-Miller classification system for stress fractures characterizes these injuries based on the patient's symptoms as well as their position on a radiologic continuum of severity. A holistic approach to treatment that takes into account the importance of nutritional, hormonal, psychologic, and biomechanical factors is necessary for treatment success. Stress fracture management should be individualized to the patient or athlete by taking into consideration injury site (low versus high risk), grade (extent of microdamage accumulation), the individual's activity level, competitive situation, and risk tolerance. High-risk stress fractures are primarily loaded in tension, have a poor natural history, and commonly require surgical intervention. Low-risk fractures are most often those loaded in compression, have a better prognosis, and are unlikely to progress to complete fracture. The recommended treatment algorithm stratifies these injuries based upon injury severity and the biomechanical environment in which they are located. In addition to the traditional treatment strategies of rest, immobilisation, and surgical stabilization, recent modalities for enhancing healing potential have been utilized with some success from further research being required to fully confirm their efficacy.

Clinical Pearls

- Stress fractures are overuse injuries of bone that occur most commonly in the lower extremities of distance runners and military personnel.
- Stress fractures occur in three stages: Crack initiation, crack propagation, and complete fracture.
- Radiographs are rarely able to identify a stress fracture. MRI is the gold standard for identifying and grading stress fractures.
- The management of stress fractures requires a holistic approach that includes rest from the causative activity, proper nutritional support, hormonal balance, and possibly surgical stabilization.
- High risk sites require aggressive treatment to prevent fracture progression, recurrence, and nonunion.

Review

Questions

1. Which of the following levels of stress fracture progression is a normal part of homeostasis in healthy bone?
   (a) Crack initiation
   (b) Crack propagation
   (c) Complete or final fracture
   (d) Cumulative microtrauma
   (e) Insufficiency fracture
2. Which of the following sites is considered to be low risk for stress fracture progression?
   (a) Anterior tibial cortex
   (b) Dorsal navicular

(c) Mid femoral diaphysis
(d) Olecranon
(e) Tension side femoral neck

3. Which of the following imaging modalities has the greatest specificity for identifying and grading stress fractures?
(a) Bone Scintigraphy
(b) CT scan
(c) MRI
(d) Plain radiographs
(e) Ultrasound

Answers

1. a.
2. c.
3. c.

References

1. Kaeding CC, Miller TL. The comprehensive description of stress fractures: a new classification system. J Bone Joint Surg. 2013;95(13):1214–20.
2. Kaeding CC, Yu JR, Wright R, et al. Management and return to play of stress fractures. Clin J Sports Med. 2005;15(6):442–7.
3. Kaeding CC, Spindler KP, Amendola A. Management of troublesome stress fractures. Am Acad Orthop Surgeons Instr Course Lect. 2004;53:455–69.
4. Kaeding CC, Najarian R. Stress fractures—classification and management. Physician Sports Med. 2010;38(3):45–54.
5. Boden BP, Osbahr DC, Jimenez C. Low-risk stress fractures. Am J Sports Med. 2001;29(1):100–11.
6. Boden BP. High-risk stress fractures: evaluation and treatment. J Am Acad Orthop Surg. 2000;8:344–53.
7. McInnis KC, Ramey LN. High-risk stress fractures: diagnosis and management. PMR. 2016;8(3 Suppl):S113–24.
8. Lappe J, Cullen D, Haynatzki G, Recker R, Ahlf R, Thompson K. Calcium and vitamin D supplementation decreases incidence of stress fractures in female navy recruits. J Bone Miner Res. 2008;23(5):741–9.
9. Pouilles JM, Bernard J, Tremollières F, Louvet JP, Ribot C. Femoral bone density in young male adults with stress fractures. J Bone. 1989;10:105–8.
10. Rettig AC, Shelbourne KD, McCarroll JR, Bisesi M, Watts J. The natural history and treatment of delayed union stress fractures of the anterior cortex of the tibia. Am J Sports Med. 1988;16(3):250–5.
11. Brukner P, Bennell K, Matheson G. Stress fractures of the trunk. In: Stress fractures. Victoria: Blackwell Science; 1999. p. 119–38.
12. Tenforde AS, Carlson JL, Chang A, Sainani KL, Shultz R, Kim JH, Cutti P, Golden NH, Fredericson M. Association of the female athlete triad risk assessment stratification to the development of bone stress injuries in collegiate athletes. Am J Sports Med. 2017;45(2):302–10.
13. Eller DJ, Katz DS, Bergman AG, et al. Sacral stress fractures in long-distance runners. Clin J Sports Med. 1997;7:222–5.
14. Jones BH, Harris JM, Vinh TN, Rubin C. Exercise-induced stress fractures and stress reactions of bone: epidemiology, etiology, and classification. Exerc Sport Sci Rev. 1989;17:379–422.
15. Jamieson M, Everson S, Siegel C, Miller TL. Expected time to return to athletic participation following stress fracture in Division I collegiate athletes. Sports Health. 2018;10(4):340–4.
16. Jamieson M, Schroeder A, Day J, et al. Time to return to running after tibial stress fracture in female Division I collegiate track and field. Curr Orthop Pract. 2017;31(4):393–7.
17. Hosey RG, Fernandez MM, Johnson DL. Evaluation and management of stress fractures of the pelvis and sacrum. Orthopedics. 2008;31(4):383–5.
18. Krauss MR, Garvin NU, Boivin MR, Cowan DN. Excess stress fractures, musculoskeletal injuries, and health care utilization among unfit and overweight female army trainees. Am J Sports Med. 2017;45(2):311–6.
19. Miller TL, Harris JD, Kaeding CC. Stress fractures of the ribs and upper extremities: causation, evaluation, and management. Sports Med. 2013;43(8):665–74.
20. Bennell K, Brukner P. Epidemiology and site specificity of stress fractures. Clin Sports Med. 1997;16:179–96.
21. Miller TL, Best TM. Taking a holistic approach to managing difficult stress fractures. J Orthop Surg Res. 2016;11(1):98.
22. Toney CM, Games KE, Winkelmann ZK, Eberman LE. Using tuning-fork tests in diagnosing fractures. J Athl Train. 2016;51(6):498–9.
23. Coughlin MJ, Grimes JS, Traughber PD, Jones CP. Comparison of radiographs and CT scans in the prospective evaluation of the fusion of hindfoot arthrodesis. Foot Ankle Int. 2006;27(10):780–7.
24. Wall J, Feller JF. Imaging of stress fractures in runners. Clin Sports Med. 2006;25(4):781–802.
25. Brukner P, Bradshaw C, Khan KM, White S, Crossley K. Stress fractures: a review of 180 cases. Clin J Sports Med. 1996;6(2):85–9.
26. Dobrindt O, Hoffmeyer B, Ruf J, Seidensticker M, Steffen IG, Zarva A, Fischbach F, Wieners G, Furth C, Lohmann CH, et al. MRI versus bone scintigraphy. Evaluation for diagnosis and grading of stress injuries. Nuklearmedizin. 2012;51(3):88–94.
27. Dutton J. Clinical value of grading the scintigraphic appearances of tibial stress fractures in military recruits. Clin Nucl Med. 2002;27(1):18–21.
28. Gaeta M, Minutoli F, Vinci S, Salamone I, D'Andrea L, Bitto L, Magaudda L, Blandino A. High-resolution CT grading of tibial stress reactions in distance runners. Am J Roentgenol. 2006;187:789–93.
29. Bradshaw C, Khan K, Brukner P. Stress fracture of the body of the talus in athletes demonstrated with computer tomography. Clin J Sports Med. 1996;6:48–51.
30. Standaert CJ. Spondylolysis in the adolescent athlete. Clin J Sport Med. 2002;12(2):119–22.
31. Arendt EA, Griffiths HJ. The use of MR imaging in the assessment and clinical management of stress reactions of bone in high-performance athletes. Clin Sports Med. 1997;16:291–306.
32. Papalada A, Malliaropoulos N, Tsitas K, Kiritsi O, Padhiar N, Del Buono A, Maffulli N. Ultrasound as a primary evaluation tool of bone stress injuries in elite track and field athletes. Am J Sports Med. 2012;40(4):915–9.
33. Miller T, Kaeding CC, Flanigan D. The classification systems of stress fractures: a systematic review. Phys Sportsmed. 2011;39(1):93–100.
34. Cabarrus MC, Ambekar A, Lu Y, Link TM. MRI and CT of insufficiency fractures of the pelvis and the proximal femur. AJR Am J Roentgenol. 2008;191(4):995–1001.
35. Jensen J. Stress fracture in the world class athlete: a case study. Med Sci Sports Exerc. 1998;30:783–7.
36. Longhino V, Bonora C, Sansone V. The management of sacral stress fractures: current concepts. Clin Cases Miner Bone Metab. 2011;8(3):19–23.

37. Massar L, Caruso G, Sollazzo V, Setti S. Pulsed electromagnetic fields and low intensity pulsed ultrasound in bone tissue. Clin Cases Miner Bone Metab. 2009;6(2):149–54.
38. Martinez de Albornoz P, Khanna A, Longo UG, Forriol F, Maffulli N. The evidence of low-intensity pulsed ultrasound for in vitro, animal and human fracture healing. Br Med Bull. 2011;100:39–57.
39. Malliaropoulos N, Alaseirlis D, Konstantinidis G, Papalada A, Tsifountoudis I, Petras K, Maffulli N. Therapeutic ultrasound in navicular stress injuries in elite track and field athletes. Clin J Sport Med. 2017;27(3):278–82.
40. Aspenberg P, Johansson T. Teriparatide improves early callus formation in distal radial fractures. Acta Orthop. 2010;81(2):234–6.
41. O'Loughlin PF, Cunningham ME, Bukata SV, et al. Parathyroid hormone (1–34) augments spinal fusion, fusion mass volume, and fusion mass quality in a rabbit spinal fusion model. Spine. 2009;34(2):121–30.
42. Cohen SB, Sharkey PF. Subchondroplasty for the treating bone marrow lesions. J Knee Surg. 2016;29(7):555–63.
43. Bonadio MB, Giglio PN, Helito CP, et al. Subchondroplasty for treating bone marrow lesions in the knee—initial experience. Rev Bras Ortop. 2017;52(3):325–30.
44. Hyer CF, Berlet GC, Bussewitz BW, Hankins T, Ziegler HL, Philbin TM. Quantitative assessment of the yield of osteoblastic connective tissue progenitors in bone marrow aspirate from the iliac crest, tibia, and calcaneus. J Bone Joint Surg Am. 2013;95(14):1312–6.
45. Murawski CD, Kennedy JG. Percutaneous internal fixation of proximal fifth metatarsal jones fractures (Zones II and III) with Charlotte Carolina screw and bone marrow aspirate concentrate: an outcome study in athletes. Am J Sports Med. 2011;39(6):1295–301.
46. Lee DH, Ryu KJ, Kim JW, Kang KC, Choi YR. Bone marrow aspirate concentrate and platelet-rich plasma enhanced bone healing in distraction osteogenesis of the tibia. Clin Orthop Relat Res. 2014;472(12):3789–97.
47. Jäger M, Jelinek EM, Wess KM, Scharfstädt A, Jacobson M, Kevy SV, Krauspe R. Bone marrow concentrate: a novel strategy for bone defect treatment. Curr Stem Cell Res Ther. 2009;4(1):34–43.
48. Miller TL, Kaeding CC, Rodeo SA. Emerging options for biologic enhancement of stress fracture healing in athletes. J Am Acad Ortho Surg. 2020;28(1):1–9.

Models for Understanding and Preventing Fractures in Sport

5

L. V. Fortington and N. H. Hart

Learning Objectives
- Describe the three levels of injury prevention.
- Identify non-modifiable and modifiable risk factors for fractures in sport.
- Describe basic skeletal pathology of children, adolescents and adults in sport.
- Generate potential prevention strategies and discuss the strengths and weaknesses of each strategy.

5.1 Introduction

Injuries and fractures are classically considered an inevitable part of sports participation. Yet, in most settings—from workplaces to roads and waterways—injuries can be prevented or controlled. In this chapter, we demonstrate that the long-standing principles from injury prevention science, using a structured and systematic approach, can be successfully applied to the problem of injuries in sports, including acute fractures and stress fractures.

Injury prevention is often addressed at three levels:

- **Primary prevention**—preventing new injuries.
- For example, wearing protective guards in skateboarding to prevent wrist fractures [1]. Primary prevention is exemplified through the various targeted neuromuscular exercise programs designed to prepare players for their sport, targeting mainly the prevention of lower limb and knee injuries [2].
- **Secondary prevention**—reducing severity and avoiding subsequent injury. Subsequent injury (injury occurring after an initial injury) is common in many athletes [3].
- **Tertiary prevention**—reducing the consequences of injuries.
- What happens after the injury can impact the clinical outcome for an individual [4]. This means that, if managed poorly, a fracture in sport could result in permanent disability or fatality. For example, jockeys, who sustain a spinal fracture after falling from their horse, risk sustaining further damage to their spinal cord [5]. Tertiary prevention would seek to minimise long-term neurological consequences to the injured individual.

This chapter focuses on primary and secondary prevention, presenting several theoretical and applied models that can assist in understanding and preventing fractures in sport.

5.2 What Is the Problem That Needs Addressing?

The World Health Organisation (WHO) public health model has been widely used in injury and violence prevention research (Fig. 5.1) [7]. The model is well known in sports medicine through the work of van Mechelen, who demonstrated application to the problem of sports injury [6]. At its essence, the first stage of the model seeks to establish the extent of the problem. This step was covered in the opening chapters of this book, covering the epidemiology of different types of fractures by addressing questions that sought to answer how many, in whom, when and where.

Step 1 can establish what the main problems are in a particular sporting population, addressing broad questions such as:

- For junior cricketers in Sri Lanka, what injuries are most common? [8]
- Do men and women experience different injuries in rugby sevens? [9].
- Which athletes sustain the most bone stress injuries in an elite sports environment? [10];

L. V. Fortington (✉) · N. H. Hart
School of Medical and Health Sciences, Edith Cowan University, Joondalup, Australia
e-mail: l.fortington@ecu.edu.au; n.hart@ecu.edu.au

G. A. J. Robertson, N. Maffulli (eds.), *Fractures in Sport*, https://doi.org/10.1007/978-3-030-72036-0_5

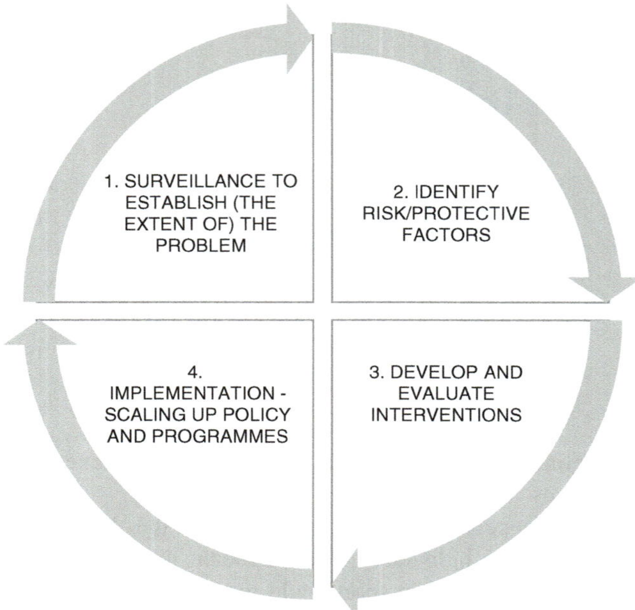

Fig. 5.1 Public health approach to injury and violence prevention. (Adapted from [6])

Step 1 can also be used to narrow focus on a particular known issue—surveillance to establish *the extent of* the problem. For this second element (*the extent of the problem*), the need to consider injury severity and burden of injury, not just incidence, is crucial [11]. A simple example of focusing on burden can be understood through the problem of wrist and hand fractures. Wrist, hand and finger fractures have a consistently high incidence rate in team ball sports [12–14]. Based on incidence alone, wrist, hand and finger fractures would be a priority if seeking to prevent the injuries that occur most often. Arguably, however, the severity of wrist and hand fractures is low, at least for the individual who can generally resume their regular activities after a period of recovery, generally with little long-term impact. Finding a balance of incidence and severity requires knowledge of the sport, the risks in the sport and its participants, and the potential consequences of the injury.

Quantifying injury incidence and severity in sports medicine is easier in theory than practice. This is because the highest quality injury data favours the capture of certain injury types. These data-favoured injuries are easily recognized: they occur suddenly, require medical attention and generally result in an athlete missing several weeks of training or competition. Acute fracture is a good example of a measurable time-loss injury. Methods to record non-acute injury in sports settings (such as bone-stress injury) continue to improve [15, 16]. Concurrently, there has been increased attention and understanding of the severity of injury, moving beyond the measure of expected or actual return to play. As these approaches to recording and reporting different types of injury becoming further established and applied more widely, quantification of the incidence and severity of fractures, inclusive of both acute and stress fractures, will become more accurate.

5.3 Identifying Risk Factors That Lead to the Problem

With an understanding of the scale and burden of the injury (fracture) problem, attention turns to risk factors and aetiology. Identifying what the risks for sustaining a fracture are, whether acute or stress related, allows measures to be put in place that can remove or reduce their impact.

Risk factors and events that predispose individuals to a heightened propensity to fracture (incidence, type, severity and location) are commonly categorised into modifiable or non-modifiable domains of internal and external origin (Fig. 5.2). Whether traumatic (impact) or fatigue (overuse), such risk factors contribute to the threshold by which physiological adaptation or pathophysiological maladaptation may occur through isolated or repetitive internal and external mechanical loads [19]. While non-modifiable risk factors are of interest to understand an individuals' risk profile, it is perhaps most helpful to examine modifiable risk factors that may form the basis of systems-based and individual-based injury prevention and reduction models [20]. In their own right, the establishment and implementation of prophylactic training programs and physical interventions (strength, power, aerobic, movement, flexibility, and balance) together with behavioural approaches (diet, nutrition, and psychology) provide compelling avenues of intervention to address many of the modifiable risk factors in athletes and their respective athletic pursuits. However, to simply establish and acknowledge internal and external risk factors is inadequate. Injury prevention models should also appreciate inciting events that merge with risk factors to produce pathology and injurious outcomes in sport [21]. That is, the causes and mechanisms leading to fracture incidence (traumatic and overuse), which typically result from a complex interaction of numerous risk factors and events.

5.3.1 Musculoskeletal Structure and Function

An individual's underlying musculoskeletal structure and function (anatomy, physiology and tissue mechanics) provides the central foundation through which human movement and adaptation occurs [22], thus plays a critically important role towards establishing robustness and resilience versus fragility and susceptibility to injury. Specifically, bone material, structure and strength are determined by genetic (non-modifiable) and environmental (modifiable) influences. Thus, targeted interventions or programs across an athlete's lifespan, which aim to optimise musculoskeletal strength (material and structural adaptations), are essential (Fig. 5.3).

Bone material and structure co-adapt in response to the routine mechanical loads placed on them throughout growth, development and adulthood [23], with a direct influence on an individual's mechanical behaviour of bone and their susceptibility to fracture [24, 25]. For example, individuals with slender phenotypes (low cross-sectional areas) primarily develop strength through disproportionate increases in density relative to a robust phenotypes (large cross-sectional areas). Accordingly, slender bones are materially more brittle and mechanically less flexible than their robust counterparts. Thus, internal and external forces transmitted during athletic pursuits lead to heightened acquisition and accumulation of microdamage at lower relative thresholds [19]. This renders individuals with a slender skeletal phenotype at higher risk of impact fracture and stress fracture [26] because of their reduced load-repetition tolerability prior to injury (Fig. 5.2).

Fig. 5.2 Modifiable and non-modifiable, internal and external risk factors of stress fractures that may increase athlete injury susceptibility across a continuum in response to an inciting event. [1] Sex (biological) and gender (identity, inclusive of transition) are distinct in definition and influence. A transitioning male or female undergoing cross-sex hormone therapy or gender-affirming surgery will have altered endocrine function that will modify an individuals' risk of fracture [17, 18]

	Non-Modifiable	Modifiable
Internal Factors	• Biological Age • Race / Ethnicity • Sex[1] • Anatomy • Anthropometry • Genetics • Previous Injury	• Body Composition • Weight • Gender[1] • Biomechanics • Physical Fitness • Training Programs • Diet and Nutrition
External Factors	• Weather Conditions • Ground / Surface • Opponent Behaviour	• Personal Protective Equipment • Sports Equipment • Footwear and Clothing • Competition Scheduling • Playing Position

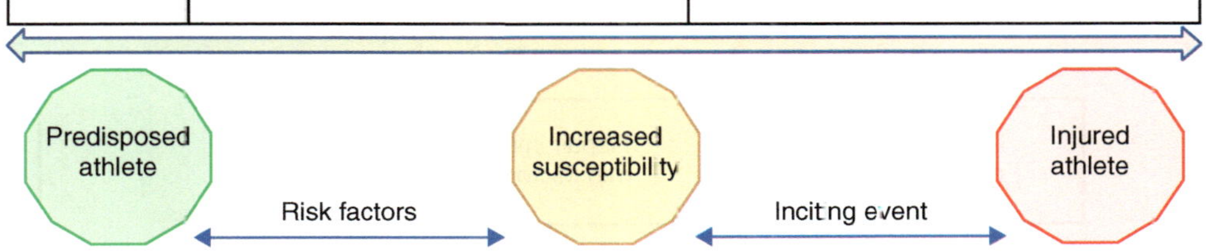

Fig. 5.3 Relationship between mechanical load (magnitude × repetition) and injury (left) and influence of targeted interventions or programs that improve resilience and musculoskeletal strength (right), highlighting the protective effect of increasing bone strength [19]

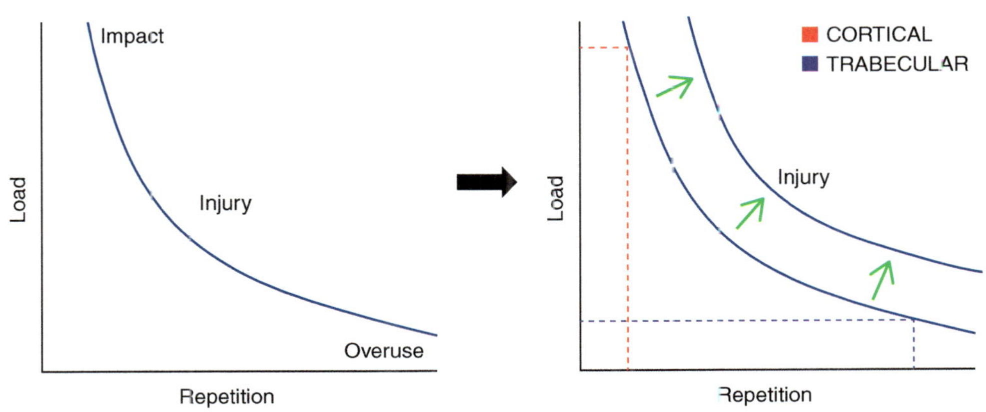

5.3.2 Skeletal Pathology

Fractures are broadly categorised as traumatic (acute onset from isolated events or events with close temporal proximity) and overuse (gradual onset from repetitious or cyclical events degenerating over time). Specifically, traumatic skeletal fractures result from an applied external force which exceeds the maximum durability (fracture load) of a given bone on a single occasion (i.e. from events such as tackling, impacts and collision in sport). On the other hand, overuse injuries are produced by repetitive low-grade and often cyclical forces (i.e. walking, running, kicking, jumping, changing direction) which exceed the tolerance of bone tissue over time in the absence of adequate repair and recovery. Pathologically, stress fractures are considered to be preventable relative to impact fractures, and are endemic in running athletes or military recruits [26], given the often unpredictable and inescapable scenarios observed in some athletic pursuits or combat scenarios [27]. Visually, the cascade of events for skeletal osteogenesis (positive response), modelling and remodelling (maintenance response) or stress reaction, stress fracture or complete fracture (pathological response) over time in response to mechanical loading [28], repair and recovery is provided (Fig. 5.4).

Skeletal pathology not only influences hard-tissue structures, but also negatively affects surrounding soft-tissue structures (muscle, tendon and ligament). The converse is also true, as pathology in nearby or neighbouring soft tissues negatively influences skeletal health. Beyond evident physical disruption and damage to a given biological tissue is the presence of catabolic endocrine-paracrine cross-talk, whereby catabolic secretomes are released and distributed into the microenvironment, leading to cellular disruption and tissue dysfunction elsewhere during the healing process [19]. For example, skeletal stress fractures, with no concomitant damage to surrounding muscle, will still lead to muscle weakness and muscle atrophy in the absence of voluntary anabolic stimuli, owing to an altered tissue microenvironment produced by the mere presence of localised circulatory catabolic cytokines. Accordingly, the prevention, reduction, and effective rehabilitation of fractures in athletic pursuits and sports participation requires more than a singular approach or individual model. Instead, an ipsative research

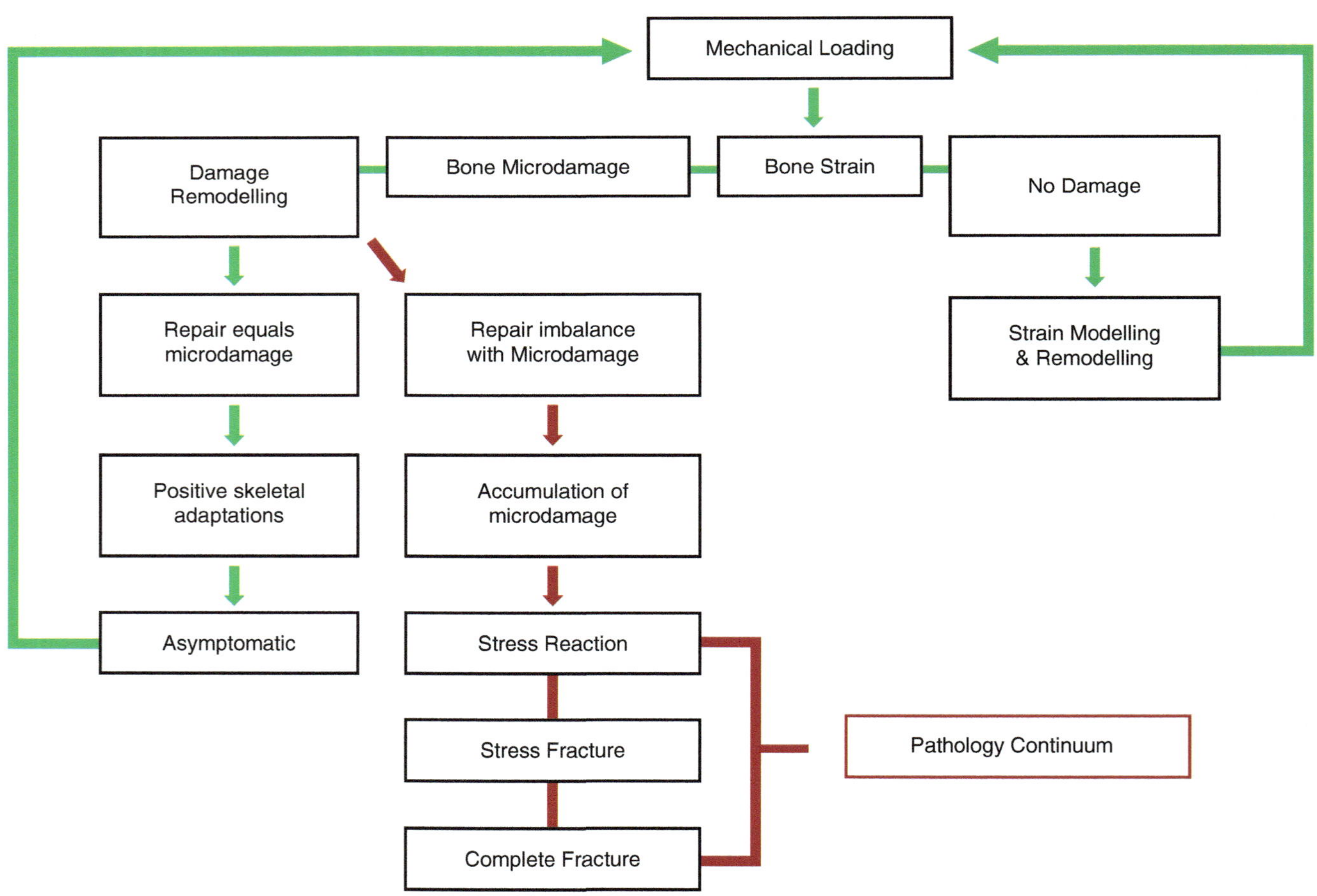

Fig. 5.4 A pathophysiological overview of overuse and fatigue fractures [19, 29, 30]

and systems-based implementation approach to protect athletes from all forms of injury is essential. This is exemplified by the recently proposed, dynamic and cyclical Team-sport Injury Prevention (TIP) model [31]. Furthermore, it is necessary to delineate between the age and stage of biological and intellectual maturity of athletes and the corresponding prevention of injury strategies.

5.3.3 Children, Adolescence and Youth

Children and adolescents have an altered injury risk and inciting event profile relative to their adult peers, owing to the ontogenic immaturity of their skeleton combined with their less developed motor skills and coordinated movement patterns. During this period of life, the underlying physiology and biomechanics of youth are highly dynamic and rapidly evolving, which often predisposes them to an increased risk of traumatic or overuse injuries, inclusive of skeletal fractures, during periods of intense or prolonged physical activity. For example, during growth and development, their particularly diverse hormonal and growth spurt phase of adolescence means that their bones undergo longitudinal and radial expansion at a rate whereby elongation exceeds mineral deposition. Accordingly, their bones are more porous and consequently more prone to fracture during this time. Similarly, immature bone is highly cartilaginous, thus it is able to withstand greater deformation before failure. Child and adolescent bones do subsequently sustain larger numbers of incomplete or partial fractures ("green stick fractures") which also heal faster than mature and biomineralised adult bone.

Given the evolving composition of bone microarchitecture and morphology, and the subsequently altered mechanical behaviour of immature and developing bone that this produced, the causes of fracture can be rather varied among children and adolescents across a variety of athletic or sporting conquests. Most prominently, youth athletes sustain fractures from impact and trauma (i.e. tackles, collisions, and falls), and thus acquire upper limb fractures at a higher rate than lower limb fractures regardless of their sex [32], likely to be more prevalent in those with low motor competence or movement coordination [33]. This is one of several reasons junior sporting programs and athletic events outlaw tackling and deliberate physical contact (i.e. creating non-contact, modified versions of the same sport or activity), and serves to exemplify the effective invocation of a modifiable, external risk mitigation strategy in an injury prevention or reduction model.

Beyond impact or traumatic causes, the skeletally immature adolescent athlete may develop injuries through repeated mechanical stresses imposed upon their musculoskeletal structures during athletic pursuits. Stress fractures are themselves a prevalent feature of injury in both immature youth and mature adult athletes from overuse and fatigue. However, what is perhaps unique to the adolescent athlete, given their open and active growth plates, are apophysitic (tuberosity stressed in traction), epiphysitic (compression or shear stress) and epiphyseolysic (growth plate widening under stress) injuries [34]. Accordingly, avulsion fractures of the epiphysis with potential for metaphysis co-involvement (as per the *Salter and Harris Classification* system) may occur, primarily from non-contact causes, through rotational and angular forces resulting from powerful muscle contraction, twisting or pivoting forces, or ground reaction forces during intense periods of physical activity.

Importantly, musculoskeletal injuries in child and adolescent athletes are typically non-permanent and without complication during the healing process with conservative rehabilitation. While premature closure of fractured growth plates following excessive, poorly rehabilitated or neglected apophysitic, epiphysitic or epiphyseolysic injuries can occur [34], this categorically should not preclude youth participation in athletic pursuits or sporting competition. For example, among 113,382 paediatric athletes presenting with injuries across 13 cohort studies, only 3.3% were from fractures, of which 8.6% of these fractures were physeal, approximating 0.3% of injuries reported [35]. Furthermore, among 260 paediatric athletes presenting with sports-related physeal fractures across 12 case series studies, 17% were associated with growth disturbance [35]. Taken together, these episodic injuries with suboptimal rehabilitation that lead to growth disturbances of poor prognoses are exceedingly small (~0.05% attributable to sports-related mechanisms), while the benefits of physical activity when young are broad-spectrum, and confer demonstrably lifelong benefits to the skeleton in older age [30, 36]. Nevertheless, where risks can be mitigated, it is incumbent upon all members of the athletic and sporting community to focus on injury prevention and harm minimisation, and, if injury does occur, optimal injury healing and rehabilitation.

5.3.4 Adults

Skeletal maturity is achieved in early adulthood. At that time, the material composition of bone transitions into a predominantly biomineralised state post-adolescence, prior to the establishment of peak mass in the third decade of life [19]. However, the adult skeleton remains both responsive and adaptive to its mechanical environment following peak bone mass acquisition, through morphological changes (site specific co-adaptive material and structural adjustments) as a mechanism to strengthen the skeleton and increase its tolerability to athletic and sporting tasks. While 40–60% of bone mineral density is genetically determined [37, 38], the remainder is modifiable, together with structural adaptation, to improve an individual's intrinsic risk of fracture. In this regard, an adult's established skeletal phenotype during ontogeny (slender-to-robust continuum) will influence the stiffness, ductility and susceptibility to accumulate micro-damage to routine physiological loading demands [25]. This is one example where sex differences between males and females currently exist, as females are not only skeletally slender relative to males, but also have less cortical cross-sectional area relative to body size and bone size [39]. This underpins their relatively weaker bones and heightened vulnerability to fracture in sporting and athletic contexts, supported epidemiologically under both impact [40] and stress [10, 41] conditions.

Athletic and sporting endeavours in adult populations are characteristically less refined, usually faster, and with greater intensity, volatility and risky behaviours, particularly as focus of intent turns towards competitiveness, success and athletic acumen instead of fun, play, skill and competency as observed in the child and adolescent populations [42]. Accordingly, while fracture mechanisms may be inherently similar, their inciting events may markedly differ in adults, producing different injury patterns and fracture causes. Indeed, adult athletes can encounter impact factures to all regions of the skeleton depending on their activity of engagement, though are most prominently observed in the hands, wrists, ribs, vertebrae and distal upper- and lower- appendicular long bones [40, 43–45]. Of course, the seriousness and potential life-threatening or life-altering nature of some fracture sites is dependent upon the location, with skull, spinal, tibial and pelvic fractures noted as major traumatic injuries with potentially significant lifelong consequences. Accordingly, injury prevention and minimisation models should prioritise combinations of internal and external modifiable risk factors, together with structural controls, in order to reduce the potential for inciting events as plausible targets at the individual and system-based level.

Lastly, adult athletes are predisposed to stress reactions and stress fractures, primarily of the weight-bearing lower limbs (tarsals, metatarsals, tibia and fibula), but also the load-bearing upper limbs and vertebrae in sports such as cricket, tennis or gymnastics, where repetitive and rotational forces are observed [10]. A myriad of nutritional, hormonal, and biomechanical factors contribute to the development of bone stress injuries in adults, which is particularly true for military recruits and sports where load carriage (body vests, equipment or apparatus) is necessary, or where high running volumes and frequencies are characteristic features [26, 27, 46]. Energy availability or relative energy deficiency in sport (RED-S) are critical nutrition-driven and endocrine altering factors influencing male and female athletes and their susceptibility to injuries and illness, inclusive of bone health and stress fracture, recently addressed as a priority issue through an *International Olympic Committee* consensus statement [47]. Thus, injury prevention and minimisation of stress fractures in adults requires more than a narrowly focused lens focused on load management paradigms (i.e. mechanical loading, microdamage, rest and recovery), but rather a multifactorial and holistic approach which also includes consideration of biomechanics (customary versus obscure movement), nutrition (quality of meals, meal timing, and energy availability), sleep quality and endocrine function (as a primary driver of homeostasis and skeletal regulation, adaptation or maladaptation).

5.4 From Understanding to Prevention

With an understanding of the problem, or more detailed insight to the extent of a problem, and having established the relevant risk and protective factors, the different injury prevention models now turn to developing measures for prevention.

In 2006, building on the four-stage Sequence of Prevention model from van Mechelen, the Translating Research into Injury Prevention Practice (TRIPP) model was published (Fig. 5.5) [48]. The TRIPP model arose from a recognition that an oversimplified understanding of the setting in which a sports injury occurs was leading to one-dimensional, and largely ineffective, measures for prevention. Thus, there was a shift in focus proposed to ensure the broader context of injury prevention was considered. Two new themes were incorporated into the original four-stage model, with revised text to more strongly promote the elements required for successful injury prevention in sporting conditions.

To provide team sports researchers and practitioners a more readily applicable tool, O'Brien et al. proposed the Team-sports Injury Prevention (TIP) model (Fig. 5.6) [31]. The TIP model focuses on a setting of a team sport training program, clarifying parts of the theory from TRIPP into a more relatable process for practitioners by reflecting on their current situation. The TIP model is cyclical, moving to re-evaluate on subsequent applications. The stages are:

1. injury and injury prevention (evaluate);
2. risk factors and injury prevention delivery (identify); and
3. content, planning and injury prevention strategies (intervene).

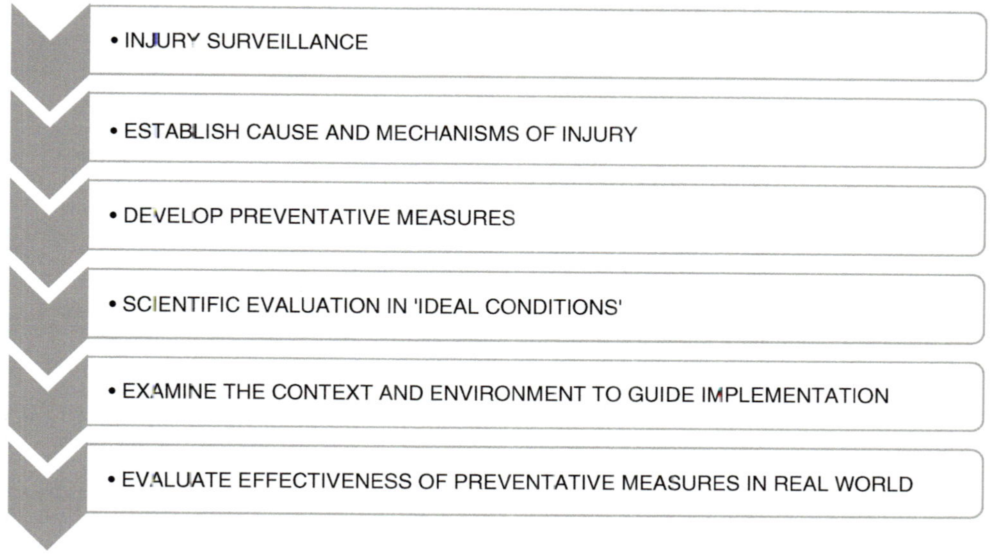

Fig. 5.5 Translating research into injury prevention practice (TRIPP) model, modified from [48]

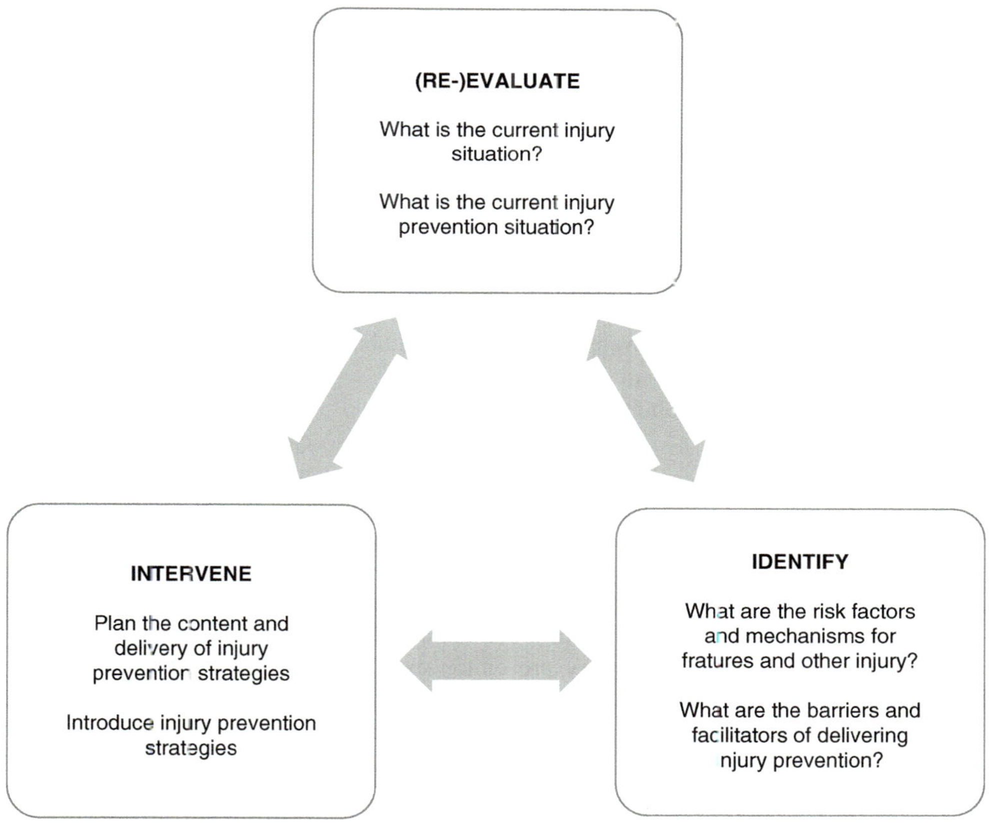

Fig. 5.6 Cyclical process of the Team-sport Injury Prevention (TIP) cycle, modified from [31]

5.5 Determining What Interventions Can Best Address the Problem

With an understanding of the injury prevention priorities and known key factors for fracture occurrence, solutions and prevention measures then need to be considered. Because of the potential range of injuries and fractures that can occur in sport, there is no single recipe for success when it comes to the actual development of prevention measures. The considered use of different models for injury prevention, in conjunction with thorough knowledge of the risk factors, is recommended. Injury prevention models embedded in wider socio-ecological principals, as opposed to addressing individual-factors, are recognised as critical to success. In 1973, Haddon published a seminal paper describing how to systematically think through potential intervention points to injury, commonly referred to as Haddon's ten countermeasures [49]:

1. Prevent the creation of the hazard
2. Reduce the amount of the hazard
3. Prevent the release of a hazard that already exists
4. Modify the rate or spatial distribution of the hazard from its source
5. Separate, by time or space, the hazard from that which can be protected
6. Separate the hazard and what is to be protected by a material barrier
7. Modify relevant basic qualities of the hazard
8. Make what is to be protected more resistant to damage from the hazard
9. Move rapidly to detect and evaluate the damage that has occurred and counter its continuation and extension
10. Stabilise, repair and rehabilitate the damage or injured person

Within the sports context, injury prevention measures tend toward use of protective equipment, or, increasingly, injury prevention exercise training programs. This negates several opportunities to intervene at earlier points outlined by Haddon in 1973, a problem that has been identified in sports medicine research [50]. Injury prevention exercise programs address stage 8 (damage resistance) while equipment addresses stage 6 (separation through a barrier). Ideally, the higher up the list, the more effective the prevention outcome will be, particularly with respect to primary prevention.

Another way to brainstorm injury prevention measures are the E's of injury prevention. Originally, the '3 E's' focused on Engineering, Enforcement and Education, which all apply to the prevention of fractures in sport (Table 5.1). Several authors have expanded on the list to introduce variants including equity, economics, environment, encouragement, emergency services, empowerment, exposure and evaluation [55].

Table 5.1 Broad approaches to consider for injury prevention

Injury prevention approach	Description	Example of application
Engineering	Products and designs that protect participants.	Several engineering solutions have been used in sport from the person-level (such as foot orthoses and footwear design [51]) through to changing surfaces and equipment used for play [52].
Education	Player development through coaching and practice Sport participants can learn behaviours to protect themselves and others	A survey of 260 Paralympic athletes, reported 9% as having a history of at least one bone stress injury [53]. This same study, also showed awareness of relative energy deficiency syndrome (REDs) was very low. Education to enhance knowledge of REDs and associated conditions in para athletes could be a helpful intervention against BSI in this population.
Enforcement	Sport regulations, and policies to ensure compliance.	Rugby provides several examples of rules, review of rules and enforcement of rules to ensure player safety, including reduce fracture risk. One example is the World Rugby Head Injury Assessment (HIA) protocol requiring players be assessed for concussion by independent medical officers [54].

Another valuable approach to development of injury prevention measures widely used in injury science is the Haddon matrix. This can be used when brainstorming if it is not yet clear what the main causes of injury are or what the best measures for prevention might be. The Haddon matrix encourages users to put thought to all potential factors involved in the event itself (i.e. how the fracture occurs) but also to the pre- and post-event factors. The model also raises the need to think through person-related factors, environmental factors (physical and social) and the 'agent' or 'vector' involved in the event, which for sports is commonly sporting equipment or another participant. Timpka et al. [56] provide a detailed description of the Haddon matrix (phase-factor matrix) applied to sports settings.

5.6 Conclusions

Fractures are debilitating and disruptive to an athlete's well-being, engagement in sport, and sporting aspirations. Fractures are also costly to the athlete, sporting organisations and healthcare systems to medically manage and rehabilitate. Accordingly, the prevention of fractures, whether acute through trauma, or chronic through overuse, remains centrally important to all persons involved at the individual, organisational and community level. Primary, secondary, and tertiary injury prevention requires investment and adoption by all stakeholders. With the extent of the problem established (incidence, recurrence and prevalence) and nature of the problem defined (aetiology and mechanisms of fractures), the most relevant injury prevention measures can be designed. Moving from concept to action is an undervalued component of preventing sports injury, with a stronger focus given toward injury surveillance to date. There are indications in the literature of stronger integration of implementation approaches into the design of prevention strategies, particularly in the application to injury prevention programs, for example, "*Seven steps for developing and implementing a preventive training program: lessons learned from JUMP-ACL and beyond*" [57], and, "*We have the programme, what next? Planning the implementation of an injury prevention programme*" [58]. Implementation remains an emerging yet integral field within sports injury prevention, to successfully transition prevention strategies into action. As noted earlier, no single model, to shape the process and practices for injury prevention, is applicable for all sports injury (or fracture) settings. However, injury prevention is the responsibility of all involved. With thoughtful, determined and creative planning, the incidence and severity of fractures in sport can be reduced.

References

1. Lewis LM, West OC, Standeven J, Jarvis HE. Do wrist guards protect against fractures? Ann Emerg Med. 1997;29:766–9.
2. Finch CF, Twomey DM, Fortington LV, Doyle TLA, Elliott BC, Akram M, Lloyd DG. Preventing Australian football injuries with a targeted neuromuscular control exercise programme: comparative injury rates from a training intervention delivered in a clustered randomised controlled trial. Inj Prev. 2016;22(2):123–8.
3. Toohey L, Drew MK, Fortington LV, Finch CF, Cook J. An updated subsequent injury categorisation model (SIC-2.0): data-driven categorisation of subsequent injuries in sport. Sports Med. 2018;48(9):2199–210.
4. Pless IB, Hagel BE. Injury prevention: a glossary of terms. J Epidemiol Community Health. 2005;59:182–5.
5. Ball JE, Ball CG, Mulloy RH, Datta I, Kirkpatrick AW. Ten years of major equestrian injury: are we addressing functional outcomes? J Trauma Manag Outcomes. 2009;3(1):2.
6. van Mechelen W, Hlobil H, Kemper HCG. Incidence, severity, aetiology and prevention of sports injuries. Sports Med. 1992;14:82–99.
7. Mercy JA, Rosenberg ML, Powell KE, Broome CV, Roper WL. Public health policy for preventing violence. Health Aff (Millwood). 1993;12:7–29.
8. Gamage PJ, Fortington LV, Kountouris A, Finch CF. Match injuries in Sri Lankan junior cricket: a prospective, longitudinal study. J Sci Med Sport. 2019;22(6):647–52.
9. Toohey LA, Drew MK, Finch CF, Cook JL, Fortington LV. A 2-year prospective study of injury epidemiology in elite Australian rugby sevens: exploration of incidence rates, severity, injury type, and subsequent injury in men and women. Am J Sports Med. 2019;47(6):1302–11.
10. Ruddick GK, Lovell GA, Drew MK, Fallon KE. Epidemiology of bone stress injuries in Australian high performance athletes: a retrospective cohort study. J Sci Med Sport. 2019;22(10):1114–8.
11. Bahr R, Clarsen B, Ekstrand J. Why we should focus on the burden of injuries and illnesses, not just their incidence. Br J Sports Med. 2018;52:1018–21.
12. Cairns MA, Hasty EK, Herzog MM, Ostrum RF, Kerr ZY. Incidence, severity, and time loss associated with collegiate football fractures, 2004-2005 to 2013-2014. Am J Sports Med. 2018;46(4):987–94.
13. Fortington LV, Finch CF. Priorities for injury prevention in women's Australian football: a compilation of national data from different sources. BMJ Open Sport Exerc Med. 2016;2:e000101.
14. O'Connor S, Leahy R, Whyte E, O'Donovan P, Fortington LV. Understanding injuries in the gaelic sport of camogie: the first national survey of self-reported worst injuries. Int J Athl Ther Train. 2019;24(6):243–8.
15. Clarsen B, Bahr R, Heymans MW, Engedahl M, Midtsundstad G, Rosenlund L, et al. The prevalence and impact of overuse injuries in five Norwegian sports: application of a new surveillance method. Scand J Med Sci Sports. 2014;25(3):323–30.
16. Docking SI, Rio E, Cook J, Orchard JW, Fortington LV. The prevalence of Achilles and patellar tendon injuries in Australian football players beyond a time-loss definition. Scand J Med Sci Sports. 2018;28(9):2016–22.
17. Fighera TM, Ziegelmann PK, Rasia da Silva T, Spritzer PM. Bone mass effects of cross-sex hormone therapy in transgender people: updated systematic review and meta-analysis. J Endocrine Soc. 2019;3(5):943–64.
18. Rothman MS, Iwamoto SJ. bone health in the transgender population. Clin Rev Bone Miner Metab. 2019;17(2):77–85.
19. Hart NH, Nimphius S, Rantalainen T, Ireland A, Siafarikas A, Newton RU. Mechanical basis of bone strength: influence of bone material, bone structure and muscle action. J Musculoskelet Neuronal Interact. 2017;17(3):114–35.
20. Hanlon C, Krzak JJ, Prodoehl J, Hall KD. Effect of injury prevention programs on lower extremity performance in youth athletes: a systematic review. Sports Health. 2020;12(1):12–22.
21. Bahr R, Krosshaug T. Understanding injury mechanisms: a key component of preventing injuries in sport. Br J Sports Med. 2005;39(6):324–9.
22. Hart NH, Newton RU, Tan J, Rantalainen T, Chivers P, Siafarikas A, Nimphius S. Biological basis of bone strength: anatomy, physiology and measurement. J Musculoskelet Neuronal Interact. 2020;20(3):347–71.
23. Rantalainen T, Weeks BK, Nogueira RC, Beck BR. Long bone robustness during growth: a cross-sectional pQCT examination of children and young adults aged 5–29 years. Bone. 2016;93:71–8.
24. Jepsen KJ, Evans R, Negus CH, Gagnier JJ, Centi A, Erlich T, Hadid A, Yanovich R, Moran DS. Variation in tibial functionality and fracture susceptibility among healthy, young adults arises from the acquisition of biologically distinct sets of traits. J Bone Miner Res. 2013;28(6):1290–300.
25. Tommasini SM, Nasser P, Hu B, Jepsen KJ. Biological co-adaptation of morphological and composition traits contributes to mechanical functionality and skeletal fragility. J Bone Miner Res. 2008;23(2):236–46.
26. Popp KL, Frye AC, Stovitz SD, Hughes JM. Bone geometry and lower extremity bone stress injuries in male runners. J Sci Med Sport. 2020;23(2):145–50.

27. Hart NH, Newton RU. Testosterone replacement for male military personnel—a potential countermeasure to reduce injury and improve performance under extreme conditions. EBioMedicine. 2019;47:16–7.
28. Hughes JM, Popp KL, Yanovich R, Bouxsein ML, Matheny RW Jr. The role of adaptive bone formation in the etiology of stress fracture. Exp Biol Med (Maywood). 2017;242(9):897–906.
29. Warden SJ, Burr DB, Brukner PD. Stress fractures: pathophysiology, epidemiology, and risk factors. Curr Osteoporos Rep. 2006;4(3):103–9.
30. Warden SJ, Davis IS, Fredericson M. Management and prevention of bone stress injuries in long distance runners. J Orthop Sports Phys Ther. 2014;44(10):749–65.
31. O'Brien J, Finch CF, Pruna R, McCall A. A new model for injury prevention in team sports: the Team-sport Injury Prevention (TIP) cycle. Sci Med Football. 2019;3(1):77–80.
32. Jenkins M, Nimphius S, Hart NH, Chivers P, Rantalainen T, Rueter K, Borland ML, McIntyre F, Stannage K, Siafarikas A. Appendicular fracture epidemiology of children and adolescents: a 10-year case review in Western Australia (2005 to 2015). Arch Osteoporos. 2018;13(1):63.
33. Jenkins M, Hart NH, Nimphius S, Chivers P, Rantalainen T, Rothacker KM, Beck BR, Weeks BK, McIntyre F, Hands B, Beeson BP, Siafarikas A. Characterisation of peripheral bone mineral density in youth at risk of secondary osteoporosis-a preliminary insight. J Musculoskel Neuronal Interact. 2019. Ahead of Print.
34. Frush TJ, Lindenfeld TN. Peri-epiphyseal and overuse injuries in adolescent athletes. Sports Health. 2009;1(3):201–11.
35. Caine D, DiFiori J, Maffulli N. Physeal injuries in children's and youth sports: reasons for concern?. Br J Sports Med. 2006;40(9):749–60.
36. Warden SJ, Roosa SM, Kersh ME, Hurd AL, Fleisig GS, Pandy MG, Fuchs RK. Physical activity when young provides lifelong benefits to cortical bone size and strength in men. Proc Natl Acad Sci. 2014;111(14):5337–42.
37. Havill LM, Mahaney MC, Binkley T, Specker BL. Effects of genes, sex, age, and activity on BMC, bone size, and areal and volumetric BMD. J Bone Miner Res. 2007;22(5):737–46.
38. Paternoster L, Lorentzon M, Lehtimäki T, Eriksson J, Kähönen M, Raitakari O, Laaksonen M, Sievänen H, Viikari J, Lyytikäinen LP, Mellström D. Genetic determinants of trabecular and cortical volumetric bone mineral densities and bone microstructure. PLoS Genet. 2013;9(2):e1003247.
39. Schlecht SH, Bigelow EM, Jepsen KJ. How does bone strength compare across sex, site, and ethnicity? Clin Orthopaed Relat Res. 2015;473(8):2540–7.
40. Court-Brown CM, Wood AM, Aitken S. The epidemiology of acute sports-related fractures in adults. Injury. 2008;39(12):1365–72.
41. Wentz L, Liu PY, Haymes E, Ilich JZ. Females have a greater incidence of stress fractures than males in both military and athletic populations: a systemic review. Mil Med. 2011;176(4):420–30.
42. Brown KA, Patel DR, Darmawan D. Participation in sports in relation to adolescent growth and development. Transl Pediatr. 2017;6(3):150.
43. Aiken SA, Watson BS, Wood AM, Court-Brown CM. Sports-related fractures in South East Scotland: an analysis of 990 fractures. J Orthop Surg (Hong Kong). 2014;22:313–7.
44. Robertson GA, Wood AM, Aitken SA, Court BC. Epidemiology, management, and outcome of sport-related ankle fractures in a standard UK population. Foot Ankle Int. 2014;35(11):1143–52.
45. Robertson GA, Wood AM. Return to sport after tibial shaft fractures: a systematic review. Sports Health. 2016;8(4):324–30.
46. Dixon S, Nunns M, House C, Rice H, Mostazir M, Stiles V, Davey T, Fallowfield J, Allsopp A. Prospective study of biomechanical risk factors for second and third metatarsal stress fractures in military recruits. J Sci Med Sport. 2019;22(2):135–9.
47. Mountjoy M, Sundgot-Borgen JK, Burke LM, Ackerman KE, Blauwet C, Constantini N, Lebrun C, Lundy B, Melin AK, Meyer NL, Sherman RT. IOC consensus statement on relative energy deficiency in sport (RED-S): 2018 update. Br J Sports Med. 2018;52(11):687–97.
48. Finch C. A new framework for research leading to sports injury prevention. J Sci Med Sport. 2006;9(1–2):3–9.
49. Haddon WJ. Energy damage and the 10 countermeasure strategies. J Trauma. 1973;13:321–31.
50. Fortington LV, Twomey D, Finch CF. Concussion in community Australian football—epidemiological monitoring of the causes and immediate impact on play. Inj Epidemiol. 2015;2:20.
51. Altman AR, Davis IS. Prospective comparison of running injuries between shod and barefoot runners. Br J Sports Med. 2016;50:476–80.
52. Drakos MC, Taylor SA, Fabricant PD, Haleem AM. Synthetic playing surfaces and athlete health. JAAOS J Am Acad Orthop Surgeons. 2013;21(5):293–302.
53. Brook EM, Tenforde AS, Broad EM, et al. Low energy availability, menstrual dysfunction, and impaired bone health: a survey of elite para athletes. Scand J Med Sci Sports. 2019;29:678–85.
54. Fuller GW, Tucker R, Starling L, et al. The performance of the World Rugby Head Injury Assessment Screening Tool: a diagnostic accuracy study. Sports Med Open. 2020;6:2.
55. Giles A, Bauer MEE, Jull J. Equity as the fourth 'E' in the '3 E's' approach to injury prevention. Injury Prev. 2019;26(1):82–4.
56. Timpka T, Ekstrand J, Svanström L. From Sports injury prevention to safety promotion in sports. Sports Med. 2006;36:733–45.
57. Padua DA, Frank B, Donaldson A, et al. Seven steps for developing and implementing a preventive training program: lessons learned from JUMP-ACL and beyond. Clin Sports Med. 2014;33(4):615–32.
58. Donaldson A, Lloyd DG, Gabbe BJ, et al. We have the programme, what next? Planning the implementation of an injury prevention programme. Inj Prev. 2017;23:273–80.

Orthobiologics for Fracture Healing in the Athlete

6

Nicola Poeta, Rocco Aicale, Greg A. J. Robertson, and Nicola Maffulli

6.1 Introduction

Optimal fracture healing remains a key determining factor for the athlete following a sport-related fracture: if achieved, this can ensure a timely return to play, with the minimum side effect profile possible. The term orthobiologics embraces the association of biological materials and substrates (including bone grafts, bone graft substitutes, growth factors, cell-signaling proteins) and cell based therapies to promote bone, ligament, muscle and tendon healing [1]. Giannoudis et al. described the "diamond concept" of fracture healing as made by mechanical stability, osteoconduction, osteoinduction, and osteogenesis [2] (Table 6.1): the latter three are the major properties of orthobiologics used in bone healing [3]. In orthobiologics, the choice of a graft may be influenced by cost, size of bone defect and comorbidities of the patient [1].

Osteoconduction properties allow cells, tissues and vasculature, aided by a natural scaffold, to integrate at the site of injury, giving possibility for the host response to heal or form new bone [4–6].

N. Poeta (✉) · R. Aicale
Department of Musculoskeletal Disorders, Faculty of Medicine and Surgery, University of Salerno, Baronissi, Italy

Clinica Ortopedica, Ospedale San Giovanni di Dio e Ruggi D'Aragona, Salerno, Italy

G. A. J. Robertson
Edinburgh Orthopaedic Trauma Unit, Royal Infirmary of Edinburgh, Edinburgh, UK

N. Maffulli
Department of Musculoskeletal Disorders, Faculty of Medicine and Surgery, University of Salerno, Baronissi, Italy

Clinica Ortopedica, Ospedale San Giovanni di Dio e Ruggi D'Aragona, Salerno, Italy

Queen Mary University of London, Barts and the London School of Medicine and Dentistry, Centre for Sports and Exercise Medicine, Mile End Hospital, London, UK

Keele University, Faculty of Medicine, School of Pharmacy and Bioengineering, Guy Hilton Research Centre, Stoke-on-Trent, UK
e-mail: n.maffulli@qmul.ac.uk

Table 6.1 Essential characteristics in orthobiologics for the bone regeneration

Osteogenesis	The direct ability to facilitate the new bone formation
Osteoinduction	The ability to stimulate the development of the cells which form new bone
Osteoconduction	The structural ability to allow cells, growth factors and vascularization to integrate at the site of the injury

Osteoinduction stimulates the development of the cells that support generation of the bone [4–6]. This stimulation occurs through substances such as growth factors, promoting differentiation of mesenchymal stem cells to osteoblasts and chondroblasts [4–6]. Osteogenesis is defined as the presence of active cellular elements within the graft, which can facilitate new bone formation [1].

There are different type of bone healing. One of these is endochondral ossification, which is the characteristic example of fracture repair [7], a cartilaginous template is first produced, to provide initial stability, and then this is substituted with bone tissue. Following fracture, bleeding in the periphery and in the intramedullary area forms a hematoma, containing mesenchymal stem cells (MSCs) and various cytokines, that stimulate a local inflammatory response with a wide range of effects, including chemotaxis, mitogenesis, and the production of vascular endothelial growth factor (VEGF) with angiogenesis [7]. The hematoma itself becomes a natural scaffold for callus formation within the medullary canal and around the fracture ends [7]. MSCs become chondrocyte cells, and the deposition of cartilaginous matrix allows the development of the soft callus, that provisionally stabilises the fracture site. The chondrocytes undergo apoptosis, while the migration of osteoblasts, into the soft callus, allow for the replacement of the cartilaginous template with hard callus, comprising of woven bone [7]. The healing process is completed with the subsequent remodelling of the hard callus, by osteoblastic and osteoclastic action, to form mature lamellar bone [7] (Fig. 6.1).

G. A. J. Robertson, N. Maffulli (eds.), *Fractures in Sport*, https://doi.org/10.1007/978-3-030-72036-0_6

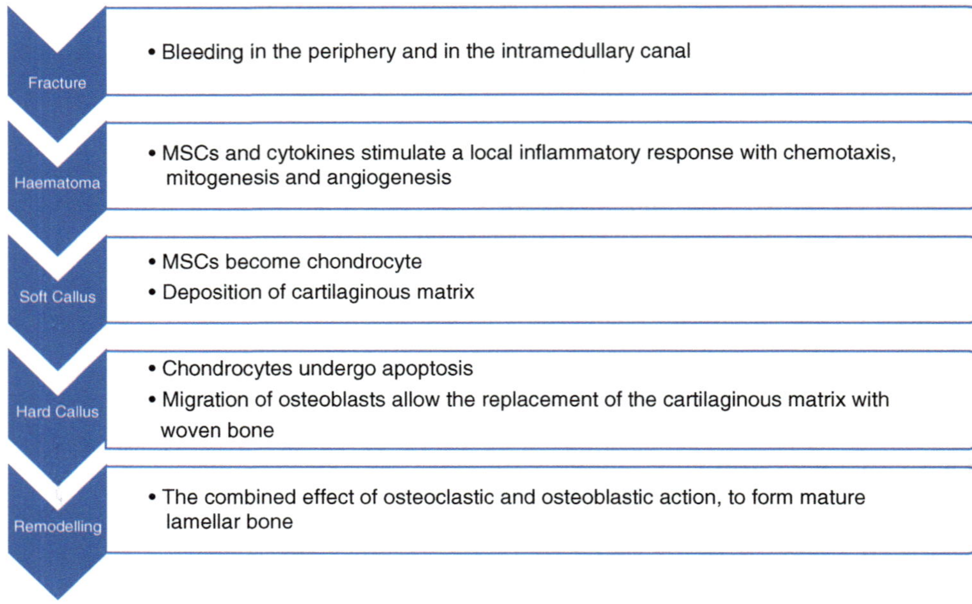

Fig. 6.1 Elementary representation of bone healing phases after fracture

Progenitor cells and local growth factors are required for proliferation, differentiation and deposition of matrix, to provide structural solidity and a scaffold for bone formation [7]. Fibroblasts, chondroblasts and osteogenic precursors in the fracture site are fundamental for the formation of callus, bone repair and bone union [7]. Diabetes and other metabolic diseases, that alter cell proliferation, may compromise and increase the fracture healing time [8]. Thus, MSCs, growth factors and matrix substitutes can potentially be effective and used as adjuvants to conventional treatments for fracture repair [7]. The proliferation, differentiation and migration of MSCs are influenced by the chemotactic and mitogenetic properties of cytokines and growth factors. Platelets contain these cytokines and growth factors and release them when they form a fibrin clot at the fracture site. Fracture healing capacity is clinically related to the presence of these growth factors, such as platelet-derived growth factor (PDGF-AB), transforming growth factor (TGF-β1), insulin-like growth factor 1 (IGF-1) and vascular endothelial growth factor (VEGF) [9, 10]. PDGF acts with an autocrine feedback mechanism, stimulating the production and release of other facilitating factors, promoting neovascularization through the interaction between VEGF and supporting cells, and facilitating cell migration and proliferation [11]. Hydroxyapatite and collagen largely form the extracellular matrix of the bone and provide a structure for osteogenic progenitor adhesion, cell migration and mechanical integrity. In the case of fracture, these substances provide osteoconductive properties; however, a large bone defect may result in matrix discontinuity, with secondary atrophy and non-union, rather than bone healing [12, 13]. Commonly, normal bone healing requires intercellular signalling through the matrix and the intervention of osteocytes which, through mechano-sensory stimuli across the bone matrix, regulate bone resorption and formation [14–16]. Bone needs proper stimulation to maintain normal structure and density [14], and excessive or insufficient stresses will cause problems with excessive bone release and resorption [14].

The stress forces if excessive can negatively influence the healing process of the bone [14, 17, 18]. In the case of bone defects, it has been reported, both in '*in vivo*' and '*in vitro*' studies, that the use of allograft and autograft increases the probability of callus formation [16]. Regarding the type of graft, the literature highlights more the importance of adequate filling of the defect, than the type of graft [7]. Within the current literature, the role of allografts in fracture healing has not been extensively defined yet, and more studies are needed to better guide their use [7].

6.2 Applications of Orthobiologics

Several biomechanical and biological factors can determine the outcome of fracture healing, with each a potential cause for delayed union or non-union. Union delay occurs when the fracture movement can be found after four months [1] . Non-union is defined as a non-healed fracture after 9 months, without signs of progressive healing for the proceeding 3 months, or, according to another definition, when healing has not been achieved at 6 months [6]. Orthobiologics can be a valid therapeutic approach in patients with fracture non-union or delayed unions [6, 19, 20]. Non-unions may be classified as hypertrophic and atrophic [1]. In the former, callus is formed but is incomplete; the consequent motion permissible at the fracture site does not allow achievement of union. In this case, the goal of management is to improve mechani-

Table 6.2 Orthobiologics characteristics for each item which can be use

	Osteogenetic	Osteoinductive	Osteoconductive
Autologous bone graft	YES	YES	YES
Allogenic bone graft	NO	YES	YES
Demineralised bone matrix (DBM)	NO	YES	YES
Bone graft substitutes	NO	NO	YES
Stem cell allografts	YES	YES	YES
Bone marrow aspirate concentrate	YES	YES	NO
Platelet-rich plasma	YES	YES	NO
Bone morphogenetic protein	NO	YES	NO
Platelet-derived growth factor	NO	YES	NO
Parathyroid hormone	NO	YES	NO
Vitamin D and calcium	NO	YES	NO
Bioabsorbable implants	NO	YES	YES
miRNA	NO	YES	NO

cal skeletal fixation [1]. Atrophic non-union is associated with a lack of callus formation, due to poor vascularity or poor metabolic conditions; these may be improved by changing the biological environment of the fracture site [19, 20].

Depending on the patient and their comorbidities, orthobiological treatments, with cells, growth factors or bone graft, can be used to facilitate healing process for such delayed unions and non-union [1]. To the best of our knowledge, the gold standard orthobiologic agent remains bone autograft, due to its osteoinductive, osteoconductive and osteogenic properties; however, low availability and complications from harvest, can result in it being a sub-optimal choice in the management of large bone defects [1] (Table 6.2).

Stress fractures are another area in the orthopaedics and sports medicine, in which the role of orthobiologics is developing Orthobiologic agents (Fig. 6.2) which can be used in the management of stress fractures include bone graft, synthetic bone graft substitutes, growth factors, stem-cell based treatments; further agents such as platelet-rich plasma and platelet-derived growth factor may also be potential safe adjuncts in stress fracture surgery.

6.3 Bone Grafts

6.3.1 Autologous Bone Grafts

Autologous bone grafts have osteoconductive, osteoinductive and osteogenesis properties [3, 6, 21], and can be used without the risk of transmission disease. For this reason, these have long been considered the gold standard choice of bone graft [22]. There are various types of autologous bone graft including cortical or cancellous graft, and vascularised or non-vascularised graft. Cancellous bone graft has the greatest osteogenic, osteoinductive and osteoconductive potential, but this does not provide immediate mechanical support [4].

Cortical autologous graft is usually preferred if, immediate mechanical support is required, but harvesting of such grafts can have considerable morbidity [23] .The gold standard autologous graft remains the iliac crest bone graft, due to the presence of both cortical and cancellous components, providing mechanical support and abundant osteogenic potential respectively [24]. Disadvantages of this type of graft include infection and pain at the donor site, longer operating times, and blood loss [6, 25].

Within the field of sports medicine, autologous bone graft has been reported for use in the treatment of stress fractures of the tibial diaphysis [22, 26–29], navicular [30–33] metatarsal [34–36], lumbar spine [37–40], and femoral neck [41–43].

6.3.2 Bone Allograft

Allografts can be cortical, cancellous, osteochondral or demineralised bone matrix. Following harvest, this is routinely processed prior to use. Allograft processing can comprise removal of graft cells, using ethanol, or sterilizing the material through irradiation. The structural properties of the allograft are dependent on its composition (cortical vs. cancellous); though this can often afford mechanical support, especially in compression, along with, osteoinductive and osteoconductive capacities, to facilitate bone healing post-implantation [6, 24].

6.3.3 Demineralised Bone Matrix (DBM)

DBM is an allogenic bone graft, that has been purged of its inorganic materials; it has osteoinductive potential, due to the presence of Bone Morphogenetic Proteins (BMP) and VEGF. The most important properties are its osteoinductive and osteoconductive capacities. The lack of donor site morbidity, the reduction of blood loss and the reduced operating

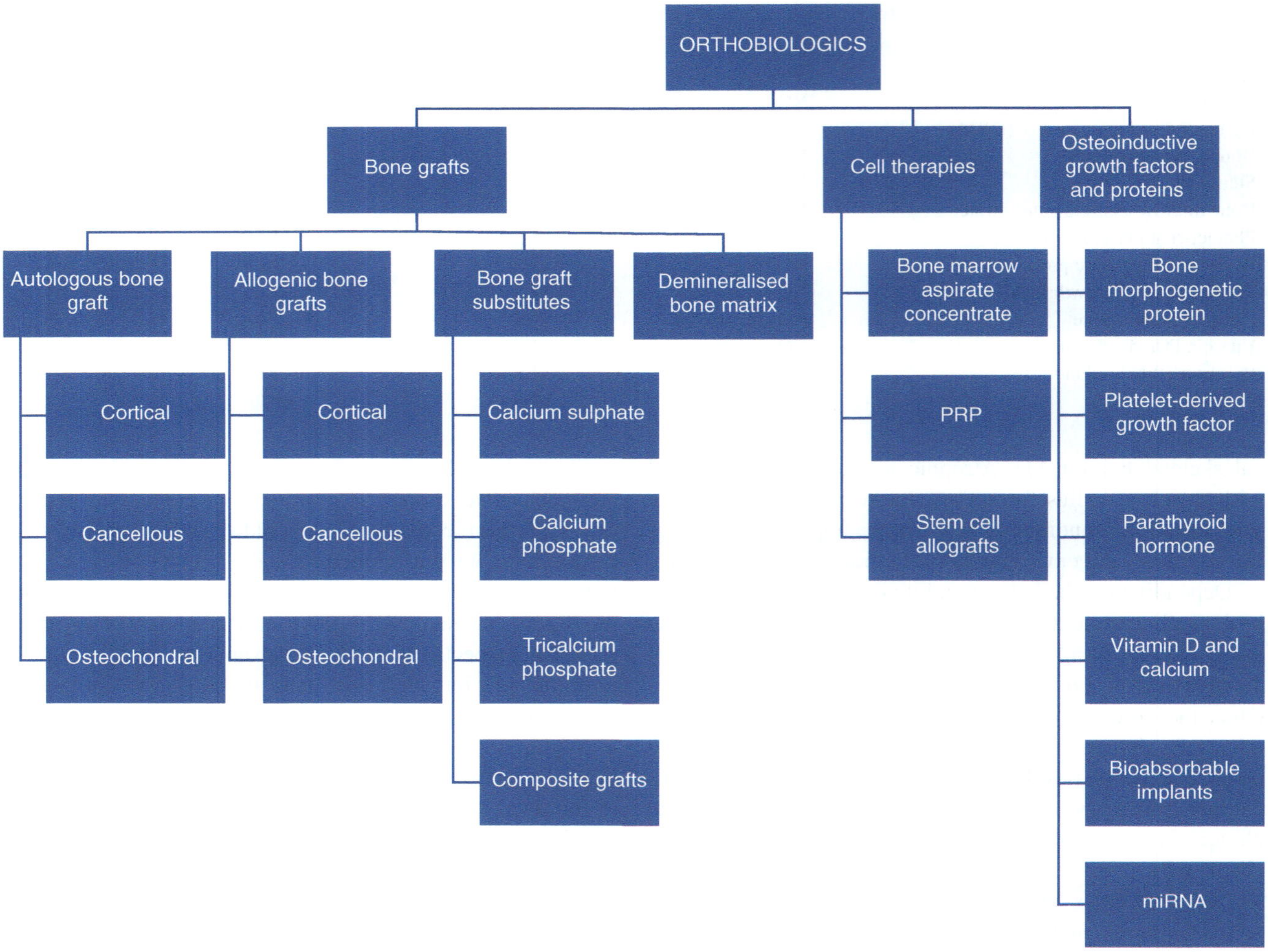

Fig. 6.2 Classification of orthobiologic agents

times make these grafts advantageous. However, its high costs and the possibility for transmission of bacteria and viruses are significant limitations [6, 25]. In sport medicine, its use has been described for the management of stress fracture of tibial diaphysis, in elite dancers [29] and in athletes [26], with both reporting favourable outcomes.

6.3.4 Bone Graft Substitutes

Various synthetic substitutes, such as calcium sulphate, calcium phosphate, tricalcium phosphate and coral hydroxyapatite, have been developed to fill large bone defects, or to manage infected fracture sites, through the combined used with antibiotics. These substances all have good resistance to compression, similar to cancellous bone, except calcium phosphate, which is ten times stronger, with a notably slower bone resorption time [6].

6.3.4.1 Calcium Sulphate

Calcium Sulphate (CS) has osteoinductive potential, as its ability to create a local acidic environment, can stimulate the release of BMPs, which in turn stimulates bone apposition [44–46]. Disadvantages of this substitute include the rapid reabsorption of the scaffold, which exceeds the speed of bone formation, causing a decrease in the resistance of the bone. CS is considered useful in the management of fractures, tumours and osteomyelitis, due to the possibility of combining it with antibiotics [47, 48]. Earlier loading, reduced stiffness and better patient satisfaction were noted in cases of calcaneal fractures, treated with percutaneous fixation and CS cement, compared to conventional open reduction internal fixation (ORIF) [49]. In cases of pathological fracture, the management with percutaneous fixation and augmentation with CS shown satisfactory results in terms of fracture healing, defect recurrence and soft tissue complications [50].

6.3.4.2 Calcium Phosphate

Calcium Phosphate (CP) is reabsorbed between 26 and 86 weeks post-insertion, providing sufficient time for bone formation; this is in contrast to CS, which is degraded much quicker. Crystalline CP comprises a structure similar to bone mineral matrix; this is formed by an isothermal reaction, with hardening of the inorganic calcium phosphate salts, often applied as cement [51, 52]. Advantage of CP are that its compressive strength is up to ten times greater than cancellous bone with the same resistance to tension, while demonstrating good biocompatibility, with no inflammation and or similar reaction *in vivo* [53]. This type of substitute provides good structural support and improves the use of internal fixation devices, such as screws; it may be used in case of fractures with large bone defects [54].

Studies on the management of intraarticular calcaneal fractures have found CP to be a useful adjunct to achieving anatomical reduction of the articular surface [54]. By comparison, cancellous bone grafting has been shown to fail in supporting post-surgical reduction and preventing calcaneal fracture collapse, with subsequent loss of height and joint congruency [54].

6.3.4.3 Tricalcium Phosphate

Another absorbable ceramic material is tricalcium phosphate (TCP) ($Ca_3(PO_4)_2$). This may have two crystalline forms: a polygonal alpha-TCP form and a spherical beta-TCP form [55]. In orthopaedic surgery, the most used form is the beta-TCP, which has a microporous structure that imitates the architecture of cancellous bone and undergoes rapid reabsorption [51]. TCP has good biocompatibility, does not produce inflammation *in vivo*, and usually integrates within 6–12 months. It is normally available in granule or block form [56]. TCP and cancellous bone have similar resistance to compression [56]. Coral hydroxyapatite, produced by marine corals, has very similar characteristics to TCP [56, 57]. In a recent study, the use of TCP, in association with ORIF, for patients with long bone and calcaneus fractures, was found to result in an increase in union rates, up to 85–90%, at 12 months follow-up [57].

6.3.4.4 Composite Grafts

The use of monophasic grafts has many advantages; however, adverse reactions can occur, such as complications at the wound site, insufficient mechanical support, inflammatory reactions in vivo, and slow or incomplete osseointegration [7]. Composite grafts have therefore been developed, to combine the properties of various materials. A composite graft comprising CP and CS, promotes angiogenic invasion and bone integration, through the rapid absorption of CS, while CP provides adequate structural support [58]. In recent studies, the management of proximal humeral tumours and vertebral fractures with biphasic bone grafts, such as Cerament (Bonesupport, Lund, Sweden) and Pro-Dense (Wright Medical Technology Inc., Memphis, Tennessee), has been described with good clinical and radiological results, without a notable increase in complication rates. Specifically, the use of such composite grafts in 14 patients with cysts and benign solid tumours of the proximal humerus (with an average size of 40 mL), found a decrease in the average lesion size of 18 mL, at 12 month follow-up [59]. In another study, with 33 patients undergoing vertebroplasty, on a total of 66 vertebrae [60] (osteoporotic fractures in 86% of cases), good cement distribution with fracture stabilization, and no new vertebral fractures were reported, at 1 month CT scan follow-ups [61]. Furthermore, VAS pain scores were found to decrease from 8.4 points to 2.7 points, at 6 months follow-up [61, 62].

6.3.5 Stem Cell Allografts

MSCs allografts, which can be used as an isolated agent, or in combination with a supportive substrate, such as demineralised cortical bone and Β-TCP/collagen, is characterised by its osteogenic, osteoinductive and osteoconductive properties [63, 64]. This type of allograft is new, and it is proposed to decrease the rate of non-union, in at-risk subjects. Furthermore, in high-risk patients undergoing arthrodesis procedures of the foot and ankle region, an increase in the success rate has been found with the use of this graft type [63, 65, 66].

6.4 Cell Therapies

6.4.1 Bone Marrow Aspirate Concentrate

Bone marrow has two types of stem cells, hematopoietic and mesenchymal (MSCs) [67]. It is the MSCs, specifically, which can be utilized in orthopaedic practice. The Mesenchymal and Tissue Stem Cell Committee of the International Society for Cellular Therapy has outlined the minimum criteria for identifying MSCs:

- in standard culture, they must remain adherent to plastic
- they must express CD105, CD73 and CD90, and must not express surface molecules CD45, CD34, CD14 or CD11b, CD79alpha or CD19 and HLA-DR
- in vitro, MSCs must differentiate into osteoblasts, adipocytes and chondroblasts [68]

The interest in Bone Marrow Aspirate Concentrate (BMAC) for musculoskeletal diseases, fractures care and fusion procedures, is due to its osteogenic potential. Research has focussed on how to increase the number of

MSCs at fracture sites or infection sites, through the influence of specific cytokines and growth factors [69]. BMAC has angiogenetic properties, that allows the development of normal blood flow at the site, and paracrine action, that may influence the cell population at the fracture site, through the action of cytokines [6]. The combined use of BMAC with DBM, allograft, or ceramic grafts is recommended, to provide the BMAC with a carrier agent, and to give structural support to the graft [5, 6]. In a clinical trial, BMAC was used for the treatment of Jones's fracture of the fifth metatarsal in athletes, with good functional results; however, data on return to sport and risk of refracture, in comparison with standard fixation, was not obtained [70, 71]. BMAC shows promising results, even in patients with diabetes or at high risk of non-union, when compared with iliac crest autografts; specific advantages include less invasive harvest techniques, and fewer numbers of complications, with reduced morbidity [6, 70]. There is a growing evidence to support its use for the surgical management of stress fractures of the fifth metatarsal [34], medial malleolus [72], tibial diaphysis [29] and cuneiform [73]. Specifically regarding fifth metatarsal stress fractures, in a retrospective review of 37 elite level professional soccer players, who were managed with intramedullary screw fixation, autologous cancellous bone grafting and BMAC fracture-site injection, for fifth metatarsal stress fractures, Miller et al. [34] recorded a mean return time to sport of 10.5 weeks, with an union rate of 97% and a mean time to complete radiological union of 12.7 weeks.

6.4.2 Platelet-Rich Plasma

Megakaryocytes, in the medulla, form platelets which contain granules named alpha, beta and delta. There are about 50–80 alpha granules per platelet, and each contain many factors, including TGF-ß (ß1 and ß2 isomers), IGF, interleukin-1 (IL-1), epidermal growth factor (EGF), PDGF, platelet factor 4 (PF4), platelet-derived angiogenesis factor (PDAF), VEGF, platelet-derived endothelial growth factor (PDEGF) and epithelial cell growth (ECGF). Mishra et al. evaluated platelet count, activation methods and white blood cell count to classify different types of PRP [74]. This study, together with others, showed that a leukocyte-deplete PRP is better than a leukocyte-rich PRP. The leukocytes, injected together with the PRP, can increase the inflammatory response at the site of use, causing an increase in pain; for this reason, it is preferable to use PRP low in leukocytes. Regardless of the presence of leukocytes, all studies to-date have shown no negative effects of PRP, in any type [75, 76]. PRP can be administered as either an activated or an inactivated form: the activation of the PRP takes place with the addition of calcium chloride, that forms an applicable gelatinous substance; if the non-activated PRP is used, it will be mixed with the collagen of the tissues to produce activation [77]. The use of PRP has been proposed for numerous applications in the orthopaedic field, including as treatment of atrophic non-union [1] and stress fractures [78]. One study found that the addition of PRP facilitated fracture union in 87% of cases, at 4 months follow-up [79]. Another study found that the combination of PRP and intramedullary nailing showed an increase in the rate of fracture union, compared to the use of intramedullary nailing alone [80]. In the management of acute fractures, PRP has proven useful, both in clinical and functional outcomes, and in terms of union of the bone segments [81–83]. In the treatment of displaced intra-articular calcaneal fractures, the combination of PRP with bone allograft has been shown to give clinical and radiological results similar to those using bone autograft, and better than those using bone allograft alone, when assessed using the American Orthopaedic Foot and Ankle Society (AOFAS) score [84]. However, despite this developing evidence in the literature, further robust research is required to validate the clinical use of PRP as routine therapy [29, 34, 71–73]. Similarly, the combination of PRP with MSCs has been hypothesised to promote fracture healing: yet further evidence and randomized controlled trials (RCTs) are necessary, to validate the safety and effectiveness of this treatment option [74].

6.5 Osteoinductive Growth Factors and Proteins

6.5.1 Bone Morphogenetic Protein

The TGF-β family also includes bone morphogenetic proteins (BMPs), which present osteoinductive properties, mediated by inducted differentiation of osteoblasts; they also have an osteogenic and angiogenetic activity [6]. BMPs are injected in a liquid form, and need structural support, such as collagen sponges and calcium ceramics, to be inserted and maintained at the site of action [48].

The U.S. Food and Drug Administration (FDA) has authorised the use of BMP-2 and BMP-7 for the management of open tibial fractures, fracture non-unions and for spinal fusions [6, 56, 82]. There are several drawbacks to the use of BMPs, which include heterotopic bone formation, excessive cost, low probability of carcinogenesis, compartment syndrome and the possibility to develop liver or kidney failure [5, 25]. The use of BMP for the management of sport-related stress fractures remains limited, with reports of use in the treatment of stress fractures of the tibial diaphysis and in the treatment of spondylolysis [29, 85].

6.5.2 Platelet-Derived Growth Factor

PDGF plays an important role in chemotaxis, and has five isoforms: PDGF-AA (PDGFA), -BB (PDGFB), -CC (PDGFC), and -DD (PDGFD), and -AB [86]. These are different forms of the same protein, deriving from a family of genes, and have similar biological functions [87]. The most effective in bone is the isomer PDGF-BB type, which has the properties of stimulating chemotaxis, recruiting inflammatory cells at the site of action, and increasing collagen deposition by promoting angiogenesis [11, 88–90]. The FDA has approved recombinant human platelet-derived growth factor-BB (rhPDGF-BB), for use in foot and ankle arthrodesis procedures, due to its useful osteoinductive properties [91].

The most important risk associated with the use of rhPDGF-BB, is potential carcinogenicity, associated with topical use; however, no correlation has been found between the use of rhPDGF-BB in ankle and foot procedures, and carcinogenesis [92].

6.5.3 Parathyroid Hormone

Calcium metabolism is regulated by numerous factors, one of which is parathyroid hormone (PTH). The FDA approved the use of the recombinant form of PTH (rhPTH), for a number of orthopaedics diseases, including osteoporosis and fracture healing [93, 94]. RhPTH is the only FDA approved anabolic agent for patients with osteoporosis or with a decrease in bone mineralization [93, 94]. RhPTH increases bone density and reduces the risk of fractures. Several studies have shown an increase in the speed of fracture healing and bone formation with this substance [93–96]. Aspenberg et al. compared the use of daily injections of rhPTH versus placebo, in a RCT, which assessed the healing of distal radial fractures in 102 postmenopausal women, and found faster fracture healing rates in the rhPTH group [97].

6.5.4 Vitamin D and Calcium

Vitamin D is essential for bone remodelling and healing. The integration of vitamin D promotes osteoblastogenesis, increases the production of osteocalcin and osteopontin, and stimulates bone reabsorption mediated by osteoclasts [98–100]. In the case of fractures of the proximal humerus and distal radius, the use of vitamin D has been shown, in many studies, to offer beneficial effects in terms of increase in bone mineral density and callus formation [101, 102]. A Cochrane review found Vitamin D to be ineffective in preventing hip fractures when used alone; however, good results were reported, for hip fracture prevention, when Vitamin D was combined with calcium [103].

6.5.5 Bioabsorbable Implants

The use of absorbable implants, especially in childhood orthopaedics, has been designed to avoid the requirement for plate removal after fracture healing. Fixation removal surgery is very common in paediatric orthopaedics and is associated with various risks. The use of plates is essential for the stabilization of the fracture, to maintain reduction and alignment during the healing process; as such, absorbable plates could replace steel and titanium implants, in the future [104, 105].

6.5.6 miRNA

Numerous non-coding RNAs have recently been identified, including small interfering RNA (siRNA), Piwi-interacting RNA (piRNA), long non-coding RNAs (lncRNA) and MicroRNA (miRNA) [85, 92]. MiRNAs may influence gene expression, by silencing the activity of some genes and blocking the production of specific proteins, therefore influencing the production of essential factors for the fracture healing [106]. The levels of six miRNAs (miR-16, miR-19b-1, miR-25, miR-92a, miR-101, and miR-129-5p) were found to be altered in per-trochanteric fracture models [107, 108]. A recent study on mice showed that miR-92a influenced the volume of callus and neovascularization at the fracture site [108]. One study found that the injection of osteoblastic cells, which overexpressed miR-21, to the fracture site of transverse femur fractures in mice, resulted in an increase in endo-chondral ossification, a greater volume of fracture callus and a stronger biomechanical fracture repair, at 7 days follow-up. These results suggest the potential of miR-21 as a therapeutic approach to improve the fracture healing process [109].

Another mi-RNA, miR-29b, was analysed, and was found to promote osteoblasts differentiation, influencing the regulation of HDAC4 (histone deacetylase 4), TFG-ß3, ACVR2A (Activin A Receptor Type 2A), CTNNBIP1 (Catenin Beta Interacting Protein 1), and DUSP2 proteins (Dual Specificity Phosphatase 2) [110]. MiR-29b injected into the fracture site of transverse femoral fractures in mice, showed significantly increased bone callus volume and fracture union, at 2 weeks post-injection [88, 109].

6.6 Influence of Systemic Factors

Many systemic factors may influence orthobiologic treatments and fracture healing. These include nonsteroidal anti-inflammatory drugs (NSAIDs), which are widely used in sports medicine and have been linked to decreased bone healing [7]. NSAIDs work by inhibiting the COX-2 pathway and decreasing prostaglandin production, an important part of the inflammatory process in the acute phase of bone healing [7]. Studies conducted in animal models confirmed that the use of NSAIDs inhibits the acute phase of bone healing, increasing the likelihood of delayed union and non-union [7, 111]. However, a recent systematic review has reported that those studies which found NSAIDs to be safe to consume during fracture healing, were of higher methodological quality than those which advised against the use of NSAIDS during fracture healing [112]. The dose of nicotine, contained within a single cigarette, may reduce mesenchymal cells differentiation and proliferation, resulting in a reduced rate of fracture repair [113, 114]. Smoking has been found to result in an increased rate of superficial and deep infections, as well as an increase in non-union and delayed union rates [115]. Smoking cessation, even for a short time, improves bone and soft tissue healing, decreasing possible complications [116]. An increased risk of impaired fracture healing is also observed in patients with diabetes. Diabetes promotes the development of a systemic inflammatory state, which in conjunction with the resultant hyperglycaemia, results in an increase in oxygen reactive species and an increase in bone resorption, secondary to a decrease in the number and function of osteoblasts and an increase in the activity of osteoclasts [117, 118]. This causes a high risk of complications such as infections, non-union and delayed union [119].

6.7 Conclusions

Orthobiologics research is characterised by the search for cellular, molecular and biomechanical components that may influence bone physiology and repair: this can facilitate optimal fracture healing in the athlete, allowing the earliest return to play possible. The study of the structural composition and repair processes of bone opens new scientific research and future innovations. Well established treatments exist to facilitate the process of bone healing, such as autologous and allogenic bone graft. However, the therapeutic use of bone substitutes, stem cells and growth factors, has shown promising results for the management of fractures, as well as for the treatment of non-unions, stress fractures, bone cysts, and bone defects created during surgery. In order to facilitate the routine use of more innovative orthobiologic materials in clinical practice, there is the need for further research, particularly well-designed RCTs, to properly define treatment indications, treatment benefits, costs, and possible adverse reactions, to maintain safe and effective practice in this field.

References

1. Calcei JG, Rodeo SA. Orthobiologics for bone healing. Clin Sports Med. 2019;38(1):79–95.
2. Giannoudis PV, Einhorn TA, Marsh D. Fracture healing: the diamond concept. Injury. 2007;38:S3–6.
3. Egol K, Nauth A, Lee M, Pape H-C, Watson J, Borrelli J. Bone grafting: sourcing, timing, strategies, and alternatives. J Orthop Trauma [Internet]. 2015 Dec [cited 2020 Mar 27];29. insights.ovid.com.
4. Finkemeier CG. Bone-grafting and bone-graft substitutes. J Bone Joint Surg Am. 2002;84(3):454–64.
5. Bray CC, Walker CM, Spence DD. Orthobiologics in pediatric sports medicine. Orthop Clin North Am. 2017;48(3):333–42.
6. Roberts TT, Rosenbaum AJ. Bone grafts, bone substitutes and orthobiologics: the bridge between basic science and clinical advancements in fracture healing. Organogenesis. 2012;8(4):114–24.
7. Lin SS, Yeranosian MG. The role of orthobiologics in fracture healing and arthrodesis. Foot Ankle Clin. 2016;21(4):727–37.
8. Beam HA, Parsons JR, Lin SS. The effects of blood glucose control upon fracture healing in the BB Wistar rat with diabetes mellitus. J Orthop Res. 2002;20(6):1210–6.
9. Gandhi A, Doumas C, Dumas C, O'Connor JP, Parsons JR, Lin SS. The effects of local platelet rich plasma delivery on diabetic fracture healing. Bone. 2006;38(4):540–6.
10. Street JT, Wang JH, Wu QD, Wakai A, McGuinness A, Redmond HP. The angiogenic response to skeletal injury is preserved in the elderly. J Orthop Res. 2001;19(6):1057–66.
11. Al-Zube L, Breitbart EA, O'Connor JP, Parsons JR, Bradica G, Hart CE, et al. Recombinant human platelet-derived growth factor BB (rhPDGF-BB) and beta-tricalcium phosphate/collagen matrix enhance fracture healing in a diabetic rat model. J Orthop Res. 2009;27(8):1074–81.
12. Langer R, Vacanti JP. Tissue engineering. Science. 1993;260(5110):920–6.
13. Azad V, Breitbart E, Al-Zube L, Yeh S, O'Connor JP, Lin SS. rhBMP-2 enhances the bone healing response in a diabetic rat segmental defect model. J Orthop Trauma. 2009;23(4):267–76.
14. Beaupré GS, Orr TE, Carter DR. An approach for time-dependent bone modeling and remodeling—theoretical development. J Orthop Res. 1990;8(5):651–61.
15. Hart RT, Davy DT, Heiple KG. A computational method for stress analysis of adaptive elastic materials with a view toward applications in strain-induced bone remodeling. J Biomech Eng. 1984;106(4):342–50.
16. Weinans H, Huiskes R, Grootenboer HJ. The behavior of adaptive bone-remodeling simulation models. J Biomech. 1992;25(12):1425–41.
17. Crowder C, Stout S. Bone histology: an anthropological perspective. Boca Raton: CRC Press; 2011. 410 p.
18. Recker RR. Bone histomorphometry techniques & interpretation. 1st ed. Boca Raton, FL: CRC Press; 1983. 312 p.
19. Gómez-Barrena E, Rosset P, Lozano D, Stanovici J, Ermthaller C, Gerbhard F. Bone fracture healing: cell therapy in delayed unions and nonunions. Bone. 2015;70:93–101.

20. Antonova E, Le TK, Burge R, Mershon J. Tibia shaft fractures: costly burden of nonunions. BMC Musculoskelet Disord. 2013;14:42.
21. Nauth A, Lane J, Watson JT, Giannoudis P. Bone graft substitution and augmentation. J Orthop Trauma. 2015;29(Suppl 12):S34–8.
22. Miller CP, Chiodo CP. Autologous bone graft in foot and ankle surgery. Foot Ankle Clin. 2016;21(4):825–37.
23. Berkes MB, Little MTM, Schottel PC, Pardee NC, Zuiderbaan A, Lazaro LE, et al. Outcomes of Schatzker II tibial plateau fracture open reduction internal fixation using structural bone allograft. J Orthop Trauma. 2014;28(2):97–102.
24. Sen MK, Miclau T. Autologous iliac crest bone graft: should it still be the gold standard for treating nonunions? Injury. 2007;38(Suppl 1):S75–80.
25. Gross RH. The use of bone grafts and bone graft substitutes in pediatric orthopaedics: an overview. J Pediatr Orthop. 2012;32(1):100–5.
26. Borens O, Sen MK, Huang RC, Richmond J, Kloen P, Jupiter JB, et al. Anterior tension band plating for anterior tibial stress fractures in high-performance female athletes: a report of 4 cases. J Orthop Trauma. 2006;20(6):425–30.
27. Orava S, Hulkko A. Stress fracture of the mid-tibial shaft. Acta Orthop Scand. 1984;55(1):35–7.
28. Orava S, Karpakka J, Hulkko A, Väänänen K, Takala T, Kallinen M, et al. Diagnosis and treatment of stress fractures located at the mid-tibial shaft in athletes. Int J Sports Med. 1991;12(4):419–22.
29. Miyamoto RG, Dhotar HS, Rose DJ, Egol K. Surgical treatment of refractory tibial stress fractures in elite dancers: a case series. Am J Sports Med. 2009;37(6):1150–4.
30. Torg JS, Pavlov H, Cooley LH, Bryant MH, Arnoczky SP, Bergfeld J, et al. Stress fractures of the tarsal navicular. A retrospective review of twenty-one cases. J Bone Joint Surg Am. 1982;64(5):700–12.
31. Saxena A, Fullem B. Navicular stress fractures: a prospective study on athletes. Foot Ankle Int. 2006;27(11):917–21.
32. Khan KM, Fuller PJ, Brukner PD, Kearney C, Burry HC. Outcome of conservative and surgical management of navicular stress fracture in athletes. Eighty-six cases proven with computerized tomography. Am J Sports Med. 1992;20(6):657–66.
33. McCormick JJ, Bray CC, Davis WH, Cohen BE, Jones CP, Anderson RB. Clinical and computed tomography evaluation of surgical outcomes in tarsal navicular stress fractures. Am J Sports Med. 2011;39(8):1741–8.
34. Miller D, Marsland D, Jones M, Calder J. Early return to playing professional football following fixation of 5th metatarsal stress fractures may lead to delayed union but does not increase the risk of long-term non-union. Knee Surg Sports Traumatol Arthrosc. 2019;27(9):2796–801.
35. Lee KT, Park YU, Young KW, Kim JS, Kim JB. The plantar gap: another prognostic factor for fifth metatarsal stress fracture. Am J Sports Med. 2011;39(10):2206–11.
36. Muscolo L, Migues A, Slullitel G, Costa-Paz M. Stress fracture nonunion at the base of the second metatarsal in a ballet dancer: a case report. Am J Sports Med. 2004;32(6):1535–7.
37. Nozawa S, Shimizu K, Miyamoto K, Tanaka M. Repair of pars interarticularis defect by segmental wire fixation in young athletes with spondylolysis. Am J Sports Med. 2003;31(3):359–64.
38. Debnath UK, Freeman BJC, Gregory P, de la Harpe D, Kerslake RW, Webb JK. Clinical outcome and return to sport after the surgical treatment of spondylolysis in young athletes. J Bone Joint Surg Br. 2003;85(2):244–9.
39. Sutton JH, Guin PD, Theiss SM. Acute lumbar spondylolysis in intercollegiate athletes. J Spinal Disord Tech. 2012;25(8):422–5.
40. Raudenbush BL, Chambers RC, Silverstein MP, Goodwin RC. Indirect pars repair for pediatric isthmic spondylolysis: a case series. J Spine Surg Hong Kong. 2017;3(3):387–91.
41. Biz C, Berizzi A, Crimì A, Marcato C, Trovarelli G, Ruggieri P. Management and treatment of femoral neck stress fractures in recreational runners: a report of four cases and review of the literature. Acta Bio-Medica Atenei Parm. 2017;88(4S):96–106.
42. Lee C-H, Huang G-S, Chao K-H, Jean J-L, Wu S-S. Surgical treatment of displaced stress fractures of the femoral neck in military recruits: a report of 42 cases. Arch Orthop Trauma Surg. 2003;123(10):527–33.
43. Neubauer T, Brand J, Lidder S, Krawany M. Stress fractures of the femoral neck in runners: a review. Res Sports Med Print. 2016;24(3):185–99.
44. Walsh WR, Morberg P, Yu Y, Yang JL, Haggard W, Sheath PC, et al. Response of a calcium sulfate bone graft substitute in a confined cancellous defect. Clin Orthop. 2003;406:228–36.
45. Urban RM, Turner TM, Hall DJ, Infanger S, Cheema N, Lim TH. Healing of large defects treated with calcium sulfate pellets containing demineralized bone matrix particles. Orthopedics. 2003;26(5 Suppl):s581–5.
46. Turner TM, Urban RM, Gitelis S, Haggard WO, Richelsoph K. Resorption evaluation of a large bolus of calcium sulfate in a canine medullary defect. Orthopedics. 2003;26(5 Suppl):s577–9.
47. Borrelli J, Prickett WD, Ricci WM. Treatment of nonunions and osseous defects with bone graft and calcium sulfate. Clin Orthop. 2003;411:245–54.
48. McKee MD, Wild LM, Schemitsch EH, Waddell JP. The use of an antibiotic-impregnated, osteoconductive, bioabsorbable bone substitute in the treatment of infected long bone defects: early results of a prospective trial. J Orthop Trauma. 2002;16(9):622–7.
49. Chen L, Zhang G, Hong J, Lu X, Yuan W. Comparison of percutaneous screw fixation and calcium sulfate cement grafting versus open treatment of displaced intra-articular calcaneal fractures. Foot Ankle Int. 2011;32(10):979–85.
50. Chen L, Zhang G, Li S, Wu Z, Yuan W, Hong J. Percutaneous treatment of calcaneus fractures associated with underlying bone cysts. Foot Ankle Int. 2012;33(5):424–9.
51. Wiltfang J, Merten HA, Schlegel KA, Schultze-Mosgau S, Kloss FR, Rupprecht S, et al. Degradation characteristics of alpha and beta tri-calcium-phosphate (TCP) in minipigs. J Biomed Mater Res. 2002;63(2):115–21.
52. Eriksson F, Mattsson P, Larsson S. The effect of augmentation with resorbable or conventional bone cement on the holding strength for femoral neck fracture devices. J Orthop Trauma. 2002;16(5):302–10.
53. Goodman SB, Bauer TW, Carter D, Casteleyn PP, Goldstein SA, Kyle RF, et al. Norian SRS cement augmentation in hip fracture treatment. Laboratory and initial clinical results. Clin Orthop. 1998;348:42–50.
54. Longino D, Buckley RE. Bone graft in the operative treatment of displaced intraarticular calcaneal fractures: is it helpful? J Orthop Trauma. 2001;15(4):280–6.
55. Frankenburg EP, Goldstein SA, Bauer TW, Harris SA, Poser RD. Biomechanical and histological evaluation of a calcium phosphate cement. J Bone Joint Surg Am. 1998;80(8):1112–24.
56. Moore WR, Graves SE, Bain GI. Synthetic bone graft substitutes. ANZ J Surg. 2001;71(6):354–61.
57. Cameron HU. Tricalcium phosphate as a bone graft substitute. Contemp Orthop. 1992;25(5):506–8.
58. Wee J, Thevendran G. The role of orthobiologics in foot and ankle surgery: allogenic bone grafts and bone graft substitutes. EFORT Open Rev. 2017;2(6):272–80.
59. Abramo A, Geijer M, Kopylov P, Tägil M. Osteotomy of distal radius fracture malunion using a fast remodeling bone substitute consisting of calcium sulphate and calcium phosphate. J Biomed Mater Res B Appl Biomater. 2010;92(1):281–6.
60. Kaczmarczyk J, Sowinski P, Goch M, Katulska K. Complete twelve month bone remodeling with a bi-phasic injectable bone

substitute in benign bone tumors: a prospective pilot study. BMC Musculoskelet Disord. 2015;16:369.

61. Marcia S, Boi C, Dragani M, Marini S, Marras M, Piras E, et al. Effectiveness of a bone substitute (CERAMENT™) as an alternative to PMMA in percutaneous vertebroplasty: 1-year follow-up on clinical outcome. Eur Spine J. 2012;21(Suppl 1):112–8.
62. Iundusi R, Gasbarra E, D'Arienzo M, Piccioli A, Tarantino U. Augmentation of tibial plateau fractures with an injectable bone substitute: CERAMENT™. Three year follow-up from a prospective study. BMC Musculoskelet Disord. 2015;16:115.
63. Jones CP, Loveland J, Atkinson BL, Ryaby JT, Linovitz RJ, Nunley JA. Prospective, multicenter evaluation of allogeneic bone matrix containing viable osteogenic cells in foot and/or ankle arthrodesis. Foot Ankle Int. 2015;36(10):1129–37.
64. Harford JS, Dekker TJ, Adams SB. Bone marrow aspirate concentrate for bone healing in foot and ankle surgery. Foot Ankle Clin. 2016;21(4):839–45.
65. Rush SM, Hamilton GA, Ackerson LM. Mesenchymal stem cell allograft in revision foot and ankle surgery: a clinical and radiographic analysis. J Foot Ankle Surg. 2009;48(2):163–9.
66. Scott RT, Hyer CF. Role of cellular allograft containing mesenchymal stem cells in high-risk foot and ankle reconstructions. J Foot Ankle Surg. 2013;52(1):32–5.
67. Hernigou P, Poignard A, Manicom O, Mathieu G, Rouard H. The use of percutaneous autologous bone marrow transplantation in nonunion and avascular necrosis of bone. J Bone Joint Surg Br. 2005;87(7):896–902.
68. Dominici M, Le Blanc K, Mueller I, Slaper-Cortenbach I, Marini F, Krause D, et al. Minimal criteria for defining multipotent mesenchymal stromal cells. The International Society for Cellular Therapy position statement. Cytotherapy. 2006;8(4):315–7.
69. Crane JL, Cao X. Bone marrow mesenchymal stem cells and TGF-β signaling in bone remodeling. J Clin Invest. 2014;124(2):466–72.
70. Murawski CD, Kennedy JG. Percutaneous internal fixation of proximal fifth metatarsal jones fractures (Zones II and III) with Charlotte Carolina screw and bone marrow aspirate concentrate: an outcome study in athletes. Am J Sports Med. 2011;39(6):1295–301.
71. Carney D, Chambers MC, Kromka JJ, LaBaze D, West RV, Musahl V, et al. Jones fracture in the elite athlete: patient reported outcomes following fixation with BMAC. Orthop J Sports Med [Internet]. 2018 Jul 27 [cited 2020 Jan 31];6(7 Suppl 4). https://www.ncbi.nlm.nih.gov/pmc/articles/PMC6102760/.
72. Nguyen A, Beasley I, Calder J. Stress fractures of the medial malleolus in the professional soccer player demonstrate excellent outcomes when treated with open reduction internal fixation and arthroscopic spur debridement. Knee Surg Sports Traumatol Arthrosc. 2019;27(9):2884–9.
73. Adams SB, Lewis JS Jr, Gupta AK, Parekh SG, Miller SD, Schon LC. Cannulated screw delivery of bone marrow aspirate concentrate to a stress fracture nonunion: technique tip. Foot Ankle Int. 2013;34(5):740–4.
74. Le ADK, Enweze L, DeBaun MR, Dragoo JL. Current clinical recommendations for use of platelet-rich plasma. Curr Rev Musculoskelet Med. 2018;11(4):624–34.
75. Mishra A, Harmon K, Woodall J, Vieira A. Sports medicine applications of platelet rich plasma. Curr Pharm Biotechnol. 2012;13(7):1185–95.
76. McCarrel TM, Minas T, Fortier LA. Optimization of leukocyte concentration in platelet-rich plasma for the treatment of tendinopathy. J Bone Joint Surg Am. 2012;94(19):e143(1–8).
77. Sánchez M, Anitua E, Azofra J, Andía I, Padilla S, Mujika I. Comparison of surgically repaired Achilles tendon tears using platelet-rich fibrin matrices. Am J Sports Med. 2007;35(2):245–51.
78. Miller TL, Kaeding CC, Rodeo SA. Emerging options for biologic enhancement of stress fracture healing in athletes. JAAOS - J Am Acad Orthop Surg. 2020;28(1):1–9.
79. Duramaz A, Ursavaş HT, Bilgili MG, Bayrak A, Bayram B, Avkan MC. Platelet-rich plasma versus exchange intramedullary nailing in treatment of long bone oligotrophic nonunions. Eur J Orthop Surg Traumatol Orthop Traumatol. 2018;28(1):131–7.
80. Dülgeroglu TC, Metineren H. Evaluation of the effect of platelet-rich fibrin on long bone healing: an experimental rat model. Orthopedics. 2017;40(3):e479–84.
81. Hutchinson ID, Rodeo SA, Perrone GS, Murray MM. Can platelet-rich plasma enhance anterior cruciate ligament and meniscal repair? J Knee Surg. 2015;28(1):19–28.
82. Radice F, Yánez R, Gutiérrez V, Rosales J, Pinedo M, Coda S. Comparison of magnetic resonance imaging findings in anterior cruciate ligament grafts with and without autologous platelet-derived growth factors. Arthrosc J Arthrosc Relat Surg. 2010;26(1):50–7.
83. Marcazzan S, Taschieri S, Weinstein RL, Del Fabbro M. Efficacy of platelet concentrates in bone healing: a systematic review on animal studies—Part B: large-size animal models. Platelets. 2018;29(4):338–46.
84. Wei L-C, Lei G-H, Sheng P, Gao S-G, Xu M, Jiang W, et al. Efficacy of platelet-rich plasma combined with allograft bone in the management of displaced intra-articular calcaneal fractures: a prospective cohort study. J Orthop Res. 2012;30(10):1570–6.
85. Gillis CC, Eichholz K, Thoman WJ, Fessler RG. A minimally invasive approach to defects of the pars interarticularis: restoring function in competitive athletes. Clin Neurol Neurosurg. 2015;139:29–34.
86. Tischer E, Gospodarowicz D, Mitchell R, Silva M, Schilling J, Lau K, et al. Vascular endothelial growth factor: a new member of the platelet-derived growth factor gene family. Biochem Biophys Res Commun. 1989;165(3):1198–206.
87. Schlüter H, Apweiler R, Holzhütter H-G, Jungblut PR. Finding one's way in proteomics: a protein species nomenclature. Chem Cent J. 2009;3:11.
88. Lieberman JR, Daluiski A, Einhorn TA. The role of growth factors in the repair of bone. Biology and clinical applications. J Bone Joint Surg Am. 2002;84(6):1032–44.
89. Barnes GL, Kostenuik PJ, Gerstenfeld LC, Einhorn TA. Growth factor regulation of fracture repair. J Bone Miner Res. 1999;14(11):1805–15.
90. Frey C, Halikus NM, Vu-Rose T, Ebramzadeh E. A review of ankle arthrodesis: predisposing factors to nonunion. Foot Ankle Int. 1994;15(11):581–4.
91. DiGiovanni CW, Petricek JM. The evolution of rhPDGF-BB in musculoskeletal repair and its role in foot and ankle fusion surgery. Foot Ankle Clin. 2010;15(4):621–40.
92. Lin SS, Montemurro NJ, Krell ES. Orthobiologics in foot and ankle surgery. J Am Acad Orthop Surg. 2016;24(2):113–22.
93. Neer RM, Arnaud CD, Zanchetta JR, Prince R, Gaich GA, Reginster JY, et al. Effect of parathyroid hormone (1-34) on fractures and bone mineral density in postmenopausal women with osteoporosis. N Engl J Med. 2001;344(19):1434–41.
94. Hodsman AB, Bauer DC, Dempster DW, Dian L, Hanley DA, Harris ST, et al. Parathyroid hormone and teriparatide for the treatment of osteoporosis: a review of the evidence and suggested guidelines for its use. Endocr Rev. 2005;26(5):688–703.
95. Alkhiary YM, Gerstenfeld LC, Krall E, Westmore M, Sato M, Mitlak BH, et al. Enhancement of experimental fracture-healing by systemic administration of recombinant human parathyroid hormone (PTH 1-34). J Bone Joint Surg Am. 2005;87(4):731–41.
96. Andreassen TT, Ejersted C, Oxlund H. Intermittent parathyroid hormone (1-34) treatment increases callus formation and

mechanical strength of healing rat fractures. J Bone Miner Res. 1999;14(6):960–8.
97. Aspenberg P, Genant HK, Johansson T, Nino AJ, See K, Krohn K, et al. Teriparatide for acceleration of fracture repair in humans: a prospective, randomized, double-blind study of 102 postmenopausal women with distal radial fractures. J Bone Miner Res. 2010;25(2):404–14.
98. Gorter EA, Hamdy NAT, Appelman-Dijkstra NM, Schipper IB. The role of vitamin D in human fracture healing: a systematic review of the literature. Bone. 2014;64:288–97.
99. Zhou S, Glowacki J, Kim SW, Hahne J, Geng S, Mueller SM, et al. Clinical characteristics influence in vitro action of 1,25-dihydroxyvitamin D(3) in human marrow stromal cells. J Bone Miner Res. 2012;27(9):1992–2000.
100. van Leeuwen JP, van Driel M, van den Bemd GJ, Pols HA. Vitamin D control of osteoblast function and bone extracellular matrix mineralization. Crit Rev Eukaryot Gene Expr. 2001;11(1–3):199–226.
101. Doetsch AM, Faber J, Lynnerup N, Wätjen I, Bliddal H, Danneskiold-Samsøe B. The effect of calcium and vitamin D3 supplementation on the healing of the proximal humerus fracture: a randomized placebo-controlled study. Calcif Tissue Int. 2004;75(3):183–8.
102. Kolb JP, Schilling AF, Bischoff J, Novo de Oliveira A, Spiro A, Hoffmann M, et al. Calcium homeostasis influences radiological fracture healing in postmenopausal women. Arch Orthop Trauma Surg. 2013;133(2):187–92.
103. Avenell A, Mak JCS, O'Connell D. Vitamin D and vitamin D analogues for preventing fractures in post-menopausal women and older men. Cochrane Database Syst Rev. 2014;(4):CD000227.
104. Bassuener SR, Mullis BH, Harrison RK, Sanders R. Use of bioabsorbable pins in surgical fixation of comminuted periarticular fractures. J Orthop Trauma. 2012;26(10):607–10.
105. Ahmad J, Jones K. Randomized, prospective comparison of bioabsorbable and steel screw fixation of lisfranc injuries. J Orthop Trauma. 2016;30(12):676–81.
106. Treiber T, Treiber N, Meister G. Regulation of microRNA biogenesis and its crosstalk with other cellular pathways. Nat Rev Mol Cell Biol. 2019;20(1):5–20.
107. Murata K, Ito H, Yoshitomi H, Yamamoto K, Fukuda A, Yoshikawa J, et al. Inhibition of miR-92a enhances fracture healing via promoting angiogenesis in a model of stabilized fracture in young mice. J Bone Miner Res. 2014;29(2):316–26.
108. Sun Y, Xu L, Huang S, Hou Y, Liu Y, Chan K-M, et al. mir-21 overexpressing mesenchymal stem cells accelerate fracture healing in a rat closed femur fracture model. BioMed Res Int. 2015;2015:412327.
109. Lee WY, Li N, Lin S, Wang B, Lan HY, Li G. miRNA-29b improves bone healing in mouse fracture model. Mol Cell Endocrinol. 2016;430:97–107.
110. Li Z, Hassan MQ, Jafferji M, Aqeilan RI, Garzon R, Croce CM, et al. Biological functions of miR-29b contribute to positive regulation of osteoblast differentiation. J Biol Chem. 2009;284(23):15676–84.
111. Giannoudis PV, MacDonald DA, Matthews SJ, Smith RM, Furlong AJ, De Boer P. Nonunion of the femoral diaphysis. The influence of reaming and non-steroidal anti-inflammatory drugs. J Bone Joint Surg Br. 2000;82(5):655–8.
112. Marquez-Lara A, Hutchinson ID, Nuñez F, Smith TL, Miller AN. Nonsteroidal anti-inflammatory drugs and bone-healing: a systematic review of research quality. JBJS Rev. 2016;4(3).
113. Kim DH, Liu J, Bhat S, Benedict G, Lecka-Czernik B, Peterson SJ, et al. Peroxisome proliferator-activated receptor delta agonist attenuates nicotine suppression effect on human mesenchymal stem cell-derived osteogenesis and involves increased expression of heme oxygenase-1. J Bone Miner Metab. 2013;31(1):44–52.
114. Ng TK, Carballosa CM, Pelaez D, Wong HK, Choy KW, Pang CP, et al. Nicotine alters microRNA expression and hinders human adult stem cell regenerative potential. Stem Cells Dev. 2013;22(5):781–90.
115. Adams CI, Keating JF, Court-Brown CM. Cigarette smoking and open tibial fractures. Injury. 2001;32(1):61–5.
116. Lee JJ, Patel R, Biermann JS, Dougherty PJ. The musculoskeletal effects of cigarette smoking. J Bone Joint Surg Am. 2013;95(9):850–9.
117. Jiao H, Xiao E, Graves DT. Diabetes and its effect on bone and fracture healing. Curr Osteoporos Rep. 2015;13(5):327–35.
118. Folk JW, Starr AJ, Early JS. Early wound complications of operative treatment of calcaneus fractures: analysis of 190 fractures. J Orthop Trauma. 1999;13(5):369–72.
119. Loder RT. The influence of diabetes mellitus on the healing of closed fractures. Clin Orthop. 1988;232:210–6.

Fracture Rehabilitation

7

Kyle Wentz, Austin Marcolina, and Lindsay Ramey Argo

Learning Objectives

- Review the principles of immobilisation following traumatic fracture with a goal of using the least restrictive device for the shortest duration possible to insure stability.
- Understand the common terminology related to weight-bearing status that affects rehabilitation after a fracture
- Provide an overview of assistive devices to maintain appropriate weightbearing precautions
- Discuss evidence-based rehabilitation protocols following traumatic and stress fractures
- Review factors that affect fracture healing

7.1 Rehabilitation Principles for Acute Fractures

The general treatment protocol for fracture management and rehabilitation involves (1) insuring alignment of the bone to anatomic or near-anatomic position; (2) immobilisation to prevent displacement or sequelae; (3) weight bearing and loading restrictions to support bone healing; and (4) therapeutic approaches to restore function, including maximal joint range of motion, full weight bearing capacity and return to pre-fracture activity levels, as able.

7.1.1 Fracture Alignment and Surgical Fixation

The same principles apply to fracture alignment for fractures of the upper extremity, lower extremity or axial skeleton. Non-displaced and minimally displaced fractures can typically be managed non-operatively with a period of immobilisation and weight bearing restrictions until hard callus is formed.

Displaced fractures without any of the features noted below can typically be managed with closed reduction or traction to realign the bone in an anatomic position and counter the forces of the surrounding musculature. This will require post-reduction immobilisation and weight bearing restrictions to maintain alignment until healing can occur.

Operative intervention should be considered in the following instances, as surgical interventions have demonstrated improved functional outcomes [1]:

1. Unstable fractures that cannot be maintained in a reduced position
2. Displaced intra-articular fractures
3. Fracture sites that are known to heal poorly and yield poor outcomes non-operatively (Ex: Femoral neck fracture)
4. Fractures that cause significant disruption of the muscle-tendon or ligament function of an affected joint (Ex: Patellar fracture disrupting the extensor mechanism)
5. Displaced pathologic fractures in non-terminal patients, fractures in growth areas in skeletally immature individuals with high risk for growth arrest (Ex: Salter Harris III–V)
6. Nonunion or malunion that have failed non-operative treatment.
7. Open fractures
8. Unstable fractures of the spine, long bones or pelvis—especially in the setting of polytrauma
9. Impending pathologic fractures

K. Wentz · A. Marcolina
Department of Physical Medicine and Rehabilitation, University of Texas Southwest Medical Center, Dallas, TX, USA
e-mail: Kyle.wentz@phhs.org; Austin.marcolina@phhs.org

L. R. Argo (✉)
Department of Physical Medicine and Rehabilitation, University of Texas Southwest Medical Center, Dallas, TX, USA

Musculoskeletal Medicine, WellMed Medical Group, San Antonio, TX, USA
e-mail: lnr8t@virginia.edu

G. A. J. Robertson, N. Maffulli (eds.), *Fractures in Sport*, https://doi.org/10.1007/978-3-030-72036-0_7

10. Fractures in individuals who would poorly tolerate prolonged immobilisation required for non-operative management (Ex: Elderly individual with hip fracture)
11. Fractures associated with vascular or neurologic deficits

While the details of surgical interventions are outside of the scope of this chapter, the surgical approach affects the rehabilitation protocol utilized. For example, patients treated with intramedullary (IM) fixation can typically tolerate earlier weightbearing and ambulation, as compared to plate fixation [2].

7.1.2 Immobilisation

The benefits of immobilisation include minimizing pain and risk of dislocation while supporting fracture healing. General principles are as follows:

1. Immobilisation should include the fracture site and the joint distal to the fracture. If there is rotational instability along the long axis, the joint above and below the fracture should be immobilized.
2. Joints should be immobilized in a functional position with efforts to minimize risk of contractures and optimize function
3. Choose the least restrictive type and means of immobilisation and move to a less restrictive option as early as possible to optimize functional outcomes

Immobilisation can be achieved in a number of ways, including traditional casts, adjustable casts, boots, splints and braces. Casts are made of fiberglass or plaster of Paris. They are non-removable, circumferential immobilizers and provide the greatest stability but cannot accommodate swelling. This increases the risk for skin breakdown, compartment syndrome, or need for re-casting if applied during the inflammation phase. Removable devices, such as splints, are commonly employed during the first 1–2 weeks to minimize this risk, with casts applied after acute swelling has resolved [3]. Newer alternatives to traditional casts, including casts made of polymer and foam that can be reshaped, tightened or removed to accommodate swelling, can be considered with close monitoring.

Upper extremity immobilisation is often accomplished using a short or long arm cast. Short arm casts begin at the proximal 1/3 of the forearm and extend to the distal palmar crease, and should stabilize the forearm and wrist in a neutral, "hand-shake" position [4]. They are used to restrict movement at the wrist following distal forearm and carpal bone fractures (excluding the scaphoid). They permit range of motion (ROM) of the elbow and fingers. Variations of the short arm cast immobilize specific fingers, including the thumb spica cast for scaphoid fractures or the ulnar gutter cast for fourth and fifth metatarsal fractures. In more proximal forearm fractures, fractures involving the radius and ulna with rotational instability along the long axis or fractures involving the elbow joint, a long arm cast immobilizing the elbow joint at 90° of flexion should be considered. If only pronation and supination immobilisation is required, a Munster cast (i.e. is a cast which immobilizes the arm, hand, and sometimes the thumb, and extends proximally past the elbow laterally and posteriorly, thus preventing supination and pronation. The cast leaves the antecubital space free, allowing partial flexion of the elbow) may be used. Fractures requiring elbow immobilisation are often worn in a sling for the first 1–2 weeks to accommodate initial swelling.

Similar principles apply to lower extremity immobilisation. Short leg casts stabilize the ankle at 90° of flexion with a subtalar neutral position, while permitting flexion and extension of the knee [3]. Short leg casts typically begin just distal to the fibular head while extending to include the tarsals and metatarsals. A short leg is appropriate in the management of distal fibula, mid foot, or malleolar fractures. A long leg cast is helpful when greater stability is needed, such as proximal tibia, fibula, patella, or distal femoral fractures [3]. Long leg casts tend to be heavier and produce more of a burden for patient mobility, and should only be used when a short leg cast provides insufficient stability.

When casts are not safe, available or necessary, removable devices, such as slings, splints or boots, can be used. For example, minimally displaced mid-clavicle fractures heal well with a period of shoulder immobilisation using a figure-eight sling [5]. Patients have demonstrated good outcomes following use of a short leg walking boot, rather than a cast, when treating non-displaced distal fibular or metatarsal fractures [3]. In compliant patients, these adjustable and removable devices are often more comfortable and better tolerated.

The length of immobilisation varies depending on injury type, site, severity, surgical intervention, and patient risk factors. Following operative fixation, this timeline should be determined in conjunction with the surgeon. Following non-operative fixation, mobilization can typically begin once callus is demonstrated on follow-up imaging, typically ranging from 4 to 8 weeks. A recent review of 213 rehabilitation protocols for operative and non-operative foot and ankle fractures found that the mean time for immobilisation was 6 weeks [6]. Newer studies support improved outcomes with earlier mobilization following uncomplicated fractures at the foot and ankle [7–9]. Discontinuation of the method of immobilisation or transition to less aggressive immobilisation means should be considered as early as possible to minimize atrophy, joint stiffness or contracture [5]. In addition, early and regular ROM of the joints adjacent to the site of immobilisation should be initiated.

7.1.3 Weight Bearing Status, Assistive Devices and Activity Modifications

To minimize the risk of displacement and support fracture healing, restricted weight bearing status (WBS) is often recommended

- Non weight bearing (NWB): the affected limb should be completely offloaded without any contact with the ground or other surface
- Toe touch weight bearing (TTWB) or touch down weight bearing (TDWB); the affected limb is allowed to support itself on the ground or a surface, but is not yet cleared to bear weight in functional tasks
- Partial weight bearing (PWB): the affected limb can bear up to 50% body weight
- Weightbearing as tolerated (WBAT): the affected limb can bear as much weight as tolerated without pain. If pain occurs, they should decrease the weight until pain-free
- Full weightbearing (FWB): the affected extremity can bear weight unrestricted

The terms PWB and TTWB are often interpreted differently [10]. Patients often put more weight on the extremity than they realize and demonstrate poor compliance with such recommendations [11].

Surgically treated patients with traumatic lower extremity fractures, particularly peri-articular and intra-articular fractures, typically require a period of NWB and/or PWB precautions. Traditional postoperative management consisted of NWB for up to 6–12 weeks, followed by PWB with a 25% increase in weight loading every week [12]. However, research on early permissive WBS is under investigation with early results supporting improved functional outcomes with minimal to no negative effects [7, 13–16]. Patients who are treated with IM fixation can typically undertake immediate WBAT.

For the upper extremity, the same principles and definitions apply regarding WBS. Such precautions should be considered among individuals who regularly use an assistive device (ADs), such as a cane, crutch, walker or rollator, for daily ambulation.

Several ADs are available to aid patients with daily mobility needs while maintaining WBS, including wheelchairs, walkers, crutches and canes. Manual wheelchairs are commonly required to maintain lower extremity NWB status in patients at high fall risk or among individuals with bilateral lower extremity NWB or PWB restrictions. There are several adaptations to manual wheelchairs that can accommodate various patient situations, including elevated leg rests, removable or fixed foot plates, removable or adjustable arm troughs, specialized seat cushions to adjust seat height and prevent skin irritation, adjustable lumbar support and various wheel types for different terrains. Details regarding advanced wheelchair prescription are beyond the scope of this chapter but wheelchair modifications should be considered to help facilitate immobilisation and WBS recommendations.

Axillary crutches can often be used by patients with good strength and balance to maintain NWB, TTWB or PWB of a single lower extremity. The crutches should be properly fitted, and patient should be taught how to use them on flat surface and stairs. Axillary crutches should be fitted so the top of the crutch is approximately two finger widths below the axilla. In patients who have difficulty tolerating axillary crutches, a forearm or Loftstrand crutch can be considered. Other alternatives in patients at low fall risk with distal lower extremity fracture include knee scooters and knee crutches. While research on such devices is limited, small pilot studies have shown improved assisted ambulation and decreased perceived exertion using such devices compared to traditional axillary crutches [17, 18]. For older individuals with less-restrictive weight bearing precautions (WBAT), rolling walkers and/or canes should be considered. A walker can provide stability for patients during ambulation and decrease risk of falls and reinjury by providing a wider base of support. Canes are the least support of all ADs reviewed, and will provide limited weight bearing supporting or stability following a fracture. However, they can be useful as a patient is transitioning from more supportive ADs to unassisted ambulation.

Additional options are available for individuals who require an AD for safe mobility but need to maintain NWB or PWB restrictions for the upper extremity following fracture. A platform crutch or walker can be used to maintain NWB or PWB following distal upper extremity fracture while providing support of the lower extremities to facilitate earlier ambulation in the rehabilitation process.

7.1.4 Therapy: Restoring Range of Motion, Strength and Function

Exercises to maintain ROM of the joints surrounding the fracture site should begin early in the recovery process. For example, exercises to promote elbow and finger ROM and strength should be encouraged while a patient is in a short arm cast to minimize disuse atrophy and prevent contracture development. In addition, early ROM and strengthening improve functional outcomes in patients treated with ORIF [7, 15, 16]. Early ROM and strengthening following distal radius fractures managed with ORIF resulted in earlier return to work and sporting activities than implementing delayed ROM and strengthening [15]. Following unstable ankle fractures treated with ORIF, patients exhibit improved functional outcomes with post-operative ROM and WBAT at 2 weeks without cast immobilisation, compared to those treated with cast immobilisation followed by ROM and WBAT beginning at 6 weeks [7]. Other studies champion the benefits of early ROM to include pain relief, decreased edema, and faster return to work [8].

Such protocols can be done with a detailed home exercise program provided by the supervising healthcare provider or by initiating physical or occupation therapy early in the recovery process. The choice is often individualized based on patient age, risk factors, compliance, fracture site and stability, and healthcare provider comfort. Once immobilisation and weight bearing restrictions are lifted, a formal rehabilitation program to maintain or restore full ROM of the involved joint, rebuild strength, improve neuromuscular control and oversee gradual return to pre-injury activity level is recommended.

Overall, there continues to be a lack of evidence surrounding specific rehabilitation protocols following non-operative and surgical intervention of fractures [6, 19]. However, it is generally believed that adhering to the above principles of appropriate stabilization, proper weight bearing precautions and early mobilization and ROM, as able, will lend to better clinical outcomes.

There are some relative controversies regarding modalities and techniques to promote healing and functional recovery following traumatic fractures, including continuous passive motion (CPM), blood flow restriction (BFR), and bone stimulator use:

1. CPM has been proposed to maintain full ROM, promote healing and improve functional outcomes following peri-articular fractures. CPM hastens the clearance of hemarthrosis during the inflammatory response [20] and to improve hyaline cartilage healing in animal models [21]. Literature is largely limited to use following total knee arthroplasty (TKA) for degenerative joint disease with mixed results in vivo. One study found no improvement in outcomes in patients who underwent CPM after TKA for osteoarthritis compared to those who did not [22]. Little research is available on the use of CPM following articular fractures, and most studies involve small sample sizes with mixed surgical approaches, making it difficult to assess the added value of CPM in this context [21]. Further, high quality research is needed to determine evidence-based guidelines for the use of CPM following articular and peri-articular fractures.
2. BFR has been proposed as a mechanism to speed functional recovery following fractures by helping to maintain strength and minimize muscle atrophy. One theory suggests that when low intensity exercise occurs with compression of the associated musculature, we induce a hypermetabolic state that can reduce muscle atrophy during rehabilitation [23]. Others suggest that BFR can cause increased cellular swelling that will stimulate muscular hypertrophy. Some studies suggest that BFR, when combined with exercise, can provide benefits in fracture rehabilitation [24]. One study suggests that compressive knee wraps after knee injury can promote bone health [25]. Another study suggests that low intensity exercise when combined with moderate vascular occlusion can improve rate of return of muscular strength [26]. While there is a paucity of strong research regarding this modality, the use of BFR combined with an individualized exercise program shows promise in promoting recovery after a fracture.
3. Bone stimulators are devices which use energy fields to promote bone healing and have been proposed as adjunctive treatment following a fracture. Modalities for non-invasive bone stimulation include pulsed electromagnetic field (PEMF) and low intensity pulsed ultrasound (LIPUS) with no clear benefit of one modality over another. Both types of stimulation require regular, daily use for maximal benefit [27].

   LIPUS has been shown to stimulate osteogenesis, with accelerated healing time and improved strength, in vitro and animal models [28]. The evidence for the use of LIPUS in human trials following fresh fracture has provided inconsistent results with low-quality and/or heterogenous studies limiting conclusions [28–30]. When applied to non-union fractures, LIPUS has demonstrated more consistent benefit, with similar healing rates to surgical interventions [31].

   PEMF has been shown to stimulate human osteoblast cell proliferation and differentiation, with the potential to accelerate healing times, in vitro studies [32]. Similar to LIPUS, there are limited, high-quality studies with inconsistent results regarding the benefit of PEMF following acute fractures. More consistent evidence supports the use of PEMF in non-union fractures [27, 29, 31, 33].

   Regardless of modality, the functional benefit of bone stimulators following fresh fractures remains unclear, but evidence suggests potential benefit when applied to non-union fractures.

7.2 Rehabilitation of Stress Fractures

Stress fractures are common, overuse injuries from repetitive, sub-maximal loading without appropriate rest [34–36]. Typically seen in athletes and military personnel, repetitive overload produces recurring microtrauma and an imbalance between bone resorption and repair [36]. Symptoms, including pain, usually begin after the initiation of an increased intensity in physical activity or training regimen [34]. Both intrinsic and extrinsic factors are associated with stress fractures, including female gender, poor biomechanics, Vitamin

Table 7.1 High and low-risk stress fracture sites

High-risk	Low-risk
Lower extremity: • Femoral neck: tension side • Patella • Anterior tibia • Medial malleolus • Talus • Tarsal navicular • Fifth metatarsal (proximal) • Sesamoids of the great toe	Upper extremity: • Clavicle • Scapula • Humerus • Olecranon • Ulna • Radius • Metacarpals Axial Skeleton: • Ribs • Pars interarticularis • Sacrum • Pubic rami Lower extremity: • Femoral neck: compression side • Femoral shaft • Posteromedial tibia • Fibula • Calcaneus • First–fourth metatarsals

D deficiency, strength imbalance, high volume training regimen, and inappropriate footwear [37].

Stress fractures can be subclassified into high and low-risk based on location (Table 7.1) [34, 35, 38, 39]. High-risk stress fractures have a tendency for prolonged recovery, progression to complete fracture, and/or increased potential for delayed or non-union. The bones associated with high-risk stress fractures are under high tensile load with diminished vascular supply. This can lead to sub-optimal healing and increased morbidity, if they are not identified early and treated appropriately. In contrast, low-risk stress fractures occur in areas with good blood supply and/or low tensile load with decreased risk for progression to a complete fracture or delayed/nonunion fracture [34, 40]. Low-risk fractures can be managed more conservatively and typically have a favorable prognosis when treated with activity and/or WBS restrictions [34].

Rehabilitation protocols for stress fracture management are outlined below. Site specific protocols will be discussed in detail in subsequent chapters.

7.2.1 Fracture Alignment and Surgical Fixation

Low-risk stress fractures rarely require surgical intervention. The initial management should focus on off-loading the bone using conservative, non-operative measures. Surgical evaluation should only occur if symptoms persistent or worsening despite appropriate conservative care [34].

The need for surgical intervention varies greatly for high risk stress fractures and is typically based on fracture site, level of athletic participation, anticipated recovery time and mutual physician-patient decision making. High-risk stress fractures may require surgical intervention, as detailed in Table 7.4 and subsequent chapters. Early evaluation by an orthopedic surgeon is recommended [35, 39].

7.2.2 Immobilisation

The use of immobilisation for low-risk, lower extremity stress fractures is controversial. Low-risk fractures tend to heal well with or without immobilisation, but a shorter recovery period has been documented with adjunctive use of pneumatic bracing for 3–6 weeks, as dictated by pain [40]. However, use of such devices has been associated with muscle atrophy, restricted ROM and/or diminished neuromuscular control [42]. We use a controlled ankle motion (CAM) boot if there is pain limiting daily walking among athletes with a time-sensitive recovery. The shortest duration of immobilisation and early, regular NWB ROM exercises should be encouraged. The benefit of immobilisation of upper extremity and axial stress fractures has not been well-studied [35, 39].

Immobilisation should be considered, as able, among high-risk stress fractures managed non-operatively due to their increased risk for delayed or non-union. If there are worsening symptoms despite immobilisation and activity restriction, surgical evaluation is recommended [35, 43].

7.2.3 Weight Bearing Status, Assistive Devices and Activity Restrictions

Low-risk stress fractures can typically be managed with restricted activity and WBS, as dictated by symptoms. The removal of the repetitive microtrauma will allow for healing to occur though an increase in bone repair, as opposed to the predominate bone resorption that occurs during intensive activity.

In patients with low-risk lower extremity stress fractures who present with pain on weight bearing, a period of NWB or PWB with AD followed by a gradual progression to pain-free FWB is recommended [34, 40]. In patients with pain during impact activities only, WBAT without AD can typically be permitted but specific activity restriction guidelines are recommended. At minimum, impact activity should be restricted for 4–6 weeks. As pain allows, the patient can begin with non-impact activity (swimming) followed by low-impact activity (cycling, elliptical). Full impact exercises can begin after the appropriate recovery period and as pain permits [34]. The same principles should be applied to low-risk upper extremity and axial stress fractures. Tables 7.2, 7.3, and 7.4 describe general protocols, by site, for low-risk stress fractures in the axial skeleton, upper and lower extremity.

Table 7.4 Overview of lower extremity stress fracture rehabilitation protocols

Lower extremity	Surgical Intervention	Immobilisation	WBS/activity	Rehabilitation progression
Low-risk				
Femur [34, 41] – Shaft – Neck, Compression	Rare; only for delayed/ non-union or if the fracture spans greater than half of the neck width	No supporting evidence	TTWB 1–4 weeks; progress to FWB as tolerated by pain over 6–12 weeks	1. Full active hip ROM 2. Pain free strengthening of hip musculature with limited weight bearing 3. Gradual return to full activity and weight bearing – Light jogging at 6 weeks – Sport-specific activity by 12 weeks
Posteromedial tibial shaft [34]	Rare; exchange intermedullary nailing for delayed or non-union	Consider adjunctive pneumatic brace during limited activity	WBAT; no running/ high-impact exercise for 4–8 weeks with limited activity for a total of 8–12 weeks	1. Full active knee/ankle ROM 2. Begin low-impact activity such as stationary bikes and elliptical machines once asymptomatic 3. Gradual return to full sport at 8–12 weeks
Fibula [34]	Rare; only for non-union	CAM or aircast boot for 3–6 weeks	WBAT; limited activity for 3–6 weeks as tolerated	1. Full active knee/ankle ROM 2. Pain free strengthening of lower leg musculature with limited weight bearing 3. Gradual return to full activity and weight bearing
Calcaneus [34]	Rare; percutaneous screw fixation vs. ORIF for delayed or non-union	Short leg walking boot for 3–6 weeks	WBAT; limited activity for 3–6 weeks as tolerated	1. Full active foot ROM 2. Pain free strengthening of foot and ankle musculature with limited weight bearing 3. Gradual return to full activity and weight bearing – Consider heel pads
First–fourth metatarsals [34]	Not indicated	Short leg walking boot for 4 weeks; below-the-knee walking cast for persistent symptoms	WBAT; no impact activities for 4–6 weeks as tolerated	1. Full active foot ROM 2. Pain free strengthening of foot and ankle musculature with limited weight bearing 3. Gradual return to full activity and weight bearing – Consider metatarsal insert pads
High-risk				
Femur [35, 39, 41] – Neck, tension	Evaluation for ORIF; percutaneous screw for widening displacement	Pneumatic bracing for 6–12 weeks	NWB 0–6 weeks; PWB 6–12 weeks; limited activity for a total of 6–12 weeks	1. Full active hip ROM 2. Pain free strengthening of hip stabilization musculature with limited weight bearing 3. Gradual return to full activity and weight bearing
Patella [35, 39]	Evaluation in setting of high level athletes widening displacement despite immobilisation	Extension immobilisation for 4–6 weeks for non or minimally displaced fractures	PWB with limited activity for 6 weeks to 6 months	1. Full active hip ROM 2. Pain free strengthening of foot and ankle musculature with limited weight bearing 3. Gradual return to full activity and weight bearing – Average length of return to full sport is 6 months post-surgery
Anterior tibia [35, 39]	Consider IM nail for delayed/ non-union fractures or persistent symptoms	Pneumatic bracing for 3–6 months	NWB for 3–6 months; limited activity for 3–4 months	1. Full active hip ROM 2. Pain free strengthening of foot and ankle musculature with limited weight bearing 3. Gradual return to full activity and weight bearing
Medial malleolus [35, 39]	Early surgical intervention with malleolar screws or ORIF in high-level athletes and delayed/non-union fractures	Short leg cast or CAM boot for 6–8 weeks	NWB 4–8 weeks, followed by PWB and limited activity for an additional 4–6 weeks	1. Full active foot and ankle ROM 2. Pain free strengthening of foot and ankle musculature with limited weight bearing 3. Gradual return to full activity and weight bearing

Table 7.4 (continued)

Lower extremity	Surgical Intervention	Immobilisation	WBS/activity	Rehabilitation progression
Talus [35, 39]	Evaluation for ORIF if symptoms persist despite non-operative management	Cast immobilisation or CAM boot for 4–6 weeks, depending upon symptom severity	NWB for 6 weeks, followed by PWB and limited activity with for 4–6 weeks	1. Full active foot and ankle ROM 2. Pain free strengthening of foot and ankle musculature 3. Gradual return to full activity and weight bearing – Poor outcomes are associated with return to full activity prior to 6 weeks – Orthotics can be used as an adjunct to correct subtalar pronation
Tarsal navicular [35, 39]	Rare; evaluation for ORIF if symptoms persist despite non-operative management	Cast immobilisation for 6–8 weeks	NWB for 6–8 weeks, followed by PWB and limited activity for an additional 4–6 weeks	1. Full active foot and ankle ROM 2. Pain free strengthening of foot and ankle musculature 3. Gradual return to full activity and weight bearing
Proximal fifth metatarsal [35, 39]	Evaluation for intramedullary screw fixation in those with positive XR	Cast immobilisation for 6 weeks, followed by CAM boot for 3–6 weeks	NWB for 6 weeks, followed by progressive weight bearing for 3–6 weeks	1. Full active foot and toe ROM 2. Pain free strengthening of foot and toe musculature 3. Gradual return to full activity and weight bearing
Sesamoids of the Great Toe [35, 39]	Evaluation for partial excision, sesamoidectomy, or grafting if symptoms persist	Toe spica short leg cast for 6–8 weeks, followed by CAM boot for 3–6 weeks	NWB for 6–8 weeks, followed by protected weight bearing for an additional 3–6 weeks	1. Full active foot and toe ROM 2. Pain free strengthening of foot and toe musculature during protected weight bearing with use of a removable boot 3. Gradual return to full activity and weight bearing – Modified orthotics with forefoot offloading and limited dorsiflexion can be used for future prevention

High-risk stress fractures often require a dedicated period of NWB with AD, followed by a similar, but more gradual, progression to FWB and return to activity. The period of weight-bearing restriction has been documented to last from 4 weeks to 6 months, depending on the site and severity of the stress fracture. Similar to low-risk stress fractures, as the pain subsides, the patient can begin the progression of non-impact to low-impact to full activity, using protocols as detailed in Table 7.4 [50,70]. Given the increased likelihood for delayed or non-union, the authors recommend using a lower threshold for reimaging should symptoms persist for longer than 6–12 weeks.

The duration of weight-bearing and activity restriction has been associated with specific features on advanced imaging which can be used to predict severity of injury (Table 7.5). MR imaging, in particular, shows a positive association between image severity and time to full return to sport [41, 49, 51, 52]. In general, high-grade injuries with a visible fracture line or marrow edema on T1 sequences require a longer recovery period than low-grade injuries with no visible fracture line and marrow edema only on the T2 or short tau inversion recovery (STIR) sequences [41, 49, 51, 52]. Recovery prediction has the strongest correlation when combining features of fracture risk with fracture severity to help predict recovery time [53]. Other forms of advanced imaging, such as CT and bone scans, can also be used in the evaluation of stress fractures, but the appearance of the images is not a consistent prognostic indicator for recovery time [51, 52].

7.2.4 Therapy: Restoring Range of Motion, Strength and Function

The common steps in stress fracture rehabilitation include optimizing bone healing while maintaining full ROM of the adjacent joints, restoring strength and gradually returning to pre-injury activity level, as detailed in Tables 7.2, 7.3, and 7.4. There is limited evidence behind specific rehabilitation protocols following stress fractures, and guidelines are largely based on case reports, case series or anecdotal experience.

Table 7.2 Overview of upper extremity, low-risk stress fracture rehabilitation protocols

Upper extremity	Surgical intervention	Immobilisation	WBS/activity	Rehabilitation progression
Clavicle [44]	Not indicated	No supporting evidence	NWB for 4–6 weeks, as tolerated by pain	1. Full active shoulder ROM 2. Pain-free strengthening without body weight 3. Gradual return to activity: – Throwers: Progressive interval throwing program – Gymnasts: Gradual return to FWB stunts
Scapula [45]	Not indicated	No supporting evidence	WBAT; limit overhead motion for 6–8 weeks	1. Full active shoulder ROM 2. Pain-free strengthening without body weight 3. Gradual return to overhead activity, as tolerated by pain
Humerus [34] – *Shaft* – *Proximal growth plate*	Not indicated	No supporting evidence	WBAT; limit throwing and weightlifting for 6–8 weeks (adults) and up to 12 weeks (adolescents)	1. Full active shoulder & elbow ROM 2. Pain-free strengthening without body weight 3. Gradual return to throwing and lifting, as tolerated by pain – Throwers: Insure adequate rest days, monitor pitch counts
Olecranon [46, 47]	Rare; surgical referral for skeletally immature affecting growth plate	No supporting evidence	WBAT; limiting throwing and valgus motion for ≥6 weeks	1. Full active elbow ROM 2. Pain-free strengthening without body weight 3. Gradual return to throwing at 6–8 weeks: – Throwers: Progressive interval throwing program
Ulna [47]	Not indicated	No supporting evidence	WBAT; activity restriction as dictated by pain for 6–8 weeks.	1. Full active elbow ROM 2. Pain-free strengthening without body weight 3. Gradual return to sport at 6–8 weeks
Radius [47]	Not indicated	Short arm cast × 3 weeks; posterior wrist splint × 3 weeks	WBAT; limited activity for 6–8 weeks	1. Full active elbow, wrist and finger ROM 2. Pain-free strengthening of the wrist and forearm at 6–8 weeks 3. Gradual return to pain-free weightbearing activity. Progress to full sport return.
Metacarpals [48]	Not indicated	Reserved for refractory cases	WBAT; limited activity for 6–12 weeks	1. Full active finger ROM 2. Pain-free strengthening of the wrist and fingers 3. Gradual return to pain-free weightbearing activity and sport

The rehabilitation protocol should also focus on identifying and correcting modifiable risk factors for future bone stress injuries. One of the strongest predictors for future stress fracture is a history of a prior stress fracture. In a recent meta-analysis, athletes with a history of stress fracture had a five-fold higher risk of developing a new stress fracture as compared to individuals with no prior history [54]. This rehabilitation period should be viewed as an opportunity to education and train athletes to minimize future risk. This should include assessment of internal risk factors for bone health, including adequate nutrient and energy supply and/or regular menses as components of relative-energy deficiency syndrome (RED-S). External risk factors, including poor biomechanics, improper equipment or footwear and/or poor training habits, should be reviewed and discussed (Table 7.6).

Debated topics in stress fracture rehabilitation include use of bone stimulators and alterations in running mechanics:

Table 7.3 Overview of axial, low-risk stress fracture rehabilitation protocols

Axial	Surgical intervention	Immobilisation	WBS/activity	Rehabilitation progression
First Rib [34]	Not indicated	No supporting evidence	WBAT; limited activity for 4 weeks	1. Full active shoulder ROM 2. Pain free strengthening of shoulder stabilizing musculature 3. Gradual return to full activity
Middle Ribs [34]	Not indicated	No supporting evidence	WBAT; limited activity for 4–6 weeks, especially limiting extreme shoulder flexion followed by extension	1. Full active shoulder and thoracic ROM 2. Pain-free strengthening of shoulder/thoracic stabilizing musculature, with a specific focus on serratus anterior 3. Gradual return to full activity
Pars interarticularis [34]	Rare; lumbar interbody fusion in cases of severe spondylolisthesis	Lumbosacral anti-lordotic orthosis in setting of spondylolisthesis while symptomatic	WBAT; limited activity for 6 weeks to 6 months, dictated by pain	1. Full active spine ROM 2. Pain-free strengthening of abdominal and paraspinal musculature 3. Gradual return to full activity and weight bearing
Sacrum [34]	Not indicated	No supporting evidence	WBAT; limited activity for 4 weeks	1. Full active hip and lumbar spine ROM 2. Pain-free strengthening of pelvic musculature 3. Gradual return to full activity and weight bearing
Pubic Rami [34]	Not indicated	No supporting evidence	WBAT; limited activity for 6–10 weeks	1. Full active hip and lumbar spine ROM 2. Pain free strengthening of pelvic and hip musculature 3. Gradual return to full activity and weight bearing – Future prevention through increased rest periods, decreased intensity of exercise, and shortened stride length

1. As discussed in more detail in the traumatic fracture section, bone stimulators are a popular adjunctive therapy used to promote bone healing after a fracture. There is no evidence to support the use of bone stimulators in the management of low-risk stress fractures. Two randomized, controlled trials found no difference in recovery time following low-risk stress fractures of the lower extremity [55, 56]. No studies have been identified assessing the role of bone stimulators in the treatment of high-risk stress fractures. The authors of this chapter limit bone stimulator use to superficial stress fractures refractory to standard care.
2. Modification of running patterns is also a commonly debated adjunct in the management and prevention of lower extremity stress fractures, particularly among athletes with recurrent stress fractures. While supportive studies are small and/or of low quality, they suggest that adjustments in running mechanics, including modifying foot strike pattern from heel to mid- or fore-foot strike, shortening stride length, and/or increasing cadence, can influence loading rates and stress at particular bony sites, particularly the tibia [72.73]. Contradictory evidence argues that the impact forces that are adjusted for with the above changes, may not directly correlate with stress, and may not change the risk of developing a stress fracture [74,75]. While high quality research is needed to determine the efficacy of such strategies on the management and/or prevention of lower extremity stress reactions, early research shows promise.

7.3 Additional Factors Affecting Bone Healing

Many factors contribute to the efficacy and speed of bone healing, including characteristics of the fracture and the patient. See Table 7.2 for details [57, 58]. Such factors should be reviewed by the treating physician when creating an individualize rehabilitation plan and anticipated recovery timeline. When able, modifiable variables should be addressed during the recovery period to optimize fracture healing. For

Table 7.5 Stress fracture grading systems using MRI

Grade	Grade	Fredericson scale [49]	Arendt scale [50]	Nattiv scale [51]
Low grade	1	Mild to moderate periosteal edema on T2; normal marrow on T2 and T1	Positive signal change on STIR imaging	Mild marrow or periosteal edema on T2b; T1 normal
	2	Moderate to severe periosteal edema on T2; marrow edema on T2 but not T1	Positive STIR + positive T2	Moderate marrow or periosteal edema plus positive T2; T1 normal
High grade	3	Moderate to severe periosteal edema on T2; marrow edema on T2 and T1	Positive T1 and T2 but without definite cortical break	Severe marrow or periosteal edema on T2 and T1
	4	Moderate to severe periosteal edema on T2; marrow edema on T2 and T1; + fracture line	Positive T1 and T2 with fracture line	Severe marrow or periosteal edema on T2 and T1 plus fracture line on T2 or T1

Table 7.6 Factors that adversely affect bone healing

Osseous factors	Patient factors
• Poor blood supply • Intra-articular fractures • Mechanically unstable fractures • Increased degree of bone loss • Inappropriate or ineffective bone stabilization	• Older age • Nutritional deficiencies (Vitamin C, D, and calcium) • Previous gastric bypass • Diabetes mellitus • Hormone imbalance • Smoking • HIV positive • Excessive alcohol consumption • Medication: see below • Pathologic bone: osteoporosis, metastatic bone disease

a review of the basic science involved in fracture healing, please refer to Chap. 4.

Several medications slow bone healing both *in vivo* and animal models, including non-steroidal anti-inflammatory drugs (NSAIDs) [59–63], methotrexate [64] and bisphosphonates [65–67]. However, there is conflicting or unclear evidence in human studies to draw conclusions regarding clinical practice. Oral corticosteroids, particularly when used long-term, can compromise fracture healing, and patients on these medications long-term are at increased risk of fractures [68]. Caution should be used with oral or injectable corticosteroids during fracture healing and rehabilitation.

Clinical Pearls

- Initial management of both traumatic and stress fractures should focus on supporting bone healing via surgery, immobilisation, altered weight bearing status and/or activity restrictions, while minimizing risk for sequela from the fracture itself or its treatment protocol and optimizing functional recovery.
- Immobilisation is associated with muscle atrophy and joint stiffness. The least restrictive immobilisation device should be used for the shortest period necessary to stabilize the fracture. When immobilisation is required, ROM and strengthening of adjacent structures should begin early under the guidance of a healthcare professional.
- Emerging literature has demonstrated improved outcomes with early mobilization and permissive weight bearing following certain fractures (ankle, radial) without articular involvement managed with ORIF.
- Following any fracture, a graded return-to-activity program, progressing from non-impact, to partial and finally full impact exercise, is advised.
- Further research is needed to establish evidence-based fracture rehabilitation protocols and to better understand the role of emerging treatment options in functional recovery.

Review

Questions (and Answers in bold)

1. True or **False**. Patients with a low-grade stress fracture of the posteromedial tibia should be immobilized on crutches for 4–6 weeks.
2. Which of the following features can be used to predict recovery time following a stress fracture?
   (a) Grade of stress fracture on advanced imaging
   (b) Stress fracture risk group based on location
   (c) Size of stress fracture on advanced imaging
   (d) **A and B**
   (e) All of the Above
3. An 18 year old male unstable bi-malleolar ankle fracture without articular involvement and undergoes ORIF. Currently literature suggests improved short-term functional outcomes with the following:
   (a) Immediate WBAT and ROM
   (b) **NWB and Immobilisation in a short leg boot for 2 weeks followed by progressive ROM and WBAT**
   (c) NWB and Immobilisation in a short leg boot for 6 weeks followed by progressive ROM and WBAT

(d) NWB and Immobilisation in a short leg boot for 8 weeks followed by progressive ROM and WBAT

4. What factors are associated with prolonged recovery and/or poor healing following fracture?
   (a) Older Age
   (b) Poor Blood Supply
   (c) History of Gastric Bypass Surgery
   (d) A and B
   (e) **All of the Above**

References

1. Whittle AP. General principles of fracture treatment. In: Azar FM, Canale ST, Beaty JH, editors. Campbell's operative orthopaedics. Philadelphia, PA: Elsevier/Mosby; 2017. p. 2656–711.
2. Hoyt BW, Pavey GJ, Pasquina PF, Potter BK. Rehabilitation of lower extremity trauma: a review of principles and military perspective on future directions. Curr Trauma Rep. 2015;1:50–60.
3. Boyd AS, Benjamin HJ, Asplund C. Splints and casts: indications and methods. Am Fam Physician. 2009;80(5):491–9.
4. Garcia-Rodriguez JA, Longino PD, Johnston I. Short arm cast: casting immobilization series for primary care. Can Fam Physician. 2018;64(10):746–9.
5. Stracciolini A. In: Wiley JF, Fields KB, Stack AM, Wolfson AB, editors. Basic techniques for splinting of musculoskeletal injuries. Waltham, MA: UpToDate, UpToDate; 2019.
6. Pfeifer CG, Grechenig S, Frankewycz B, Ernstberger A, Nerlich M, Krutsch W. Analysis of 213 currently used rehabilitation protocols in foot and ankle fractures. Injury. 2015;46(Suppl 4):S51–7.
7. Dehghan N, McKee MD, Jenkinson RJ, et al. Early weight-bearing and range of motion versus non-weight-bearing and immobilization after open reduction and internal fixation of unstable ankle fractures: a randomized controlled trial. J Orthop Trauma. 2016;30(7):345–52.
8. Jansen H, Jordan M, Frey S, Holscher-Doht S, Meffert R, Heintel T. Active controlled motion in early rehabilitation improves outcome after ankle fractures: a randomized controlled trial. Clin Rehabil. 2018;32(3):312–8.
9. Vioreanu M, Dudeney S, Hurson B, Kelly E, O'Rourke K, Quinlan W. Early mobilization in a removable cast compared with immobilization in a cast after operative treatment of ankle fractures: a prospective randomized study. Foot Ankle Int. 2007;28(1): 13–9.
10. Thompson SG, Phillip RD, Roberts A. How do orthopaedic surgeons and rehabilitation professionals interpret and assess 'toe touch' weight bearing and 'partial' weight bearing status in the rehabilitation setting? BMJ Open Sport Exerc Med. 2018;4(1):e000326.
11. Hurkmans HL, Bussmann JB, Selles RW, Benda E, Stam HJ, Verhaar JA. The difference between actual and prescribed weight bearing of total hip patients with a trochanteric osteotomy: long-term vertical force measurements inside and outside the hospital. Arch Phys Med Rehabil. 2007;88(2):200–6.
12. Ruedi T, editor. AO principles of fracture management. New York: Thieme; 2007.
13. Kalmet PHS, Meys G, YY VH, et al. Permissive weight bearing in trauma patients with fracture of the lower extremities: prospective multicenter comparative cohort study. BMC Surg. 2018;18(1):8.
14. Thewlis D, Fraysse F, Callary SA, et al. Postoperative weight bearing and patient reported outcomes at one year following tibial plateau fractures. Injury. 2017;48(7):1650–6.
15. Brehmer JL, Husband JB. Accelerated rehabilitation compared with a standard protocol after distal radial fractures treated with volar open reduction and internal fixation: a prospective, randomized, controlled study. J Bone Joint Surg Am. 2014;96(19):1621–30.
16. Dehghan N, Mitchell SM, Schemitsch EH. Rehabilitation after plate fixation of upper and lower extremity fractures. Injury. 2018;49(S1):S72–7.
17. Kocher BKCR, Lobez DM, Kirk KL. Comparative study of assisted ambulation and perceived exertion with the wheeled knee walker and axillary crutches in health subjects. Foot Ankle Int. 2016;37(11):1232–7.
18. Martin KD, Unangst AM, Huh J, Chisholm J. Patient preference and physical demand for hands-free single crutch vs standard axillary crutches in foot and ankle patients. Foot Ankle Int. 2019;40(10):1203–8.
19. Schnackers M, van Horn YY, Meys GHH, Brink PRG, Smeets R, Seelen HAM. Evidence-based rehabilitation therapy following surgery for (peri-)articular fractures: a systematic review. J Rehabil Med. 2019;51(9):638–45.
20. Ferretti M, Srinivasan A, Deschner J, et al. Anti-inflammatory effects of continuous passive motion on meniscal fibrocartilage. J Orthop Res. 2005;23(5):1165–71.
21. O'Driscoll SW, Giori NJ. Continuous passive motion (CPM): theory and principles of clinical application. J Rehabil Res Dev. 2000;37(2):179–88.
22. Boese CK, Weis M, Phillips T, Lawton-Peters S, Gallo T, Centeno L. The efficacy of continuous passive motion after total knee arthroplasty: a comparison of three protocols. J Arthroplast. 2014;29(6):1158–62.
23. Fry CS, Glynn EL, Drummond MJ, et al. Blood flow restriction exercise stimulates mTORC1 signaling and muscle protein synthesis in older men. J Appl Physiol (1985). 2010;108(5):1199–209.
24. Fujita S, Abe T, Drummond MJ, et al. Blood flow restriction during low-intensity resistance exercise increases S6K1 phosphorylation and muscle protein synthesis. J Appl Physiol (1985). 2007;103(3):903–10.
25. Loenneke JP, Young KC, Wilson JM, Andersen JC. Rehabilitation of an osteochondral fracture using blood flow restricted exercise: a case review. J Bodyw Mov Ther. 2013;17(1):42–5.
26. Takarada Y, Takazawa H, Sato Y, Takebayashi S, Tanaka Y, Ishii N. Effects of resistance exercise combined with moderate vascular occlusion on muscular function in humans. J Appl Physiol (1985). 2000;88(6):2097–106.
27. Xix Congresso Nazionale S.I.C O.O.P. Società Italiana Chirurghi Ortopedici Dell'Ospedalità Privata A, Verdoni F, Compagnone D, et al. Chemical and physical influences in bone and cartilage regeneration: a review of literature. J Biol Regul Homeost Agents. 2019;33(2 Suppl 1):89–95.
28. Martinez de Albornoz P, Khanna A, Longo UG, Forriol F, Maffulli N. The evidence of low-intensity pulsed ultrasound for in vitro, animal and human fracture healing. Br Med Bull. 2011;100:39–57.
29. Schandelmaier S, Kaushal A, Lytvyn L, et al. Low intensity pulsed ultrasound for bone healing: systematic review of randomized controlled trials. BMJ. 2017;356:j656.
30. Griffin XL, Parsons N, Costa ML, Metcalfe D. Ultrasound and shockwave therapy for acute fractures in adults. Cochrane Database Syst Rev. 2014;(6):CD008579.
31. Leighton R, Watson JT, Giannoudis P, Papakostidis C, Harrison A, Steen RG. Healing of fracture nonunions treated with low-intensity pulsed ultrasound (LIPUS): a systematic review and meta-analysis. Injury. 2017;48(7):1339–47.
32. Barnaba S, Papalia R, Ruzzini L, Sgambato A, Maffulli N, Denaro V. Effect of pulsed electromagnetic fields on human osteoblast cultures. Physiother Res Int. 2013;18(2):109–14.

33. Aleem IS, Aleem I, Evaniew N, et al. Efficacy of electrical stimulators for bone healing: a meta-analysis of randomized sham-controlled trials. Sci Rep. 2016;6:31724.
34. Boden BP, Osbahr DC, Jimenez C. Low-risk stress fractures. Am J Sports Med. 2001;29(1):100–11.
35. Boden BP, Osbahr DC. High-risk stress fractures: evaluation and treatment. J Am Acad Orthop Surg. 2000;8(6):344–53.
36. Astur DC, Zanatta F, Arliani GG, Moraes ER, Pochini Ade C, Ejnisman B. Stress fractures: definition, diagnosis and treatment. Rev Bras Ortop. 2016;51(1):3–10.
37. Ramey L, Kasitinon D. Risk factors for developing stress fractures. In: Miller T, Keading C, editors. Stress fractures in athletes: diagnosis and management. 2nd ed. Basel: Springer International Publishing; 2015.
38. Murray SR, Reeder MT, Udermann BE, Pettitt RW. High-risk stress fractures: pathogenesis, evaluation, and treatment. Compr Ther. 2006;32(1):20–5.
39. McInnis KC, Ramey LN. High-risk stress fractures: diagnosis and management. PM R. 2016;8(3 Suppl):S113–24.
40. Robertson GA, Wood AM. Lower limb stress fractures in sport: optimising their management and outcome. World J Orthop. 2017;8(3):242–55.
41. Ramey LN, McInnis KC, Palmer WE. Femoral neck stress fracture: can MRI grade help predict return-to-running time? Am J Sports Med. 2016;44(8):2122–9.
42. Grosset JF, Onambele-Pearson G. Effect of foot and ankle immobilization on leg and thigh muscles' volume and morphology: a case study using magnetic resonance imaging. Anat Rec Adv Integr Anat Evol Biol. 2008;291(12):1673–83.
43. Abbott A, Bird M, Brown SM, Wild E, Stewart G, Mulcahey MK. Part II: presentation, diagnosis, classification, treatment, and prevention of stress fractures in female athletes. Phys Sportsmed. 2020;48(1):25–32.
44. Fallon KE, Fricker PA. Stress fracture of the clavicle in a young female gymnast. Br J Sports Med. 2001;35(6):448–9.
45. Donaldson LD. Scapular stress fracture in water polo: a case report. Sports Health. 2012;4(6):502–3.
46. Fujioka H, Tsunemi K, Takagi Y, Tanaka J. Treatment of stress fracture of the olecranon in throwing athletes with internal fixation through a small incision. Sports Med Arthrosc Rehabil Ther Technol. 2012;4(1):49.
47. Jones GL. Upper extremity stress fractures. Clin Sports Med. 2006;25(1):159–74, xi
48. Duarte ML, Nobrega RRD, Prado J, Scoppetta LCD. Metacarpal stress fracture in amateur tennis player—an uncommon fracture. Rev Bras Ortop. 2017;52(5):608–11.
49. Fredericson M, Bergman AG, Hoffman KL, Dillingham MS. Tibial stress reaction in runners. Correlation of clinical symptoms and scintigraphy with a new magnetic resonance imaging grading system. Am J Sports Med. 1995;23(4):472–81.
50. Arendt EA, Griffiths HJ. The use of MR imaging in the assessment and clinical management of stress reactions of bone in high-performance athletes. Clin Sports Med. 1997;16(2):291–306.
51. Nattiv A, Kennedy G, Barrack MT, et al. Correlation of MRI grading of bone stress injuries with clinical risk factors and return to play: a 5-year prospective study in collegiate track and field athletes. Am J Sports Med. 2013;41(8):1930–41.
52. Beck BR, Bergman AG, Miner M, et al. Tibial stress injury: relationship of radiographic, nuclear medicine bone scanning, MR imaging, and CT severity grades to clinical severity and time to healing. Radiology. 2012;263(3):811–8.
53. Dobrindt O, Hoffmeyer B, Ruf J, et al. Estimation of return-to-sports-time for athletes with stress fracture—an approach combining risk level of fracture site with severity based on imaging. BMC Musculoskelet Disord. 2012;13:139.
54. Wright AA, Taylor JB, Ford KR, Siska L, Smoliga JM. Risk factors associated with lower extremity stress fractures in runners: a systematic review with meta-analysis. Br J Sports Med. 2015;49(23):1517–23.
55. Gan TY, Kuah DE, Graham KS, Markson G. Low-intensity pulsed ultrasound in lower limb bone stress injuries: a randomized controlled trial. Clin J Sport Med. 2014;24(6):457–60.
56. Rue JP, Armstrong DW 3rd, Frassica FJ, Deafenbaugh M, Wilckens JH. The effect of pulsed ultrasound in the treatment of tibial stress fractures. Orthopedics. 2004;27(11):1192–5.
57. Marsell R, Einhorn TA. The biology of fracture healing. Injury. 2011;42(6):551–5.
58. Stevenson S, Emery SE, Goldberg VM. Factors affecting bone graft incorporation. Clin Orthop Relat Res. 1996;324:66–74.
59. Borgeat A, Ofner C, Saporito A, Farshad M, Aguirre J. The effect of nonsteroidal anti-inflammatory drugs on bone healing in humans: a qualitative, systematic review. J Clin Anesth. 2018;49:92–100.
60. Fader L, Whitaker J, Lopez M, et al. Tibia fractures and NSAIDs. Does it make a difference? A multicenter retrospective study. Injury. 2018;49(12):2290–4.
61. Garcia-Martinez O, De Luna-Bertos E, Ramos-Torrecillas J, Manzano-Moreno FJ, Ruiz C. Repercussions of NSAIDS drugs on bone tissue: the osteoblast. Life Sci. 2015;123:72–7.
62. van Esch RW, Kool MM, van As S. NSAIDs can have adverse effects on bone healing. Med Hypotheses. 2013;81:343–6.
63. Wheatley BM, Nappo KE, Christensen DL, Holman AM, Brooks DI, Potter BK. Effect of NSAIDs on bone healing rates: a meta-analysis. J Am Acad Orthop Surg. 2019;27(7):e330–6.
64. Pountos I, Giannoudis PV. Effect of methotrexate on bone and wound healing. Expert Opin Drug Saf. 2017;16(5):535–45.
65. Kates S, Ackert-Bicknell C. How do bisphosphonates affect fracture healing? Injury. 2016;47(Supp 1):S65–8.
66. Li YT, Cai HF, Zhang ZL. Timing of the initiation of bisphosphonates after surgery for fracture healing: a systematic review and meta-analysis of randomized controlled trials. Osteoporos Int. 2015;26(2):431–41.
67. Xue D, Li F, Chen G, Yan S, Pan Z. Do bisphosphonates affect bone healing? A meta-analysis of randomized controlled trials. J Orthop Surg Res. 2014;9:45.
68. van Staa TP, Leufkens HG, Abenhaim L, Zhang B, Cooper C. Use of oral corticosteroids and risk of fractures. J Bone Miner Res. 2000;15(6):993–1000.

Bone Health in Athletes

8

Karen Hind and Jennifer Hamer

8.1 Introduction

Building and maintaining good bone health in the athlete is crucial to longevity of career, protection against bone stress injury and reducing the risk of osteoporosis. Bone health in the athlete should not be taken for granted and while the benefits of regular exercise across the lifespan are well-recognised, there are numerous factors concerning training, nutrition and hormones that need to be considered. High levels of endurance exercise, and participation in sports that emphasise leanness, have been associated with low bone strength, bone loss and elevated bone injury risk in both males and females. Such skeletal problems are often reported in athletes displaying conditions of relative energy deficit in sports (RED-S) and the Female Athlete Triad. Participation in sports that involve high levels of physical contact are associated with fracture risk regardless of bone density. In this chapter, we give an overview of skeletal physiology which provides the basis for understanding how bone responds to loading through exercise, and examine bone strength in athletes from sports with different loading and physical characteristics. We address low bone density and fracture which are issues that the athlete may encounter, often because of relative energy deficit (purposeful or inadvertent), hormonal alterations or overtraining. This chapter concludes with steps for supporting good bone health in the athlete.

K. Hind (✉)
Department of Sport and Exercise Sciences, Durham University, Durham, UK
e-mail: karen.hind@durham.ac.uk

J. Hamer
Griffith University, Queensland, Australia

8.2 Bone Physiology

There are two types of bone tissue—cortical and trabecular, which differ according to structure, function and location. In cortical bone, the structural unit is the Haversian system, which runs the length of the bone, and consists of concentric layers or lamellae. Cortical bone has a high resistance to torque, and has a slow bone turnover rate. It is found on the outer surfaces of most bones and in the shaft of long bones. Trabecular bone has a mesh-like design which allows bone to withstand the sudden stresses that occur through the joints during loading. Bone remodelling takes place predominantly within trabecular bone, which is the main site of bone metabolism. Trabecular bone is more sensitive to hormonal alterations, and bone turnover is faster [1]. This is likely to explain why bone loss in athletes with nutritional or hormonal deficiencies is likely to be first observed at a trabecular-dominant site, such as the lumbar spine [2].

Throughout the lifespan, bone is in a constant state of remodelling through bone resorption and bone formation. The whole remodelling cycle takes approximately 3 months. Bone remodelling is influenced primarily by mechanical stress on the bone, alterations in levels of hormones and the maintenance of normal calcium levels in the extracellular fluid. Following bone resorption, osteoblast cells direct to the resorption pit, and secrete collagen and proteins which result in uncalcified bone tissue, osteiod. Osteoblasts assist with the calcification of the osteoid, involving the secretion of osteocalcin, alkaline phosphatase and osteonectin [3].

Bone turnover is modulated by a wide variety of hormones. Of primary importance to bone health is oestrogen, which is produced by the ovaries in women, and in small amounts by the male testes and adrenal cortex. Oestrogen has an essential role in the development and maintenance of bone strength, exerting positive influences on bone formation and limiting osteoclastic activity. Oestrogen also exerts its influence on bone formation through an increase in pro-inflammatory cytokines. Deficiencies, such as that arising from the menopause,

G. A. J. Robertson, N. Maffulli (eds.), *Fractures in Sport*, https://doi.org/10.1007/978-3-030-72036-0_8

can bring rapid bone loss. Oestrogen deficiency can also occur in young female athletes, who have high training loads and inadequate dietary energy intake, leading to hypothalamic amenorrhoea. Primary hypothalamic amenorrhea is present when a female has not commenced her menstrual cycle by age 16 years. Secondary hypothalamic amenorrhea is present when a female with previously normal menstrual cycles has fewer than three menstrual cycles per year. There are several other hormones, relevant to females, which can influence bone metabolism. Increases in follicle-stimulating hormone (FSH) can impact bone metabolism through osteoclast FSH receptors and FSH increased expression of RANKL [4]. Reductions in testosterone promote osteoclastogenesis and reduce bone formation and calcium absorption. In both men and women, androgens have independent effects on bone development [5].

8.3 Skeletal Loading

Bone adapts to its loading environment, and responds to a wide range of biochemical and physical stimuli. In particular, the musculoskeletal loading sustained during exercise training is a major osteogenic stimulus. The mechanism by which bone adapts to loading is well described in the mechanostat theory [6], which proposes that survival of the skeleton depends on the functional coordination of bone modelling and remodelling, and that, when all else is equal, individuals who are physically active will possess stronger bones than their less active peers. The process by which bone responds to loading occurs via the osteocyte bone cells and through plasma membrane disruption [7]. The movement of interstitial fluid produces shear stress on osteocyte cell membrane, instigating mechanotransduction [8]. Osteocytes respond through calcium signalling to the bone cells [9]. Loading of bone also increases bone formation through regulation of osteoprogeterin, which suppresses the resorptive activity of osteoclasts [10].

The key components of an optimal exercise programme for bone strength have been identified through animal studies. Dynamic rather than static loads, high strain magnitudes, high strain rates, rapid strain reversal, and unusual frequency distributions provide optimal osteogenic stimuli [11, 12]. The duration of load and the number of loading cycles appear to be of minor importance, whereas rest periods bring a positive role [13]. In humans, exercise that mimics the loading patterns identified in animal studies have been successful in increasing bone health. For instance, jumping movements are particularly efficacious for improving femoral bone strength, especially if undertaken as short-discrete bouts [14, 15]. In contrast, walking brings about relatively modest improvements in bone health [16], likely reflecting the habituation and desensitisation to the continuous loading and repetitive nature of these activities.

8.4 Bone Strength in Athletes

High impact and multidirectional loading is important for bone strength, and athletes from sports such as rugby, soccer, volleyball and hockey have greater bone density than those who participate in non-impact or repetitive endurance sports, such as swimming and cycling [17, 18]. For cyclists in particular, the deficits can be significant, with an increased risk for osteoporosis. The skeletal response to loading is localised to the focus of strain. This localisation can be seen through the greater bone strength in the dominant versus nondominant forearms of racquet sports' players [19, 20], the increased bone strength in the upper body of gymnasts [21], and the greater lower limb bone density compared to the spine in long-distance runners [2]. Furthermore, interesting comparisons in loading distribution can be made between runners and field-based athletes. Distance running generates a pattern of repetitive loading in one direction with moderately high ground reaction forces, and loading of the foot and leg in a repetitive manner, which may provide lower body site-specific benefits, but not overall total body benefits to bone strength [22]. In field sports, greater ground reaction forces are produced and applied in multiple directions during jumping, starting and stopping. For example, rugby and soccer players are exposed to high intensity intermittent activities including sprinting, jumping and transverse and torsional loads, all of which are beneficial for bone strength [23]. As well as gravitational loading, significant forces are applied to bone from localised muscle.

8.5 Low Energy Availability and Bone Health in Athletes

Low energy availability (LEA) or relative energy deficit occurs when there is a failure to match calorific energy intake with exercise energy expenditure. Situations of LEA can arise unintentionally when an athlete is unaware of the energy requirements to fuel training or are unable to consume enough energy to support a high volume training load. Alternatively, LEA can also occur intentionally with a goal to optimise body size and composition for competitive success. Some athletes may also show signs of disordered eating including fasting, skipping meals, avoiding certain food groups, purging, using laxatives and diet pills [24, 25].

Energy deficit can negatively affect bone health in both male and female athletes, associated with bone loss and bone injury. Several well controlled trials inducing short term LEA demonstrate unfavourable alterations to bone turnover, in both male and female athletes [26]. The Female Athlete Triad and the Relative Energy Deficiency (RED-S) models both describe the interrelationship between LEA and bone health in athletes. The Female Athlete Triad consists of three interrelated components: LEA with or without disordered eating, menstrual dysfunction and low bone mineral density [27]. The RED-S model expands on the Triad model, acknowledging that male athletes and athletes with a disability are also affected [28]. RED-S also describes sports performance risks such as reduced training response, impaired judgement, decreased coordination and concentration [28].

In females, when energy availability [energy intake (kcal) − exercise energy expenditure (kcal)/fat free mass (FFM, kg)] falls below 30 kcal/kg FFM/day, perturbation of reproductive function and bone metabolism occurs [26]. This suppression in reproductive function presents in female athletes as functional hypothalamic amenorrhea (FHA), whereby there is the loss of menses without any identifiable organic cause [29]. FHA manifests with a downregulation of the hypothalamic pituitary ovarian axis, causing an inhibition of gonadotropin realising hormone and abnormal secretions of follicle stimulating hormone and luteinizing hormone, resulting in a decreased production of oestradiol and progesterone. Athletes with longstanding functional hypothalamic amenorrhoea benefit less from the osteogenic effects of exercise [30, 31]. Even subtle alterations in the oestrogen/progesterone imbalance (e.g., regular menstruation but alterations in luteinising hormone), as seen in subclinical ovulatory disturbances, may adversely impact bone, particularly at trabecular-bone-dominant sites, such as the spine [32]. In male athletes, the reproductive hormones can also be negatively impacted and indicated through reductions in testosterone and other metabolic hormones [33].

Additional endocrine disturbances arise from LEA, including hypercortisolaemia, growth hormone resistance, reductions in insulin-like growth factor-1 (IGF-1) and suppressed 3,5,3 triiodothyronine (TT_3) [34]. Each influence bone turnover; for example, hypercortisolaemia limits osteoblastic function and increases bone resorption [35], while reductions in IGF-1 limit the activity of osteoblasts and bone collagen synthesis [36]. Notably, in studies where an energy deficit has been experimentally induced in exercising females, significant reductions in IGF-1 and TT_3, with corresponding reductions in bone formation, have been demonstrated, indicating direct effects of low energy availability on bone metabolism [26]. Prolonged LEA also disrupts the body's nitrogen balance [34], which can lead to further negative effects on skeletal integrity through a loss of muscle mass and muscle strength. The long-term effects of LEA and negated bone strength during an athletic career are unclear. Several studies have reported bone loss is not reversible, thereby increasing risk of osteoporosis and fragility fracture [37]. Although recovery of bone density through weight gain and resumption of menses has been demonstrated, this may be limited to the years of peak bone mass accrual, up to the age of around 30 years [38].

8.6 Bone Stress Injury and Fracture

Stress fractures are common athletic injuries arising from repetitive skeletal loading which causes the physical breakdown of bone microstructure. Excessive running or jumping, together with additional factors such as LEA, hormone deficiencies, or decreased sun exposure (vitamin D), may increase an athlete's risk for sustaining this overuse injury [33, 39, 40]. Amenorrhoeic female athletes are two to four times more likely to sustain a stress fracture than menstruating athletes [33, 41]. Similarly, male athletes with LEA and suppressed testosterone levels are over four times more likely to sustain a stress fracture, compared with athletes in adequate energy availability [33]. The bone stress injuries can be severe, and there have been case reports of displaced femoral neck fractures in amenorrhoeic female long-distance runners [42]. High volume training can also increase the risk of stress fracture, if the increase in volume does not follow an appropriate progression, with sufficient periods of recovery [43].

While stress fractures are a major indicator of low bone strength, this is not the case for athletes in weight-assisted sports such as cycling. In cycling, most fractures are traumatic, for example from a bike crash. Amongst professional cyclists, traumatic fractures are the most commonly reported injury, with vertebral fracture requiring the longest time off training. In one study of 50 elite male cyclists, 2 cyclists had previously experienced a fracture to the spine requiring internal fixation and bone grafting. Another cyclist reported a pelvic fracture after commencing running training. This cyclist also had signs of chronic LEA and osteoporosis that had not previously been identified (lumbar spine Z score −3.2), suggesting that this cyclist had sustained a fragility fracture [44].

8.7 Management of Bone Health in the Athlete

Athletes suffering a fracture or suspected LEA require early intervention given the risk to long term bone health and continued interruptions to training, which in severe cases, might end an athlete's career. A multidisciplinary team approach is recommended: this may include a sports clinician, dietician, physiologist and psychologist, and the primary goal should be to increase energy availability, and in female athletes, to restore menstrual function [28].

8.7.1 Bone Health Assessment

If an athlete has sustained a bone stress injury/fracture and/or is displaying signs of LEA, and/or menstrual disturbances, a bone density assessment is indicated. The most widely used and universally recognised method for bone health assessment is dual energy X-ray absorptiometry (DXA). This method provides a highly precise measurement of bone mineral density (BMD) [45, 46], and uses low iodising radiation with bone density evaluations typically equivalent to, or less, than 2 days of natural background radiation. A bone density assessment by DXA usually includes scans of both the lumbar spine and total hip, with each scan only taking several minutes. The Z-score measures the deviation from mean age-, sex- and race-matched values, while the T-score measures deviation from mean sex- and race-matched values in a young adult population. The threshold for diagnosis indicates the level of fracture risk. In postmenopausal females and males aged over 50 years, osteoporosis is defined as a BMD T-score that is −2.5 or less, and osteopenia as a BMD T-score that is between −1.0 and −2.4 [47]. In those aged under 50 years, low BMD is identified as a Z-score that is equal to or less than −2.0, although −1.0 might be a more useful threshold of suboptimum BMD for male and female athletes, who require stronger bones for repetitive or higher impact activities. In agreement, the International Olympic Committee consensus statement on RED-S recommends that an athlete with a BMD Z-score of less than −1.0 requires a treatment plan if they are to continue training, due to increased injury risk [28]. The definitions of osteoporosis and low BMD for age, are further described in the official Positions of the International Society of Clinical Densitometry [48].

8.7.2 Nutrition

Bone formation is suppressed when energy availability falls below 30 kcal/kg FFM/day [26], and a target of 45 kcal/kg FFM/day is recommended for athletes [27]. Athletes should avoid fasted training at high intensities to minimise the risk of negative skeletal effects. Some elite athletes may be involved in small amounts of fasted training or participate in training with low carbohydrate availability to enhance the utilisation of fat as a fuel source. This approach generally is appropriate for low intensity training sessions [49]. If an athlete has a history of disordered eating, RED-S or low BMD, this practice should be avoided.

There are several further nutritional considerations for athlete bone health. Protein supports muscle protein synthesis and there is some evidence for benefits to bone strength [50]. This is potentially through an effect from leucine, which stimulates insulin secretion and the production of IGF-1 promoting osteoblast function [51]. Current data supports the intake of 1.2–2 g/kg/day of protein for athletes involved in heavy training, which is higher than the 0.8 g/kg/day recommended for the general population. There is little evidence to suggest that higher protein intakes will have harmful effects on bone health. However, it is advisable that athletes ensure they maintain adequate calcium intakes during periods of high protein intake [52]. Calcium is vital for growth, maintenance and repair of bone tissue and regulation of muscle contraction. Athletes are advised to consume 1500 mg of calcium/day to support bone health [28]. Vitamin D regulates serum calcium and has been demonstrated to affect bone mineralisation, thus making it essential for skeletal strength and adaptation to mechanical stress. Vitamin D insufficiency is diagnosed at levels of 50–75 nmol/L, and a deficiency is diagnosed when levels drop to <50 nmol/L. Athletes are at risk for vitamin D deficiency, particularly over winter months, and in such scenarios, supplementation of 1500–2000 IU/day of vitamin D is recommended [52].

8.7.3 Resistance Exercise

An athlete's training programme can include small modifications to promote bone strength, namely through the inclusion of resistance exercise, which develops whole body muscle and bone strength. Studies have shown that regular strength training is associated with higher BMD in female distance runners, regardless of amenorrhoea [2]. In intervention studies, improved BMD in premenopausal women and prematurely menopausal women have been reported following resistance training interventions [53, 54]. In male high-performance cyclists with low BMD, regular skeletal loading exercises such as Pilates, was associated with significant increases in BMD over a 6 month intervention period [55]. For athletes who specialise in sports associated with lower BMD, it is advisable to incorporate high impact loading and resistance training into their programme 2–3 days per week, to provide the stimulus required to support bone health [28].

8.7.4 Hormone Therapy

In female amenorrheic athletes, hormone interventions can be considered as an adjunct, alongside increasing energy availability [56]. The oral contraceptive pill can regulate or manipulate menses and associated symptoms, but does not provide protection to bone strength in amenorrheic women. The combined oral contraceptive (OC) pill has been found to have no beneficial effect on bone density [57, 58], and there have also been several reports of lower bone density in OC users compared to those who do not use the OC pill [59, 60]. There is also some evidence that OCs might lower the set-point for skeletal mechanical adaptation as a result of exercise [61, 62]. Progesterone-only contraception, in particular Depot Medroxyprogesterone Acetate (DMPA), also known as DepoProvera®, can decrease bone density, especially with long term use [63, 64]. Furthermore, the findings of a recent systematic review and meta-analysis do not support oestrogen therapy as a treatment for low BMD in premenopausal women with functional hypothalamic amenorrhea [65]. The primary approach should be to resolve the underlying issue of LEA. This will involve increases in energy intake, reduction in training load and increased recovery periods, ultimately leading to a restoration of hormone function [66].

8.8 Summary

- Bone responds to its loading environment—gravitational and impact loading, as well as muscle forces provide osteogenic stimulus.
- Athletes should ensure that energy needs are well balanced with sufficient energy intake to support bone health.
- RED-S brings about negative consequences for bone strength and therefore athletes, their coaches and support teams, should recognise signs and seek positive interventions.
- Small modifications to an athlete's training programme can increase osteogenic loading, for example, whole body resistance exercise.

References

1. Beerthuizen R, van Beek A, Massai R, Mäkäräinen L, Hout JIT, Bennink HC. Bone mineral density during long-term use of the progestagen contraceptive implant Implanon® compared to a non-hormonal method of contraception. Hum Reprod. 2000;15(1):118–22.
2. Hind K, Truscott JG, Evans JA. Low lumbar spine bone mineral density in both male and female endurance runners. Bone. 2006;39(4):880–5.
3. Florencio-Silva R, Sasso GRDS, Sasso-Cerri E, Simões MJ, Cerri PS. Biology of bone tissue: structure, function, and factors that influence bone cells. BioMed Res Int. 2015;2015:421746.
4. Colaianni G, Cuscito C, Colucci S. FSH and TSH in the regulation of bone mass: the pituitary/immune/bone axis. Clin Dev Immunol. 2013;2013:382698.
5. Manolagas SC, O'Brien CA, Almeida M. The role of estrogen and androgen receptors in bone health and disease. Nat Rev Endocrinol. 2013;9(12):699.
6. Frost H. Bone "mass" and the "mechanostat": a proposal. Anat Rec. 1987;219(1):1–9.
7. Yu K, Sellman DP, Bahraini A, Hagan ML, Elsherbini A, Vanpelt KT, Marshall PL, Hamrick MW, McNeil A, McNeil PL, McGee-Lawrence ME. Mechanical loading disrupts osteocyte plasma membranes which initiates mechanosensation events in bone. J Orthop Res. 2018;36(2):653–62.
8. Robling AG, Turner CH. Mechanical signaling for bone modeling and remodeling. Crit Rev Eukaryot Gene Exp. 2009;19(4):319.
9. Marques EA, Mota J, Viana JL, Tuna D, Figueiredo P, Guimarães JT, Carvalho J. Response of bone mineral density, inflammatory cytokines, and biochemical bone markers to a 32-week combined loading exercise programme in older men and women. Arch Gerontol Geriatr. 2013;57(2):226–33.
10. Galea GL, Lanyon LE, Price JS. Sclerostin's role in bone's adaptive response to mechanical loading. Bone. 2017;96:38–44.
11. Ehrlich PJ, Lanyon LE. Mechanical strain and bone cell function: a review. Osteoporos Int. 2002;13(9):688–700.
12. Rubin CT, Sommerfeldt DW, Judex S, Qin YX. Inhibition of osteopenia by low magnitude, high-frequency mechanical stimuli. Drug Discov Today. 2001;6(16):848–58.
13. Robling AG, Burr DB, Turner CH. Partitioning a daily mechanical stimulus into discrete loading bouts improves the osteogenic response to loading. J Bone Miner Res. 2000;15(8):1596–602.
14. Martyn-St James M, Carroll S. Effects of different impact exercise modalities on bone mineral density in premenopausal women: a meta-analysis. J Bone Miner Metab. 2010;28(3):251–67.
15. Zhao R, Zhao M, Zhang L. Efficiency of jumping exercise in improving bone mineral density among premenopausal women: a meta-analysis. Sports Med. 2014;44(10):1393–402.
16. Martyn-St James M, Carroll S. Meta-analysis of walking for preservation of bone mineral density in postmenopausal women. Bone. 2008;43(3):521–31.
17. Hind K, Gannon L, Whatley E, Cooke C, Truscott J. Bone cross-sectional geometry in male runners, gymnasts, swimmers and non-athletic controls: a hip-structural analysis study. Eur J Appl Physiol. 2012;112(2):535–41.
18. Tenforde AS, Fredericson M. Influence of sports participation on bone health in the young athlete: a review of the literature. PM&R. 2011;3(9):861–7.
19. Ducher G, Tournaire N, Meddahi-Pellé A, Benhamou CL, Courteix D. Short-term and long-term site-specific effects of tennis playing on trabecular and cortical bone at the distal radius. J Bone Miner Metab. 2006;24(6):484–90.
20. Kontulainen S, Sievänen H, Kannus P, Pasanen M, Vuori I. Effect of long-term impact-loading on mass, size, and estimated strength of humerus and radius of female racquet-sports players: a peripheral quantitative computed tomography study between young and old starters and controls. J Bone Miner Res. 2003;18(2):352–9.
21. Burt LA, Greene DA, Ducher G, Naughton GA. Skeletal adaptations associated with pre-pubertal gymnastics participation as determined by DXA and pQCT: a systematic review and meta-analysis. J Sci Med Sport. 2013;16(3):231–9.
22. Fredericson M, Chew K, Ngo J, Cleek T, Kiratli J, Cobb K. Regional bone mineral density in male athletes: a comparison of soccer players, runners and controls. Br J Sports Med. 2007;41(10):664–8.
23. Robling AG, Hinant FM, Burr DB, Turner CH. Shorter, more frequent mechanical loading sessions enhance bone mass. Med Sci Sports Exerc. 2002;34(2):196–202.
24. Manore MM, Kam LC, Loucks AB. The female athlete triad: components, nutrition issues, and health consequences. J Sports Sci. 2007;25(S1):S61–71.

25. Melin AK, Heikura IA, Tenforde A, Mountjoy M. Energy availability in athletics: health, performance, and physique. Int J Sport Nutr Exerc Metab. 2019;29(2):152–64.
26. Ihle R, Loucks AB. Dose-response relationships between energy availability and bone turnover in young exercising women. J Bone Miner Res. 2004;19(8):1231–40.
27. De Souza MJ, Nattiv A, Joy E, Misra M, Williams NI, Mallinson RJ, Gibbs JC, Olmsted M, Goolsby M, Matheson G, Female Athlete Triad Coalition, American College of Sports Medicine, American Medical Society for Sports Medicine, American Bone Health Alliance. 2014 Female Athlete Triad Coalition consensus statement on treatment and return to play of the female athlete triad: 1st International Conference held in San Francisco, CA, May 2012, and 2nd International Conference held in Indianapolis, IN, May 2013. Clin J Sport Med. 2014;24(2):96–119.
28. Mountjoy M, Sundgot-Borgen J, Burke L, Carter S, Constantini N, Lebrun C, Meyer N, Sherman R, Steffen K, Budgett R, Ljungqvist A. The IOC consensus statement: beyond the female athlete triad—relative energy deficiency in sport (RED-S). Br J Sports Med. 2014;48(7):491–7.
29. Gordon CM, Ackerman KE, Berga SL, Kaplan JR, Mastorakos G, Misra M, Murad MH, Santoro NF, Warren MP. Functional hypothalamic amenorrhea: an endocrine society clinical practice guideline. J Clin Endocrinol Metabol. 2017;102(5):1413–39.
30. Ackerman KE, Putman M, Guereca G, Taylor AP, Pierce L, Herzog DB, Klibanski A, Bouxsein M, Misra M. Cortical microstructure and estimated bone strength in young amenorrheic athletes, eumenorrheic athletes and non-athletes. Bone. 2012;51(4):680–7.
31. Bonis M, Loftin M, Speaker R, Kontos A. Body composition of elite, eumenorrheic and amenorrheic, adolescent cross-country runners. Pediatr Exerc Sci. 2009;21(3):318–28.
32. Li D, Hitchcock CL, Barr SI, Yu T, Prior JC. Negative spinal bone mineral density changes and subclinical ovulatory disturbances—prospective data in healthy premenopausal women with regular menstrual cycles. Epidemiol Rev. 2014;36(1):137–47.
33. Heikura IA, Uusitalo AL, Stellingwerff T, Bergland D, Mero AA, Burke LM. Low energy availability is difficult to assess but outcomes have large impact on bone injury rates in elite distance athletes. Int J Sport Nutr Exerc Metab. 2018;28(4):403–11.
34. Zanker CL, Cooke CB. Energy balance, bone turnover, and skeletal health in physically active individuals. Med Sci Sports Exerc. 2004;36(8):1372–81.
35. Bressot C, Meunier P, Chapuy M, Lejeune E, Edouard C, Darby A. Histomorphometric profile, pathophysiology and reversibility of corticosteroid-induced osteoporosis. Metab Bone Dis Relat Res. 1979;1(4):303–11.
36. Yakar S, Rosen CJ, Beamer WG, Ackert-Bicknell CL, Wu Y, Liu J-L, et al. Circulating levels of IGF-1 directly regulate bone growth and density. J Clin Investig. 2002;110(6):771–81.
37. Keen AD, Drinkwater BL. Irreversible bone loss in former amenorrheic athletes. Osteoporos Int. 1997;7:311–5.
38. Hind K, Zanker C, Truscott J. Five-year follow-up investigation of bone mineral density by age in premenopausal elite-level long-distance runners. Clin J Sport Med. 2011;21(6):521–9.
39. Barrack MT, Gibbs JC, De Souza MJ, Williams NI, Nichols JF, Rauh MJ, Nattiv A. Higher incidence of bone stress injuries with increasing female athlete triad–related risk factors: a prospective multisite study of exercising girls and women. Am J Sports Med. 2014;42(4):949–58.
40. Tenforde AS, Carlson JL, Chang A, Sainani KL, Shultz R, Kim JH, Cutti P, Golden NH, Fredericson M. Association of the female athlete triad risk assessment stratification to the development of bone stress injuries in collegiate athletes. Am J Sports Med. 2017;45(2):302–10.
41. Nattiv A. Stress fractures and bone health in track and field athletes. J Sci Med Sport. 2000;3(3):268–79.
42. Okamoto S, Arai Y, Hara K, Tsuzihara T, Kubo T. A displaced stress fracture of the femoral neck in an adolescent female distance runner with female athlete triad: a case report. BMC Sports Sci Med Rehabil. 2010;2(1):6.
43. Fredericson M, Jennings F, Beaulieu C, Matheson GO. Stress fractures in athletes. Top Magn Reson Imaging. 2006;17(5):309–25.
44. Keay N, Francis G, Hind K. Low energy availability assessed by a sport-specific questionnaire and clinical interview indicative of bone health, endocrine profile and cycling performance in competitive male cyclists. BMJ open sport & exercise medicine. 2018;4(1):p.e000424.
45. Carey JJ, Delaney MF. Utility of DXA for monitoring, technical aspects of DXA BMD measurement and precision testing. Bone. 2017;104:44–53.
46. Hind K, Oldroyd B, Truscott JG. In vivo precision of the GE Lunar iDXA densitometer for the measurement of total-body, lumbar spine, and femoral bone mineral density in adults. J Clin Densitom. 2010;13(4):413–7.
47. Kanis JA, Kanis JA. Assessment of fracture risk and its application to screening for postmenopausal osteoporosis: synopsis of a WHO report. Osteoporos Int. 1994;4(6):368–81.
48. Schousboe JT, Shepherd JA, Bilezikian JP, Baim S. Executive summary of the 2013 International Society for Clinical Densitometry Position Development Conference on bone densitometry. J Clin Densitom. 2013;16(4):455–66.
49. Burke LM, Jeukendrup AE, Jones AM, Mooses M. Contemporary nutrition strategies to optimize performance in distance runners and race walkers. Int J Sport Nutr Exerc Metab. 2019;29(2):117–29.
50. Ispoglou T, White H, Preston T, McElhone S, McKenna J, Hind K. Double-blind, placebo-controlled pilot trial of L-Leucine-enriched amino-acid mixtures on body composition and physical performance in men and women aged 65–75 years. Eur J Clin Nutr. 2016;70(2):182–8.
51. Yang J, Zhang X, Wang W, Liu J. Insulin stimulates osteoblast proliferation and differentiation through ERK and PI3K in MG-63 cells. Cell Biochem Funct. 2010;28(4):334–41.
52. Sale C, Elliott-Sale KJ. Nutrition and athlete bone health. Sports Med. 2019;49(Suppl 2):139–51.
53. Watson SL, Weeks BK, Weis LJ, Harding AT, Horan SA, Beck BR. High-intensity resistance and impact training improves bone mineral density and physical function in postmenopausal women with osteopenia and osteoporosis: the LIFTMOR randomized controlled trial. J Bone Miner Res. 2018;33(2):211–20.
54. Winters-Stone KM, Dobek J, Nail LM, Bennett JA, Leo MC, Torgrimson-Ojerio B, et al. Impact + resistance training improves bone health and body composition in prematurely menopausal breast cancer survivors: a randomized controlled trial. Osteoporos Int. 2013;24(5):1637–46.
55. Keay N, Francis G, Entwistle I, Hind K. Clinical evaluation of education relating to nutrition and skeletal loading in competitive male road cyclists at risk of relative energy deficiency in sports (RED-S): 6-month randomised controlled trial. BMJ open sport & exercise medicine. 2019;5(1):p.e000523.
56. Kandemir N, Slattery M, Ackerman KE, Tulsiani S, Bose A, Singhal V, Baskaran C, Ebrahimi S, Goldstein M, Eddy K, Klibanski A, Misra M. Bone parameters in anorexia nervosa and athletic amenorrhea: comparison of two hypothalamic amenorrhea states. J Clin Endocrinol Metab. 2018;103(6):2392–402.
57. Hind K, Truscott J, Carroll S. Case report: female athlete triad in monozygotic twins. Phys Sportsmed. 2008;36(1):119–24.

58. Nappi C, Bifulco G, Tommaselli GA, Gargano V, Di Carlo C. Hormonal contraception and bone metabolism: a systematic review. Contraception. 2012;86(6):606–21.
59. Hartard M, Kleinmond C, Wiseman M, Weissenbacher ER, Felsenberg D, Erben RG. Detrimental effect of oral contraceptives on parameters of bone mass and geometry in a cohort of 248 young women. Bone. 2007;40(2):444–50.
60. Prior JC, Kirkland SA, Joseph L, Kreiger N, Murray TM, Hanley DA, et al. Oral contraceptive use and bone mineral density in premenopausal women: cross-sectional, population-based data from the Canadian Multicentre Osteoporosis Study. Can Med Assoc J. 2001;165(8):1023–9.
61. Hartard M, Bottermann P, Bartenstein P, Jeschke D, Schwaiger M. Effects on bone mineral density of low-dose oral contraceptives compared to and combined with physical activity. Contraception. 1997;55:87–90.
62. Weaver CM, Teegarden D, Lyle RM, McCabe GP, McCabe LD, Proulx W, et al. Impact of exercise on bone health and contraindication of oral contraceptive use in young women. Med Sci Sports Exerc. 2001;33(6):873–80.
63. Curtis KM, Martins SL. Progestogene-only contraception and bone mineral density: a systematic review. Contraception. 2006;73:470–87.
64. Shaarawy M, El-Mallah SY, Seoudi S, Hassan M, Mohsen IA. Effects of the long-term use of depot medroxyprogesterone acetate as hormonal contraceptive on bone mineral density and biochemical markers of bone remodeling. Contraception. 2006;74(4):297–302.
65. Aalberg K, Stavem K, Norheim F, Russell MB, Chaibi A. Effect of oral and transdermal oestrogen therapy on bone mineral density in functional hypothalamic amenorrhoea: a systematic review and meta-analysis. BMJ Open Sport & Exercise Medicine. 2021;7(3):p. e001112.
66. Keay N. What's so good about menstrual cycles. BJSM. 2018. https://blogs.bmj.com/bjsm/2019/02/08/whats-so-good-about-menstrual-cycles/. Last accessed 4 Jun 2019

Part II

Acute Fractures in Sport: Upper Limb

Acute Fractures in Sport: Shoulder

9

Iain D. M. Brown, Samuel P. Mackenzie, William M. Oliver, Jamie A. Nicholson, and Oisin J. F. Keenan

Learning Objectives

- Contrast the different types of clavicle fracture and the rationale for operative treatment.
- Appreciate the spectrum of injuries to the acromioclavicular joint, and how this guides their management.
- Understand the pathoanatomy of glenohumeral dislocation.
- Appreciate the indications for surgical fixation of a greater tuberosity fracture.
- Recall the absolute and relative indications for primary operative fixation of humeral shaft fractures.

9.1 Clavicle Fractures

9.1.1 Epidemiology

Clavicle fractures account for 35% of shoulder girdle injuries and 4% of all fractures in adults [1, 2]. There is a bimodal distribution of injuries with the majority of injuries sustained in young males, and a smaller proportion in the elderly [1]. The incidence has increased over the last decade, corresponding with the popularity of cycling [3, 4].

9.1.2 Classification

The Edinburgh classification, developed by Robinson *et al.*, is commonly used and based on fracture location (1-medial, 2-middle and 3-lateral) followed by displacement (A-undisplaced or B-displaced). The final number reflects each fracture sub-type [1].

- ***Type 1: Medial fractures*** are uncommon (5%). A peculiarity of this bony region is the late fusion of the growth plate (between 23 and 26 years of age). As a result, a physeal disruption can occur, even in early adulthood.
- ***Type 2: Midshaft fractures*** are the most common (80%) and the main focus of this chapter.
- ***Type 3: Lateral-end fractures*** (15%) share a spectrum of soft tissue injury with acromioclavicular joint disruption. In displaced fractures, there is often avulsion of the coracoclavicular ligaments, which results in instability and a high incidence of nonunion if treated non-operatively.

9.1.3 Diagnosis

Patients will typically present following a direct blow to the shoulder during contact sport or a fall. Swelling, crepitus at the fracture site and inability to move the shoulder are typical presenting features [5]. Skin tenting is relatively common as the sternocleidomastoid pulls the medial portion of a midshaft fracture superiorly. True skin compromise and breakdown is rare. If the skin is not blanched and has normal capillary refill, it is not considered to be under threat. Occasionally puncture wounds in the dermis can occur resulting in an open fracture. Continuous venous ooze (the expressed fracture haematoma) or exposed fat at the base of wound are typical features. If suspected, the patient should be provided with immediate intravenous antibiotics, the consideration of tetanus booster and referral to an orthopaedic surgeon. Careful consideration should be given to associated chest or other serious traumatic injuries as a high incidence is reported with open clavicle fractures [6].

An anteroposterior radiograph of the shoulder or clavicle is sufficient to make a diagnosis. Upright radiographs may indicate displacement more accurately [7]. A modified axial view will demonstrate posterior displacement, which is often

I. D. M. Brown (✉) · S. P. Mackenzie · W. M. Oliver
Edinburgh Orthopaedics, The Royal Infirmary of Edinburgh, Edinburgh, UK

J. A. Nicholson
Trauma and Orthopaedic Surgery, University of Edinburgh, Edinburgh, UK

O. J. F. Keenan
Edinburgh Orthopaedic Trauma Unit, Edinburgh, UK

G. A. J. Robertson, N. Maffulli (eds.), *Fractures in Sport*, https://doi.org/10.1007/978-3-030-72036-0_9

underappreciated in injures involving the lateral-third. Assessment of displacement and shortening is not possible on plain radiographs due to variation in beam angle and patient position between films [8]. Computed tomography (CT) is superior but is reserved for complex fracture or cases of nonunion [9]. Medial fractures are difficult to visualize on plain radiographs, and may be confused with physeal injuries or sternoclavicular dislocations. A CT is recommended if there is clinical suspicion [10].

9.1.4 Treatment

9.1.4.1 Emergency Department

Closed reduction will not improve the deformity and is contraindicated. The arm should be immobilized in a broad arm sling and referred to a fracture clinic. Figure of eight bandaging/bracing is uncomfortable and does not reduce the risk of malunion or nonunion [11]. Patients are encouraged to attain a normal range of elbow movement at the earliest opportunity. The sling can be discarded when pain allows (usually within 2 weeks).

9.1.4.2 Surgical Decision-Making

The decision to perform surgical fixation of clavicle injures is based largely on fracture configuration and displacement. Consideration needs to be given to the inherent risk of nonunion associated with the fracture pattern. Nonunion carries significant morbidity in clavicle fractures and usually mandates delayed fixation; this is best avoided where possible in the athlete. The need for accelerated rehabilitation and potential malunion risk are perhaps even more relevant in the athletic population. The effect of shortening and malunion is, however, contentious: With respect to midshaft fractures, it is unclear whether this significantly affects long-term shoulder performance.

When operative fixation is undertaken there is good evidence for plate fixation, which appears to be superior to intramedullary techniques. Occasionally supplementary coraco-clavicular fixation is needed for lateral-end fractures. We will consider each fracture configuration respectively in this section with regards to the treatment and benefit.

9.1.4.3 Midshaft Fractures

Undisplaced fractures (2A1) heal without intervention and are expected to have an excellent outcome [11]. Displaced (2B) or angulated (2A2) fractures in skeletally immature adults (under 16 years of age) should be managed non-operatively, as nonunion is exceptionally rare (<1%) and there is excellent remodelling and recovery potential [12–14].

Optimal treatment of completely displaced midshaft fractures (2B) in adults is contentious and has been subject of extensive investigation. Symptomatic nonunion occurs in approximately 12% of cases following nonoperative management; acute plate fixation reduces this to less than 3% [15–17]. However, it is accepted that athletes are more likely to be younger and non-smokers, and therefore the nonunion risk with non-operative management is likely to be lower in reality. A degree of malunion is to be expected after non-operative management of a displaced midshaft fracture. Although scapulothoracic kinematics are subtly altered by a malunion [18], convincing evidence of a significant deleterious effect on shoulder function has not been proven [19–21]. It is unclear from the current literature whether high-level athletes would be more susceptible to functional impairment as a result of malunion. Beyond the reduction of nonunion risk, plate fixation allows the earlier return of shoulder function which may be advantageous to athletes particularly in the first 3 month following injury [22–24]. Even if better reduction can be achieved with operative management, long-term shoulder function is likely be excellent, regardless of treatment, provided union occurs [15].

If a patient is undecided on operative management and there is time for some rehabilitation before competition, an alternative option is delayed fixation. When surgery is performed in the first 3–12 weeks following injury it appears to have a similar risk profile to acute fixation [25–27]. Additionally, a lack of early functional recovery at 6 weeks post-injury (defined by a combination of QuickDASH score above 40, fracture mobility on exam and no callus on radiograph) appears to be a strong predictor of nonunion following non-operative management, and may avoid a prolonged delay to diagnosis [28]. When fixation is undertaken in skeletally mature adults, open reduction and internal fixation with an anatomic contoured site-specific plate has a large evidence-base, and is the technique of choice. Although minimally invasive techniques have been described using intramedullary nail devices [29], they are associated with an increased risk of major complications and nonunion [30].

9.1.4.4 Lateral-Third Fractures

Fractures with cortical alignment (3A1 and 3A2) should be managed conservatively. Clinical examination and axial radiograph should be undertaken to ensure posterior displacement is not under-appreciated. Displaced lateral fractures (3B1 and 3B2) have a significant nonunion rate, and therefore primary operative fixation should be considered. Although the hook plate is the historical implant of choice in many centres, this can cause irritation to the rotator cuff and requires a secondary removal procedure. More recently, pre-contoured site-specific locking plates have been employed in an attempt to optimise fixation of the small lateral segment (Fig. 9.1). Suspensory ligament techniques, which anchor the medial segment to the coracoid, can be used in isolation in the case of a very small lateral segment, or in conjunction with a locking plate (Fig. 9.2) [31, 32].

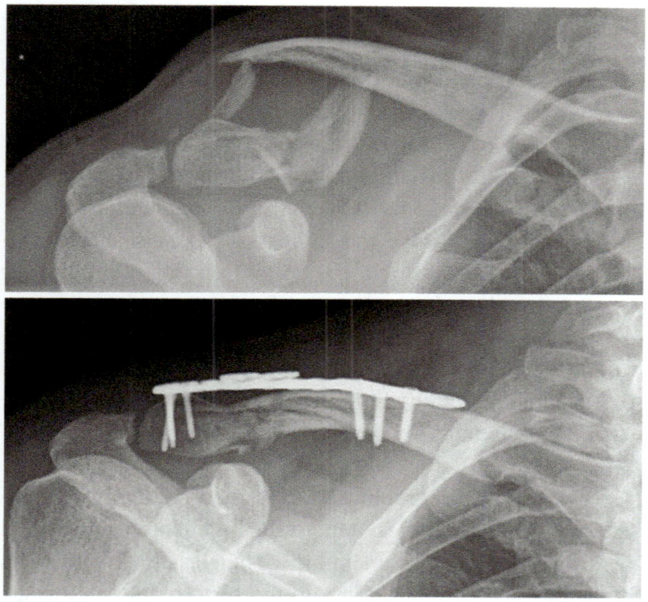

Fig. 9.1 Lateral end clavicle fracture with comminution, stabilised with a lateral end plate with coraco-clavicular sling

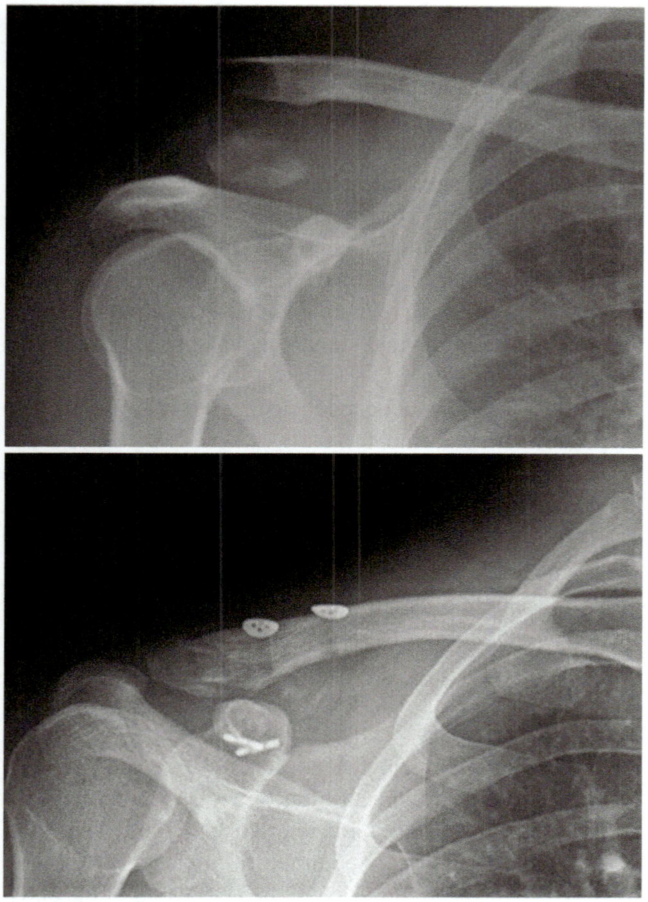

Fig. 9.2 Lateral end clavicle fracture stabilised with a suspensory ligament technique

9.1.4.5 Medial-Third Fractures

Medial third-fractures are rare in athletes. Caution should be taken when diagnosing pain around the medial clavicle as this may indicate sternoclavicular joint dislocation or transphyseal injury. If posterior displacement is suspected this requires urgent advanced cross sectional imaging (normally CT) and Orthopaedic consultation [10] [11].

There is little evidence to guide treatment of these injuries. Probably only posteriorly displaced fractures with no cortical contact (1B1 and 1B2), akin to a SCJ dislocation, mandate surgical action. If there is adequate bone stock, fixation could be with a conventional clavicle contoured plate. However, in the context of comminution or transphyseal fracture, with little medial bone stock for screw purchase, a soft tissue reconstruction (e.g. figure of 8 hamstring allograft) may be required. Such cases should be performed by Orthopaedic surgeons with experience operating in this anatomical region, or with the assistance of a Cardiothoracic specialist.

9.1.5 Rehabilitation

Most randomized trials adopt a similar approach to clavicle fracture rehabilitation regardless of the treatment chosen:

- Sling for 2–3 weeks, followed by active strengthening and mobilisation with physiotherapy.
- Full contact and return to play from 3 months [33–36], however earlier return has been reported in professional athletes at 6 weeks without an increase in complications [37].

9.1.5.1 Evidence for Return to Function

Following an undisplaced midshaft fracture, 95% of athletes can be expected to return to normal activity in a mean of 10.6 weeks. Patients with a displaced midshaft fractures return to sport quicker after operative management (9.3 weeks) when compared to non-operative management (21.5 weeks) [33, 34, 38]. Return to high level performance is expected and has been demonstrated in professional American football players [35, 36, 39], cyclists [40] and ice hockey players [34].

9.1.6 Complications

- ***Refracture***: Athletes are arguably more prone to repeat injuries compared to the general public, but the risk of refracture is difficult to quantify. Evidence from randomized trials suggests refracture is exceptionally rare when union occurs [15]. A small cohort of professional American football players did find refracture incidence of

57% following non-operative management at 1 year, but it is unclear if this is generalisable [39].

- ***Periprosthetic fracture***: Following fixation, the rigid construct of plate and screws may produce a stress riser and periprosthetic fracture has been reported in up to 5% of cases following operative management [22]. It is unclear if removal of the plate would decrease this risk.
- ***Infection***: Deep infections following plate fixation can be associated with osteomyelitis and nonunion, and although rare, they are devastating when encountered. When combined with superficial wound infection, the incidence is around 4–5%: this is potentially higher compared to other common fracture fixation procedures.
- ***Fixation failure***: A secondary operation, to revise a plate fixation for acute pull-out of the construct or to address nonunion, may be required in approximately 8% of cases.
- ***Neurovascular injuries***: Intra-operative damage to the subclavian vessels or brachial plexus is rare at approximately 0–1.5% [11, 16, 41].

9.1.7 Preventative Measures

For athletes undertaking contact sports, protective 'shock-absorbing' clothing may reduce the risk of clavicle fractures resulting from direct impact. However, the evidence of benefit is lacking, and the ability to wear protective equipment will depend on the given sport.

9.2 Acromioclavicular Joint Injuries

9.2.1 Epidemiology

Acromioclavicular joint (ACJ) injuries occur in 1.8 people per 10,000 population, and account for 40–50% of shoulder injuries in contact sports [42] [43]. There is a strong male preponderance (8:1), with injuries predominantly affecting young patients (20–39 years) involved in sports such as cycling, American football and rugby [42, 44]. The vast majority represent minor sprains, with relatively few involving a complete disruption of the supporting ligaments [45].

9.2.2 Classification

The acromioclavicular articulation has little bony conformity and thus relies on the surrounding soft tissues for stability. An appreciation of the soft tissue restraints is essential when considering the injury and treatment. These include:

- ***The acromioclavicular (AC) ligament***: this envelopes the joint capsule on all surfaces. The superior component is thought to be most important and is responsible for resistance to horizontal movement.
- ***The coracoclavicular (CC) ligaments***: the conoid (more medial) and trapezoid (more lateral) ligaments run from the base of the coracoid to the under-surface of the lateral clavicle. These resist both horizontal and superior displacement of the lateral clavicle.
- ***Deltotrapezial fascia***: a thickened layer of fascia that traverses the junction between the deltoid and trapezius. Both muscles bridge the ACJ, the trapezius on the posterosuperior aspect and the deltoid on the anteroinferior aspect, with both muscles and fascia conferring a degree of stability.
- ***The ACJ capsule and intra-articular disc***: the joint capsule and intervening intra-articular disc form the structure of the joint and provide a degree of stability.

Rockwood radiographically classified ACJ injuries into six grades, based on the extent of the ligamentous injury and the direction of displacement [45]. The classification depicts an increasing degree of injury to the surrounding soft tissue restraints and hopes to guide management, although significant interobserver variation is reported. Full appreciation of the injury can only be attained after scrutiny of both anteroposterior and axillary radiographs. The grades are:

1. ACJ ligament sprain. No radiographic displacement but the patient has localised tenderness.
2. ACJ ligament rupture but intact coracoclavicular ligaments. Displacement (superior to inferior) is less than the width of the lateral clavicle.
3. Both ACJ and coracoclavicular ligaments ruptured. Displacement is more than the width of the clavicle, but no anteroposterior displacement is present. Clinically, type III injuries are reducible with downward pressure on the lateral clavicle and simultaneous upward pressure on the arm.
4. Both ACJ and coracoclavicular ligaments ruptured, with posterior displacement.
5. Both ACJ and coracoclavicular ligaments ruptured, with gross displacement and injury to the deltotrapezial fascia. 100–300% superior displacement is seen (Fig. 9.3). Type V injures are not reducible.
6. Displacement beneath the coracoid. This injury is often mentioned, but rarely seen.

9.2.3 Diagnosis

ACJ injuries typically occur after direct trauma to the point of the shoulder with the arm in adduction [46]. Abrasions, swelling and bruising are common. In higher grade injures there will be clear prominence of the lateral end of the clavicle. The 'piano-key sign' can be elicited in higher grade injuries, where the clavicle can be depressed so that it resides in a reduced position next to the acromion. The 'scarf test' (pain during flexion and adduction of the shoulder, as if

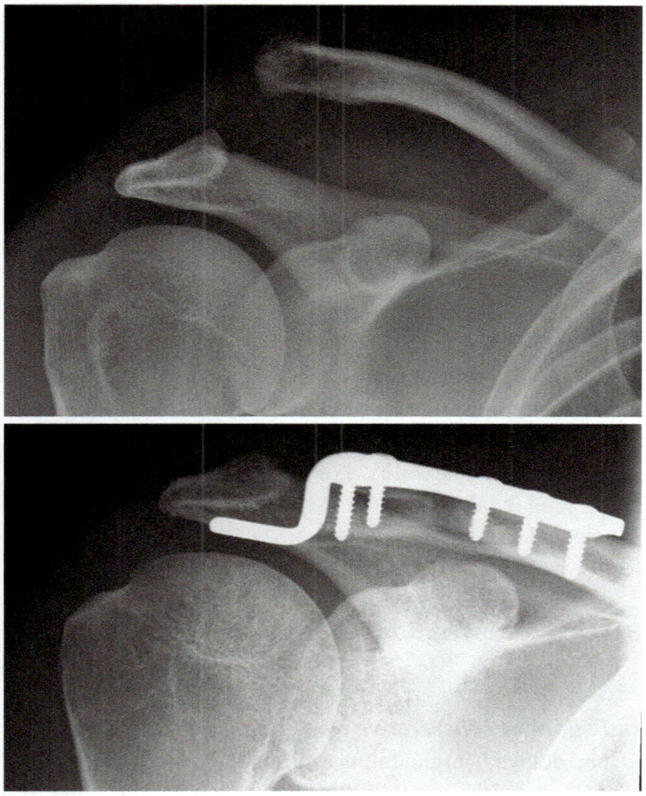

Fig. 9.3 Grade V ACJ disruption subsequently stabilised by a hook plate

throwing a scarf over the opposite shoulder) is positive, although this test is usually reserved for examination in the chronic setting [47]. The position of the clavicle during the test should be noted; posterior movement may suggest instability and the need for stabilisation surgery.

Radiographs are obtained in the form of an anteroposteior view of the clavicle at a ten degree cephalad angle (the Zanca view) [48]. This is optimal for the interpretation of incongruity. In addition, an axillary view permits an assessment of posterior displacement, to differentiate grade III and IV injuries. Cross-sectional imaging is rarely indicated but may offer assessment of the deltotrapezial fascia and, in chronic injuries, of cartilage degeneration [49].

9.2.4 Treatment

9.2.4.1 Surgical Decision-Making

The goal of treatment is expeditious return of normal shoulder function with minimal intervention. For injures at either end of the Rockwood criteria, the optimal treatment is clear:

- Grade I and II injuries are treated conservatively. A broad arm sling is applied but intermittently removed to allow elbow movements and discarded once pain allows.
- Grade V and VI injuries commonly require surgical stabilisation.

Considerable debate surrounds the treatment of grade III and IV disruptions. Traditionally these injures were treated surgically, however, there is mounting evidence to support non-operative management [50, 51]. A recently published randomised control trial found that patients with grade III and IV injuries achieved similar functional outcomes at 1 year whether they were treated with acute stabilisation or conservatively [52]. Furthermore, those treated non-surgically attained final outcome at an earlier stage than those who underwent stabilisation. At 6 weeks post-injury, 33% of the nonoperative group had returned to sport compared to 15% of the operative group. This evidence is countered by the small number of patients treated conservatively, in whom outcome is poor and delayed surgery is therefore required [52].

Optimal management must take into account the sporting endeavour, the level of participation and the preference of the player. Some may prefer to defer surgery in an effort to return to play as early as possible. Others, particularly those involved in professional sport, may opt for early intervention for fear of a failed rehabilitation and the need for a second period of convalescence after surgery. Early surgery is commonly offered to those involved in overhead or throwing sports, who are particularly vulnerable to issues of scapular dyskinesia and ACJ pain. In most cases, decreasing pain and improved range of movement at 2–4 weeks will herald a successful outcome without surgery. Delaying surgery for this period does not increase the risk or challenge of an operation.

9.2.4.2 Surgical Techniques

There is a myriad of surgical techniques available for stabilisation of the ACJ. Regardless of the implant choice or technique, the surgeon should ensure stability of the ACJ to allow scarring and healing of the surrounding soft tissues. Surgical treatments are therefore described in terms of their mechanical and biological components.

Mechanical Stability

This is achieved by anchoring the distal clavicle to the acromion or the coracoid.

- **Hook plate**: This device indirectly reduces the clavicle to the acromion, with the lateral end of the plate residing under the posterior acromion (Fig. 9.3). While this technique is considered robust and is supported by level 1 evidence, issues include rotator cuff impingement and the requirement of a secondary procedure for metalwork removal [53].
- **Coracoclavicular suspensory devices**: These techniques aim to re-establish the pull of the CC ligaments by secur-

ing the clavicle to the coracoid. Various methods have been described, and these can be grouped according to the method of fixation to the clavicle and to the coracoid; either looped around the bone or tunnelled through (Fig. 9.2). Looped devices (e.g. Lockdown; Surgicraft/Infinity-Lock; Neoligaments) involve the passage of a braided suture material of varying width around the coracoid followed by fixation to the clavicle with a screw. Detractors of this technique point to the high rates of osteolysis around the clavicle: however this appears to have been addressed with newer generation implants. Perhaps more common are tunnelled implants, which provide stability via the use of suture buttons through the clavicle and coracoid (TightRope; Arthrex). This technique has been optimised with the use of multiple buttons and suture tapes to improve contruct strength.
- **Acromioclavicular devices**: Adjunct stabilisation of the lateral clavicle and acromion can be considered to limit translational movement of the ACJ during healing. This can be achieved with tunnelled sutures or suture anchors (Internal Brace; Arthrex).

Biological Healing

In the acute setting, the biological repair is achieved through healing of the recently injured local soft tissues. In a chronic injury such a response is not expected, and consideration should be given to soft tissue repair and/or adjuncts.

- **The Weaver-Dunn procedure**: This involves excision of the distal clavicle and transfer of the coraco-acromial (CA) ligament to the osteotomy site. While this was previously performed in isolation, it is now often employed along with CC stabilisation.
- **Soft tissue reconstruction of the CC ligaments**: This can be achieved with cadaveric allograft (hamstring, flexor hallucis longus) or hamstring autograft. The tendon is looped around the coracoid and secured to the clavicle through a drill hole or passed as a loop.
- **Acromioclavicular ligament reconstruction:** This involves the identification, preservation and subsequent repair of the superior ligament and capsule. These structures will have been damaged but an attempt at repair should be routinely performed.
- **Deltotrapezial fascia repair**: The degree of disruption of this layer will be defined by the grade of injury. However, plication of the fascia provides further support and is recommended in all cases.

9.2.4.3 Authors' Preferred Technique

Acute Injury (Within 4 Weeks)

Acute fixation is recommended in overhead athletes with scapular malpositioning, irrespective of Rockwood grading. Restoration of function is vitally important. Reconstruction of the CC ligaments and acute suturing of the AC ligament capsule is the authors' preferred mode of treatment. This involves using braided, artificial ligament (Infinity-Lock; Neoligaments) looped around the coracoid, with fixation to the clavicle via a drilled bony tunnel, directly superior to the base of the coracoid, and tied over a metal button. This, in turn, is wrapped circumferentially around the clavicle and tied to itself.

Chronic Injury

The authors' preferred treatment is similar to that for acute injury, using the Infinity-Lock device, with or without tendon allograft augmentation and the Internal Brace to address anteroposterior instability. For additional stability, augmentation with the CA ligament to the distal clavicle can be used in selected cases.

9.2.5 Complications

- ***Failure of conservative management***: This may necessitate delayed surgical intervention.
- ***ACJ arthritis***: Instability-related degeneration of the ACJ may require subsequent surgical intervention.
- ***Surgical complications***: These include infection (thought due to the relative subcutaneous nature of the ACJ), re-displacement (partial or full), symptomatic metalwork (especially with the Hook plate), coracoid stress fractures, neurovascular injury and ongoing pain.

9.2.6 Rehabilitation

With non-surgical management, sling use is typically recommended for 1–2 weeks. Following surgery, rehabilitation usually involves sling immobilisation for 4 weeks, with early with active assisted movements. As pain improves the patient will progress to active range of movement. Strapping or bracing is of limited use [54].

Contact athletes can expect to return sport around 3–6 months after injury. Those involved in overhead sports will require a longer period of convalescence, approximately 6–9 months.

9.2.7 Preventative Measures

For athletes undertaking contact sports, protective 'shock-absorbing' clothing may reduce the risk of ACJ injuries resulting from direct impact. However, the evidence of benefit is lacking, and the ability to wear protective equipment will depend on the given sport.

9.3 Glenohumeral Instability

9.3.1 Epidemiology

The incidence of glenohumeral dislocations is 23.9/100,000 person-years, with the vast majority displacing anteriorly [55]. The 'rule of halves' provides an aide memoire to some of the common demographics:

- ½ (45%) of all dislocations occur at the glenohumeral joint.
- ½ (46%) are the result of sporting endeavours.
- ½ (46%) occur in patients between the ages of 15 and 29 years [55, 56].

Males are affected 2.5 times more than women; however, this is due to the greater participation in contact sports rather than a true predilection to injury. Contact sports account for the majority of dislocations with activities such as American football, basketball, ice hockey and rugby most often implicated [56–59]. Posterior dislocation is rare, accounting for only 5% of all glenohumeral dislocations with only 6% of these occurring during a sporting exposure [60].

9.3.1.1 Recurrent Instability

Recurrent instability is common, occurring in 66% of young patients within the first 5 years after the primary injury [61]. Adolescents are at particular risk, with only 7% of patients predicted to have a stable shoulder 10 years after the initial incident [62]. Over 60% of this cohort will develop recurrent instability within 2 years of the primary dislocation.

9.3.2 Classification

The classification of glenohumeral instability is challenging due to the heterogenicity of the patient population and the spectrum of injury. Numerous classification systems have been developed, none of which are comprehensive, definitively guide treatment or are in common use in the literature [63–70]. One of the first, and initially popular, depictions was developed by Thomas and Matsen who described two groups of patients:

- **TUBS**—***T***raumatic ***U***ndirectional instability that requires ***B***ankart ***S***tabilisation.
- **AMBRI**—***A***trauamtic ***M***ulti-directional instability, which is commonly ***B***ilateral, most commonly responds to ***R***ehabilitation but may benefit from ***I***nferior capsular shift.

This system made the important delineation between those patients with and without joint laxity. Laxity is defined as a varying degree of painless, physiological translation of the humerus on the glenoid fossa during movement. On the other hand, instability is defined as the pathological translation of the humerus within the fossa resulting in pain and disruption of constitutional anatomical restraints. These conditions are not mutually exclusive and, in practice, most athletes who suffer glenohumeral instability lie within a spectrum of laxity and instability. Due to the complexity of injury and the variation between patients, descriptive methods are now most commonly used to define the features of instability and generally include six characteristics:

- The ***direction*** of the humeral head in relation to the glenoid (anterior, posterior, inferior, multi-directional).
- The ***degree*** of movement (subluxation or dislocation).
- The ***frequency*** (number of occurrences).
- The ***aetiology*** (traumatic, atraumatic or neuromuscular).
- The ***chronicity*** (acute, chronic, acute-on-chronic).
- The ***volition*** (voluntary or involuntary).

These descriptions draw from elements of the patient history, clinical examination and radiological evaluation, and when considered together, offer a clear means of communication regarding a patient's pathology between clinicians in the multidisciplinary team.

9.3.3 Diagnosis

Patients invariably present in one of two clinical scenarios; to the emergency department during an acute episode of dislocation, or to the outpatient department after a reduced primary dislocation or due to ongoing or recurrent instability.

9.3.3.1 Emergency Department

In the former group, rapid clinical assessment aims to identify the direction of dislocation, to allow expeditious closed manipulation and the relief of discomfort. Important clinical features include: the injury mechanism, the presence of shoulder girdle pain, the appearance of a squared shoulder (prominence of the acromion due to anterior shoulder dislocation), and limited shoulder range of movement. The clinician should always be wary of the patient with shoulder pain who holds the forearm firmly to the abdomen and does not tolerate any external rotation, for these are the classic features of a posterior dislocation. A careful neurovascular examination of the axillary (sensory only as pain will limit motor assessment), median, radial and ulnar nerves, and palpation of the radial pulse is mandatory.

Plain radiographs in two planes are required to make an accurate diagnosis. Due to discomfort, an axillary view is rarely possible and therefore a modified axial (Velpeau) view is used to compliment the anteroposterior image. A reduction manoeuvre should only be undertaken after the exclusion of a humeral neck fracture. Other important radiological features include fractures of the greater tuberosity and the presence of an anterior glenoid rim fracture (Bony Bankart lesion). Post-reduction radiographs and neurovascular examinations are essential.

9.3.3.2 Outpatient Department

For those patients who present to the outpatient department, clinical history should focus on the six features listed in the previous section. Clinical examination should include: an assessment of the range of movement (in flexion, abduction, internal and external rotation), an evaluation of rotator cuff integrity, the identification of anterior or posterior apprehension, documentation of any hypermobility (Beighton score), and the exclusion of any neurological injury, particularly to the axillary nerve.

Plain radiographs (anteroposterior and axillary views) ensure joint congruity, allow initial assessment of humeral or glenoid bone loss and can identify joint degeneration. Multiplanar imaging is ubiquitous and aims to define the pathoanatomy of the injury. Computed Tomography (CT) offers the definitive assessment of bone loss, whilst Magnetic Resonance Imaging-Arthrogram (MRI-A) images the soft tissue envelope and therefore, depending on clinician preference, both may be performed. Plain MRI will demonstrate a rotator cuff tear but cannot exclude labral pathology, and is therefore used less frequently. Numerous eponymous names or acronyms are used in the orthopaedic literature regarding glenohumeral pathology found using CT/MRI-A.

Glenoid Lesions

- ***Bankart lesion***: a detachment of the anteroinferior labrum, with an anterior portion of the inferior glenohumeral ligament.
- ***Bony Bankart lesion***: as above but the anteroinferior glenoid rim is avulsed (Fig. 9.4).
- ***SLAP***: ***S***uperior ***L***abrum ***A***nterior to ***P***osterior tear. Important as this represents a lesion that can destabilise the long head of biceps anchor to the superior glenoid [71].
- ***HAGL***: ***H***umeral ***A***vulsion of the ***G***lenohumeral ***L***igaments. Rather than the more common avulsion from the glenoid side of the joint, the inferior glenohumeral ligament is detached from the medial calcar of the humerus [72].
- ***ALPSA***: ***A***nterior ***L***abrum ***P***eriosteal ***S***leeve ***A***vulsion. Rather than the complete detachment of the labrum seen in the Bankart lesion, the labrum is avulsed with a portion of the glenoid periosteum, which then becomes medialised and can heal to the glenoid neck [73].
- ***PASTA***: ***P***artial ***A***rticular ***S***upraspinatus ***T***endon ***A***vulsion. Although a finding commonly seen in rotator cuff disease, this lesion may be observed after dislocation in athletes [74].

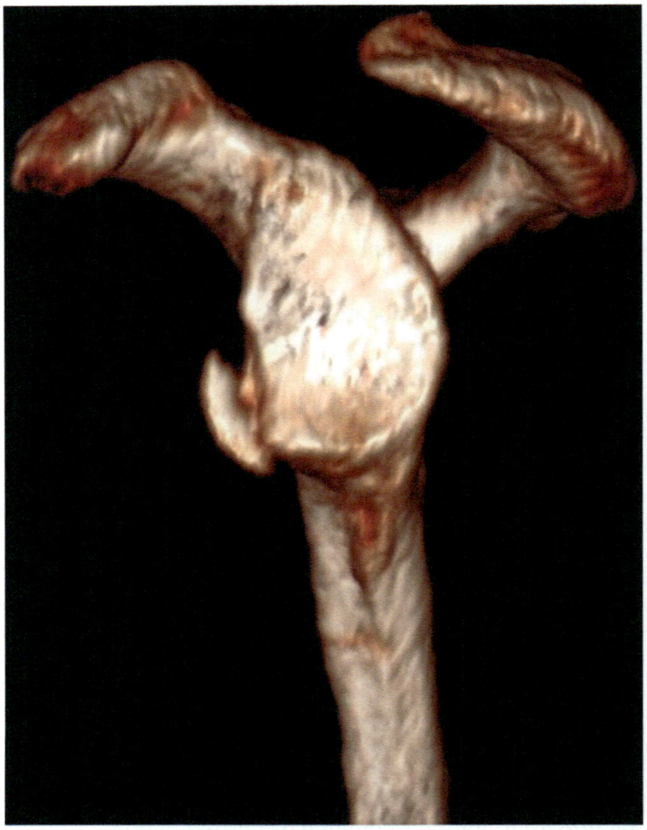

Fig. 9.4 3D CT image of a bony Bankart lesion

Humeral Lesions

- ***Hill-Sachs lesion***: a defect or groove in the posterolateral aspect of the humeral head, caused by the attrition contact of the glenoid during anterior dislocation [75] (Fig. 9.5).
- ***Reverse Hill-Sachs (McLaughlin) lesion***: a defect or groove in the anteromedial aspect of the humeral head, secondary to posterior dislocation [76].

9.3.4 Treatment

9.3.4.1 Closed Treatment of Acute Dislocations

Pitch-side relocation of a glenohumeral dislocation should be performed with caution and only by an experienced practitioner. It is generally reserved for those patients with recurrent anterior instability rather than in the setting of any primary dislocation or in the case of posterior instability [77]. The vast majority of dislocations are reduced using appropriate analgesia with or without the provision of sedation. A myriad of techniques exist for reduction, each with advocates and detractors. The two most commonly used are the Hippocratic method (in line traction/ counter-traction) or

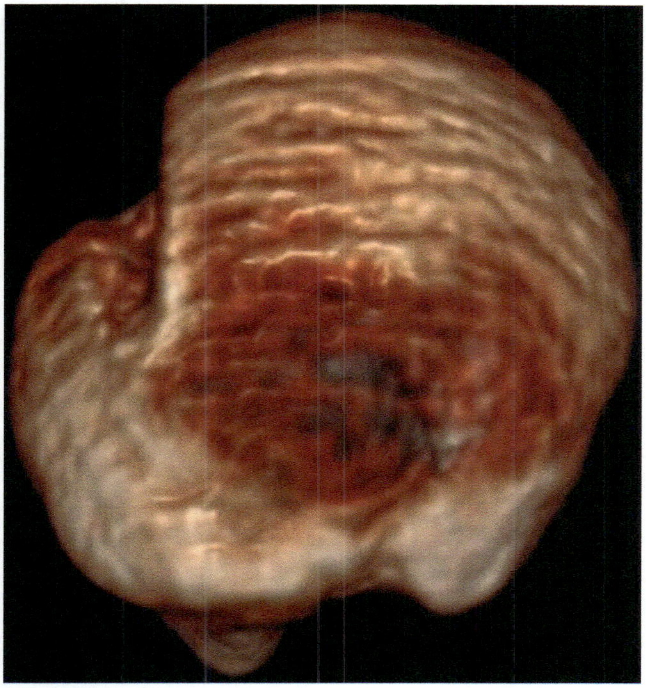

Fig. 9.5 3D CT image of the humeral head with a large Hill-Sachs lesion

the Kocher's manoeuvre (external rotation, adduction, internal rotation) [78, 79]. Regardless of the technique used, the clinician should be either experienced or supervised before making any attempt.

9.3.4.2 Conservative Management

The optimal regime for conservative management of a first-time dislocation is unclear. Prolonged immobilisation is no longer favoured [80, 81]. The majority of patients are managed in a position of internal rotation, with the forearm resting against the abdomen in a broad arm sling—the so called 'safe' position. More recently, evidence has suggested that a position of external rotation may confer benefit by limiting recurrence [82–84]. In practise, patients report difficulty adhering to this regime, limiting its use. Rehabilitation (see below) is a key component of conservative management.

9.3.4.3 Surgical Decision-Making

Management of a primary dislocation, and whether to offer early surgery, is a clinical conundrum. A period of immobilisation, followed by physiotherapy, remains the mainstay of initial treatment. However, there is high-level evidence to support primary stabilisation in those patients at risk of recurrent instability [85]. High-risk patients, in whom primary surgery may be recommended, include: males [85], patients aged <30 years of age at injury, patients who participate in contact sports, and those with radiological evidence of a bony Bankart lesion [85].

The timing of surgery is of particular importance to the professional athlete due to the competitive and financial implications of loss-of-play. Some may prefer to pursue conservative management, in an effort to return to sport before the end of a particular season. Bracing may be of benefit for in-season return [86]. It is noteworthy that while surgery reduces recurrence, it does not confer any functional benefit when compared to a non-operatively managed patient in whom the shoulder becomes stable. Patients who experience recurrent episodes of dislocation or ongoing subjective instability invariably require surgery to allow return to sport. However, it should be noted that stability can still be achieved with conservative means, even after multiple episodes of dislocation [80].

9.3.4.4 Surgical Techniques

The choice of surgical technique requires careful consideration based on the degree of instability, shoulder laxity, radiographic findings and surgeon skill-set. Scoring systems such as the Instability Severity Index Score can guide treatment [87]. The available techniques can be broadly divided into those that address defects of soft tissue, or defects of bone (Fig. 9.6). Soft tissue techniques involve repair of the glenoid capsuloligamentous complex (labrum) or advancement of the capsule and rotator cuff into a Hill-Sachs defect (remplissage). Bony procedures attempt to compensate for anteroinferior bone loss (common in recurrent instability) or humeral bone loss (Hill-Sachs lesion), through the use of either autologous or allogenic bone grafts.

The exact combination of stabilisation techniques may not be finalised until an arthroscopic examination of the shoulder is performed. This has the advantage of not only re-assessing any labral or bony lesions that may have changed since imaging, but ensures there are no concurrent injury to the biceps tendon, its anchor or the rotator cuff. More advanced analysis using multiplanar CT can offer additional pre-operative information to guide the use of soft tissue or bony procedures. A method has been popularised by Itoi et al. who advocate a combined measurement of the Hill-Sachs lesion and glenoid bone loss [88]. This allows the lesion to be described as 'on track' or 'off track. 'On track' lesions are more stable and can be treated with soft tissue stabilisation. 'Off track' lesions are more unstable and invariably require bony augmentation.

9.3.4.5 Soft Tissue Procedures

These are suitable in patients with primary or recurrent instability in whom there is limited loss of bone from the antero-inferior glenoid, with or without a small Hill-Sachs lesion.

Labral (Bankart) Repair

Suture anchors are used to re-approximate the labrum to the anterior glenoid rim. Debate surrounding the merits of open

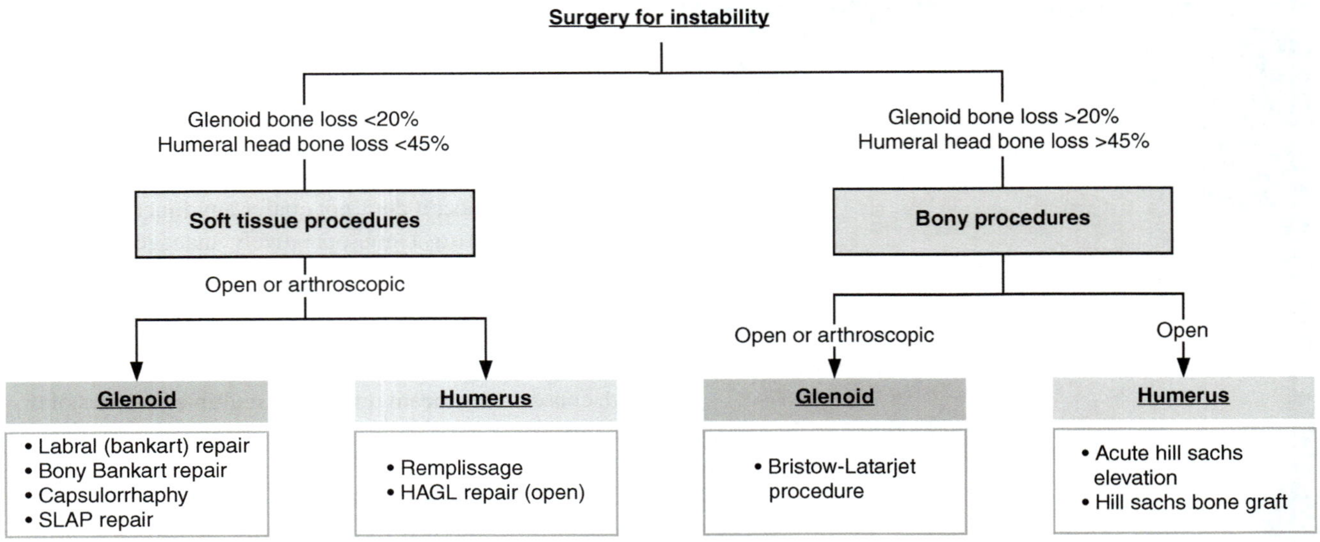

Fig. 9.6 Surgical planning for glenohumeral instability

versus arthroscopic techniques exists. Level I evidence suggests no difference in rate of recurrence, while a meta-analysis suggests marginal superiority of open methods [89, 90]. Most evidence reports recurrent instability as the sole outcome, missing any of the purported benefits of the arthroscopic repair (smaller incisions, less stiffness in external rotation, minimal deltoid injury and preservation of subscapularis). The majority of soft tissue Bankart repairs are now performed arthroscopically. Arthroscopic Bankart repair reduces recurrence after first time dislocation by 76% [91].

Bony Bankart Repair

The fixation method is determined by the size of the lesion, specifically if it is greater or less than 25% of the glenoid articular surface. Lesions comprising <25% of the glenoid articular surface can be treated arthroscopically with suture anchors. This allows return to play in professional athletes involved in collision sports [92]. Larger fragments require an open procedure to allow fracture reduction and internal fixation with screws.

SLAP Repair

A SLAP lesion is often found in athletes with shoulder instability. Treatment is dependent on the extent of the tear and the degree of detachment of the long head of biceps form the superior glenoid. In younger athletes (<35 years), simple tears can be repaired with suture anchors. In older patients, repair has a high failure rate and may result in undue stiffness. In these patients a biceps tenodesis, arthroscopically or open in the sub-pectoral region, can be performed.

Remplissage

Remplissage means ‘filling’ in French. Where there is a Hill-Sachs lesion which ‘engages’ with the anterior glenoid rim during arthroscopic examination in external rotation, arthroscopic capsulodesis and infraspinatus tenodesis may be deployed—in additional to Bankart repair—in order to ‘fill’ the Hill-Sachs defect [93]. The addition of this technique in higher risk patients limits recurrence [87].

HAGL Repair

A HAGL lesion occurs in approximately 9% of glenohumeral dislocations [72, 94]. HAGL lesions treated non-operatively are at high risk of recurrent instability. Both open and arthroscopic fixation techniques are available. Often, the concomitant lesions are addressed during initial arthroscopy, with staged open repair of the HAGL lesion.

9.3.4.6 Bony Procedures

These procedures address significant bony pathology, most commonly related to recurrent instability.

Glenoid Augmentation: The Modified Bristow-Latarjet Procedure

While fixation of an acute bony Bankart is possible in some patients, the majority with either longstanding instability or multiple dislocations will not have a suitable portion of the glenoid for re-attachment. Furthermore, the glenoid has often been eroded by multiple dislocations rather than a discrete fracture of the rim. Therefore, bony augmentation is required. First described in 1954, the Latarjet procedure involved the fusion of a resected part of the coracoid, along with the origin of the conjoint tendon, as an osteotendinous autograft to the deficient anterior rim of the glenoid [95]. Subsequent modifications by Bristow allowed preservation of the subscapularis tendon. Considered the gold standard for significant glenoid bone loss with an engaging Hill-Sachs lesion, the technique is thought to work via the "triple blocking" mechanism [96]:

- ***Bone effect***: The addition of the coracoid increases or restores the anteroposterior diameter of the glenoid.
- ***Sling effect***: The conjoint tendon (origins of the short head of biceps and the coracobrachialis muscle) acts as a sling on the inferior subscapularis and anteroinferior capsule.
- ***Capsular reinforcement***: The remnant of the coracoacromial ligament is incorporated into the capsular repair.

The Bristow-Latarjet procedure offers athletes a high chance of return to previous level of play (88%), with almost all (98%) returning to the index sport. Recurrent instability occurs in 4.9% of patients [97]. Salvage procedures for a failed Latarjet involve the use of either autologous bone graft, most commonly from the pelvic brim (Eden-Hybinette procedure) or the use of allogenic bone. Neither have the benefit of a blood supply via tendinous attachment, therefore lessening the chance of union.

Humeral Osteoplasty

Acute Hill-Sachs lesions can be elevated to restore the articular surface [98]. The favoured technique employs an anterior cruciate ligament reconstruction drill jig, which is used to identify the deepest part of the lesion fluoroscopically. After drilling, a tamp is then passed into the humeral head to elevate the depressed articular surface. Bone graft or substitute is then used to reinforce the elevated segment. When combined with soft tissue repair of the glenoid labrum, excellent results have been described [99, 100]. Although desirable, many larger Hill-Sachs lesions amenable to this technique are chronic due to multiple dislocations and are therefore not suitable. It is in the setting of a primary dislocation, within 4 weeks of injury, that a large defect can be elevated.

Humeral Head Augmentation

Reserved for refractory cases with large head defects, this can be achieved with either matched humerus/femoral allograft or a synthetic partial replacement. The evidence, albeit from small case series, suggests that functional outcome, sufficient to allow return to sport, can be achieved with allograft. However, there are substantial rates of operative complication [101].

9.3.5 Complications

9.3.5.1 Complications of Injury [102]

13.5% of patients have a neurological deficit in the affected upper limb after dislocation. The majority of lesions involve the axillary nerve (77%), however multiple nerves or plexus injures occur in 9% of dislocations. In 15% of dislocations, there is a concomitant fracture of the greater tuberosity, while rotator cuff tears occur in 10%. Eight percentage of patients suffer a dislocation in combination with a nerve palsy, and tuberosity fracture or cuff tear. Vascular injury is rare following glenohumeral dislocation [103].

9.3.5.2 Complications of Surgery

Stiffness is a significant complication after shoulder stabilisation procedure in athletes. Limited motion, particularly for those involved in throwing sports, may significantly impact performance. An external rotation deficit is most commonly reported. Stiffness after 9 months of appropriate physiotherapy may warrant arthroscopic inspection and release. Nerve injury occurs in 8% of open and 3% of arthroscopic procedures [104]. The vast majority resolve spontaneously, but pervasive symptoms which fail to improve after 6 weeks warrant nerve conduction studies. Radiographic features of joint arthropathy are found in 8–11% of patients in whom the primary dislocation occurred before the age of 40 years [105, 106]. Infection is rare after arthroscopic stabilisation [91].

9.3.6 Rehabilitation

Rehabilitation is an essential component in the successful treatment of glenohumeral instability. A full return to sport is the aim of treatment, regardless of the chosen method. Patient and injury features, such as hypermobility and the direction of instability, must be considered when planning a rehabilitation regime [107]. A supervised, goal-based protocol should be employed rather than any regime based on preset time points.

Both conservatively and operatively managed patients will require a period of sling immobilisation for pain relief and to allow soft tissue recovery. Neck pain is common after shoulder injury and mostly attributable to inappropriate strain of the trapezius, which acts to elevate the scapula in an effort to allow movement. Therefore, postural coaching consisting of scapula elevation/depression and protraction/retraction is important to minimise spasm and ensure a normal posture of the shoulder girdle.

Regaining motion is the initial goal soon after injury/surgery, followed by strengthening of the rotator cuff and periscapular muscles. Closed chain exercises concentrating on the rotator cuff are beneficial in the early phase, to re-engage the concavity compression action of these muscles. Once comfortable, submaximal isometric exercises are a safe way to allow muscle reactivation. In the intermediate phase, it is important to stress to the patient that increased number of repetitions rather than increased load will result in better engagement of the rotator cuff muscles [108]. Formal assessment of muscle strength through isokinetic testing machines, or through the use of more portable methods such as a hand held dynamometer, is helpful in assessing progress towards normal strength, particularly in rotation [109].

Return to play may be considered once the athlete regains symmetrical range of movement and strength. Return to play can be achieved after 6 weeks in cases of conservative management [86]. Return to play after surgical stabilisation can be achieved by 4 months in high-level athletes [110].

9.3.7 Preventative Measures

Due to the unique range of movement of the shoulder girdle, efforts to support the joint through taping or bracing prove challenging, as restricted movement can result in limited performance. While taping may help the athlete to gain confidence, it is ineffective in improving joint position sense, inferior laxity or handball accuracy [111]. Bracing can play a role in return to sport as part of a generalised treatment regime: however, its importance is not defined [86]. In high-level contact athletes, preventative bracing did not limit the occurrence of labral injuries [112]. Overhead athletes often exhibit sport-specific adaptations to the shoulder range of movement and musculature. Most commonly, this manifests as weak external rotation and restriction in internal rotation [113–115]. These issues should be addressed with physical therapy, in order to avoid potential injury.

9.4 Proximal Humerus Fractures

Fractures of the proximal humerus are complex injuries that can involve the humeral head, neck, the greater and lesser tuberosities, or these components in combination. Fractures of the head and neck are rarely implicated in sporting injuries, and are most commonly the result of a high energy transfer such as a road traffic accident, or low energy transfer in elderly patients. Fractures of the greater tuberosity, which can complicate anterior glenohumeral dislocation, may be related to sporting endeavours, and are the focus of this chapter. Isolated lesser tuberosity fractures are rare, and are considered beyond the scope of this text.

The importance of greater tuberosity fractures lies with the insertion of the supraspinatus and infraspinatus muscles. Two of the four rotator cuff muscles, these are essential for optimal shoulder function and therefore sporting performance. A displaced fracture of the tuberosity will compromise the action of these muscles, resulting in weakness and limited range of active movement. Therefore, this bony injury can be regarded as analogous to a rotator cuff tear.

9.4.1 Epidemiology

The incidence of proximal humerus fractures is 82 per 100,000 patient-years [114]. Twenty percentage of these injures are isolated to the greater tuberosity [116]. Fifteen percentage of all anterior glenohumeral dislocations are complicated by a greater tuberosity fracture [102].

9.4.2 Classification

Two classifications relate to the fractures of the greater tuberosity, the Neer and Mutch systems. The Neer system relates to all proximal humerus fractures, and defines the number of parts involved (the head, the shaft, the lesser and greater tuberosity) and whether they are displaced more than 1 cm [117]. It offers no description of the morphology or size of the tuberosity component. More recently, Mutch et al. offered a more detailed description of greater tuberosity fractures [118]:

- ***Type I***: A small component that has displaced superiorly and medially—this represents a rotator cuff avulsion.
- ***Type II***: A vertical split with a large tuberosity component. This is likely caused by impaction on the anterior surface of glenoid during dislocation or subluxation.
- ***Type III***: A depressed fracture involves a fragment that is displaced inferiorly. This is probably due to impaction beneath the inferior surface of the glenoid when the humerus is dislocated, or beneath the inferior surface of the acromion during extreme abduction.

9.4.3 Diagnosis

Patients with greater tuberosity fractures invariably present soon after injury, with features of shoulder discomfort and the inability to move the upper limb. The examination will be limited by pain and may mimic a simple glenohumeral dislocation. Only limited assessment, focussing on the neurovascular function of the affected limb, should be performed before plain radiography.

Anteroposterior and modified axial radiographs will demonstrate the tuberosity fracture and any glenohumeral dislocation (Fig. 9.7). CT imaging best defines the size, morphology and displacement of the tuberosity fragment. MRI can identify a concomitant rotator cuff tear [119].

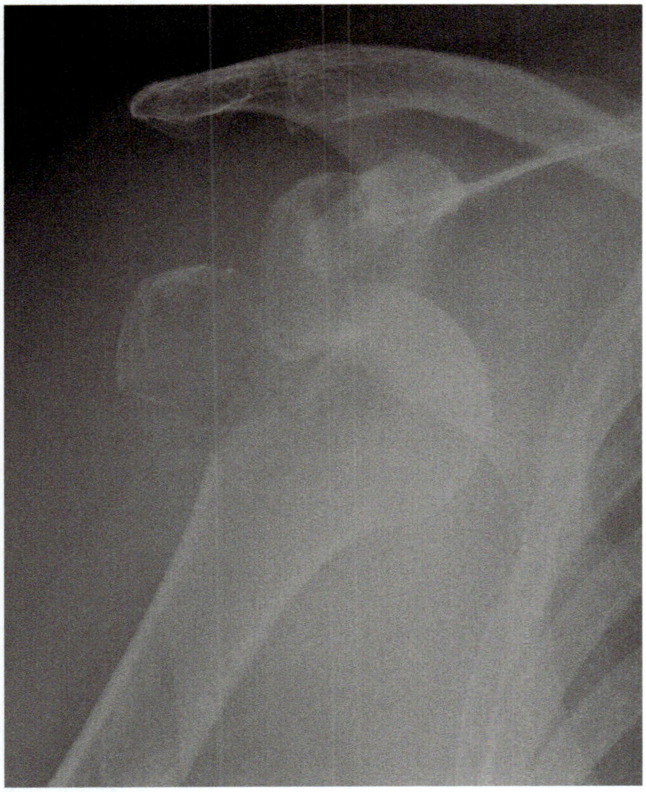

Fig. 9.7 Anterior glenohumeral dislocation with greater tuberosity fracture

9.4.4 Treatment

Emergency department treatment involves the reduction of any dislocation and the provision of a broad arm sling. Treatment is defined by the degree of displacement of the tuberosity component (Fig. 9.8). Traditionally the arbitrary value of >1 cm, as defined by Neer, was an indication for surgery. More recent work has demonstrated that the function of the rotator cuff is significantly diminished if there is displacement >5 mm [120]. This would be of particular importance in the athlete, and therefore the authors advocate surgery when displacement is >5 mm. Late displacement of the tuberosity can occur, and therefore weekly radiographic review is recommended for the first month after injury.

The method of surgical fixation is defined by the size of the fragment. Small bony avulsions should be secured with bone anchors, most commonly achieved in an open manner. Larger fragments can be secured with multiple partially threaded cancellous screws or with a pre-contoured plate and screws. Secondary complications include cuff tear, subacromial impingement and adhesive capsulitis.

9.4.5 Preventative Measures

The authors are not aware of any relevant literature addressing the prevention of greater tuberosity fractures in athletes.

9.5 Humeral Shaft Fractures

9.5.1 Epidemiology

Humeral diaphyseal fractures constitute approximately 1% of all adult fractures [121]. In the general population, these

Fig. 9.8 Authors' suggested algorithm for treatment of greater tuberosity fractures

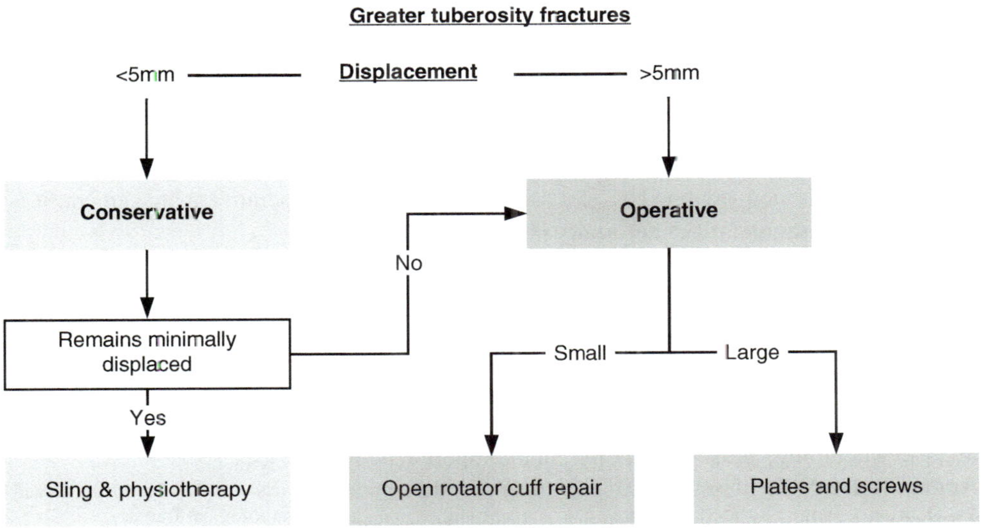

injuries most frequently occur in the middle- and older aged (mean age at injury 54–62 years) [121–124]. Published literature indicates that approximately 1–7% of all humeral diaphyseal fractures are sport-related [121–123, 125, 126]. Adolescent and young adult males are disproportionately affected [122], probably due to a greater participation in contact sports.

9.5.2 Classification

9.5.2.1 Descriptive Classification

This is based upon the anatomical location within the humeral diaphysis, which is divided into: proximal-third (12–41% of injuries), middle-third (53–66%), and distal-third (11–22%) [122, 123, 125, 126].

9.5.2.2 AO-OTA Classification [127]

This is based upon fracture configuration. Simple fractures (type **A**, 54–68%) [122–126] may be spiral (**A1**), oblique (**A2**, fracture line ≥30° perpendicular to the long axis of the humerus) or transverse (**A3**, fracture line <30° perpendicular to the long axis of the humerus). In addition to the main proximal and distal fracture fragments, 'wedge fractures' (type **B**, 25–34%) involve a separate fragment, which may be intact (**B2**) or fragmented (**B3**). Segmental fractures (type **C**, 4–16%)—in which there is no contact between the proximal and distal fractures—may also be either intact (**C2**) or fragmented (**C3**). Note that **B1** and **C1** fractures no longer exist as part of the AO-OTA classification.

9.5.2.3 Other Radiographic Features

Humeral shaft fractures are invariably mobile in the days following injury, and early fracture deformity and displacement are largely dependent upon the deforming forces present and the quality of the immobilisation. Fracture gap has been suggested as a possible risk factor for nonunion [128], although this may be difficult to quantify in spiral or multifragmentary fracture patterns. The radiographic aims of treatment are:

1. To achieve fracture union—defined as bridging callus across all fracture cortices;
2. To avoid malunion—defined as ≥30° of valgus deformity and ≥20° of sagittal plane deformity [129].

9.5.3 Diagnosis

Sport-related injuries commonly result from a direct blow to the upper arm or elbow, either during a high-energy fall (skiing, snowboarding, horse-riding) or contact sport (rugby, American football). The injured arm may be deformed, shortened, swollen or bruised; abrasions should be assessed and an open fracture excluded. Neurovascular status should be assessed and documented. Vascular injuries are rare following a closed humeral shaft fracture, but neurological injuries are relatively common—these may involve the radial nerve (8–12%), ulnar nerve (2–4%) or median nerve (1–2%) [123, 125, 126, 130–132]. Exclude associated injuries: to the shoulder, including humeral neck fracture (5%), glenohumeral dislocation or soft tissue injury (e.g. rotator cuff injury (18%) or acromioclavicular joint injury (12%) [133]); and to the elbow, including elbow dislocation or ipsilateral forearm fracture (resulting in a 'floating elbow').

Plain radiographs including two orthogonal views that visualise the shoulder and elbow are required to properly assess a humeral shaft fracture. Doppler ultrasound scanning or CT angiography may be indicated in cases of suspected vascular injury.

9.5.4 Management

9.5.4.1 Surgical Decision-Making

The principal determinants of a good outcome after a humeral shaft fracture are achievement of union and recovery of functional shoulder and elbow range of motion. Regardless of the treatment modality, a good outcome can be expected if the fracture heals in a timely fashion and without significant deformity. For the majority of patients conservative management will be appropriate, although clear indications exist for early surgery (Table 9.1). Athletes provide a particular challenge as the expediency with which complete recovery is attained is of greater importance than in the general population. As is frequently the case in sporting injures of the shoulder, the clinician must provide adequate information and counsel so that the optimal treatment for a particular patient is chosen. For athletes with a humeral shaft fracture, three key factors drive the decision for surgery: the potential risks of operative intervention (see below); the risk of nonunion or malunion; and the risk of shoulder or elbow stiffness.

Humeral shaft fracture nonunion may result in persistent pain and impaired functional recovery, and invariably leads to secondary surgical intervention. Compared with non-operative management, it is accepted that operative fixation

Table 9.1 Indications for operative management of a humeral diaphyseal fracture

Absolute indications	Relative indications
Significant vascular injury	Open fracture
Progressive neurological deficit	Segmental fracture
Intra-articular fracture extension	Obesity or large breasts
Polytrauma	Periprosthetic fracture
Loss of reduction during closed treatment	Patient preference
Pathological fracture	

results in lower rates of nonunion [134–137]—this also explains why surgery is performed when patients fail to achieve union after functional bracing. Malunion, particularly when it involves rotational malalignment [138], or shoulder/elbow stiffness, related to brace immobilisation, are likely to impair return to sport for throwing or overhead athletes [139, 140]; treatment should therefore be selected to best avoid these complications. However the potential advantages of operative fixation need to be weighed against the inherent risks associated with surgery.

9.5.4.2 Non-operative Protocol

Non-operative management varies by treatment centre, but typically involves:

- ***Temporary immobilisation***, using a plaster of Paris 'U-slab' applied in the Emergency Department—although this is often technically challenging, the resulting cast may be heavy and uncomfortable for patients and severely limits shoulder and elbow mobility.
- ***Definitive immobilisation***, using a functional humeral brace [141] applied in the Outpatient Department (usually within 2 weeks of injury); note that in some centres patients are placed directly into a humeral brace in the Emergency Department.

Immobilisation is continued until clinical and/or radiographic union is achieved—the total period of cast/brace immobilisation is usually ***8–12 weeks***.

9.5.4.3 Surgical Techniques

Indications for primary operative management of a patient with a humeral shaft fracture are summarised in Table 9.1.

Potential operative techniques include:

- Open reduction and internal fixation (ORIF)—which may be performed via an anterolateral (Fig. 9.9) or posterior approach
- Minimally-invasive plate osteosynthesis (MIPO)
- Intramedullary (IM) nailing—may be antegrade (through the humeral head) or retrograde (through the supracondylar region of the distal humerus)
- External fixation—usually reserved for severe open injuries involving extensive soft tissue or bone loss.

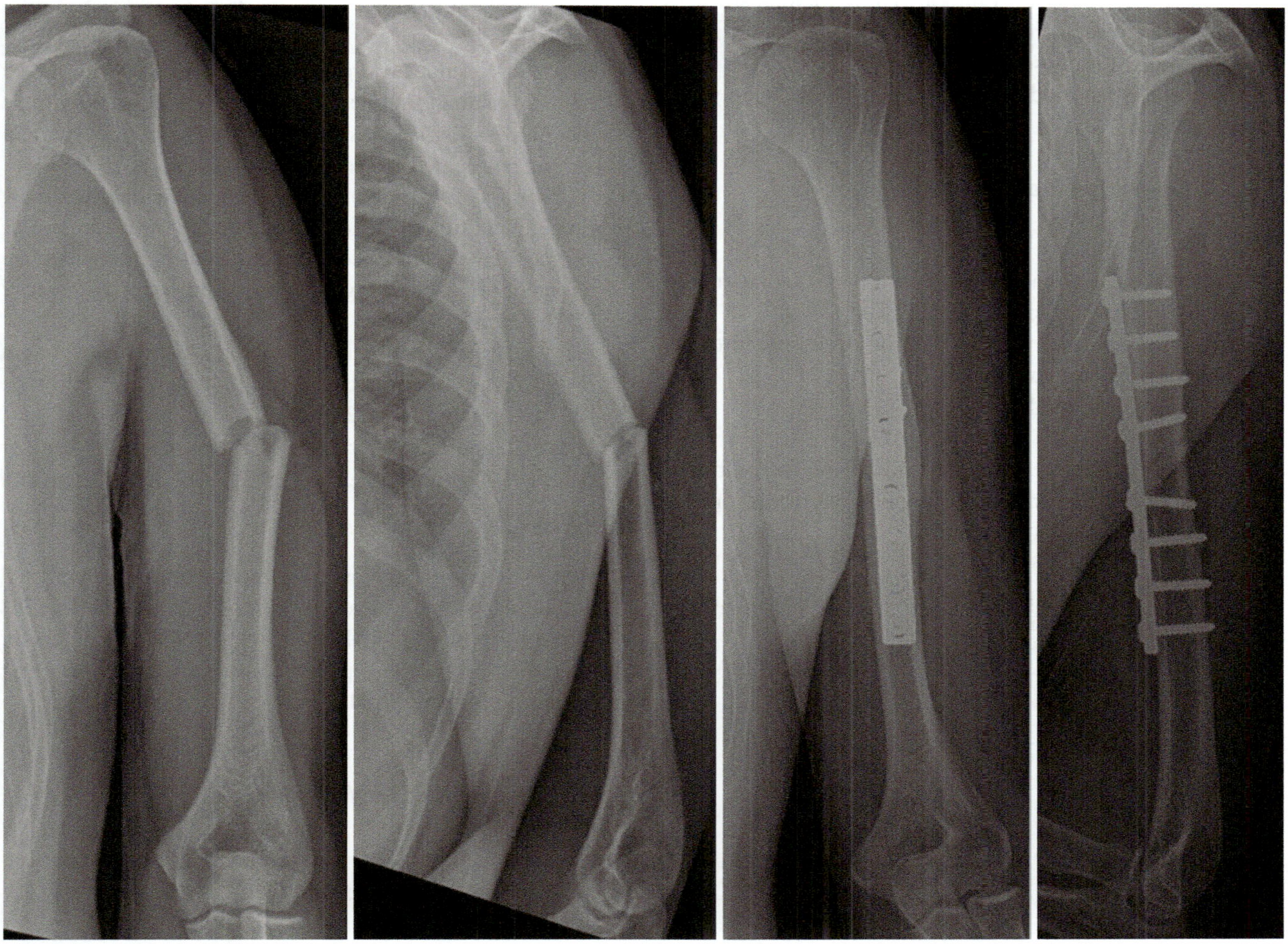

Fig. 9.9 Pre- and post-operative anteroposterior and lateral views of a left humeral shaft fracture, managed with open reduction and internal fixation using a plate and screws via an anterolateral approach (the ***authors' preferred technique***)

9.5.4.4 Authors' Preferred Technique

Although the preferred method of operative fixation varies by treatment centre, published case series [142], reviews [143, 144] and randomised controlled trials [145, 146] have consistently recommended ORIF as the strategy of choice when surgery is indicated. Accordingly, ORIF is the preferred fixation technique for uncomplicated, traumatic humeral shaft fractures in our centre.

9.5.5 Complications

9.5.5.1 Non-operative Management

Potential complications of non-operative management include:

- ***Skin irritation***—reported in 4–10% [137, 147], and may result in superficial infection or necessitate early brace removal
- ***Malunion***—historically, coronal deformity <30° and sagittal deformity <20° have been considered acceptable [129]; however malrotation occurs in up to 38% of patients and may impair shoulder rotation [138]
- ***Shoulder stiffness***—reported in up to 42–60% [148, 149]
- ***Elbow stiffness***—less common than shoulder stiffness, and has been shown to improve with normal activity without the need for physiotherapy [150]
- ***Nonunion***—reported nonunion rates vary widely, but may be up to 33% in some series (Table 9.2).

9.5.5.2 Operative Management

Potential complications of ORIF include:

- ***Neurological injury***—most commonly radial neurapraxia, reported in up to 16% [157]
- ***Infection***—approximately 1–2% for closed fractures and 2–5% for open fractures
- ***Nonunion***—reported in up to 9% [134]

Further to the above, MIPO carries an increased risk of ***neurological injury***, particularly involving the radial or musculocutaneous nerves [158, 159].

Table 9.2 Reported nonunion rates following non-operative management of humeral shaft fractures

Nonunion < 10%	Nonunion 10–20%	Nonunion > 20%
Sarmiento et al. 1977 [141]	Naver et al. 1986 [153]	Toivanen et al. 2005 [156]
Balfour et al. 1982 [151]	Koch et al. 2002 [148]	Harkin et al. 2017 [136]
Zagorski et al. 1988 [152]	Rutgers/Ring 2006 [147]	
Fjalestadt et al. 2000 [138]	Ekholm et al. 2006 [154]	
Sarmiento et al. 2000 [131]	Ali et al. 2015 [155]	
Rosenberg et al. 2006 [149]		

Additional potential complications of IM nailing include:

- Violation of the ***rotator cuff***—resulting in pain and weakness during shoulder movements
- ***Intra-operative fracture***—usually in the supracondylar region of the distal humerus during retrograde nail insertion
- ***Metalwork prominence***—which may result in subacromial impingement and require subsequent metalwork removal [160]
- ***Nonunion***—compared with ORIF, IM nailing carries a slightly higher risk of nonunion, which is reported in up to 15% [161]

9.5.6 Rehabilitation

Regardless of treatment strategy or level of sporting participation, early physiotherapy is paramount in order to avoid subsequent shoulder and elbow stiffness. The appropriate physiotherapy regime is dependent upon the athlete and the sport they play, but typically involves graduated shoulder and elbow rehabilitation—for example:

- Pendular shoulder exercises, in combination with active elbow/wrist/hand range of motion exercises, begin once the humeral brace has been applied, and the surgical wound has healed ***(~2 weeks post-injury)***
- Active shoulder range of motion and gentle passive elbow range of motion exercises (with humeral brace in situ, if appropriate) begin once pain has abated and there are clinical/radiographic signs of fracture healing ***(~6 weeks post-injury)***
- Passive/resistance shoulder and elbow exercises begin once fracture union is confirmed (and the humeral brace has been removed) ***(~12 weeks post-injury)***
- Patients should be instructed to not lift anything heavier than 0.5 kg with their affected limb for 12 weeks post-injury.

Return to play may begin once fracture union is confirmed and shoulder/elbow range of motion are restored [140] ***(4–6 months post-injury)***. Following operative management, it is reported that 90% of patients return to normal sporting activity within 4 months [162].

9.5.7 Preventative Measures

The authors are not aware of any relevant literature addressing the prevention of humeral shaft fractures in athletes.

Clinical Pearls

- Midshaft clavicle fracture fixation results in a lower incidence of nonunion and can facilitate earlier rehabilitation.
- The majority of acromioclavicular joint dislocations can be effectively managed conservatively. However surgery does have a role in the management of some injuries, with various operative options available.
- The rate of glenohumeral re-dislocation in young athletes is high but surgical management should be timed within a season to minimise loss of play.
- In contrast to the general population, there should be a lower threshold for operative fixation of humeral shaft fractures in athletes.

Review

Questions

1. What is the rate of nonunion of a midshaft clavicle fracture following non-operative management?
2. Which grade of ACJ disruption displaces inferiorly (and is rarely seen)?
3. What is the rate of recurrence following a primary glenohumeral dislocation in young adult males?
4. What are the absolute indications for primary operative management of a displaced, traumatic humeral shaft fracture?

Answers

1. 16%
2. Grade VI
3. 66%
4. Significant/progressive neurovascular injury; intra-articular extension; polytrauma; loss of closed reduction

Referrences

1. Robinson CM. Fractures of the clavicle in the adult: epidemiology and classification. J Bone Jt Surg. 1998;80:476–84.
2. Postacchini F, Gumina S, De Santis P, Albo F. Epidemiology of clavicle fractures. J Shoulder Elb Surg. 2002;11:452–6.
3. Huttunen TT, Launonen AP, Berg HE, Lepola V, Felländer-Tsai L, Mattila VM. Trends in the incidence of clavicle fractures and surgical repair in Sweden: 2001–2012. J Bone Joint Surg Am. 2016;98:1837–42.
4. Herteleer M, Winckelmans T, Hoekstra H, Nijs S. Epidemiology of clavicle fractures in a level 1 trauma center in Belgium. Eur J Trauma Emerg Surg. 2018;44:717–26.
5. Van Lancker HP, Martineau PA. (i) The diagnosis and treatment of shoulder injuries in contact and collision athletes. Orthop Trauma. 2012;26:1–11.
6. Taitsman LA, Nork SE, Coles CP, Barei DP, Agel J. Open clavicle fractures and associated injuries. J Orthop Trauma. 2006;20:396–9.
7. Backus JD, Merriman DJ, McAndrew CM, Gardner MJ, Ricci WM. Upright versus supine radiographs of clavicle fractures: does positioning matter? J Orthop Trauma. 2014;28:636–41.
8. Plocher EK, Anavian J, Vang S, Cole PA. Progressive displacement of clavicular fractures in the early postinjury period. J Trauma Inj Infect Crit Care. 2011;70:1263–7.
9. Smekal V, Deml C, Irenberger A, Niederwanger C, Lutz M, Blauth M, Krappinger D. Length determination in midshaft clavicle fractures: validation of measurement. J Orthop Trauma. 2008;22:458–62.
10. MacDonald PB, Lapointe P. Acromioclavicular and sternoclavicular joint injuries. Orthop Clin North Am. 2008;39:535–45.
11. Khan LAK, Bradnock TJ, Scott C, Robinson CM. Fractures of the clavicle. J Bone Jt Surg Ser A. 2009;91:447–60.
12. Bae DS, Shah AS, Kalish LA, Kwon JY, Waters PM. Shoulder motion, strength, and functional outcomes in children with established malunion of the clavicle. J Pediatr Orthop. 2013;33:544–50.
13. Schulz J, Moor M, Roocroft J, Bastrom TP, Pennock AT. Functional and radiographic outcomes of nonoperative treatment of displaced adolescent clavicle fractures. J Bone Joint Surg Am. 2013;95:1159–65.
14. Robinson L, Gargoum R, Auer R, Nyland J, Chan G. Sports participation and radiographic findings of adolescents treated nonoperatively for displaced clavicle fractures. Injury. 2015;46:1372–6.
15. Lenza M, Buchbinder R, Johnston RV, Ferrari BA, Faloppa F. Surgical versus conservative interventions for treating fractures of the middle third of the clavicle. Cochrane Database Syst Rev. 2019; https://doi.org/10.1002/14651858.CD009363.pub3.
16. Amer K, Smith B, Thomson JE, Congiusta D, Reilly MC, Sirkin MS, Adams MR. Operative versus nonoperative outcomes of middle-third clavicle fractures. J Orthop Trauma. 2020;34:e6–e13.
17. Murray IR, Foster CJ, Eros A, Robinson CM. Risk factors for nonunion after nonoperative treatment of displaced midshaft fractures of the clavicle. J Bone Jt Surg Ser A. 2013;95:1153–8.
18. Stegeman SA, De Witte PB, Boonstra S, De Groot JH, Nagels J, Krijnen P, Schipper IB. Posttraumatic midshaft clavicular shortening does not result in relevant functional outcome changes. Acta Orthop. 2015;86:545–52.
19. Rasmussen JV, Jensen SL, Petersen JB, Falstie-Jensen T, Lausten G, Olsen BS. A retrospective study of the association between shortening of the clavicle after fracture and the clinical outcome in 136 patients. Injury. 2011;42:414–7.
20. Figueiredo GSDL, Tamaoki MJS, Dragone B, Utino AY, Netto NA, Matsumoto MH, Matsunaga FT. Correlation of the degree of clavicle shortening after non-surgical treatment of midshaft fractures with upper limb function. BMC Musculoskelet Disord. 2015; https://doi.org/10.1186/s12891-015-0585-3.
21. Goudie EB, Clement ND, Murray IR, Lawrence CR, Wilson M, Brooksbank AJ, Robinson CM. The influence of shortening on clinical outcome in healed displaced midshaft clavicular fractures after nonoperative treatment. J Bone Jt Surg Am. 2017;99:1166–72.
22. Robinson CM, Goudie EB, Murray IR, et al. Open reduction and plate fixation versus nonoperative treatment for displaced midshaft clavicular fractures. J Bone Jt Surg Ser A. 2013;95:1576–84.
23. Woltz S, Stegeman SA, Krijnen P, Van Dijkman BA, Van Thiel TPH, Schep NWL, De Rijcke PAR, Frölke JPM, Schipper IB. Plate fixation compared with nonoperative treatment for displaced midshaft clavicular fractures a multicenter randomized controlled trial. J Bone Jt Surg Am. 2017;99:106–12.
24. Ahrens PM, Garlick NI, Barber J, Tims EM. The clavicle trial. J Bone Jt Surg Am. 2017;99:1345–54.
25. Das A, Rollins KE, Elliott K, Johnston P, Van-Rensburg L, Tytherleigh-Strong GM, Ollivere BJ. Early Versus Delayed

Operative Intervention in Displaced Clavicle Fractures. J Orthop Trauma. 2014;28:119–23.
26. Sawalha S, Guisasola I. Complications associated with plate fixation of acute midshaft clavicle fractures versus non-unions. Eur J Orthop Surg Traumatol. 2018;28:1059–64.
27. Nicholson JA, Gribbin H, Clement ND, Robinson CM. Open reduction and internal fixation of clavicular fractures after a delay of three months is associated with an increased risk of complications and revision surgery. Bone Jt J. 2019;101-B:1385–91.
28. Nicholson JA, Clement ND, Clelland AD, MacDonald D, Simpson AHRW, Robinson CM. Displaced midshaft clavicle fracture union can be accurately predicted with a delayed assessment at 6 weeks following injury: a prospective cohort study. J Bone Joint Surg Am. 2020; https://doi.org/10.2106/JBJS.19.00955.
29. King PR, Ikram A, Eken MM, Lamberts RP. The effectiveness of a flexible locked intramedullary nail and an anatomically contoured locked plate to treat clavicular shaft fractures: a 1-year randomized control trial. J Bone Jt Surg Am. 2019;101:629–34.
30. Asadollahi S, Hau RC, Page RS, Richardson M, Edwards ER. Complications associated with operative fixation of acute midshaft clavicle fractures. Injury. 2016;47:1248–52.
31. Robinson CM, Akhtar MA, Jenkins PJ, Sharpe T, Ray A, Olabi B. Open reduction and endobutton fixation of displaced fractures of the lateral end of the clavicle in younger patients. J Bone Jt Surg Ser B. 2010;92:811–6.
32. Robinson CM, Bell KR, Murray IR. Open reduction and tunneled suspensory device fixation of displaced lateral-end clavicular fractures: medium-term outcomes and complications after treatment. J Bone Jt Surg Am. 2019;101:1335–41.
33. Robertson GA, Wood AM, Oliver CW. Displaced middle-third clavicle fracture management in sport: still a challenge in 2018. Should you call the surgeon to speed return to play? Br J Sports Med. 2018;52:348–9.
34. Hebert-Davies J, Agel J. Return to elite-level sport after clavicle fractures. BMJ Open Sport Exerc Med. 2018; https://doi.org/10.1136/bmjsem-2018-000371.
35. Vora D, Baker M, Pandarinath R. Impact of clavicle fractures on return to play and performance ratings in NFL athletes. Clin J Sport Med. 2019;29:459–64.
36. Jack RA, Sochacki KR, Navarro SM, McCulloch PC, Lintner DM, Harris JD. Performance and return to sport after clavicle open reduction and internal fixation in national football league players. Orthop J Sport Med. 2017; https://doi.org/10.1177/2325967117720677.
37. Meisterling SW, Cain EL, Fleisig GS, Hartzell JL, Dugas JR. Return to athletic activity after plate fixation of displaced midshaft clavicle fractures. Am J Sports Med. 2013;41:2632–6.
38. Souza NASM de, Belangero PS, Figueiredo EA de, Pochini A de C, Andreoli CV, Ejnisman B (2018) Displaced midshaft clavicle fracture in athletes – should we operate? Rev Bras Ortop (English Ed 53:171–175.
39. Morgan RJ, Bankston LS, Hoenig MP, Connor PM. Evolving management of middle-third clavicle fractures in the national football league. Am J Sports Med. 2010;38:2092–6.
40. van der Ven DJC, Timmers TK, Broeders IAMJ, van Olden GDJ. Displaced clavicle fractures in cyclists. Clin J Sport Med. 2019;29:465–9.
41. Clitherow HDS, Bain GI. Major neurovascular complications of clavicle fracture surgery. Shoulder Elb. 2015;7:3–12.
42. Chillemi C, Franceschini V, Dei Giudici L, Alibardi A, Salate Santone F, Ramos Alday LJ, Osimani M. Epidemiology of Isolated acromioclavicular joint dislocation. Emerg Med Int. 2013; https://doi.org/10.1155/2013/171609.
43. Mazzocca AD, Arciero RA, Bicos J. Evaluation and treatment of acromioclavicular joint injuries. Am J Sports Med. 2007; https://doi.org/10.1177/0363546506298022.
44. Webb J, Bannister G. Acromioclavicular disruption in first class rugby players. Br J Sports Med. 1992; https://doi.org/10.1136/bjsm.26.4.247.
45. Rockwood CA, Jr YD. Disorders of the acromioclavicular joint. Philadelphia, PA: The Shoulder; 1998. p. 483–553.
46. Hudson VJ. Evaluation, diagnosis, and treatment of shoulder injuries in athletes. Clin Sports Med. 2010;29:19–32.
47. Bin PH, Yokota A, Gill HS, El Rassi G, EG MF. Diagnostic accuracy of clinical tests for the different degrees of subacromial impingement syndrome. J Bone Jt Surg A. 2005;87:1446–55.
48. Zanca P. Shoulder pain: involvement of the acromioclavicular joint. (analysis of 1,000 cases). Am J Roentgenol Radium Ther Nucl Med. 1971;1971:493–506.
49. Ernberg LA, Potter HG. Radiographic evaluation of the acromioclavicular and sternoclavicular joints. Clin Sports Med. 2003; https://doi.org/10.1016/S0278-5919(03)00006-1.
50. Schlegel TF, Burks RT, Marcus RL, Dunn HK. A prospective evaluation of untreated acute grade III acromioclavicular separations. Am J Sports Med. 2001; https://doi.org/10.1177/03635465010290060401.
51. Spencer EE. Treatment of grade III acromioclavicular joint injuries: a systematic review. Clin. Orthop. Relat. Res. 2007;2007:38–44.
52. Murray IR, Robinson PG, Goudie EB, Duckworth AD, Clark K, Michael Robinson C. Open reduction and tunneled suspensory device fixation compared with nonoperative treatment for type-III and type-IV acromioclavicular joint dislocations: the ACORN prospective, randomized controlled trial. J Bone Jt Surg Am. 2018; https://doi.org/10.2106/JBJS.18.00412.
53. McKee M, Pelet S, McCormack RG, et al. Multicenter randomized clinical trial of nonoperative versus operative treatment of acute acromio-clavicular joint dislocation. J Orthop Trauma. 2015; https://doi.org/10.1097/BOT.0000000000000437.
54. Bergfeld JA, Andrish JT, Clancy WG. Evaluation of the acromioclavicular joint fol lowi ng first- and second-degree sprains. Am J Sports Med. 1978; https://doi.org/10.1177/036354657800600402.
55. Zacchilli MA, Owens BD. Epidemiology of shoulder dislocations presenting to emergency departments in the United States. J Bone Joint Surg Am. 2010;92:542–9.
56. Owens BD, Agel J, Mountcastle SB, Cameron KL, Nelson BJ. Incidence of glenohumeral instability in collegiate athletics. Am J Sports Med. 2009;37:1750–4.
57. Wagstrom E, Raynor B, Jani S, Carey J, Cox CL, Wolf BR, Gao Y, Kuhn JE, Hettrich CM. Epidemiology of glenohumeral instability related to sporting activities using the FEDS (frequency, etiology, direction, and severity) classification system: a multicenter analysis. Orthop J Sport Med. 2019;7:232596711986103.
58. Kaplan LD, Flanigan DC, Norwig J, Jost P, Bradley J. Prevalence and variance of shoulder injuries in elite collegiate football players. Am J Sports Med. 2005;33:1142–6.
59. Gil JA, Goodman AD, DeFroda SF, Owens BD. Characteristics of operative shoulder injuries in the National Collegiate Athletic Association, 2009–2010 through 2013–2014. Orthop J Sport Med. 2018; https://doi.org/10.1177/2325967118790764.
60. Robinson CM, Seah M, Akhtar MA. The epidemiology, risk of recurrence, and functional outcome after an acute traumatic posterior dislocation of the shoulder. J Bone Jt Surg Ser A. 2011;93:1605–13.
61. Robinson CM, Howes J, Murdoch H, Will E, Graham C. Functional outcome and risk of recurrent instability after primary traumatic anterior shoulder dislocation in young patients. J Bone Jt Surg Ser A. 2006;88:2326–36.

62. Roberts SB, Beattie N, McNiven ND, Robinson CM. The natural history of primary anterior dislocation of the glenohumeral joint in adolescence. Bone Jt J. 2015;97-B:520–6.
63. Thomas SC, Matsen FA. An approach to the repair of avulsion of the glenohumeral ligaments in the management of traumatic anterior glenohumeral instability. J Bone Joint Surg Am. 1989;71:506–13.
64. Silliman JF, Hawkins RJ. Classification and physical diagnosis of instability of the shoulder. Clin Orthop Relat Res. 1993;1993:7–19.
65. Protzman RR. Anterior instability of the shoulder. J Bone Joint Surg Am. 1980;62:909–18.
66. Joseph TA, Williams JS, Brems JJ. Laser capsulorrhaphy for multidirectional instability of the shoulder: an outcomes study and proposed classification system. Am J Sports Med. 2003;31:26–35.
67. Gerber C, Nyffeler RW. Classification of glenohumeral joint instability. Clin. Orthop. Relat. Res. 2002;2002:65–76.
68. Cofield RH, Irving JF. Evaluation and classification of shoulder instability. With special reference to examination under anesthesia. Clin Orthop Relat Res. 1987;1987:32–43.
69. Stein DA, Jazrawi L, Bartolozzi AR. Arthroscopic stabilization of anterior shoulder instability: a review of the literature. Arthrosc J Arthrosc Relat Surg. 2002;18:912–24.
70. Kuhn JE. Shoulder injuries in athletes. A new classifi cation system for shoulder instability. Br J Sport Med. 2010;44:341–6.
71. Grossman MG, Tibone JE, McGarry MH, Schneider DJ, Veneziani S, Lee TQ. A cadaveric model of the throwing shoulder: a possible etiology of superior labrum anterior-to-posterior lesions. J Bone Jt Surg Ser A. 2005;87:824–31.
72. Bui-Mansfield LT, Banks KP, Taylor DC. Humeral avulsion of the glenohumeral ligaments: the HAGL lesion. Am J Sports Med. 2007;35:1960–6.
73. Neviaser TJ. The anterior labroligamentous periosteal sleeve avulsion lesion: a cause of anterior instability of the shoulder. Arthroscopy. 1993;9:17–21.
74. Waibl B, Buess E. Partial-thickness articular surface supraspinatus tears: a new transtendon suture technique. Arthroscopy. 2005;21:376–81.
75. Hill HA, Sachs MD. The Grooved defect of the humeral head. Radiology. 1940;35:690–700.
76. Mclaughlin H. Posterior dislocation of the shoudler. J Bone Jt Surg Am. 1952;34:584–90.
77. Shah R, Chhaniyara P, Wallace WA, Hodgson L. Pitch-side management of acute shoulder dislocations: a conceptual review. BMJ Open Sport Exerc Med. 2017; https://doi.org/10.1136/bmjsem-2016-000116.
78. Chitgopkar SD, Khan M. Painless reduction of anterior shoulder dislocation by Kocher's method. Injury. 2005;36:1182–4.
79. Hippocrates. Injuries of the shoulder. Dislocations Clin Orthop Relat Res. 1989;1989:4–7.
80. Hovelius L, Olofsson A, Sandström B, et al. Nonoperative treatment of primary anterior shoulder dislocation in patients forty years of age and younger: a prospective twenty-five-year follow up. J Bone Jt Surg Ser A. 2008;90:945–52.
81. Liavaag S, Brox JI, Pripp AH, Enger M, Soldal LA, Svenningsen S. Immobilization in external rotation after primary shoulder dislocation did not reduce the risk of recurrence: a randomized controlled trial. J Bone Jt Surg Ser A. 2011; https://doi.org/10.2106/JBJS.J.00416.
82. Heidari K, Asadollahi S, Vafaee R, Barfehei A, Kamalifar H, Chaboksavar ZA, Sabbaghi M. Immobilization in external rotation combined with abduction reduces the risk of recurrence after primary anterior shoulder dislocation. J Shoulder Elb Surg. 2014;23:759–66.
83. Murray JC, Leclerc A, Balatri A, Pelet S. Immobilization in external rotation after primary shoulder dislocation reduces the risk of recurrence in young patients. A randomized controlled trial. Orthop Traumatol Surg Res. 2018; https://doi.org/10.1016/j.otsr.2018.10.007.
84. Itoi E, Hatakeyama Y, Sato T, Kido T, Minagawa H, Yamamoto N, Wakabayashi I, Nozaka K. Immobilization in external rotation after shoulder dislocation. J Bone Jt Surg Am. 2007;89:2124–31.
85. Robinson MC, Howes J, Helen M, Will E, Graham C. Functional outcome and risk of recurrent instability dislocation in young patients. J Bone Jt Surg Am. 2006;88-A:2326–36.
86. Buss DD, Lynch GP, Meyer CP, Huber SM, Freehill MQ. Nonoperative management for in-season athletes with anterior shoulder instability. Am J Sports Med. 2004;32:1430–3.
87. Balg F, Boileau P. The instability severity index score: a simple pre-operative score to select patients for arthroscopic or open shoulder stabilisation. J Bone Jt Surg Ser B. 2007;89:1470–7.
88. Itoi E. "On-track" and "off-track" shoulder lesions. EFORT Open Rev. 2017;2:343–51.
89. Mohtadi NGH, Bitar IJ, Sasyniuk TM, Hollinshead RM, Harper WP, Orth FRACS. Arthroscopic versus open repair for traumatic anterior shoulder instability: a meta-analysis. 2005; https://doi.org/10.1016/j.arthro.2005.02.021.
90. Hobby J, Griffin D, Dunbar M, Boileau P. Is arthroscopic surgery for stabilisation of chronic shoulder instability as effective as open surgery? A systematic review and meta-analysis of 62 studies including 3044 arthroscopic operations. J Bone Jt Surg Ser B. 2007;89:1188–96.
91. Robinson CM, Jenkins PJ, White TO, Ker A, Will E. Primary arthroscopic stabilization for a first-time anterior dislocation of the shoulder. a randomized, double-blind trial. J Bone Joint Surg Am. 2008;90:708–21.
92. Shah N, Nadiri MN, Torrance E, Funk L. Arthroscopic repair of bony Bankart lesions in collision athletes. Shoulder Elb. 2018;10:201–6.
93. Purchase RJ, Wolf EM, Hobgood ER, Pollock ME, Smalley CC. hill-sachs "remplissage": an arthroscopic solution for the engaging Hill-Sachs lesion. Arthrosc J Arthrosc Relat Surg. 2008;24:723–6.
94. Longo UG, Rizzello G, Ciuffreda M, Locher J, Berton A, Salvatore G, Denaro V. Humeral avulsion of the glenohumeral ligaments: a systematic review. Arthrosc J Arthrosc Relat Surg. 2016;32:1868–76.
95. Kamihira M, Takata K. Treatment of recurrent dislocation of the shoulder. Orthop Traumatol. 1975;24:432–4.
96. Young AA, Maia R, Berhouet J, Walch G. Open Latarjet procedure for management of bone loss in anterior instability of the glenohumeral joint. J Shoulder Elb Surg. 2011;20:S61–9.
97. Burkhart SS, De Beer JF, Barth JRH, Criswell T, Roberts C, Richards DP. Results of modified Latarjet reconstruction in patients with anteroinferior instability and significant bone loss. Arthrosc J Arthrosc Relat Surg. 2007;23:1033–41.
98. Sandmann GH, Ahrens P, Schaeffeler C, et al. Balloon osteoplasty—a new technique for minimally invasive reduction and stabilisation of Hill-Sachs lesions of the humeral head: a cadaver study. Int Orthop. 2012;36:2287–91.
99. Re P, Gallo RA, Richmond JC. Transhumeral head plasty for large Hill-Sachs lesions. Arthrosc J Arthrosc Relat Surg. 2006;22:798.e1–4.
100. Miniaci A, Gish MW. Management of anterior glenohumeral instability associated with large Hill–Sachs defects. Tech Shoulder Elb Surg. 2004;5(3):170–5.
101. Saltzman BM, Riboh JC, Cole BJ, Yanke AB. Humeral head reconstruction with osteochondral allograft transplantation. Arthroscopy. 2015;31:1827–34.
102. Robinson CM, Shur N, Sharpe T, Ray A, Murray IR. Injuries associated with traumatic anterior glenohumeral dislocations. J Bone Jt Surg Ser A. 2012;94:18–26.

103. Stayner LR, Cummings J, Andersen J, Jobe CM. Shoulder dislocations in patients older than 40 years of age. Orthop Clin North Am. 2000;31:231–9.
104. Kim S-H, Ha K-I, Cho Y-B, Ryu B-D, Oh I. Arthroscopic anterior stabilization of the shoulder: two to six-year follow-up. J Bone Joint Surg Am. 2003;85:1511–8.
105. Ogawa K, Yoshida A, Ikegami H. Osteoarthritis in shoulders with traumatic anterior instability: preoperative survey using radiography and computed tomography. J shoulder Elb Surg. 2006;15:23–9.
106. Hovelius L, Augustini BG, Fredin H, Johansson O, Norlin R, Thorling J. Primary anterior dislocation of the shoulder in young patients: a ten-year prospective study. J Bone Jt Surg Ser A. 1996;78:1677–84.
107. Kuhn JE. Treating the initial anterior shoulder dislocation – an evidence-based medicine approach. Sports Med Arthrosc. 2006;14:192–8.
108. Bitter NL, Clisby EF, Jones MA, Magarey ME, Jaberzadeh S, Sandow MJ. Relative contributions of infraspinatus and deltoid during external rotation in healthy shoulders. J Shoulder Elb Surg. 2008;16:563–8.
109. Johansson FR, Skillgate E, Lapauw ML, Clijmans D, Deneulin VP, Palmans T, Engineer HK, Cools AM. Measuring eccentric strength of the shoulder external rotators using a handheld dynamometer: reliability and validity. J Athl Train. 2015;50:719–25.
110. Jaggi A, Lambert S. Rehabilitation for shoulder instability. Br J Sports Med. 2010;44:333–40.
111. Bradley T, Baldwick C, Fischer D, Murrell GAC. Effect of taping on the shoulders of Australian football players. Br J Sports Med. 2009;43:735–8.
112. Baker HP, Tjong VK, Dunne KF, Lindley TR, Terry MA. Evaluation of shoulder-stabilizing braces: can we prevent shoulder labrum injury in collegiate offensive linemen? Orthop J Sport Med. 2016; https://doi.org/10.1177/2325967116673356.
113. Cools AM, Palmans T, Johansson FR. Age-related, sport-specific adaptions of the shoulder girdle in elite adolescent tennis players. J Athl Train. 2014;49:647–53.
114. Saccol MF, Gracitelli GC, da Silva RT, Laurino CF de S, Fleury AM, Andrade M dos S, da Silva AC (2010) Shoulder functional ratio in elite junior tennis players. Phys Ther Sport 11:8–11.
115. Ellenbecker T, Roetert EP. Age specific isokinetic glenohumeral internal and external rotation strength in elite junior tennis players. J Sci Med Sport. 2003;6:63–70.
116. Gruson KI, Ruchelsman DE, Tejwani NC. Isolated tuberosity fractures of the proximal humeral: current concepts. Injury. 2008;39:284–98.
117. Neer CS. Four-segment classification of proximal humeral fractures: purpose and reliable use. J Shoulder Elb Surg. 2002;11:389–400.
118. Mutch J, Laflamme GY, Hagemeister N, Cikes A, Rouleau DM. A new morphological classification for greater tuberosity fractures of the proximal humerus: validation and clinical implications. Bone Jt J. 2014;96(B):646–51.
119. Rouleau DM, Laflamme GY, Mutch J. Fractures of the greater tuberosity of the humerus: a study of associated rotator cuff injury and atrophy. Shoulder Elb. 2016;8:242–9.
120. Nyffeler RW, Seidel A, Werlen S, Bergmann M. Radiological and biomechanical assessment of displaced greater tuberosity fractures. Int Orthop. 2019;43:1479–86.
121. Court-Brown CM, Caesar B. Epidemiology of adult fractures: a review. Injury. 2006;37:691–7.
122. Tytherleigh-Strong G, Walls N, Mcqueen MM. The epidemiology of humeral shaft fractures. J Bone Jt Surg Br. 1998;80:249–53.
123. Ekholm R, Adami J, Tidermark J, Hansson K, Tornkvist H, Ponzer S. Fractures of the shaft of the humerus: an epidemiological study of 401 fractures. J Bone Jt Surg Br. 2006;88-B:1469–73.
124. Bergdahl C, Ekholm C, Wennergren D, Nilsson F, Möller M. Epidemiology and patho-anatomical pattern of 2,011 humeral fractures: data from the Swedish Fracture Register. BMC Musculoskelet Disord. 2016;17:1–10.
125. Tsai CH, Fong YC, Chen YH, Hsu CJ, Chang CH, Hsu HC. The epidemiology of traumatic humeral shaft fractures in Taiwan. Int Orthop. 2009;33:463–7.
126. Belangero WD, Zublin CM, Martinez Siekavizza SN, et al. Demographics and clinical features of humeral shaft fractures: the Latin American multicentre prospective study (HSF-LAMPS). J Orthop Surg (Hong Kong). 2019;27:1–8.
127. Meinberg EG, Agel J, Roberts CS, Karam MD, Kellam JF. Fracture and dislocation classification compendium–2018. J Orthop Trauma. 2018;32:S1–S170.
128. Neuhaus V, Menendez M, Kurylo JC, Dyer GS, Jawa A, Ring D. Risk factors for fracture mobility six weeks after initiation of brace treatment of mid-diaphyseal humeral fractures. J Bone Jt Surg. 2014;96:403–7.
129. Klenerman L. Fractures of the shaft of the humerus. J Bone Jt Surg Br. 1966;48:105–11.
130. Noble J, Munro CA, Prasad VSSV, Midha R. Analysis of upper and lower extremity peripheral nerve injuries in a population of patients with multiple injuries. J Trauma. 1998;45:116–22.
131. Sarmiento A, Zagorski JB, Zych GA, Latta LL, Capps CA. Functional bracing for the treatment of fractures of the humeral diaphysis. J Bone Jt Surg Am. 2000;82:478–86.
132. Shao YC, Harwood P, Grotz MRW, Limb D, Giannoudis PV. Radial nerve palsy associated with fractures of the shaft of the humerus. A systematic review. J Bone Jt Surg Br. 2005;87:1647–52.
133. O'Donnell TMP, McKenna JV, Kenny P, Keogh P, O'Flanagan SJ. Concomitant injuries to the ipsilateral shoulder in patients with a fracture of the diaphysis of the humerus. J Bone Jt Surg Br. 2008;90:61–5.
134. Denard A, Richards JE, Obremskey WT, Tucker MC, Floyd M, Herzog GA. Outcome of nonoperative vs operative treatment of humeral shaft fractures: a retrospective study of 213 patients. Orthopedics. 2010; https://doi.org/10.3928/01477447-20100625-16.
135. Clement ND. Management of humeral shaft fractures; non-operative versus operative. Arch Trauma Res. 2015;4:e28013.
136. Harkin FE, Large RJ. Humeral shaft fractures: union outcomes in a large cohort. J Shoulder Elb Surg. 2017;26:1881–8.
137. Matsunaga FT, Tamaoki MJS, Matsumoto MH, Netto NA, Faloppa F, Belloti JC. Minimally invasive osteosynthesis with a bridge plate versus a functional brace for humeral shaft fractures: a randomized controlled trial. J Bone Jt Surg [Am]. 2017;99:583–92.
138. Fjalestad T, Strømsøe K, Salvesen P, Rostad B. Functional results of braced humeral diaphyseal fractures: why do 38% lose external rotation of the shoulder? Arch Orthop Trauma Surg. 2000;120:281–5.
139. Werner SL, Suri M, Guido JA, Meister K, Jones DG. Relationships between ball velocity and throwing mechanics in collegiate baseball pitchers. J Shoulder Elb Surg. 2008;17:905–8.
140. Burnier M, Barlow JD, Sanchez-Sotelo J. Shoulder and elbow fractures in athletes. Curr Rev Musculoskelet Med. 2019;12:13–23.
141. Sarmiento A, Kinman PB, Galvin EG, Schmitt RH, Phillips JG. Functional bracing of fractures of the shaft of the humerus. J Bone Jt Surg Am. 1977;59:596–601.
142. Bell MJ, Beauchamp CG, Kellam JK, McMurtry RY. The results of plating humeral shaft fractures in patients with multiple injuries. The Sunnybrook experience. J Bone Jt Surg [Br]. 1985;67:293–6.

143. Gregory PR, Sanders RW. Compression plating versus intramedullary fixation of humeral shaft fractures. J Am Acad Orthop Surg. 1997;5:215–23.
144. Bhandari M, Devereaux PJ, McKee MD, Schemitsch EH. Compression plating versus intramedullary nailing of humeral shaft fractures – a meta-analysis. Acta Orthop. 2006;77:279–84.
145. Chapman JR, Henley MB, Agel J, Benca PJ. Randomized prospective study of humeral shaft fracture fixation: intramedullary nails versus plates. J Orthop Trauma. 2000;14:162–6.
146. McCormack RG, Brien D, Buckley RE, McKee MD, Powell J, Schemitsch EH. Fixation of fractures of the shaft of the humerus by dynamic compression plate or intramedullary nail. J Bone Jt Surg [Br]. 2000;82:336–9.
147. Rutgers M, Ring D. Treatment of diaphyseal fractures of the humerus using a functional brace. J Orthop Trauma. 2006;20:597–601.
148. Koch PP, Gross DFL, Gerber C. The results of functional (Sarmiento) bracing of humeral shaft fractures. J Shoulder Elb Surg. 2002;11:143–50.
149. Rosenberg N, Soudry M. Shoulder impairment following treatment of diaphysial fractures of humerus by functional brace. Arch Orthop Trauma Surg. 2006;126:437–40.
150. Pehlivan O. Functional treatment of the distal third humeral shaft fractures. Arch Orthop Trauma Surg. 2002;122:390–5.
151. Balfour GW, Mooney V, Ashby ME. Diaphyseal fractures of the humerus treated with a ready-made fracture brace. J Bone Jt Surg Am. 1982;64:11–3.
152. Zagorski JB, Latta LL, Zych GA, Finnieston AR. Diaphyseal fractures of the humerus. Treatment with prefabricated braces. J Bone Jt Surg Am. 1988;70:607–10.
153. Naver L, Aalberg JR. Humeral shaft fractures treated with a ready-made fracture brace. Arch Orthop Trauma Surg. 1986;106:20–2.
154. Ekholm R, Tidermark J, Törnkvist H, Adami J, Ponzer S. Outcome after closed functional treatment of humeral shaft fractures. J Orthop Trauma. 2006;20:591–5.
155. Ali E, Griffiths D, Obi N, Tytherleigh-Strong G, Van Rensburg L. Nonoperative treatment of humeral shaft fractures revisited. J Shoulder Elb Surg. 2015;24:210–4.
156. Toivanen JAK, Nieminen J, Laine H-J, Honkonen SE, Järvinen MJ. Functional treatment of closed humeral shaft fractures. Int Orthop. 2005;29:10–3.
157. Jawa A, McCarty P, Doornberg J, Harris M, Ring D. Extra-articular distal-third diaphyseal fractures of the humerus. A comparison of functional bracing and plate fixation. J Bone Jt Surg [Am]. 2006;88:2343–7.
158. Livani B, Belangero WD. Bridging plate osteosynthesis of humeral shaft fractures. Injury. 2004;35:587–95.
159. Apivatthakakul T, Patiyasikan S, Luevitoonvechkit S. Danger zone for locking screw placement in minimally invasive plate osteosynthesis (MIPO) of humeral shaft fractures: a cadaveric study. Injury. 2010;41:169–72.
160. Kurup H, Hossain M, Andrew JG. Dynamic compression plating versus locked intramedullary nailing for humeral shaft fractures in adults. Cochrane Database Syst Rev. 2011;2011:CD005959.
161. Mahabier KC, Vogels LMM, Punt BJ, Roukema GR, Patka P, Van Lieshout EMM. Humeral shaft fractures: retrospective results of non-operative and operative treatment of 186 patients. Injury. 2013;44:427–30.
162. Niall DM, O'Mahony J, McElwain JP. Plating of humeral shaft fractures – has the pendulum swung back? Injury. 2004;35:580–6.

Acute Fractures in Sport: Elbow

10

Brandon J. Erickson, Daniel A. Seigerman, and Anthony A. Romeo

10.1 Epidemiology of Elbow Fractures in Sport

The elbow joint is a complex hinge joint that is made up of three distinct articulations: ulno-trochlear (between the distal humerus and proximal ulna), radio-capitellar (between the distal humerus and radial head), and the proximal radio-ulnar joint (PRUJ) (between the proximal radius and ulna). Unlike the shoulder, which is a relatively unstable ball and socket joint that relies on soft tissue restraints to provide the majority of its stability, the congruity of the elbow afford this joint a significant amount of stability. Stability of the elbow is provided by both bony and soft tissue restraints, of which both account for approximately 50% of elbow stability.

Fractures about the elbow are much less common than soft tissue injuries (ulnar collateral ligament tears, triceps tendonitis, flexor-pronator tears, etc.) in athletes [1, 2]. There are two primary etiologies of fractures about the elbow in sport: macrotrauma and overuse. Macro-traumatic injuries involve a high-energy collision of the player with another object (another player, the ground, etc.) where a tremendous amount of force is placed through the elbow. This can result in an elbow dislocation, fracture, or both. The magnitude and direction of the force play a role in the ultimate injury (rotational, bending, etc.).

B. J. Erickson (✉) · D. A. Seigerman
Rothman Orthopaedic Institute, New York, NY, USA
e-mail: brandon.erickson@rothmanortho.com

A. A. Romeo
DuPage Medical Group, DuPage, IL, USA

10.2 Specific Elbow Fractures in Sport

10.2.1 Distal Humerus

10.2.1.1 Epidemiology

Fractures of the distal humerus are not common in athletes. While the "thrower's fracture of the humerus" (Fig. 10.1a–d) has been previously described as a spiral fracture of the mid to distal third of the humerus, there is very limited literature on distal humeral fractures in athletes [3]. These fracture typically occur from a macrotrauma with either a rotational or bending moment that causes the humerus to fail. The fracture pattern is dictated by the imparted force with spiral fractures seen in rotational injuries and transverse fractures seen following a bending moment.

10.2.1.2 Diagnosis

Diagnosis of distal humeral fractures is made from history and physical exam. The history can involve a trauma of an opponent landing on the patient's arm, the patient falling onto an outstretched arm, or the patient hearing a crack when throwing a baseball or other overhead object. Aside from associated pain, there may be paresthesia in the hand from nerve injury, especially to the radial nerve. A physical exam is undertaken, although this can be somewhat limited, due to the patient's pain. A complete neurovascular exam is performed to rule out any associated nerve injury. It is imperative to evaluate the radial nerve: this can be injured either from the trauma or swelling, or from a fracture where the nerve is interposed between the fragments (Holstein–Lewis fracture). Often there will be swelling and tenderness around the fracture site. Wrist motion should be pain free, but elbow motion is often painful. Radiographs of the elbow including an anteroposterior (AP), lateral (Fig. 10.1e, f), and oblique are ordered. These will often show the fracture. However, if there is any question of fracture extension intra-articularly, a computed tomography (CT) scan of the elbow is ordered with 3D reconstructions (Fig. 10.1g). The CT scan can also

G. A. J. Robertson, N. Maffulli (eds.), *Fractures in Sport*, https://doi.org/10.1007/978-3-030-72036-0_10

help with fracture pattern recognition and to look for any areas of comminution.

10.2.1.3 Classification

There are several classification systems for distal humeral fractures including Jupiter, Milch and AO/OTA. The AO/OTA is one of the most commonly utilized classification systems and classifies these fractures into 3 types: Type A—extra-articular: (supracondylar fracture); Type B—intra-articular—single column fracture; Type C—intra-articular—both medial and lateral columns are fractured (i.e. the joint is not contiguous with the shaft) [4].

10.2.1.4 Treatment

Treatment of distal third humeral fractures is based on fracture alignment and timing of return to sport (RTS). If a patient suffers a spiral distal humeral fracture that is well aligned, this fracture can often be treated effectively in a Sarmiento brace. However, if the fracture is not well aligned or the athlete needs to return to sport more expeditiously, then the fracture can be fixed with open reduction internal fixation (ORIF) (Fig. 10.1e–j). The authors will offer athletes the option of operative fixation if they wish to RTS more quickly than can be achieved with non-operative management. While a humeral nail can be used in some fracture patterns, we do not commonly treat our athletes with a nail for fear of injury to their rotator cuff and the potential for subsequent post-operative shoulder pain. When performing an ORIF for distal humeral fractures, the location of the fracture often dictates the surgical approach. If the fracture extends proximally, then an anterolateral approach is often required. However, if the fracture is isolated to the distal third of the humerus, a posterior approach is often used to gain access to the fracture. Similarly, if the fracture extends into the joint, a posterior approach is used, most commonly with an olecranon osteotomy. There are several approaches to the posterior

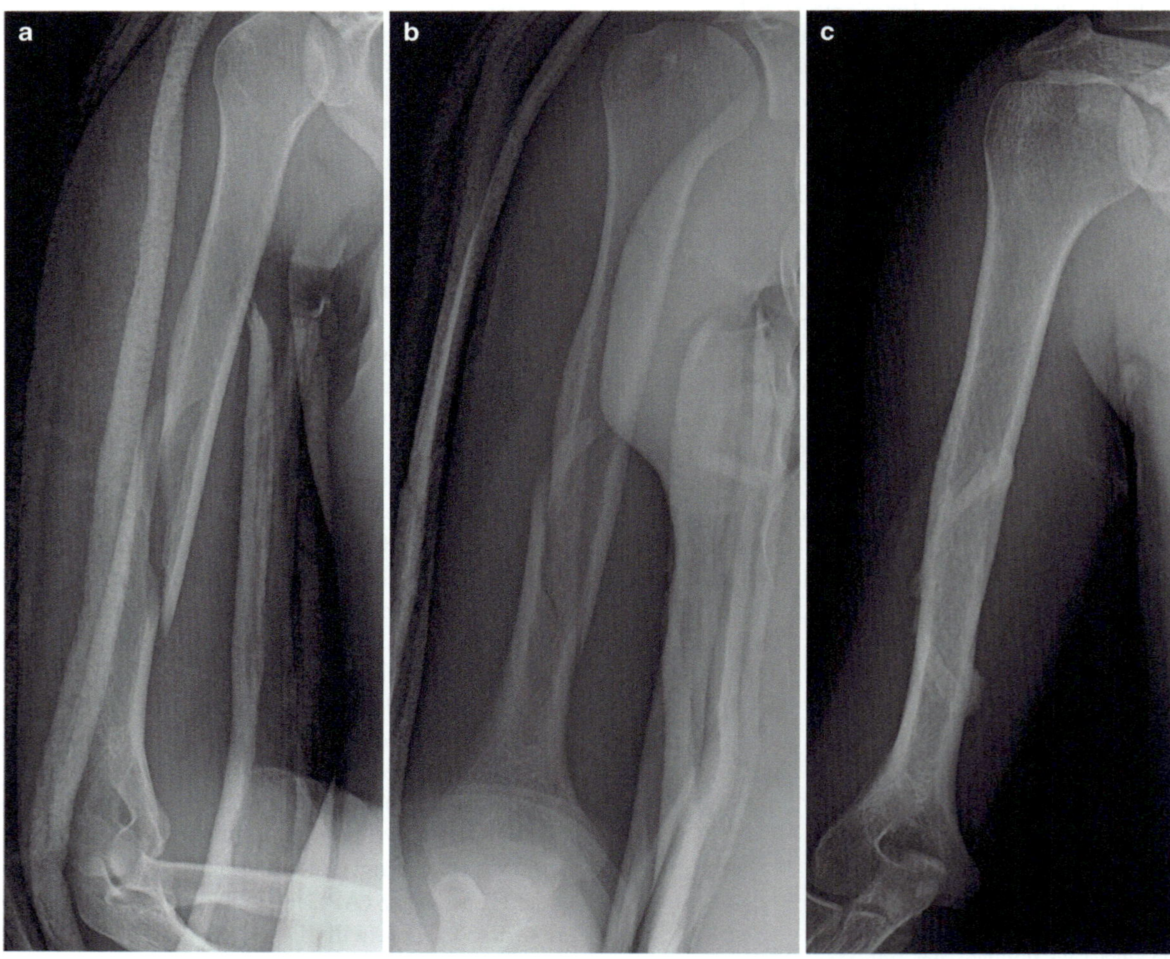

Fig. 10.1 (**a**–**d**) Radiographs of a 25 year old male who sustained a mid to distal third spiral humeral shaft fracture while throwing a baseball at initial presentation (**a**, **b**) and after 10 weeks of conservative treatment (**c**, **d**). (**e**–**j**) Images of a 16 year old male who sustained a distal humeral fracture after landing on his arm during a lacrosse game. (**e**, **f**) Are the radiographs at initial presentation that demonstrate the distal third humeral fracture, while **g** is the 3D reconstruction of the elbow CT that was obtained to ensure the fracture did not extend into the joint. Figures **h**–**j** are radiographs following open reduction internal fixation at 3 month follow-up demonstrating union of the fracture

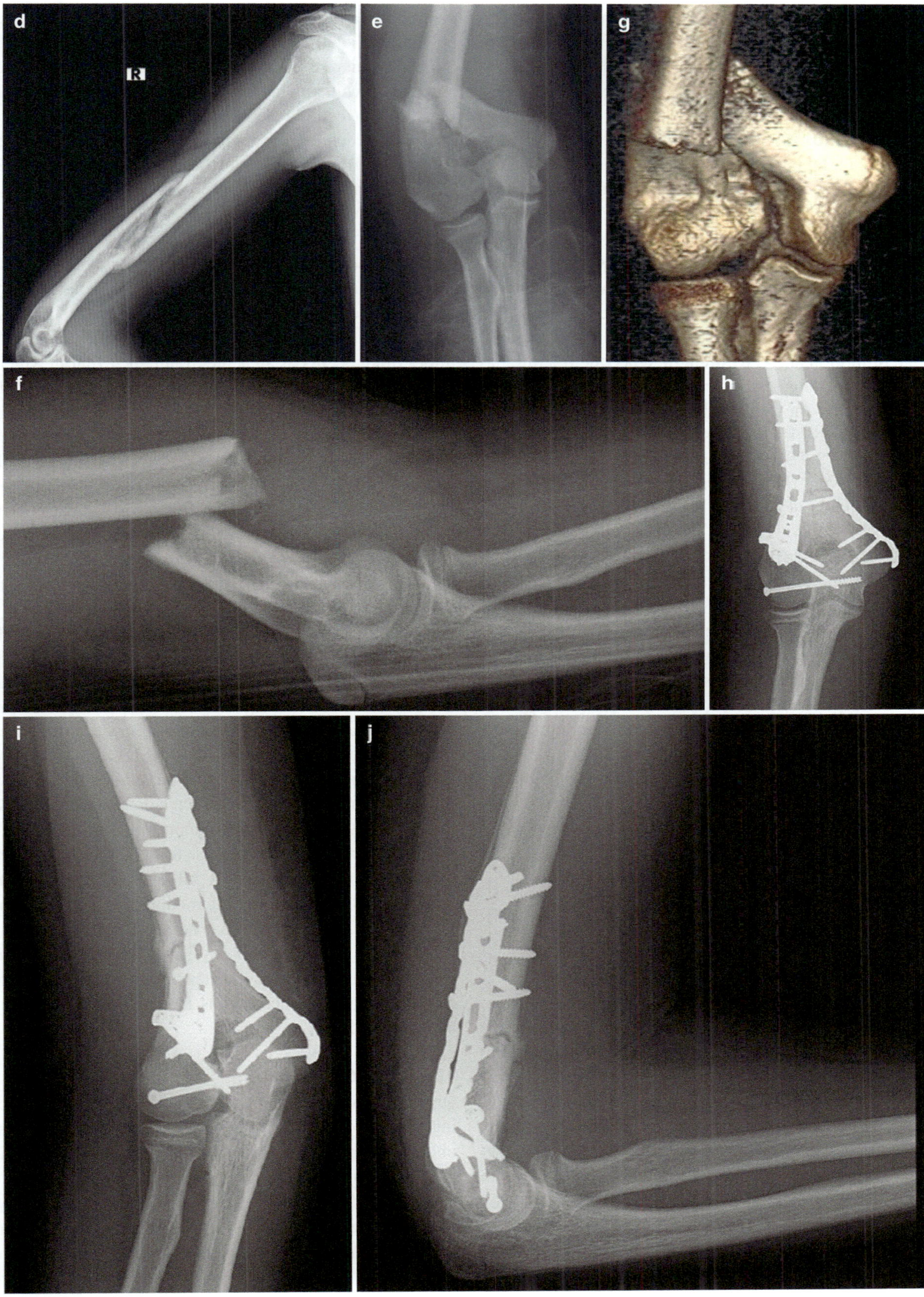

Fig. 10.1 (continued)

humerus, including a triceps split, para-tricipital and others. The surgeon should use the approach with which they are most comfortable when performing an ORIF of the distal humerus.

10.2.1.5 Rehabilitation

This involves a brief period of protection and immobilisation followed by elbow and shoulder ROM. Stiffness can be a problem in these athletes, so a balance between immobilisation to allow fracture healing and mobilization to prevent stiffness is extremely important. No lifting with the injured upper extremity is permitted for the first 6 weeks while the fracture unites. During this period the athlete is encouraged to work out their legs as well as work on their shoulder and hip range of motion and core strength. Once the fracture has healed, a gentle strengthening program is begun followed by a sport-specific return to play program. Athletes who compete in contact or collision sports (American football, rugby) are often able to RTS faster than overhead athletes as the stress placed on the elbow by an overhead athlete is more significant than that of a contact athlete.

10.2.1.6 Complications

Depending on the fracture pattern and treatment, patients with distal humeral fractures are at risk for non-union, malunion, nerve injury (either from the fracture or iatrogenically at the time of surgery), or elbow stiffness depending on the exact fracture. Hardware here is typically not symptomatic unless it encroaches into the joint, or in the case of plating the olecranon for an olecranon osteotomy. If symptomatic, this hardware can be removed after a minimum of 6 months if the fracture has successfully united. However, the athlete must be held out of competition following hardware removal, to prevent a fracture through one of the screw holes while these consolidate.

10.2.2 Medial Epicondyle Fractures

10.2.2.1 Epidemiology

Medial epicondyle fractures are most commonly seen in overhead athletes (typically pitchers) and gymnasts, as the amount of stress placed across the medial epicondyle with activities in these sports is significant [5, 6].· These injuries can often be separated based on the status of the medial epicondylar growth plate, which commonly fuses around age 14–18, and is typically the last growth plate of the elbow to fuse. The growth plate commonly fuses at an earlier age in females than males, as females often reach skeletal maturity at a younger age. Athletes who are still growing, and whose medial epicondyle growth plate has not yet closed, are susceptible to apophysitis and avulsion injures of the medial epicondyle, with repeated valgus stress of the elbow. Skeletally mature athletes, however, can injure the medial epicondyle with an elbow subluxation/dislocation or following surgery (medial epicondyle fracture following ulnar collateral ligament reconstruction (UCLR)) [7–10]. Medial epicondyle fractures account for approximately 10–20% of all elbow fractures in adolesscents and adults [11].

10.2.2.2 Diagnosis

Athletes who present with a medial epicondyle fracture will often complain of pain in and around the medial elbow, that is exacerbated by passive wrist extension and forearm supination, and active wrist flexion and forearm pronation. The injury often occurs as an acute, traumatic event in which the player felt a "pop": report of increasing pain around the medial epicondyle secondary to repetitive valgus loads over time, should raise the suspicion of a medial epicondylar stress fracture. It is important to ask the patient if they have any ulnar nerve symptoms such as numbness/tingling on the pinky or ulnar half of the ring finger, or weakness of their hand. This can indicate involvement of the ulnar nerve, which will influence how these injuries are treated. On inspection there may or may not be bruising present around the medial elbow depending on the chronicity of the injury. On palpation, pain should be located to the medial elbow, specifically on the medial epicondyle. The elbow should be meticulously palpated to ensure there are no other sites of tenderness, such as along the course of the ulnar collateral ligament. Range of motion of the elbow is first assessed including flexion/extension and forearm supination/pronation. Stress placed across the medial epicondyle will cause pain, so exam maneuvers that stretch or activate the common flexor-pronator mass will be uncomfortable for the patient. Similarly, a moving valgus stress test or 'milking' maneuver will often cause pain in these athletes as these maneuvers impart significant stress on the medial elbow. A neurovascular exam, focused on the ulnar nerve, including ulnar nerve compression test at the elbow, Tinel's testing at the elbow, ulnar nerve instability assessment, and testing for weakness of the first dorsal interosseous is critical to document any ulnar nerve deficit.

10.2.2.3 Classification

Once the exam is complete, radiographs of the elbow including an anteroposterior (AP), oblique, and lateral views are obtained (Fig. 10.2a–c). In skeletally immature individuals it is helpful to X-ray the contralateral, uninjured elbow as a baseline to determine the normal radiographic anatomy for that particular patient's elbow. Depending on the severity of injury, the radiographs can be normal, can show widening of

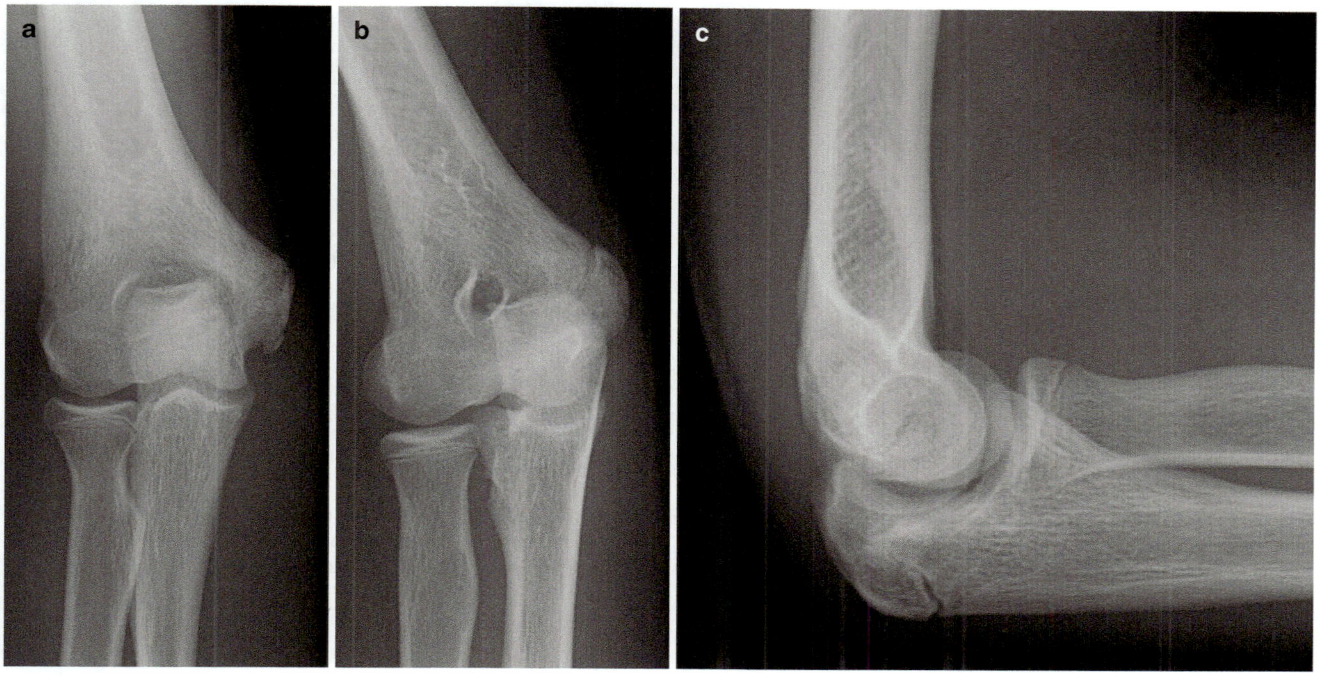

Fig. 10.2 (**a–c**) Anteroposterior (**a**), oblique (**b**), and lateral (**c**) radiographs of the elbow of a 15 year old male. Several of the growth plates are still open. There is also evidence of a calcification within the proximal aspect of the ulnar collateral ligament

the medial epicondyle physis, or can show a discrete fracture through the medial epicondyle with displacement. A magnetic resonance imaging (MRI) can be obtained in patients with normal X-Rays who have a suspected medial epicondyle fracture. If positive, the MRI will show edema within the medial epicondyle and possibly a discrete fracture line. The MRI is also useful to rule out other pathologies within the elbow including injuries to the flexor pronator mass, ulnar collateral ligament (UCL), cartilage, and others.

10.2.2.4 Treatment

Treatment of these injuries is based on the severity of the injury as well as the athlete's activity level and sport. For skeletally immature patients with a minimally displaced fracture of the medial epicondyle on MRI, but no significant (<5 mm) widening of the physis on X-Ray, conservative management with a period of rest and immobilisation followed by regaining range of motion (ROM) and strength, and finally a RTS program [12, 13]. These injuries are most common in baseball players, and a 4–6 week shutdown period with no throwing followed by a return to throwing program once the elbow is asymptomatic is often effective in allowing these athletes to RTS. When there is more than 10 mm of widening of the medial epicondyle physis in an overhead athlete, these players often benefit from open reduction internal fixation (ORIF) of the fracture [14]. There are several techniques for fixation of the fracture fragment, including cannulated screws, tension band, suture anchors, and others (Fig. 10.3a–d). The fracture often translates anterior and distal, so fluoroscopy is helpful to evaluate and confirm the reduction before the fracture is fixed. We typically use one or two cannulated screws provided the fracture fragment is large enough to afford fixation without splintering. It is imperative to identify and protect the ulnar nerve when preforming this surgery, to prevent any damage to this critical structure.

Finally, in older athletes who have a history of an UCLR, a fracture through the humeral drill tunnel can occur, especially if the tunnel was created too medial (close to the medial cortex). These injuries are significant and often warrant surgical intervention with ORIF using a cannulated screw or suture anchors.

A recent study evaluated medial epicondyle fractures in professional baseball players using the major league baseball (MLB) injury tracking system [9]. In total, 15 professional baseball pitchers underwent open reduction internal fixation for a medial epicondyle fracture between 2010–2016. All of these players had a history of UCLR and the majority of these players were starting pitchers (80%). Overall 55% were able to RTS at the same or higher level, and for players who were able to RTS, their performance upon RTS was not significantly different from that of a matched control group or compared to their own pre-operative performance.

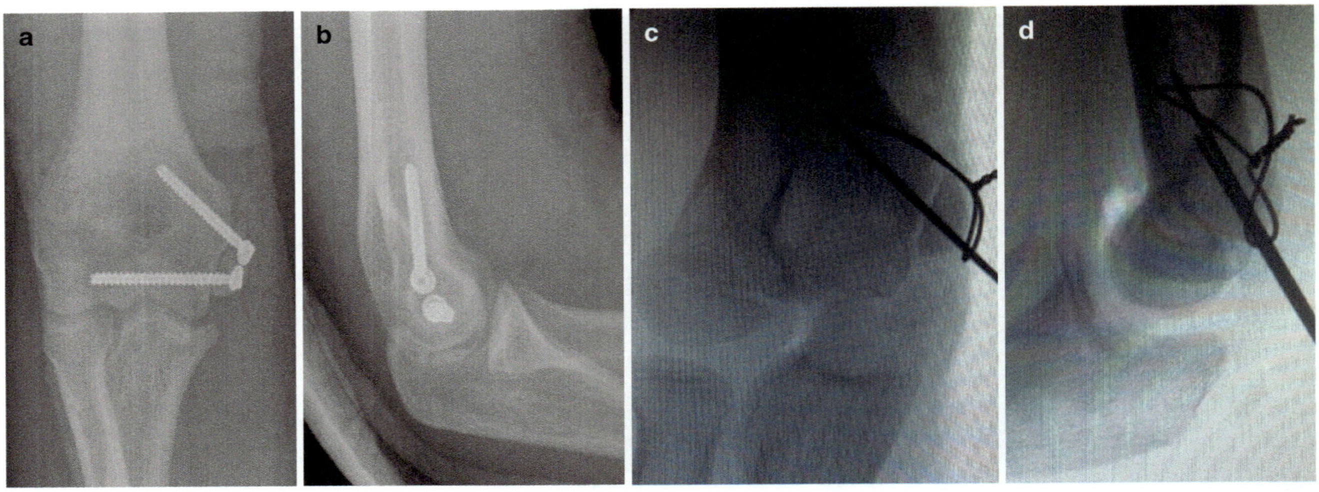

Fig. 10.3 (**a–d**) Anteroposterior (**a**) ad lateral (**b**) radiograph following open reduction internal fixation of a displaced medial epicondyle fracture in a skeletally immature adolescent baseball player using a two screw construct. Anteroposterior (**c**) and lateral (**d**) radiograph following open reduction internal fixation of a medial epicondyle fracture in a skeletally immature baseball player using a tension band construct

10.2.2.5 Rehabilitation

Rehabilitation following non-operative and operative treatment of medial epicondyle fractures is specific to each patient. A brief period of immobilisation is typically afforded (7–10 days) followed by controlled elbow movement. Strengthening is started after fracture healing has occurred and timing of return to sport is based on the particular sport (shorter time for contact athletes, longer time for overhead athletes).

10.2.2.6 Complications

While patients who undergo ORIF of the medial epicondyle fracture typically do well, there are several complications that can occur. Non-union or mal-union of the fracture, infection, hardware irritation, failure of the construct, and ulnar nerve irritation are all potential complications following ORIF of the medial epicondyle. Treatment of each complication is on an individual basis.

10.2.3 Isolated Elbow Dislocations

10.2.3.1 Epidemiology

Simple or isolated elbow dislocations make up approximately 10–25% of elbow injuries [15]. Simple elbow dislocations involve a dislocation of the ulnohumeral and radiocapitellar joint without an associated fracture. These injuries are commonly seen from a fall onto an outstretched hand, with a load placed on the athlete while falling. There is often a valgus load with some hyperextension, that causes the elbow to dislocate. This causes varying degrees of injury to the lateral ulnar collateral ligament (LUCL), elbow capsule, medial ulnar collateral ligament (UCL), and other structures. While isolated elbow dislocations do not involve an associated fractures, studies have found that nearly 100% of elbow dislocations result in some form of osteochondral injury [16].

10.2.3.2 Diagnosis

The diagnosis of a simple elbow dislocation is often made by history, physical exam, and radiographic imaging. If the physician is covering a game and a player dislocates his or her elbow, or the physician is called to the emergency department to review a player because of an elbow deformity, the diagnosis is often obvious. There will be a deformity to the elbow, with significant pain on any attempted elbow movement. It is extremely important to assess neurovascular status of the extremity both before and after reduction. Radiographs confirm the diagnosis and the elbow is reduced in a timely manner. If the athlete presents to the office, the elbow has typically already been reduced and the diagnosis is made by history as well as prior radiographs. Physical exam following reduction of an elbow dislocation should determine the position of stability for the elbow (the amount of extension where the elbow becomes unstable), as the elbow should be protected from this range of motion initially. Finally, the physician should also examine the shoulder and wrist for any concomitant pathology.

10.2.3.3 Classification

As simple elbow dislocations do not involve a fracture, these injures are classified based on the direction of the elbow dislocation. Posterolateral dislocations are the most common direction of dislocation.

10.2.3.4 Treatment

The mainstay of treatment for isolated elbow dislocations is brief immobilisation followed by early range of motion. Prolonged immobilisation has been shown to have poor outcomes [15]. The elbow is most stable in flexion and least stable in extension, so the elbow should be splinted in 90° of flexion to begin with for approximately 10 days. The splint can be changed to a hinged elbow brace or removable splint that allows complete flexion but prevents extension to the point of instability for the next 2–3 weeks. Once the elbow has become stable, full extension can be allowed, as long as there is no evidence of instability. Full ROM should be achieved at the 4–6 week mark. While surgery is uncommon in these patients, if the elbow does not remain concentrically reduced, or if the elbow is not stable at 50° of extension or less, repair of the UCL and LUCL is recommended.

10.2.3.5 Rehabilitation

Rehabilitation following simple elbow dislocations is based on the stability of the joint. The more stable the joint, the more aggressive the rehabilitation can be. Following the initial period of immobilisation, therapy is initiated to help the patient regain full ROM while avoiding any positions of instability. Once ROM is achieved at the 4- to 6-week mark, gentle strengthening is begun with the elbow at the side. Varus and valgus stress on the elbow is avoided for at least 8–10 weeks.

10.2.3.6 Complications

Elbow stiffness is the most common complication that occurs following elbow dislocation. This may necessitate an arthroscopic or open elbow release, if a functional ROM cannot be achieved. Persistent elbow instability requiring UCL or LUCL repair is a possible complication as well. Finally, delayed instability, such as posterolateral rotatory instability, is a potential complication. This may require a LUCL reconstruction in the future, if the athlete complains of persistent elbow discomfort or a sense of instability.

10.2.4 Fracture Dislocations of the Elbow

10.2.4.1 Epidemiology

Elbow instability injuries have been reported to occur at an incidence of 0.04 per 10,000 athlete exposures (i.e. one athlete participating in one game or practice session, regardless of time duration, within which they are exposed to a risk of sport-related injury) [17]. While most of these are simple dislocations (i.e. do not involve a concomitant fracture), an associated fracture is seen with elbow dislocations in approximately 26% of cases [18, 19]. The treatment of complex elbow dislocations varies greatly from simple dislocations.

10.2.4.2 Diagnosis

Similar to a simple elbow dislocation, the diagnosis is made via history, exam, and radiographs. Acutely there will be a significant deformity present, with radiographic evidence of the dislocation. However, unlike simple elbow dislocations, an associated fracture about the elbow is often appreciated. The mechanism of injury (axial load, valgus stress, direct impact, etc.) will often determine the associated fracture. While the associated fracture may not be clearly visible on initial radiographs, advanced imaging in the form of a CT scan can be useful to identify and characterize the fracture. As before, a thorough exam of the entire upper extremity is necessary including a complete neurovascular exam and an exam of the shoulder and wrist to rule out concomitant pathology.

10.2.4.3 Classification

Complex elbow dislocations are classified by the direction of the dislocation as well as the associated fracture. The associated fracture of the proximal radius or proximal ulna can be further classified using the AO classification system. Fractures of the radial head and neck region can be classified as complete articular, partial articular, or extra-articular. The extra-articular radial fractures can be divided into avulsion of the bicipital tuberosity, simple radial neck, multi-fragmentary radial neck. The partial articular radial fractures can be divided into simple and fragmentary. The complete articular radial fractures can be divided into simple and multi-fragmentary. The extra-articular proximal ulnar fractures can be divided into avulsion of the triceps insertion, metaphyseal simple fracture, and metaphyseal fragmentary fracture. The partial articular proximal ulnar fractures can be further divided into olecranon and coronoid fractures. The complete articular fractures are divided into coronoid and olecranon fractures, that are simple, multi-fragmentary involving the olecranon, or multi-fragmentary involving coronoid process. Finally, coronoid fractures can be classified based on the size of the fragment where a type I involves avulsion of the tip of the coronoid, type II involves a single or comminuted fragment of 50% of the process or less, and type III involves a single or comminuted fragment involving more than 50% of the coronoid process [20, 21].

10.2.4.4 Treatment

Treatment of complex elbow dislocations is based on the associated fracture pattern. A complex elbow dislocation with an isolated non-displaced radial head fracture or isolated small coronoid fracture can be managed non-operatively. However, this injury pattern is rare. More commonly these injuries involve olecranon fractures, communited radial head fractures, or large coronoid fractures. In these cases, surgical intervention is required for reduction and stabilization of the fracture and repair of the lateral collateral ligament (LCL).

The elbow is commonly approached from the lateral side, unless there is a concomitant olecranon fracture. The olecranon is often reduced and plated with a posterior plate, while treatment for the coronoid and radial head is more variable. Coronoid fractures can be treated with suture lasso fixation or lag screws depending on the size of the fragment [22]. Radial head fractures can be treated with ORIF or radial head replacement, with radial head replacement reserved for older individuals or in the setting of significant comminution (more than 3–4 fracture fragments) [23–25].

10.2.4.5 Rehabilitation

Rehabilitation following surgical intervention is often dictated by the type of surgery performed. If an ORIF of the olecranon or radial head was performed, these structures must be protected in the initial rehabilitation phase. Conversely, if a radial head replacement was performed, the rehabilitation program can be slightly more aggressive with ROM. Regardless, rehabilitation is a balance between allowing the surgically repaired structures to heal, while attempting to minimize concomitant stiffness of the elbow. Once the patient has regained full ROM, a strengthening program is regularly initiated at the 8-week mark, followed by sport specific training.

10.2.4.6 Complications

The most common complications following major trauma to the elbow are stiffness and post-traumatic arthritis [26, 27]. Symptomatic hardware, infection, and wound issues can also be seen in the patient population. Specific complications are often dictated by the fracture pattern and are discussed in the individual sections of the text involving isolated fractures.

10.2.5 Olecranon Fractures

10.2.5.1 Epidemiology

Olecranon fractures are relatively uncommon injuries in the overall athletic population and can occur from acute, traumatic injuries or, more commonly, from repetitive overload leading to a stress fracture. In the athlete, acute olecranon fractures most commonly occur following a fall onto the elbow [28]. Acute sport-related olecranon fractures have an incidence of 0.01 per 1000 general population [29].

10.2.5.2 Diagnosis

Athletes presenting with acute olecranon fractures will complain of pain and swelling in the elbow, with possible numbness in their hand, depending on nerve compression from the swelling, and pain with elbow movement. These injuries will often occur from either a direct blow to the posterior elbow or a fall on an outstretched hand. The acute event is often accompanied by a "pop" or "crack" and significant pain. On examination, the patient will have pain with elbow flexion/extension accompanied by bruising and swelling. A detailed neurovascular exam of the injured limb is mandatory.

10.2.5.3 Classification

Radiographic evaluation begins with the standard elbow series. Acute, traumatic olecranon fractures can be classified using several different systems including the Mayo classification system, AO classification system, and many others [30]. The Mayo classification system can be divide into 3 types: Type 1: non-displaced; Type II: displaced but with a stable elbow (A = non-communited; B = communited); Type III: displaced with an unstable elbow (A = non-communited; B = communited). The AO classification system divides these fractures into three types: Type A: extra-articular; Type B intra-articular; Type C intra-articular fractures of both the radial head and olecranon [30]. In acute fractures, a computed tomography (CT) scan may be necessary to better characterize the fracture and any associated comminution.

10.2.5.4 Treatment

Treatment of olecranon fractures is dictated by patient age, type of fracture, and activity level. Acute, traumatic, displaced olecranon fractures are treated with ORIF using either a tension band or plate and screw construct. The authors typically use an olecranon specific plate to minimize hardware irritation, although in some athletes the plate is symptomatic and needs to be removed in the off-season. This is followed by a brief period of immobilisation after which supervised passive ROM is begun in an effort to prevent stiffness. Patients with non-displaced olecranon fractures, where the joint is well-aligned, can be trialed with non-operative management. This involves a posterior splint with the elbow in 45–60° for 10–14 days, followed by transition to a hinged elbow brace, with passive elbow extension and active elbow flexion. Full motion is obtained by 4 weeks, but the elbow is not loaded until 6–8 weeks depending on healing. One can consider obtaining advanced imaging with either a CT or magnetic resonance image (MRI) to verify fracture union before allowing these athletes to RTS.

A recent study evaluated 52 olecranon fractures treated with ORIF in professional baseball players between 2010 and 2016 [31]. To note, the majority of these were primary olecranon stress fractures (73%) and were treated with a single screw (60%). The authors reported an overall RTS rate of 67.5% (57.9% returned to the same or higher level of play) with no significant decline in performance upon RTS compared to a group of matched controls and to the player's individual preoperative performance. Interestingly, it took players an average of 314 days to return to their same level of play.

10.2.5.5 Rehabilitation

Following ORIF of olecranon fractures, patients are typically immobilized in a posterior moulded spin for 7–10 days. Passive elbow extension and active elbow flexion are then begun, with care taken to avoid passively hyperflexing the elbow or forcefully extending the elbow, in the immediate post-operative period. This minimizes stress on the fracture fixation. Once the fracture has healed and the patient has regained their elbow motion, a strengthening program is begun. This is followed by a sport specific rehabilitation protocol and gradual RTS. Those patients with non-displaced olecranon fractures that are managed non-operatively will remain in the splint longer as there is no hardware in place. Once ROM is regained at 4 weeks, flexor pronator strengthening is begun but no triceps strengthening is undertaken for 6–8 weeks to prevent distraction of the fracture. Once the patient has reached the 6–8 week mark, they are typically cleared to begin a RTS program.

10.2.5.6 Complications

The skin around the posterior elbow does not have a robust blood supply and there is minimal sub-cutaneous fat to protect the hardware. Hence, skin breakdown and hardware irritation are two of the most common complications following olecranon ORIF. Other complications include non-union, mal-union, loss of reduction, ulnar nerve irritation, elbow stiffness, and continued pain. Each complication is managed on a case by case basis.

10.2.6 Proximal Radius Fractures

10.2.6.1 Epidemiology

Fractures of the proximal radius are relatively common, occurring in an athlete following significant trauma. The proximal radius includes the articular surface of the radial head, the radial neck, and up to the bicipital tuberosity. The significant majority of these injuries occur at the radial head and neck region. The radial head is a component of the elbow joint, and comprises the radio-capitellar articulation. The radial head has a major role in elbow pronation and supination, and affords bony stability to the lateral aspect of the elbow joint. Injury to the radial head and neck can occur as a result of two mechanisms. The first is from an instability pattern. The radial head fracture is a component to the terrible triad injury pattern (radial head fracture, elbow dislocation, and coronoid process fracture of the ulna). The second mechanism is a direct injury with a fall or blunt trauma to the proximal radius.

10.2.6.2 Diagnosis

Patients who sustain a proximal radius fracture often present with pain and swelling at the elbow. Range of motion of the elbow is typically reduced, secondary to pain in flexion/extension, as well as supination/pronation. Often, patients are focally tender over the proximal radius. There can be associated neurological deficit on exam if there was significant trauma or substantial subsequent swelling; however, most patients who sustain these injuries are neurovascularly intact.

Radiographs of the elbow will commonly demonstrate a posterior fat pad sign, indicating intra-articular swelling. However, secondary to displacement, they do not always demonstrate the radial head/neck fracture clearly. If the radiographs are non-diagnostic and the patient demonstrates a block to motion, a CT scan is obtained to better characterize the bony anatomy of the radial head/neck region.

10.2.6.3 Classification

The Mason classification, used to classify radial head fractures, is divided into four types: Type I: Nondisplaced or minimally displaced (<2 mm), no mechanical block to rotation; Type II: Displaced >2 mm or angulated, possible mechanical block to forearm rotation; Type III: Comminuted and displaced, mechanical block to motion; Type IV: Radial head fracture with associated elbow dislocation [32].

10.2.6.4 Treatment

The treatment of radial head and neck fractures is based upon the number of articular fragments, presence of a block to motion, and overall stability of the elbow joint. Isolated radial neck fractures, and radial head fractures that are minimally displaced without a block to motion, can be treated with an early active motion protocol. Typically, these patients are placed into a sling for 2–3 days followed by immediate active and passive assisted-motion with structured physical therapy [33]. Regular flexion, extension, pronation, and supination exercises are encouraged immediately to prevent long-term stiffness.

Fractures, with a subsequent block to motion, and those that are comprised of multiple fragments can be treated with either open reduction and internal fixation or radial head arthroplasty. Ring and Jupiter have simplified treatment planning, recommending that fractures involving three or less fragments are amenable to fixation with osteosynthesis, while fractures with more than three fragments are better treated with arthroplasty [34]. Fractures of the proximal radius that occur from instability patterns of injury, such as terrible triad injuries, are commonly amenable to radial head arthroplasty. It is imperative to evaluate and treat any injuries to the LCL, as there is often an associated injury. In the athletic population there is no data to dictate whether an ORIF or radial head replacement is the preferred method of treatment. One concern with a radial head replacement is earlier wear in the athlete population and the possibility for implant loosening given the stresses they place on their elbow. It is for this reason the authors typically favor ORIF over radial head replacement, for the athletic patient, when possible.

10.2.6.5 Rehabilitation

For isolated radial head or neck fractures, rehabilitation begins with a brief period of immobilisation followed by regaining elbow ROM. Strengthening of the elbow is avoided until full elbow ROM has been achieved. The timing of RTS is based on how quickly patients regain their motion and strength, and is typically longer for overhead athletes than contact athletes.

10.2.6.6 Complications

One of the most important complications of proximal radius fractures is an acute block to elbow rotation for these patients. Many of these fractures can be managed non-operatively, but if they develop a mechanical block to motion they often necessitate surgical intervention. Patients can also develop stiffness, continued pain, or iatrogenic posterolateral rotator instability (PLRI) if they undergo an ORIF and the LUCL is damaged. The posterior interosseous nerve (PIN) is at risk during ORIF, and as such can be damaged during surgery. Furthermore, there can be post-traumatic arthritis associated with this injury pattern.

10.2.7 Radial Diaphyseal Fractures

10.2.7.1 Epidemiology

Fractures of the radial shaft are known as the "fracture of necessity" as proper length and rotation of the bone is critical for elbow and wrist function. The mechanism of injury is typically a direct blow to the forearm causing fracture of both the radius and ulna (Fig. 10.4a, b), or the radius in isolation. Due to the importance of the radial bow, and its critical involvement with forearm rotation, anatomic alignment is

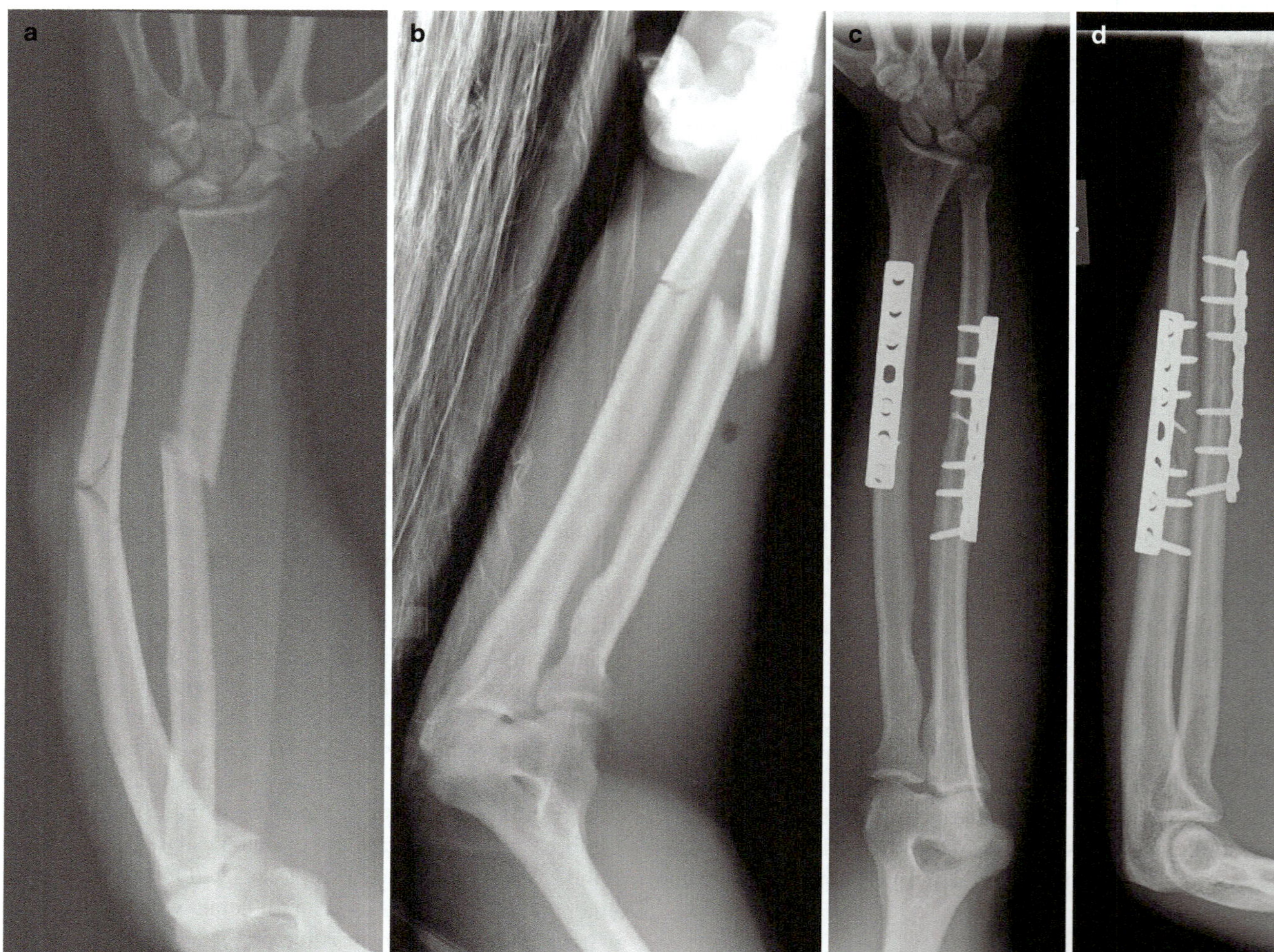

Fig. 10.4 (**a**, **b**) Anteroposterior (**a**) and lateral (**b**) views of a displaced both bone forearm fracture sustained from a sporting injury. (**c**, **d**) Anteroposterior (**c**) and lateral (**d**) views following open reduction internal fixation of a both bone forearm fracture

paramount. In addition to the bony fracture, it is important to consider the soft tissue injuries as well. Profound swelling can lead to compartment syndrome necessitating immediate release.

10.2.7.2 Diagnosis

Patients who have sustained acute radial diaphyseal fractures will present with pain and swelling in the forearm. This can be accompanied neurological symptoms in the patient's hand, secondary to the swelling. There will be tenderness around the fracture site and significant pain with forearm rotation.

It is important to consider the wrist and elbow joints when evaluating radial shaft fractures. A distal third radial shaft fracture may cause a dislocation of the distal radioulnar joint (DRUJ), known as a Galeazzi fracture-dislocation. It is important to obtain anatomic reduction and stable fixation of the fracture to establish reduction and stability of the DRUJ.

Routine x-ray assessment should image the forearm, the wrist and the elbow, to assess for concomitant proximal or distal injuries.

10.2.7.3 Classification

Classification of these fractures is largely descriptive, and should include any concomitant injuries to the elbow and/or wrist. The AO classification of radial diaphysis fractures divides these fractures into proximal, middle, and distal fractures as well as fracture type (simple, wedge, multi-fragmentary). Simple fractures can be further classified as spiral, oblique, or transverse. Wedge fractures can be further classified as intact or fragmentary wedge. Finally, multi-fragmentary fractures can be further classified as an intact segmental or fragmentary segmental fractures.

10.2.7.4 Treatment

A fracture of the radial shaft should be treated with surgical stabilization. Fixation for radial shaft fractures is typically done through plate and screw fixation using 3.5 mm compression plating systems (Fig. 10.4c, d). Other techniques do include flexible nailing in length stable fractures [35]. It is important to start early motion to avoid stiffness and contracture. The DRUJ must be evaluated at the time of surgery after the radial fracture is fixed to ensure stability. If the DRUJ is unstable, this may require temporary screw or K-Wire fixation.

10.2.7.5 Rehabilitation

Similar to previous protocols, rehabilitation comprises of an initial period of fracture immobilisation, followed by progressive ROM of the elbow, wrist and hand. This is followed by forearm strengthening and gradual RTS.

10.2.7.6 Complications

Complications include non-union, mal-union, nerve injury (specifically to the PIN and the superficial branch of the radial nerve), elbow or wrist stiffness, or hardware issues.

10.2.8 Ulnar Diaphyseal Fractures

10.2.8.1 Epidemiology

The ulnar shaft is a cutaneous bone that is palpable on the dorsal and ulnar aspect of the forearm. It is at risk to fracture when forces are aimed directly to this region. While ulnar shaft fractures are rare in the contact athlete, this patient population is at higher risk than the general population for such injuries. Some term this fracture the "nightstick" injury as this injury can occur from a direct blow to the ulna (such as when a person raises their forearm to block someone who is trying to hit them with a nightstick).

10.2.8.2 Diagnosis

Patients presenting with acute ulnar diaphyseal fractures will complain of pain and swelling in the forearm. This can be accompanied by paresthesia in the patient's hand, secondary to the swelling. There will be tenderness around the fracture site and significant pain with forearm rotation. Wrist and elbow motion may or may not be painful. X-Rays of the forearm are reviewed, and if there is any question for concomitant proximal or distal injuries, elbow and wrist films should be ordered.

10.2.8.3 Classification

Classification of these fractures is largely descriptive, and should include any concomitant injuries to the elbow and/or wrist. The AO classification for ulnar diaphysis fractures divides these fractures into proximal, middle, and distal fractures as well as fracture type (simple, wedge, multi-fragmentary). Simple fractures can be further classified as spiral, oblique, or transverse. Wedge fractures can be further classified as intact or fragmentary wedge. Finally, multi-fragmentary fractures can be further classified as an intact segmental or fragmentary segmental fractures.

10.2.8.4 Treatment

Since the ulna is a fixed structure, and remains relatively stable during pronation and supination of the forearm, not all ulnar diaphyseal fractures require operative treatment. If satisfactory fracture length, translational alignment, and rotational alignment are noted on clinical and radiological assessment (i.e. $<50\%$ translational displacement and $<10°$ of angulation), short arm splinting, short arm casting or long arm casting are acceptable means of treatment. Short arm splinting can facilitate an accelerated rehabilitation over both short and long arm casting, and should be considered. However, in the athletic population, these fractures are often fixed to allow earlier RTS. This is a shared decision between the athlete and surgeon, but if the player wished to RTS as quickly as possible, an ORIF is typically offered. If the fracture is not length stable, or significantly displaced, fracture fixation using a 3.5 mm compression technique should be performed, often with excellent results [36]. Finally, injuries to the radius and ulna can occur concomitantly with one another. When the athlete has a radius and ulna fracture, this is typically treated with open reduction and internal fixation of both fractures. The careful management of concomitant soft tissue injuries, when present, is also paramount.

10.2.8.5 Rehabilitation

The fracture is immobilized initially to allow appropriate healing. For both non-operative and operative management, short arm splinting is preferable, with gentle elbow and wrist motion exercises commenced, as early as possible to prevent stiffness. Graduated progression is then made towards strengthening as fracture healing permits. This is followed by sport-specific rehabilitation exercises with a gradual RTS.

10.2.8.6 Complications

Patients with operatively-managed ulna fractures are at risk for non-union, mal-union, construct failure, fracture proximal or distal to the plate, hardware irritation (necessitating future hardware removal) or tendon irritation from the plate. Those patients treated conservatively are at risk for loss of reduction, non-union, and mal-union. Typically, ulnar shaft fractures are treated conservatively if there is$<50\%$ displacement and $<10^\circ$ of angulation. Hence, if subsequent X-rays demonstrate an increase in angulation or displacement, these fractures may need operative intervention, as their risk of non-union or mal-union, with secondary displacement, is significantly increased.

10.3 Preventative Measures

Prevention of fractures about the elbow in sport is difficult. There are many sports where fractures about the elbow occur from a macro-traumatic events. In these instances, the injuries cannot usually be prevented. Maintaining a proper strengthening program in these athletes and encouraging a complete diet to augment bone health is the mainstay for prevention. Proprioceptive training programs in which the players learn how to take a hit, and how to properly land once they are hit, may be beneficial although further studies are needed in this area. There is no evidence to recommend the use of protective equipment for the athlete to reduce the incidence of fractures about the elbow.

References

1. Erickson BJ, Gupta AK, Harris JD, Bush-Joseph C, Bach BR, Abrams GD, et al. Rate of return to pitching and performance after Tommy John surgery in major league baseball pitchers. Am J Sports Med. 2013;42(3):536–43.
2. Camp CL, Dines JS, van der List JP, Conte S, Conway J, Altchek DW, et al. Summative report on time out of play for major and minor league baseball: an analysis of 49,955 injuries from 2011 through 2016. Am J Sports Med. 2018;46(7):1727–32.
3. Miller A, Dodson CC, Ilyas AM. Thrower's fracture of the humerus. Orthop Clin North Am. 2014;45(4):565–9.
4. Gradu G, Jupiter JB. Current concepts review – fractures of the shaft of the humerus. Acta Chir Orthop Traumatol Cechoslov. 2013;80(5):321–7.
5. Morrey BF, Tanaka S, An KN. Valgus stability of the elbow. A definition of primary and secondary constraints. Clin Orthopaed Relat Res. 1991;265:187–95.
6. Morrey BF. Applied anatomy and biomechanics of the elbow joint. Instr Course Lect. 1986;35:59–68.
7. Schwartz ML, Thornton DD, Larrison MC, Cain EL, Aaron DG, Wilk KE, et al. Avulsion of the medial epicondyle after ulnar collateral ligament reconstruction: imaging of a rare throwing injury. AJR Am J Roentgenol. 2008;190(3):595–8.
8. Osbahr DC, Chalmers PN, Frank JS, Williams RJ 3rd, Widmann RF, Green DW. Acute, avulsion fractures of the medial epicondyle while throwing in youth baseball players: a variant of Little League elbow. J Shoulder Elb Surg. 2010;19(7):951–7.
9. Erickson BJ, Chalmers PN, D'Angelo J, Ma K, Romeo AA. Open reduction internal fixation of medial epicondyle fractures after ulnar collateral ligament reconstruction in professional baseball pitchers. Orthop J Sports Med. 2019;7(6):2325967119852896.
10. Cain EL Jr, Dugas JR, Wolf RS, Andrews JR. Elbow injuries in throwing athletes: a current concepts review. Am J Sports Med. 2003;31(4):621–35.
11. Gottschalk HP, Eisner E, Hosalkar HS. Medial epicondyle fractures in the pediatric population. J Am Acad Orthop Surg. 2012;20(4):223–32.
12. Axibal DP, Carry P, Skelton A, Mayer SW. No difference in return to sport and other outcomes between operative and nonoperative treatment of medial epicondyle fractures in pediatric upper-extremity athletes. Clin J Sports Med. 2018;30(6):e214–8.
13. Axibal DP, Ketterman B, Skelton A, Carry P, Georgopoulos G, Miller N, et al. No difference in outcomes in a matched cohort of operative versus nonoperatively treated displaced medial epicondyle fractures. J Pediatr Orthop B. 2018;28(6):520–5.
14. Lawrence JT, Patel NM, Macknin J, Flynn JM, Cameron D, Wolfgruber HC, et al. Return to competitive sports after medial epicondyle fractures in adolescent athletes: results of operative and nonoperative treatment. Am J Sports Med. 2013;41(5):1152–7.
15. Mehlhoff TL, Noble PC, Bennett JB, Tullos HS. Simple dislocation of the elbow in the adult. Results after closed treatment. J Bone Joint Surg Am. 1988;70(2):244–9.
16. Durig M, Muller W, Ruedi TP, Gauer EF. The operative treatment of elbow dislocation in the adult. J Bone Joint Surg Am. 1979;61(2):239–44.
17. Goodman AD, Lemme N, DeFroda SF, Gil JA, Owens BD. Elbow Dislocation and Subluxation Injuries in the National Collegiate Athletic Association, 2009–2010 through 2013–2014. Orthop J Sports Med. 2018;6(1):2325967117750105.
18. Stoneback JW, Owens BD, Sykes J, Athwal GS, Pointer L, Wolf JM. Incidence of elbow dislocations in the United States population. J Bone Joint Surg Am. 2012;94(3):240–5.
19. Josefsson PO, Nilsson BE. Incidence of elbow dislocation. Acta Orthop Scand. 1986;57(6):537–8.

20. Doornberg JN, Ring D. Coronoid fracture patterns. J Hand Surg Am. 2006;31(1):45–52.
21. Regan W, Morrey B. Fractures of the coronoid process of the ulna. J Bone Joint Surg Am. 1989;71(9):1348–54.
22. Garrigues GE, Wray WH III, Lindenhovius AL, Ring DC, Ruch DS. Fixation of the coronoid process in elbow fracture-dislocations. J Bone Joint Surg Am. 2011;93(20):1873–81.
23. Eyberg BA, McKee MD. Indications and clinical results of radial head replacement: has anything changed? J Orthop Trauma. 2019;33(Suppl 8):S1–6.
24. Swensen SJ, Tyagi V, Uquillas C, Shakked RJ, Yoon RS, Liporace FA. Maximizing outcomes in the treatment of radial head fractures. J Orthopaed Traumatol. 2019;20(1):15.
25. Leigh WB, Ball CM. Radial head reconstruction versus replacement in the treatment of terrible triad injuries of the elbow. J Shoulder Elb Surg. 2012;21(10):1336–41.
26. Wyrick JD, Dailey SK, Gunzenhaeuser JM, Casstevens EC. Management of complex elbow dislocations: a mechanistic approach. J Am Acad Orthop Surg. 2015;23(5):297–306.
27. Cohen MS, Hastings H 2nd. Acute elbow dislocation: evaluation and management. J Am Acad Orthop Surg. 1998;6(1):15–23.
28. Robertson GA, Wood AM, Bakker-Dyos J, Aitken SA, Keenan AC, Court-Brown CM. The epidemiology, morbidity, and outcome of soccer-related fractures in a standard population. Am J Sports Med. 2012;40(8):1851–7.
29. Aitken SA, Watson BS, Wood AM, Court-Brown CM. Sports-related fractures in South East Scotland: an analysis of 990 fractures. J Orthop Surg (Hong Kong). 2014;22(3):313–7.
30. Benetton CA, Cesa G, El-Kouba Junior G, Ferreira AP, Vissoci JR, Pietrobon R. Agreement of olecranon fractures before and after the exposure to four classification systems. J Shoulder Elb Surg. 2015;24(3):358–63.
31. Erickson BJ, Chalmers PN, D'Angelo J, Ma K, Ahmad CS, Romeo AA. Performance and return to sport after open reduction and internal fixation of the olecranon in professional baseball players. Am J Sports Med. 2019;47(8):1915–20.
32. Ayyaswamy B, Howell L, Anand A, Charalambous CP. Interobserver and intraobserver variations in radial head fracture classification-assessment of two classification systems. J Orthop. 2019;16(6):463–7.
33. Paschos NK, Mitsionis GI, Vasiliadis HS, Georgoulis AD. Comparison of early mobilization protocols in radial head fractures. J Orthop Trauma. 2013;27(3):134–9.
34. Ring D, Quintero J, Jupiter JB. Open reduction and internal fixation of fractures of the radial head. J Bone Joint Surg Am. 2002;84(10):1811–5.
35. Huang YC, Renn JH, Tarng YW. The titanium elastic nail serves as an alternative treatment for adult proximal radial shaft fractures: a cohort study. J Orthop Surg Res. 2018;13(1):10.
36. Ali M, Clark DI, Tambe A. Nightstick fractures, outcomes of operative and non-operative treatment. Acta Med (Hradec Kralove). 2019;62(1):19–23.

11 Acute Fractures in Sport: Wrist

P. G. Robinson, Andrew D. Duckworth, and D. A. Campbell

Learning Objectives

- Understand the prevalence of wrist fractures sustained secondary to sporting activities
- Understand key features in the history and examination of the wrist to guide the diagnosis and when further imaging is beneficial
- Recognise the management and rehabilitation options available for each fracture in the wrist
- Learn specific complications and treatment pitfalls with sports related fractures of the wrist

11.1 Distal Radius Fractures

11.1.1 Epidemiology

Fracture of the distal radius is the most common fracture of the upper limb with an incidence of 22 fractures per 10,000 persons/year [1]. Sports related distal radius fractures account for 12.5% of all upper limb fractures in adults [2] and 23% in adolescents [3]. The average age of athletes sustaining distal radius fractures is notably younger (less than 18 years old) compared to the general population (greater than 50 years old) [4]. Sports-related distal radius fractures are more common in males (76%) than females (24%), and males are reported to be, on average, 19 years younger than females at the time of the injury.

P. G. Robinson
Edinburgh Orthopaedics - Trauma, Royal Infirmary of Edinburgh, Edinburgh, UK

A. D. Duckworth (✉)
Usher Institute, University of Edinburgh, Edinburgh, UK

Edinburgh Orthopaedics - Trauma, Royal Infirmary of Edinburgh, Edinburgh, UK
e-mail: Andrew.Duckworth@ed.ac.uk

D. A. Campbell
Orthopaedics, Spire Leeds Hospital, Leeds, UK

Sports contributing to the greatest number of distal radius fractures include rugby, soccer and skiing or snowboarding. This may vary with geographical location. Lawson et al. [5] reviewed 225 sports-related distal radius fractures over a 5-year period from a single institution in the United Kingdom and found 50% occurred in soccer. Of these, 79% occurred from a fall and 21% occurred secondary to the ball striking the players hand. They also reported more fractures occurring on synthetic pitches (54%) than grass pitches (28%). Athletes typically have better bone quality than the general population [6] and subsequently the force required to fracture the distal radius is higher than in non athletes. Fractures in this region are often sustained following high energy falls onto the hand, resulting in a greater proportion being intra-articular (and a smaller proportion being extra-articular) than the general non-athlete population [7–9].

11.1.2 Classification

Classification of distal radius fractures has been well described in the orthopaedic literature and several systems exist including those described by Gartland and Werley, Mayo, Melone, AO, Fernandez and Frykman.

Simple terms are initially helpful to describe distal radius fractures such as:

- intra-articular
- extra-articular
- displacement
- angulation
- comminution

These terms are informative and often help guide management. The updated AO/OTA Fracture and Dislocation Classification (2018) is commonly used (Fig. 11.1). The original AO Classification System was known to reduce in reliability when subclassified [10] and a recent review of distal radius classification described poor reproducibility and reliability [11].

G. A. J. Robertson, N. Maffulli (eds.), *Fractures in Sport*, https://doi.org/10.1007/978-3-030-72036-0_11

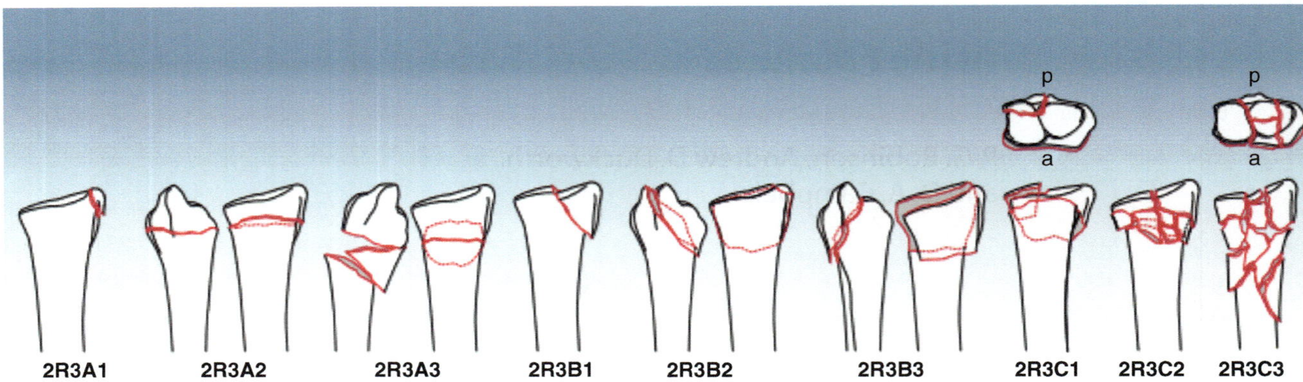

Fig. 11.1 The AO/OTA Fracture and Dislocation Classification (2018) system for distal radius fractures (*AO/OTA Fracture and Dislocation Classification. Introduction to the classification of long bone fractures. Radius. Pages 9–12*)

Published studies have found differences in fracture types amongst different sports. Lawson et al. described more complex fracture patterns of the distal radius in higher energy mechanisms such as horseback riding and skiing [5], with more simple fracture configurations seen in athletes injured during soccer [4] and rugby [12]. Interestingly, variations in fracture configuration have also been reported within individual sports. In a 2004 study, novice snowboarders were more likely to sustain extra-articular distal radius fractures and less likely to sustain intra-articular fractures than their professional counterparts. In the same retrospective review of 740 snowboarders with distal radius fractures, 54.1% were type A (extra-articular fractures), 4.3% were type B (partial articular) and 41.6% were type C (complete articular) [7].

11.1.3 Diagnosis

11.1.3.1 History

The evaluation of the injured wrist begins with a detailed history that includes the mechanism of injury, the amount of energy involved and the potential for associated injuries (intrinsic ligament, triangular fibrocartilage complex [TFCC], neural injury). The timing of the injury will distinguish between acute and chronic pathology. Establishing the direction of fall can also be useful. For example, when someone falls with their hand in front of them the wrist is typically in a pronated and extended position, which tends to impact upon the radial structures of the wrist. If someone falls with their hand behind them, the forearm is supinated and the wrist extended, which tends to load the ulnar structures of the wrist. Tanabe et al. [13] studied 91 patients with intra-articular distal radius fractures in three different wrist positions (extension, neutral and flexion). With the wrist in an extended position, fractures of the sigmoid notch and dorsal ulnar corner of the radius were most frequently involved. In a neutral position, the sigmoid notch, dorsal radial, and volar radial corners were most commonly involved and in wrist flexion, fractures of the sigmoid notch and dorsal radial corner were most commonly seen.

Hand dominance is of relative importance and knowledge of the sport and the demands of the athlete are essential. For example, the position of a diver's wrist when entering the water, the range of movements in the trailing and leading wrists of a golfer, or the type of grip a tennis player uses when playing each shot will all affect load and the likelihood of certain injury patterns. Other relevant aspects of the history include previous injury or surgery to the wrist as well as a past medical and social history.

11.1.3.2 Physical Examination

There should be full exposure from the fingertips to above the elbow and the contralateral limb should be visible for comparison. Inspect for bruising, pallor and deformity (for example, the classic 'dinner fork' deformity seen in dorsally displaced distal radius fractures). Palpation should include the distal radius and ulna, distal radioulnar joint (DRUJ), the carpus (particularly the scaphoid), metacarpals and phalanges, along with the elbow. It is important to consider associated ligamentous injuries of the carpus. The thumb and base should be assessed. Movement at the wrist joint should be recorded actively and then passively. Movements include radial/ulnar deviation, flexion/extension and pronation/supination. Limb asymmetry in the place of reaching active end-range can be a reflection of subtle pathology. A detailed neurovascular assessment of the motor and sensory function of the median, radial and ulnar nerves must be performed. The capillary refill time should be assessed as a well as radial and ulnar pulses.

11.1.3.3 Radiological Investigations

First line radiological investigations for distal radius fractures are posteroanterior (PA) and lateral plain radiographs.

The radiographs should be scrutinised for radiocarpal alignment, volar tilt, radial height and inclination. Computer topography (CT) scans can be helpful to further assess intra-articular or comminuted fractures improving decision-making and surgical planning. Magnetic resonance imaging (MRI) scans play a role in the diagnosis of associated ligamentous injuries and assessment of the TFCC as well as in revealing occult fractures.

Hanker et al. arthroscopically assessed the wrists of 173 athletes with distal radius fractures [14]. They found TFCC tears in 61% of cases, carpal instability in 20%, scapholunate ligament tears in 8%, lunotriquetral ligament tears in 12%, perilunate injuries in 8% and DRUJ instability in 9%. Osteochondral fractures were found in 22% of cases and intra-articular loose bodies in 18% of cases. It is important that clinicians identify associated soft tissue injuries at the time of distal radius fractures as failing to recognise these can lead to poor outcomes.

11.1.4 Treatment

The goal of early return to maximum function is paramount in all patients, but particularly in the athlete. Fractures need to heal in an acceptable position. The factors predictive of stability previously described by LaFontaine [15] and MacKenney [16] should be considered in decision-making when formulating a management plan. Mackenney et al. followed up over 4000 distal radius fractures and concluded advanced age, dorsal comminution and loss of radial height were predictive of radiographic outcome. LaFontaine et al. concluded that four main factors increased the risk of secondary fracture displacement:

- dorsal comminution
- intra-articular fracture
- associated ulnar fracture
- dorsal angulation >20°.

The authors reported that each factor had a linear correlation with loss of reduction and if ≥3 were present, close radiographic follow up and/or surgery should be considered because displacement was almost inevitable.

11.1.4.1 Non-operative

Non-operative management of distal radius fractures in the athlete should be considered in the case of undisplaced intra-articular or extra-articular fractures. Displaced intra-articular fractures are a relative indication for surgery [17]. Patients with displaced extra-articular fractures with instability following manipulation should be considered for surgery to avoid delay in definitive treatment and return to sport. Non-operative management includes a short arm cast for four to six weeks. In some cases, where pain is well controlled and there are no concerns regarding stability, a wrist splint may suffice. For fractures that have undergone primary manipulation, a below elbow back slab is routinely used, with check radiographs at 7–10 days to ensure there is no displacement that would warrant surgical intervention. If there is no displacement after two weeks, the backslab can be exchanged for a lightweight short arm cast for a further four weeks. Finger, elbow and shoulder range of movement exercises should start while in cast.

11.1.4.2 Operative

Recognition of the relevant fracture patterns is imperative when considering operative management, as failure to address these at the time of surgery can lead to loss of reduction, radiocarpal subluxation and a poor outcome. There is conflicting evidence regarding restoration of radiological anatomy of the distal radius and functional outcome, although younger athletic patients are less likely to tolerate malunion [18, 19]. Fixation choices include Kirschner wires, locked volar plating (Fig. 11.2), dorsal plating, fragment specific plating, bridging or nonbridging external fixation or rarely internal bridging fixation.

Undisplaced Extra Articular Fractures

Athletes may perceive there will be an advantage with early internal fixation even in situations where the fracture is undisplaced. In these circumstances, a full explanation should be given regarding the relative risks and benefits of such an aggressive approach. It is not recommended to treat such injuries in this way and the athlete must be made aware that fracture healing could even be delayed if surgery is undertaken.

Extra-articular, Unstable (AO Type A or Frykman Type I)

Unstable extra-articular fractures can be treated successfully with a variety of fixation options. In a study comparing Kirschner wire fixation to open reduction and internal fixation (ORIF) for well reduced extra-articular distal radius fractures, no difference in functional outcome in the short and medium term was reported [20, 21]. However, 6 weeks of plaster immobilisation is typically required after Kirschner wire fixation which will limit activities. In comparison, after ORIF, the patient can rapidly wean from immobilisation within 2 weeks, which facilitates early range of movement and progressive post-operative activities. Furthermore, secondary loss of reduction is less frequent when fractures are treated with ORIF using a volar locking plate [22]. Volar and dorsal plating techniques appear to be biomechanically equivalent. However volar locking plates are associated with improved functional outcome in intra-articular fractures [23, 24]. Dorsal plating has an increased

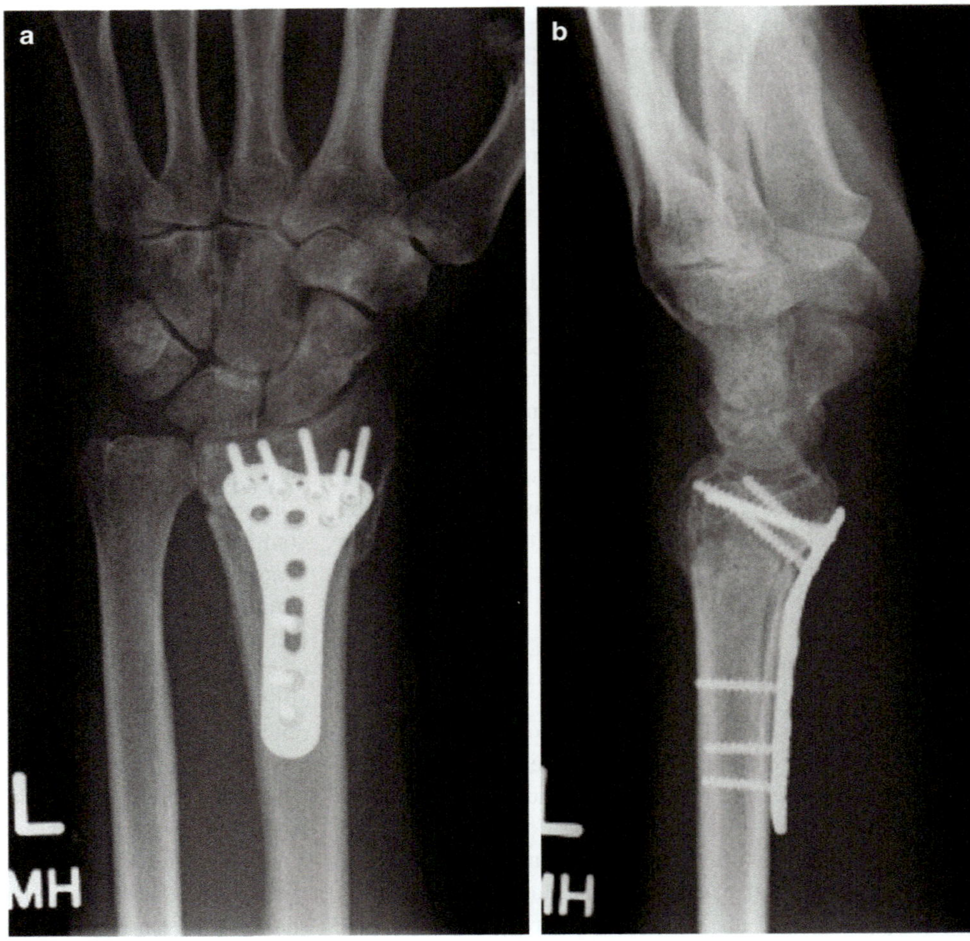

Fig. 11.2 PA (**a**) and lateral (**b**) radiographs of a volar plating of a distal radius fracture

risk of extensor tendon irritation and need for removal of metalwork [25, 26].

Partial-Articular, Unstable (AO Type B)

Shear fractures exist when the main fragment involves only part of the articular surface. These patterns demand a buttress (anti-glide) plating technique. Emphasis must be placed on capturing the ulnar corner of the volar cortex in this specific fracture pattern, as this acts as a primary stabiliser to carpal subluxation and partly stabilises the DRUJ [27]. Displaced fractures of the radial styloid (chauffeur's fracture) can be treated with a single lag screw (Fig. 11.3) or a fixed angle plate. These particular injuries are associated with scapholunate ligament disruption and there is evidence to support arthroscopic-assisted assessment and reduction in these cases [28]. Dorsal rim fractures should be approached from the dorsal surface and fixed with a dorsal or a fragment specific plate.

Intra-articular, Unstable (AO Type C1 and C2)

Many of these fractures can be managed successfully with volar locking plates. However, some studies have advocated the use of fragment specific plating using two or more low profile plates to capture individual fracture fragments and this has been reported to achieve good functional results [29–31] They have also been found in some studies to yield superior biomechanical strength compared to dorsal [32] or volar plating [33, 34].

Intra-articular, Comminuted (AO Type C3 or Frykman Type III)

The method of surgical fixation for these fractures depends greatly on the fracture configuration and severity of comminution. CT scanning preoperatively can be helpful to delineate the fracture fragments. Volar locking plates can be used for these fractures provided all intra-articular fragments can be reduced and stabilised. Fragment specific plating may be indicated in more complex patterns, using dorsoradial double plating or dorsoradiopalmar triple plating techniques [35]. External fixation or internal bridging fixation may be considered in the presence of severe intra-articular comminution. There is recent literature supporting the use of wrist arthroscopy in intra-articular distal radius fracture fixation to ensure adequate reduction of the articular

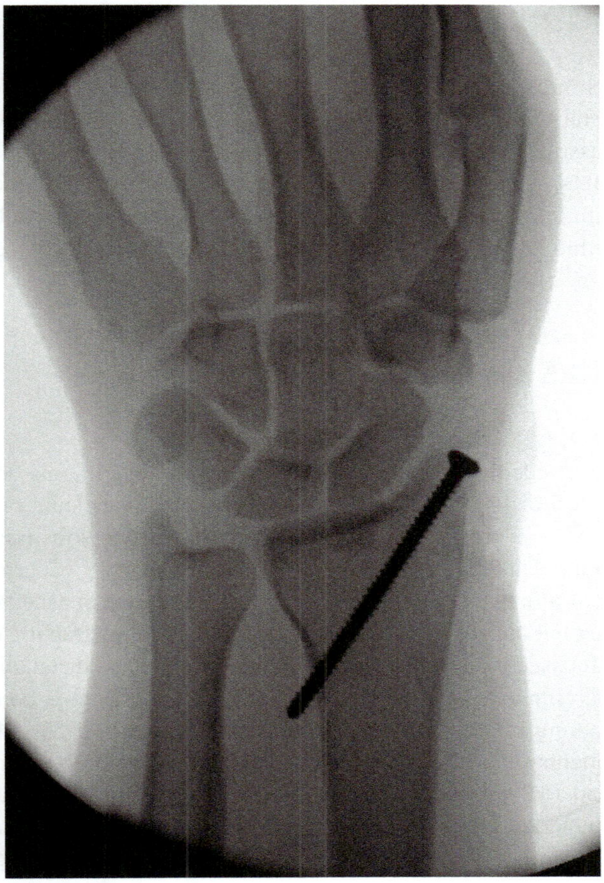

Fig. 11.3 Lag screw fixation of a radial styloid fracture

surface is achieved. Arthroscopy also allows detection of more subtle soft tissue injuries which can be treated if required [36].

11.1.5 Complications

Complications associated with conservative management of distal radius fractures include symptomatic malunion, non-union (rare), tendon rupture, and less commonly persistent pain, stiffness and complex regional pain syndrome. Post-traumatic osteoarthritis can occur in poorly reduced intra-articular fractures (>2 mm step). Additional complications associated with surgical management include infection and nerve/blood vessel injury. Flexor or extensor tendon ruptures can occur, particularly when internal fixation devices are prominent. This risk can be reduced by placing the implant proximal to the transverse ridge of the radius (watershed), distal to pronator quadratus [37] as well as by seating the plate flush to the bone and ensuring the appropriate length of screws [38, 39] . The pros and cons of metal work removal and the future risk of periprosthetic fractures should be discussed with the patient.

11.1.6 Rehabilitation

There is no current consensus on rehabilitation protocol for distal radius fractures. However, most clinicians would agree that early range of movement improves outcome [40], particularly in the athlete population. The additional benefit of continuing mobilisation of uninjured joints and muscles in the affected limb should also be considered. Surgically treated distal radius fractures may allow early range of motion exercises with the use of a removable splint. Return to light activities can be considered two months following the injury. Range of movement exercises of the fingers, wrist and elbow should begin immediately as pain allows. Factors affecting the clinician's decision to allow an athlete to return to sport include ongoing symptoms, radiographic bone healing (possibly confirmed by CT scan) and the level of contact/risk the patient will be exposed to.

The decision on when to allow an athlete to return to sport can be challenging. There are no firm rules and current evidence is limited to expert opinion and small case series. Henn and Wolfe suggest at least of 80% of baseline range of movement and strength should be demonstrated along with radiographic healing prior to returning to play [41], while Beleckas and Calfee allowed return to sport in a cast prior to fracture healing in sports such as soccer or running [42]. The decision about a return to sport involves unique considerations. A playing cast can be used if delay to return to sport is critical, although this can breach playing safety rules and may not be allowed in certain sports. On all occasions, the risks and benefits of a return to training and playing before radiological union has been confirmed must be discussed and recorded. Time lost to injury following distal radius fractures can be significant. One study reported the average loss of playing time in professional American football players to be 42 days, which was equivalent to one third of the season [43].

11.1.7 Preventative Measures

At present, there is no evidence to recommend the use of protective equipment, by the athlete, as a primary preventative measure against distal radial fractures.

Prevention of re-injury in healing distal radius fractures is difficult for athletes who return to collision or contact sports before radiological healing. Wrist splints or short arm casts can be considered in the early return to play period in sports where this will not interfere with performance [41, 42]. Unlike the elderly patient sustaining a distal radius fracture with underlying osteopenia or osteoporosis, it is likely that the bone quality of the athlete is adequate. Prevention of future re-fractures can focus on adequate imaging, rehabilitation and correct timing for return to sport. A discussion between the clinician and the patient should occur regarding the removal of metalwork in patients who have undergone plate fixation, as there is a risk of future periprosthetic fracture [44, 45] both with metalwork in place and also in the weeks after metal removal.

11.2 Distal Ulna Fractures

11.2.1 Epidemiology

Fractures of the distal ulna are categorised into

1. Ulna styloid fractures in association with a distal radius fracture.
2. Isolated distal ulna fractures.

Ulnar fractures occur in conjunction with approximately 58% of distal radius fractures [46]. Styloid fractures can be associated with distal radio ulnar joint (DRUJ) instability due to triangular fibrocartilage complex (TFCC) disruption. Distal ulnar shaft fractures can occur in isolation (without radial injury) and are described as 'nightstick' type injuries if sustained from a direct blow. Less commonly stress fractures of the ulna can occur in association with sports such as tennis and golf [47–49].

11.2.2 Classification

The most commonly recognised classifications system for distal ulna fractures are the AO classification [50] and the classification described by Biyani et al. [51]. The latter refers to distal ulna metaphyseal fractures in concurrence with distal radius fractures. These can be considered to be within 5 cm of the distal dome of the ulnar head [52] (Fig. 11.4).

11.2.3 Diagnosis

11.2.3.1 History

Ulnar sided wrist pain and tenderness following trauma or a known distal radius fracture should raise the suspicion of a distal ulna fracture or an associated ulnar sided soft tissue injury. The clinician should establish if the injury occurred from a direct blow to the wrist (likely fracture) or whether they fell onto an outstretched hand (equally likely fracture or soft tissue injury). Stress fractures can occur at the distal ulna and clinical suspicion should be raised if a patient is complaining of atraumatic ulnar sided wrist pain [48, 53, 54]. Patients suffering from a concurrent dislocation of the radial head (Monteggia fracture patterns) may complain of pain around the elbow joint as well. However, this is more common with more proximal ulnar fractures and high energy injuries.

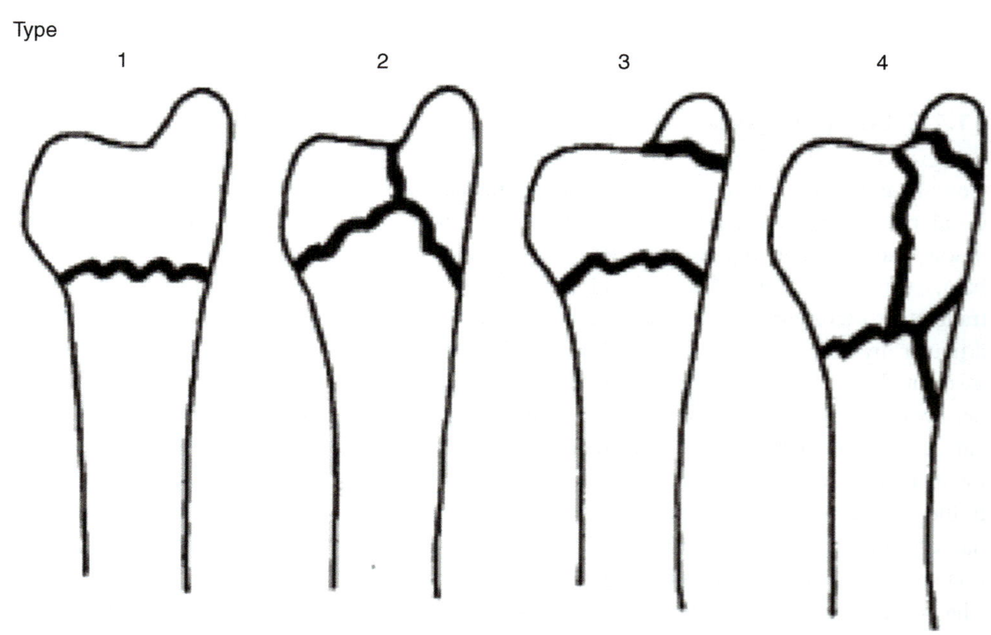

Fig. 11.4 Classification of distal ulnar fractures from *Biyani A, Simison AJ, Klenerman L. Fractures of the distal radius and ulna. 1995 Jun;20(3):357–64* [51]

11.2.3.2 Physical Exam

Careful examination of the wrist is important for detection of instability at the DRUJ or subluxation of the extensor carpi ulnaris tendon. Inspection of the distal ulna may show bruising, swelling or deformity. Range of active movement in pronation and supination should also be assessed. Dorsal prominence of the distal ulna may represent an injury to the DRUJ and stability can be assessed with the ballotment test. This involves stabilising the distal radius between the thumb and forefinger with one hand, while using the other hand to move the distal ulna dorsally and volarly assessing for excess movement or a palpable clunk. The DRUJ is most stable in supination. Comparing the injured and non-injured sides is always helpful. This may be too painful in an acute fracture. Inspection and palpation of the elbow should also be performed to assess for an associated radial head dislocation.

11.2.3.3 Radiological Investigations

PA and lateral radiographs of the distal radius and ulna should be performed. The clinician should also carefully inspect the DRUJ for any widening or malalignment on both views. CT scanning with the forearm in pronation, neutral and supination can be useful to detect cases of subtle DRUJ instability and an MRI scan can be performed if a TFCC tear is suspected. Modern 3T scanners can be as accurate as MR Arthrography in diagnosing TFCC or intrinsic ligament defects, particularly in an acute situation. Bombaci et al. found a strong correlation between distal radius fractures extending into the DRUJ (with associated distal ulnar styloid fracture) and the presence of a TFCC tear seen on MRI scanning [55].

11.2.4 Treatment

11.2.4.1 Non-operative

In the absence of DRUJ instability following reduction of any concurrent distal radius fracture, ulnar styloid fractures are usually managed non-operatively. There is a risk of non-union of the ulna (55–70%) [56, 57] but the literature would suggest this does not negatively impact on functional outcomes [58, 59]. One study demonstrated that the presence of an ulnar styloid fracture at the time of distal radius fracture in association with a stable DRUJ did not affect subjective postoperative outcomes up to 1 year. Furthermore, the size of the fragment, the degree of displacement or the presence or absence of nonunion did not affect the outcome [60]. However, in a case series of eight patients with symptomatic ulnar styloid fracture nonunions, five patients with TFCC tears diagnosed on MRI arthrogram who went on to have excision of the non-union and arthroscopic TFCC repair had significant improvements in pain and DASH scores [61]. With regards to distal ulna shaft fractures, it is appropriate to leave these fractures to heal in an above elbow cast for 2 weeks followed by 4 weeks in a below elbow cast, provided they are undisplaced or minimally displaced.

11.2.4.2 Operative

If following volar plate fixation of a distal radius fracture, the DRUJ remains unstable, ulnar styloid fractures may warrant operative fixation ± stabilisation of the DRUJ. The ulnar styloid may also warrant fixation if it is comminuted and extending into the DRUJ. Stabilisation of an ulnar styloid fracture can be performed with a Kirschner wire, headless screw, transosseous suture or plate fixation [62]. If the TFCC remains intact, there should be resultant stability of the DRUJ. If this is not the case, then two 2 mm Kirschner wires can transfix the distal radius and ulna with the forearm in supination for 6 weeks, although efforts should be made to identify and repair the cause of instability. If the distal ulna is irreducible, it may indicate soft tissue interposition (most likely the extensor carpi ulnaris tendon) and open reduction is indicated.

The limited literature would suggest that isolated distal ulna fractures which are displaced by >50% of translation and/or 10° of angulation, should undergo fixation to avoid disruption of the interosseous membrane and loss of longitudinal stability of the forearm [63]. Distal ulnar fractures can be challenging to fix and metalwork is often better tolerated on the volar aspect. The dorsal sensory branch of the ulnar

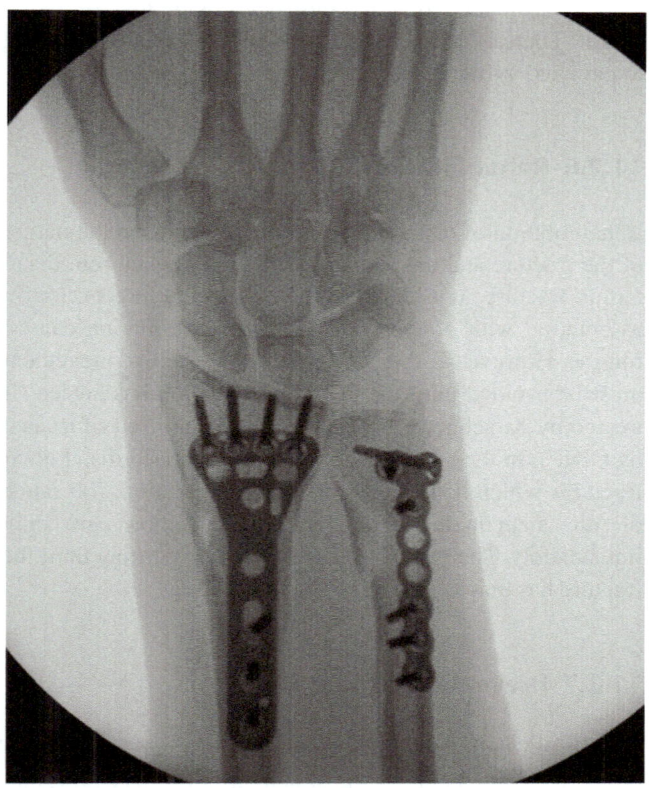

Fig. 11.5 Anteroposterior radiograph of fixation of a distal ulnar fracture during distal radius open reduction internal fixation

nerve must be protected as it passes from volar to dorsal at around the level of the ulnar styloid [64]. Fixation methods in this region include Kirschner wires, tension band wiring, intraosseous wiring or plate fixation (Fig. 11.5) [65]. Ring et al. reported the results of 24 unstable distal ulnar fractures (in association with distal radius fractures) using mini-condylar plates [62]. Satisfactory range of motion, grip strength and radiographic measurements were achieved at an average follow up of 26 months. Both bone fractures (except those involving ulnar styloid injury) are mechanically similar to forearm fractures. Consideration should be given to stabilising both bones.

In the case of severely comminuted distal ulna fractures it may be very challenging to achieve fixation. Excision of the distal ulna (Darrach's procedure) is not recommended in the active athlete.

11.2.5 Complications

Ongoing pain with a conservatively managed, ununited ulnar styloid fracture can occur in up to 14% of patients [66]. Due to the lack of soft tissue coverage, wound healing and infection can be problematic and metalwork removal is common [67]. Furthermore, injury to the dorsal sensory branch of the ulnar nerve can occur. Ulnar impaction can be seen if an associated distal radial fracture heals with loss of radial height. There is also a risk of arthrosis of the DRUJ leading to pain and stiffness.

11.2.6 Rehabilitation

Rehabilitation of distal ulna fractures depends on the nature of the fracture and the management of any concurrent distal radius fracture. If a distal ulnar styloid fracture occurs in association with a stable DRUJ then rehabilitation can be routine. However, if the DRUJ is unstable, active movement must be avoided until the DRUJ stabilisation has healed (if treated by Kirschner wires) or has been stabilised (if treated by ORIF). In the presence of isolated, displaced distal ulnar fractures which have undergone internal fixation, full range of movement at the wrist, forearm and elbow can begin immediately. The patient should avoid heavy lifting until the fracture has united [68].

11.2.7 Preventative Measures

At present, there is no evidence to recommend the use of protective equipment, by the athlete, as a primary preventative measure against distal ulna fractures.

A wrist splint will offer some protection from further fracture. The risk is minimised by allowing the distal ulna to heal before returning to sport. In cases of distal ulna plating, discussion should be had with the patient regarding plate removal against the risk of future periprosthetic fractures.

11.3 Carpal Fractures

11.3.1 Scaphoid

11.3.1.1 Epidemiology

The scaphoid is the most commonly fractured carpal bone contributing to approximately 70% of all carpal fractures [69, 70]. Fractures typically occur in young males aged 20–29 yrs [69, 70] and the overall incidence is thought to be 12 per 100,000 of the general population [71]. However, this is known to vary between countries [70–74]. Males sustain scaphoid fractures more commonly than females with an incidence of 38 per 100,000 in males compared to 8 per 100,000 in women [72]. However, the incidence of scaphoid fractures is increasing in females and this is thought to be secondary to greater participation in athletic activities [75, 76]. In American college football the incidence has been reported to be as high as 1 in 100 players [77].

The typical mechanism of injury is a fall onto an outstretched hand with the forearm pronated and the wrist in radial deviation with extension of greater than 90°. Less common mechanisms include a direct blow or axial loading with the wrist in a neutral position, for example when throwing a punch [78]. A quarter to a third of scaphoid fractures are reported to be related to sporting activities [2, 70, 75] and the most prevalent sports involved depend entirely on the geographical location of the patient. Duckworth et al. found contact sports to be the second most common mechanism of injury (23.5%), with soccer injuries making up over two-thirds of these [70].

The scaphoid is predominantly covered in articular cartilage. Blood supply is from distal to proximal via the dorsal carpal branch of the radial artery, which means proximal pole vascularity is at risk following a fracture. The waist of the scaphoid is the most common fracture location. A study of 513 scaphoid fractures reported 64% at the waist, 31% in

Table 11.1 Herbert classification of scaphoid fractures

Type	Stability	Description
A	Stable	A1 Tubercle fracture
		A2 Incomplete waist fracture
B	Unstable	B1 Distal oblique fracture
		B2 Complete waist fracture
		B3 Proximal pole fracture
		B4 Trans-scaphoid-perilunate fracture/dislocation of carpus
C		C Delayed union
D		D1 Fibrous union
		D2 Pseudoarthrosis

the distal pole and 5% in the proximal pole [71]. Duckworth et al. reported the most common pattern to be Herbert B2 fractures (36.4%), with 31.1% of all scaphoid fractures being type A fractures and 68.9% being type B [70].

11.3.1.2 Classification

Scaphoid

There are many classifications used to describe fractures of the scaphoid. The Herbert classification [79] is popular and is based on fracture stability and rate of union (Table 11.1). Type A fractures are defined as stable and type B as unstable. Type C fractures are those that have a delayed union and D describe a fibrous union (that is sometimes thought of as a stable non-union). The Russe and Mayo classifications are also used. The Russe classification defines fractures based on the orientation of the fracture line (horizontal, transverse, oblique or vertical oblique) [80]. Horizontal fractures are most stable and vertical oblique are the most unstable. The Mayo classification describes scaphoid fractures based on their anatomical location (distal, middle or proximal), whilst further dividing distal into distal tubercle and distal articular. They also use a variety of parameters to define instability (Table 11.2).

Table 11.2 Mayo criteria for instability

Indicators of instability
>1 mm of fracture displacement
Lateral intrascaphoid angle >35°
Bone loss of comminution
Fracture malalignment
Proximal pole fractures
Dorsal intercalated segment instability (DISI) deformity
Perilunate fracture dislocation

11.3.1.3 Diagnosis

Scaphoid

As previously mentioned, the mechanism of injury is often either a fall onto an outstretched hand (with the wrist in extension and radial deviation) or a violent twisting injury. Patients can present late, with an occult fracture or an established non-union. They may complain of a dull aching pain over the radial aspect of the wrist, pain on loading, subjective stiffness and weakened grip strength after an injury perceived as minor [81–83].

On inspection of the wrist there may be bruising, swelling or fullness at the anatomical snuffbox but often there are few signs. Tenderness over the scaphoid tubercle and in the anatomical snuffbox as well as pain on axial loading of the thumb can be detected and should be sought diligently. The presence of all three of these findings have been reported to be 100% sensitive and 74% specific for the diagnosis scaphoid fractures [84]. Other examination findings may include a weakened grip and reduced range of motion.

The sensitivity of initial radiographs in detecting a scaphoid fracture is reported to be between 59% and 79% [85]. The views used are PA and lateral radiographs with the wrist in neutral, an oblique radiograph at 45–60° of pronation and a PA radiograph of the wrist in 45° of radial deviation. A PA radiograph of the wrist in 45° of ulnar deviation is also performed. It has been suggested that visible fracture lines on plain radiographs of the scaphoid signify some degree of displacement of the fracture. If initial radiographs are negative but the patient has positive symptoms or signs, a repeat radiograph in 10–14 days should be performed. The patient must be treated with appropriate immobilisation until a fracture can be excluded.

MRI scanning has been shown to have 100% sensitivity for diagnosing scaphoid fractures [86]. However, this has been reported to be lower in a recent Cochrane review with a sensitivity of only 88% (range 67–100%) (Table 11.2). The review found bone scintigraphy to be the most sensitive

Table 11.3 Computed tomography versus magnetic resonance imaging versus bone scintigraphy for clinically suspected scaphoid fractures in patients with negative plain radiographs (Mallee et al., Cochrane Database of Systematic Reviews 2015, Issue 6)

Test	Number of studies	Number of suspected fractures	Summary sensitivity (95% CI)	Summary specificity (95%)	Summary LR+ (95% CI)	Summary LR− (95% CI)	Consequences in cohort of 1000 patients	
							Missed fractures	Overtreated
CT	4	277	0.72 (0.36–0.92)	0.99 (0.71–1.00)	119.98 (1.49–9655.66)	0.28 (0.10–0.85)	56	8
MRI	5	221	0.88 (0.64–0.97)	1.00 (0.38–1.00)	826.64 (0.51–1,334,596)	0.12 (0.03–0.42)	24	0
BS	6	543	0.99 (0.69–1.00)	0.86 (0.73–0.94)	7.35 (3.51–15.37)	0.01 (0.00–0.49)	2	112

The confidence intervals for summary estimates are wide for all three tests.

imaging modality although a significant number of patients were over-treated after this more invasive diagnostic method [87]. MRI is advised in high-risk patients when there is uncertainty regarding the presence of a fracture on initial radiographs, despite clinical findings consistent of a fracture.

A recent study by Gidwani et al. showed immediate MRI scanning in clinically suspected scaphoid fractures with negative radiographs was cost effective in a UK healthcare setting [88]. It can also detect other occult injuries including an associated ligamentous injury. CT scanning is helpful in determining the amount of fracture displacement. Finally, MRI scanning can also be useful in the diagnosis of avascular necrosis (AVN). Athlete patients will return to their sport quicker if diagnostic certainty is obtained at an early stage (Table 11.3).

11.3.1.4 Treatment

Scaphoid

The goal of scaphoid fracture management is to achieve fracture union and prompt functional recovery while avoiding the complications of malunion or particularly nonunion. The management strategy depends on a number of factors, but the most important of these are the location of the fracture and the degree of displacement. Undisplaced fractures, particularly in the distal pole and waist have a high union rate with conservative or operative management. However, displaced fractures are at risk of further displacement and nonunion. Time to healing is related to fracture location. Distal pole fractures heal on average at eight weeks, waist fractures at nine weeks, and proximal pole fractures can take 16 weeks [89].

Nonoperative

Undisplaced fractures of the distal pole and waist can be routinely managed in a short arm cast. There is no clinical advantage in immobilising the thumb in the cast [90]. In fact, one study has even shown higher union rates in patients without thumb immobilisation [91]. Conservative management for these fractures is cost effective with low risk and cast immobilisation should continue until fracture union. Clementson et al. performed a randomised controlled trial of conservative treatment versus arthroscopically assisted screw fixation of undisplaced or minimally displaced scaphoid waist fractures. The authors found significantly better range of movement at 26 weeks in the conservative cohort and fewer radiographic signs of arthritis at median follow up of 6 years [92]. However, for the athlete, it may be inconvenient to be placed in a cast for 4–6 weeks and there is some evidence to suggest that surgical management with percutaneous fixation (Fig. 11.6) of undisplaced or minimally displaced waist fractures may help athletes return to activities sooner [92–94]. Proximal pole

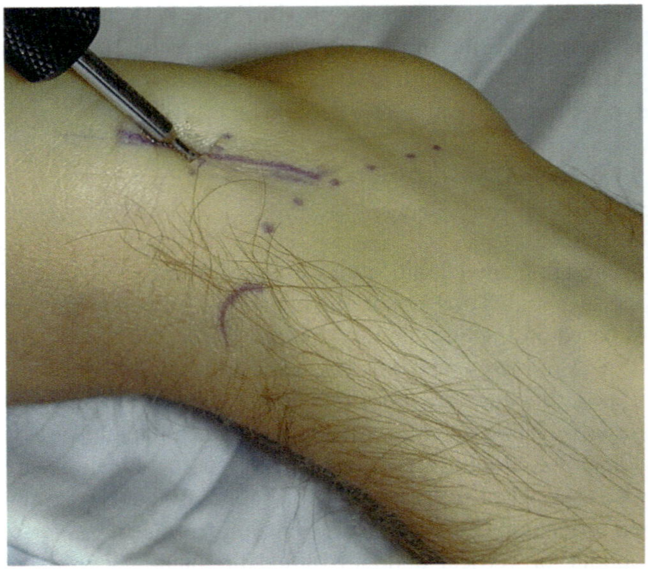

Fig. 11.6 Percutaneous volar approach to the scaphoid

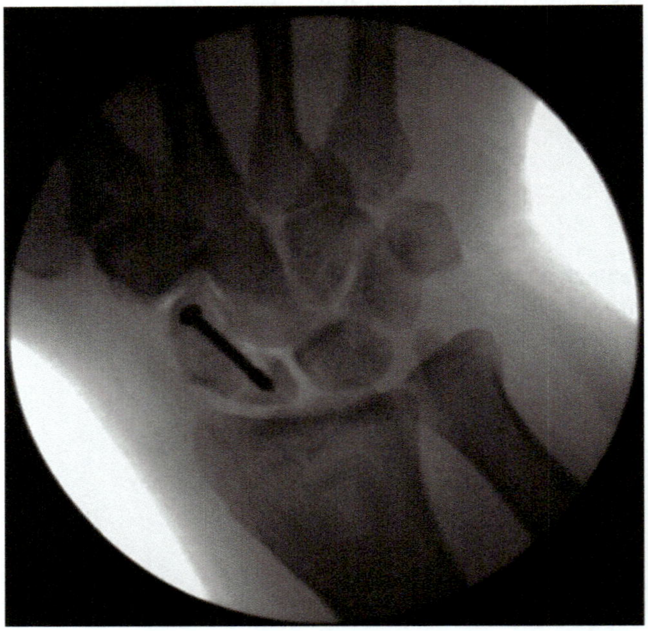

Fig. 11.7 Anteroposterior radiograph of scaphoid fixation

fractures are rarely appropriate for conservative treatment and have a nonunion rate ranging between 20% and 40% with this method of treatment [90, 95–98]. Screw fixation is recommended for these fracture patterns.

Operative

Operative fixation should be considered for patients with displaced and unstable fractures to avoid the risk of malunion and nonunion. Due to the risk of avascular necrosis and nonunion, all proximal pole fractures in athletes should also be considered for surgical fixation [99, 100] (Fig. 11.7). This can be performed either through a small dorsal approach for proximal pole fractures using a headless compression screw, or through a volar approach for waist fractures. If scaphoid waist fractures are displaced by >1 mm they are considered unstable and consideration should be made to fix these surgically. Reduction can be difficult without opening the fracture and reducing directly. A meta-analysis by Singh et al. showed displaced waist fractures are 17 times more likely to go onto non-union with cast immobilisation compared to operative management [101].

Controversy exists in the management of undisplaced scaphoid waist fractures. Both surgical and non-surgical management of these fractures is acceptable and achieve high rates of union. However, a number of studies [102, 103] have reported a faster return to work and sport following percutaneous fixation.

A recent systematic review by Robertson et al. analysed 160 fractures in 11 studies comparing operative and nonoperative treatment. The mean time to return to sport for operative patients was 7.9 weeks compared to 9.6 weeks in the conservative cohort. It is worth noting that the patients allowed to return to sport with a 'playing cast' (in the conservative cohort) did so in an average time of 1.9 weeks. Regarding fracture union, 97% of patients united in the operative cohort at a mean time of 9.8 weeks compared to 85% in the conservative cohort at a mean time of 14.0 weeks. If open fixation is required, where possible, a volar approach is utilised in order to correct any deformity and to avoid injury to the dorsal blood supply to the scaphoid.

Five of six recent systematic reviews with meta-analysis have compared non-operative and operative management for waist fractures and found that neither method is clearly superior. Surgical management is known to be associated with improved functional outcome, a more rapid return to function, sports and work, and superior union rates, but with a significantly higher rate of complications [102–107].

11.3.1.5 Complications

Scaphoid

Conservative management has few complications but does affect lifestyle during treatment. Stiffness, delayed union and nonunion are the most significant drawbacks to treating patients in cast. A recent meta-analysis of randomised controlled trials reported that patients undergoing surgery had an odds ratio of 6.96 for complications compared to nonoperative patients [104]. The most prevalent complication was related to metal work. However, less common risks from surgery include infection, intraoperative technical difficulties, complex regional pain syndrome and scarring. Symptoms related to these complications eventually resolved in most cases. Non-union can eventually lead to scaphoid nonunion advanced collapse (SNAC).

11.3.1.6 Rehabilitation

If there is doubt regarding union of conservatively or operatively treated scaphoid fractures, a CT scan should be performed [108, 109]. Once 50% of the fracture has bridging bone, the patient can be taken out of cast and given a removable splint for comfort while beginning range of movement and strengthening exercises [109, 110]. With regards to operatively treated fractures, return to sport can be considered at 4–6 weeks for low impact sports such as tennis, golf and baseball provided there is fracture healing on plain radiographs or CT scans [111]. Complete fracture healing should be present prior to allowing athletes to return to high energy contact sports such as American football, rugby and ice hockey. Time to union is longer in proximal pole fractures and this should be taken into consideration when deciding on return to sport.

11.3.1.7 Preventative Measures

Fractures of the carpus are difficult to prevent. However, a high index of suspicion and further imaging can avoid a missed diagnosis and the complications of this, as well as unnecessary immobilisation for the patient.

11.4 Other Carpal Bones

11.4.1 Epidemiology

Triquetral fractures account for approximately 15% of carpal fractures [112–114]. These fractures typically occur with a fall onto an extended and ulnar deviated wrist caus-

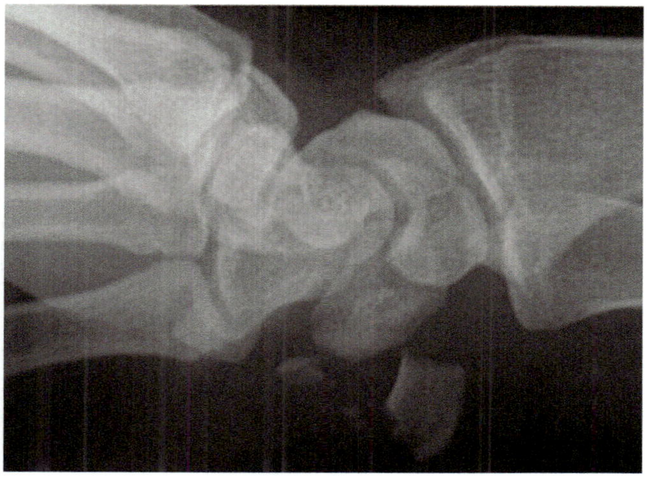

Fig. 11.8 Lateral radiograph of the wrist showing an avulsion fracture dislocation of the pisiform

ing impaction of the ulnar styloid on the triquetrium. Hyperflexion/radial deviation injuries can lead to dorsal rim avulsion fractures. **Trapezial fractures** account for the third most common carpal bone fractures and comprise approximately 3% of carpal fractures [115]. They typically occur with axial compression of the thumb. **Capitate fractures** may occur in isolation, be part of a greater arc perilunate fracture dislocation, or occur in combination with a fracture of the scaphoid (Fenton's Syndrome). The mechanism is often axial load of the third metacarpal or a fall onto an extended and ulnarly deviated wrist. Certain patterns of capitate fracture, like scaphoid fracture, are prone to non union. **Pisiform fractures** typically occur when falling backwards onto a supinated and extended wrist (i.e. when snowboarding or ice skating). They can also arise from repetitive trauma or a sudden contraction of the flexor carpi ulnaris tendon (Fig. 11.8).

The incidence of **lunate fractures** is likely confounded by mis-diagnosis of a congenital bi-partite lunate or the presence of Kienböck's disease. However, when the bone is acutely injured, it is commonly due to the capitate being driven into the lunate during axial load.

Hook of **hamate fractures** are classically seen in racquet sports, baseball and golf. They are thought to occur as a consequence of repetitive load from the flexor tendons of the little and ring finger. Fractures of the body occur in conjunction with subluxation of the fourth and fifth metacarpal bases. **Trapezoid fractures** are extremely rare in isolation due to their keystone anatomy and the protected position within the distal row. They are typically seen in carpometacarpal dislocations.

11.4.2 Classification

Triquetral fractures have been described to occur in three typical patterns

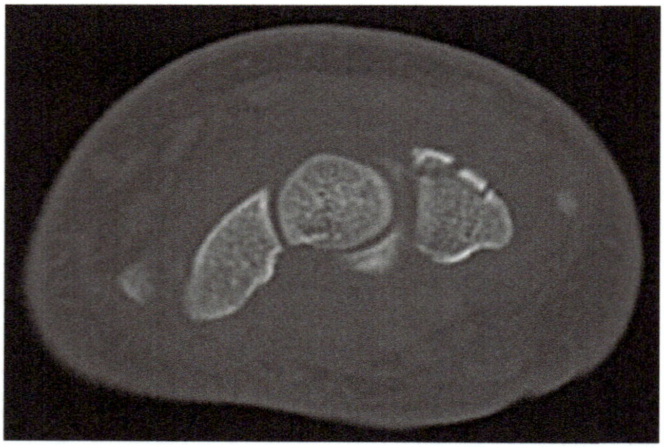

Fig. 11.9 CT scan demonstrating a dorsal 'chip' avulsion fracture of the triquetrum

1. dorsal 'chip' avulsion fractures (93%)
2. body fractures (3%) or
3. volar avulsions (4%) [116].

Dorsal 'chip' avulsion fractures are the most common type and occur after avulsion of the radiotriquetral and triquetroscaphoid ligament insertions at their apex (Fig. 11.9). **Trapezial fractures** have been classified as:

1. vertical intra-articular,
2. horizontal,
3. dorsal radial tuberosity,
4. anterior medial ridge and
5. comminuted [117].

Capitate fractures can be described by their fracture pattern:

1. transverse pole,
2. transverse body,
3. verticofrontal and
4. parasagittal fractures.

Transverse fractures are the most common.

Pisiform fractures are described as:

1. transverse,
2. parasagittal,
3. comminuted and
4. pisiform-triquetral impaction fractures.

Avulsions fractures can occur from sudden flexor carpi ulnaris contraction.

Lunate fractures can be classified as:

1. palmar pole,
2. transverse,
3. osteochondral, and
4. transarticular body fractures.

Hamate fractures are typically defined as occurring at the hook or the body. **Trapezoid fractures** are classified as:

1. dorsal rim or
2. body fractures.

11.4.3 Diagnosis

Triquetral fractures usually present with focal tenderness on the dorsal ulnar surface of the carpus. Lateral or 45° oblique radiographs are most helpful and can show the 'pooping duck' sign. Fractures to the body of the triquetrum can be detected with PA radiographs, although CT will better delineate the fracture. Lunotriquetral ligament injuries should also be considered, because they may benefit from surgical management. Volar avulsion injuries are best detected by radial deviation radiographs. These injuries, whilst rare, are associated with carpal instability. Further imaging with MRI scanning is recommended if this is the case. **Trapezial fractures** present with tenderness over the thumb base (volarly, radially or dorsally) and bruising is typically evident. PA, pronated AP, lateral and Bett's (or Gedda's) views are helpful in the diagnosis. CT scanning is useful to assess displacement and intra-articular involvement. **Capitate fractures** are usually high energy injuries and are often associated with other carpal fractures or ligamentous injuries. The wrist is notably swollen. More advanced imaging with CT (usually) and, on occasions MRI, is useful.

Pisiform fractures present with pain focally over the palmar ulnar surface of the hand but also deep hypothenar eminence pain. There may be sensory or motor symptoms from ulnar neuropraxia. Supinated views (30° or 45°) of the carpus are helpful in detecting these fractures. **Lunate fractures** usually present with dorsal wrist pain. Standard PA and lateral radiographs can diagnose the fracture. Dorsal or volar translation of the capitate is classical of dorsal or volar lip fractures. CT or MRI scans may be helpful if there is any question regarding fractures in the presence of possible Keinbock's disease.

Hamate fractures present with pain at the base of the hypothenar eminence which increases with direct palpation or gripping. Resisted flexion of the little and ring finger can exacerbate symptoms. Ulnar neuropraxia can also be present. Carpal tunnel views and supinated, oblique carpal plain radiographs are useful adjuncts. A CT scan is almost always recommended (Fig. 11.10). **Trapezoid fractures** may present with pain in the anatomical snuffbox and at the base of the first metacarpal. Pain is made worse by pinch gripping. PA and lateral radio-

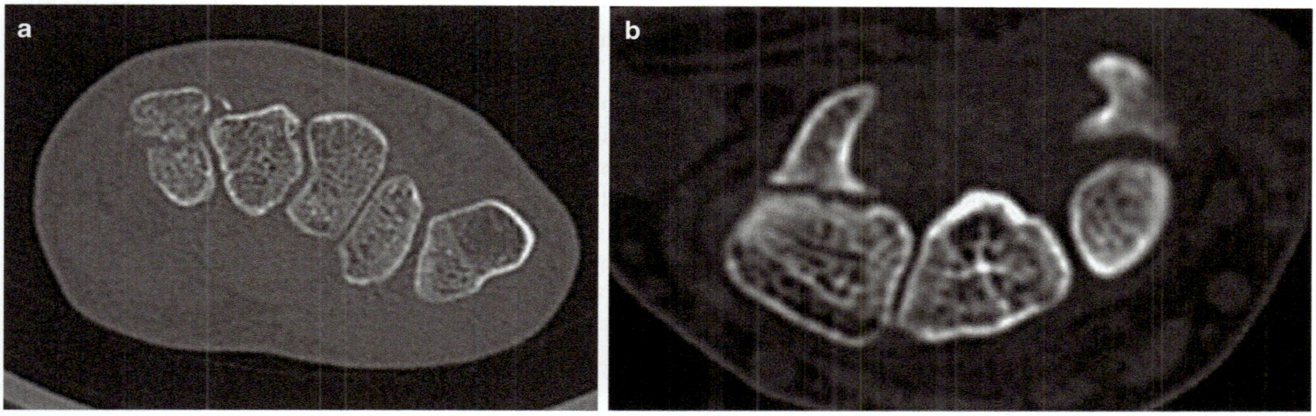

Fig. 11.10 CT scans demonstrating (**a**) hamate body fracture and (**b**) hamate hook non union

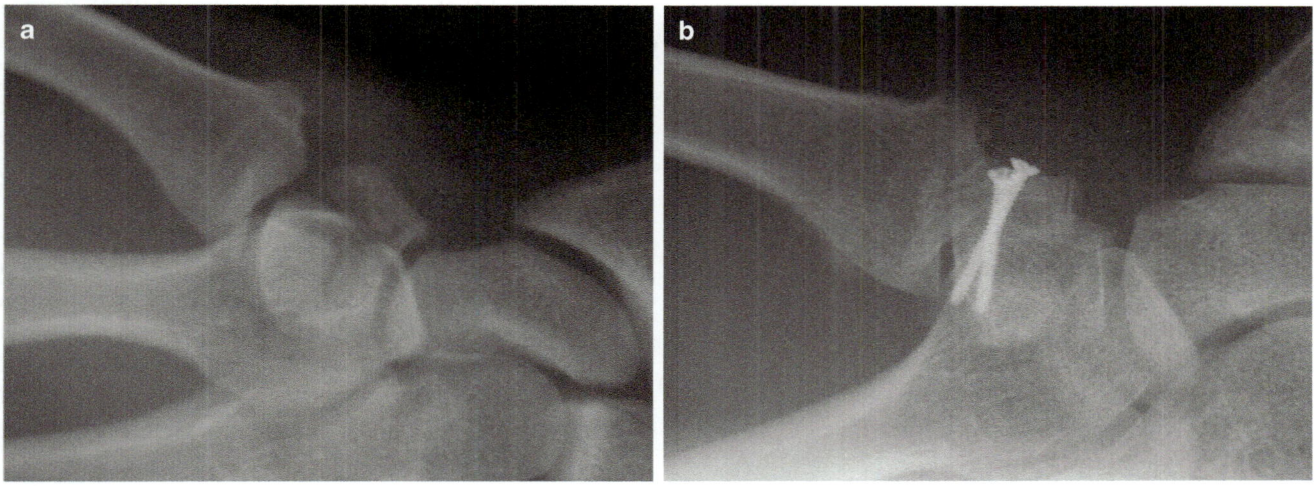

Fig. 11.11 Plain radiographs demonstrating a trapezial fracture (**a**) and subsequent management with screw fixation (**b**)

graphs can diagnose the fracture. Unstable fractures can lead to proximal and dorsal subluxation of the first metacarpal.

11.4.4 Treatment

Triquetral fracture management is dictated by the degree of displacement, the presence of associated injuries and the demands of the patient. Cast immobilisation for 4–6 weeks for isolated body fractures is advisable. However, the majority of avulsion fractures do not require treatment other than pain relief [118]. **Trapezial fractures** often required surgical fixation (Fig. 11.11) and only undisplaced fractures should be treated conservatively.

Immobilisation can take the form of a short arm cast with thumb extension for 4–6 weeks. Displaced **capitate fractures** should be reduced and stabilised with headless compression screws. **Pisiform fracture** patterns do not routinely dictate their management and can often be treated with cast immobilisation. Indications for later excision include comminution, significant displacement or flexor carpi ulnaris dysfunction. Undisplaced **lunate fractures** can be treated with cast immobilisation for 4–6 weeks. Displaced fractures should be managed with ORIF and good results have been reported [119]. Kirschner wire stabilisation to adjacent bones can be used if ORIF is not achievable. Dorsal avulsion fractures should raise the suspicion of scapholunate ligament injuries and primary repair must be considered if diagnosed, particularly in the athlete. **Hamate fractures** affecting the hook have a high nonunion rate [120]. These fractures occur through abnormal bone after a stress response. Symptomatic non union of the hamate hook is best treated with excision. This is an effective treatment in athletes and non-athletes with excellent postoperative grip strength and range of movement reported [121, 122]. Fractures to the body of the hamate should undergo ORIF or Kirschner wire fixation if they are displaced or affecting the stability of the ring finger or little finger carpometacarpal joints (CMCJs). **Trapezoid fractures** can be routinely managed with cast immobilisation if undisplaced. However, if they are displaced or there is subluxation of the CMCJ, fixation should be performed with Kirschner wires or, occasionally, ORIF. Primary arthrodesis of the second CMC joint is a reasonable treatment for comminuted frcatures.

11.4.5 Complications

Complications of **triquetral fractures** are adjacent ligamentous laxity, nonunion or pisotriquetral arthritis. **Trapezial fractures** can be complicated by carpometacarpal joint or scaphotrapezial arthritis, as well as nonunion, carpal tunnel syndrome, flexor carpi ulnaris tendinopathy (and/or rupture) and loss of pinch strength. **Capitate fractures** are often complicated by non-union, typically due to a delayed diagnosis. Avascular necrosis of the bone can also occur leading to carpal collapse and pancarpal arthritis. **Pisiform fractures** rarely cause persistent pain—even if they progress to nonunion or pisotriquetral arthritis. Late excision is a reasonable treatment in symptomatic cases. **Lunate fractures** may suffer similar complications to the capitate including avascular necrosis, carpal instability and arthritis. **Hamate fractures** can be complicated by a persistently painful non-union (hook) and carpometacarpal joint arthritis (body). Complications of **trapezoid fractures** include nonunion, delayed union or posttraumatic arthritis.

11.4.6 Rehabilitation

Fractures to other carpal bones will undergo a similar rehabilitation process to that of scaphoid fractures. Understanding the biomechanics of the wrist is crucial to advising patients on restrictions during fracture healing. For example, athlete patients who are in cast can be allowed to continue ipsilateral arm strengthening programmes provided they avoid gripping with the injured hand. Running should be allowed with the wrist in neutral and the fingers in extension. This wrist positioning avoids longitudinal loading of the carpus [123].

11.5 Perilunate Dislocations and Fracture-Dislocations

11.5.1 Epidemiology

Perilunate (PLI) dislocations and fracture-dislocations are high energy injuries that occur after landing onto a hyperflexed, ulnar deviated wrist with intercarpal supination [124, 125]. The mechanism often involves a fall from a height, at speed in sports, or in a road traffic accident [126, 127]. These injuries can be purely ligamentous (called 'lesser arc' injuries and known as perilunate dislocations) or combined ligamentous and bony (called 'greater arc' injuries and known as perilunate fracture dislocations). Ligament injuries progress from radial to ulnar and involve (in sequence) the scapholunate ligament, disruption of the lunocapitate joint, lunotriquetrial ligament injury and dissociation of the carpus from the lunate. The lunate may then finally dislocate into the carpal tunnel when there is failure of the dorsal radiolunate ligament [128].

11.5.2 Classification

The most commonly used classification for perilunate injuries is the Mayfield classification [129]. The four stages are:

1. Scapholunate ligament disruption leading to scapholunate dissociation
2. Capitolunate ligament disruption and capitate dislocation dorsally
3. Lunotriquetrial ligament disruption and triquetrum dislocation dorsally
4. Dorsal radiolunate ligament rupture and volar dislocation of the lunate

Herzberg et al. described a classification where stage 1 was when the lunate remained in the fossa, stage 2A was when it was dislocated but rotated less than 90° and stage 2B was when it was dislocated and rotated more than 90° [126].

11.5.3 Diagnosis

Due to the high energy required to produce a perilunate dislocation or fracture-dislocation, a high index of suspicion exists when patients complain of wrist pain and swelling after significant trauma. Up to 26% of perilunate injuries are associated with polytrauma and 11% with another upper limb injury [126]. On examination, there is significant pain and tenderness at the wrist. In Mayfield type 1 injuries, the tenderness is typically dorsally over the scapholunate ligament [68]. There may be swelling, bruising or blanching of the skin volarly at the wrist crease where the lunate has been extruded. Clinical features of median nerve compression are frequent and can result in irreversible loss of function if not identified and managed urgently.

Standard PA and lateral radiographs (Fig. 11.12) are usually sufficient to diagnose the injury. More subtle injury types can be detected on scaphoid views. PA views may demonstrate disruption of Gilula's lines and loss of carpal height. A scaphoid 'ring' sign may be seen when the scaphoid is flexed. Lateral views demonstrate the capitate dislocated from the lunate articulation or the lunate dislocated from the fossa (lunate dislocation). Examination under anaesthetic with fluoroscopy may help determine any subtle fractures or ligamentous injuries [130].

11.5.4 Treatment

Immediate treatment of an isolated perilunate dislocaton or fracture-dislocation includes neurovascular assessment (with particular attention to the median nerve) and an attempt at closed reduction under procedural sedation. Tavernier's manoeuvre can be performed which involves direct volar thumb pressure over the lunate, wrist extension with traction to bring the capitate forwards, and finally flexion of the wrist to reduce the capitatolunate joint. Closed reduction and nonoperative management has been shown to yield poor long-term results and should be avoided as definitive treatment [131, 132]. The most com-

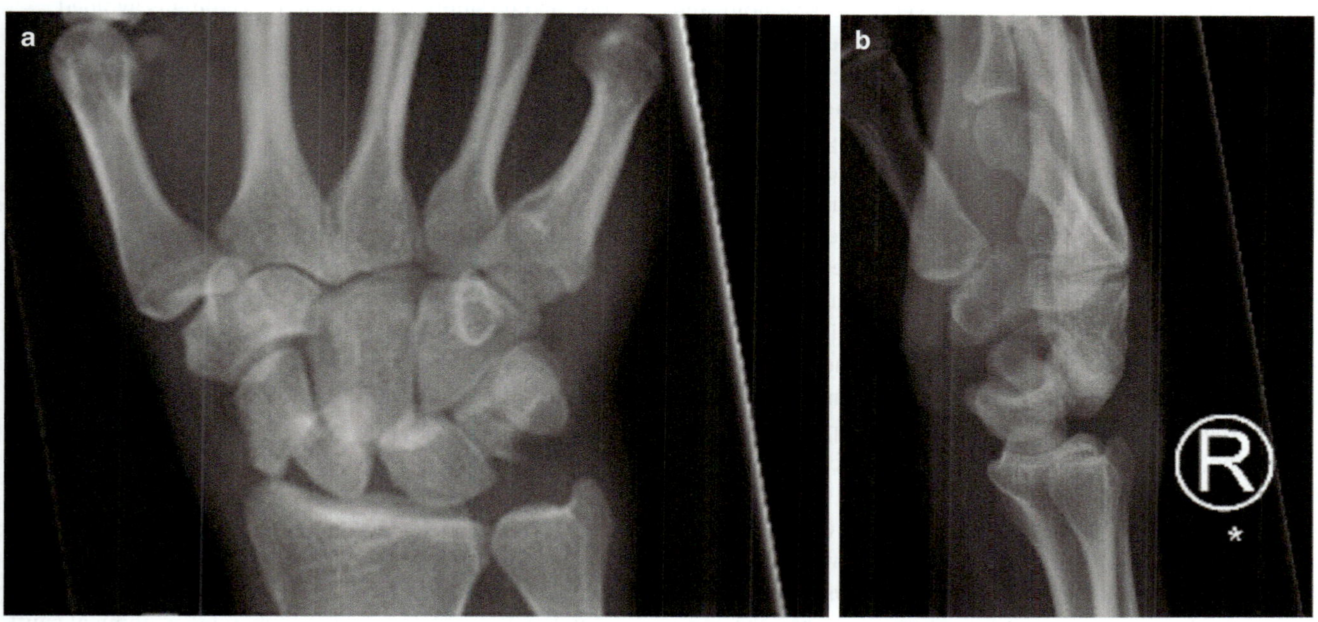

Fig. 11.12 PA (**a**) and lateral (**b**) radiographs of a perilunate dislocation

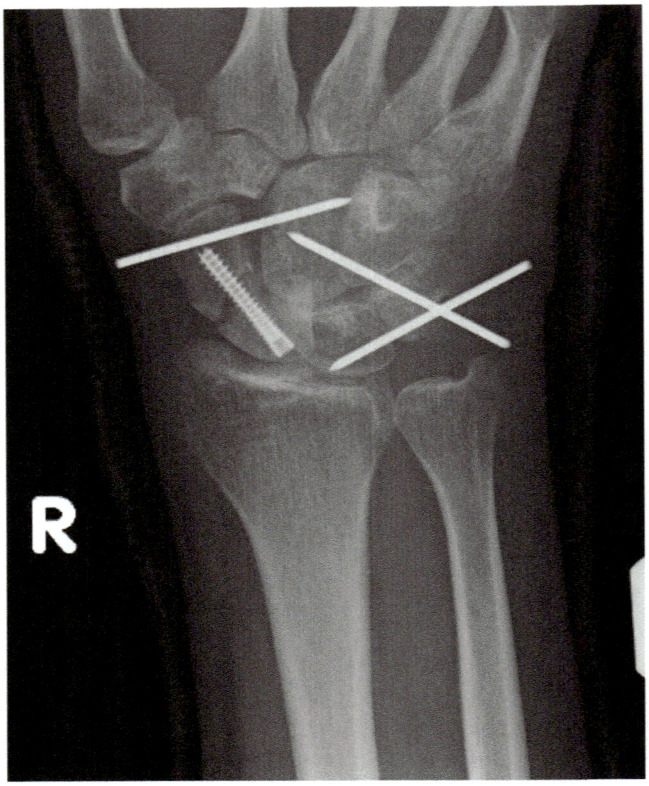

Fig. 11.13 Kirschner wire stabilisation and scaphoid open reduction internal fixation of a transcaphoid perilunate fracture dislocation

mon treatment is through a dorsal (or combined dorsal and volar) approach with open reduction, repair of the injured ligaments and Kirschner wire stabilisation of the scapholunate and lunotriquetral articulations (Fig. 11.13). A Kirschner wire is also placed between the scaphoid and capitate to suspend the latter bone above the repaired ligament. Much of the literature describing outcomes after different methods of surgical treatment are limited to small retrospective series. Functional and radiographic results vary significantly amongst these studies [133–135]. Uncertainty remains regarding the importance of repairing the lunotriquetral ligament in the presence of perilunate fracture dislocations. Some surgeons believe that Kirschner wire stabilisation may be inadequate and increase the risk of volar intercalated instability deformity [136]. In some greater arc injuries, (trans-scaphoid PLI) the scapholunate ligament is not injured and therefore does not require stabilisation/repair. In lesser arc injuries, scapholunate ligament repair is recommended to restore carpal stability [137, 138].

Raab et al. retrospectively reviewed ten cases of lunate and perilunate dislocations in athletes. Six were treated by closed reduction and percutaneous pin fixation. Nine athletes (90%) returned to play, with five returning during the same season as injury (four of which underwent closed reduction and percutaneous pinning) [139].

11.5.5 Complications

The most recognised early complication is acute carpal tunnel syndrome. This can occur in up to 45% of cases [126, 136, 140–142] and may be due to direct compression from the dislocated lunate or increased pressure from haematoma or oedema [143]. Later complications include stiffness, midcarpal instability, avascular necrosis, scapholunate advanced collapse (SLAC) and midcarpal arthrosis [144–146].

11.5.6 Rehabilitation

After reduction and stabilisation of perilunate injuries, cast immobilisation is advised for 10 weeks until Kirschner wires are removed. Wrist physiotherapy can begin at 12 weeks [68, 147–149] but stiffness persists for many months. Cast immobilisation should avoid inclusion of the metacarpophalangeal, proximal interphalangeal and distal interphalangeal joints to allow movement of the fingers during casting.

Clinical Pearls

- The stability of the distal radio ulnar joint (DRUJ) must be assessed in all distal radius fractures, with early surgical repair of the triangular fibrocartilage complex (TFCC) when indicated to ensure maintained stability and wrist function.
- Surgical management of undisplaced or minimally displaced scaphoid waist fractures can produce a faster return to sport than conservative management
- Maintaining strength and conditioning of athletes during cast immobilisation can avoid asymmetrical deconditioning, and be safely undertaken, if gripping is avoided

Review

Questions

1. What is the rate of concurrent ulnar styloid fractures with distal radius fractures?
2. What three examination findings in combination have been shown to be most sensitive for predicting scaphoid fractures?
3. What is the best treatment choice for persistent pain following non union of the hook of the hamate?

Answers

1. 58%
2. Tenderness over the scaphoid tubercle, anatomical snuffbox and on axial thumb compression
3. Hook of hamate excision

References

1. Ali M, Eiriksdottir A, Murtadha M, Åkesson A, Atroshi I. Incidence of distal radius fracture in a general population in southern Sweden in 2016 compared with 2001. Osteoporos Int. 2020;31(4):715–20.
2. Aitken S, Court-Brown CM. The epidemiology of sports-related fractures of the hand. Injury. 2008;39(12):1377–83.
3. Wood AM, Robertson GA, Rennie L, Caesar BC, Court-Brown CM. The epidemiology of sports-related fractures in adolescents. Injury. 2010;41(8):834–8.
4. Robertson GA, Wood AM, Bakker-Dyos J, Aitken SA, Keenan AC, Court-Brown CM. The epidemiology, morbidity, and outcome of soccer-related fractures in a standard population. Am J Sports Med. 2012;40(8):1851–7.
5. Lawson GM, Hajducka C, McQueen MM. Sports fractures of the distal radius--epidemiology and outcome. Injury. 1995;26(1):33–6.
6. Schipilow JD, Macdonald HM, Liphardt AM, Kan M, Boyd SK. Bone micro-architecture, estimated bone strength, and the muscle-bone interaction in elite athletes: an HR-pQCT study. Bone. 2013;56(2):281–9.
7. Matsumoto K, Sumi H, Sumi Y, Shimizu K. Wrist fractures from snowboarding: a prospective study for 3 seasons from 1998 to 2001. Clin J Sport Med. 2004;14(2):64–71.
8. Brogren E, Petranek M, Atroshi I. Incidence and characteristics of distal radius fractures in a southern Swedish region. BMC Musculoskelet Disord. 2007;8:48.
9. Flinkkila T, Sirnio K, Hippi M, Hartonen S, Ruuhela R, Ohtonen P, et al. Epidemiology and seasonal variation of distal radius fractures in Oulu, Finland. Osteoporos Int. 2011;22(8):2307–12.
10. Plant CE, Hickson C, Hedley H, Parsons NR, Costa ML. Is it time to revisit the AO classification of fractures of the distal radius? Inter- and intra-observer reliability of the AO classification. Bone Joint J. 2015;97-b(6):818–23.
11. Shehovych A, Salar O, Meyer C, Ford DJ. Adult distal radius fractures classification systems: essential clinical knowledge or abstract memory testing? Ann R Coll Surg Engl. 2016;98(8):525–31.
12. Robertson GA, Wood AM, Heil K, Aitken SA, Court-Brown CM. The epidemiology, morbidity and outcome of fractures in rugby union from a standard population. Injury. 2014;45(4):677–83.
13. Tanabe K, Nakajima T, Sogo E, Denno K, Horiki M, Nakagawa R. Intra-articular fractures of the distal radius evaluated by computed tomography. J Hand Surg Am. 2011;36(11):1798–803.
14. Hanker GJ. Radius fractures in the athlete. Clin Sports Med. 2001;20(1):189–201.
15. Lafontaine M, Hardy D, Delince P. Stability assessment of distal radius fractures. Injury. 1989;20(4):208–10.
16. Mackenney PJ, McQueen MM, Elton R. Prediction of instability in distal radial fractures. J Bone Joint Surg Am. 2006;88(9):1944–51.
17. Ng CY, McQueen MM. What are the radiological predictors of functional outcome following fractures of the distal radius? J Bone Joint Surg Br. 2011;93(2):145–50.
18. Karnezis IA, Fragkiadakis EG. Association between objective clinical variables and patient-rated disability of the wrist. J Bone Joint Surg Br. 2002;84(7):967–70.
19. Wilcke MK, Abbaszadegan H, Adolphson PY. Patient-perceived outcome after displaced distal radius fractures. A comparison between radiological parameters, objective physical variables, and the DASH score. J Hand Ther. 2007;20(4):290–8. quiz 9
20. Costa ML, Achten J, Parsons NR, Rangan A, Griffin D, Tubeuf S, et al. Percutaneous fixation with Kirschner wires versus volar locking plate fixation in adults with dorsally displaced fracture of distal radius: randomised controlled trial. BMJ. 2014;349:g4807.
21. Costa ML, Achten J, Rangan A, Lamb SE, Parsons NR. Percutaneous fixation with Kirschner wires versus volar locking-plate fixation in adults with dorsally displaced fracture of distal radius: five-year follow-up of a randomized controlled trial. Bone Joint J. 2019;101-B(8):978–83.
22. Orbay JL, Fernandez DL. Volar fixed-angle plate fixation for unstable distal radius fractures in the elderly patient. J Hand Surg Am. 2004;29(1):96–102.
23. Ruch DS, Papadonikolakis A. Volar versus dorsal plating in the management of intra-articular distal radius fractures. J Hand Surg Am. 2006;31(1):9–16.
24. Jakubietz MG, Gruenert JG, Jakubietz RG. Palmar and dorsal fixed-angle plates in AO C-type fractures of the distal radius: is there an advantage of palmar plates in the long term? J Orthop Surg Res. 2012;7(1):8.
25. Kambouroglou GK, Axelrod TS. Complications of the AO/ASIF titanium distal radius plate system (pi plate) in internal fixation of the distal radius: a brief report. J Hand Surg Am. 1998;23(4):737–41.
26. Carter PR, Frederick HA, Laseter GF. Open reduction and internal fixation of unstable distal radius fractures with a low-profile plate: a multicenter study of 73 fractures. J Hand Surg Am. 1998;23(2):300–7.
27. O'Shaughnessy MA, Shin AY, Kakar S. Stabilization of volar ulnar rim fractures of the distal radius: current techniques and review of the literature. J Wrist Surg. 2016;5(2):113–9.
28. Geissler WB, Freeland AE. Arthroscopic management of intra-articular distal radius fractures. Hand Clin. 1999;15(3):455–65viii.
29. Saw N, Roberts C, Cutbush K, Hodder M, Couzens G, Ross M. Early experience with the TriMed fragment-specific fracture fixation system in intraarticular distal radius fractures. J Hand Surg Eur Vol. 2008;33(1):53–8.
30. Gavaskar AS, Muthukumar S, Chowdary N. Fragment-specific fixation for complex intra-articular fractures of the distal radius: results of a prospective single-centre trial. J Hand Surg Eur Vol. 2012;37(8):765–71.
31. Benson LS, Minihane KP, Stern LD, Eller E, Seshadri R. The outcome of intra-articular distal radius fractures treated with fragment-specific fixation. J Hand Surg Am. 2006;31(8):1333–9.
32. Peine R, Rikli DA, Hoffmann R, Duda G, Regazzoni P. Comparison of three different plating techniques for the dorsum of the distal radius: a biomechanical study. J Hand Surg Am. 2000;25(1):29–33.
33. Taylor KF, Parks BG, Segalman KA. Biomechanical stability of a fixed-angle volar plate versus fragment-specific fixation system: cyclic testing in a C2-type distal radius cadaver fracture model. J Hand Surg Am. 2006;31(3):373–81.
34. Cooper EO, Segalman KA, Parks BG, Sharma KM, Nguyen A. Biomechanical stability of a volar locking-screw plate versus fragment-specific fixation in a distal radius fracture model. Am J Orthop (Belle Mead NJ). 2007;36(4) E46–9.
35. Fricker R JJ, Kastelec M. Distal forearm. AO Foundation; 2019. https://www2.aofoundation.org/wps/portal/surgery?showPage=diagnosis&bone=Radius&segment=Distal. Accessed 1 Oct 2019.
36. Smeraglia F, Del Buono A, Maffulli N. Wrist arthroscopy in the management of articular distal radius fractures. Br Med Bull. 2016;119(1):157–65.
37. Orbay J. Volar plate fixation of distal radius fractures. Hand Clin. 2005;21(3):347–54.
38. Dardas AZ, Goldfarb CA, Boyer MI, Osei DA, Dy CJ, Calfee RP. A prospective observational assessment of unicortical distal screw placement during volar plate fixation of distal radius fractures. J Hand Surg Am. 2018;43(5):448–54.
39. Soong M, Earp BE, Bishop G, Leung A, Blazar P. Volar locking plate implant prominence and flexor tendon rupture. J Bone Joint Surg Am. 2011;93(4):328–35.
40. Handoll HH, Elliott J. Rehabilitation for distal radial fractures in adults. Cochrane Database Syst Rev. 2015;9:CD003324.
41. Henn CM, Wolfe SW. Distal radius fractures in athletes: approaches and treatment considerations. Sports Med Arthrosc Rev. 2014;22(1):29–38.

42. Beleckas C, Calfee R. Distal radius fractures in the athlete. Curr Rev Musculoskelet Med. 2017;10(1):62–71.
43. Carlisle JC, Goldfarb CA, Mall N, Powell JW, Matava MJ. Upper extremity injuries in the National Football League: part II: elbow, forearm, and wrist injuries. Am J Sports Med. 2008;36(10):1945–52.
44. Clement ND, Yousif F, Duckworth AD, Teoh KH, Porter DE. Retention of forearm plates: risks and benefits in a paediatric population. J Bone Joint Surg Br. 2012;94(1):134–7.
45. Bauer D, Schweizer A, Nagy L. Periprosthetic fracture of the ulna-a case report. J Wrist Surg. 2015;4(2):134–8.
46. May MM, Lawton JN, Blazar PE. Ulnar styloid fractures associated with distal radius fractures: incidence and implications for distal radioulnar joint instability. J Hand Surg Am. 2002;27(6):965–71.
47. Rettig AC. Stress fracture of the ulna in an adolescent tournament tennis player. Am J Sports Med. 1983;11(2):103–6.
48. Fragniere B, Landry M, Siegrist O. Stress fracture of the ulna in a professional tennis player using a double-handed backhand stroke. Knee Surg Sports Traumatol Arthrosc. 2001;9(4):239–41.
49. Koskinen SK, Mattila KT, Alanen AM, Aro HT. Stress fracture of the ulnar diaphysis in a recreational golfer. Clin J Sport Med. 1997;7(1):63–5.
50. Muller ME, Koch P, et al. Comprehensive classification of fractures of long bones. New York, NY: Springer; 1990.
51. Biyani A, Simison AJ, Klenerman L. Fractures of the distal radius and ulna. J Hand Surg Br. 1995;20(3):357–64.
52. Logan AJ, Lindau TR. The management of distal ulnar fractures in adults: a review of the literature and recommendations for treatment. Strat Trauma Limb Reconstr. 2008;3(2):49–56.
53. Tornese D, Curci D, Nardo A, Cuccia A, Pozzi G. Stress fracture of the ulna in an elite ice dancer. J Sports Sci Med. 2015;14(1):37–40.
54. Wiltfong RE, Carruthers KH, Popp JE. Completed ulnar shaft stress fracture in a fast-pitch softball pitcher. Orthopedics. 2017;40(2):e360–e2.
55. Bombaci H, Polat A, Deniz G, Akinci O. The value of plain X-rays in predicting TFCC injury after distal radial fractures. J Hand Surg Eur Vol. 2008;33(3):322–6.
56. Buijze GA, Ring D. Clinical impact of united versus nonunited fractures of the proximal half of the ulnar styloid following volar plate fixation of the distal radius. J Hand Surg Am. 2010;35(2):223–7.
57. Kim JK, Yun YH, Kim DJ, Yun GU. Comparison of united and nonunited fractures of the ulnar styloid following volar-plate fixation of distal radius fractures. Injury. 2011;42(4):371–5.
58. Lindau T, Arner M, Hagberg L. Intraarticular lesions in distal fractures of the radius in young adults. A descriptive arthroscopic study in 50 patients. J Hand Surg Br. 1997;22(5):638–43.
59. Catalano LW 3rd, Cole RJ, Gelberman RH, Evanoff BA, Gilula LA, Borrelli J Jr. Displaced intra-articular fractures of the distal aspect of the radius. Long-term results in young adults after open reduction and internal fixation. J Bone Joint Surg Am. 1997;79(9):1290–302.
60. Sammer DM, Shah HM, Shauver MJ, Chung KC. The effect of ulnar styloid fractures on patient-rated outcomes after volar locking plating of distal radius fractures. J Hand Surg Am. 2009;34(9):1595–602.
61. Protopsaltis TS, Ruch DS. Triangular fibrocartilage complex tears associated with symptomatic ulnar styloid nonunions. J Hand Surg Am. 2010;35(8):1251–5.
62. Ring D, McCarty LP, Campbell D, Jupiter JB. Condylar blade plate fixation of unstable fractures of the distal ulna associated with fracture of the distal radius. J Hand Surg Am. 2004;29(1):103–9.
63. Dymond IW. The treatment of isolated fractures of the distal ulna. J Bone Joint Surg Br. 1984;66(3):408–10.
64. Hazel A, Nemeth N, Bindra R. Anatomic considerations for plating of the distal ulna. J Wrist Surg. 2015;4(3):188–93.
65. Dennison DG. Open reduction and internal locked fixation of unstable distal ulna fractures with concomitant distal radius fracture. J Hand Surg Am. 2007;32(6):801–5.
66. Reeves B. Boomerang bone disease: bilateral dysplasia of ulna and fibula. Proc R Soc Med. 1966;59(8):711–2.
67. Corea JR, Brakenbury PH, Blakemore ME. The treatment of isolated fractures of the ulnar shaft in adults. Injury. 1981;12(5):365–70.
68. White TMSG. A. McRae's orthopaedic trauma and emergency management. 3rd ed. Amsterdam: Elsevier; 2016. p. 216–127.
69. Bohler L, Trojan E, Jahna H. The results of treatment of 734 fresh, simple fractures of the scaphoid. J Hand Surg Br. 2003;28(4):319–31.
70. Duckworth AD, Jenkins PJ, Aitken SA, Clement ND, Court-Brown CM, McQueen MM. Scaphoid fracture epidemiology. J Trauma Acute Care Surg. 2012;72(2):E41–5.
71. Garala K, Taub NA, Dias JJ. The epidemiology of fractures of the scaphoid: impact of age, gender, deprivation and seasonality. Bone Joint J. 2016;98-B(5):654–9.
72. Larsen CF, Brondum V, Skov O. Epidemiology of scaphoid fractures in Odense, Denmark. Acta Orthop Scand. 1992;63(2):216–8.
73. Hove LM. Epidemiology of scaphoid fractures in Bergen, Norway. Scand J Plast Reconstr Surg Hand Surg. 1999;33(4):423–6.
74. Sward EM, Schriever TU, Franko MA, Bjorkman AC, Wilcke MK. The epidemiology of scaphoid fractures in Sweden: a nationwide registry study. J Hand Surg Eur Vol. 2019;44(7):697–701.
75. Van Tassel DC, Owens BD, Wolf JM. Incidence estimates and demographics of scaphoid fracture in the U.S. population. J Hand Surg Am. 2010;35(8):1242–5.
76. Kawamura K, Chung KC. Treatment of scaphoid fractures and nonunions. J Hand Surg Am. 2008;33(6):988–97.
77. Geissler WB. Arthroscopic management of scaphoid fractures in athletes. Hand Clin. 2009;25(3):359–69.
78. Horii E, Nakamura R, Watanabe K, Tsunoda K. Scaphoid fracture as a "puncher's fracture". J Orthop Trauma. 1994;8(2):107–10.
79. Herbert TJ, Fisher WE. Management of the fractured scaphoid using a new bone screw. J Bone Joint Surg Br. 1984;66(1):114–23.
80. Russe O. Follow-up study results of 22 cases of operated old fractures and pseudarthroses of the scaphoid bone of the hand. Z Orthop Ihre Grenzgeb. 1960;93:5–14.
81. Pandit S, Wen DY. Scaphoid fractures with unusual presentations: a case series. Cases J. 2009;2:7220.
82. Winston MJ, Weiland AJ. Scaphoid fractures in the athlete. Curr Rev Musculoskelet Med. 2017;10(1):38–44.
83. Grover R. Clinical assessment of scaphoid injuries and the detection of fractures. J Hand Surg Br. 1996;21(3):341–3.
84. Parvizi J, Wayman J, Kelly P, Moran CG. Combining the clinical signs improves diagnosis of scaphoid fractures. A prospective study with follow-up. J Hand Surg Br. 1998;23(3):324–7.
85. Blum A, Sauer B, Detreille R, Zabel JP, Pierrucci F, Witte Y, et al. The diagnosis of recent scaphoid fractures: review of the literature. J Radiol. 2007;88(5 Pt 2):741–59.
86. Gaebler C, Kukla C, Breitenseher M, Trattnig S, Mittlboeck M, Vecsei V. Magnetic resonance imaging of occult scaphoid fractures. J Trauma. 1996;41(1):73–6.
87. Mallee WH, Wang J, Poolman RW, Kloen P, Maas M, de Vet HC, et al. Computed tomography versus magnetic resonance imaging versus bone scintigraphy for clinically suspected scaphoid fractures in patients with negative plain radiographs. Cochrane Database Syst Rev. 2015;6:Cd010023.
88. Rua T, Malhotra B, Vijayanathan S, Hunter L, Peacock J, Shearer J, et al. Clinical and cost implications of using immediate MRI in the management of patients with a suspected scaphoid fracture and negative radiographs results from the SMaRT trial. Bone Joint J. 2019;101-b(8):984–94.
89. Grewal R, Suh N, Macdermid JC. Use of computed tomography to predict union and time to union in acute scaphoid fractures treated nonoperatively. J Hand Surg Am. 2013;38(5):872–7.
90. Clay NR, Dias JJ, Costigan PS, Gregg PJ, Barton NJ. Need the thumb be immobilised in scaphoid fractures? A randomised prospective trial. J Bone Joint Surg Br. 1991;73(5):828–32.

91. Buijze GA, Goslings JC, Rhemrev SJ, Weening AA, Van Dijkman B, Doornberg JN, et al. Cast immobilization with and without immobilization of the thumb for nondisplaced and minimally displaced scaphoid waist fractures: a multicenter, randomized, controlled trial. J Hand Surg Am. 2014;39(4):621–7.
92. Clementson M, Jorgsholm P, Besjakov J, Thomsen N, Bjorkman A. Conservative treatment versus arthroscopic-assisted screw fixation of scaphoid waist fractures—a randomized trial with minimum 4-year follow-up. J Hand Surg Am. 2015;40(7):1341–8.
93. Schernberg F. Recent scaphoid fractures (within the first three weeks). Chir Main. 2005;24(3–4):117–31.
94. Inoue G, Shionoya K. Herbert screw fixation by limited access for acute fractures of the scaphoid. J Bone Joint Surg Br. 1997;79(3):418–21.
95. Gellman H, Caputo RJ, Carter V, Aboulafia A, McKay M. Comparison of short and long thumb-spica casts for non-displaced fractures of the carpal scaphoid. J Bone Joint Surg Am. 1989;71(3):354–7.
96. Terkelsen CJ, Jepsen JM. Treatment of scaphoid fractures with a removable cast. Acta Orthop Scand. 1988;59(4):452–3.
97. Steinmann SP, Adams JE. Scaphoid fractures and nonunions: diagnosis and treatment. J Orthop Sci. 2006;11(4):424–31.
98. Gholson JJ, Bae DS, Zurakowski D, Waters PM. Scaphoid fractures in children and adolescents: contemporary injury patterns and factors influencing time to union. J Bone Joint Surg Am. 2011;93(13):1210–9.
99. Krimmer H. Management of acute fractures and nonunions of the proximal pole of the scaphoid. J Hand Surg Br. 2002;27(3):245–8.
100. Arsalan-Werner A, Sauerbier M, Mehling IM. Current concepts for the treatment of acute scaphoid fractures. Eur J Trauma Emerg Surg. 2016;42(1):3–10.
101. Singh HP, Taub N, Dias JJ. Management of displaced fractures of the waist of the scaphoid: meta-analyses of comparative studies. Injury. 2012;43(6):933–9.
102. Buijze GA, Doornberg JN, Ham JS, Ring D, Bhandari M, Poolman RW. Surgical compared with conservative treatment for acute nondisplaced or minimally displaced scaphoid fractures: a systematic review and meta-analysis of randomized controlled trials. J Bone Joint Surg Am. 2010;92(6):1534–44.
103. Symes TH, Stothard J. A systematic review of the treatment of acute fractures of the scaphoid. J Hand Surg Eur Vol. 2011;36(9):802–10.
104. Ibrahim T, Qureshi A, Sutton AJ, Dias JJ. Surgical versus nonsurgical treatment of acute minimally displaced and undisplaced scaphoid waist fractures: pairwise and network meta-analyses of randomized controlled trials. J Hand Surg Am. 2011;36(11):1759–68.e1.
105. Alshryda S, Shah A, Odak S, Al-Shryda J, Ilango B, Murali SR. Acute fractures of the scaphoid bone: systematic review and meta-analysis. Surgeon. 2012;10(4):218–29.
106. Shen L, Tang J, Luo C, Xie X, An Z, Zhang C. Comparison of operative and non-operative treatment of acute undisplaced or minimally-displaced scaphoid fractures: a meta-analysis of randomized controlled trials. PLoS One. 2015;10(5):e0125247.
107. Al-Ajmi TA, Al-Faryan KH, Al-Kanaan NF, Al-Khodair AA, Al-Faryan TH, Al-Oraini MI, et al. A systematic review and meta-analysis of randomized controlled trials comparing surgical versus conservative treatments for acute undisplaced or minimally-displaced scaphoid fractures. Clin Orthop Surg. 2018;10(1):64–73.
108. Kovacic J, Bergfeld J. Return to play issues in upper extremity injuries. Clin J Sport Med. 2005;15(6):448–52.
109. Belsky MR, Leibman MI, Ruchelsman DE. Scaphoid fracture in the elite athlete. Hand Clin. 2012;28(3):269–78,vii.
110. Slade JF 3rd, Gillon T. Retrospective review of 234 scaphoid fractures and nonunions treated with arthroscopy for union and complications. Scand J Surg. 2008;97(4):280–9.
111. Dy CJ, Khmelnitskaya E, Hearns KA, Carlson MG. Opinions regarding the management of hand and wrist injuries in elite athletes. Orthopedics. 2013;36(6):815–9.
112. Garcia-Elias M. Dorsal fractures of the triquetrum-avulsion or compression fractures? J Hand Surg Am. 1987;12(2):266–8.
113. van Onselen EB, Karim RB, Hage JJ, Ritt MJ. Prevalence and distribution of hand fractures. J Hand Surg Br. 2003;28(5):491–5.
114. Hey HW, Chong AK, Murphy D. Prevalence of carpal fracture in Singapore. J Hand Surg Am. 2011;36(2):278–83.
115. Hove LM. Fractures of the hand. Distribution and relative incidence. Scand J Plast Reconstr Surg Hand Surg. 1993;27(4):317–9.
116. Hocker K, Menschik A. Chip fractures of the triquetrum. Mechanism, classification and results. J Hand Surg Br. 1994;19(5):584–8.
117. Walker JL, Greene TL, Lunseth PA. Fractures of the body of the trapezium. J Orthop Trauma. 1988;2(1):22–8.
118. Chen NC, Jupiter JB, Jebson PJ. Sports-related wrist injuries in adults. Sports Health. 2009;1(6):469–77.
119. Hsu AR, Hsu PA. Unusual case of isolated lunate fracture without ligamentous injury. Orthopedics. 2011;34(11):e785–9.
120. Failla JM. Osteonecrosis associated with nonunion of the hook of the hamate. Orthopedics. 1993;16(2):217–8.
121. Stark HH, Chao EK, Zemel NP, Rickard TA, Ashworth CR. Fracture of the hook of the hamate. J Bone Joint Surg Am. 1989;71(8):1202–7.
122. Devers BN, Douglas KC, Naik RD, Lee DH, Watson JT, Weikert DR. Outcomes of hook of hamate fracture excision in high-level amateur athletes. J Hand Surg Am. 2013;38(1):72–6.
123. Gislason MKS, Nash BW. Loading on the Scapho-Trapezium-Trapezoid joint during gripping. In: 22nd Congress of the international society of biomechanics. 2009.
124. Johnson RP. The acutely injured wrist and its residuals. Clin Orthop Relat Res. 1980;149:33–44.
125. Fisk GR. Carpal instability and the fractured scaphoid. Ann R Coll Surg Engl. 1970;46(2):63–76.
126. Herzberg G, Comtet JJ, Linscheid RL, Amadio PC, Cooney WP, Stalder J. Perilunate dislocations and fracture-dislocations: a multicenter study. J Hand Surg Am. 1993;18(5):768–79.
127. Wickramasinghe NR, Duckworth AD, Clement ND, Hageman MG, McQueen MM, Ring D. Acute median neuropathy and carpal tunnel release in perilunate injuries can we predict who gets a median neuropathy? J Hand Microsurg. 2015;7(2):237–40.
128. Mayfield JK, Johnson RP, Kilcoyne RK. Carpal dislocations: pathomechanics and progressive perilunar instability. J Hand Surg Am. 1980;5(3):226–41.
129. Melone CP Jr, Murphy MS, Raskin KB. Perilunate injuries. Repair by dual dorsal and volar approaches. Hand Clin. 2000;16(3):439–48.
130. Weil WM, Slade JF 3rd, Trumble TE. Open and arthroscopic treatment of perilunate injuries. Clin Orthop Relat Res. 2006;445:120–32.
131. Adkison JW, Chapman MW. Treatment of acute lunate and perilunate dislocations. Clin Orthop Relat Res. 1982;164:199–207.
132. Apergis E, Maris J, Theodoratos G, Pavlakis D, Antoniou N. Perilunate dislocations and fracture-dislocations. Closed and early open reduction compared in 28 cases. Acta Orthop Scand Suppl. 1997;275:55–9.
133. Minami A, Kaneda K. Repair and/or reconstruction of scapholunate interosseous ligament in lunate and perilunate dislocations. J Hand Surg Am. 1993;18(6):1099–106.
134. Palmer AK, Dobyns JH, Linscheid RL. Management of post-traumatic instability of the wrist secondary to ligament rupture. J Hand Surg Am. 1978;3(6):507–32.
135. Forli A, Courvoisier A, Wimsey S, Corcella D, Moutet F. Perilunate dislocations and transscaphoid perilunate fracture-dislocations: a retrospective study with minimum ten-year follow-up. J Hand Surg Am. 2010;35(1):62–8.

136. Knoll VD, Allan C, Trumble TE. Trans-scaphoid perilunate fracture dislocations: results of screw fixation of the scaphoid and lunotriquetral repair with a dorsal approach. J Hand Surg Am. 2005;30(6):1145–52.
137. Budoff JE. Treatment of acute lunate and perilunate dislocations. J Hand Surg Am. 2008;33(8):1424–32.
138. Kremer T, Wendt M, Riedel K, Sauerbier M, Germann G, Bickert B. Open reduction for perilunate injuries—clinical outcome and patient satisfaction. J Hand Surg Am. 2010;35(10):1599–606.
139. Raab DJ, Fischer DA, Quick DC. Lunate and perilunate dislocations in professional football players. A five-year retrospective analysis. Am J Sports Med. 1994;22(6):841–5.
140. Hildebrand KA, Ross DC, Patterson SD, Roth JH, MacDermid JC, King GJ. Dorsal perilunate dislocations and fracture-dislocations: questionnaire, clinical, and radiographic evaluation. J Hand Surg Am. 2000;25(6):1069–79.
141. Sotereanos DG, Mitsionis GJ, Giannakopoulos PN, Tomaino MM, Herndon JH. Perilunate dislocation and fracture dislocation: a critical analysis of the volar-dorsal approach. J Hand Surg Am. 1997;22(1):49–56.
142. Trumble T, Verheyden J. Treatment of isolated perilunate and lunate dislocations with combined dorsal and volar approach and intraosseous cerclage wire. J Hand Surg Am. 2004;29(3):412–7.
143. Herzberg G. Perilunate and axial carpal dislocations and fracture-dislocations. J Hand Surg Am. 2008;33(9):1659–68.
144. Lutz M, Arora R, Kammerlander C, Gabl M, Pechlaner S. Stabilization of perilunate and transscaphoid perilunate fracture-dislocations via a combined palmar and dorsal approach. Oper Orthop Traumatol. 2009;21(4–5):442–58.
145. Wilke B, Kakar S. Delayed avascular necrosis and fragmentation of the lunate following perilunate dislocation. Orthopedics. 2015;38(6):e539–42.
146. Minami A, Ogino T, Ohshio I, Minami M. Correlation between clinical results and carpal instabilities in patients after reduction of lunate and perilunar dislocations. J Hand Surg Br Eur. 1986;11(2):213–20.
147. Sauder DJ, Athwal GS, Faber KJ, Roth JH. Perilunate injuries. Orthop Clin North Am. 2007;38(2):279–88, vii.
148. Komurcu M, Kurklu M, Ozturan KE, Mahirogullari M, Basbozkurt M. Early and delayed treatment of dorsal transscaphoid perilunate fracture-dislocations. J Orthop Trauma. 2008;22(8):535–40.
149. Leung YF, Ip SP, Wong A, Ip WY. Transscaphoid transcapitate transtriquetral perilunate fracture-dislocation: a case report. J Hand Surg Am. 2006;31(4):608–10.

Acute Fractures in Sport: Hand

12

Kyle W. Morse and Michelle G. Carlson

12.1 Metacarpal Fractures

Hand injuries are common throughout recreational, amateur and professional sports. These injuries require special consideration and management in the athlete. Bartels et al. [1] reported a total of 725 hand and wrist injuries between 2009 and 2014 in National Collegiate Athletic Association American football players with the majority of injuries occurring during competitive games. Amongst high school athletes, Swenson et al. [2] reported that hand and finger fractures were most commonly reported fracture with an incidence of 28.3% in that population. Hand fractures are especially devastating as it can affect a player's dexterity and performance as nearly all sports require the hands for effective play. This chapter will discuss the relevant epidemiology, classification, diagnosis, treatment, complications, rehabilitation and preventative measures for metacarpal and phalangeal fractures.

12.1.1 Epidemiology

Metacarpal fractures are common in the general population as they comprise 18% of all fractures below the elbow, occur with an incidence rate of 13.6 per 100,000 person-years in the US, and are the most commonly occurring fracture in the young male athlete population, most often occurring between the ages of 10–40 [3–6]. These fractures usually occur in contact sports such as basketball, American football and hockey due to either a fall or a direct impact on the hand by an opposing player, but have also been reported in baseball following a baseball strike to the dorsum of the hand while batting [7]. Nakashian et al. [4] reported metacarpal fractures occurring most commonly during basketball, American football and cycling. Cairns et al. [8] reported that finger metacarpal fractures made up 17% and thumb metacarpal fractures 5.7% of all fractures reported amongst NCAA American football players between 2004 and 2014, and 22.4% and 46.4% respectively required surgery. Amongst National Football League (NFL) players, Mall et al. [9] reported metacarpal fractures were the most common injury to the hand at 17% of all injuries between 1996 and 2005 with a mean loss of 16 days or play. Additionally, fractures about the thumb metacarpal made up 10% of all injuries with Bennett fractures comprising 2% with mean loss of play time of 14 and 30 days respectively. Etier et al. [10] reported on metacarpal fractures in American football players and found that the middle finger was the most frequently reported finger and the metacarpal shaft was the most common location. Morse et al. [11] identified 26 metacarpal fractures that occurred in professional basketball players in the National Basketball Association (NBA) between January 2009 and May 2014 with fracture of the fourth metacarpal being the most commonly fractured.

12.1.2 Classification

The metacarpal bone is comprised of four main sections: the base, shaft, neck, and head and furthermore each metacarpal has unique characteristics that affect both fracture morphology and management. The base provides articulation with the carpus and forms the carpometacarpal joint (CMCJ). Fractures through the metacarpal base can extend proximally to become intra-articular fractures at the CMCJ, which can affect joint stability. The CMCJs of the radial sided fingers are more stable due to soft tissue attachments and the broader bases of the metacarpals. This increase in stability results in reduced range of motion, which is contrasted to the ring and little finger metacarpals, as their CMCJs allow larger degrees of flexion to permit mobility during grip. Due to these differences, more displacement can be tolerated with the two ulnar metacarpals as compensation occurs through the CMCJs [12].

K. W. Morse (✉) · M. G. Carlson (✉)
Hospital for Special Surgery, New York, NY, USA
e-mail: morsek@hss.edu; carlsonm@hss.edu

G. A. J. Robertson, N. Maffulli (eds.), *Fractures in Sport*, https://doi.org/10.1007/978-3-030-72036-0_12

The metacarpal shaft is the diaphyseal section of the bone and represents the second most common location for a metacarpal fracture. The index metacarpal is the longest with the widest base while the little finger metacarpal is the shortest [3]. Multiple intrinsic and extrinsic soft tissue structures connect to the metcarpal shaft and provide stability. The index, long, ring, and little finger metacarpals are interconnected by the intermetacarpal ligament and the deep transverse metacarpal ligament distally. The dorsal and palmar interossei provide additional stability. Isolated metacarpal shaft fractures are inherently stable given these soft tissue restraints, especially, in the long and ring metacarpals. The border metacarpals (index and little) have less soft tissue support due to the lack of the deep intermetacarpal ligaments and are therefore more susceptible to shortening, but they are able to tolerate more malrotation because they do not easily impinge on the other fingers [13, 14]. The flexor and extensor tendons originating outside of the hand provide the extrinsic attachments. Following a fracture, these tendinous attachments provide a deforming force to the metacarpal shaft, placing it an apex dorsal angulation due to shortening from the intrinsic muscles [6].

The metacarpal neck is the metadiaphyseal region of the bone and is the most common location for a metacarpal fracture as the volar portion of the metacarpal neck is one of the weakest regions along the bone [3, 5, 6, 14]. A boxer's fracture is a common eponym used to describe the little finger metacarpal neck fracture. This fracture typically results from a punching injury in non-professional boxers, as trained boxers impact the index and middle fingers causing a fracture at the base of the index metacarpal [3, 6, 13].

The metacarpal head is the distal end of the bone that articulates with the proximal phalanx to create the condyloid metacarpophalangeal joint (MCPJ). Metacarpal head fractures are the least common type of metacarpal fracture [5, 6]. The unique osseous structure and ligamentous attachments about the metacarpal head enable a cam mechanism at the MCPJ. The volar surface of the head is wider with a greater radius of curvature than the dorsal surface and additionally, the head is positioned volar to the long axis of the metacarpal shaft [13]. Multiple soft tissue constraints stabilize the MCPJ, most notably the proper collateral ligaments, which originate dorsally on the metacarpal head and span volarly to the proximal phalanx base. Given the oblique trajectory of these ligaments, range of motion is associated with a change of ligament length, with maximum length and tension occurring with MCPJ flexion. The position of maximum stability of the joint is therefore in flexion, which has implications for long term immobilisation—if the MCPJ is mobilized in extension, a contracture can develop [3].

Lastly special consideration is given to the thumb, given its importance to hand function. The thumb provides range of motion in multiple axes compared to the other four metacarpals, provides up to 40% of hand function and the thumb metacarpal is pronated compared to the rest of the hand [15]. Given this large range of motion, a large amount of deformity can be tolerated by thumb fractures distal to the base, however, the lack of interossei muscles leads to instability [3].

Metacarpal fractures are best classified descriptively by location and fracture morphology and are described by the anatomic region for which the fracture occurs—base, shaft, neck and head. They are further described by dorsal or volar angulation. Lastly, the fracture pattern is defined, which can be transverse, spiral, oblique, or comminuted.

12.1.3 Diagnosis

Potential metacarpal fractures can present on the sideline and in the physician's office. Regardless of the treatment setting, a focused history and physical examination of the hand should be performed. The injury should be identified as occurring on the dominant or non-dominant hand. The mechanism of injury as well as the location of the patient's pain should be obtained. For athletes, the history should focus on the player's sport, position, and activity level.

Patients will generally present with edema, ecchymosis, and tenderness to palpation over the affected metacarpal. The skin is inspected and the presence of an open fracture is noted. Examination focuses on crepitus as well as the examination of surrounding fingers. Range of motion of the MCPJ is assessed. The patient is asked to make a fist and the finger cascade is observed to assess for malrotation. The fingers should point towards the scaphoid tubercle and any overlapping digits or malrotation should be noted [3]. Comparison to the contralateral hand may also be useful to fully compare the deformity.

Following history and examination, a standard hand radiograph series is obtained, which includes posteroanterior, oblique, and lateral views of the hand and the fracture is described as detailed above. Portable radiographs are utilized for game day assessments. Computed tomography (CT) scans are useful to better define complex fracture patterns and metacarpal base fractures that have intra-articular extension.

12.1.4 Treatment

Following assessment, an athlete may be able to return to protected play immediately if splinted, depending on their pain, position, and requirements for hand use. The affected metacarpal can be splinted with a hand-based splint or club cast. Some splints may be worn under a glove.

Following acute treatment or after evaluation in the clinical setting, an athlete with a metacarpal fracture is splinted in either a volar gutter or ulnar gutter splint depending on the location of the fracture in the intrinsic plus position, with the wrist held in slight extension of 30°, with the injured finger and adjacent digit placed in 45° of flexion at the MCPJ, with both the proximal interphalangeal joints (PIPJs) and the distal interphalangeal joints (DIPJs) free. As described in the previous section, splinting in this position relaxes the intrinsic muscles and prevents proper collateral ligament contracture. There is no need to include the PIPJs as it will just cause them to become stiff.

Goals of treatment are to provide a stable environment for fracture healing, an anatomic reduction to prevent permanent deformity and restore proper hand function, and allow an athlete to return to play at their pre-injury level without lasting consequences later in life. Operative or non-operative treatment and timing depends on a number of factors, both patient-specific and fracture-specific. Patient-specific factors include the athlete's sport, position, and necessary hand use for their given sport and position. In addition, the athletic level of performance and professional demands must be taken into consideration. Fracture-specific factors include location along the metacarpal, pattern, amount of displacement and angulation, malrotation, and intra-articular extension with involvement of an adjacent joint.

12.1.5 Metacarpal Base Fractures

Anatomic reduction should be attained when treating metacarpal base fractures to prevent CMCJ incongruity. CMCJ stability must be assessed to determine the best treatment course [5]. Due to the increased range of motion about the ring and little finger CMCJs, fractures with intra-articular extension are more common about these fingers. Fractures about the ulnar base of the little finger are commonly referred to as baby or reverse Bennett fractures [3, 6]. The volar-radial fragment of the reverse Bennett fracture is held in place by the ring metacarpal's deep transverse carpal ligament while the little finger metacarpal shaft is displaced proximally, dorsally, and ulnarly due to the extensor carpi ulnaris and the hypothenar musculature [3, 6, 15].

Fracture patterns with stable CMCJs can undergo non-operative management with splinting. Non-surgical management can be attempted for non-displaced reverse Bennett fractures with the wrist splinted in 30° of extension to reduce the deforming force from the extensor carpi ulnaris, but this situation is rare [6, 12].

Unstable metacarpal base fractures should undergo surgical management and reverse Bennett fractures usually require closed reduction and percutaneous pinning, and occasionally open reduction. Multiple constructs can be utilized for their treatment to include crossed k-wire fixation and low-profile plates that cross the CMCJ. When surgically repairing ring and little finger metacarpal base fractures, care must be taken to visualize and protect the dorsal ulnar sensory nerve [5, 6]. For reverse Bennett fractures, the extensor carpi ulnaris is retracted to expose the joint capsule and either k-wires or 1.0–1.5 mm screws can be utilized for fixation (Fig. 12.1) [6]. If a plate and screw type construct is chosen, intra-articular penetration from the screws must be avoided and this is confirmed utilizing intra-operative fluoroscopy [5]. Highly comminuted fractures may be more amenable to k-wire fixation that can cross both the CMCJ and adjacent metacarpals (Fig. 12.2). When CMCJ instability is present or there was a CMCJ dislocation, the joint is reduced and stabilized [5]. The post-surgical splint following a CMCJ injury includes a splint

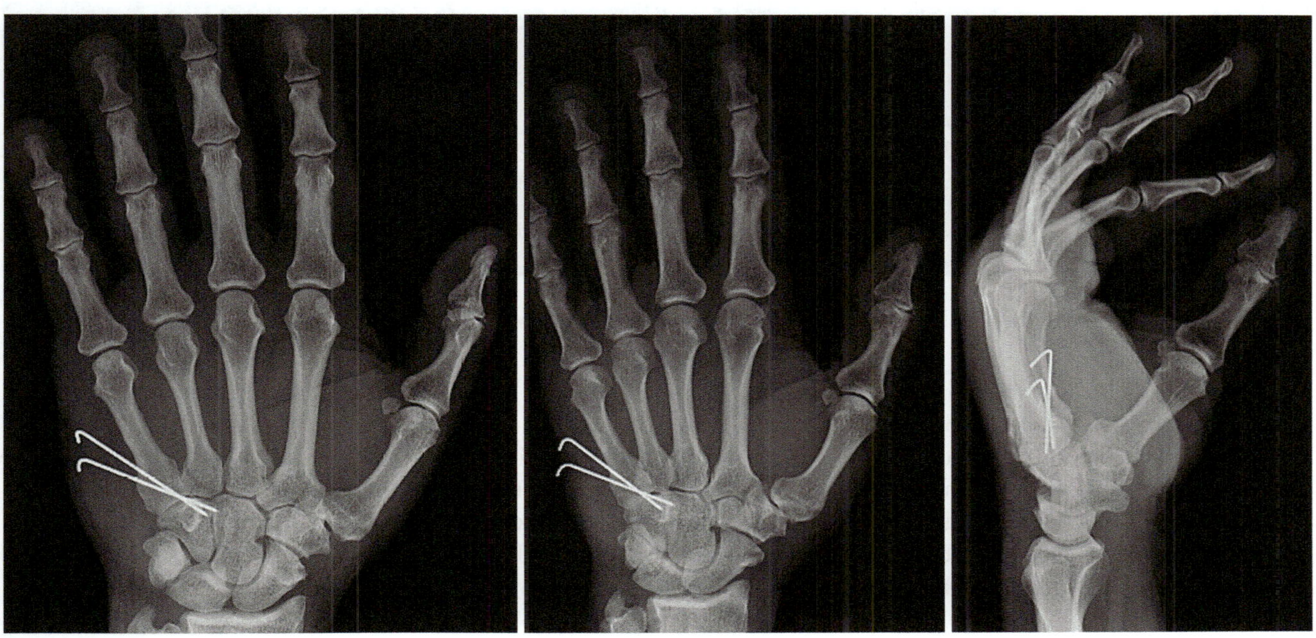

Fig. 12.1 Reverse Bennett Fracture treated with k-wire fixation

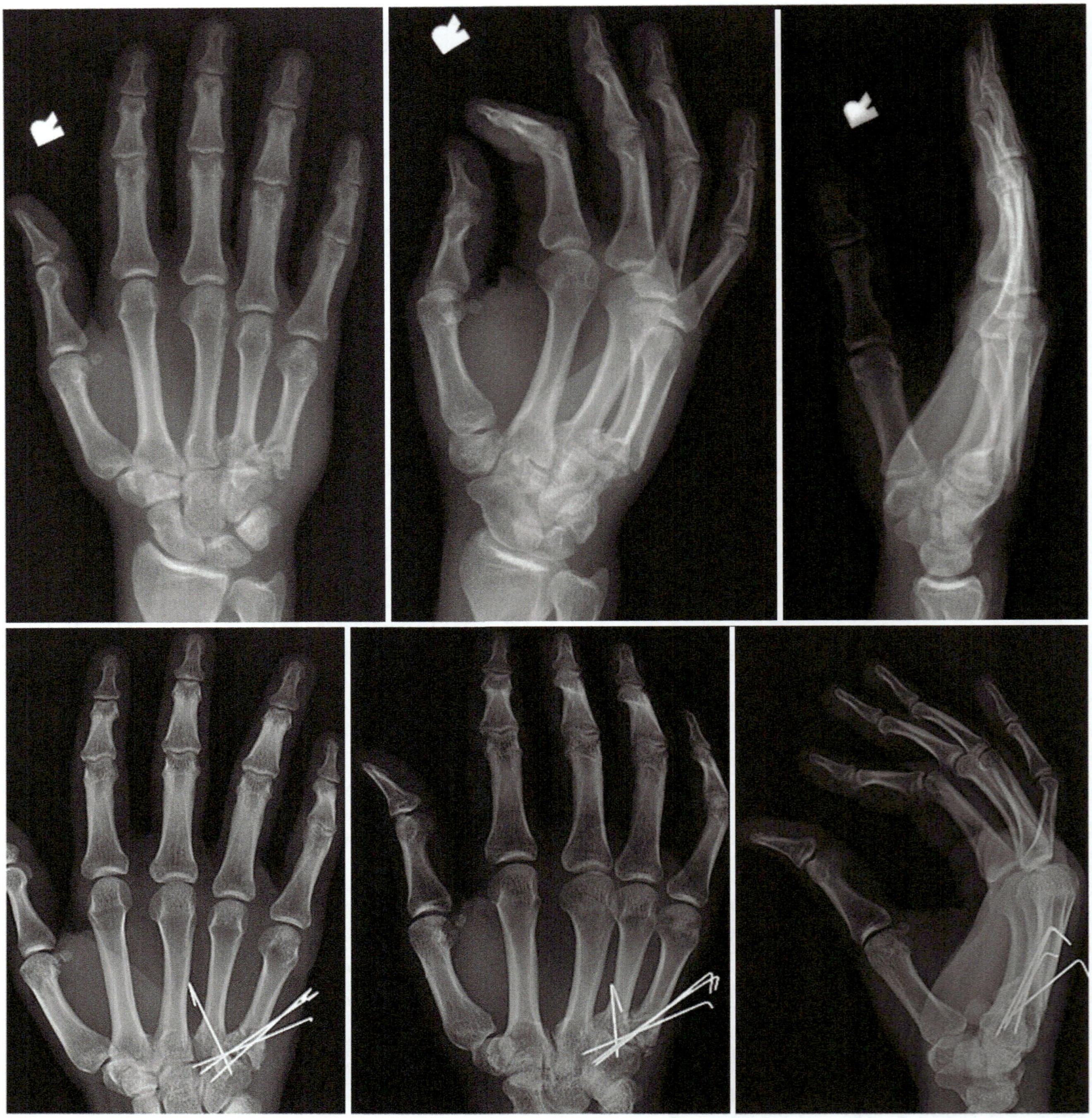

Fig. 12.2 Comminuted fractures of the ring and little finger metacarpal bases treated with crossed k-wire fixation

that spans the MCPJ and the wrist. A digit is included on either side of the affected metacarpal. For CMCJ fracture dislocations, pins are usually left in for six weeks to ensure that the joint will be stable with pin removal.

Athletes that have persistent pain following non-operative or operative management can elect to undergo CMCJ fusion, which may improve their pain at the cost of decreased range of motion. As there is very little motion in the CMCJs, arthrodesis usually does not lead to significant loss of function, especially since secondary post-traumatic degenerative changes often result in joint stiffness without further treatment. Of course, any hand surgery can affect sports performance and serious consideration and counseling should occur before proceeding with this treatment [5].

12.1.6 Metacarpal Shaft Fractures

Metacarpal shaft fractures present with a characteristic apex dorsal angulation due to intrinsic muscle shortening. Most metacarpal shaft fractures can be treated non-operatively due to the stabilizing effects of the deep transverse metacarpal ligaments and transverse metacarpal ligaments. To note, however, the index and little finger metacarpals are not stabilized by these ligaments.

Despite these stabilizing attachments, accurately assessing the amount of angulation and malrotation is paramount when treating metacarpal shaft fractures as it varies across the metacarpals. Typically accepted degrees of angulation include 10° at the index finger, 20° for the middle finger and 30° in the ring and little fingers respectively [5, 13]. The amount of acceptable angulation however for the treatment of a high-performance athlete is often less at 10° of dorsal angulation across all metacarpals as residual deformity can severely affect player performance (Table 12.1) [6].

Malrotation can also result in severe deformity and have a profound impact on hand function as 10° of malrotation can lead to a 2 cm overlap with an adjacent finger [5, 16]. In addition to angulation and malrotation, other authors have noted that excessive shortening should not be tolerated and can lead to a severe extensor lag and loss of intrinsic muscle power [17, 18]. Fractures of two adjacent metacarpals may be at a greater risk of shortening due to loss of stabilization from the interconnecting intermetacarpal ligament. In a cadaveric model of index and little finger short oblique fracture patterns, Strauch et al. [18] found a maximum shortening of 5 mm and postulated that the deep transverse intermetacarpal ligament and interosseous muscles prevented further shortening. The authors also report that for every 2 mm of shortening, 7° of extensor lag was created, but concluded that due to the ability of the MCPJ to hyperextend, the shortening and subsequent extensor lag can be compensated and allow the MCPJ to extend to neutral [18].

Operative indications for metacarpal shaft fractures in the athlete include open fractures, dorsal angulation greater than 10°, any malrotation, palpable dorsal fracture spike placing the skin at risk and spiral oblique fractures. Metacarpal shaft fractures that are stable and do not meet the above criteria can be treated non-operatively in a radial gutter or ulnar gutter splint in the intrinsic plus position with the wrist in 30° of extension, the MCPJ between 45° of flexion and the IPJs free. The splint is maintained until there is evidence of clinical healing and radiographic union [6].

Several operative techniques have been described to treat metacarpal shaft fractures, which focuses on stability for a given fracture pattern. These fractures typically require open reduction and internal fixation to aim for anatomic reduction under direct visualization and closed reduction is not routinely used. The metacarpal is approached dorsally utilizing a longitudinal incision centered on the fracture. The extensor tendon is then identified and carefully retracted and protected throughout the procedure either radially or ulnarly depending on the direction that allows direct access to the fracture. Periosteal flaps are then elevated off the fracture and subsequently repaired following fixation, to cover the construct and protect the extensor tendon.

Multiple fixation constructs have been proposed depending on the fracture pattern. Crossed k-wire fixation is not routinely utilized given the difficulty of insertion, inadequate stability, and potential for tendon irritation [5, 6]. For transverse fractures, intramedullary k-wires can be used but this is a less stable construct and does not control rotation [5]. Oblique and spiral fractures can be treated with interfragmentary lag screws, an intramedullary compression screw, and low-profile plate and screw constructs, or a combination depending on the length of the fracture. 2.0 or 2.5 mm interfragmentary screws offer a stable construct for long spiral oblique fractures that are three times the diameter length [6]. A spanning plate with 2.5 mm screws proximal and distal to the fracture will increase the immediate strength of the construct and allow for earlier return to play (Fig. 12.3). Short oblique fractures may be better suited to an intramedullary compression screw, which are inserted retrograde through the MCPJ (Fig. 12.4). Care is taken to protect the extensor mechanism and the joint capsule should be repaired with non-absorbable suture for closure. Berg et al. [19] found minimal subchondral and sagittal plane intrusion for headless intramedullary screws and del Pinal et al. [20] reported that all patients returned to work or sporting activities at an average of 76 days but recommended the use of plate and screw constructs for comminuted fracture patterns. Ozer et al. [21] reported similar post-surgical functional outcome measures for patients treated with a 1.6 mm intramedullary nail compared to plate and screw constructs. While the functional outcomes were similar, there was a greater loss of reduction (13%), a higher penetration of the MCPJ (15%), and tendon irritation requiring hardware removal (39%) in the intramedullary nail group [21]. 1.5–2.0 mm plate and screw constructs can be utilized in neutralization fashion to add stability when required for comminuted fractures or for short oblique fractures, but are prone to tendon irritation and scarring and should be avoided unless necessary [5, 6].

Table 12.1 Acceptable degrees of dorsal angulation between athletes and non-athletes for metacarpal shaft and neck fractures

	Metacarpal shaft fractures		Metacarpal neck fractures	
	Non-athlete (°)	Athlete (°)	Non-athlete (°)	Athlete (°)
Index	10	10	10	5
Middle	20	10	20	10
Ring	30	10	30–70	25–30
Little	30	10	40–70	40–45

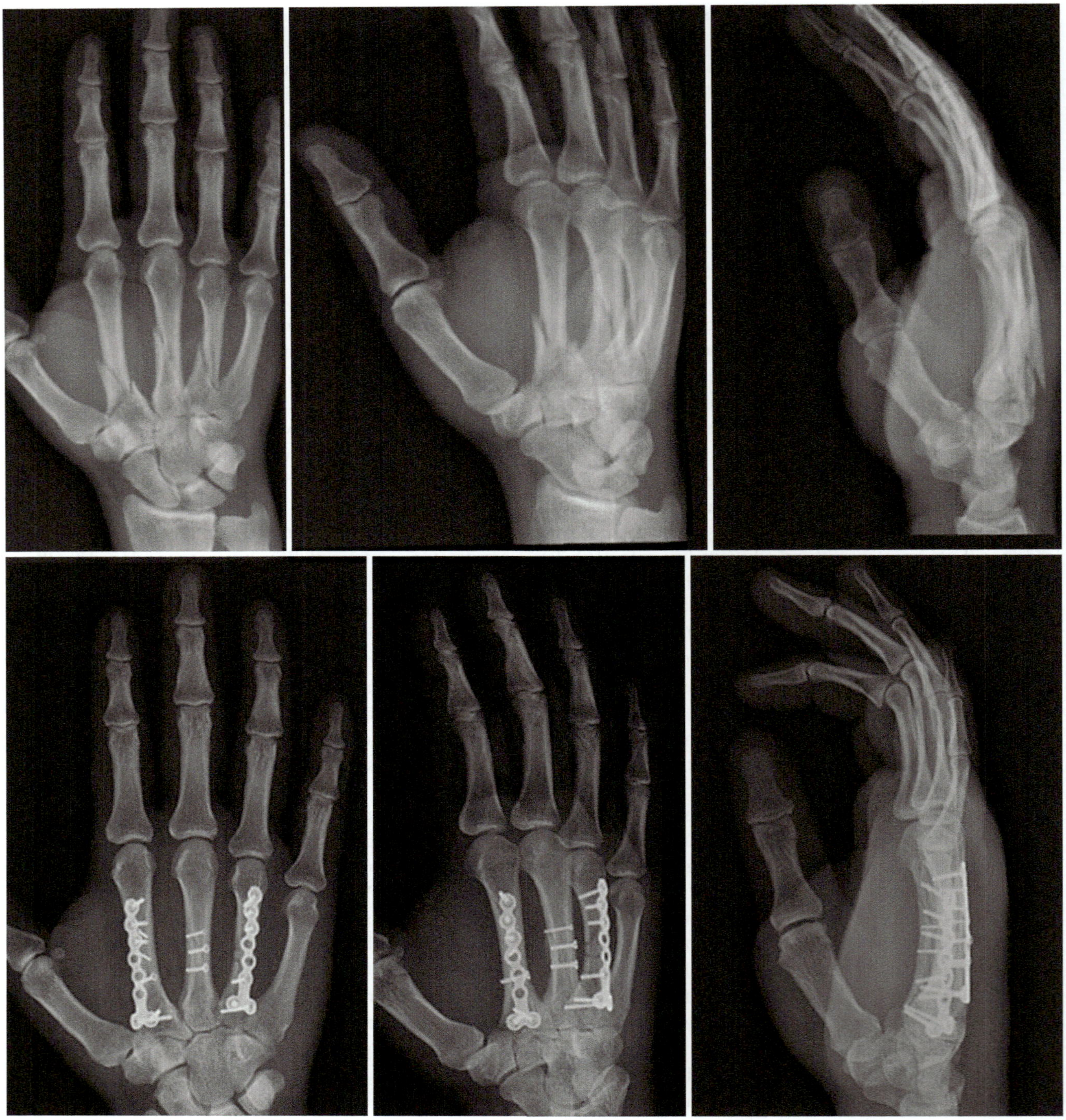

Fig. 12.3 Oblique fractures of the index, middle and ringer metacarpal shafts treated with open reduction and internal fixation utilizing both plate and screw constructs and lag screw technique

Following surgery, athletes are placed into a clamshell splint for post-operative protection and begin immediate range of motion the day after surgery. Depending on construct stability, and ability to wear protective equipment, return to play is between several days and 4 weeks.

12.1.7 Metacarpal Neck Fractures

Metacarpal neck fractures represent the most frequent location of metacarpal fractures and commonly occur in the ulnar fingers [6]. As the intrinsic muscles lay volar to the axis of rota-

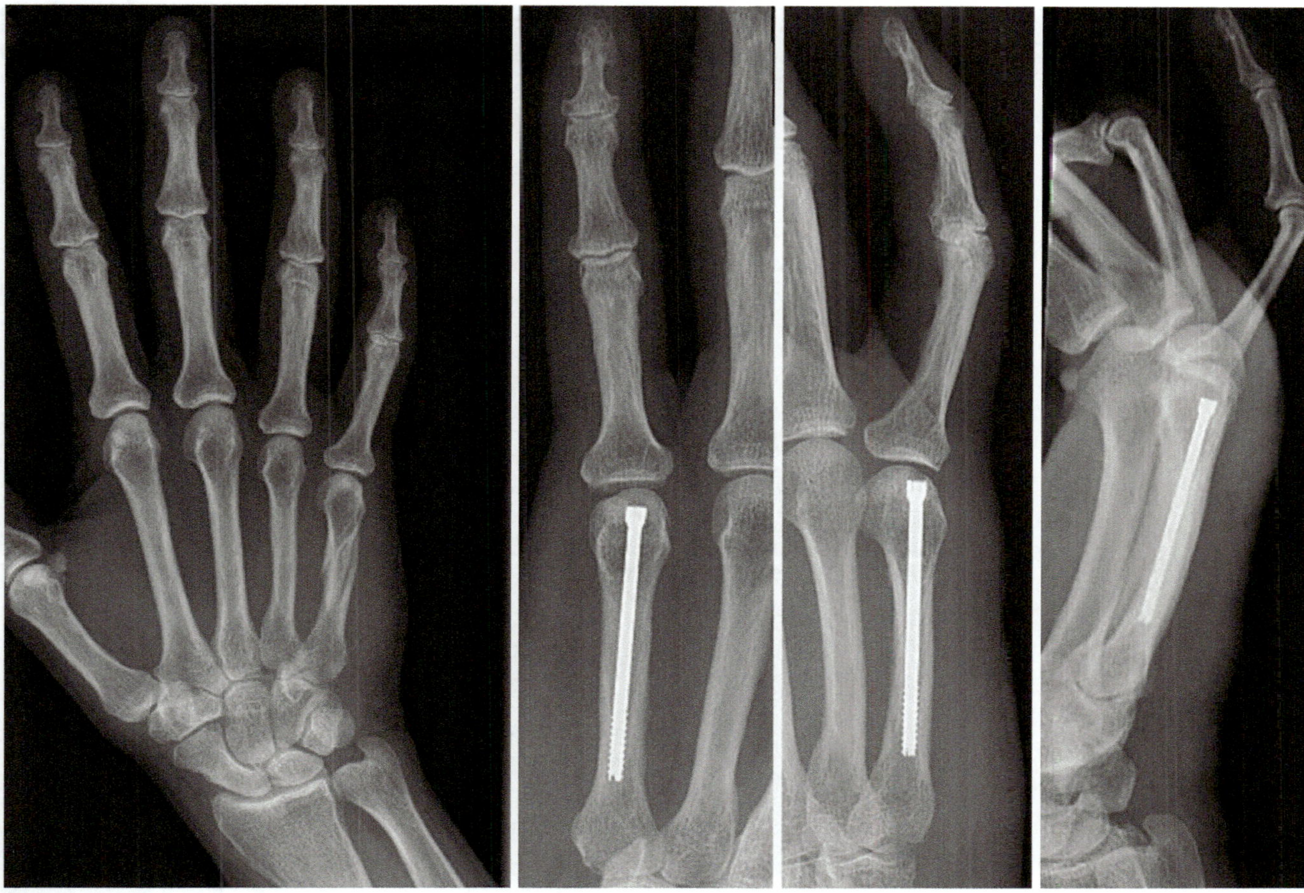

Fig. 12.4 Short oblique fracture of the little finger metacarpal shaft treated with an intramedullary screw

tion of the metacarpal, their shortening results in the characteristic apex dorsal deformity. In addition, pseudoclawing may result from intrinsic and extrinsic muscle imbalance. This deformity is characterized by MCPJ hyperextension with PIPJ flexion, with an inability to fully extend the PIPJ [6].

Proper management depends on the amount of angulation and rotational deformity present. Similar to metacarpal shaft fractures, the amount of angulation that can be tolerated increases ulnarly across the hand due to increased CMCJ mobility in the ring and little fingers [22]. Multiple degrees of angulation have been cited as acceptable. Commonly used values included 10° degrees for the index finger, 20° in the middle finger, 30° in the ring finger and 40° in the little finger [5, 13]. Some studies advocate as high as 70° in the ring and little fingers, but these guidelines may not be applicable for high performing athletes who depend on their ulnar fingers for grasp and grip strength [5, 6, 23]. Ball and racquet sport athletes such as baseball players and tennis players may suffer significant performance deficits if this amount of rotational deformity remains uncorrected. Similarly, a basketball player may have difficulty dribbling, if the metacarpal head remains prominent in their palm [7, 13]. For high performance athletes, surgical management is generally indicated for dorsal angulation of 5° in the index finger, 10° in the middle finger, 25–30° in the ring finger and 40–45° in the little finger (Table 12.1) [6]. Fractures that have rotational deformity should also be treated operatively to correct finger overlap.

Fractures that do not meet the above criteria can be treated non-operatively. The Jahss maneuver was historically described for reduction of acute dorsally angulated neck and shaft fractures. The fracture is reduced by applying counterpressure on the fracture and flexing the MCPJ to 90°, while simultaneously applying a dorsal force through the joint [5, 6]. This maneuver has fallen out of recent favor and is not commonly performed for the treatment of non-operative fractures [6]. For non-operatively treated fractures, patients are placed in either a radial or ulnar gutter splint, which is maintained until clinical and radiographic evidence of healing. In baseball players, Goldfarb advocates for a cuff splint to protect the long, ring and little fingers while allowing finger range of motion [7].

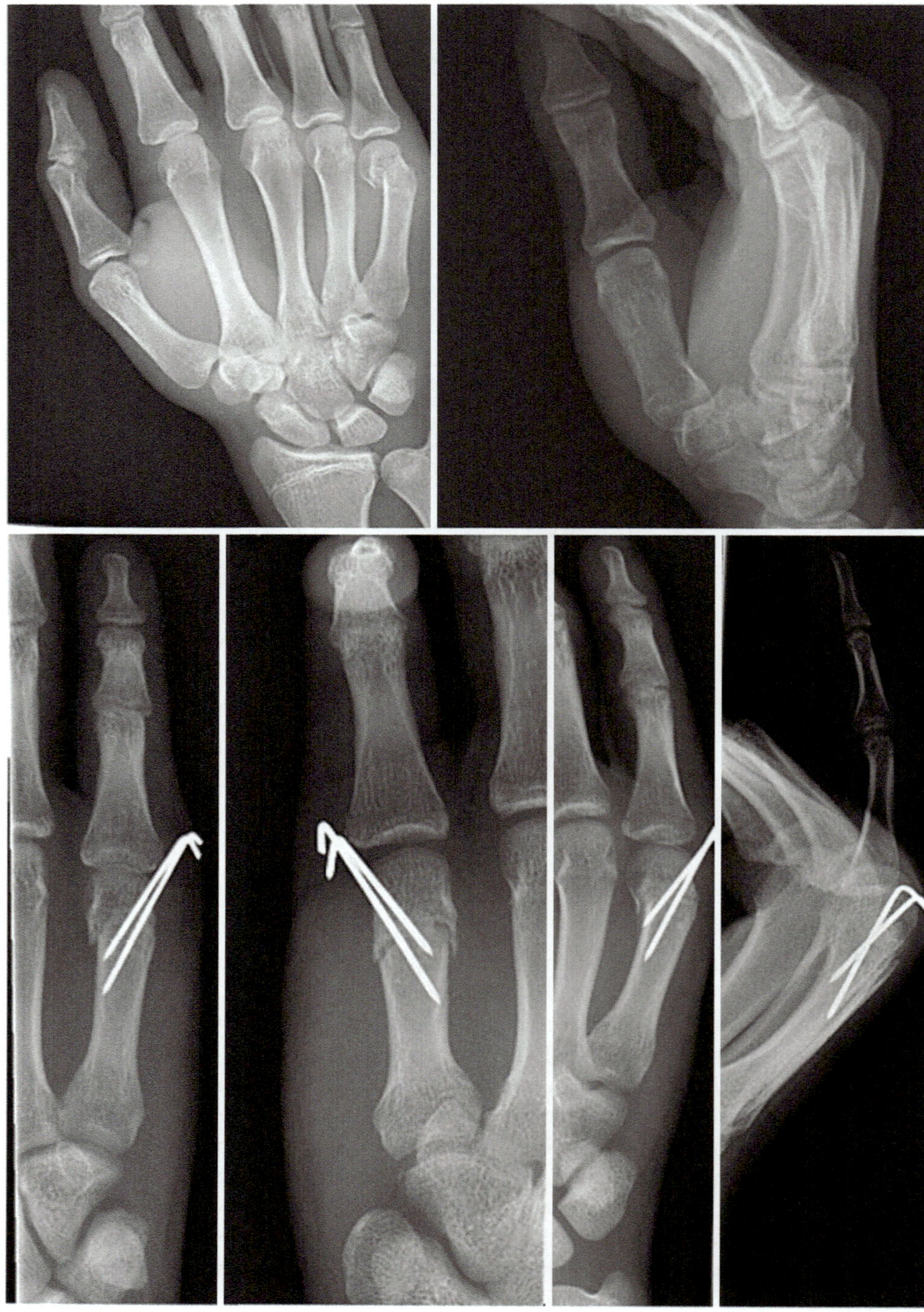

Fig. 12.5 Metacarpal neck fracture treated with crossed k-wire fixation

Multiple fixation techniques and constructs can be utilized for fractures that require operative intervention. Closed reduction and percutaneous pinning utilizing the Jahss maneuver followed by placing 1.1–1.6 mm k-wires in a crossed or intramedullary fashion has been described (Fig. 12.5). Placing intramedullary wires can be accomplished either anterograde or retrograde. When passing the wires antegrade, the starting point is the ulnar aspect of the metacarpal base, while the collateral recess can be utilized to place them retrograde [5]. The intramedullary k-wires can be buried to allow for earlier return to play. More preferably, an intramedullary screw can be utilized, which provides a more biomechanically stable construct to avoid pin breakage and pin site infection (Fig. 12.6). Open reduction is required when closed reduction results in unacceptable fracture reduction. This gives the most biomechanically stable construct.

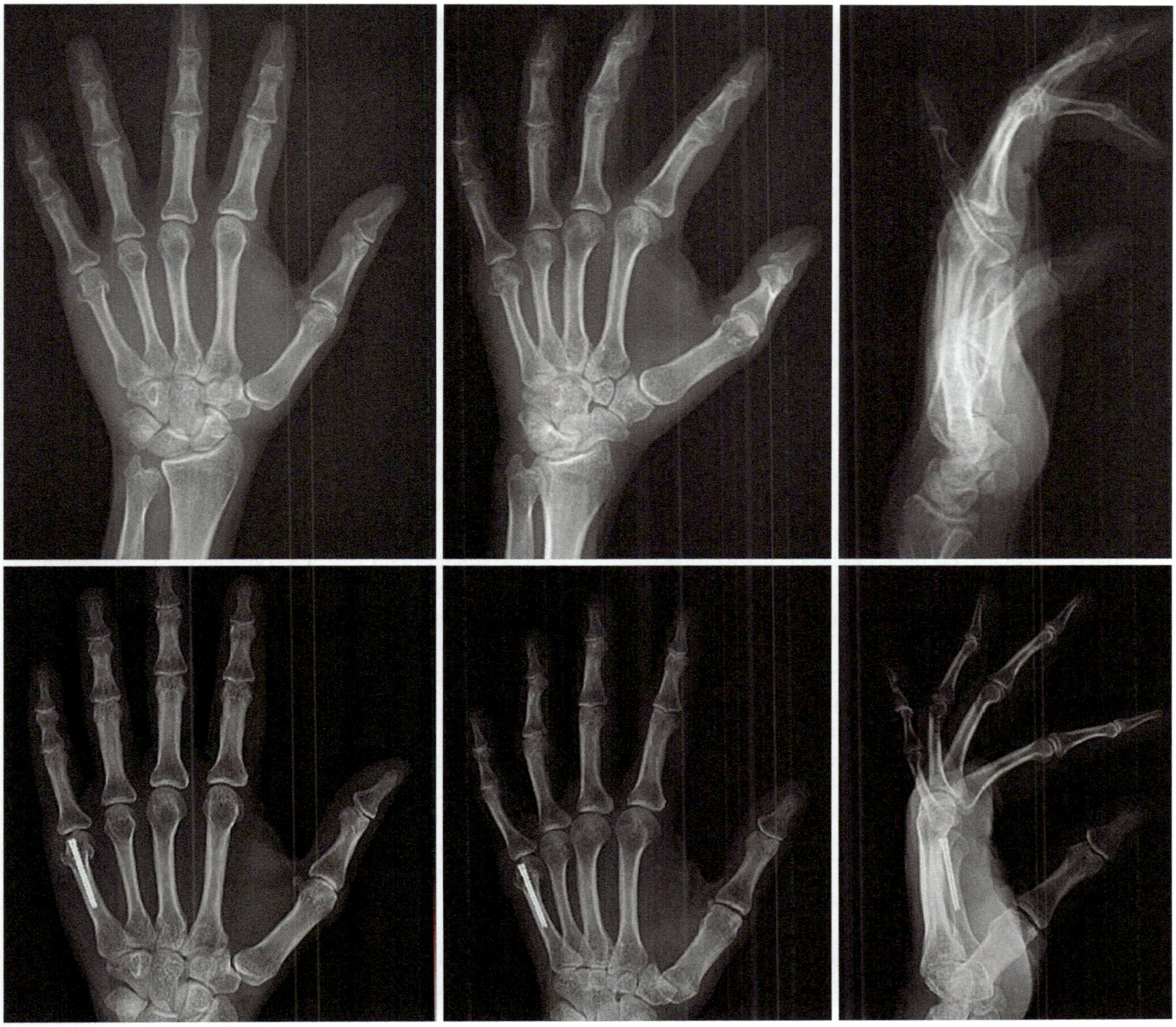

Fig. 12.6 Metacarpal neck fracture treated with retrograde intramedullary screw fixation

Plating fractures in this location is challenging, given the proximity of the collateral ligaments, the joint capsule, and the extensor tendon. A low profile T plate can be selected, to avoid interference with these structures [5, 6]. Fujitani et al. [24] retrospectively compared intramedullary k-wire fixation with two 1.2 mm k-wires with plate and screw constructs and reported that the post-operative finger range of motion was greater in the intramedullary group but post-operative grip strength was greater for those patients treated with plate and screw constructs. Following operative management, immediate motion is undertaken focusing on the PIPJs and MCPJs to reduce post-operative stiffness.

12.1.8 Metacarpal Head Fractures

Metacarpal head fractures often have intra-articular extension and proper reduction of the metacarpal head is often necessary to prevent MCPJ incongruity. Therefore, most metacarpal head fractures require operative management given the small amount of rotational deformity that can be tolerated at this joint. In addition, comminution and ligamentous avulsions of the collateral ligaments must be taken into consideration. Non-operative management may be indicated for extra-articular collateral ligament avulsion fractures with clinical evidence of MCPJ stability.

For non-operative management, a radial or ulnar gutter splint is applied with the wrist in 30° of extension, the MCPJs in 45° of flexion, with the IPJs free. The splint is maintained until there is clinical evidence of healing and radiographic evidence of fracture union.

The aim of operative management for metacarpal head fractures is to provide stable internal fixation, restore MCPJ congruity, and enable early range of motion. The recommended approach depends on the fractured finger. For the index and little fingers, a dorsal approach to the MCPJ with a longitudinal midline division of the extensor mechanism is performed to preserve the sagittal band attachments. A longitudinal capsulotomy is then performed to the access the MCPJ. For the middle and ring fingers, the ulnar sagittal band is incised to allow dissection of the MCPJ capsule [6].

The fixation construct depends on the fracture morphology and amount of comminution. Headless compression screws, 1.0–1.5 mm countersunk cortical screws and bioabsorbable screws have all been described for fixation [5, 6]. Patients with excessive comminution carry a poor prognosis with a high likelihood for joint instability and development of post traumatic arthritis [5]. Internal fixation is still preferred for severely comminuted fractures in the athlete given the negative impact that other fixation methods carry. The use of external fixation, MCPJ arthroplasty and MCPJ fusion have been advocated, but would severely limit and negatively impact a player's return to play, performance, and career.

12.1.9 Thumb Metacarpal Fractures

The thumb can tolerate a large degree of angular deformity given the considerable range of motion at the thumb CMCJ. Thumb webspace narrowing and MCPJ hyperextension may occur with dorsal angulation exceeding 30° and operative intervention is recommended [5, 15]. Similar fixation methods for the lesser digits are utilized for thumb metacarpal head, neck, and shaft fractures. These are less common than base fractures, due to force transmission to the base, secondary to a lack of stabilizing forces about the metacarpal [15]. Reduction can be performed by applying direct pressure on the base of the thumb with concurrent application of pressure over the fracture and axial traction, extension, and pronation [15]. A thumb spica splint or cast is used during non-operative management. For fractures requiring operative management, a dorsal approach can be utilized between the intramuscular interval of the extensor pollicis longus and the extensor pollicis brevis. Similar to fractures of the lesser digits, multiple constructs to include k-wires and 1.5–2.5 mm screws and plates can be utilized [5].

12.1.10 Thumb Metacarpal Base Fractures

Fractures about the base of the thumb pose a special challenge given the thumb's importance to hand function. Malreduction can result in the development of arthritis, pain, decreased motion, and reduced grip strength, and the restoration of these is paramount in the athlete.

Two types of intra-articular fractures have been described at the base of the thumb: The Bennett Fracture and the Rolando Fracture [5, 6, 15]. The Bennett fracture is an intra-articular fracture through the base of the thumb that consists of two parts: a constant volar-ulnar fragment and the remaining metacarpal shaft. The volar-ulnar joint fragment is stabilized by the volar oblique ligament while the remaining metacarpal shaft is displaced dorsally, radially, and proximally by the abductor pollicis longus, adductor pollicis, and extensor pollicis brevis respectively [6, 15].

Rolando fractures now generally refer to all comminuted intra-articular fractures about the thumb metacarpal base but were originally described at T-Type and Y-Type fractures in which there was both a volar ulnar fragment and a dorsal-radial fragment [5, 6, 13, 15].

Non-displaced Bennett fractures may be treated in a thumb spica cast followed by protected play splinting for 4–6 weeks [25]. If return to play is attempted the athlete should be followed weekly with repeat radiographs to assess for likely displacement. Often prophylactic pinning of the CMCJ is warranted to prevent displacement. Displaced Bennett and Rolando fractures require surgical intervention as the deforming forces about the thumb hold the fracture fragments in an unacceptable position. Bennett fractures can typically be treated by closed reduction and percutaneous pinning. Reduction is accomplished by the application of axial traction, abduction, and pronation while simultaneously applying force over the metacarpal base [15]. Two 1.1–1.6 mm k-wires are then introduced into the trapezium and/or index finger and the other into the volar-ulnar fragment [5, 6]. If a residual 2 mm articular stepoff remains of a large fragment after attempted closed reduction, open reduction is performed utilizing the Wagner approach with 1.0–1.5 mm screw fixation. The Wagner approach involves an incision along the glabrous portion of the thumb, extra-periosteal elevation of the thenar muscles and a capsulotomy [6, 15]. Following fixation and closure, a thumb spica is applied until evidence of clinical healing and radiographic union [6].

Surgical management of Rolando fractures is similar to Bennett fractures, however, the amount of comminution makes the outcome less predictable [5, 15]. A Wagner approach is again used and screw fixation is utilized. The outcome of these fractures is more variable and supplementary methods such as bone grafting metaphyseal voids, external fixation and arthrodesis may be required. However, this should be a method of last resort in the athlete, as it will increase time to return to play, and impede athletic performance [5, 6].

12.1.11 Complications

Complications following metacarpal fractures include non-union, malunion, infection, and post-operative stiffness. Fusetti et al. [26] reported a 35% total complication rate in their treatment of metacarpal fractures with 15% related to fracture healing, 10% to stiffness, and 8% to plate loosening or breakage [6]. Malunion may result in dorsal angulation, shortening, and malrotation. Most commonly, the angular deformity is dorsal, which can secondarily result in MCPJ hyperextension and PIPJ flexion [6]. For non-operatively treated metacarpal head and neck fractures, athletes may be sensitive to apex dorsal angulation as the metacarpal head will be prominent in the palm and patients should be adequately counseled appropriately before being treated non-operatively. For the treatment of mal-union, open reduction with internal fixation and concurrent dorsal wedge osteotomy can be used to correct the deformity. Malrotation can also cause significant performance effects as 1° of malrotation can produce 5° of malrotation at the fingertips [6, 16]. An osteotomy through the base of the metacarpal can be used to correct malrotation deformity up to 25° [6, 27].

Pin-site infection may also occur. Infections are treated with pin removal, irrigation and debridement, deep hardware removal and the use of either oral or intravenous antibiotics. Stiffness is an unwanted complication as it can affect performance in the athletic population. Early range of motion should be emphasized as soon as fracture stability is achieved. In addition, plate fixation should be avoided when possible to reduce the potential for scarring and tendon adhesion [6].

Intra-articular fractures at the metacarpal base carries a higher complication rate with persistence of pain in approximately 40% [5, 12]. Improperly reduced thumb metacarpal base fractures can result in instability, which may have to be managed with arthrodesis.

12.1.12 Rehabilitation

Attainting fracture stability is paramount to begin rehabilitation and decrease post-operative stiffness from extensor tendon adhesion and scarring. Dressings are typically removed 2–3 days following surgery and patients are placed into a removable thermoplastic splint. At this time, finger range of motion is begun with formal hand therapy while post-operative swelling is controlled with ice and elevation. Sutures are removed 2 weeks following surgery. Hand therapy for range of motion is continued throughout this time until 3–4 weeks post-operatively, at which time strengthening is begun to improve grip strength. The thermoplastic splint can be removed when there is clinical evidence of healing and radiographic union, usually at 3–4 weeks. For surgically-managed Bennett fractures, range of motion can begin 7–10 days following plate and screw fixation, and 4 weeks following k-wire fixation. K-wires should be removed 4–6 weeks post-operatively, as long as there is evidence of clinical and radiographic healing [25].

Return to play is dependent on player position, sport, athletic participation, fracture pattern, and fracture stability. A professional athlete may have increased incentive for a quicker return to play compared to a recreational athlete, and appropriate counseling and goals should be established during the treatment course. The player's pain level, ability to adequately perform, and ability to protect themselves without risking worsening of the injury or additional injury need to be assessed [28]. In professional basketball players, Morse et al. [11] reported an average of 26 days between injury and return to play for non-operatively managed fractures, while operatively managed fractures returned at an average of 57 days. Therefore, surgical management may not always result in a quicker return to play, likely due to more severe fracture patterns [11]. Guss et al. [29] reported no significant differences in reported performance metrics between operative and non-operative management for NBA players who sustained a metacarpal fracture. They also found no difference in outcome between shooting versus non-shooting hand injuries, as well as no decline in post-injury performance, compared to matched controls. The authors concluded that these players can return to their pre-injury level of performance. Etier et al. [10] reported on the return to play for 20 metacarpal fractures in high school, NCAA and recreational American football players. Twelve of these athletes required surgery. The authors reported a mean return to protected play of 16.9 days, with in-season athletes having a mean return to play of 6.3 days.

For fractures treated non-operatively, a player may remain casted for up to 3–4 weeks, with range of motion exercises beginning following cast removal [25]. The player usually can return to sport at two weeks, if they can play protected in the cast. For these athletes, their fractured hand should not be required for their sport specific activities, such as: gripping a bat, racquet or club; or throwing, striking or catching a ball, as in baseball or volleyball. Players may also have a splint that is worn during athletic activities, and another for use outside of sporting activities, as additional foam padding may be required for in-game activities, to protect the player and opposing athletes [30]. Some athletes may be able to wear a splint or brace inside their gloves [7]. Bracing is continued for four to six weeks. For fractures treated operatively, most athletes return after 4–6 weeks, when they have regained their range of motion and grip strength. Fractures that were operatively managed with k-wire fixation should wait until the k-wires have been removed prior to returning to sport. This allows them to return at a higher performance level.

12.1.13 Preventative Measures

Few measures have been reported in the literature with regards to prevention as a unique balance exists between dexterity and player protection. In some cases, protective gloves and taping can be utilized to prevent injury to the hands. Technique modification to included maintaining the hands closed during blocking can also be focused upon.

12.2 Phalangeal Fractures

12.2.1 Epidemiology

Phalangeal fractures are common in athletes. Morse et al. [11] reported 33 phalangeal fractures in the NBA between January 2009 to May 2014, 13 of which required surgical treatment. In college American football players, Cairns et al. [8] reported 83 finger phalangeal fractures and 30 thumb phalangeal fractures in NCAA American football players between 2004 and 2014, making up 5.7% and 3.0% of all fractures in this population respectively. In addition, they reported that 46.4% and 43.3% of these injuries required surgery [8]. In NFL players, Mall et al. [9] reported finger fractures as the third most common fracture about the hand accounting for 14% of all hand injuries, with a mean loss of play of 10 days.

12.2.2 Classification

Similar to the metacarpal, the phalanges consist of a base, shaft, neck, and head. The proximal phalanx base articulates with the metacarpal head to form the MCPJ. The bases of the middle and distal phalanges form the PIPJ and DIPJ with the heads of the proximal and middle phalanges respectively. The heads of the proximal and middle phalanx contain two condyles separated by an intercondylar notch to provide additional stability [3]. The distal phalanx is covered by the nail plate. The collateral ligaments maintain uniform tension throughout range of motion and therefore can remain in extension during immobilisation without risk of contracture [3].

The soft tissue attachments surrounding the phalanges apply deforming forces and result in various fracture orientations. Phalangeal fractures adopt several typical fracture patterns. A characteristic apex volar angulation is typically adopted in proximal phalanx shaft fractures as the lumbricals and interossei flex the proximal phalanx base while the central slip inserting onto the dorsal base of the middle phalanx pulls the distal fragment into extension. Middle phalanx fractures do not display a consistent fracture pattern, as the terminal slips of the flexor digitorum superficialis insert into the volar base of the middle phalanx and can act as a balancing force to the extensor mechanism [3]: however, these fractures often displace apex volarly. Similarly, in distal phalanx fractures, balanced forces typically result in minimal deformity, as the extensor mechanism inserts dorsally at the base, while the flexor digitorum profundus inserts volarly [3].

Phalangeal fractures are classified based upon the location of the fracture and both its pattern and displacement. The mechanism of injury is often indicative of the resulting fracture pattern: spiral and oblique fractures occur with torsion, resulting in angular deformities; transverse patterns occur with direct impact such as a fall onto a closed fist [3]. London described three types of phalangeal fractures that involve the condyles, with Type I being nondisplaced and stable, Type II as unstable and Type III as being either bicondylar or comminuted [14, 31]. Furthermore, PIPJ fracture-dislocations are described as dorsal lip or volar lip and will be described below.

12.2.3 Diagnosis

A history and focused hand exam is performed when evaluating potential phalangeal fractures. The athlete's sport, position, time of season, and activity level are assessed as these factors can help dictate management. For instance, a phalangeal fracture in the non-dominant hand may be treated differently from a similar fracture in the throwing hand of a quarterback or baseball player [32]. The mechanism of injury is sought as it can elucidate common fracture patterns such as a jersey finger or mallet finger. A focused hand exam is performed. The skin integrity is evaluated for the possibility of an open fracture, which can also occur at the nail bed in tuft fractures. Edema and ecchymosis are evaluated as well as any obvious deformities. Malrotation of the fingers is assessed. Standard antero-posterior, lateral, and oblique radiographs are obtained and portable fluoroscopy can also be utilized if available at the site of a game. CT scans can also be utilized to better define the fracture morphology and determine the amount of intra-articular extension.

12.2.4 Treatment

Depending on the fracture pattern, the athlete's sport, position, and the requirements of the hand during play, the athlete may return to the game with the injury. Simple fracture patterns can be splinted with an aluminum foam splint or buddy taped to an adjacent finger and may be protected under gloves.

Unstable and intra-articular fracture patterns usually necessitate surgical treatment. General indications include open fractures, intra-articular fractures, those with rotational malalignment, greater than 15° of angulation, and shortening greater than 6 mm [3]. Apex volar angulated shaft fractures that are not properly reduced can lead to both extensor lag and pseudoclawing [3].

As in metacarpal fractures, both patient-specific and fracture-specific factors guide treatment decisions. Goals of surgical treatment are: to provide mechanical stability to enable fracture healing; to restore length, alignment and rotation to decrease deformity; and to restore proper function and allow return to play at the athlete's pre-injury level, without lasting consequences.

12.2.5 Phalangeal Head Fractures

Fractures involving the phalangeal bases and head are typically intra-articular and anatomic reduction of the articular surface should be sought to ensure joint congruency, maximize joint function at the MCPJ, PIPJ and DIPJ, and minimize the potential to develop post-traumatic arthritis [3, 33]. Some fractures may be treated with closed reduction and percutaneous k-wire stabilization. Fractures that can not be anatomically reduced should undergo open reduction to allow for direct visualization (Fig. 12.7). Unicondylar fractures are unstable and require fixation [14]. During open reduction, careful dissection is necessary to preserve the collateral ligament attachments and the vascular supply to prevent the development of avascular necrosis to the condyles [3]. Low profile plate and screw constructs can be utilized as well as k-wires to stabilize the fracture or a combination of both [3, 14]. A cannulated headless compression screw may be used when treating unicondylar or bicondylar fractures as they can be placed entirely within the cortex and prevent irritation from surrounding soft tissues although they are often too large [14].

12.2.6 Phalangeal Base Fractures

For phalangeal base fractures, a dorsal approach may be used to access the fracture. The MCPJ capsule is incised and the joint can be inspected. Some base fractures may have severe comminution and are referred to as pilon-type fractures. An external fixation frame may be applied to these to provide distraction ligamentotaxis and maintain the reduction (Fig. 12.8) [3]. Use of an external fixation frame is cautioned in the athlete however as it can prevent early return to play. Alternatively, a dorsal T-Plate with bone grafting behind fracture fragments can be successful, although often later plate removal is necessary.

12.2.7 Proximal Interphalangeal Joint Dislocations and Fractures

Dislocations and fractures involving the PIPJ are common in athletes and often viewed as minor injuries. However, these can have severe consequences, if improperly diagnosed or treated, as the PIPJ provides 85% of fingertip flexion and up to 110° of flexion [34–37]. The PIPJ is constrained by both bony and soft tissue constraints, and functions as a hinge joint with the bony constraints described above. The volar plate as well as the proper and accessory collateral ligaments provide the soft tissue constraints to the joint, with the volar plate preventing excessive hyperextension [34]. These constraints prevent excessive lateral or rotational motion and given that the PIPJ remains unprotected in most sporting activities, the PIPJ is prone to injury [34, 35]. Often, these injuries are reduced on the sideline: thus, it is important to obtain an accurate history, with physical exam and AP and lateral radiograph views of the PIPJ to facilitate a proper diagnosis [34].

Dorsal dislocations of the PIPJ are more common than lateral or volar dislocations. Dorsal dislocations typically include injury to the volar plate. They may also include a bony avulsion and collateral ligament injury. Lateral dislocations can occur radially or ulnarly and involve injury to the collateral ligament on the side from which the force of injury occurred. Volar dislocations are the rarest form of PIPJ injuries and typically involves an avulsion to the central slip. PIPJ fracture dislocations also occur and are typically described as volar lip, dorsal lip, or pilon type fractures. Pilon-type fractures are described above and occur from excessive axial loading. Volar lip fractures occur most commonly with an accompanying dorsal dislocation due to an axial load on a flexed PIPJ [34].

Management goals for PIPJ fractures are similar to those of phalangeal base and head fractures and should ensure joint congruency and allow early range of motion to decrease stiffness [34]. Treatment of PIPJ fractures depends on the stability of the joint. In addition, the amount of articular surface involvement is considered before proceeding with a given treatment modality. Volar lip fractures are generally considered stable if less than 30% of the articular surface is involved [34]. Fractures that involve 30–50% of the articular surface but maintain reduction with less than or equal to 30° of flexion are classified as tenuous and require constant re-evaluation as these fractures may progress to becoming unstable [34, 36]. Lastly, fractures involving greater than

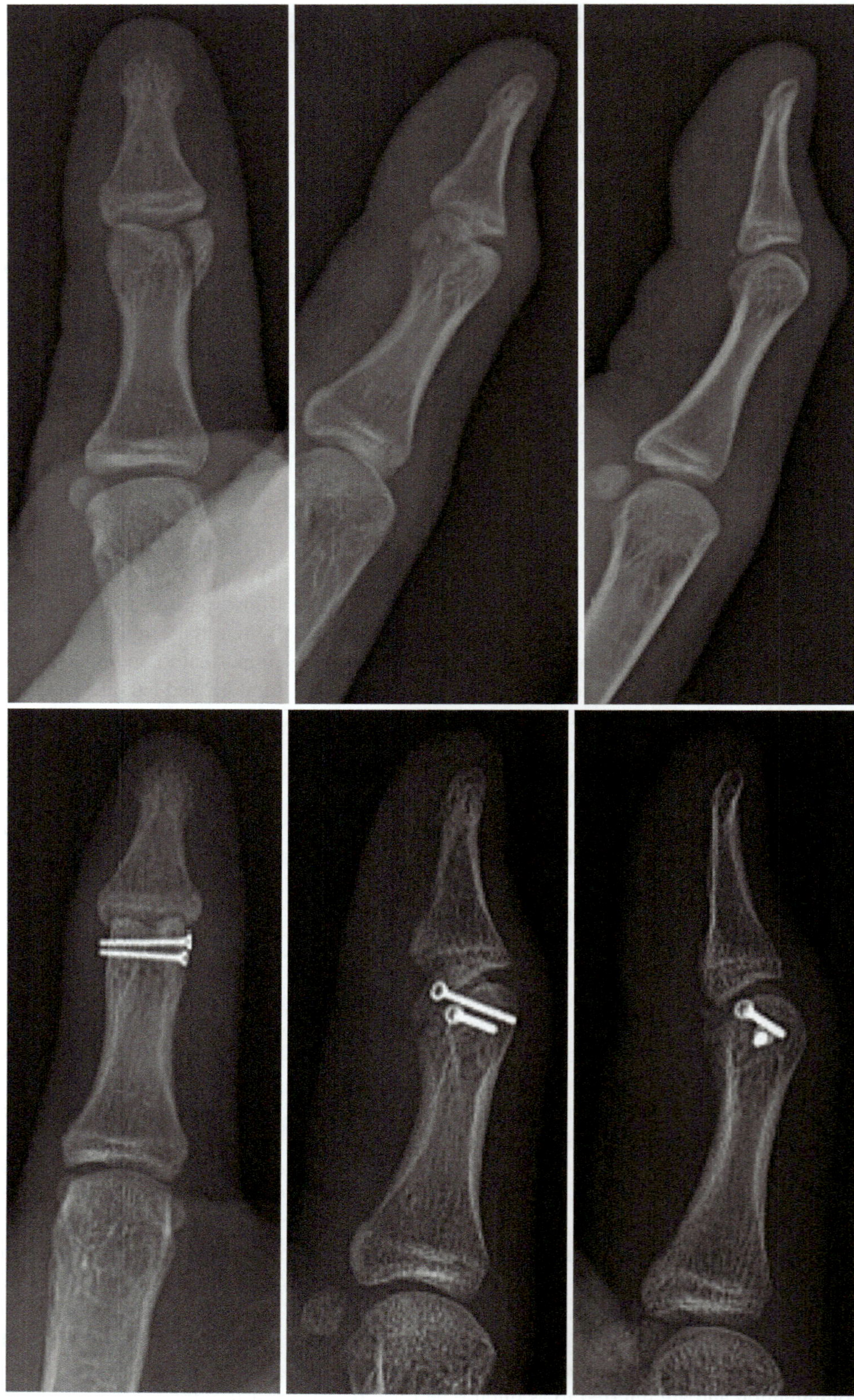

Fig. 12.7 Phalangeal head fracture of the thumb proximal phalanx treated with open reduction and interfragmentary screws

50% of the articular surface or requiring more than 30° of flexion are considered unstable [34]. For dorsal lip fractures, stable fractures typically involve less than 50% of the joint surface and are stable in full extension. Those fractures that are greater than 50% of the joint surface or do not remain reduced in extension are considered unstable [34, 36].

Non-operative treatment can be pursued if the joint is stable, and this treatment course includes closed reduction, buddy taping, splinting, and early range of motion [34]. Closed reduction is performed under digital 'local anaesthetic' blockage, with the reduction method dependent on the direction of the dislocation. It is important to note that several soft tissue structures may become entrapped within the joint and prevent reduction [36]. These include the volar plate in the setting of dorsal dislocations; in volar dislocations, the phalanx may become buttonholed through the flexor tendon sheath, with the extensor tendon sheath entrapped within the joint. Following reduction, a splint is applied and radiographs are performed to ensure reduction. Patients are followed with serial radiographs to ensure the joint remains reduced. The patient continues buddy taping for approximately three weeks [34]. Dorsal blocking splints are utilized when excessive extension must be prevented and is used in volar lip fractures that are stable in less than 30° of flexion, as buddy taping only prevents hyperextension [34]. These splints maintain joint stability between 30 and 90° and allow the patient to immediately mobilize the joint [36]. The splint is changed weekly, decreasing flexion by 10° per week. These patients then progress to buddy taping, when the fracture dislocation is stable in full extension [34, 36]. For volar fracture dislocations, the PIPJ is splinted in full extension for 3–4 weeks, with the DIPJ free to allow for DIPJ range of motion. Following this time period, dynamic PIPJ extension splinting occurs for a further two weeks and passive flexion and strengthening occurs. There are several indications for surgical management. This includes unstable injuries as above. In addition, dislocations that were unable to be primarily reduced, those that failed non-operative management, and open fractures should proceed to surgical management. In addition, fractures that have excessive deformity such as rotational malalignment, shortening of more than 6 mm, and angulation greater than 15° should be considered for surgical management [34].

Similar to other phalangeal fractures, a multitude of surgical options exist, which include closed reduction percutaneous pinning, hinged external fixation, and open reduction internal fixation [34, 38]. For severely comminuted fractures, volar plate arthroplasty and osteochondral allograft may be considered. K-wires may be utilized in players, who have a low demand of their injured hand. Open reduction with internal fixation can be utilized for fractures with minimal comminution and large fragments [36]. Fixation materials include intramedullary screws, as well as plate and screw constructs. Multiple surgical approaches are utilized to include the shotgun volar, midaxial lateral, and dorsal [34]. The shotgun volar approach is most commonly utilized for volar lip fractures. A volar based incision is made along the digit, extending from the proximal flexion crease to the DIPJ crease. The neurovascular bundles are identified and gently retracted. The flexor tendon sheath is then incised between the A2 and A4 pulleys. The flexor tendons are then retracted and the volar plate is exposed, and released distally and laterally. The collateral ligaments are then released, which allow the joint to be hyperextended, exposing both the middle and proximal phalangeal joint surfaces [34]. The midaxial approach is made along either the ulnar or radial border of the digit and can be used for fixation of unicondylar fractures or pilon type fractures as described above [34]. Dorsal lip fractures can be approached from the dorsal approach, which utilizes a curved dorsally based incision over the PIPJ. The lateral bands are identified and the joint capsule is incised between the lateral bands and the central slip [34].

Multiple studies have reported various dynamic external fixation constructs with good results. Ellis et al. [37] described a construct consisting of a combination of 1.4 and 0.9 mm k-wires and dental grade rubber bands. The authors reported that all patients maintained a congruent joint and had an average range of motion in flexion between 1° and 89° with grip strength being 92% of the contralateral side [37]. At an average follow up of 26 months, five patients in the cohort had evidence of arthritis [37]. Ruland et al. [39] reported outcomes on 34 patients utilizing a similar construct and reported average flexion of 88° at a mean follow up of 16 months. The authors reported a complication rate of 29%, with superficial pin site infections affecting 8 patients [39]. In addition to the pin site infections, one patient had extensor tendon adhesions that required surgical lysis, and one patient, with a pilon fracture, went on to develop a swan neck deformity [39].

12.2.8 Phalangeal Shaft Fractures

Extra-articular fractures that have minimal displacement and rotation can be treated non-operatively. Protective orthoplast splints incorporating the joint below and above the fracture as well as the adjacent digit can be used to enable protected return to play. Fractures that have excessive angulation and significant malrotation require surgery. For athletes, minor malrotation may significantly affect their performance due to finger overlap, and negatively impacts on grasp and grip strength. Extra-articular phalangeal fractures about the thumb can typically be treated non-operatively due to the ability of the thumb MCPJ to compensate for deformity. In the proximal phalanx, up 20° of angular deformity and 30° of lateral deformity may be tolerated [15].

Multiple fixation constructs are available for shaft fractures which include k-wire stabilization, plate and screw constructs, lag screws and cerclage wiring. Closed reduction and percutaneous k-wire stabilization can be used for simple fracture patterns (Figs. 12.8 and 12.9). The MCPJ is flexed to reduce pull of the flexor tendons and crossed k-wires are introduced anterograde starting at the condyles. A pointed reduction clamp can be applied percutaneously and aid reduction as necessary. If open reduction is required, a mid-

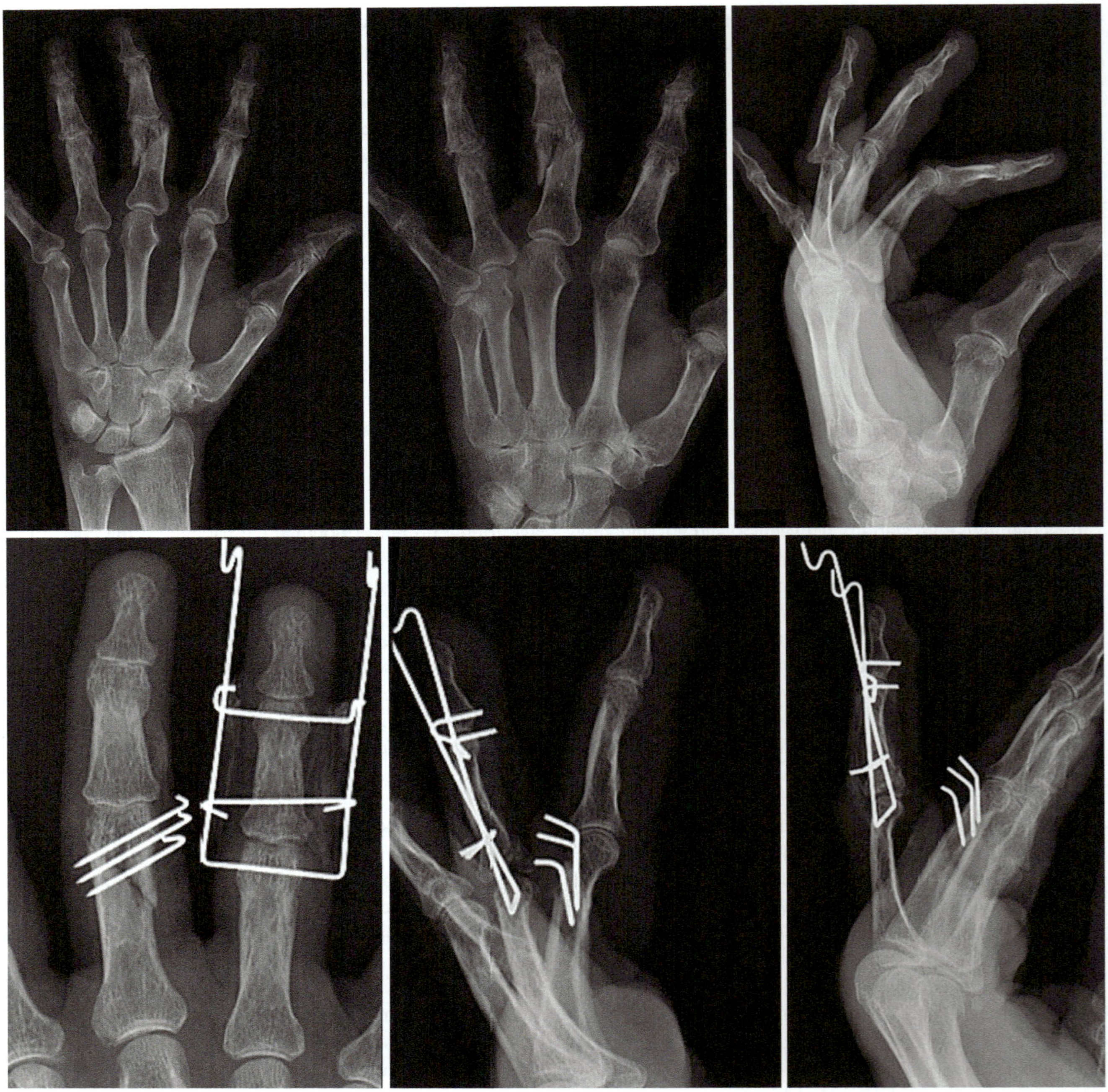

Fig. 12.8 Phalangeal base fracture treated with k-wire external fixation frame. Also noted is a middle phalangeal oblique shaft fracture treated with closed reduction and percutaneous k-wire fixation

axial incision is preferred and plates or screws may be placed laterally (Fig. 12.10). Lateral placement may result in less extensor tendon adhesion formation [14, 40]. During the dorsal approach, dissection is carried down to the extensor tendon and a longitudinal incision is made in the sagittal band either radial or ulnar to the extensor tendon. This can then be repaired with non-absorbable suture following fixation. For the mid-axial approach, blunt dissection is carried down to the level of the fracture to protect the neurovascular bundle and the ulnar side may be preferable to protect the lumbrical's insertion [14]. The volar aspect of the lateral band and the extensor tendon are retracted dorsally [14]. Tendon adhesions may occur following these approaches. For oblique and spiral fractures, a suture cerclage can be utilized, with non-absorbable suture to aid in reduction. This mimics cerclage wire fixation and is performed by passing a non-absorbable suture around the fracture and tightly tying it to provide provisional fracture reduction.

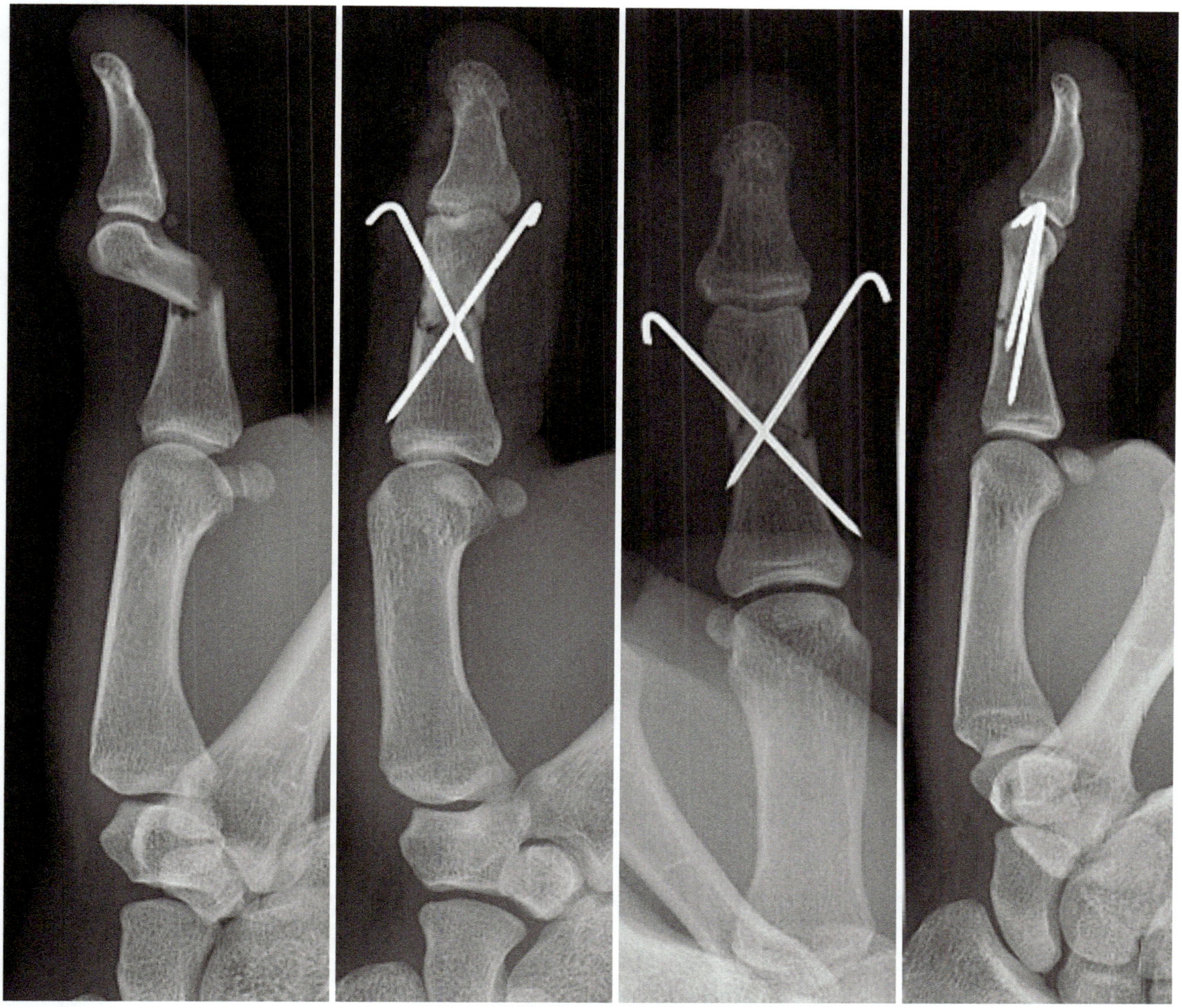

Fig. 12.9 Transverse fracture of the little phalangeal shaft treated with closed reduction and percutaneous k-wire fixation

12.2.9 Distal Phalanx Fractures

Multiple common fracture patterns occur around the distal phalanx. Tuft fractures involve the overlaying nail plate and result from a crush mechanism [22]. These fractures typically have an associated subungual hematoma. If there is a displaced distal phalanx fracture and large subungual hematoma, the nail should be removed and repair of the germinal or sterile matrix performed with an absorbable suture such as 6-0 vicryl rapide (Ethicon, Summerville, New Jersey), to prevent nail deformity. Following suture repair, the nail or a prosthetic nail can be fashioned and placed under the nail fold to prevent closure. A volar based aluminum splint or plastic fingertip protection splint can then be placed [22]. Careful attention must be given to children who present with tuft fractures as the fracture can involve the distal growth plate. A Seymour fracture requires open reduction, given the open fracture at the growth plate, and interposition of the germinal matrix in the fracture gap. In addition, k-wire stabilization may be indicated in displaced or unstable diaphyseal fractures. The k-wire is placed longitudinally across the fracture and through the extended DIPJ [40, 41].

Mallet fractures are dorsal avulsions of the terminal tendon insertion due to forced flexion when the finger is in hyperextension [22, 42]. Patients present with the distal phalanx in flexion and are unable to extend at the DIPJ [22, 42]. Most of these fractures can be treated non-operatively with immobilisation. However, these fractures may result in joint incongruency, and operative indications include volar subluxation and articular involvement greater than 40% [3, 22].

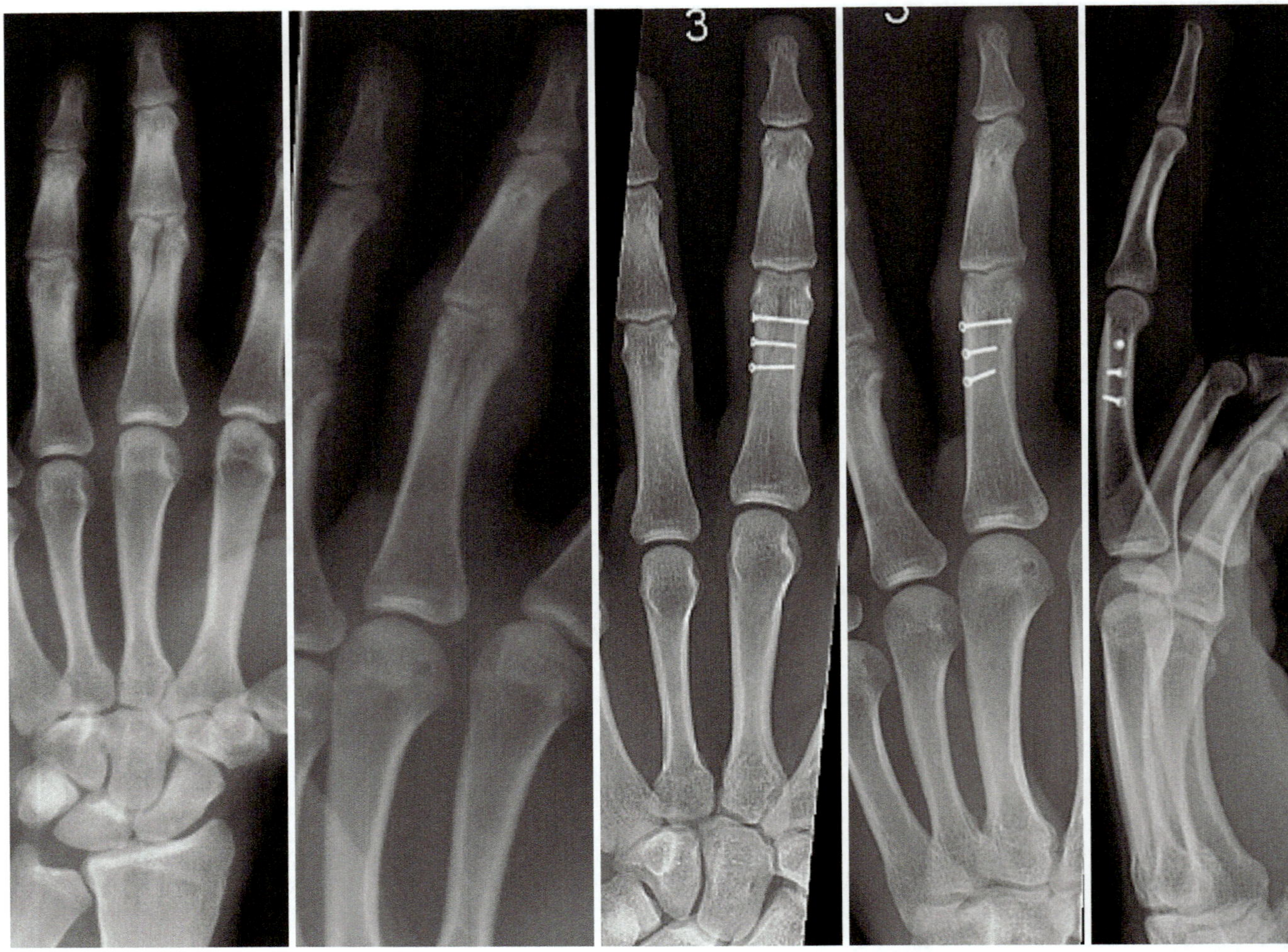

Fig. 12.10 Oblique fracture of the middle phalangeal shaft with extension into the phalangeal head treated with open reduction and interfragmentary screws

Improperly treated fractures may progress to either developing osteoarthritis or a swan neck deformity with the PIPJ hyperextended, due to proximal retraction of the central slip resulting in imbalanced extension force, and the DIPJ remaining in flexion [42]. These fractures can be fixed with k-wire fixation, in a variety of constructs such as k-wire dorsal block pinning, or screw fixation. Typically, a retrograde axial K wire holding the DIPJ reduced with concomitant DIPJ splinting is all that is necessary for 6–8 weeks.

12.2.10 Complications

There are several complications that may occur following a phalangeal fracture. Fractures treated non-operatively may result in a rotational deformity and loss of motion, both of which could be detrimental to an athlete. Malunion and non-union may also occur following improperly reduced or stabilized fractures. Non-union occurs if there is no evidence of clinical or radiographic healing after 4 months and typically result from angular or rotational deformity [3].

Hardware irritation and wound infection are unique to operatively treated fractures. Fractures that are treated with lag screws or plate and screw constructs can irritate surrounding extensor and flexor tendons as there is less space between the bone and construct compared to metacarpals [14]. This can result in residual pain and stiffness. Proper screw length should be ensured on intraoperative fluoroscopy to ensure smooth tendon gliding. Wound infection can occur following both open and closed reduction. Superficial pin site infections may occur, and can be treated with oral antibiotics and pin removal. K-wire breakage can also occur. When utilizing dynamic external fixators, arthritis, pin site infections and adhesions may occur.

Stiffness is a common complication following both operative and non-operative treatment of phalangeal fractures. Following a dorsal or mid-axial approach to the phalanx, tendon adhesions can result in decreased ROM. Early rehabilitation should be sought for fractures with stable constructs, to prevent post-operative stiffness, which is particularly detrimental in the athlete. Most finger phalangeal fractures are healed within 4 weeks, so should be stable by this stage. For PIPJ fracture dislocations, chronic instability, presenting as joint subluxation, can occur [34].

12.2.11 Rehabilitation

The restoration of range of motion and function is vital when managing phalangeal fractures. Stable fractures that are treated non-operatively may return to protected play immediately with a joint-immobilizing splint with range of motion exercises beginning at 3 weeks [40]. Following surgical management, the patient is transitioned to a thermoplastic removable splint at 2–3 days. At this time, range of motion exercises with formal hand therapy exercises are begun, in conjunction with ice and elevation to reduce swelling. Sutures are removed at two weeks and range of motion activity is begun. Strengthening is increased, four weeks post-injury, as long as there is clinical evidence of healing and radiographic union. Exercises that require gripping are restarted at this time [43, 44]. In Major League Baseball players, Graham [43] reported that 25% of athletes returned at 7 weeks, 50% between week 7 and 9 and 25% between 9 and 12. Amongst professional basketball players in the National Basketball Association, Morse et al. [11] reported a total of 33 days missed for phalangeal fractures treated non-operatively compared to 46 days for those treated operatively, likely reflecting sequelae of surgery and complex fracture patterns. For professional American football players, Gaston [32] recommended immediate return to play for stable factures treated non-operatively. For fractures treated operatively, he recommended return to play at 1–2 weeks following surgery, with range of motion exercises beginning 2–3 days post-operatively. For such fractures, he recommended return to noncontact practice following the resolution of swelling, and return to protected play with contact 1–3 weeks depending on the fracture type [32]. For distal phalanx fractures, Evans and Pervaiz [40] recommended immediate return to play with a splint for stable fractures and range of motion beginning at 3 weeks. For distal phalanx fractures that require k-wire stabilization, the pins are removed when there is evidence of healing, usually at 4 weeks. At this stage, players may begin range of motion exercises, with return to protected play over the following 2 weeks [40].

12.2.12 Preventative Measures

Similar to metacarpal fractures, protective hand gear can be utilized to prevent phalangeal fractures. This includes appropriate wear of gloves during athletic activities and buddy taping. Technique medication may include closed fist and proper striking techniques in contact sports.

References

1. Bartels DW, Hevesi M, Wyles C, Macalena J, Kakar S, Krych AJ. Epidemiology of Hand and Wrist Injuries in NCAA Men's Football: 2009–2010 to 2013–2014. Orthop J Sports Med. 2019;7(4):2325967119835375. https://doi.org/10.1177/2325967119835375.
2. Swenson DM, Yard EE, Collins CL, Fields SK, Comstock RD. Epidemiology of US high school sports-related fractures, 2005–2009. Clin J Sport Med. 2010;20(4):293–9. https://doi.org/10.1097/JSM.0b013e3181e8fae8.
3. Cotterell IH, Richard MJ. Metacarpal and phalangeal fractures in athletes. Clin Sports Med. 2015;34(1):69–98. https://doi.org/10.1016/j.csm.2014.09.009.
4. Nakashian MN, Pointer L, Owens BD, Wolf JM. Incidence of metacarpal fractures in the US population. Hand N Y N. 2012;7(4):426–30. https://doi.org/10.1007/s11552-012-9442-0.
5. Fufa DT, Goldfarb CA. Fractures of the thumb and finger metacarpals in athletes. Hand Clin. 2012;28(3):379–88. https://doi.org/10.1016/j.hcl.2012.05.028.
6. Suh N, Weiland AJ. Metacarpal fractures in the athlete. In: The athlete's hand and wrist. Chicago, IL: A Master Skills Publication; 2014. p. 115–20.
7. Goldfarb CA. Commentary metacarpal fracture in the professional baseball player. Hand Clin. 2012;28(3):389. https://doi.org/10.1016/j.hcl.2012.05.029.
8. Cairns MA, Hasty EK, Herzog MM, Ostrum RF, Kerr ZY. Incidence, severity, and time loss associated with collegiate football fractures, 2004–2005 to 2013–2014. Am J Sports Med. 2018;46(4):987–94. https://doi.org/10.1177/0363546517749914.
9. Mall NA, Carlisle JC, Matava MJ, Powell JW, Goldfarb CA. Upper extremity injuries in the National Football League: part I: hand and digital injuries. Am J Sports Med. 2008;36(10):1938–44. https://doi.org/10.1177/0363546508318197.
10. Etier BE, Scillia AJ, Tessier DD, et al. Return to play following metacarpal fractures in football players. Hand N Y N. 2015;10(4):762–6. https://doi.org/10.1007/s11552-015-9769-4.
11. Morse KW, Hearns KA, Carlson MG. Return to play after forearm and hand injuries in the National Basketball Association. Orthop J Sports Med. 2017;5(2):2325967117690002. https://doi.org/10.1177/2325967117690002.
12. Bushnell BD, Draeger RW, Crosby CG, Bynum DK. Management of intra-articular metacarpal base fractures of the second through fifth metacarpals. J Hand Surg. 2008;33(4):573–83. https://doi.org/10.1016/j.jhsa.2007.11.019.
13. Soong M, Chase S, George KN. Metacarpal fractures in the athlete. Curr Rev Musculoskelet Med. 2017;10(1):23–7. https://doi.org/10.1007/s12178-017-9380-0.
14. Geissler WB. Operative fixation of metacarpal and phalangeal fractures in athletes. Hand Clin. 2009;25(3):409–21. https://doi.org/10.1016/j.hcl.2009.05.005.
15. Carlsen BT, Moran SL. Thumb trauma: Bennett fractures, Rolando fractures, and ulnar collateral ligament injuries. J Hand Surg. 2009;34(5):945–52. https://doi.org/10.1016/j.jhsa.2009.03.017.
16. Royle SG. Rotational deformity following metacarpal fracture. J Hand Surg Edinb Scotl. 1990;15(1):124–5. https://doi.org/10.1016/0266-7681(90)90068-f.
17. Meunier MJ, Hentzen E, Ryan M, Shin AY, Lieber RL. Predicted effects of metacarpal shortening on interosseous muscle func-

tion. J Hand Surg. 2004;29(4):689–93. https://doi.org/10.1016/j.jhsa.2004.03.002.
18. Strauch RJ, Rosenwasser MP, Lunt JG. Metacarpal shaft fractures: the effect of shortening on the extensor tendon mechanism. J Hand Surg. 1998;23(3):519–23. https://doi.org/10.1016/S0363-5023(05)80471-X.
19. ten Berg PWL, Mudgal CS, Leibman MI, Belsky MR, Ruchelsman DE. Quantitative 3-dimensional CT analyses of intramedullary headless screw fixation for metacarpal neck fractures. J Hand Surg. 2013;38(2):322-330.e2. doi:https://doi.org/10.1016/j.jhsa.2012.09.029
20. del Piñal F, Moraleda E, Rúas JS, de Piero GH, Cerezal L. Minimally invasive fixation of fractures of the phalanges and metacarpals with intramedullary cannulated headless compression screws. J Hand Surg. 2015;40(4):692–700. https://doi.org/10.1016/j.jhsa.2014.11.023.
21. Ozer K, Gillani S, Williams A, Peterson SL, Morgan S. Comparison of intramedullary nailing versus plate-screw fixation of extra-articular metacarpal fractures. J Hand Surg. 2008;33(10):1724–31. https://doi.org/10.1016/j.jhsa.2008.07.011.
22. Halim A, Weiss A-PC. Return to play after hand and wrist fractures. Clin Sports Med. 2016;35(4):597–608. https://doi.org/10.1016/j.csm.2016.05.005.
23. Ford DJ, Ali MS, Steel WM. Fractures of the fifth metacarpal neck: is reduction or immobilisation necessary? J Hand Surg Edinb Scotl. 1989;14(2):165–7. https://doi.org/10.1016/0266-7681(89)90119-8.
24. Fujitani R, Omokawa S, Shigematsu K, Tanaka Y. Comparison of the intramedullary nail and low-profile plate for unstable metacarpal neck fractures. J Orthop Sci. 2012;17(4):450–6. https://doi.org/10.1007/s00776-012-0223-y.
25. Evans P, Pervaiz K. Sport-specific commentary on Bennett and metacarpal fractures in football. Hand Clin. 2012;28(3):393–4. https://doi.org/10.1016/j.hcl.2012.05.031.
26. Fusetti C, Meyer H, Borisch N, Stern R, Santa DD, Papaloïzos M. Complications of plate fixation in metacarpal fractures. J Trauma. 2002;52(3):535–9. https://doi.org/10.1097/00005373-200203000-00019.
27. Weckesser EC. Rotational osteotomy of the metacarpal for overlapping fingers. J Bone Joint Surg Am. 1965;47:751–6.
28. Clinkscales C. Sports-specific commentary on Bennett's fractures in professional basketball players: Bennett fractures and metacarpal fractures. Hand Clin. 2012;28(3):391–2. https://doi.org/10.1016/j.hcl.2012.05.030.
29. Guss MS, Begly JP, Ramme AJ, Hinds RM, Karia RJ, Capo JT. Performance outcomes after metacarpal fractures in National Basketball Association Players. Hand N Y N. 2016;11(4):427–32. https://doi.org/10.1177/1558944716628500.
30. Carruthers KH, O'Reilly O, Skie M, Walters J, Siparsky P. Casting and splinting management for hand injuries in the in-season contact sport athlete. Sports Health. 2017;9(4):364–71. https://doi.org/10.1177/1941738117700133.
31. London PS. Sprains and fractures involving the interphalangeal joints. The Hand. 1971;3(2):155–8. https://doi.org/10.1016/0072-968x(71)90035-0.
32. Gaston RG. Football commentary: phalangeal fractures—displaced/nondisplaced. Hand Clin. 2012;28(3):407–8. https://doi.org/10.1016/j.hcl.2012.05.035.
33. Kiefhaber TR, Stern PJ. Fracture dislocations of the proximal interphalangeal joint. J Hand Surg. 1998;23(3):368–80. https://doi.org/10.1016/S0363-5023(05)80454-X.
34. Gaston RG. Proximal interphalangeal joint fractures and dislocations in the athlete. In: The athlete's hand and wrist. Chicago, IL: A Master Skills Publication; 2014. p. 107–14.
35. Bindra RR, Foster BJ. Management of proximal interphalangeal joint dislocations in athletes. Hand Clin. 2009;25(3):423–35. https://doi.org/10.1016/j.hcl.2009.05.008.
36. Caggiano NM, Harper CM, Rozental TD. Management of proximal interphalangeal joint fracture dislocations. Hand Clin. 2018;34(2):149–65. https://doi.org/10.1016/j.hcl.2017.12.005.
37. Ellis SJ, Cheng R, Prokopis P, et al. Treatment of proximal interphalangeal dorsal fracture-dislocation injuries with dynamic external fixation: a pins and rubber band system. J Hand Surg. 2007;32(8):1242–50. https://doi.org/10.1016/j.jhsa.2007.07.001.
38. Kodama N, Takemura Y, Ueba H, Imai S, Matsusue Y. Operative treatment of metacarpal and phalangeal fractures in athletes: early return to play. J Orthop Sci. 2014;19(5):729–36. https://doi.org/10.1007/s00776-014-0584-5.
39. Ruland RT, Hogan CJ, Cannon DL, Slade JF. Use of dynamic distraction external fixation for unstable fracture-dislocations of the proximal interphalangeal joint. J Hand Surg. 2008;33(1):19–25. https://doi.org/10.1016/j.jhsa.2007.07.018.
40. Evans P, Pervaiz K. Sports specific commentary: phalangeal fractures in basketball. Hand Clin. 2012;28(3):405. https://doi.org/10.1016/j.hcl.2012.05.034.
41. Chen F, Kalainov DM. Phalanx fractures and dislocations in athletes. Curr Rev Musculoskelet Med. 2017;10(1):10–6. https://doi.org/10.1007/s12178-017-9378-7.
42. Lamaris GA, Matthew MK. The diagnosis and management of mallet finger injuries. Hand N Y N. 2017;12(3):223–8. https://doi.org/10.1177/1558944716642763.
43. Graham T. Care of phalangeal fractures in the elite athlete's hand. In: The athlete's hand and wrist. Chicago, IL: A Master Skills Publication; 2014. p. 95–105.
44. Shin SS. Phalangeal fractures in baseball: commentary. Hand Clin. 2012;28(3):403. https://doi.org/10.1016/j.hcl.2012.05.033.

Part III

Acute Fractures in Sport: Lower Limb

Acute Fractures in Sport: Hip

13

Blake J. Schultz and Kenneth A. Egol

Learning Objectives

- To review the etiology of acute hip fractures in athletes, including the need for work-up of concomitant injuries and relevant risk factors.
- To review the clinical examination findings and peri-operative imaging required for accurate diagnosis and optimal management for various fractures about the hip.
- To discuss specific surgical treatment options, including approaches and implant choice relevant to treating different types of athletes.
- To review post-operative expectations and rehabilitation protocols.

13.1 Introduction

Acute hip fractures in athletics are rare. They can occur either through a low energy stress mechanism secondary to excessive loading or from high energy trauma. The latter group requires a thorough evaluation following the Advanced Trauma Life Support (ATLS) protocols looking for associated injuries [1–3]. Given differences in the osseous and vascular anatomy, injury mechanisms, fracture patterns and goals of treatment, hip fractures in young, active sporting patients should be managed differently than geriatric hip fractures [1]. These injuries are associated with significant morbidity, including avascular necrosis (AVN), post-traumatic arthritis and decreased range of motion (ROM) and strength, which can have both short and long-term implications for athletes. This chapter reviews fractures of the hip, femoral head, neck, peritrochanteric region and shaft, (Fig. 13.1) with brief discussions on pertinent anatomy, common classification systems, diagnosis and management with special considerations for the athletic patient.

Goal (from email): *Provide a concise description of the epidemiology, contemporary management principles, predicted outcome and preventative measures of sport-related acute fractures of the femoral head, femoral neck, proximal femur and femoral diaphysis.*

B. J. Schultz · K. A. Egol (✉)
Department of Orthopedic Surgery, NYU Langone Orthopedic Hospital, New York, NY, USA
e-mail: Kenneth.Egol@nyulangone.org

13.2 Avulsion Fractures

13.2.1 Epidemiology

Avulsion fractures can affect any of the muscular insertion sites around the hip. The most common sites are the abductors on the greater trochanter (GT) and the iliopsoas insertion on the lesser trochanter (Fig. 13.2) [4–6]. These injuries typically occur in adolescent athletes because of the timing of secondary ossification of the apophyses coinciding with the hormonally induced increase in muscle strength [6].

These injuries usually present acutely, after sudden forceful eccentric contraction of the muscle such as sprinting or kicking, and have a high prevalence in gymnastics, soccer and track and field athletes.

13.2.2 Classification

Fracture displacement is the most relevant prognostic factor for acute fractures, and can classified according to McKinney et al. [7] (Table 13.1). The degree of fracture displacement is important to point towards operative versus non-operative management. The specific location of the avulsion may also be more or less relevant for athletes in different sports depending on functional demands, and may in itself be an indication of operative or non-operative management.

G. A. J. Robertson, N. Maffulli (eds.), *Fractures in Sport*, https://doi.org/10.1007/978-3-030-72036-0_13

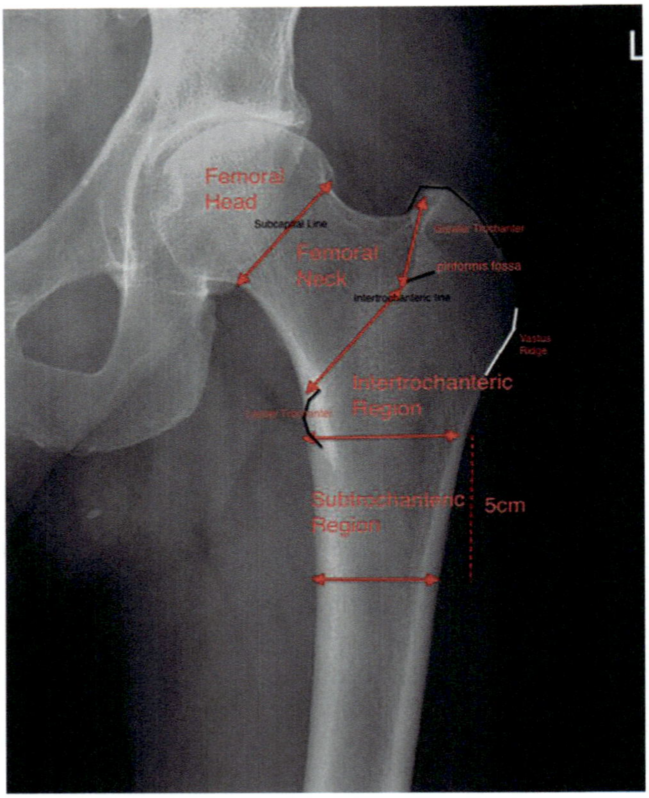

Fig. 13.1 AP radiograph of the left hip demonstrating various anatomic regions *(Fig. 1.4, page 5 in Egol, Kenneth, and Philipp Leucht, eds. 2017. Proximal Femur Fractures An Evidence-Based Approach to Evaluation and Management. Cham: Springer)*

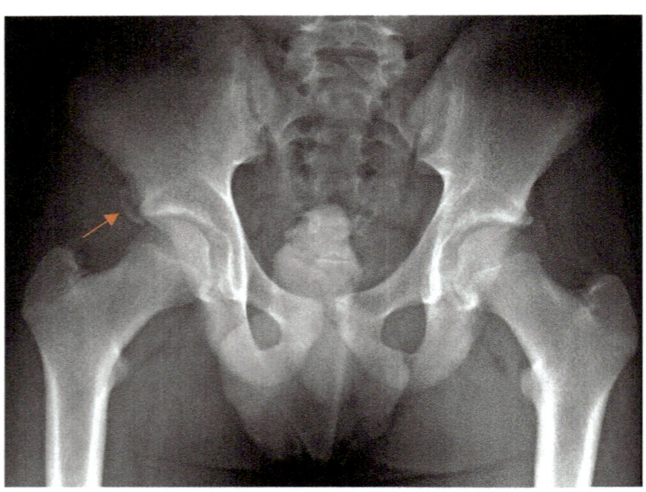

Fig. 13.2 Antero-posterior (AP) pelvis radiograph of a 15 year male who felt a pop in his hip after kicking a rugby ball. Minimally displaced avulsion fracture of the Anterior Inferior Iliac Spine (AIIS) that was treated non-operatively

Table 13.1 Classification of avulsion fractures of the hip described by McKinney et al. [7]

Type I: Non-displaced avulsions
Type II: Avulsions displaced ≤2 cm
Type III: Avulsions displaced >2 cm
Type IV: Symptomatic non-unions and painful exostoses

13.2.3 Diagnosis

13.2.3.1 Physical Exam

Athletes will often report a pop or snap at the time of the injury, and will present with acute onset of pain and tenderness at the muscle insertion. Pain is typically exacerbated by passive stretch of the muscle. Athletes will generally exhibit decreased muscle function, though other muscle groups may compensate [3].

13.2.3.2 Imaging

Standard AP pelvis radiographs can be used to identify displaced fractures, (Fig. 13.2) but smaller, non-displaced fractures may be difficult to visualize. Oblique and axial radiographic views can help assess displacement. Computed tomography (CT) can be used to detail displaced fragments and magnetic resonance imaging (MRI) can be used to evaluate apophysitis and avulsions in young athletes whose ossification centers have not yet ossified [7].

13.2.4 Treatment

Most avulsion fractures can be treated with rest, protected weight bearing and early range ROM and stretching [5, 8].

Operative fixation is less common, [9] but may be required for fractures of the GT that are displaced more than 2–3 cm or have painful non-unions. In a large meta-analysis, Eberach et al. showed a higher rate of return to sport in patients treated surgically (92%) versus non-operatively (80%), indicating a lower threshold for surgical fixation in athletes with high functional demand, [6] GT avulsions may produce dysfunction of the abductor mechanism and Trendelburg gait with extra-articular impingement if the fracture is not reduced [10, 11].

Fixation options depend on location and the size of the fragment. Displaced greater trochanter fractures require open reduction with substantial fixation to counter the pull of the abductors. Hook plates supplemented with cerclage wires can be used to capture the avulsed fragment (Fig. 13.3).

13.2.5 Complications

Most avulsion fractures heal well, but there are a few described complications, especially non-unions and exosto-

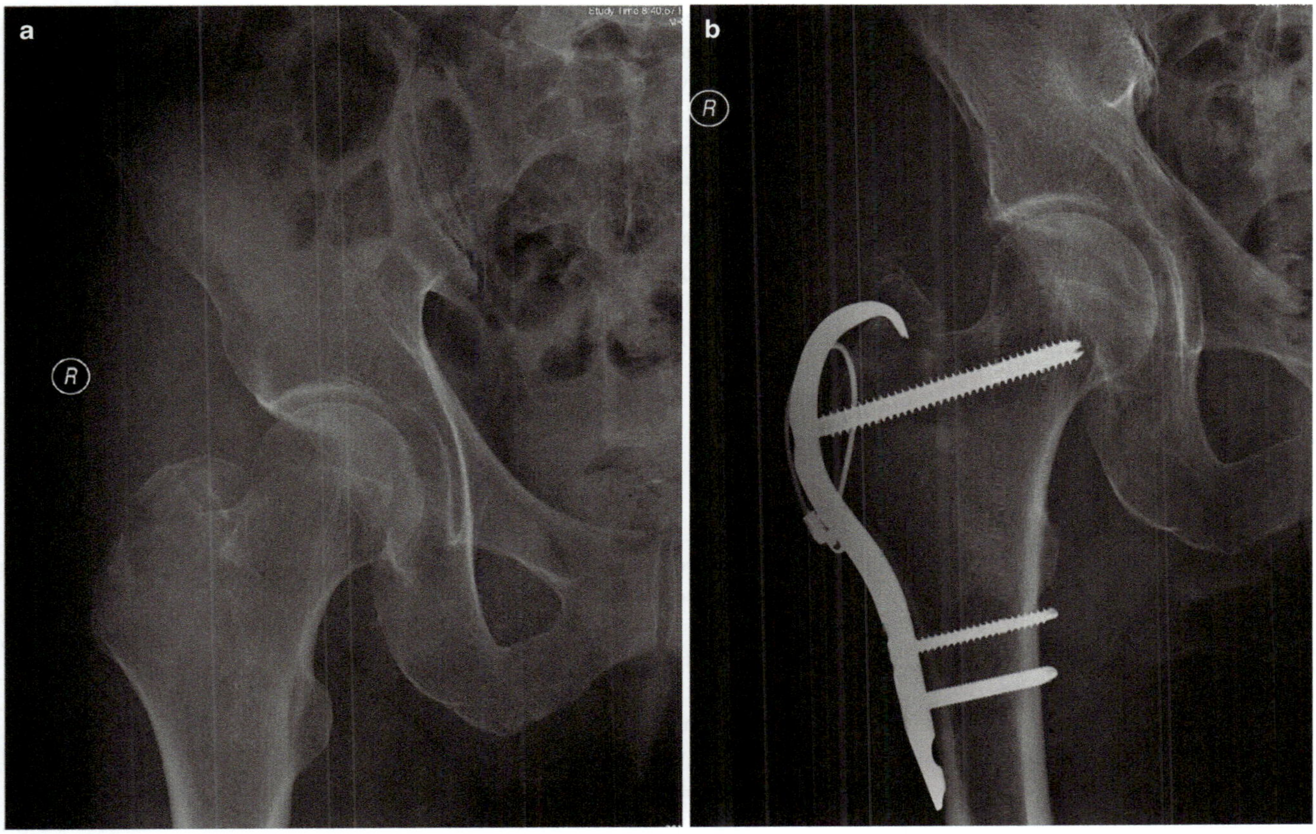

Fig. 13.3 (**a**) AP radiograph showing a displaced greater trochanter fractures. (**b**) Treatment with a hook plate and cerclage wires

sis [7]. Both can be painful and limit the functional strength of the affected muscle. Non-unions can be treated with operative fixation, and symptomatic exostosis can be excised. A rarer, but devastating complication of greater trochanter avulsion fractures is avascular necrosis of the femoral epiphysis, described after both operative and non-operative treatment [12].

13.2.6 Rehabilitation

Metzmaker and Pappas described a 5-phase non-operative protocol to manage acute avulsion fractures. Rehabilitation starts with protected weight bearing with crutches and limited ROM, and advances to return to sport at approximately 2 months [7, 13] (Table 13.2).

Following surgery, most patients will be non-weight bearing for 7–10 days with gradual progressive weight bearing for 3–6 weeks with physical therapy. Return to sport can vary depending on the injury and surgeon preference, and range from 4 weeks to 4 months [14–16].

Table 13.2 Non-operative progression for treatment of acute avulsion injuries, initially described by Metzmaker and Pappas [7, 13]

Phase	Post-injury (days)	ROM	Activity	Radiographic appearance
I	0–7	Restricted	Protected WB	Osseous separation
II	7 to 14–20	Gentle active and passive	Protected WB	Osseous separation
III	14–20 to 30	Increase active and passive ROM	Wean crutches	Early callus
IV	30–60	No restrictions	Light athletic training	Mature callus
V	60 to return	Normal	Full activity	Mature callus

13.3 Femoral Head Fractures

13.3.1 Epidemiology

Femoral head fractures require high energy axial impaction or shear force to a flexed knee. These fractures are almost always associated with posterior hip dislocations [17, 18], and concomitant injuries including acetabular and femoral neck fractures, and ipsilateral knee injuries [19]: thorough clinical and diagnostic work-up are therefore necessary. Femoral head fractures can cause significant morbidity because of the tenuous blood supply to the femoral head, the involvement of the articular surface of the hip joint, and the extensive dissection necessary to reduce and treat these injuries anatomically. Post-traumatic changes including AVN (6–23% of patients) [20–23], heterotopic ossification (HO) (6–64%) [22–26], and post-traumatic arthritis can lead to significantly restricted hip function after injury, with particular morbidity for athletes [27].

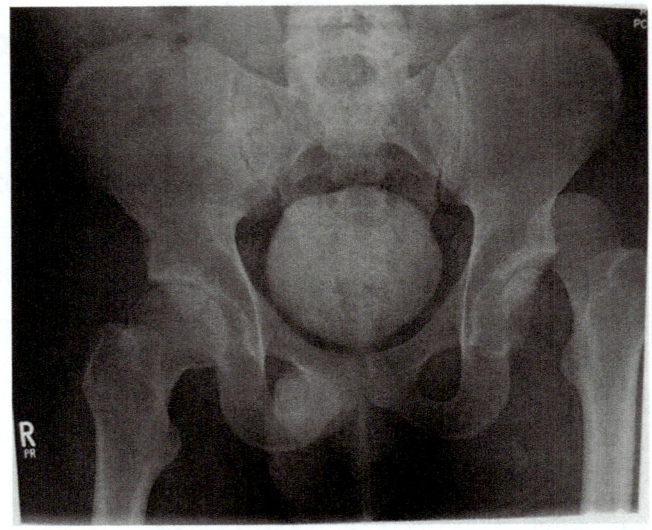

Fig. 13.4 AP radiograph of the pelvis showing a left sided femoral head fracture-dislocation with an associated femoral neck fracture (*Fig. 4.2, page 29, in Egol, Kenneth, and Philipp Leucht, eds. 2017. Proximal Femur Fractures An Evidence-Based Approach to Evaluation and Management. Cham: Springer*)

13.3.2 Diagnosis

13.3.2.1 Physical Exam

Athletes with femoral head fractures present with localized groin pain and inability to bear weight. With an associated hip dislocation, the limb will be shortened. In posterior dislocations, the limb will be flexed, adducted and internally rotated, while anterior dislocations will be often present with limb abduction and external rotation. Posterior dislocations are more common, and are associated with sciatic nerve neurapraxia, so a detailed distal neurovascular exam of all the branches of the sciatic nerve is important [22]. Posterior dislocations are also associated with posterior knee dislocations and tears of the posterior cruciate ligament, so a thorough knee exam is indicated after the hip dislocation has been reduced.

13.3.2.2 Imaging

Radiographic examination should start with anterior-posterior (AP) pelvis, AP and cross-table lateral views of the hip (Fig. 13.4) Inlet and outlet views should be obtained if acetabular fractures are suspected. CT scans help better characterize the fracture and evaluate the presence intra-articular fragments, femoral head impaction, acetabular fractures, and concentric reduction of the hip [19]. CT scans should not routinely be obtained until after closed reduction to limit radiation exposure, and should have a minimum of 2 mm cuts through the hip. MRI can identify cartilaginous lesions and labral pathology associated with hip dislocations.

13.3.3 Classification

Femoral head fractures can be classified according to the AO/OTA system, which distinguishes between avulsion and rupture of the ligamentum teres and larger fractures of the femoral head (Fig. 13.5). The Pipkin classification is most commonly used to describe fractures associated with posterior hip dislocations [28, 29] (Fig. 13.6). Type I fractures tend to be smaller and are differentiated from Type II based on involvement of the weight-bearing portion of the femoral head. Type III fractures are associated with femoral neck fractures, and have a high incidence of AVN due to the the tenuous blood supply of the femoral head [30]. The lateral epiphyseal branches of the medial circumflex artery are the primary blood supply of the femoral head (Fig. 13.7) [31, 32]. These branches are intracapsular, leading to significant risk of AVN of the femoral head with intracapsular neck fractures. Type IV fractures are associated with acetabular fractures.

13.3.4 Treatment

If there is an associated hip dislocation, urgent reduction is required. If reduction is delayed more than 6 h, there is an increased risk of AVN [33]. An associated femoral neck fracture may be a contraindication to closed reduction attempts outside of the operating room, so scrutiny of the injury radiographs is necessary. Post-reduction radiographs and CT scans with reconstructions can be used to determine reduction quality, fracture pattern and presence of loose bodies, all of which will help dictate the definitive treatment plan.

13.3.4.1 Non-operative Management

Non-operative management is an option in the general population for Pipkin I fractures or Pipkin II with <1 mm step off, no inter-articular loose bodies and a stable hip joint [19, 26]. There may be a lower threshold for operative intervention in

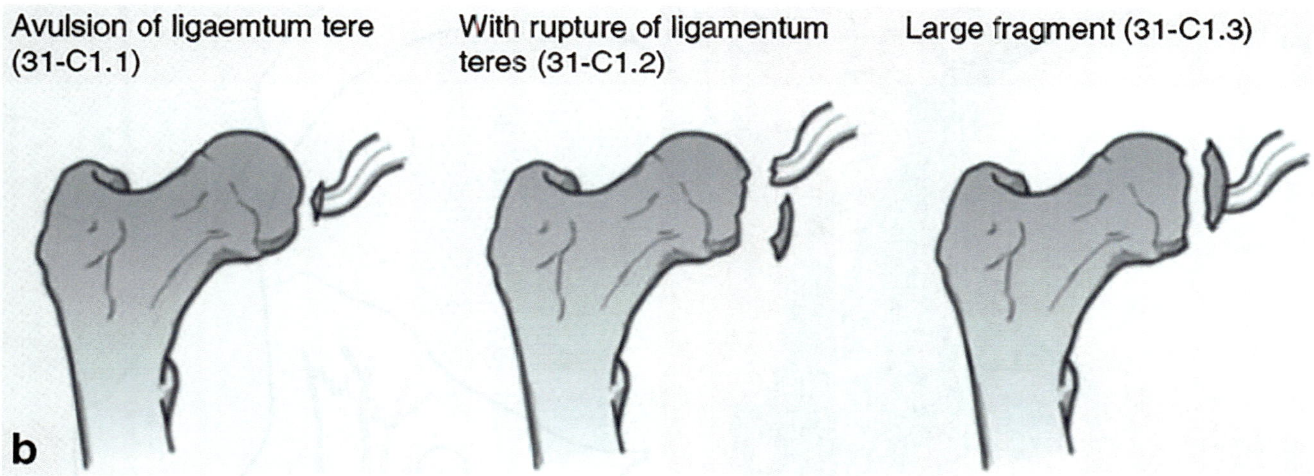

Fig. 13.5 AO/OTA classification of femoral neck fractures (*Fig. 4.6b, page 34 in in Egol, Kenneth, and Philipp Leucht, eds. 2017. Proximal Femur Fractures An Evidence-Based Approach to Evaluation and Management. Cham: Springer*)

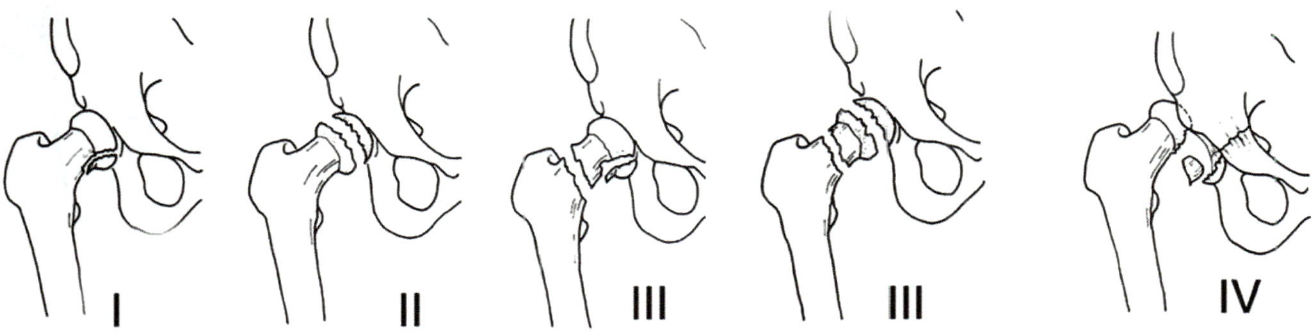

Fig. 13.6 Pipkin classification of femoral head fractures: type I femoral head fracture below the fovea; type II femoral head fracture above the fovea; type III, type I or II with additional fracture of the femoral neck; type IV additional fracture of the acetabulum (*Fig. 67.1 in Peter Giannoudis, and Nikolaos Kanakaris. 2014. "Femoral Head Fractures." In Trauma and Orthopaedic Classification, edited by Nick Lasanioanos, 303–4. Springer*)

high demand athletes, especially given the high incidence of intra-articular loose bodies not appreciated on CT scan that can lead to rapid joint degermation if not addressed [34]. Patients treated non-operatively should remain partial weight bearing for 4–6 weeks with restricted adduction and internal rotation. They should be followed with serial radiographs to confirm that reduction is maintained.

13.3.4.2 Surgical Indications

Operative indications include Pipkin II with >1–2 mm step off, intra-articular loose bodies, associated femoral neck or acetabular fractures (Pipkin III or IV), or irreducible fracture-dislocations. If urgent surgery is not possible, patients with unstable hip joints or loose intra-articular fragments should be placed in distal femur skeletal traction.

There is some controversy regarding fragment fixation versus excision [19, 27]. Any soft tissue or bony fragments in the joint space are clear indications for surgery to prevent rapid destruction of the joint. Small fragments (<1 cm^2) distal to the round ligament do not necessarily need anatomic reduction unless they interfere with joint motion [35]. If they are symptomatic, small fragments can be excised, while large fragments should be anatomically reduced and fixed [36]. These fragments are still attached to the inferior joint capsule, so reduction may help preserve the blood supply to the femoral head. Osteochondral fragments superior to the ligamentum teres involve the weight-bearing articular surface, and thus require anatomic reduction [35]. These fractures can be fixed with mini or small fragment screws (2.7 or 3.5 mm) or 3.0 mm cannulated screws, either headless or with the heads buried below the level of cartilage (Fig. 13.8) Areas with articular impaction should be elevated, and the defect backfilled with autogenous cancellous bone graft or some other bone void filler. Ipsilateral femoral neck fractures should be fixed prior to the femoral head with 7.0 or 7.3 mm cancellous screws [37] (Fig. 13.9) Arthroplasty is a reliable treatment option in older, lower demand patients, [38] but would not be appropriate for younger athletic patients.

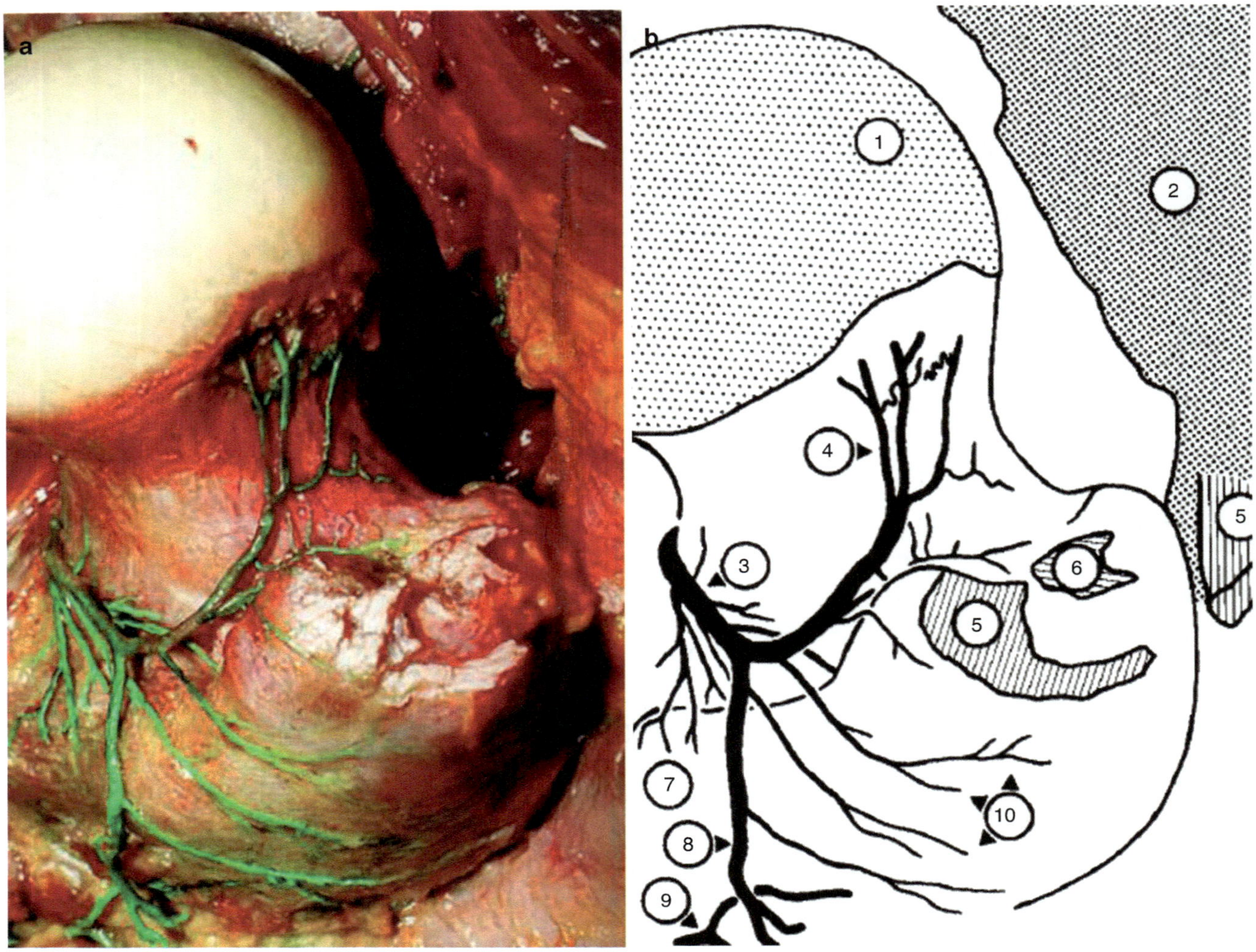

Fig. 13.7 (**a**) Photograph showing the perforation of the terminal branches of the femoral circumflex arteries on the posterior-superior femoral neck. (**b**) Illustration showing: (1) head of the femur, (2) gluteus medius, (3) deep branch of MFCA, 4 (terminal subsynovial branches of MFCA), (5) gluteus medius tendon insertion, (6) pirifomis tendon insertion, (7) less trochanter with nutrient vessel, (8) trochanteric branch, (9) branch of the first perforating artery, (10) trochanteric branches (*Fig. 1.1, page 3*. Egol, Kenneth, and Philipp Leucht, eds. 2017. *Proximal Femur Fractures An Evidence-Based Approach to Evaluation and Management*. Cham: Springer)

13.3.4.3 Arthroscopy

Traditionally, these fractures have been treated through open approaches, but recently hip arthroscopy has been used for loose body removal, chondral and labral repair and arthroscopy-assisted ORIF [39–41]. The incidence of loose bodies after hip dislocations is reported up to 91% [34], and these are not always appreciated on CT scan [40]. Even small loose bodies can cause rapid joint degeneration, so making sure they are removed is important, especially in athletes who hope to return to high-impact activity. Arthroscopy can also address chondral pathology and repair of labrum avulsions via suture anchor. There are small series and case reports of reduction and internal fixation of femoral neck fractures with arthroscopy alone, or with arthroscopy as an adjunct to an open approach [41–43]. Though not the standard of care for larger, or displaced fractures, arthroscopy is an attractive option for athletes, especially if there is concern for loose bodies in otherwise non-operatively managed fractures, and could provide quicker recovery, less blood less and less disruption of the capsuloligamentous structures than open approaches [37]. Hip arthroscopy is contraindicated if there are associated acetabular fractures: this would result in fluid extravasation into the pelvis [44].

13.3.4.4 Open Approaches

Open surgical management can be accomplished through an anterior or posterior approach. The anterior Smith-Peterson or surgical hip dislocations provide better access to the femoral head for direct visualization of fracture reduction and preservation of the joint capsule and ligamentum teres

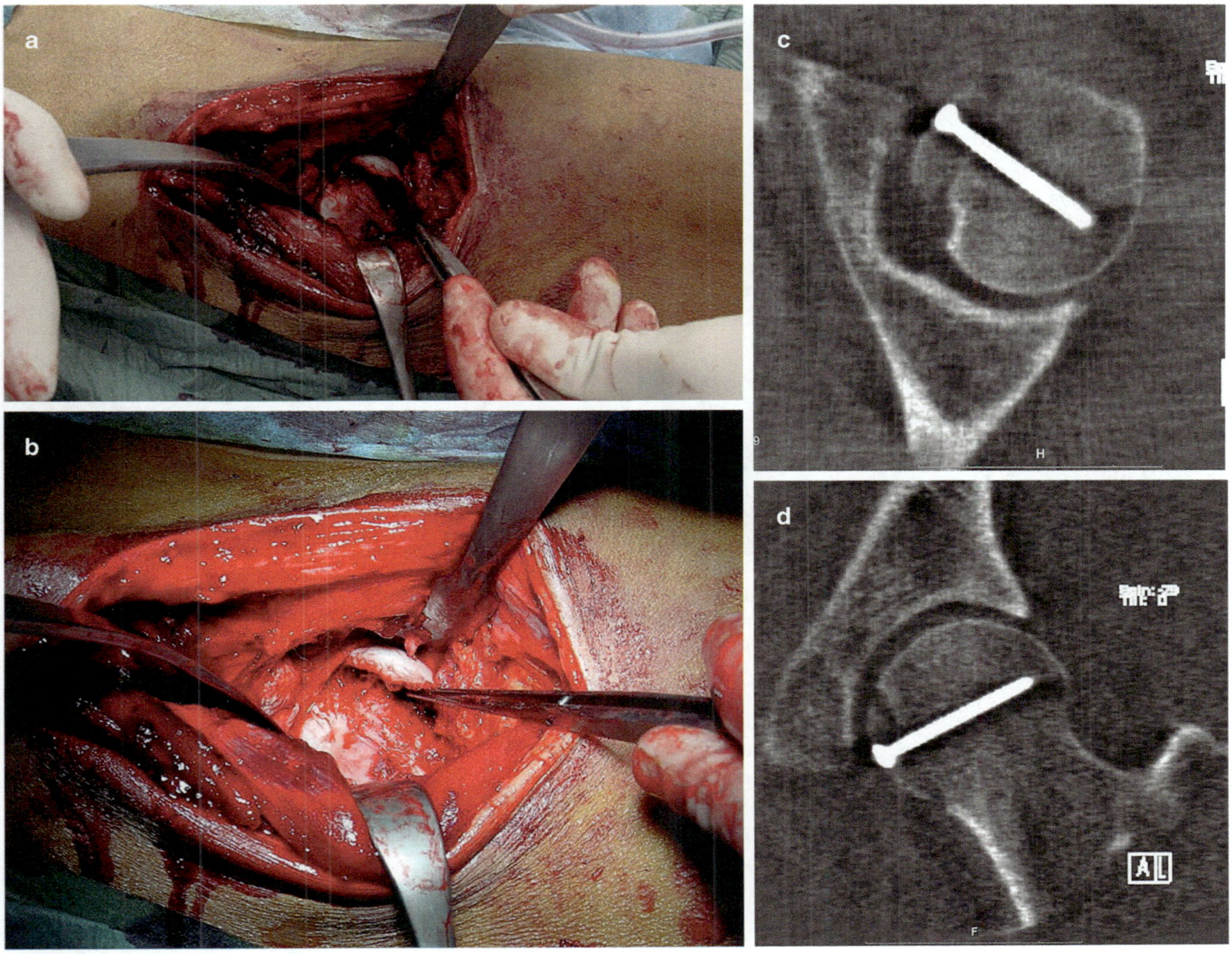

Fig. 13.8 (**a**) Anterior approach to the hip demonstrating a displaced femoral head fragment. (**b**) Mobilization and reduction of the fragment. (**c/d**) Intra-op C-arm coronal and axial views showing fracture fixation with small fragment screw (*Fig. 4.10, page 38. In Egol, Kenneth, and Philipp Leucht, eds. 2017. Proximal Femur Fractures An Evidence-Based Approach to Evaluation and Management. Cham: Springer*)

(Fig. 13.8) [45–47]. Compared to posterior approaches, anterior approaches are associated with less blood loss and operative time, without increased risk of osteonecrosis [26]. A posterior Kocher-Langenbeck may be indicated in cases of associated acetabular fractures or irreducible dislocations where either posterior bony or soft-tissue structures need to be addressed [48]. Direct anatomic reduction of the femoral head fragments is more difficult through a posterior approach. A trochanteric osteotomy has been described to facilitate femoral head dislocation and joint restoration, and may be a good option in femoral head fractures with associated posterior acetabular fractures [27, 46]. However, the osteotomy puts the deep branch of the medial femoral circumflex at risk, [32] and dislocating the femoral head can compromise the vascular supply to the fracture fragment, both of which can increase the risk of AVN. Pipkin type III fractures associated with femoral neck fractures require an anterolateral Watson-Jones approach to address the femoral neck first. Fixation of the femoral head can be performed either through the same incision or a separate anterior approach [19].

13.3.5 Complications

13.3.6 Avascular Necrosis

AVN is a major complication of femoral head fractures, with a reported incidence as high as 6–23% [20–23]. Urgent reduction is important to minimize such risk. Most cases of AVN will present within 6 months to 2 years of injury, so

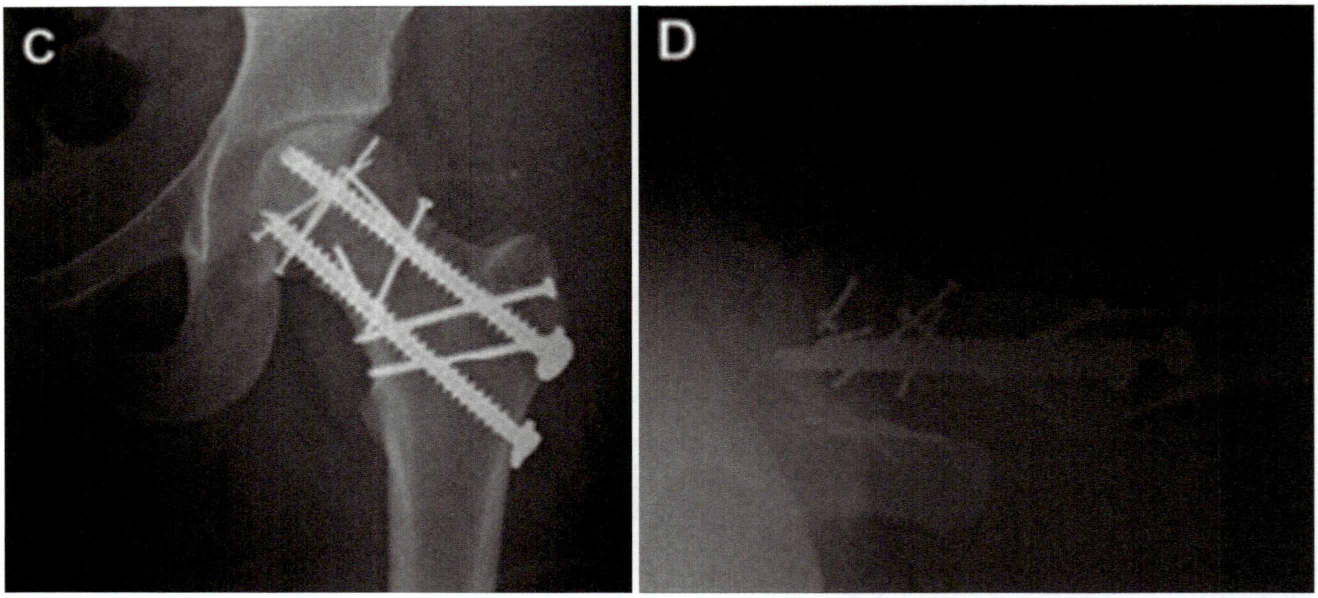

Fig. 13.9 AP and cross-table radiographs of a left sided femoral head fracture-dislocation with an associated femoral neck fracture treated with cannulated screws for the femoral neck and small-fragment screws for the femoral head (*Fig. 1C & 1D in Ross, James R., and Michael J. Gardner. 2012. "Femoral Head Fractures." Current Reviews in Musculoskeletal Medicine 5 (3): 199–205.* https://doi.org/10.1007/s12178-012-9129-8)

close post-operative monitoring is recommended [49]. Advanced imaging such as dynamic MRI (Fig. 13.10) or single-photon emission computerized tomography (SPECT) can be used if there is clinical concern [50]. Titanium implants facilitate MRI follow-up studies for femoral head viability [51].

13.3.7 Heterotopic Ossification

HO is also a common sequelae of injury and surgical treatment, with a reported incidence of 6–64% [22–26]. The posterior approach, especially when associated with acetabular fixation, carries a higher rate of HO, a likely consequence of the extensive stripping of the gluteal muscles off the ilium. HO can significantly reduce the range of motion, a major concern in athletes hoping to return to sport. Indomethacin can be used prophylactically for 6 weeks post-operatively. Prophylactic radiation therapy is also an option, but not in a young population [44].

13.3.7.1 Sciatic Neurapraxia

Sciatic nerve neurapraxia is another complication that could be particularly devastating for athletes. There is a higher reported incidence with associated posterior hip disloca-

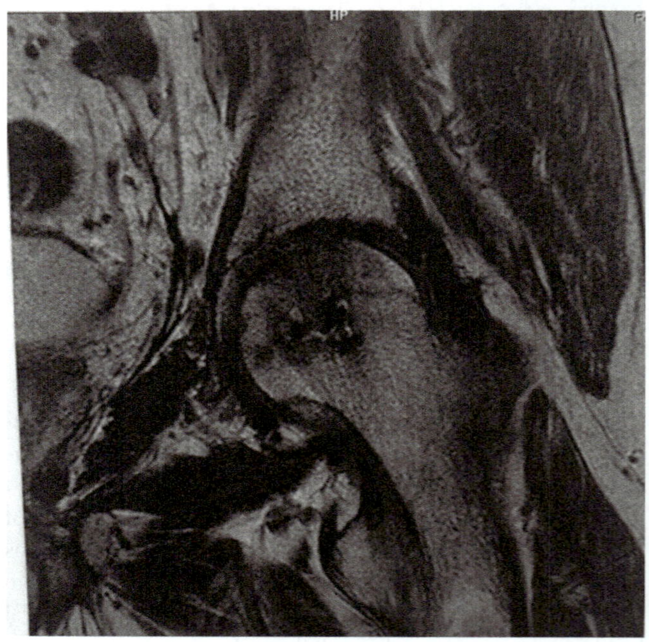

Fig. 13.10 Coronal MRI 9 months after a posterior hip dislocation showing AVN of the femoral head (*Fig. 4.12, page 40. In Egol, Kenneth, and Philipp Leucht, eds. 2017. Proximal Femur Fractures An Evidence-Based Approach to Evaluation and Management. Cham: Springer*)

tions, ranging from 10% to 23% [21–23]. The peroneal division of the sciatic nerve is most often affected. There is spontaneous recovery in 60–70% of patients, [52] so it is important to have accurate documentation of the clinical examination findings throughout the peri-operative period.

13.3.7.2 Arthritis

In the long term, femoral head fractures are associated with high rates of post-traumatic arthritis and degenerative joint disease secondary to joint incongruity and initial cartilage damage from the injury [21–23, 26, 28].

13.3.8 Rehabilitation

Patients undergoing ORIF should be prescribed protected weight bearing for 8–12 weeks post-operatively, but can undertake early range of motion (ROM) exercises. Hip flexion >90°, adduction and internal rotation should be restricted for 2 months [19]. Physical therapy should focus on strengthening of the quadriceps and abductors and low impact training such as swimming or cycling [27].

13.4 Femoral Neck Fracture

13.4.1 Epidemiology

Femoral neck fractures in young patients can occur either through high energy trauma causing acute fractures or through repetitive loading causing stress fractures. High energy fractures are less common, but often occur from an axial load with external rotation with the hip in an abducted position [53, 54]. These patients have a higher incidence of basicervical and more distal femoral neck fractures compared to the subcapital pattern often seen in geriatric patients [1]. These distal fractures tend to be more vertically oriented, and therefore more unstable: this has implications for optimal reduction and fixation techniques [55–57]. Urgent reduction is required to preserve the blood supply to femoral neck and avoid AVN of the femoral head, as described in the previous section [54].

Stress fractures of the femoral neck are more common than acute traumatic fractures in athletes, especially in female athletes and sports requiring repetitive loading such as distance running, dancing and gymnastics [58]. They occur through fatigue with excessive, repetitive strain leading to microscopic fractures that outpace the bones ability to remodel, progressing to macroscopic cracks and eventually propagating to fractures if not identified and treated promptly [59]. Even without propagation, femoral stress fractures can cause much morbidity, often with delayed diagnosis, lingering pain and significant impact on return to sport [59].

Stress fractures constitute 1–20% of athletic injuries seen in Sports Medicine clinics, of which approximately 3–33% are in the femur [58, 60, 61]. Stress fractures are generally associated with sudden increases in training volume or intensity, low baseline bone density, amenorrhea, calcium deficiency, low levels of physical fitness and poor biomechanics. The female athlete triad of osteoporosis, amenorrhea and low energy availability is classically linked with femoral stress fractures, [62] though all high-intensity athletes are at risk.

13.4.2 Classification

The Pauwels classification [55] is useful to distinguish the more vertically oriented acute femoral neck fractures seen in young patients (Fig. 13.11) [63]. Type III fractures are the least stable and most difficult to treat. The Garden classification is also used to describe whether the fracture is complete and displaced or not [64]. The traditional Garden classification has four types, but commonly this has been simplified to two types, non-displaced and displaced, which are most important to plan management [65].

Femoral stress fractures occur mostly commonly in the femoral neck, and more rarely in the trochanteric region or shaft. The mechanical axis of the leg is typically medial to the femoral neck, so repetitive strain leads to compression type fracture on the inferior-medial side and tension fractures on the superior-lateral side (Fig. 13.12). Superolateral neck fractures are considered at high risk, and are associated with more complications because of the tenuous blood supply to the femoral head. Fracture location and the extent of involvement of the femoral neck have been used to classify these injuries and guide treatment (Table 13.3) [59].

13.4.3 Diagnosis

13.4.3.1 Physical Exam

Young patients with displaced femoral neck fracture present with a shortened, flexed and externally rotated lower extremity with localized pain and inability to bear weight. Patients with non-displaced fractures may be able to walk, but with groin pain and limitation of motion. There is usually pain with hip rotation.

Athletes with stress fractures typically present with insidious onset of pain in the anterior thigh, groin or ipsilateral

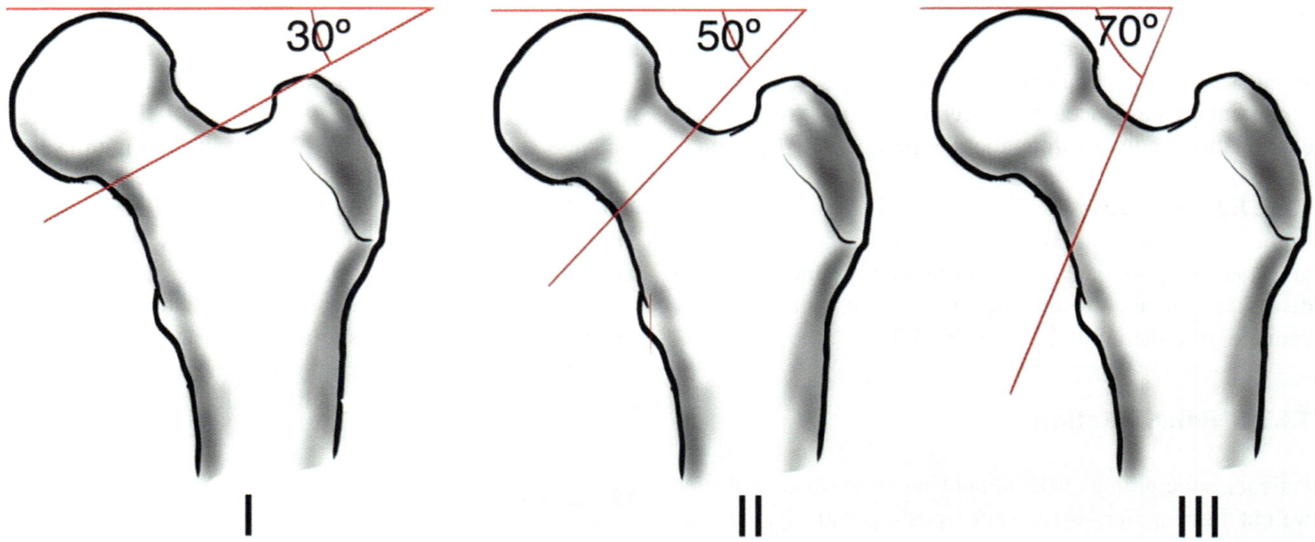

Fig. 13.11 Pauwels classification of femoral neck fractures: type I obliquity of the fracture line 0–30°; type II obliquity 30–50°; type III obliquity >70° (*Fig. 68.1 in Peter Giannoudis, and Nikolaos Kanakaris. 2014. "Femoral Neck Fractures." In Trauma and Orthopaedic Classification, edited by Nick Lasanioanos, 305–308. Springer*)

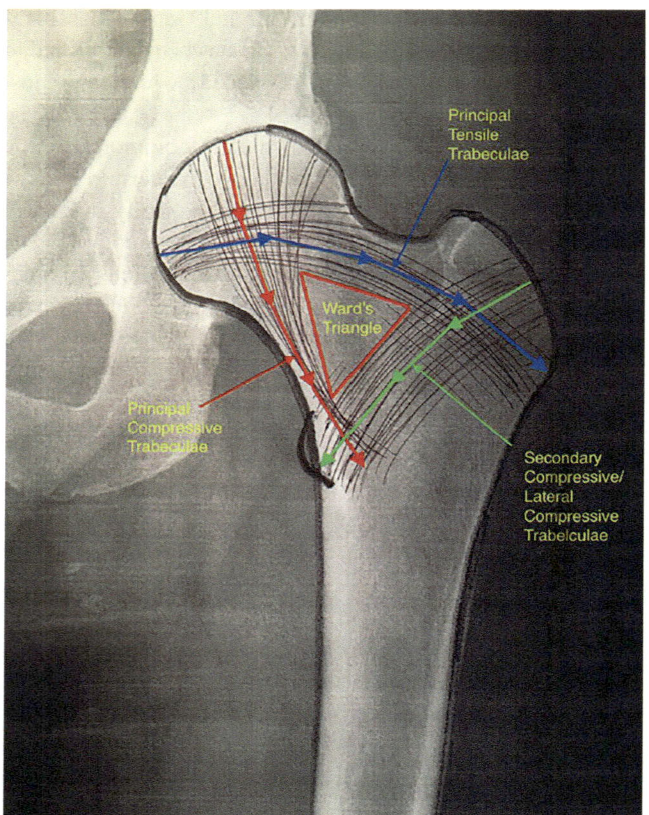

Fig. 13.12 AP radiograph demonstrating the principal compression and tension trabecular of the proximal femur (*Fig. 1.3, page 5, in Egol, Kenneth, and Philipp Leucht, eds. 2017. Proximal Femur Fractures An Evidence-Based Approach to Evaluation and Management. Cham: Springer*)

Table 13.3 Femoral neck stress fracture classification system and treatment recommendations

Type	MRI/radiographic features	Treatment
Compression	No visible fracture	Nonsurgical
	<50%	Nonsurgical
	>50%	Surgical
Tension	Any	Individually based decision
Displaced	Any	Emergent surgical fixation

Adapted from page 115 from Marc Haro, Julia Bruene, Kathleen Weber, and Bernard Bach. 2015. "Stress Fractures of the Femur." In Stress Fractures in Athletes; Diagnosis and Management, edited by Timothy Miller and Christopher Kaeding, 111–24. New York: Springer

knee. The pain is worse with high impact activity and relieved with activity cessation. These athletes often may present with remarkably few positive findings at clinical examination, with no swelling and good muscle tone and strength. They may have an antalgic gait and tenderness directly over the femoral neck or with log roll, extreme range of motion and straight leg raise [66]. The 'hop test', where the athlete hops repeatedly on the symptomatic leg, has a high sensitivity, but low specificity for identifying lower extremity stress fractures. A test is considered positive if the athletes is unable to perform repeated hops or reports worsening, localized groin or femoral shaft pain [67].

13.4.3.2 Imaging

Plain radiographs, including AP pelvis and AP and cross-table lateral of the hip, are usually sufficient to diagnose acute displaced femoral neck fractures (Fig. 13.13). In patients with a high index of suspicion and negative radiographs, advanced imaging may be necessary. MRI is more

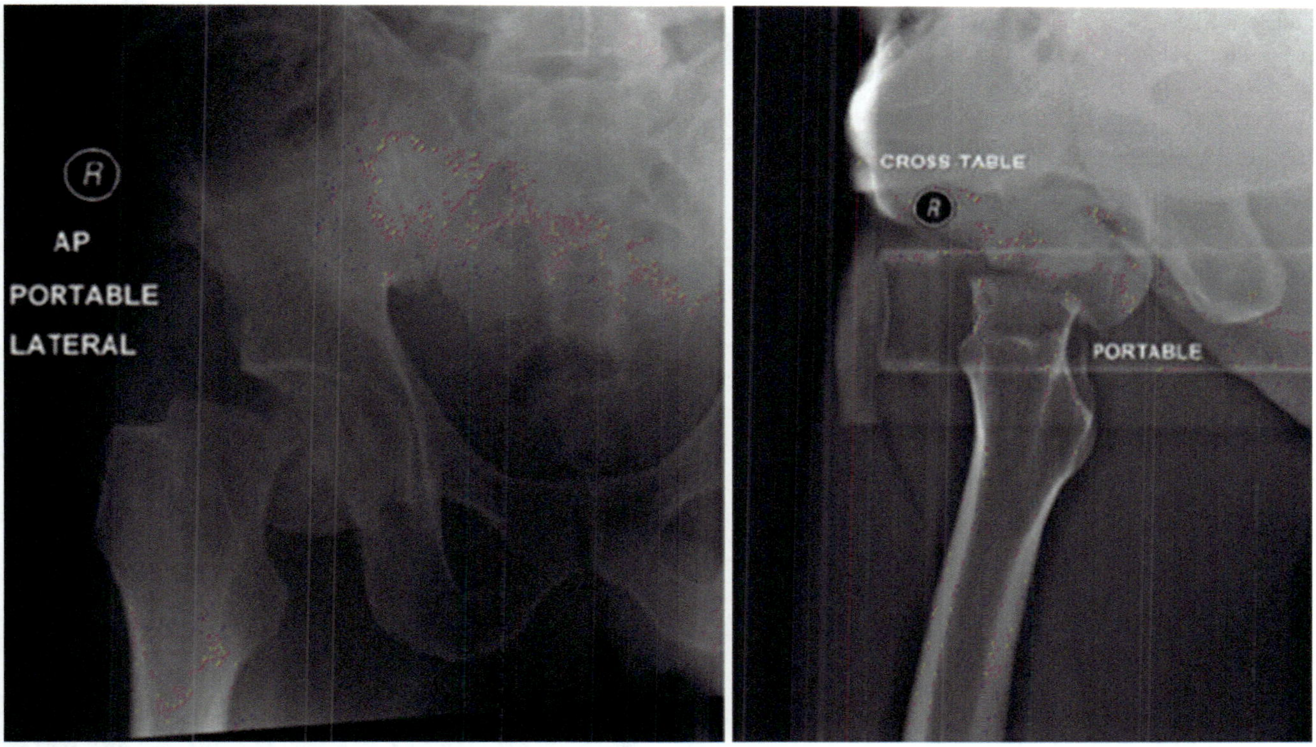

Fig. 13.13 AP and cross-table lateral radiographs of a right hip showing a displaced femoral neck fracture [143] (*Fig. 1 In Makhni, M. 2017. "Femoral Neck Fractures." In Orthopedic Emergencies, edited by Eric Swart and Charles Day, 285. Springer*)

sensitive to diagnose occult hip fractures compared to CT, [68] and limits radiation, an important consideration in young athletes [69].

Stress fractures may appear normal during the early stage of injury (up to 4 weeks), but later findings include linear lucency, periosteal reaction and sclerotic cortical changes at the fracture site (Fig. 13.14). MRI has increased sensitivity and specificity to diagnose subtle fracture lines and to better asses the percentage involvement of the femoral neck in both acute and stress fractures (Fig. 13.15) [70]. Given the high risk of complications associated with delayed diagnosis, MRI should be considered for athletes with persistent femoral pain for greater than 2 weeks without an obvious source. Bone scans have good sensitivity, but poor specificity compared to MRI, and have associated radiation exposure which may be a concern in younger athletes [71]. Laboratory studies are not necessary for diagnosis, but may help explain the etiology of suspected insufficiency fractures.

13.4.4 Treatment

13.4.4.1 Acute Traumatic Femoral Neck Fractures

There is a very limited role for nonoperative management of acute traumatic femoral neck fractures in athletes. Even nondisplaced fractures are associated with higher complication and increased displacement rates [72]. Urgent reduction of displaced fractures is required to preserve blood supply to the femoral head, with recommendation for reduction within 8–12 h of injury [54, 73]. However, anatomic reduction is the most reliable predictor of AVN, so waiting for an experienced surgeon may trump urgent surgery [3, 74]. Prior to surgery, the leg should be left in the shortened and externally rotated position to decrease the intracapsular pressure [75].

Closed Reduction

Fluoroscopically assisted closed reduction should be attempted first starting with the hip in 45° of flexion and slight abduction, then extending the internally rotating the leg with gentle axial traction. If anatomic reduction is obtained on orthogonal and oblique views, percutaneous fixation with cannulated screws is an option. This can be combined with a fluoroscopically assisted joint aspiration [76] or anterior capsulotomy through a small laterally based skin incision to decrease the intracapsular pressure [77]. This theoretically helps restore blood flow to the femoral head, though there is limited clinical outcome data regarding this. We do not recommend routine capsulotomy to decrease the intracapsular pressure.

Open Approach

If the reduction is not anatomic, there should be a low threshold for open reduction, especially in young athletes [78].

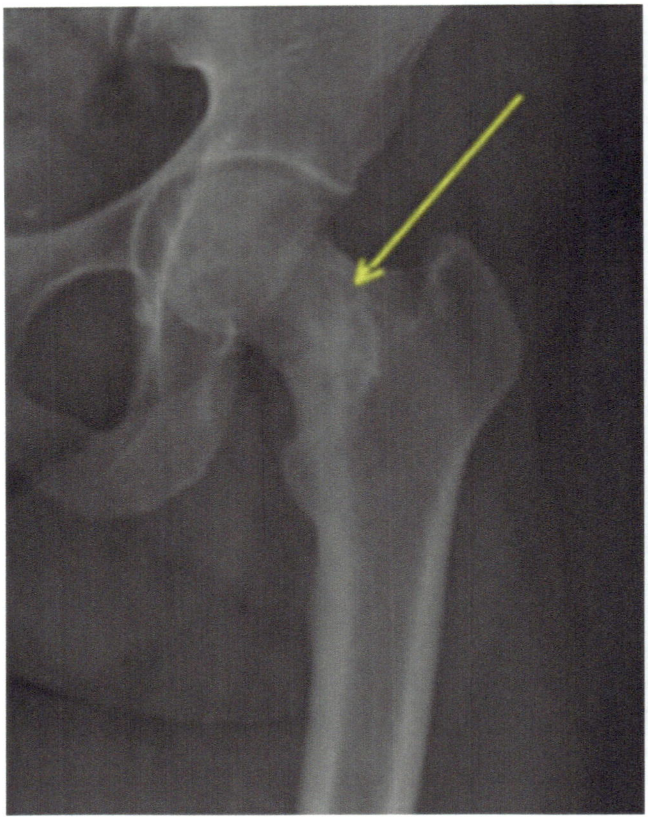

Fig. 13.14 Plain radiographs showing a compression side stress fracture of the inferomedial femoral neck. Note the linear lucency, periosteal reaction and sclerotic cortical changes at the fracture site (*Fig. 8.3 on page 114 of. Marc Haro, Julia Bruene, Kathleen Weber, and Bernard Bach. 2015. "Stress Fractures of the Femur." In Stress Fractures in Athletes; Diagnosis and Management, edited by Timothy Miller and Christopher Kaeding, 111–24. New York: Springer*)

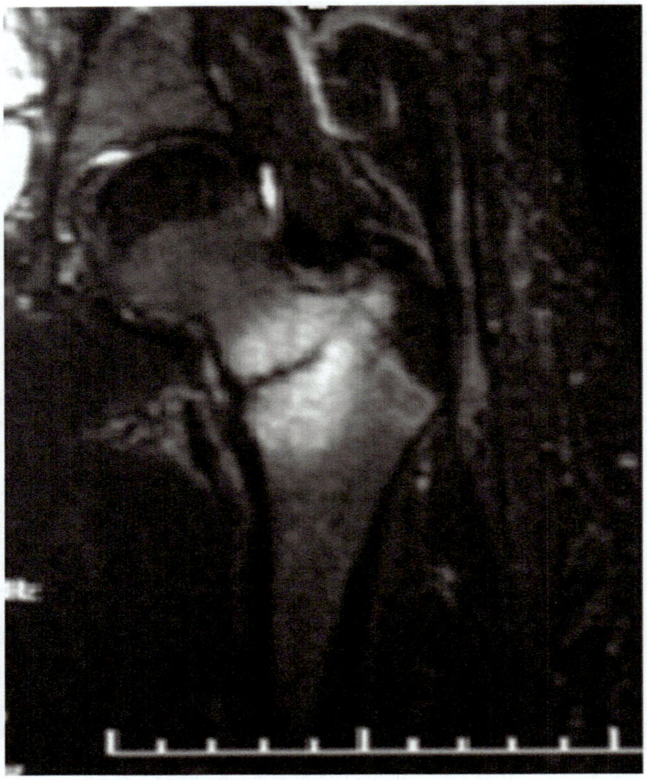

Fig. 13.15 Coronal T2 MRI showing near complete propagation of a compression sided femoral stress fracture (*Fig. 8.4 on page 115 of Marc Haro, Julia Bruene, Kathleen Weber, and Bernard Bach. 2015. "Stress Fractures of the Femur." In Stress Fractures in Athletes; Diagnosis and Management, edited by Timothy Miller and Christopher Kaeding, 111–24. New York: Springer*)

Open reduction is recommended through a two-incision approach [79]. An anterior modified Smith-Petersen approach [47] is used to expose the fracture and femoral head [45], and a second, small lateral incision is used for placement of either cannulated screws or a sliding hip screw with a short plate.

Fracture Reduction

Fracture reduction can be aided through a variety of common techniques including pointed reduction clamps, Schanz pins or large (2 mm) guide pins in the femoral neck to act as joysticks and provisional reconstruction plates. For unstable vertical fractures, often seen in high energy fractures, it is important to obtain anatomic reduction of the inferior/medial spike to improve stability and decrease displacement risk [80].

Fracture Fixation

Cannulated screw fixation is an option for transcervical fractures. Two or three parallel or divergent 6.5–7.3 mm screws placed perpendicular to the fracture site in an inverted triangle provides optimal stability and compression (Fig. 13.16) [1]. The screw insertion sites below the level of the lesser trochanter lead to stress risers that increase the risk of subtrochanteric femur fractures [81]. In high risk-patterns, such as Pauwels type III, a screw and side plate can be used [82] with the option for a medial buttress plate for supplementary fixation [83].

Fixed angle constructs such as sliding hip screws may offer increased biomechanical stability in Pauwels type III or basicervical fractures, [84] with fewer complications than cannulated screws, [85], especially when combined with an antirotation screw (Fig. 13.18) [86]. However, it is unclear whether there is a clinical difference in stability or return to function, and this approach does require a larger lateral dissection [56]. Newer femoral neck specific fixation systems

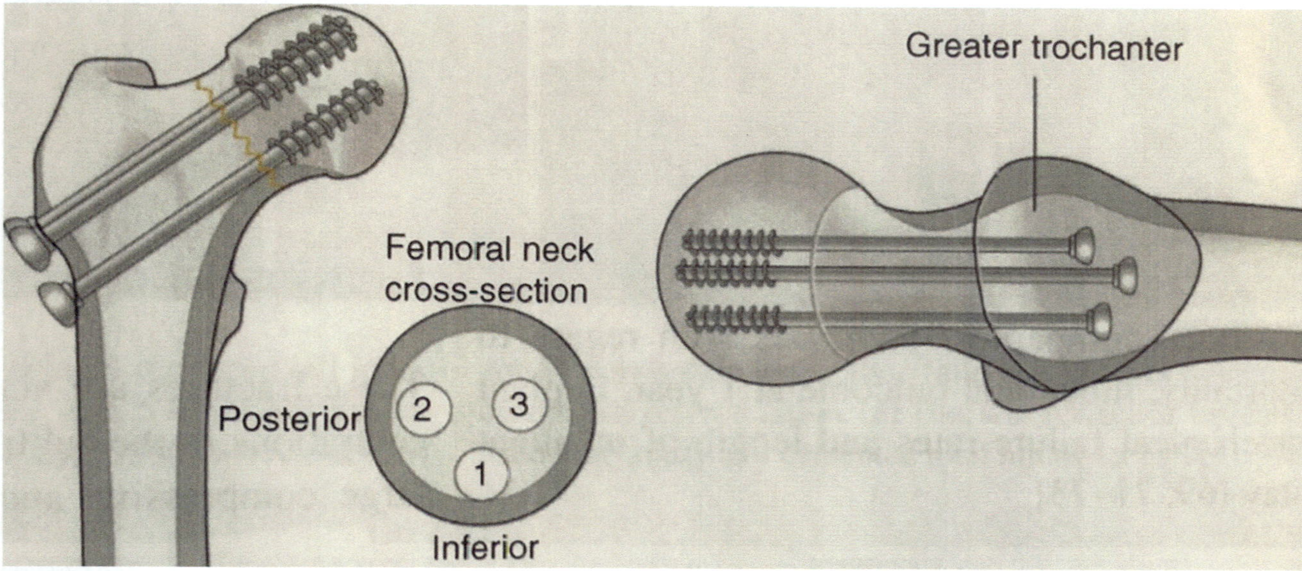

Fig. 13.16 Recommended configuration of cannulated screws for treatment of femoral neck fractures (*Fig. 5.3, page 53. In Egol, Kenneth, and Philipp Leucht, eds. 2017. Proximal Femur Fractures An Evidence-Based Approach to Evaluation and Management. Cham: Springer*)

have recently been developed with similar biomechanical properties, but clinical data are still limited for these implants. (Fig. 13.17).

With ipsilateral femoral shaft fractures, the authors recommending fixing the femoral neck first with a sliding hip screw if the neck is displaced, followed by fixing the shaft with a retrograde nail. A single antegrade implant may be used if the neck component is non displaced.

Acute arthroplasty is a reliable and effective treatment option for geriatric patients with femoral neck fractures, [38] but is not a good option for young, high demand athletes. It remains a salvage procedure when fixation fails or post traumatic complications occur.

13.5 Peritrochanteric Fractures

13.5.1 Epidemiology

Peritrochanteric fractures, including intertrochanteric and subtrochanteric fractures, in young patients usually result from high energy trauma, and are often associated with other injuries. Operative treatment, especially in young athletes, is indicated. These fractures are extra-capsular, so there is less immediate threat to the bloody supply of the femoral head. Therefore, urgent reduction is less essential, but surgery should still be performed as soon as the patient is stable, within 24–48 h [87]. Considering the high energy nature of these injuries, closed reduction is often difficult, and there is a high complication rate [88].

Though not discussed in detail here, intertrochanteric stress fractures are also seen in endurance athletes. Work-up and treatment is similar to femoral neck stress fractures described above and in the 'Stress Fractures' section of this book. In these fractures, a short dynamic hip screw is indicated, and the use of cannulated screws is proscribed.

13.5.2 Classification

Extracapsular peritrochanteric fractures can be classified according to the Modified Evans classification [89] (Fig. 13.18). In general terms, intertrochanteric fractures can be categorized as 'stable' or 'unstable'. The pertinent fracture characteristics that make a fracture unstable include the presence of posterior medical comminution (Type IV), reverse obliquity (Type IV), subtrochanteric extension of the fracture, and whether the lateral wall of the trochanter is intact or not.

Subtrochanteric fractures have traditionally been classified using the Russell and Taylor classification, which distinguishes fractures based on involvement of the lesser trochanter (medial calcar) and the greater trochanter (piriformis fossa).(Fig. 13.19) [90, 91]. Historically, this classification was used to differentiate fractures that could be treated with intramedullary nailing (IMN) (type I) versus those that needed ORIF with screw and plate devices or fixed-angle constructs. However, with modern cephalomedullary nails, this hard distinction may be less relevant, and the use of cephalomedullary nails is more prevalent.

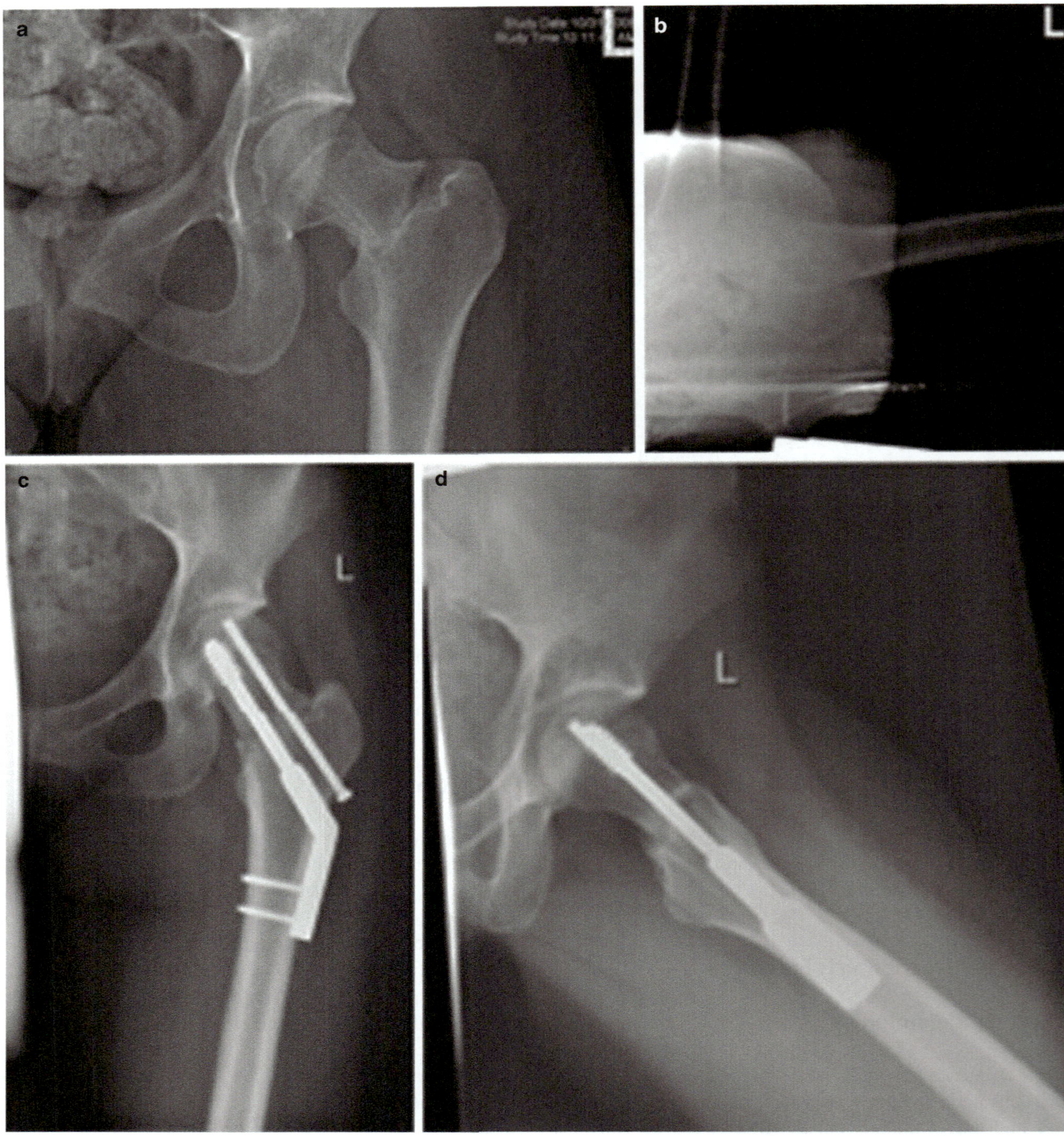

Fig. 13.17 (**a**, **b**) Anteror-posterior (AP) and cross-table lateral radiographs of a displaced femoral neck fracture at time of injury. (**c**, **d**) AP and frog-leg lateral views 6 weeks status post treatment with sliding hip screw and antirotation screw

13.5.3 Diagnosis

13.5.3.1 Physical Exam

The clinical exam will be similar to femoral neck fractures with acute pain and inability to bear weight. The injured leg will often be shortened and externally rotated if displaced.

13.5.3.2 Imaging

Standard AP pelvis and AP and cross-table lateral hip radiographs are required. Full length femur films are also indicated to look for associated injuries and to assess the inner diameter of the intramedullary canal and the antecurvature of the femur [92]. Traction-internal rotation radio-

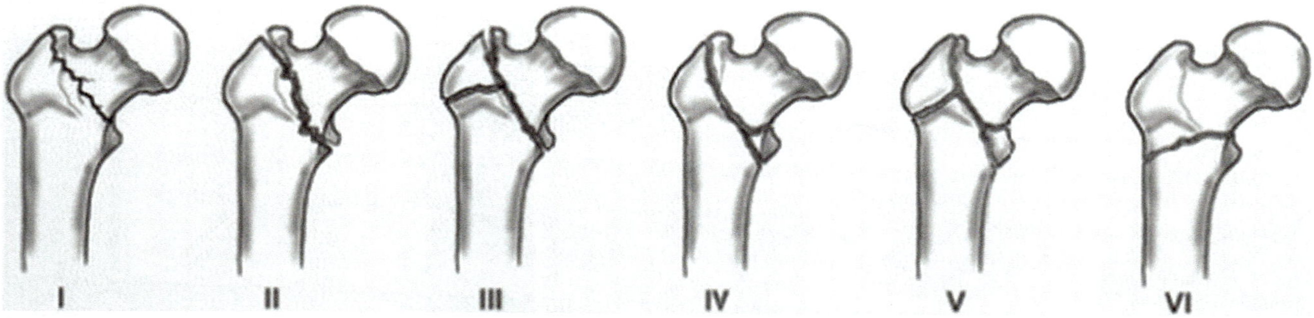

Fig. 13.18 Modified-Evans classification of intertrochanteric fractures. Type I-non-displaced 2-part; Type II-displaced 2-part; Type III-displaced 3-part fracture with posterolateral comminution; Type IV-displaced 3-part with posteromedial comminution; Type V-displaced 4-part fracture with comminution involving both trochanters; Type VI-reverse obliquity (Fig. 70.1 *in Nick Lasanioanos and Nikolaos Kanakaris. 2014. "Intertrochanteric Hip Fractures." In Trauma and Orthopaedic Classification, edited by Nick Lasanioanos, 305–308. Springer)*

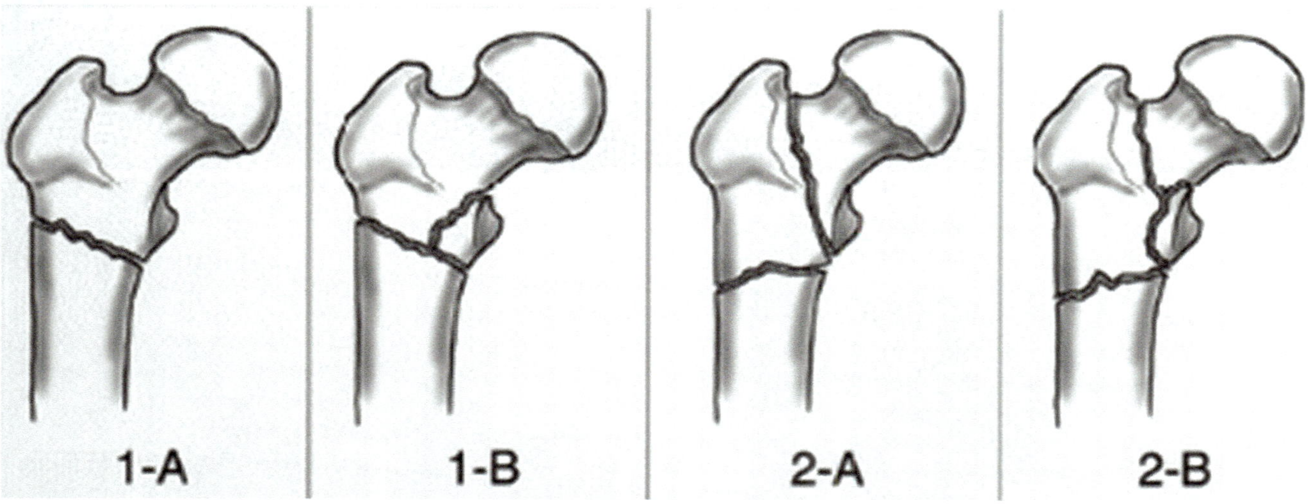

Fig. 13.19 Russell-Taylor classification of subtrochanteric fractures. Type IA—does not involve piriformis fossa below the lesser trochanter; Type IB—does not involve the piriformis fossa but does involve lesser trochanter; Type IIA—involving the piriformis fossa and stable medial buttress; Type IIB—involves piriformis fossa and the medial femoral cortex (*Fig. 71.1 in Kanakaris, Nikolaos, and P. V. Giannoudis. 2015. "Subtrochanteric Fractures." In Trauma and Orthopaedic Classifications, edited by N Lasanioanos, N.K. Kanakaris, and P.V. Giannoudis, 317–19. London: Springer)*

graphs may also be useful to help correctly identify the fracture pattern, which can impact surgical planning and implant choice (Fig. 13.20) [93]. The surrounding muscles origin and insertion sites lead to classic radiographic presentation, with the proximal fragment being abducted (glute medius and minimus), flexed (iliopsoas) and externally rotated (short external rotators), and the distal fragment being abducted and shortened (adductors). If there is high clinical suspicion for fracture despite negative radiographs, MRI or CT help to rule out occult fracture [94, 95] (Fig. 13.21). Again, MRI can limit radiation in young athletes [69].

13.5.4 Treatment

Virtually all peritrochanteric fractures require surgical reduction and fixation as soon as the patient is stable, especially in young athletes.

13.5.4.1 Intertrochanteric Fractures-Cephalomedullary Nail vs. Sliding Hip Screw

There is debate about the optimal implant for intertrochanteric fractures, but the general consensus is that stable fractures can be treated effectively with either a sliding hip screw or cephalomedullary nail [94, 96–98].

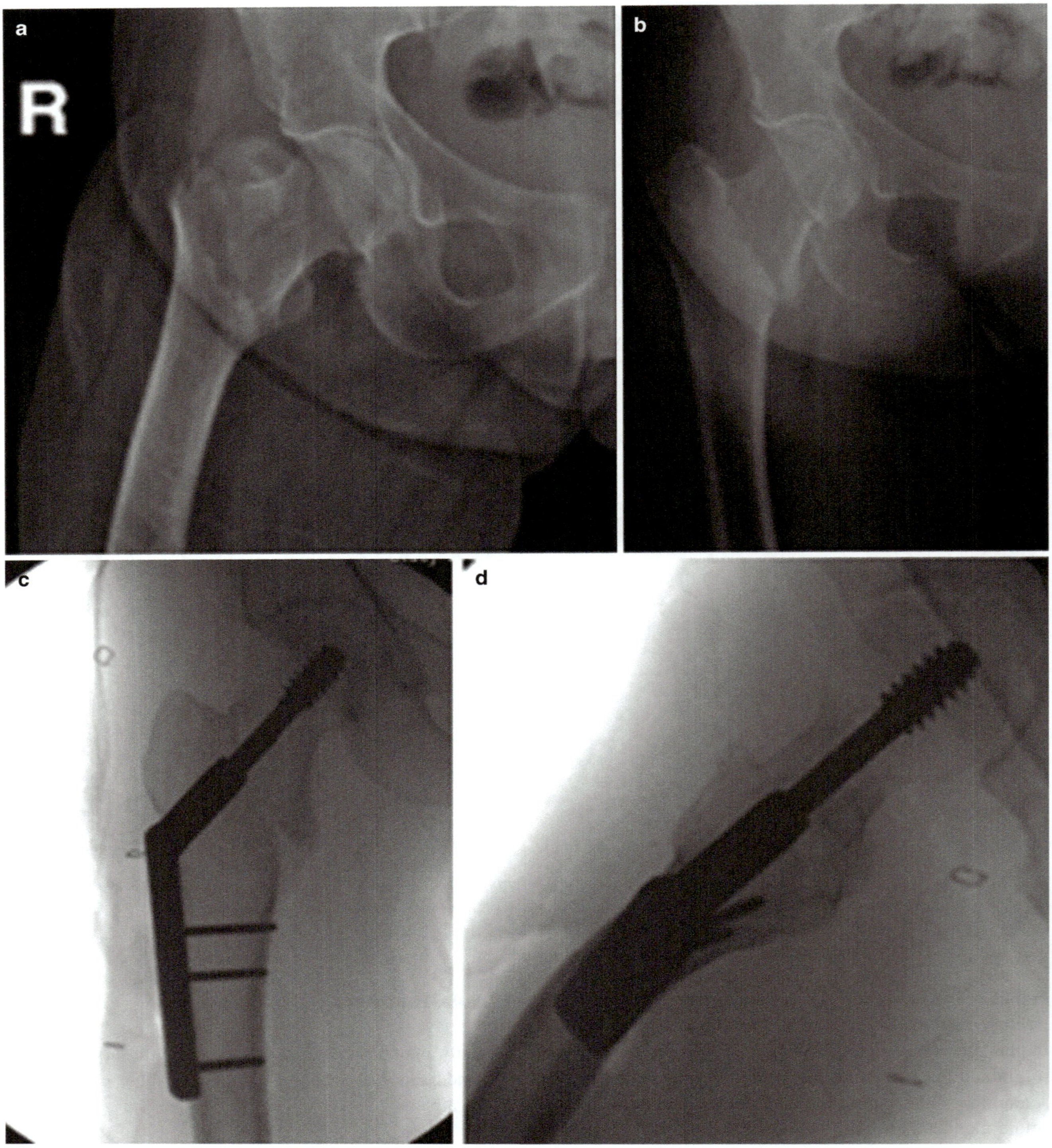

Fig. 13.20 A&B: AP and traction internal rotation view of the right hip, better characterizing the integrity of the lateral wall. C&D: Treatment with a sliding hip screw

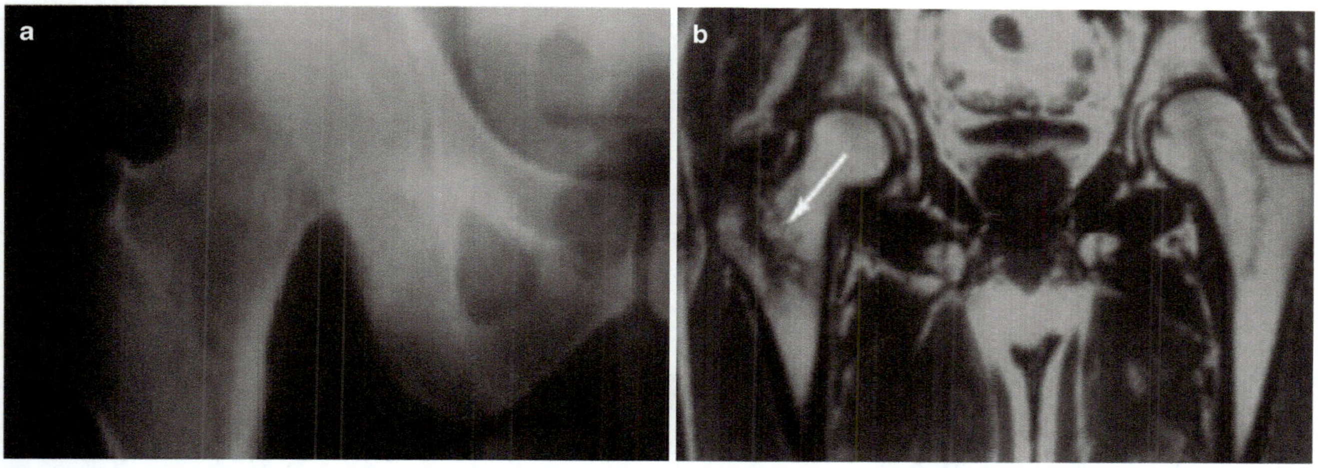

Fig. 13.21 (**a**) AP X-ray of R hip. (**b**) Coronal slice pelvic MRI. The MRI shows an occult right intertrochanteric femur fracture not visualized on plain films [144] (*Fig. 81 a & b in. Manninger, J, and K Fekete. 2007. "Diagnostic Investigations." In Internal Fixation of Femoral Neck Fractures, edited by J. Manninger, U Bosch, P. Cserháti, K Fekete, and G Kazar. Vienna: Springer*)

Sliding hip screws allow for secondary impaction of the fracture along the axis of the gliding hip screw (Fig. 13.22). Central placement of the guide wire is necessary to ensure impaction occurs along the proper trajectory, so it is important to check this on multiple views intra-operatively. An anti-rotation screw can be added parallel to the lag screw to provide increased rotational stability. In stable patterns with an intact lateral wall, even those with posteromedial comminution, sliding hip screws have shown equivalent long-term functional outcomes compared to cephalomedullary nails for stable patters with an intact lateral wall, including those with posteromedial comminution [99, 100]. Cephalomedullary nails allow superior early mobility, which may be important for athletes [100]. However, most studies focus on the geriatric population, with limited clinical data comparing the biomechanical outcomes or return to sport of these approaches in athletes specifically. For athletes specifically, sliding hip screws require dissection of the vastus lateralis, which is important for knee extension and stabilization, while cephalomedullary nails require entry through the hip abductors (see Sect. 6 for discussion on piriformis vs. lateral entry nails).

For unstable fractures, including reverse obliquity posteromedial comminution, extension into the lateral wall, with subtrochanteric extension, treatment with a sliding hip screw is contraindicated because of the risk of excessive sliding and shortening (Fig. 13.22). Treatment with an intramedullary nail is recommended in these fracture configurations [101–103]. By shortening the lever arm of force affecting the medial calcar region, intramedullary systems nearly double the failure resistance compared to extramedullary devices (Fig. 13.23) [104, 105]. There is no difference in complications or hardware failure in short vs. long nails for trochanteric fractures, but these are not specific to young, active patients [106, 107] athletes.

13.5.4.2 Subtrochanteric Fractures

Locked intramedullary nailing is the gold standard for fixation of acute subtrochanteric femur fractures [108]. Compared to plates and screws, intramedullary nails have increased stiffness and rigidity and better resist the deforming forces of medialization from the adductor muscles [109–111]. In young patients with healthy bone, a reconstruction type intramedullary nail with a smaller diameter can be used. Two smaller screws into the femoral neck provide rotational stability of the proximal fragment while avoiding a large screw tract [108] (Fig. 13.24).

Common pitfalls in treatment of subtrochanteric fractures include varus malreduction, rotational malreduction and leg length discrepancy, [108] all of which could be particularly concerning for athletes returning to high level activity. With the importance of anatomic reduction for athletes, surgeons should have a low threshold to move to open reduction techniques in fractures difficult to reduce, as this improves reduction quality in young patients with high energy injuries [112].

13.5.5 Complications

For intertrochanteric fractures, the most common complication is lag screw cut-out, often attributed to inadequate reduction and subsequent malposition of the femoral neck screw into the anterior-superior quadrant [105]. In addition to mal-reduction, tip-apex distance greater than 25 mm has also been associated with higher rates of lag screw cut out [113]. Femoral neck blades (instead of a screw) can decrease the rate of proximal cutout.

Non-union and malunion are two of the most common complications of subtrochanteric IMN, both of which can

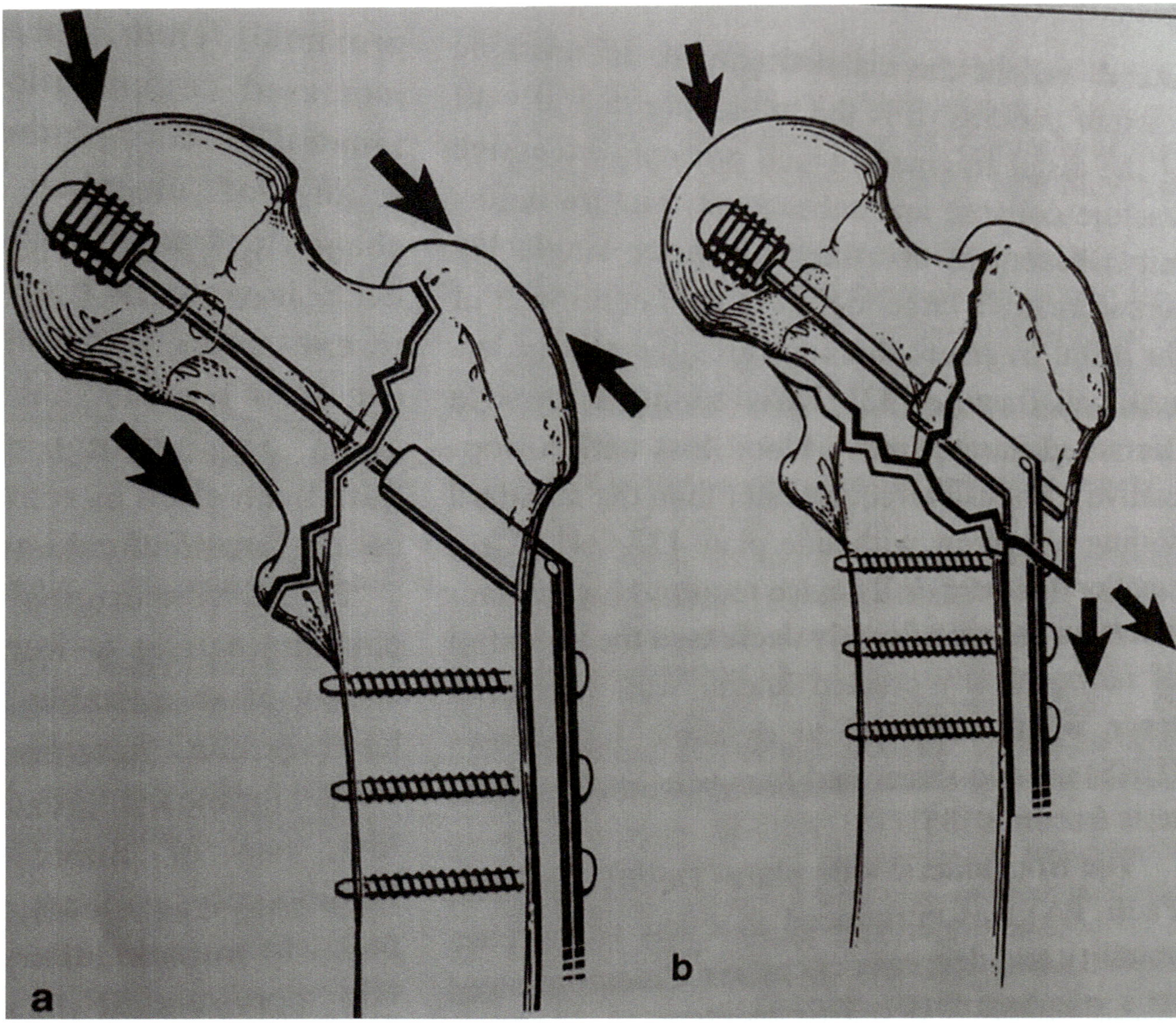

Fig. 13.22 (**a**) Illustration of standard obliquity intertrochanteric fracture treated with a sliding hip screw perpendicular to the fracture, allowing for compression. (**b**) Reverse obliquity fractures are not suitable to sliding hip screws because compression along the axis of the screw will lead to medialization of the shaft and significant shortening (*Fig. 7.3, page 81 in In Egol, Kenneth, and Philipp Leucht, eds. 2017. Proximal Femur Fractures An Evidence-Based Approach to Evaluation and Management. Cham: Springer*)

typically be traced back to non-anatomic reduction in an otherwise healthy young patient. External rotation malunion can be particularly problematic because it shifts the weight-bearing axis posteriorly, altering gait mechanics [114].

13.5.6 Rehabilitation

IMN are length stable constructs, so most younger patients without confounding injuries can normally be allowed to weight bear at tolerated (WBAT) immediately, even with comminuted fractures. Rehabilitation should focus on early mobilization, abductor strengthening and gait training.

13.6 Femoral Diaphysis Fracture

13.6.1 Epidemiology

Femoral diaphyseal fractures in athletes are associated with high-energy trauma with axial loading, torsional forces or direct trauma to the femoral shaft. As with proximal femoral fractures, health care professional must have a high suspicion for concomitant injuries, specifically ipsilateral femoral neck fractures. These injuries are more common in high impact sports such as ice hockey, football, rugby and motor sports like NASCAR and motocross.

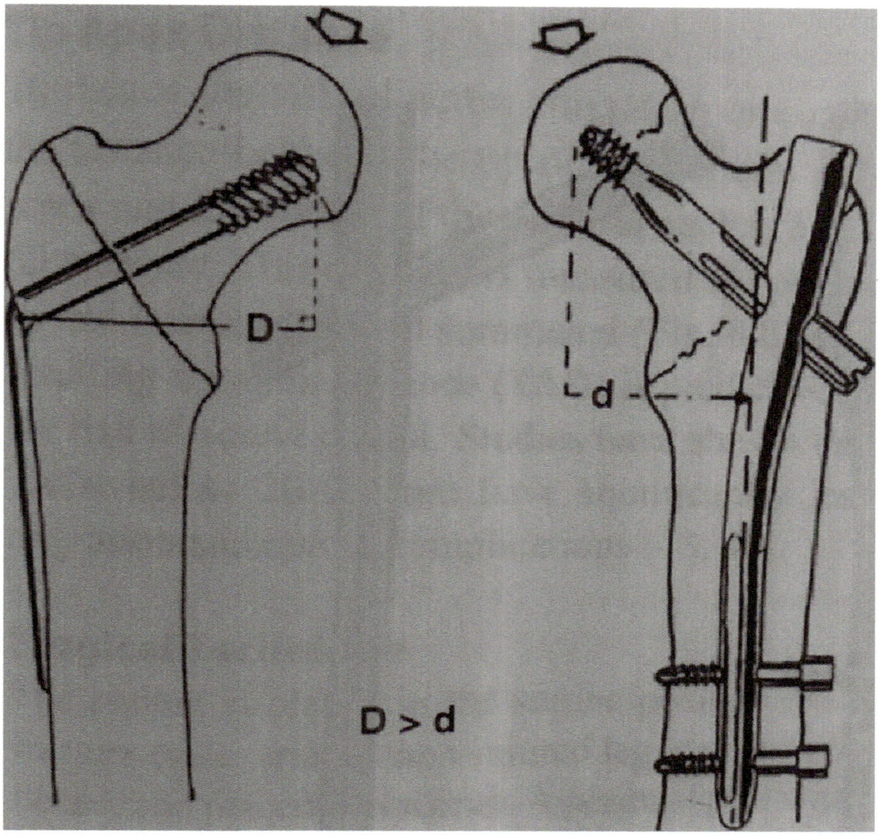

Fig. 13.23 Illustrations comparing the shorter lever arm in extramedullary fixation (left) versus intramedullary fixation (right) (Fig. 8.5, page 91 in *In Egol, Kenneth, and Philipp Leucht, eds. 2017. Proximal Femur Fractures An Evidence-Based Approach to Evaluation and Management. Cham: Springer*)

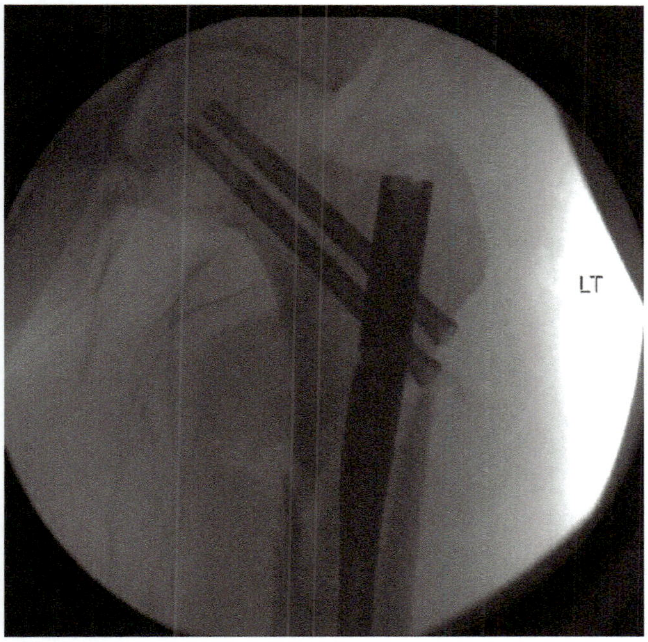

Fig. 13.24 AP radiograph showing treatment of a subtrochanteric femur fracture with an intramedullary recon nail (Fig. 9.2d, page 105 in *In Egol, Kenneth, and Philipp Leucht, eds. 2017. Proximal Femur Fractures An Evidence-Based Approach to Evaluation and Management. Cham: Springer*)

13.6.2 Classification

Diaphyseal fractures can be described using the OTA classification system (Fig. 13.25). The Winquist and Hansen classification system has previously been used to describe the comminution of diaphyseal femur fractures, but with current intramedullary nail (IMN) technology it carries little clinical implications (Fig. 13.26) [115].

13.6.3 Diagnosis

13.6.3.1 Physical Exam

Patients will present acutely, often with gross deformity of the leg. Blood loss in closed femoral shaft fractures can be between 1000 and 1500 ml athletes will often have a tense, swollen thigh [116]. It is important to document whether the injury is open or closed and perform a thorough distal neurovascular exam.

13.6.3.2 Imaging

Standard radiographs include AP and lateral views of the entire femur, as well as the ipsilateral hip and knee. The incidence of associated ipsilateral femoral neck fractures is

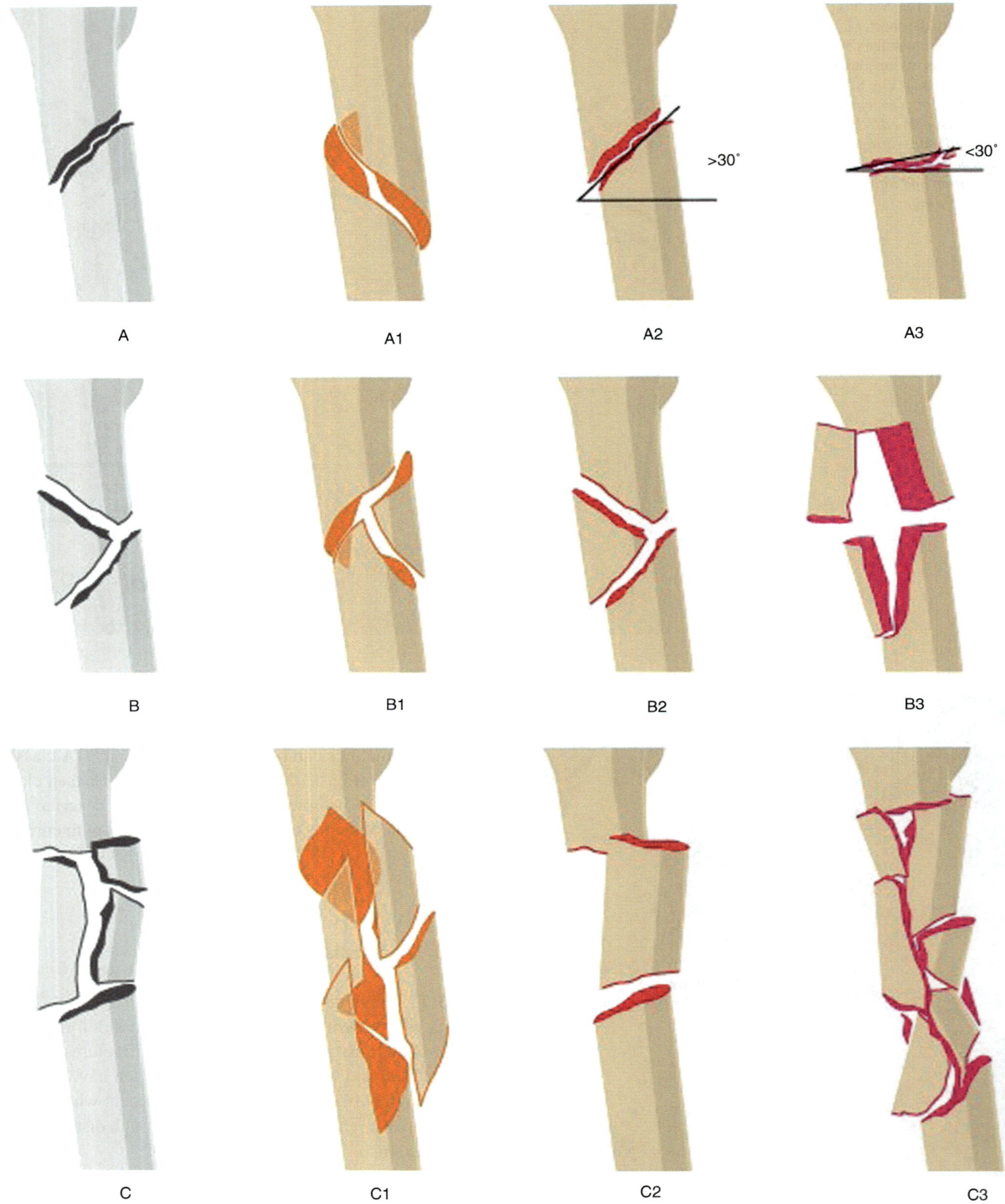

Fig. 13.25 AO/OTA classification of femoral diaphyseal fractures. Group A: Simple fractures; A1: spiral, A2: oblique ($\geq 30°$), A3: transverse ($<30°$). Group B: Wedge fractures; B1: torsion wedge, B2: bending wedge, B3: multifragmentary. Group C: Complex fractures; C1: comminuted spiral, C2: segmental; C3: irregular comminuted (*Fig. 1913.19.3 in from Krettek C., Gösling T. (2015) Femur Diaphysis. In: Rommens P., Hessmann M. (e ds) Intramedullary Nailing. Springer, London*)

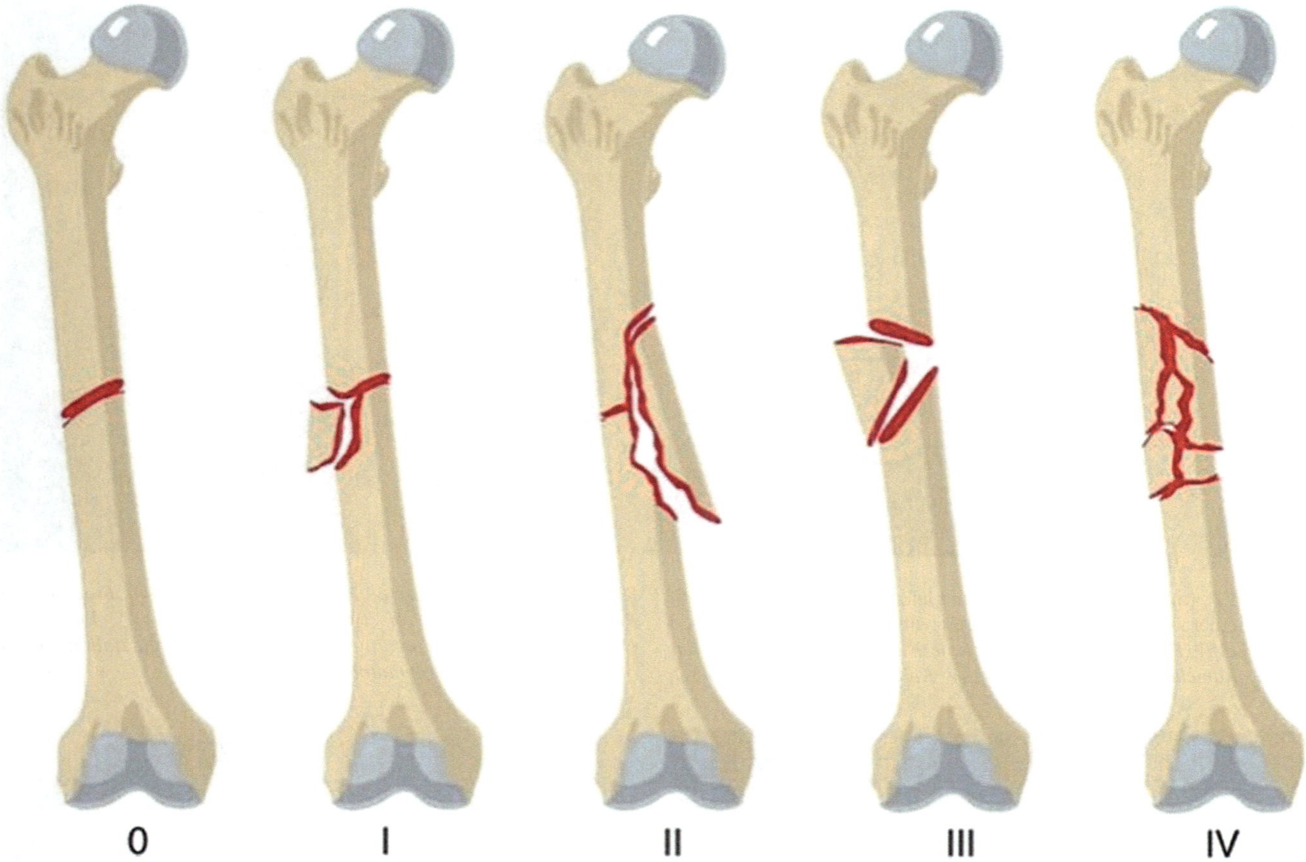

Fig. 13.26 Winquist classification for diaphyseal femur fractures. *Grade 0*: no comminution. *Grade 1*: small wedge fragment or comminution, ≥50% of intact cortical contact. *Grade II:* large wedge or comminution segment, ≥50% of intact cortical contact, *Grade III:* large wedge or comminution, <50% intact cortical contact. *Grade IV*: comminution zone without direct contact between the main fragments (*Fig. 19.3 in from Krettek C., Gösling T. (2015) Femur Diaphysis. In: Rommens P., Hessmann M. (e ds) Intramedullary Nailing. Springer, London)*

between 2% and 6% (Fig. 13.27). The diagnosis of these injuries can be delayed in 19–31% of patients, [117] prompting some institutions to prescribe CT scans and internal rotation AP radiographs a standardized part of their diagnostic protocol for diaphyseal femur fractures [118]. Prompt diagnosis of associated femoral neck fractures is important because it affects surgical management.

13.6.4 Treatment

There is a limited role for non-operative management of acute diaphyseal femoral shaft fractures in athletes, with most requiring urgent surgical fixation. Stabilization within 24 h is associated with decreased complications, decreased hospital length of stay and improved rehabilitation [119]. As in the general population, the gold standard treatment for diaphyseal femur fractures in stable patients is a reamed antegrade IMN [120].

13.6.4.1 Retrograde IMN

The type of IMN may be more relevant in athletes given specific complications associated with the different start sites. Retrograde nails have been associated with more postoperative knee pain, likely from the dissection required to reach the medial femoral condyle start site (Fig. 13.28) [121–123]. When choosing a retrograde nail, it is particularly important to ensure the nail is not prominent, as even 1 mm of prominence can significantly increase the mean contact pressure in the patellofemoral joint, leading to increased pain and delayed rehabilitation. The midline scar has also been associated with kneeling pain. Retrograde nailing is recommended for patients with ipsilateral tibial shaft or acetabular fractures, in patients with bilateral femur fractures, and in patients with ipsilateral femoral neck fractures [124]. With ipsilateral femoral neck fractures, the authors recommending fixing the femoral neck first with a sliding hip screw, then fixing the shaft with a retrograde nail (Figs. 13.29 and 13.30).

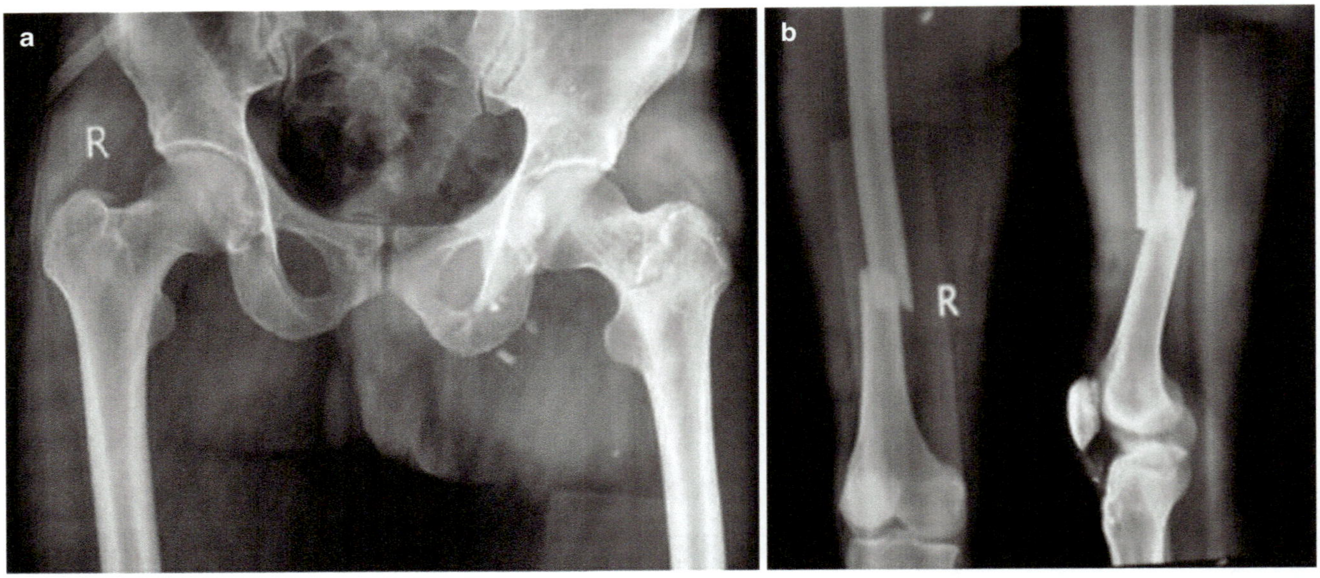

Fig. 13.27 (**a**, **b**) AP pelvis and AP and lateral L femur showing ipsilateral femoral neck and shaft fractures with extension into the distal femur [145] (*Fig. 2 in Singh, Roop, Rajesh Rohilla, Narender Kumar Magu, Ramchander Siwach, Virender Kadian, and Sukhbir Singh Sangwan. 2008. "Ipsilateral Femoral Neck and Shaft Fractures: A Retrospective Analysis of Two Treatment Methods." Journal of Orthopaedics and Traumatology: Official Journal of the Italian Society of Orthopaedics and Traumatology*)

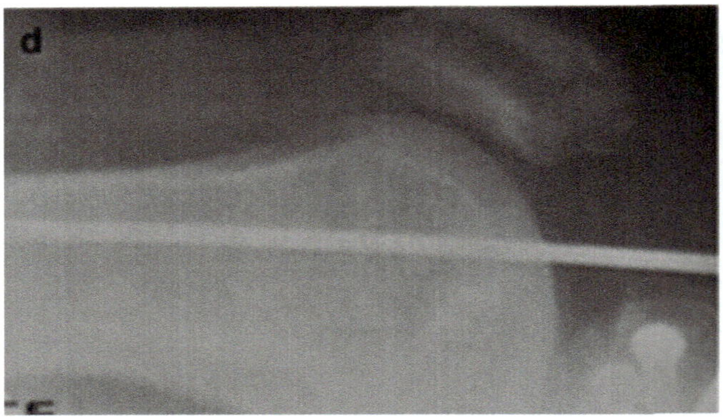

Fig. 13.28 Fluoroscopic lateral start site for retrograde IMN. It is important to be anterior to Blumensaat's line (*Fig. 19.36 from Krettek C., Gösling T. (2015) Femur Diaphysis. In: Rommens P., Hessmann M. (eds) Intramedullary Nailing. Springer, London*)

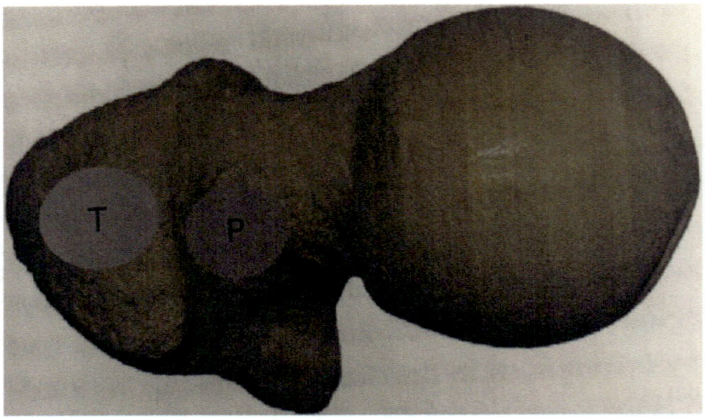

Fig. 13.29 Illustration of the superior proximal femur comparing the trochanteric (T) and piriformis (P) start sites (Fig. 8.7, page 92, in *In Egol, Kenneth, and Philipp Leucht, eds. 2017. Proximal Femur Fractures An Evidence-Based Approach to Evaluation and Management. Cham: Springer*)

13.6.4.2 Antegrade IMN

Antegrade nails require dissection of the hip abductors, especially with a piriformis start site (Figs. 13.31 and 13.32). Antegrade nails are associated with more hip pain postoperatively than retrograde nails. Using a lateral entry trochanteric start site nail may reduce the insult to the abductors compared to a piriformis start site (Fig. 13.31) [125, 126]. It may also be technically easier to find the lateral entry start site in athletes with large gluteal musculature, but the disadvantage is that there is not a straight trajectory down to the fracture in the femoral diaphysis. The literature is mixed on the clinical implications on range of motion and strength of the abductors after piriformis vs lateral entry start sites [122, 127, 128]. These studies were performed in the general population, mostly in geriatric populations, not in athletes, who may be more sensitive to slight changes in muscle strength and function.

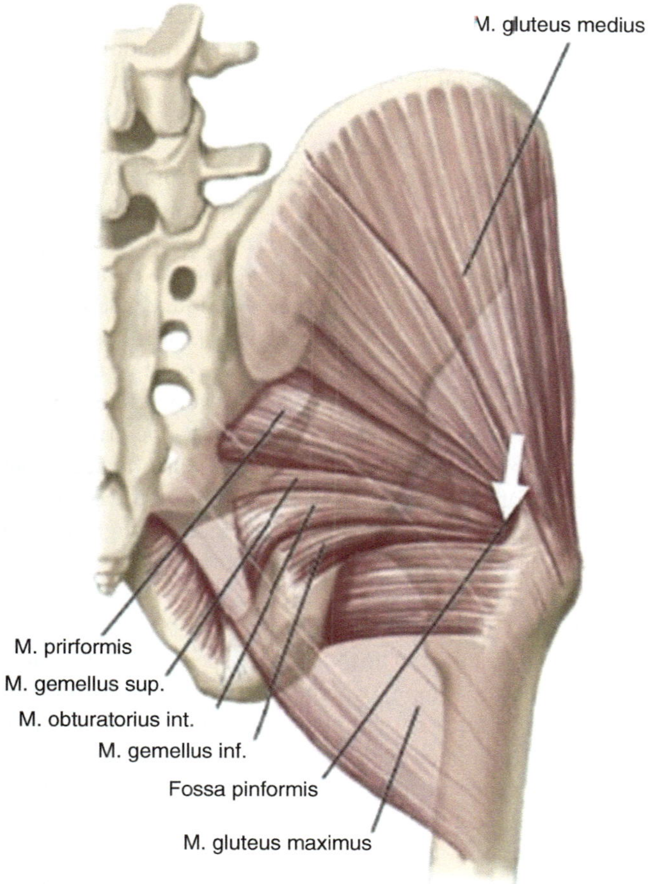

Fig. 13.30 Musculotendinous anatomy of the abductors. The white arrow represents the piriformis fossa. Note the dissection of the abductors necessary to find the appropriate start site (*Fig. 19.11 from Krettek C., Gösling T. (2015) Femur Diaphysis. In: Rommens P., Hessmann M. (eds) Intramedullary Nailing. Springer, London*)

13.6.5 Complications

13.6.5.1 Hip/Knee Pain

Hip pain associated with antegrade IMN and knee pain associated with retrograde IMN are discussed above. Sport specific requirements may help guide the surgeon's decision on antegrade vs retrograde nails and specific start sites.

13.6.5.2 Rotational Malalignment

Rotational malalignment is another complication of IMN of diaphyseal fractures pertinent to athletes, with approximately 10% incidence in distal fractures and up to 27.6% incidence in proximal fractures [129]. Malrotation up to 15° compared to the contralateral side is generally well tolerated in the general population, but can be particularly painful and impair function in high demand activities including sports [130]. Excessive external rotation is particularly limiting because it is more difficult to compensate towards neutral foot progression [130]. Risk factors for malrotation include fracture comminution and the use of a fracture table, which tends to increase the risk of internal rotation compared to manual traction [131].

The most reliable way to determine malrotation is described by Jeanmart et al., using a CT scan to determine the angle between a line drawn tangential to the femoral condyles and a line drawn through the axis of the femoral neck (Fig. 13.32) [132]. Intra-operatively, the surgeon should obtain an accurate clinical exam of the uninjured leg, specifically internal and external rotation of the leg with the hip in 90° of flexion. Comparison images of the contralateral leg should also be obtained. The surgeon should start with a perfect lateral view of the knee (super-

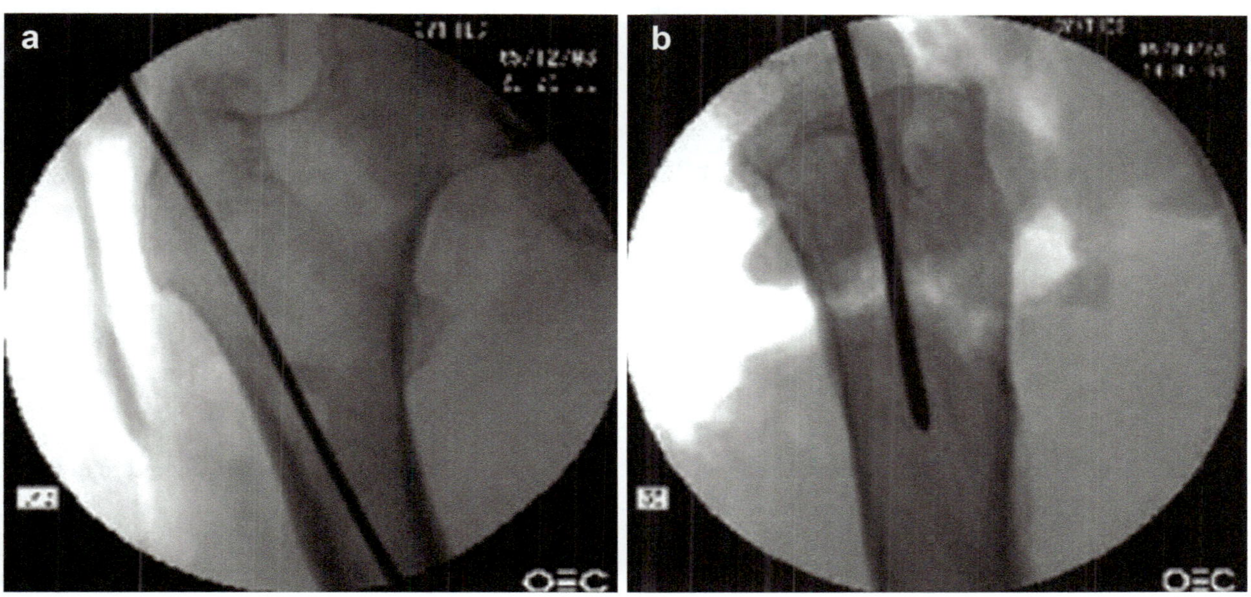

Fig. 13.31 Lateral entry start site for IMN of a diaphyseal femoral shaft fracture (*Fig. 19.16 from Krettek C., Gösling T. (2015) Femur Diaphysis. In: Rommens P., Hessmann M. (eds) Intramedullary Nailing. Springer, London, page 163*)

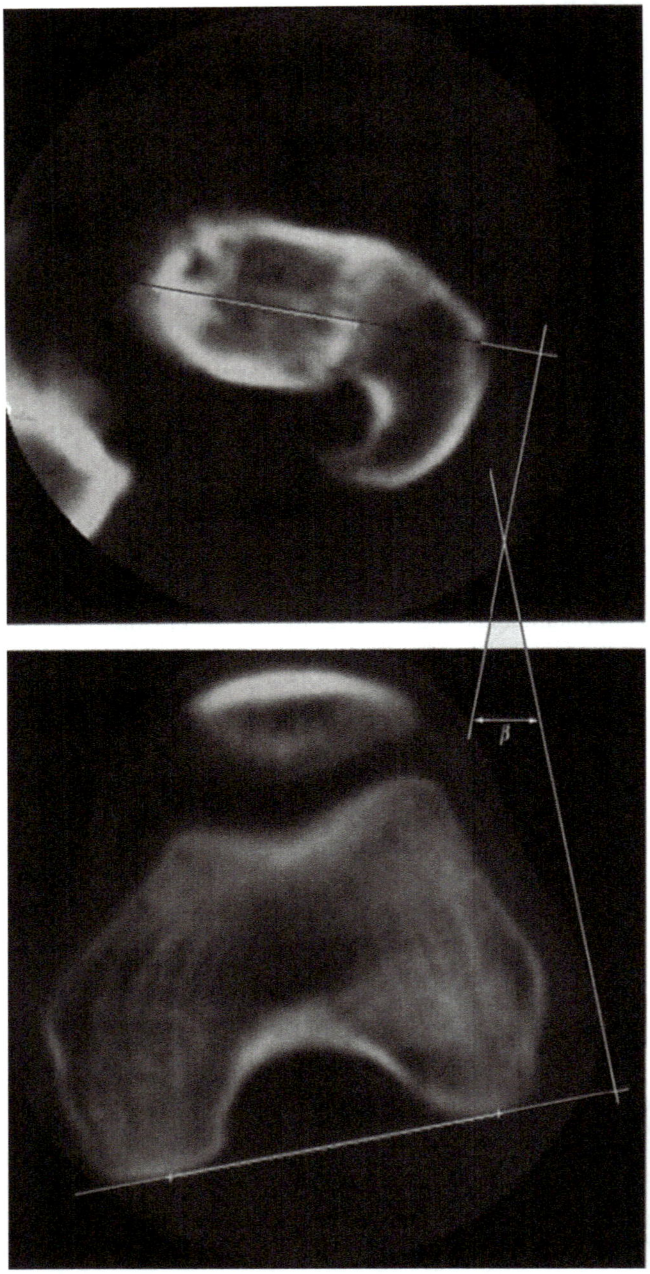

Fig. 13.32 Using CT to determine rotation after IMN of femoral diaphyseal fractures by determine an angle between a line drawn tangential to the femoral condyles and a line drawn through the axis of the femoral neck. Values should be within 15° of the contralateral side (*Fig. 6.41a & 5.41b on page 172 of Jeanmart, L, AL Baert, and A Wackenheim. n.d. Computer Tomography of Neck, Chest, Spine, and Limbs. Atlas of Pathological Computer Tomography. Vol. 3. Berlin, Heidelberg, New York: Springer*)

imposed posterior femoral condyles), then, while holding the leg in the exact same position, the C-arm should rotate 90° to obtain an AP of the hip centered on the lesser trochanter. Both images should be saved, and the same views on the injured leg should be obtained after nailing, using the version of the femoral necks to judge rotational alignment of the injured leg after nailing [80].

13.6.5.3 Leg Length Discrepancy

Leg length discrepancy (LLD) is another common complication of femur IMN, especially with comminuted fractures, with a reported incidence of >1.5 cm LLD in up to 20% of patients [133–135]. LLD can have noticeable effects on gait and increase the risk for injury when returning to sport, specifically stress fractures [136]. Post nailing clinical exam, described using the bovie cord or a ruler, is important to judge LLD, but may not be very reliable. Some institutions have instituted routine post-operative scout CTs to help judge LLD and rotation, even offering acute correction of discrepancies [134]. Intra-operative navigation techniques have also been described, though are not routinely used [137].

13.6.5.4 Delayed Union/Non-union

Other complications of IMN of diaphyseal femur fractures include delayed union, which is often treated with nail dynamization with or without bone graft, and non-union, which can be treated with reamed exchange nailing [138]. We do not recommend routine nail dynamization, and we adopt an expectant attitude to the possible lack of radiographic evidence of callus formation. In young athletic individual, unless there is malrotation and/or leg length discrepancy >1 cm, we do not in any way undertake any other procedure involving the nail.

13.6.6 Rehabilitation

Intramedullary nails provide a length stable construct that allows for immediate weight bearing for most fracture types [111, 139]. Depending on concomitant injuries, degree of comminution, or surgeon preference, patients may start with protected weight bearing for 1–2 weeks after surgery. In any case, early mobilization is important to stimulate fracture healing and limit deconditioning in athletes. Hip abductor weakness, especially after antegrade IMN, and quadriceps femoris muscle weakness are common after femur fractures, and therefore rehabilitation should focus on isometric strengthening of these muscle, range of motion of the hip and knee, patellar mobilization and gait training [140]. Athletes can expect return to sport by 6 months after surgery, but full recovery may take up to a year and professional athletes may not return to the same level of performance [141].

Table 13.1 Classification of avulsion fractures of the hip described by McKinney at al [7].

Table 13.2 Non-operative progression for treatment of acute avulsion injuries, initially described by Metzmaker and Pappas [13].

Table 13.3 Femoral neck stress fracture classification system and treatment recommendations (*Table 8.3, adapted from page 115 from Marc Haro, Julia Bruene, Kathleen Weber, and Bernard Bach. 2015. "Stress Fractures of the Femur." In Stress Fractures in Athletes; Diagnosis and Management, edited by Timothy Miller and Christopher Kaeding, 111–24. New York: Springer*)

Clinical Pearls

- Early reduction of displaced femoral head and neck fractures is important to decrease the risk of avascular necrosis of the femoral head. Anatomical reduction is required for young athletes, so surgeons should have a low threshold for open reduction.
- Provide stable fixation to allow for early rehabilitation of the affected hip.

Review

Questions

1. Femoral Neck Fracture Question Stem
   (a) A 30 year-old competitive cyclist crashed during a race and suffered an isolated, displaced basicervical femoral neck fracture. He is taken to the OR and closed reduction is attempted. There is a 5 mm step-off on the inferomedial aspect of the femoral neck. What is the neck best step in management?
   1. Additional closed reduction maneuvers
   2. Accept 5 mm of step-off and proceed with percutaneous fixation
   3. **Open reduction and internal fixation**
   4. Acute total hip arthroplasty

   Displaced femoral neck fractures are at high risk of disrupting the blood supply to femoral head. If the reduction is not anatomic, especially in young athletes, there should be a low threshold for open reduction. Open reduction can be performed through either an anterolateral Watson-Jones approach [142] or an anterior modified Smith-Petersen approach. Acute total hip arthroplasty is a reliable treatment option in older, lower demand patients, but would not be appropriate for a younger patient population.

   (b) Which of the following complications is this patient at highest risk of developing?
   1. **Osteonecrosis**
   2. Pulmonary embolism
   3. Infection
   4. Periprosthetic fracture

   The risk of avascular necrosis is reported as high as 86% in young patients with acute femoral neck fractures. AVN leads to collapse of the femoral head and osteoarthritis which are difficult problems to treat, especially in a younger, more active patients. Most cases of AVN will present within 2 months to 2 years of injury. Early diagnosis can be made with advanced imaging such as MRI or SPECT.

   (c) What factor is most associated with development of osteonecrosis?
   1. Time to surgery
   2. Verticality of fracture pattern
   3. **Reduction quality**
   4. Capsulotomy

   Urgent reduction within 8–12 h of injury is recommended to preserve blood supply to the femoral head. However, anatomical reduction is the most reliable predictor of AVN, so waiting for an experienced surgeon may trump urgent surgery. Vertical fracture patterns are more unstable, but the quality of the final reduction is more important than the fracture pattern.

References

1. Ly TV, Swiontkowski MF. Treatment of femoral neck fractures in young adults. J Bone Joint Surg Am. 2008;90:2254–66.
2. Dedrick DK, Mackenzie JR, Burney RE. Complications of femoral neck fracture in young adults. J Trauma. 1986;26:932–7.
3. O'hEireamhoin S, McCarthy T. Fractures around the hip in athletes. TOSMJ. 2010;4:58–63.
4. Rossi F, Dragoni S. Acute avulsion fractures of the pelvis in adolescent competitive athletes: prevalence, location and sports distribution of 203 cases collected. Skelet Radiol. 2001;30:127–31.
5. Schuett DJ, Bomar JD, Pennock AT. Pelvic apophyseal avulsion fractures: a retrospective review of 228 cases. J Pediatr Orthop. 2015;35:617–23.
6. Eberbach H, Hohloch L, Feucht MJ, Konstantinidis L, Südkamp NP, Zwingmann J. Operative versus conservative treatment of apophyseal avulsion fractures of the pelvis in the adolescents: a systematical review with meta-analysis of clinical outcome and return to sports. BMC Musculoskelet Disord. 2017;18:162.
7. McKinney BI, Nelson C, Carrion W. Apophyseal avulsion fractures of the hip and pelvis. Orthopedics. 2009;32:42.
8. Anduaga I, Seijas R, Pérez-Bellmunt A, Casasayas O, Alvarez P. Anterior iliac spine avulsion fracture treatment options in young athletes. J Investig Surg. 2018;2018:1–5.
9. Rajasekhar C, Kumar KS, Bhamra MS. Avulsion fractures of the anterior inferior iliac spine: the case for surgical intervention. Int Orthop. 2001;24:364–5.

10. Wood J, Rajput R, Ward A. Avulsion fracture of the greater trochanter of the femur: recommendations for closed reduction of the apophyseal. Injury Extra. 2005;36:255–8.
11. Pierannuzil LM, d'Imporzano M The hip: avulsion fractures. Pediatric and adolescent sports traumatology.
12. O'Rourke MR, Weinstein SL. Osteonecrosis following isolated avulsion fracture of the greater trochanter in children. A report of two cases. J Bone Joint Surg Am. 2003;85:2000–5.
13. Metzmaker JN, Pappas AM. Avulsion fractures of the pelvis. Am J Sports Med. 1985;13:349–58.
14. Kaneyama S, Yoshida K, Matsushima S, Wakami T, Tsunoda M, Doita M. A surgical approach for an avulsion fracture of the ischial tuberosity: a case report. J Orthop Trauma. 2006;20:363–5.
15. Pointinger H, Munk P, Poeschl GP. Avulsion fracture of the anterior superior iliac spine following apophysitis. Br J Sports Med. 2003;37:361–2.
16. Veselko M, Smrkolj V. Avulsion of the anterior-superior iliac spine in athletes: case reports. J Trauma. 1994;36:444–6.
17. Bastian JD, Turina M, Siebenrock KA, Keel MJB. Long-term outcome after traumatic anterior dislocation of the hip. Arch Orthop Trauma Surg. 2011;131:1273–8.
18. Dreinhöfer KE, Schwarzkopf SR, Haas NP, Tscherne H. Isolated traumatic dislocation of the hip. Long-term results in 50 patients. J Bone Joint Surg Br. 1994;76:6–12.
19. Droll KP, Broekhuyse H, O'Brien P. Fracture of the femoral head. J Am Acad Orthop Surg. 2007;15:716–27.
20. Stannard JP, Harris HW, Volgas DA, Alonso JE. Functional outcome of patients with femoral head fractures associated with hip dislocations. Clin Orthop Relat Res. 2000;2000:44–56.
21. Epstein HC. Posterior fracture-dislocations of the hip; long-term follow-up. J Bone Joint Surg Am. 1974;56:1103–27.
22. Roeder LF, DeLee JC. Femoral head fractures associated with posterior hip dislocation. Clin Orthop Relat Res. 1980;1980:121–30.
23. Marchetti ME, Steinberg GG, Coumas JM. Intermediate-term experience of Pipkin fracture-dislocations of the hip. J Orthop Trauma. 1996;10:455–61.
24. Hougaard K, Thomsen PB. Traumatic posterior fracture-dislocation of the hip with fracture of the femoral head or neck, or both. J Bone Joint Surg Am. 1988;70:233–9.
25. Lang-Stevenson A, Getty CJ. The Pipkin fracture-dislocation of the hip. Injury. 1987;18:264–9.
26. Swiontkowski MF, Thorpe M, Seiler JG, Hansen ST. Operative management of displaced femoral head fractures: case-matched comparison of anterior versus posterior approaches for Pipkin I and Pipkin II fractures. J Orthop Trauma. 1992;6:437–42.
27. Henle P, Kloen P, Siebenrock KA. Femoral head injuries: which treatment strategy can be recommended? Injury. 2007;38: 478–88.
28. Pipkin G. Treatment of grade IV fracture-dislocation of the hip. J Bone Joint Surg Am. 1957;39-A:1027–42.
29. Giannoudis P, Kanakaris N. Femoral head fractures. In: Lasanioanos N, Kanakaris N, Lasanioanos N, editors. Trauma and orthopaedic classification. New York, NY: Springer; 2014. p. 303–4.
30. McMahon S, Hawdon G. Vascularity of the femoral head in hip resurfacing. In: McMinn D, editor. Modern hip resurfacing. New York, NY: Springer; 2009. p. 117–24.
31. Dewar DC, Lazaro LE, Klinger CE, Sculco PK, Dyke JP, Ni AY, Helfet DL, Lorich DG. The relative contribution of the medial and lateral femoral circumflex arteries to the vascularity of the head and neck of the femur: a quantitative MRI-based assessment. Bone Joint J. 2016;98-B:1582–8.
32. Gautier E, Ganz K, Krügel N, Gill T, Ganz R. Anatomy of the medial femoral circumflex artery and its surgical implications. J Bone Joint Surg Br. 2000;82:679–83.
33. Hougaard K, Thomsen PB. Coxarthrosis following traumatic posterior dislocation of the hip. J Bone Joint Surg Am. 1987;69:679–83.
34. Epstein HC. Traumatic dislocations of the hip. Clin Orthop Relat Res. 1973:116–42.
35. Hoffmann R, Haas N. Femur, proximal. In: Ruedi T, Buckley R, Moran C, editors. AO principles of fracture management; volume 2—specific fractures. New York, NY: Thieme; 2014. p. 651–75.
36. Yoon TR, Rowe SM, Chung JY, Song EK, Jung ST, Anwar IB. Clinical and radiographic outcome of femoral head fractures: 30 patients followed for 3–10 years. Acta Orthop Scand. 2001;72:348–53.
37. Ross JR, Gardner MJ. Femoral head fractures. Curr Rev Musculoskelet Med. 2012;5:199–205.
38. Miyamoto RG, Kaplan KM, Levine BR, Egol KA, Zuckerman JD. Surgical management of hip fractures: an evidence-based review of the literature. I: femoral neck fractures. J Am Acad Orthop Surg. 2008;16:596–607.
39. Yamamoto Y, Ide T, Ono T, Hamada Y. Usefulness of arthroscopic surgery in hip trauma cases. Arthroscopy. 2003;19:269–73.
40. Mullis BH, Dahners LE. Hip arthroscopy to remove loose bodies after traumatic dislocation. J Orthop Trauma. 2006;20:22–6.
41. Matsuda DK. A rare fracture, an even rarer treatment: the arthroscopic reduction and internal fixation of an isolated femoral head fracture. Arthroscopy. 2009;25:408–12.
42. Park M-S, Her I-S, Cho H-M, Chung Y-Y. Internal fixation of femoral head fractures (Pipkin I) using hip arthroscopy. Knee Surg Sports Traumatol Arthrosc. 2014;22:898–901.
43. Deng X, Liu J, Yang S, Wang X, Li Z. Application of arthroscopic surgery combined with direct anterior approach in hip diseases. Zhongguo Xiu Fu Chong Jian Wai Ke Za Zhi. 2018;32:1167–71.
44. Ekkernkamp A, Stengel D, Wich M. Fractures of the femoral head. In: Egol K, Leucht P, editors. Proximal femur fractures an evidence-based approach to evaluation and management. Cham: Spinger; 2017. p. 36.
45. Lichstein PM, Kleimeyer JP, Githens M, Vorhies JS, Gardner MJ, Bellino M, Bishop J. Does the Watson-Jones or modified Smith-Petersen approach provide superior exposure for femoral neck fracture fixation? Clin Orthop Relat Res. 2018;476:1468–76.
46. Siebenrock KA, Gautier E, Woo AKH, Ganz R. Surgical dislocation of the femoral head for joint debridement and accurate reduction of fractures of the acetabulum. J Orthop Trauma. 2002;16:543–52.
47. Molnar RB, Routt MLC. Open reduction of intracapsular hip fractures using a modified Smith-Petersen surgical exposure. J Orthop Trauma. 2007;21:490–4.
48. McKee MD, Garay ME, Schemitsch EH, Kreder HJ, Stephen DJ. Irreducible fracture-dislocation of the hip: a severe injury with a poor prognosis. J Orthop Trauma. 1998;12:223–9.
49. Pauyo T, Drager J, Albers A, Harvey EJ. Management of femoral neck fractures in the young patient: a critical analysis review. World J Orthop. 2014;5:204–17.
50. Ehlinger M, Moser T, Adam P, Bierry G, Gangi A, de Mathelin M, Bonnomet F. Early prediction of femoral head avascular necrosis following neck fracture. Orthop Traumatol Surg Res. 2011;97:79–88.
51. Ebraheim NA, Savolaine ER, Zeiss J, Jackson WT. Titanium hip implants for improved magnetic resonance and computed tomography examinations. Clin Orthop Relat Res. 1992;1992:194–8.
52. Cornwall R, Radomisli TE. Nerve injury in traumatic dislocation of the hip. Clin Orthop Relat Res. 2000;2000:84–91.
53. Protzman RR, Burkhalter WE. Femoral-neck fractures in young adults. J Bone Joint Surg Am. 1976;58:689–95.
54. Swiontkowski MF, Winquist RA, Hansen ST. Fractures of the femoral neck in patients between the ages of twelve and forty-nine years. J Bone Joint Surg Am. 1984;66:837–46.

55. Bartonícek J. Pauwels' classification of femoral neck fractures: correct interpretation of the original. J Orthop Trauma. 2001;15:358–60.
56. Bonnaire FA, Weber AT. Analysis of fracture gap changes, dynamic and static stability of different osteosynthetic procedures in the femoral neck. Injury. 2002;33(Suppl 3):C24–32.
57. Broos PL, Vercruysse R, Fourneau I, Driesen R, Stappaerts KH. Unstable femoral neck fractures in young adults: treatment with the AO 130-degree blade plate. J Orthop Trauma. 1998;12:235–9; discussion 240.
58. Changstrom BG, Brou L, Khodaee M, Braund C, Comstock RD. Epidemiology of stress fracture injuries among US high school athletes, 2005–2006 through 2012–2013. Am J Sports Med. 2015;43:26–33.
59. Haro M, Bruene J, Weber K, Bach B. Stress fractures of the femur. In: Miller T, Kaeding C, editors. Stress fractures in athletes: diagnosis and management. New York, NY: Springer; 2015. p. 111–24.
60. Claassen J, Hu Z, Rohrbeck P. Fractures among active component, recruit trainees, and deployed service members, U.S. Armed Forces, 2003–2012. MSMR. 2014;21:2–7.
61. Snyder RA, Koester MC, Dunn WR. Epidemiology of stress fractures. Clin Sports Med. 2006;25:37–52, viii.
62. Matzkin E, Curry EJ, Whitlock K. Female athlete triad: past, present, and future. J Am Acad Orthop Surg. 2015;23:424–32.
63. Lasanioanos N, Kanakaris N. Femoral neck fractures. In: Giannoudis PV, Lasanioanos N, Kanakaris N, editors. Trauma and orthopaedic classifications. London: Springer; 2015. p. 305–8.
64. Garden RS. Low-angle fixation in fractures of the femoral neck. J Bone Joint Surg. 1961;43-B:647–63.
65. Kazley JM, Banerjee S, Abousayed MM, Rosenbaum AJ. Classifications in brief: garden classification of femoral neck fractures. Clin Orthop Relat Res. 2018;476:441–5.
66. Boden BP, Osbahr DC. High-risk stress fractures: evaluation and treatment. J Am Acad Orthop Surg. 2000;8:344–53.
67. Niva MH, Kiuru MJ, Haataja R, Pihlajamäki HK. Fatigue injuries of the femur. J Bone Joint Surg Br. 2005;87:1385–90.
68. Lubovsky O, Liebergall M, Mattan Y, Weil Y, Mosheiff R. Early diagnosis of occult hip fractures MRI versus CT scan. Injury. 2005;36:788–92.
69. Godfried D, Rahman A. Radiation exposure in the pediatric patient: what every orthopaedist should know; 2017.
70. Wright AA, Hegedus EJ, Lenchik L, Kuhn KJ, Santiago L, Smoliga JM. Diagnostic accuracy of various imaging modalities for suspected lower extremity stress fractures: a systematic review with evidence-based recommendations for clinical practice. Am J Sports Med. 2016;44:255–63.
71. DeFranco MJ, Recht M, Schils J, Parker RD. Stress fractures of the femur in athletes. Clin Sports Med. 2006;25(89–103):ix.
72. Cserháti P, Kazár G, Manninger J, Fekete K, Frenyó S. Non-operative or operative treatment for undisplaced femoral neck fractures: a comparative study of 122 non-operative and 125 operatively treated cases. Injury. 1996;27:583–8.
73. Jain R, Koo M, Kreder HJ, Schemitsch EH, Davey JR, Mahomed NN. Comparison of early and delayed fixation of subcapital hip fractures in patients sixty years of age or less. J Bone Joint Surg Am. 2002;84:1605–12.
74. Kofoed H. Femoral neck fractures in young adults. Injury. 1982;14:146–50.
75. Maruenda JI, Barrios C, Gomar-Sancho F. Intracapsular hip pressure after femoral neck fracture. Clin Orthop Relat Res. 1997;1997:172–80.
76. Christal AA, Taitsman LA, Dunbar RP, Krieg JC, Nork SE. Fluoroscopically guided hip capsulotomy: effective or not? A cadaveric study. J Orthop Trauma. 2011;25:214–7.
77. Beck M, Siebenrock KA, Affolter B, Nötzli H, Parvizi J, Ganz R. Increased intraarticular pressure reduces blood flow to the femoral head. Clin Orthop Relat Res. 2004;2014:149–52.
78. Koval K, Zuckerman J. Hip fractures: I. Overview and evaluation and treatment of femoral-neck fractures. J Am Acad Orthop Surg. 1994;2:141–9.
79. Goudie E, Duckworth A, White T. Femoral neck fractures in the young. Proximal femur fractures an evidence-based approach to evaluation and management; 2017.
80. Michael Gardner, MH. Bradford (eds) (2010) Harborview illustrated tips and tricks in fracture surgery, first. Lippincott Williams & Wilkins, Baltimore, MD.
81. Robinson CM, Adams CI, Craig M, Doward W, Clarke MCC, Auld J. Implant-related fractures of the femur following hip fracture surgery. J Bone Joint Surg Am. 2002;84:1116–22.
82. Hawks MA, Kim H, Strauss JE, Oliphant BW, Golden RD, Hsieh AH, Nascone JW, O'Toole RV. Does a trochanteric lag screw improve fixation of vertically oriented femoral neck fractures? A biomechanical analysis in cadaveric bone. Clin Biomech (Bristol, Avon). 2013;28:886–91.
83. Stacey SC, Renninger CH, Hak D, Mauffrey C. Tips and tricks for ORIF of displaced femoral neck fractures in the young adult patient. Eur J Orthop Surg Traumatol. 2016;26:355–63.
84. Panteli M, Rodham P, Giannoudis PV. Biomechanical rationale for implant choices in femoral neck fracture fixation in the non-elderly. Injury. 2015;46:445–52.
85. Hoshino CM, Christian MW, O'Toole RV, Manson TT. Fixation of displaced femoral neck fractures in young adults: fixed-angle devices or Pauwel screws? Injury. 2016;47:1676–84.
86. Kemker B, Magone K, Owen J, Atkinson P, Martin S, Atkinson T. A sliding hip screw augmented with 2 screws is biomechanically similar to an inverted triad of cannulated screws in repair of a Pauwels type-III fracture. Injury. 2017;48:1743–8.
87. Simunovic N, Devereaux PJ, Sprague S, Guyatt GH, Schemitsch E, Debeer J, Bhandari M. Effect of early surgery after hip fracture on mortality and complications: systematic review and meta-analysis. CMAJ. 2010;182:1609–16.
88. Amini MH, Feldman JJ, Weinlein JC. High complication rate in young patients with high-energy intertrochanteric femoral fractures. Orthopedics. 2017;40 e293–9.
89. Evans EM. The treatment of trochanteric fractures of the femur. J Bone Joint Surg Br. 1949;31B:190–203.
90. Kanakaris N, Giannoudis PV. Subtrochanteric fractures. In: Lasanioanos N, Kanakaris NK, Giannoudis PV, editors. Trauma and orthopaedic classifications. London: Springer; 2015. p. 317–9.
91. Russel T, Taylor J. Subtrochanteric fractures of the femur. In: Skeletal trauma. Philadephia; 1992. pp. 1832–1878.
92. Braun BJ, Veith NT, Rollmann M, Orth M, Fritz T, Herath SC, Holstein JH, Pohlemann T. Weight-bearing recommendations after operative fracture treatment-fact or fiction? Gait results with and feasibility of a dynamic, continuous pedobarography insole. Int Orthop. 2017;41:1507–12.
93. Koval KJ, Oh CK, Egol KA. Does a traction-internal rotation radiograph help to better evaluate fractures of the proximal femur? Bull NYU Hosp Jt Dis. 2008;66:102–6.
94. Gill SK, Smith J, Fox R, Chesser TJS. Investigation of occult hip fractures: the use of CT and MRI. ScientificWorldJournal. 2013; https://doi.org/10.1155/2013/830319.
95. Eggenberger E, Hildebrand G, Vang S, Ly A, Ward C. Use of CT vs. MRI for diagnosis of hip or pelvic fractures in elderly patients after low energy trauma. Iowa Orthop J. 2019;39:179–83.
96. Barton TM, Gleeson R, Topliss C, Greenwood R, Harries WJ, Chesser TJS. A comparison of the long gamma nail with the sliding hip screw for the treatment of AO/OTA 31-A2 fractures of the

proximal part of the femur: a prospective randomized trial. J Bone Joint Surg Am. 2010;92:792–8.
97. Utrilla AL, Reig JS, Muñoz FM, Tufanisco CB. Trochanteric gamma nail and compression hip screw for trochanteric fractures: a randomized, prospective, comparative study in 210 elderly patients with a new design of the gamma nail. J Orthop Trauma. 2005;19:229–33.
98. Parker MJ, Handoll HHG. Osteotomy, compression and other modifications of surgical techniques for internal fixation of extracapsular hip fractures. Cochrane Database Syst Rev. 2009;2009:CD000522.
99. Liporace F, Tejwani N. intertrochanteric femur fractures: plates and screws. Proximal femur fractures an evidence-based approach to evaluation and management; 2017.
100. Parker MJ. Sliding hip screw versus intramedullary nail for trochanteric hip fractures; a randomised trial of 1000 patients with presentation of results related to fracture stability. Injury. 2017;48:2762–7.
101. Palm H, Jacobsen S, Sonne-Holm S, Gebuhr P, Hip Fracture Study Group. Integrity of the lateral femoral wall in intertrochanteric hip fractures: an important predictor of a reoperation. J Bone Joint Surg Am. 2007;89:470–5.
102. Kregor PJ, Obremskey WT, Kreder HJ, Swiontkowski MF. Unstable pertrochanteric femoral fractures. J Orthop Trauma. 2014;28(Suppl 8):S25–8.
103. Tawari AA, Kempegowda H, Suk M, Horwitz DS. What makes an intertrochanteric fracture unstable in 2015? Does the lateral wall play a role in the decision matrix? J Orthop Trauma. 2015;29(Suppl 4):S4–9.
104. Kuzyk PRT, Lobo J, Whelan D, Zdero R, McKee MD, Schemitsch EH. Biomechanical evaluation of extramedullary versus intramedullary fixation for reverse obliquity intertrochanteric fractures. J Orthop Trauma. 2009;23:31–8.
105. Braun BJ, Holstein JH, Pohlemann T. Intertrochanteric hip fracture: intramedullary nails. Proximal femur fractures an evidence-based approach to evaluation and management; 2017.
106. Kleweno C, Morgan J, Redshaw J, Harris M, Rodriguez E, Zurakowski D, Vrahas M, Appleton P. Short versus long cephalomedullary nails for the treatment of intertrochanteric hip fractures in patients older than 65 years. J Orthop Trauma. 2014;28:391–7.
107. Dunn J, Kusnezov N, Bader J, Waterman BR, Orr J, Belmont PJ. Long versus short cephalomedullary nail for trochanteric femur fractures (OTA 31-A1, A2 and A3): a systematic review. J Orthop Traumatol. 2016;17:361–7.
108. Koval KJ, Rezaie N, Yoon R. Subtrochanteric femur fractures. Proximal femur fractures an evidence-based approach to evaluation and management; 2017.
109. Wang J, Ma X, Ma J, et al. Biomechanical analysis of four types of internal fixation in subtrochanteric fracture models. Orthop Surg. 2014;6:128–36.
110. Kraemer WJ, Hearn TC, Powell JN, Mahomed N. Fixation of segmental subtrochanteric fractures. A biomechanical study. Clin Orthop Relat Res. 1996;1996:71–9.
111. Brumback RJ, Toal TR, Murphy-Zane MS, Novak VP, Belkoff SM. Immediate weight-bearing after treatment of a comminuted fracture of the femoral shaft with a statically locked intramedullary nail. J Bone Joint Surg Am. 1999;81:1538–44.
112. DeBaun M, Gardner M. Open reduction techniques for displaced intertrochanteric femur fractures improve reduction quality in young male patients with high energy injuries; 2019.
113. Kraus M, Krischak G, Wiedmann K, Riepl C, Gebhard F, Jöckel JA, Scola A. Clinical evaluation of PFNA® and relationship between the tip-apex distance and mechanical failure. Unfallchirurg. 2011;114:470–8.
114. Gugenheim JJ, Probe RA, Brinker MR. The effects of femoral shaft malrotation on lower extremity anatomy. J Orthop Trauma. 2004;18:658–64.
115. Winquist RA, Hansen ST. Comminuted fractures of the femoral shaft treated by intramedullary nailing. Orthop Clin North Am. 1980;11:633–48.
116. Lieurance R, Benjamin JB, Rappaport WD. Blood loss and transfusion in patients with isolated femur fractures. J Orthop Trauma. 1992;6:175–9.
117. Wolinsky PR, Johnson KD. Ipsilateral femoral neck and shaft fractures. Clin Orthop Relat Res. 1995;1995:81–90.
118. Tornetta P, Kain MSH, Creevy WR. Diagnosis of femoral neck fractures in patients with a femoral shaft fracture. Improvement with a standard protocol. J Bone Joint Surg Am. 2007;89:39–43.
119. Brundage SI, McGhan R, Jurkovich GJ, Mack CD, Maier RV. Timing of femur fracture fixation: effect on outcome in patients with thoracic and head injuries. J Trauma. 2002;52:299–307.
120. Brumback RJ, Virkus WW. Intramedullary nailing of the femur: reamed versus nonreamed. J Am Acad Orthop Surg. 2000;8:83–90.
121. Ricci WM, Bellabarba C, Evanoff B, Herscovici D, DiPasquale T, Sanders R. Retrograde versus antegrade nailing of femoral shaft fractures. J Orthop Trauma. 2001;15:161–9.
122. Hussain N, Hussain FN, Sermer C, Kamdar H, Schemitsch EH, Sternheim A, Kuzyk P. Antegrade versus retrograde nailing techniques and trochanteric versus piriformis intramedullary nailing entry points for femoral shaft fractures: a systematic review and meta-analysis. Can J Surg. 2017;60:19–29.
123. Papadokostakis G, Papakostidis C, Dimitriou R, Giannoudis PV. The role and efficacy of retrograding nailing for the treatment of diaphyseal and distal femoral fractures: a systematic review of the literature. Injury. 2005;36:813–22.
124. Bedi A, Karunakar MA, Caron T, Sanders RW, Haidukewych GJ. Accuracy of reduction of ipsilateral femoral neck and shaft fractures—an analysis of various internal fixation strategies. J Orthop Trauma. 2009;23:249–53.
125. Ansari Moein CM, Verhofstad MHJ, RLW B, van der Werken C. Soft tissue injury related to choice of entry point in antegrade femoral nailing: piriform fossa or greater trochanter tip. Injury. 2005;36:1337–42.
126. Dora C, Leunig M, Beck M, Rothenfluh D, Ganz R. Entry point soft tissue damage in antegrade femoral nailing: a cadaver study. J Orthop Trauma. 2001;15:488–93.
127. Ricci WM, Schwappach J, Tucker M, Coupe K, Brandt A, Sanders R, Leighton R. Trochanteric versus piriformis entry portal for the treatment of femoral shaft fractures. J Orthop Trauma. 2006;20:663–7.
128. Stannard JP, Bankston L, Futch LA, McGwin G, Volgas DA. Functional outcome following intramedullary nailing of the femur: a prospective randomized comparison of piriformis fossa and greater trochanteric entry portals. J Bone Joint Surg Am. 2011;93:1385–91.
129. Lindsey J, Krieg J. Femoral malrotation following intramedullary nail fixation. Am Acad Orthop Surg. 2011;19:17–26.
130. Jaarsma RL, van Kampen A. Rotational malalignment after fractures of the femur. J Bone Joint Surg Br. 2004;86:1100–4.
131. Stephen DJG, Kreder HJ, Schemitsch EH, Conlan LB, Wild L, McKee MD. Femoral intramedullary nailing: comparison of fracture-table and manual traction. a prospective, randomized study. J Bone Joint Surg Am. 2002;84:1514–21.
132. Jeanmart L, Baert A, Wackenheim A. Computer tomography of neck, chest, spine, and limbs. Atlast of pathological computer tomography. Berlin: Springer; 1983.
133. Vaidya R, Anderson B, Elbanna A, Colen R, Hoard D, Sethi A. CT scanogram for limb length discrepancy in comminuted femoral shaft fractures following IM nailing. Injury. 2012;43:1176–81.
134. Gheraibeh P, Vaidya R, Hudson I, Meehan R, Tonnos F, Sethi A. Minimizing leg length discrepancy after intramedullary nailing of comminuted femoral shaft fractures: a quality improvement ini-

tiative using the scout computed tomography scanogram. J Orthop Trauma. 2018;32:256–62.
135. Winquist RA, Hansen ST, Clawson DK. Closed intramedullary nailing of femoral fractures. A report of five hundred and twenty cases. 1984. J Bone Joint Surg Am. 2001;83:1912.
136. Bennell KL, Malcolm SA, Thomas SA, Reid SJ, Brukner PD, Ebeling PR, Wark JD. Risk factors for stress fractures in track and field athletes. A twelve-month prospective study. Am J Sports Med. 1996;24:810–8.
137. Wilharm A, Gras F, Rausch S, Linder R, Marintschev I, Hofmann GO, Mückley T. Navigation in femoral-shaft fractures—from lab tests to clinical routine. Injury. 2011;42:1346–52.
138. Lynch JR, Taitsman LA, Barei DP, Nork SE. Femoral nonunion: risk factors and treatment options. J Am Acad Orthop Surg. 2008;16:88–97.
139. Arazi M, Oğün TC, Oktar MN, Memik R, Kutlu A. Early weight-bearing after statically locked reamed intramedullary nailing of comminuted femoral fractures: is it a safe procedure? J Trauma. 2001;50:711–6.
140. Paterno MV, Archdeacon MT, Ford KR, Galvin D, Hewett TE. Early rehabilitation following surgical fixation of a femoral shaft fracture. Phys Ther. 2006;86:558–72.
141. Sikka R, Fetzer G, Hunkele T, Sugarman E, Boyd J. Femur fractures in professional athletes: a case series. J Athl Train. 2015;50:442–8.
142. Watson-Jones R. Fractures of the neck of the femur. Br J Surg. 1936;23:787–808.
143. Makhni M, Shillingford J. Femoral neck fractures. In: Swart E, Day C, editors. . New York, NY: Springer; 2017. p. 383–5.
144. Manninger J, Fekete K. Diagnostic Investigations. Internal fixation of femoral neck fractures: 2007.
145. Singh R, Rohilla R, Magu NK, Siwach R, Kadian V, Sangwan SS. Ipsilateral femoral neck and shaft fractures: a retrospective analysis of two treatment methods. J Orthop Traumatol. 2008;9:141–7.

Acute Fractures in Sport: Knee

14

Stuart A. Aitken

Learning Objectives

- Describe the relevant information required when obtaining a history from an athlete with a fracture around the knee.
- Understand the salient features of the physical examination that might help in the diagnosis and subsequent treatment strategy.
- Define the overall goals of treatment of the athlete with a fracture around the knee.
- Understand the importance of acute compartment syndrome, and define the symptoms and clinical signs that accompany its development.

14.1 Distal Femur Fractures

14.1.1 Epidemiology

Fractures of the distal femur account for approximately 5% of all femoral fractures, and are most commonly seen in older patients with poor bone quality or in young adults after high energy trauma [1]. In athletes, significant axial loading is required before the distal femur will fail, and this probably explains why these injuries account for less than 1% of sports fractures [2, 3]. Nonetheless, they are severe lower limb injuries with considerable consequences in terms of future sports participation.

14.1.2 Classification

All fractures can be classified very simply as displaced or nondisplaced. In addition, the Arbeitsgemeinshaft fur Osteosynthesfragen (AO)/Orthopaedic Trauma Association (OTA) classification system separates fractures of the distal femur into three discrete morphological types [4]. Type A are extra-articular and do not involve the knee joint surface. Type B fractures are partial articular, involving injury to an isolated condyle. Type C fractures involve the joint surface and are complete articular injuries. Unfortunately, morphological classifications do not take into consideration many of the associated factors known to influence treatment and eventual outcome. These include the amount of fracture displacement and comminution, the proportion of knee joint involvement, and the accompanying soft tissue injury. However, a basic treatment plan can normally be created based upon the AO/OTA fracture type.

14.1.3 Diagnosis

A thorough history and examination is essential to evaluate the athlete presenting with a distal femur fracture. The treating physician should gather information about the causative event and the forces involved, the location of the pain, and the presence of accompanying foot symptoms such as tingling or numbness. Information provided by pre-hospital caregivers or ambulance personnel can be invaluable. It is important to establish a history of previous injury or surgery to the ipsilateral hip, thigh or knee, and the presence of any pre-existing surgical hardware in the femur.

Sports equipment and clothing should be removed to allow a thorough circumferential examination of the entire lower extremity. In particular, footwear should be removed to allow peripheral pulses and perfusion to be assessed. Most patients will present with an acute knee haemarthrosis. The direction of the causative forces producing the fracture, and the tension of the thigh musculature, leads to a typical pattern of deformity at the fracture site (Fig. 14.1).

Accordingly, the limb should be assessed clinically for shortening. If suspected, this should be promptly corrected with traction and splintage to avoid undue pressure on the deep surface of the extensor mechanism by the proximal

S. A. Aitken (✉)
MaineGeneral Orthopaedics, MaineGeneral Musculoskeletal Center, Augusta, ME, USA
e-mail: Stuart.Aitken@MaineGeneral.org

G. A. J. Robertson, N. Maffulli (eds.), *Fractures in Sport*, https://doi.org/10.1007/978-3-030-72036-0_14

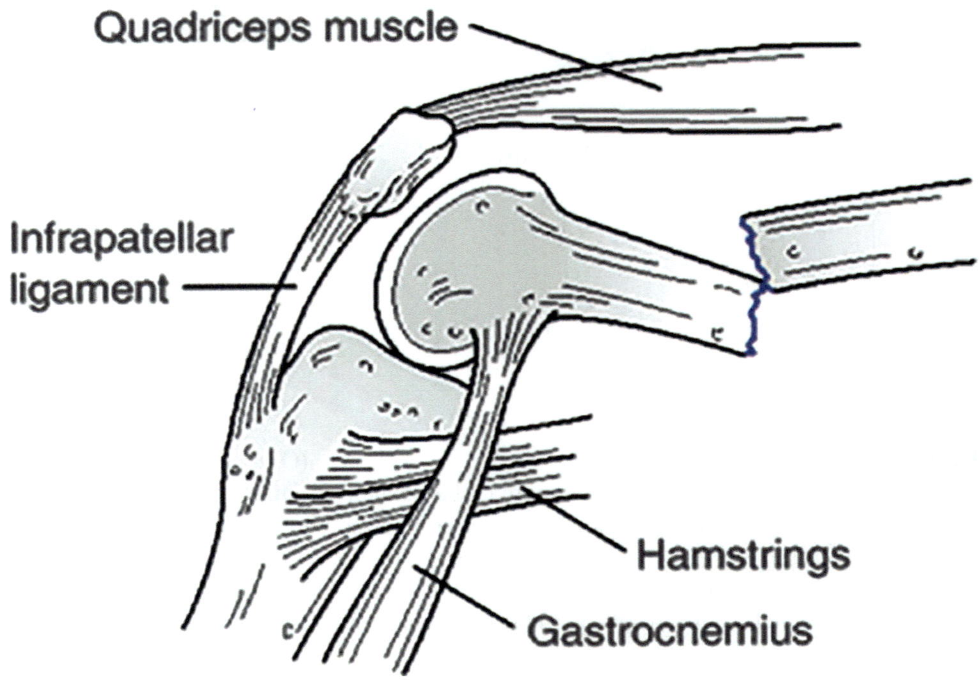

Fig. 14.1 A schematic representing the predictable deformity seen with a fracture of the distal femur. Contraction of gastrocnemius leads to fracture extension, while quadriceps and hamstrings tone causes shortening. Not seen here is the varus resulting from contraction of the adductor musculature, or the separation of the condyles seen with intra-articular injuries

fracture fragment. Vascular injury associated with distal femur fractures is surprisingly uncommon, especially given the proximity of the popliteal vessels behind the knee joint. A careful vascular examination is advisable looking for features of diminished vascular supply to the foot (prolonged capillary refill time, absent pulses, asymmetric ankle-ankle pressure indices). Cases with concerning features warrant further investigation using Doppler studies or preferably angiography.

14.1.4 Radiographic Evaluation

Initial imaging should include anteroposterior (AP) and lateral views of the knee and femur with an axial view of the patellofemoral joint. These are often sufficient, but may be supplemented by additional plain radiographs of the pelvis, hip and tibia if the clinical examination is suggestive of concomitant injury. The correction of limb shortening and the application of traction should always be followed by repeat imaging. This 'traction view' may provide a better understanding of the fracture geometry, and can reveal subtle coronal plane fracture lines between the femoral condyles. Computed tomography (CT) with multiplanar reconstruction is an important adjunct for types B and C fractures. CT provides additional information regarding the morphology of intra-articular fracture lines, and can also reveal the presence of subtle coronal plane fractures ('Hoffa' fractures) often missed on plain radiographs [5].

14.1.5 Treatment

Nonoperative methods of treatment for athletes with a fracture of the distal femur are reserved for those with nondisplaced injuries (Fig. 14.2). Typically, a brief period of knee splintage provides some pain relief, but is followed by early supervised active motion of the knee joint to prevent undue stiffness and muscle atrophy. Weight bearing is protected with crutches until symptoms improve and there is evidence of healing on repeat radiographs. The distal femur consists largely of metaphyseal bone, and nondisplaced fractures can be expected to heal in 6–8 weeks.

Advances in the design of surgical implants and techniques has led to the widespread acceptance of internal fixation as the treatment of choice for individuals with a displaced fracture of the distal femur. The goals of surgery apply to all patients, but are perhaps especially important to athletes. Anatomical reduction of the joint surface and restoration of lower limb length and alignment should be achieved and maintained using stable internal fixation methods. Adhering to these principles and using minimally invasive surgical approaches allows for rapid mobilisation of the injured extremity and accelerated knee rehabilitation.

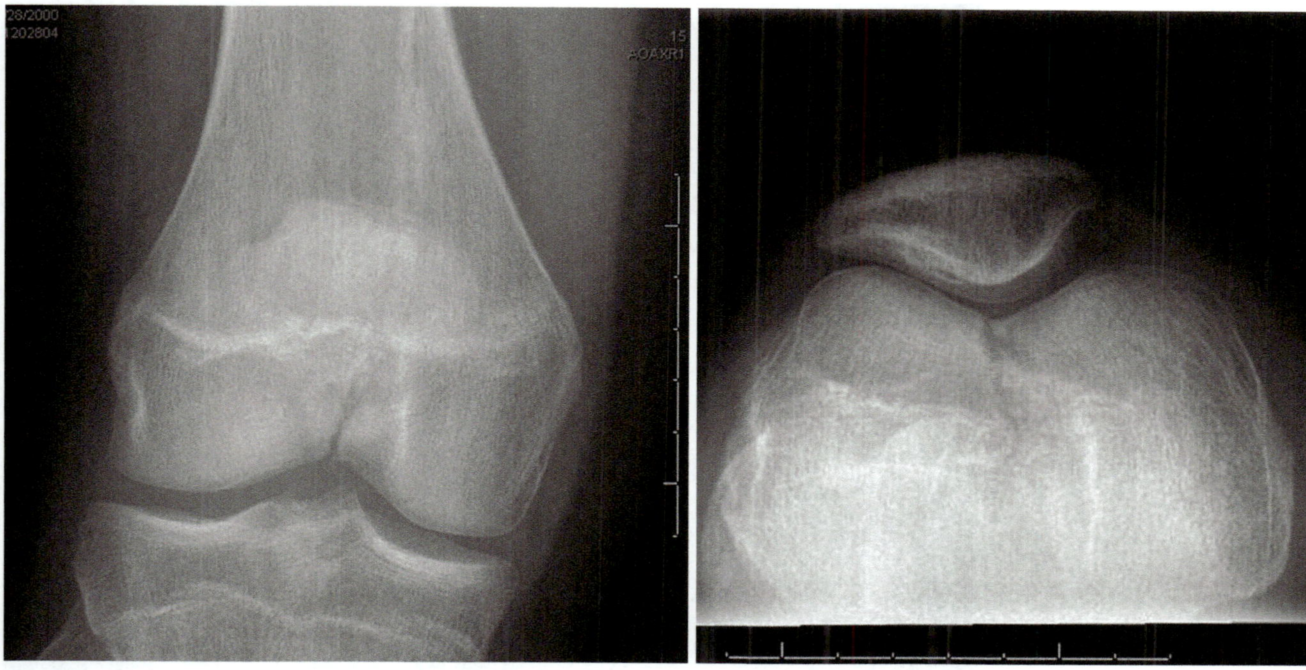

Fig. 14.2 Plain radiographs of the knee showing a nondisplaced fracture of the distal femur in a 19 year old basketball player. Protected weight bearing for 4 weeks was followed by a gradual return to full weight bearing over a further 4 week period. The athlete returned to sports participation by 10 weeks

The details of the specific surgical techniques used are beyond the scope of this chapter, but in general intra-articular fractures (types B and C) are treated with plates and screws, whereas extra-articular fractures (type A) are treated with either a long fracture specific plate or a retrograde intramedullary nail. An example of both methods of internal fixation is shown in Fig. 14.3.

14.1.6 Outcomes and Complications

Despite the advances of fracture specific implants, and knowledge of favourable surgical approaches, the treatment of displaced fractures is associated with a relatively high rate of complications. Nonunion or malunion can occur in up to 20% of cases, and infection in approximately 3% [6]. The development of knee stiffness can occur secondary to scarring beneath the quadriceps muscle, knee arthrofibrosis, or both, and is much more likely in athletes whose knees are immobilised for longer than 3 weeks. This underlines the importance of early active knee motion and rehabilitation. There are currently no data dealing with return to sport following a fracture of the distal femur.

14.1.7 Rehabilitation

Table 14.1 represents the rehabilitation protocol developed for athletes managed surgically for a distal femur fracture at the author's institution. The phases are adaptable based upon each individual's circumstances and fracture type.

14.2 Patella Fractures

14.2.1 Epidemiology

Fractures of the patella account for one third of fractures around the knee [1]. As a consequence of its position in the front of the knee joint, the patella is prone to injury by direct force. Indirect injuries can also occur, typically resulting from forceful quadriceps contraction with the knee flexed.

14.2.2 Classification

Patella fractures can be classified as displaced or nondisplaced. They are also categorised according to the geometric configuration and location of the fracture lines, as shown in

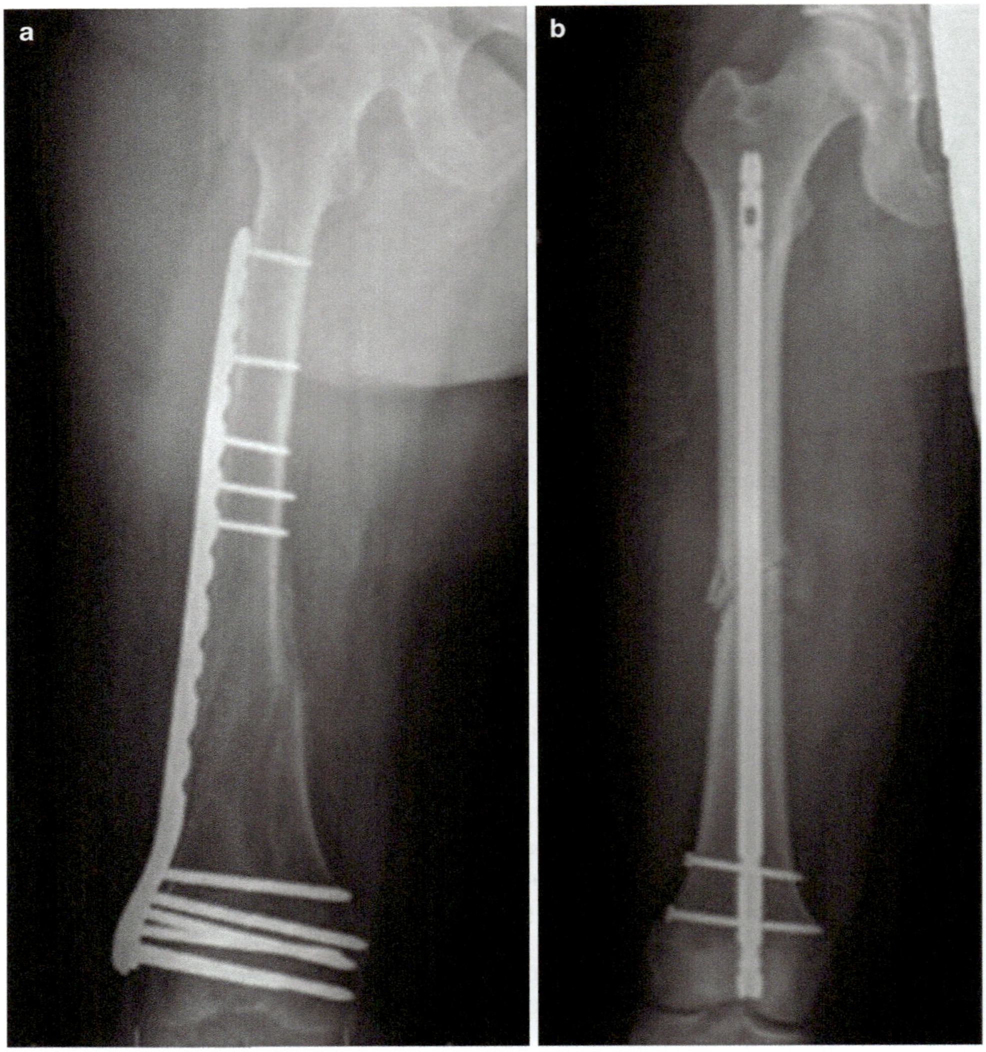

Fig. 14.3 Fractures of the distal femur can be surgically stabilised with a plate and screws (**a**). A retrograde nail can also be used, shown here used to treat a femoral shaft fracture (**b**)

Fig. 14.4. Of note, greater displacement between the fracture fragments is indicative of greater disruption to the medial and lateral patellar retinaculum, and therefore greater extensor mechanism compromise.

14.2.3 Diagnosis

The treating physician should gather information about the causative event and the forces involved. This will typically involve a fall during sports landing directly on the knee, or a near fall or stumble with forceful quadriceps contraction on a flexed knee. A high energy mechanism should prompt a search for associated injuries. A history of previous knee injury or surgery should be established.

Sports equipment and clothing should be removed to allow a thorough circumferential examination of the entire lower extremity. In athletes with displaced fractures, the acute knee haemarthrosis will be accompanied by a palpable defect between the fracture fragments. Patients with nondisplaced fractures may display neither of these signs. The examining clinician should assess the competence of the entire extensor mechanism by asking the athlete to perform a straight-leg raise. The ability to do so does not exclude patella fracture, but does suggest that the patellar retinaculum is intact.

14.2.4 Radiographic evaluation

Plain radiographs are most often sufficient. AP and lateral views are supplemented by an axial view, often known as the skyline or Merchant view. The combination of the three views allows an appreciation of fracture morphology and the degree of displacement or impaction involved. Advanced imaging by way of CT is seldom required.

Table 14.1 The typical postoperative rehabilitation protocol for athletes treated with surgical stabilisation of the distal femur

Phase 1: 0–2 weeks
Leave the surgical dressing intact and keep it dry You will need a walker or crutches to help your mobility initially **You must not put you full weight** through the injured leg Put the weight of the foot down for balance only Straight leg raises help keep your quadriceps strong Attend clinic for wound review and check x-rays at 2 weeks post-op
Phase 2: 2–6 weeks
The wounds are healed, you can get them wet in the bath or shower Begin walking on the leg, if permitted to do so (fracture specific) Start gently bending the knee 6 times daily (AROM) and **work hard to get the knee fully straight** Attend clinic for review and check x-rays at 6 weeks post-op
Phase 3: 6–12 weeks
Most athletes are permitted to start walking on the injured leg, regardless of fracture type **Work hard on getting the knee bending**, and practice this 6 times a day Gradual return to frequent walking and stair climbing, guided by your symptoms Return to 'desk based' employment only Return to some limited physical activity - e.g. stationary bike, rowing machine, upper body gym equipment, sport specific drills, non-contact drills
Phase 4: beyond 12 weeks
It is likely your fracture will be fully healed between 3 and 6 months Return to your pre-injury strength may take 6 to 12 months Return to contact sports and/or competition is advisable after both have been achieved

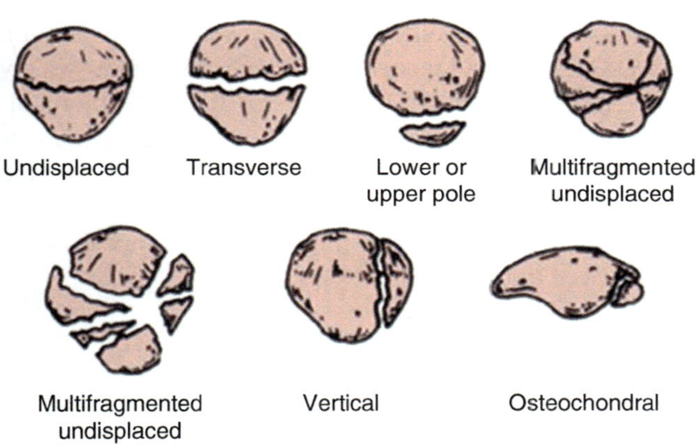

Fig. 14.4 A schematic representing the descriptive classification of patella fractures

14.2.5 Treatment

In athletic and non-athletic populations, nonoperative treatment is a viable option for nondisplaced fractures where the extensor mechanism is intact and the ability to straight-leg raise is preserved. The author allows immediate weight bearing in a splint with the knee in full extension, thereby off-loading the patella. In most cases knee flexion is not permitted for 4–6 weeks, and therefore some degree of diminished knee motion in the longer term is possible. This may not be acceptable for some athletes, depending on their sporting discipline, and operative treatment might be considered to accelerate rehabilitation.

Operative treatment in most cases allows for earlier knee motion, and is indicated in athletes with displaced fractures, those with greater than 3 mm of articular incongruity, and those with proven loss of extensor mechanism function. In high energy fractures with marked comminution, as much patellar bone as possible should be preserved. The patella increases the transmitted force of quadriceps knee extension by as much as 50% [7], and is therefore crucial in terms of athletic performance. The historical technique of patellectomy should be avoided in athletes.

Numerous variations of internal fixation techniques for patella fractures have been described. Those currently in popular use include the tension band wiring construct, cannulated screw tension band, and internal fixation with plates and screws. An example of each is provided in Fig. 14.5.

14.2.6 Outcomes and Complications

The geometric fracture pattern does not correlate well with outcome, and reported treatment results tend to be based on the type of treatment used [8]. There are currently no specific sporting data on the outcomes of patella fracture treatment. In 1972, Bostrom reported the apparent success of nonoperative treatment in the general population with 98% having a good or excellent result [9]. In contrast, the functional outcomes reported after operative treatment are less favourable. Two recent studies have shown that residual anterior knee pain is common (up to 80%) and individuals can expect reduced knee strength, power and endurance [10, 11].

14.2.7 Rehabilitation

Athletes with nondisplaced fractures will rehabilitate more quickly than those requiring surgery. In most surgical cases, the speed with which increased flexion is permitted is closely related to the stability of the fracture construct at the completion of surgery. This, in turn, will likely be dictated by the geometric configuration and location of the fracture lines as well as the bone quality. Table 14.2 is an example of a typical postoperative protocol used by this author.

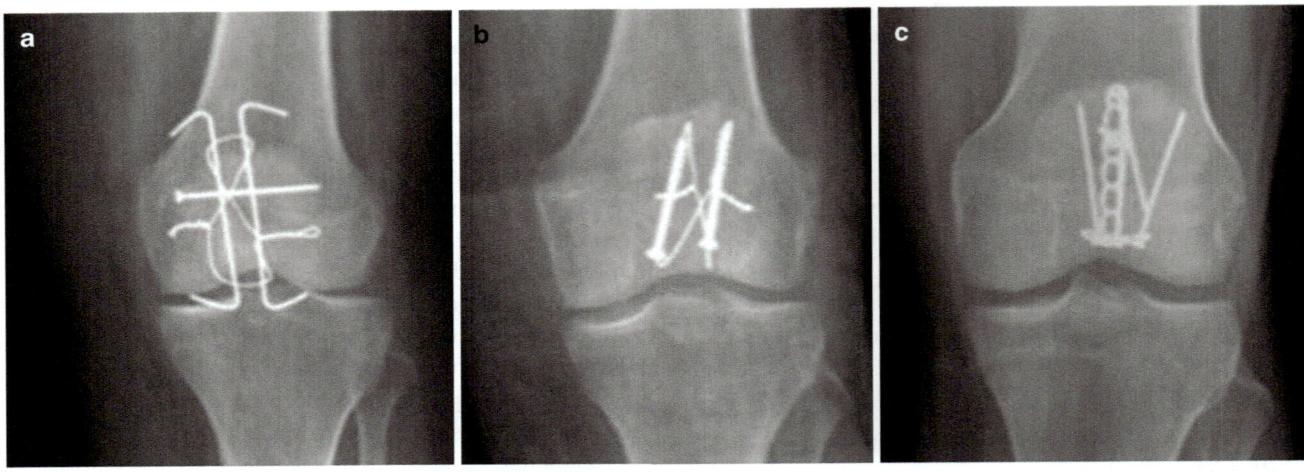

Fig. 14.5 Open reduction and stabilisation of a patella fracture using tension band wiring (**a**), cannulated screw tension band (**b**), and internal fixation with a plate and screws (**c**)

Table 14.2 The typical postoperative rehabilitation protocol for athletes treated with surgical stabilisation of a patella fracture

Phase 1: 0–2 weeks
Leave the surgical bandage intact and the knee splint on
You will need a walker or crutches to help your mobility initially
With the knee fully straight in the splint you may walk on the injured leg
Attend clinic for wound review and check x-rays at 2 weeks post-op
Phase 2: 2–4 weeks
The wound is healed, you can get it wet in the bath or shower
You will be converted to a hinged knee brace (0–30°)
You may take it off to shower and at bed time, any time you are upright you must wear it
Work hard to get the knee fully straight and bend it gently in the brace six times daily
Attend clinic for review and check X-rays at 4 weeks post-op
Phase 3: 4–12 weeks
The brace will be adjusted to allow more flexion (0–60°)
Remember, only walk on it with the knee fully straight
Work hard on getting the knee bending, and practice this six times a day
The knee should be able to straighten fully
At 8 weeks, the brace will be adjusted again (0–90°)
Phase 4: beyond 12 weeks
Discontinue the brace and work on getting full flexion back
Stretching and strengthening work are now permitted
Return to some limited physical activity
– e.g. stationary bike, rowing machine, sport specific drills, non-contact drills
Return to sports activity as you regain knee motion and strength
Return to contact sports and/or competition is advisable after both have been fully achieved

14.3 Tibial Plateau Fractures

14.3.1 Epidemiology

Fractures of the articular surface of the proximal tibia are the commonest fracture of the knee joint. In the general population, less than 10% of plateau fractures are caused by sports, as many occur in elderly women with osteoporotic bone. However, in young adults high impact sports collisions account for 20% of fractures, with the remainder occurring secondary to more traditional high energy trauma such as falls from height or road traffic accidents [1, 2].

14.3.2 Classification

The classification systems proposed by Schatzker et al. [12], the AO/OTA [4] and Luo et al. [13] are the three most widely used. They attempt to group fractures with similar morphology, with the intent of guiding treatment and predicting outcome. Fractures may involve the lateral plateau, medial plateau, or both. They are most commonly seen involving the lateral side due to the pre-existing normal anatomical valgus alignment of the knee joint.

14.3.3 Diagnosis

Tibial plateau fractures commonly occur in isolation, but associated injury to ligaments or menisci are more frequent with medial fractures or those involving both condyles. Information about the causative event and the forces involved should be gathered. Most patients are not able to weight bear. In the athletic population, injury typically results from direct impact to the lateral knee causing a valgus moment, but can also result from falls or twisting injuries. Under these circumstances, the risk of neurovascular injury or compartment syndrome is very low [14]. A history of previous ipsilateral lower limb injury or surgery should be established.

Sports equipment and clothing should be removed to allow a thorough circumferential examination of the knee. Although rare, it is important to document the presence of open wounds or findings suggestive of acute compartment syndrome (discussed in more detail in Sect. 14.5). The condition of the skin and subcutaneous tissues around the knee will influence the choice of surgical approach in operative cases. A comprehensive knee examination will be limited by pain and swelling, but the treating physician should be aware that apparent valgus instability is more likely due to damage to the lateral plateau than medial collateral ligament rupture.

14.3.4 Radiographic Evaluation

AP and lateral plain radiographs of the knee are sufficient to diagnose a displaced tibial plateau fracture. Nondisplaced fractures are not as easily identified, and advanced imaging should be considered in athletes whose history and physical examination are suggestive of plateau fracture but whose plain radiographs are normal. For most surgeons, routine CT imaging is undertaken as an aid to preoperative planning for the surgical approaches and fixation techniques used (Fig. 14.6). Magnetic Resonance Imaging (MRI) is more sensitive than CT when used to detect knee ligamentous and meniscal injury. However, controversy still exists as to whether it is strictly necessary in every case, and whether repair of injured soft tissue structures influences outcome [14].

14.3.5 Treatment

The goals of management are to restore normal limb length, alignment and knee stability and to allow early knee motion to prevent stiffness and functional deficit. Nondisplaced fractures can be managed nonoperatively with a predictably good functional outcome. The same can be said of minimally displaced lateral plateau fractures where limb alignment is

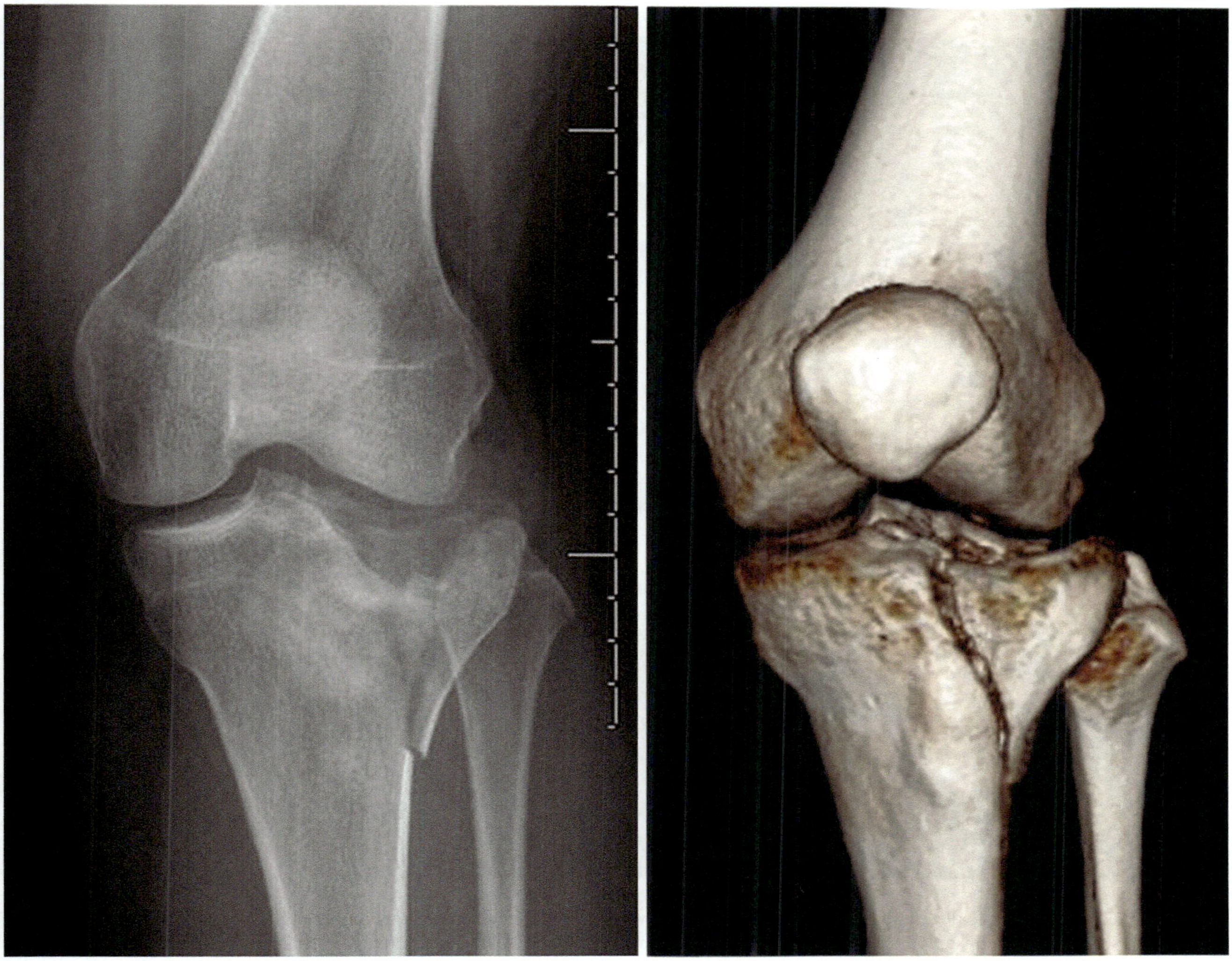

Fig. 14.6 Anteroposterior radiograph of a displaced fracture of the lateral tibial plateau, accompanied by a 3D CT reconstruction image

normal and the knee is stable. A period of protected weight bearing and knee immobilisation provides pain relief and should be followed by progressively increased range of motion exercises to prevent joint stiffness. Depending on the fracture configuration, weight bearing is typically allowed from 4 to 6 weeks onwards.

Surgery is indicated for athletes with displaced fractures. Although there is no absolute consensus as to what degree of displacement represents a threshold for surgical reduction, most surgeons consider loss of normal limb alignment, knee instability and medial plateau involvement to be absolute indications. The actual number of millimetres of fracture depression seen on CT does not predictably guide management, and the location and size of the depressed area probably exert more influence on eventual outcome.

When surgery is indicated, the specific operative plan is based upon the condition of the soft tissues and the fracture geometry. In most cases, the articular surface is elevated, reduced and supported by a plate and screws (Fig. 14.7). In some centres, arthroscopy is used as an aid to joint reduction. An external fixator may be employed to help maintain limb alignment.

14.3.6 Outcomes and Complications

In general, tibial plateau fractures have favourable outcomes if the articular surface is reduced and normal knee alignment is restored and maintained [14]. These parameters are more likely to be met in the treatment of nondisplaced sports fractures. For displaced fractures, and those with associated knee instability, favourable outcomes are not predictable. Robertson and colleagues reported a 70% return to sport rate for surgically treated athletes with tibial plateau fractures [15]. Quintens et al. examined athletes whose fracture pattern included the 'posterior column' of the plateau, and found that 68% returned to sport after a period of 9–12 months [16]. A recent report found a rate of return to amateur athlet-

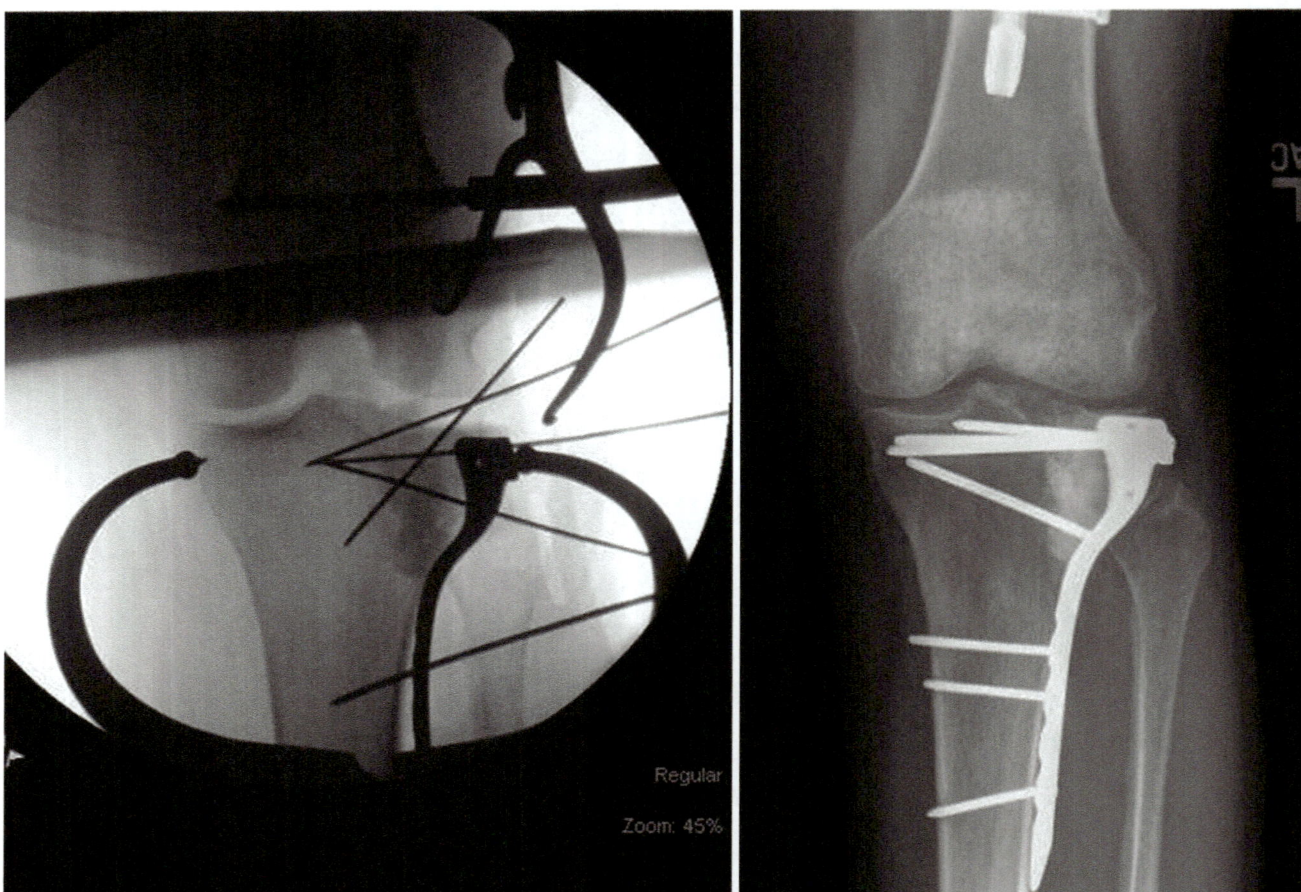

Fig. 14.7 Fluoroscopic image illustrating the concept of fracture elevation with joint reduction, temporary stabilisation with wires, backfilling of the defect, restoration of condylar width and support by a lateral plate and screws. The final radiographic appearance is also shown

ics of 52% at 15 months [17]. The eventual sporting outcome is therefore greatly influenced by the severity of the initial injury as well as the specific demands of the sporting activity to which the athlete wishes to return.

14.3.7 Rehabilitation

Table 14.3 illustrates a rehabilitation protocol developed for athletes requiring reduction and stabilisation of a tibial plateau fracture at the author's institution. Emphasis is placed on early knee joint motion while protecting weight bearing until the fracture has healed. Athletes will move through the phases at different rates depending on fracture and soft tissue characteristics.

14.3.8 Preventative Measures

At the time of writing, there is no literature specifically dealing with the prevention of tibial plateau fractures in athletes.

Table 14.3 The rehabilitation protocol developed for athletes with a surgically treated tibial plateau fracture

Phase 1: 0–2 weeks
Leave the surgical dressing intact and keep it dry You will need a walker or crutches to help your mobility initially **You must not put you full weight** through the injured leg Put the weight of the foot down for balance only Straight leg raises help keep your quadriceps strong Attend clinic for wound review and check X-rays at 2 weeks post-op
Phase 2: 2–6 weeks
The wounds are healed, you can get them wet in the bath or shower Continue with the same weight bearing precautions Start gently bending the knee six times daily (AROM) and **work hard to get the knee fully straight** Attend clinic for review and check X-rays at 6 weeks post-op
Phase 3: 6–12 weeks
Most athletes are permitted to start walking on the injured leg by 6–10 weeks **Work hard on getting the knee bending**, and practice this six times a day Gradual return to frequent walking and stair climbing, guided by your symptoms Return to 'desk based' employment only Return to some limited physical activity – e.g. stationary bike, rowing machine, upper body gym equipment, sport specific drills, non-contact drills
Phase 4: beyond 12 weeks
It is likely your fracture will be fully healed Return to your pre-injury strength may take 6–12 months Return to contact sports and/or competition is advisable when fully strong with a stable knee

14.4 Extra-articular Proximal Tibia Fractures

14.4.1 Epidemiology

Fractures of the proximal tibia occur in the metaphyseal area of the bone. They represent a watershed between tibial plateau fractures and those of the tibial shaft, and display features on history and physical examination in common with both these fracture types. In young individuals with good bone quality, a great deal of energy is required to cause the proximal tibial metaphysis to fail. In a study of almost 7000 fractures in Edinburgh, none of these fractures was caused by sports [1].

14.4.2 Classification

The AO/OTA system categorises these injuries morphologically depending on the orientation of the primary fracture line and also the presence or absence of fracture comminution [4]. They can also be described as nondisplaced or displaced. With the exception of truly nondisplaced fractures, these injuries are inherently unstable. The pull of quadriceps and gastrocnemius promotes a flexion deformity, while that of the pes anserinus and tibialis anterior causes valgus (Fig. 14.8).

14.4.3 Diagnosis

A careful assessment should be undertaken with a high index of suspicion for associated injuries from a relatively high energy mechanism. The history should aim to gather pertinent information related to the forces involved, and in the badly injured athlete this might be obtained from family members or pre-hospital providers.

Physical examination should focus on the injured knee, the leg compartments, and the foot. All sports equipment and clothing should be removed to allow a thorough circumferential examination of the extremity. A detailed vascular examination of the limb should be performed and documented. The posterior cortex of the proximal tibia is in close proximity with the popliteal artery and tibioperoneal trunk and displaced fractures may injure these structures. Any discrepancy between palpable ankle pulses and/or ankle pressure indices should prompt further investigation by way of Doppler ultrasound or angiography. The injured athlete is at risk of developing acute compartment syndrome [18], and it is important to look for findings suggestive of this potentially

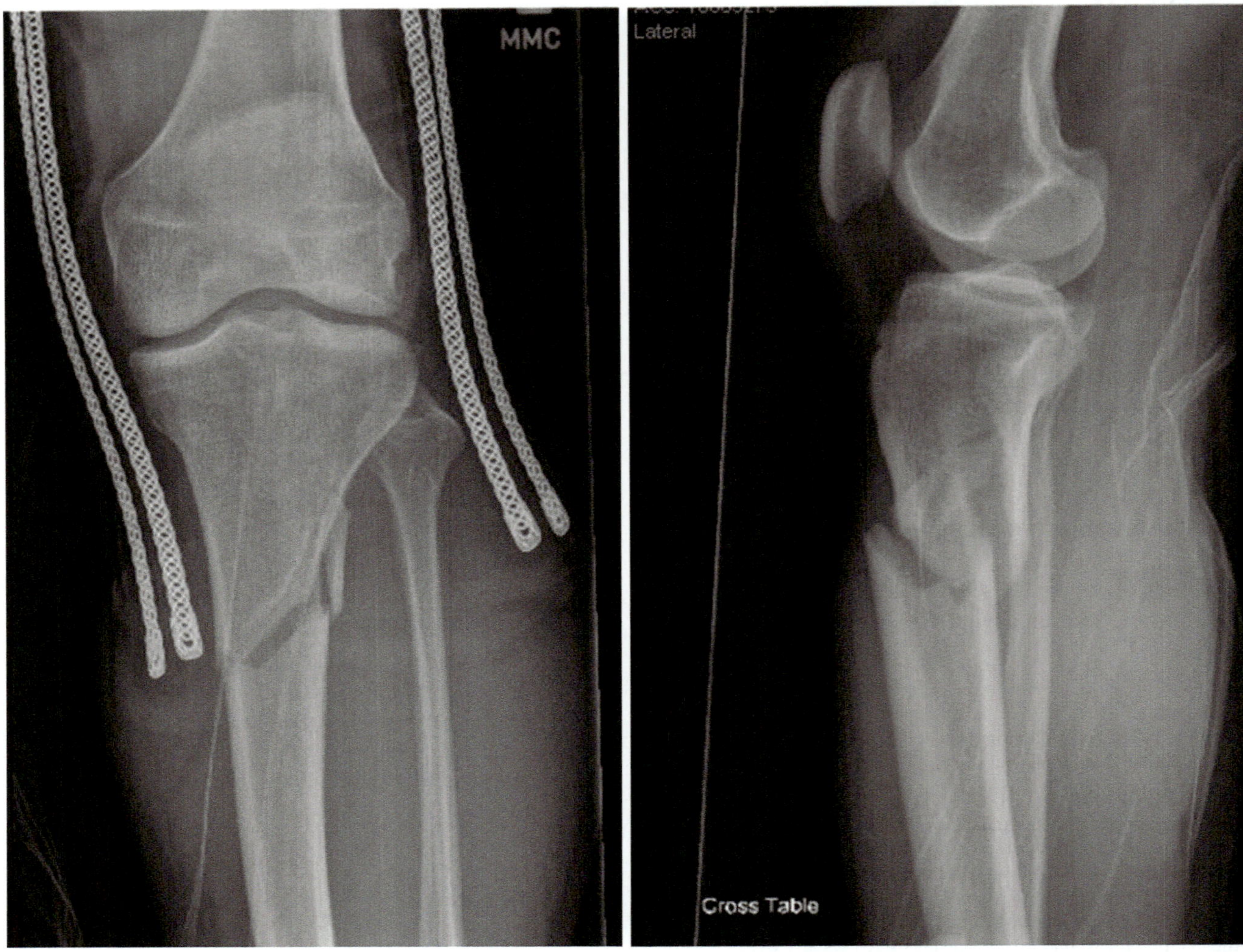

Fig. 14.8 The predictable deformity seen with an extra-articular fracture of the proximal tibia. Contraction of quadriceps and gastrocnemius leads to fracture flexion, while tibialis anterior and hamstrings tone causes valgus

devastating diagnosis. Because of the subcutaneous location of the tibia, a search for open wounds should also be undertaken. Compartment syndrome and open fractures are discussed in more detail in Sect. 14.5.

14.4.4 Radiographic Evaluation

AP and lateral plain radiographs of the knee allow for adequate evaluation of the fracture. Full length films of the tibia should also be included to evaluate for distal extension into the tibial shaft. Supplemental CT imaging of the knee might be considered if there is concern about occult fracture involving either the tibial plateau or the tibial tubercle, as both of these findings will impact the treatment strategy.

14.4.5 Treatment

In young adults, nondisplaced fracture are rare most likely to the high energy nature of the causative mechanism. However, when present these injuries should be treated with protected weight bearing and gradually increased range of motion work, in common with nondisplaced plateau fractures. Weight bearing is progressed as evidence of progression to fracture union becomes apparent.

Most proximal tibial fractures are displaced, unstable, and require surgical reduction and stabilisation. With the advancement of fracture specific implant designs, and knowledge of optimal surgical approaches, surgeons have the option of using plates and screws or an intramedullary nail (placed through a standard or suprapatellar approach) to

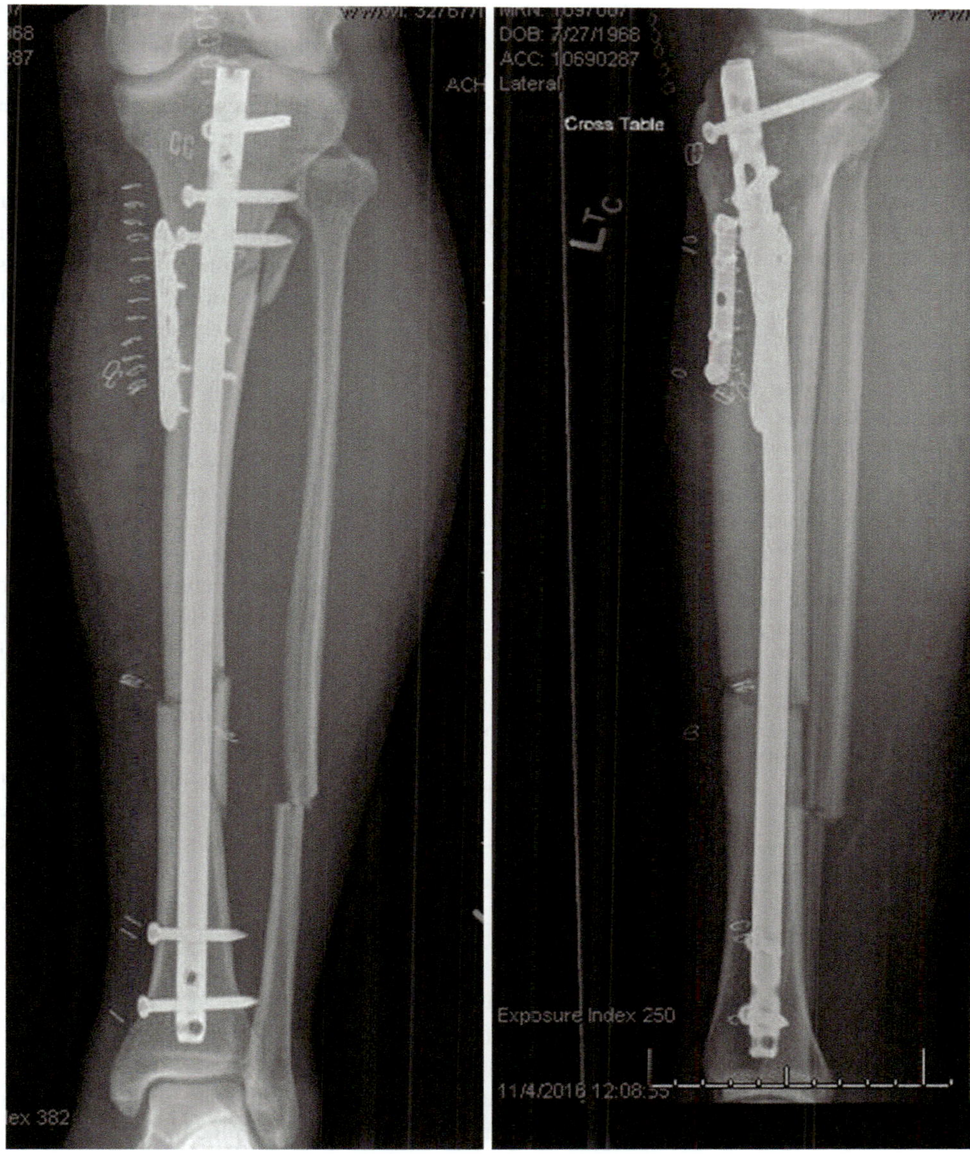

Fig. 14.9 A tibial nail used for the surgical stabilisation of a proximal tibial fracture. Careful attention has been paid to proximal fragment entry point and the stability of proximal locking screws. In this instance, a small plate and screws has been used to control flexion deformity at the fracture site

achieve these goals (Fig. 14.9). Controlling deformity at the fracture site is paramount (see Fig. 14.8). and is the main determining factor when selecting the appropriate implant and approach.

14.4.6 Outcomes and Complications

Reported outcomes for extra-articular proximal tibial fractures in the general population are more consistent with those of tibial shaft fractures than those of the tibial plateau. In a prospective trial comparing nailing with plating, the techniques were described as broadly equivalent with a mean time to union in excess of 18 weeks and a 6% nonunion rate. There is currently a lack of outcome data for proximal tibial fractures in athletes, reflecting the rarity of this injury in sport.

14.4.7 Rehabilitation

During rehabilitation emphasis is placed on early knee joint motion while protecting weight bearing until the fracture has healed, Table 14.4.

Table 14.4 The rehabilitation protocol developed for individuals with a surgically treated proximal tibia fracture

Phase 1: 0–2 weeks
Leave the surgical dressing intact and keep it dry
You will need a walker or crutches to help your mobility initially
You must not put you full weight through the injured leg
Put the weight of the foot down for balance only
Straight leg raises help keep your quadriceps strong
Attend clinic for wound review and check X-rays at 2 weeks post-op
Phase 2: 2–6 weeks
The wounds are healed, you can get them wet in the bath or shower
Continue with the same weight bearing precautions
Start gently bending the knee and **work hard to get the knee fully straight**
Attend clinic for review and check X-rays at 6 weeks post-op
Phase 3: 6–12 weeks
Work hard on getting the knee bending, and practice this six times a day
Return to 'desk based' employment only
Return to some limited physical activity may be possible – e.g. stationary bike, rowing machine, upper body gym equipment
Phase 4: beyond 12 weeks
It is likely your fracture will be fully healed between 4 and 6 months
Return to 'manual' or 'strenuous' employment as your symptoms allow
Return to your pre-injury strength may take 6–12 months
Return to contact sports and/or competition is advisable when fully strong with a stable knee

14.5 Tibial Shaft Fractures

14.5.1 Epidemiology

Fractures of the tibial shaft are the most common long bone fracture, and approximately 25% occur as a result of sport participation. They account for 4% of all sports-related fractures, with the majority found in young men [1]. In the United Kingdom, as many as 80% of these fractures result from soccer [2]. In continental Europe, injuries from skiing are commonly encountered [19]. The recovery from a fracture of the tibia is often lengthy, and can significantly impact future sports participation.

14.5.2 Classification

The systems used to describe fractures of the tibial shaft group these injuries according to the fracture morphology, the degree of accompanying soft tissue injury (skin, fat, muscle, neurovascular structures and periosteum), or both. The AO/OTA classification separates fracture morphology into three basic types: type A simple patterns; type B wedge fragment patterns; and type C complex patterns [4]. This system is predictive of the development of acute compartment syndrome [20], but a poor predictor of final functional outcome, rate of return to sports and the timing of return to athletic activity [21, 22].

The management and eventual outcome of tibial shaft fractures is more closely related to the extent of accompanying soft tissue trauma than the radiographic appearance of the fracture. The Tscherne classification describes closed fractures of the tibia according to the clinical appearance of the limb as well as the fracture morphology: C0 simple fractures with little or no soft tissue injury; C1 mild to moderately severe fractures with superficial abrasions; C2 moderately severe fracture morphology with deep contamination and skin and muscle contusion; and C3 severe fractures with extensive contusion, crushing of skin or muscle destruction [23]. Increased Tscherne grading is predictive of a decreased rate of return to sports [21], and an increase in the time taken to return to activity [22].

Open fractures are classified according to the system originally described by Gustilo and Anderson: type 1 have a clean wound <1 cm in length; type 2 have a <10 cm wound without extensive soft tissue damage; type 3 have a wound of any length with extensive soft tissue injury and a high-energy fracture pattern [24]. Type 3 injuries can be further subdivided into those with a wound that can be sutured or skin grafted (3A), those that require soft tissue flap coverage (3B) and severe limb injuries requiring revascularisation to maintain blood supply to the extremity (3C). Owing to its subcutaneous location, open fractures of the tibial shaft are relatively common following high energy trauma. In contrast, open fractures from sports trauma are less frequent, and are typically type 1 or 2.

14.5.3 Diagnosis

While these injuries commonly occur in isolation, the treating clinician should maintain an index of suspicion for fracture extension into the knee or ankle, or associated ligamentous knee injury. The identification of an associated acute compartment syndrome (ACS) is vital, and its treatment by way of leg fasciotomies is considered an orthopaedic surgical emergency. The diagnosis and treatment of compartment syndrome are discussed below.

The clinician should gather information relating to the timing and direction of injury, the location and quality of pain, the frequency and dosage of narcotic analgesia administered, and the presence of accompanying symptoms such as numbness or tingling in the foot. A history of previous injuries or surgery should be obtained. The presence of pre-existing surgical hardware, a previously united fracture or malunion may have a significant impact on subsequent management.

Physical examination should focus on the injured leg, the adjacent knee and ankle, and the foot. All sports equipment and clothing should be removed to allow a thorough circumferential examination of the extremity, paying particular attention to the presence of the following:

Skin compromise—Deformity at the fracture site can cause areas of skin puckering and tenting. If skin compromise is not addressed, full-thickness skin necrosis can occur within hours. Restoration of normal limb length and alignment, followed by the application of splintage, will relieve the pressure on 'at risk' skin areas after the initial limb assessment is completed.

Open wounds—These should be assumed to communicate with the fracture until proven otherwise. Obvious contamination should be removed, intravenous antibiotics should be administered, and the wound can be photographed to prevent repeated exposure for examinations. Emergency Department irrigation with sterile saline and coverage with a moist sterile dressing is not a substitute for formal surgical exploration in the operating room with copious irrigation, wound debridement, skeletal stabilisation and soft tissue coverage as necessary.

Vascular compromise—Athletes with displaced fractures and significant limb deformity may present with features suggestive of diminished vascular supply to the foot. A vascular examination is required before and after the restoration of normal limb length and alignment. In cases with persistent lack of foot pulses, further investigation using Doppler studies or angiography is necessary.

Motor and sensory function—Pain and skeletal instability will limit the extent and accuracy of any motor examination. A distal sensory examination of the foot should be carried out, paying particular attention to the territories of the superficial (dorsum of the foot) and deep (first dorsal web space) peroneal nerve branches, and the tibial nerve (sole of the foot). These sensory nerves travel within the muscular compartments of the leg and their dysfunction can occur secondary to elevated intra-compartmental pressures (ICP) or frank ACS.

Compartment syndrome—Examination findings suggestive of ACS include pain out of proportion to the injury, pain on passive stretch of the relevant compartment musculature, and dysfunction in the territory of the sensory nerves traversing the compartment. Notably, the absence of palpable pulses is a late finding, and the presence of 'palpably tense compartments' lacks sensitivity [25]. Athletes with an inconclusive initial examination should be serially examined frequently and a high index of suspicion for the presence of ACS should be maintained. The measurement of ICP can be of benefit in these cases, and is also useful in the evaluation of the athlete with concomitant head injury and decreased level of consciousness. The clinical and functional consequences of failing to treat ACS far outweigh the potential disadvantages of unnecessary leg fasciotomies.

14.5.4 Radiographic Evaluation

AP and lateral plain radiographs should include the entire tibia and fibula. These are supplemented by views of the ipsilateral knee and ankle, looking for periarticular fracture extension or separate bony injury. CT imaging is seldom needed but can be particularly useful in certain fracture patterns. In spiral fractures of the distal third of the tibia, CT ankle can detect occult fracture extension not easily seen on plain ankle radiographs [26].

14.5.5 Treatment

In general, surgical stabilisation of tibial shaft fractures is currently preferred over nonoperative management in a cast or brace. Tibial nailing in particular is associated with superior results with regards to nonunion rates, time to union, malunion rates, functional outcome scores and return to work. These same advantages apply to the athletic population. In addition, a faster return to sporting activity and a greater chance of returning to the same level of performance can be expected with surgical management. Additional disadvantages of management in a cast include resultant stiffness in the knee, ankle and subtalar joints as well as the loss of muscle bulk and strength associated with limited weight bearing.

14.5.5.1 Nonoperative Methods

In athletes, tibial shaft fractures should only be treated nonoperatively if adequate length and alignment can be achieved and maintained in splintage, and the individual is willing and able to avoid full weight bearing activity for 6 weeks or more. There is no absolute proven limit for acceptable length and alignment, but general expert consensus allows for up to 5° of varus or valgus, 10° of flexion or extension, 10° of rotational deformity and 10 mm of shortening [27]. The treating clinician should be aware of the tendency for tibial shaft fractures with an intact fibula to fall into varus angulation. This pattern is seen in 50% of soccer-related fractures, and so strong consideration should be given to operative treatment in this particular population.

14.5.5.2 Operative Methods

For displaced tibial shaft fractures, surgical treatment is the preferred option. It may also be used for athletes with non-displaced fractures with a strong preference for accelerated rehabilitation. Fixation with plates and screws is occasionally used in younger athletes with open physes, but the mainstay is reamed intramedullary nailing for those aged 13 years and older [28]. Nailing offers the advantages of maintaining knee and ankle motion, immediate postoperative weight bearing, preservation of the fracture site soft tissue envelope,

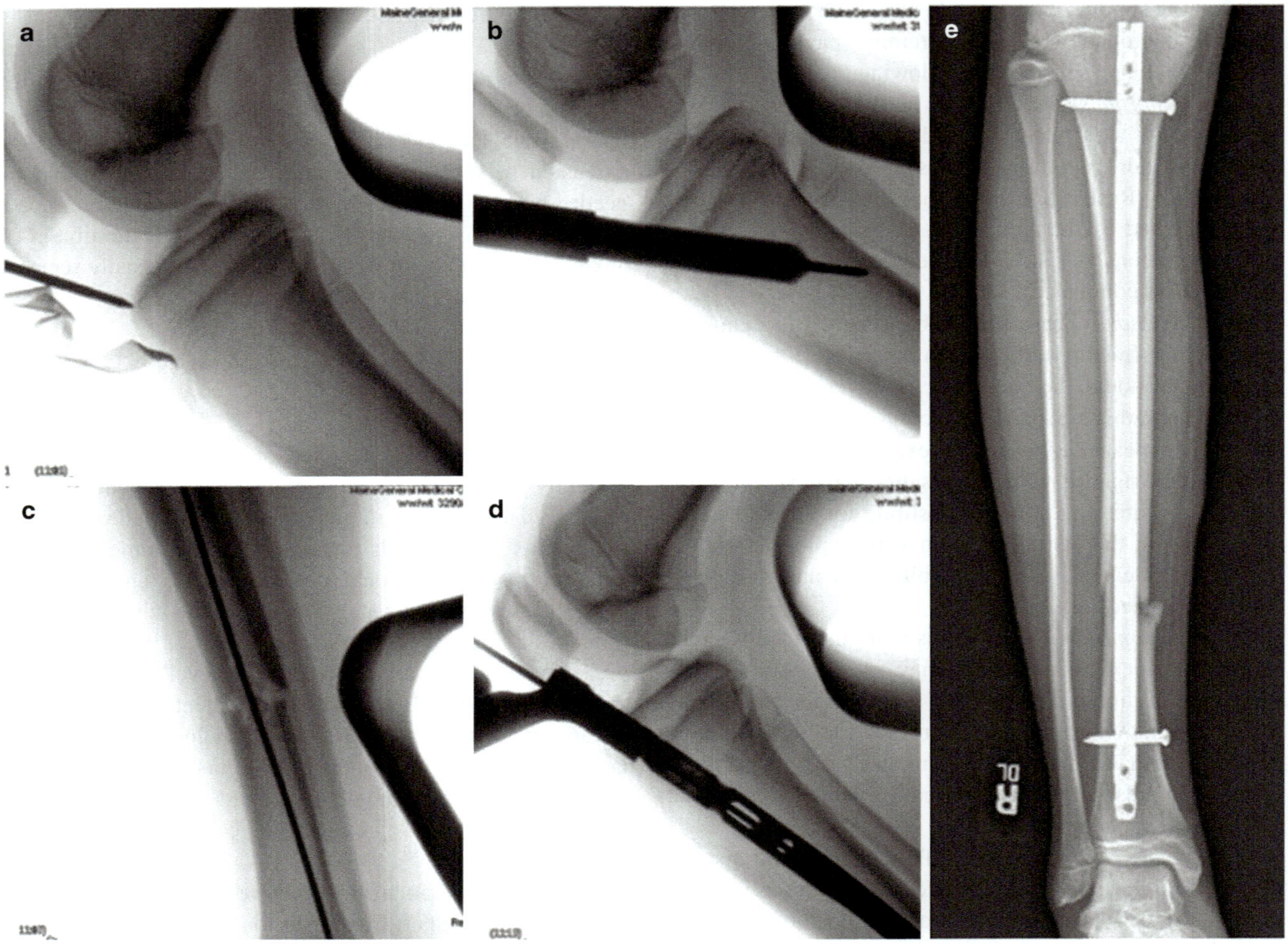

Fig. 14.10 Fluoroscopic images obtained during a tibial nailing procedure, outlining the surgical steps involved. The optimal starting point is identified using the guide pin (**a**), the opening reamer gains access to the canal (**b**), the guide wire is placed across the fracture site (**c**), canal reaming is followed by nail insertion (**d**). Proximal and distal locking screws complete the construct (**e**)

and less frequent clinic follow-up. The technical aspects of tibial nailing are beyond the scope of this chapter, but the basic principles are illustrated in Fig. 14.10.

14.5.6 Outcomes and Complications

Performance-related athletic outcomes following tibial shaft fractures have been examined in a recent systematic review [22]. Of those treated surgically, 92% returned to sports with 75% returning to the same level of competition. In contrast, 67% of those treated nonoperatively returned to sports, with only 40% achieving a similar level of competition. Unsurprisingly, the severity of the initial injury, particularly the soft tissue component, was predictive of the final sports-related outcomes.

The development of one or more complications related to the index injury or subsequent surgery can be expected to prolong the return to athletic activity. Infection is relatively uncommon following the surgical management of closed or type 1 open tibial fractures. However, its occurrence risks a poor outcome and prolonged recovery mainly from the requirement for further surgery. The median time to union for fractures of the tibial shaft in adults is 18 weeks, longer than any other sports-related fracture type. In general, persistent symptoms and radiographic signs suggestive of a lack of bony consolidation after 26 weeks are considered a nonunion [27]. In open fractures, those complicated by ACS, and in athletes who smoke tobacco, union may take longer [29]. The successful management of nonunion in the absence of infection involves an exchange nailing [30].

A systematic review of the literature in 2000 examined complications data for 895 closed tibial fractures from 13 prospective clinical trials (Table 14.5) [31], and clearly illustrated the superiority of surgery over nonoperative

Table 14.5 The results of different tibial shaft fracture treatments, combining data for 895 procedures

Result	Nailing	Plating	Nonoperative
Nonunion (%)	8	3	17
Residual displacement (%)	3	0	32
Infection (%)	3	9	0

management. The advantages of tibial nailing over plating, discussed above, come at the cost of an apparent higher rate of nonunion. The analysis of 1003 nailed tibial fractures reported a nonunion rate of 7% in closed injuries [29].

The development of ACS after tibial shaft fracture is approximately 4% [18]. The athletic population are at particular risk, as male gender, younger age and a sporting mechanism are independent risk factors for its development [32]. Even when appropriately identified and managed with surgical release of the involved compartments, athletes who suffer ACS can expect their tibial fracture to take on average 5 weeks longer to fully unite.

Soft tissue irritation from palpable screws or plates is common following the surgical stabilisation of lower extremity fractures, particularly in areas where the soft tissue envelope is thin (e.g. around the knee, ankle, anterior tibial border). Proximal and distal locking screws for tibial nails are a common source of hardware related pain. The symptoms produced are well localised, and locking screws can be removed, usually with a successful result. Poorly localised 'hardware-related' symptoms can be caused by the presence of the intramedullary nail, or occasionally long extramedullary plates. In these circumstances, removal of the implant involves a more substantial surgical insult, and is often accompanied resolution of symptoms in only 50% of cases [33].

Almost exclusively occurring after tibial nailing, anterior knee pain is common, although rarely disabling. It is associated with the proximal tibial entry point, and although the exact cause is largely unknown, it is particularly noticeable during activities involving kneeling [34]. Nail removal will often alleviate the symptoms, but this finding is inconsistent and by no means guaranteed [27].

14.5.7 Rehabilitation

Table 14.6 illustrates the rehabilitation protocol developed for athletes treated with tibial nailing at this authors institution. The protocol is divided into phases, and each phase is adaptable based on individual circumstances. Some individuals may move faster or slower through the phases based upon the specific characteristics of the fracture, the soft tissue injury and the speed of healing.

Table 14.6 The typical postoperative rehabilitation protocol for athletes treated with tibial nailing

Phase 1: 0–2 weeks
Keep the wounds covered, only remove the dressings if **absolutely necessary**
With most fractures (but not all), you can put your full weight through the injured leg, as symptoms allow
You will need crutches or a walker to help your mobility initially
You can practice flexing and extending the knee, and moving the ankle up and down
Straight leg raises help keep your quadriceps strong
Attend clinic for wound review and check X-rays at 2 weeks post-op
Phase 2: 2–6 weeks
The wounds are healed, you can get them wet in the bath or shower
Continue walking on the leg, if permitted to do so
Depending on your mobility, you may progress to using a single crutch
Attend clinic for review and check X-rays at 6 weeks post-op
Phase 3: 6–12 weeks
Gradual return to frequent walking and stair climbing, guided by your symptoms
Return to 'desk based' employment only
Return to some limited physical activity
– e.g. stationary bike, rowing machine, upper body gym equipment, sport specific drills, non-contact drills
Phase 4: beyond 12 weeks
It is likely your fracture will be fully healed between 4 and 6 months
Return to 'manual' or 'strenuous' employment as your symptoms allow
Return to your pre-injury strength may take 6–12 months
Return to contact sports and/or competition is advisable only when your fracture has healed

14.5.8 Preventative Measures

In sports such as soccer, where tibial shaft fractures commonly result from a direct blow or collision with an opponent, players are required to wear shin guards for protection purposes. Despite little clinical evidence that these measures are effective, there is good experimental evidence that shin guards are effective in reducing transmitted load to the leg [35]. In many other sports, notably skiing, tibial fractures result from twisting injury. Much work has been done on improving the design of ski boot bindings, such that the athletes leg is released from the ski prior to the transmission of substantial torsional load to the leg and knee [36].

Clinical Pearls

- Fractures around the knee are common in sports, and can have a significant impact on future athletic performance even when managed appropriately.
- The goals of treatment of all fracture types share common themes: fracture reduction and stabilisation should allow early knee motion, provide a stable joint, and maintain normal lower limb alignment.
- Management strategies that allow early weight bearing activity confer the best chance of a successful and timely return to athletic activity.

Review

Questions

1. In the evaluation of the athlete with a suspected fracture of the patella, what simple examination test can provide information about the integrity of the patellar retinaculum?
2. Following a fracture of the lateral tibial plateau, which of the following findings is the best indication for surgical management: CT imaging showing 3 mm of articular surface displacement, or a knee joint that falls into slight valgus on attempts at weight bearing?
3. A 25 year old male soccer player presents with considerable leg pain following a collision with an opponent on the pitch. What examination findings would be suggestive of an acute compartment syndrome?

Answers

1. The examining clinician should assess the competence of the entire extensor mechanism by asking the athlete to perform a straight-leg raise. The ability to do so does not exclude patella fracture but does suggest that the patellar retinaculum is intact. Athletes with an intact straight-leg raise will often be suitable for nonoperative management, unless articular incongruity exists as seen on radiographs.
2. Most surgeons consider loss of normal limb alignment, knee instability and medial plateau involvement to be absolute indications for surgery. The actual number of millimetres of fracture depression seen on CT does not predictably guide treatment.
3. Examination findings suggestive of compartment syndrome include pain out of proportion to the injury, pain on passive stretch of the relevant compartment musculature, and dysfunction in the territory of the sensory nerves traversing the compartment. Notably, the absence of palpable pulses is a late finding, and that the presence of 'palpably tense compartments' lacks sensitivity.

References

1. Aitken SA. Thesis: the epidemiology of upper limb, lower limb and pelvic fractures in adults. Edinburgh: Department of Trauma and Orthopaedics, University of Edinburgh; 2013.
2. Aitken SA, Watson BS, Wood AM, Court-Brown CM. Sports-related fractures in South East Scotland: an analysis of 990 fractures. J Orthop Surg. 2014;22(3):313–7.
3. Court-Brown CM, Wood AM, Aitken S. The epidemiology of acute sports-related fractures in adults. Injury. 2008;39(12):1365–72.
4. Meinberg EG, Agel J, Roberts CS, Karam MD, Kellam JF. Fracture and Dislocation Classification Compendium-2018. J Orthop Trauma. 2018;32(Suppl 1):S1–S170.
5. Nork SE, Segina DN, Aflatoon K, Barei DP, Henley MB, Holt S, et al. The association between supracondylar-intercondylar distal femoral fractures and coronal plane fractures. J Bone Joint Surg Am. 2005;87(3):564–9.
6. Collinge CA, Wiss DA. Distal femur fractures. In: Tornetta III P, Ricci WM, Ostrum RF, MM MQ, MD MK, Court-Brown CM, editors. Rockwood and Green's fractures in adults. 2nd ed. Philadelphia, PA: Wolters Kluwer; 2019. p. 2430–71.
7. Kaufer H. Mechanical function of the patella. J Bone Joint Surg Am. 1971;53(8):1551–60.
8. Lack WD, Karunakar MA. Patellar fractures and dislocations and extensor mechanism injuries. In: Tornetta III P, Ricci WM, Ostrum RF, McQueen MM, McKee MD, Court-Brown CM, editors. Rockwood and Green's fractures in adults. 2nd ed. Philadelphia, PA: Wolters Kluwer; 2019. p. 2537–73.
9. Bostrom A. Fracture of the patella. A study of 422 patellar fractures. Acta Orthop Scand Suppl. 1972;143:1–80.
10. Lazaro LE, Wellman DS, Sauro G, Pardee NC, Berkes MB, Little MT, et al. Outcomes after operative fixation of complete articular patellar fractures: assessment of functional impairment. J Bone Jt Surg Am. 2013;95(14):e96 1–8.
11. LeBrun CT, Langford JR, Sagi HC. Functional outcomes after operatively treated patella fractures. J Orthop Trauma. 2012;26(7):422–6.
12. Schatzker J, McBroom R, Bruce D. The tibial plateau fracture. The Toronto experience 1968–1975. Clin Orthopaed Relat Res. 1979;138:94–104.
13. Luo CF, Sun H, Zhang B, Zeng BF. Three-column fixation for complex tibial plateau fractures. J Orthop Trauma. 2010;24(11):683–92.
14. Maniar H, Kubiak EN, Horwitz DS. Tibial plateau fractures. In: Tornetta III P, Ricci WM, Ostrum RF, McQueen MM, McKee MD, Court-Brown CM, editors. Rockwood and Green's fractures in adults. 2nd ed. Philadelphia, PA: Wolters Kluwer; 2019. p. 2623–86.
15. Robertson GAJ, Wong SJ, Wood AM. Return to sport following tibial plateau fractures: a systematic review. World J Orthop. 2017;8(7):574–87.
16. Quintens L, Van den Berg J, Reul M, Van Lieshout E, Nijs S, Verhofstad M, et al. Poor sporting abilities after tibial plateau fractures involving the posterior column: how can we do better? Eur J Trauma Emerg Surg. 2019;47(1):201–9.
17. Kugelman DN, Qatu AM, Haglin JM, Konda SR, Egol KA. Participation in recreational athletics after operative fixation of tibial plateau fractures: predictors and functional outcomes of those getting back in the game. Orthop J Sports Med. 2017;5(12):2325967117743916.
18. McQueen MM, Gaston P, Court-Brown CM. Acute compartment syndrome. Who is at risk? J Bone Joint Surg. 2000;82(2):200–3.
19. Grutter R, Cordey J, Buhler M, Johner R, Regazzoni P. The epidemiology of diaphyseal fractures of the tibia. Injury. 2000;31(Suppl 3):C64–7.
20. Beebe MJ, Auston DA, Quade JH, Serrano-Riera R, Shah AR, Watson DT, et al. OTA/AO classification is highly predictive of acute compartment syndrome after tibia fracture: a cohort of 2885 fractures. J Orthop Trauma. 2017;31(11):600–5.
21. Gaston P, Will E, Elton RA, McQueen MM, Court-Brown CM. Fractures of the tibia. Can their outcome be predicted? J Bone Joint Surg. 1999;81(1):71–6.
22. Robertson GA, Wood AM. Return to sport after tibial shaft fractures: a systematic review. Sports Health. 2016;8(4):324–30.
23. Tscherne H, Oestern HJ. A new classification of soft-tissue damage in open and closed fractures (author's transl). Unfallheilkunde.

1982;85(3):111–5. Die Klassifizierung des Weichteilschadens bei offenen und geschlossenen Frakturen.
24. Gustilo RB, Anderson JT. Prevention of infection in the treatment of one thousand and twenty-five open fractures of long bones: retrospective and prospective analyses. J Bone Joint Surg Am. 1976;58(4):453–8.
25. Shuler FD, Dietz MJ. Physicians' ability to manually detect isolated elevations in leg intracompartmental pressure. J Bone Joint Surg Am. 2010;92(2):361–7.
26. Purnell GJ, Glass ER, Altman DT, Sciulli RL, Muffly MT, Altman GT. Results of a computed tomography protocol evaluating distal third tibial shaft fractures to assess noncontiguous malleolar fractures. J Trauma. 2011;71(1):163–8.
27. Boulton CL, O'Toole RB. Tibia and fibula shaft fractures. In: Tornetta III P, Ricci WM, Ostrum RF, MM MQ, MD MK, Court-Brown CM, editors. Rockwood and Green's fractures in adults. 2nd ed. Philadelphia, PA: Wolters Kluwer; 2019. p. 2687–751.
28. Court-Brown CM, Byrnes T, McLaughlin G. Intramedullary nailing of tibial diaphyseal fractures in adolescents with open physes. Injury. 2003;34(10):781–5.
29. Dailey HL, Wu KA, Wu PS, McQueen MM, Court-Brown CM. Tibial fracture nonunion and time to healing after reamed intramedullary nailing: risk factors based on a single-center review of 1003 patients. J Orthop Trauma. 2018;32(7):e263–e9.
30. Court-Brown CM, Keating JF, Christie J, McQueen MM. Exchange intramedullary nailing. Its use in aseptic tibial nonunion. J Bone Joint Surg. 1995;77(3):407–11
31. Coles CP, Gross M. Closed tibial shaft fractures: management and treatment complications. A review of the prospective literature. Can J Surg. 2000;43(4):256–62.
32. Court-Brown CM, McBirnie J. The epidemiology of tibial fractures. J Bone Joint Surg. 1995;77(3):417–21.
33. Minkowitz RB, Bhadsavle S, Walsh M, Egol KA. Removal of painful orthopaedic implants after fracture union. J Bone Joint Surg Am. 2007;89(9):1906–12.
34. MacDonald DRW, Caba-Doussoux P, Carnegie CA, Escriba I, Forward DP, Graf M, et al. Tibial nailing using a suprapatellar rather than an infrapatellar approach significantly reduces anterior knee pain postoperatively: a multicentre clinical trial. Bone Joint J. 2019;101-B(9):1138–43.
35. Tatar Y, Ramazanoglu N, Camliguney AF, Saygi EK, Cotuk HB. The effectiveness of shin guards used by football players. J Sports Sci Med. 2014;13(1):120–7.
36. Finch CF, Kelsall HL. The effectiveness of ski bindings and their professional adjustment for preventing alpine skiing injuries. Sports Med. 1998;25(6):407–16.

Acute Fractures in Sport: Ankle

15

David A. Porter, Kaitlyn Hurst, and Madison Walrod

Key Points

- Ankle fractures in athletes are common, serious, and potentially career threatening injuries.
- Displaced fractures and ligament disruptions require fracture fixation and repair of the torn ligaments.
- Recommendations are for rigid, anatomic fixation/repair with early ankle range-of-motion (ROM) and early weight bearing (where indicated)
- Ankle arthroscopy at the time of fracture fixation has gained popularity
- Repair of the deltoid ligament is recommended in athletes at the time of definitive fracture fixation
- We describe our approach using both an open procedure and arthroscopic assistance
- Cartilage injury assessment and treatment remains one of the challenges
- Rehabilitation is crucial to an optimal outcome; Our approach involves early range-of-motion and intermittent immobilisation
- Rehabilitation is enhanced and directed by ligament repair and arthroscopy, respectively.

D. A. Porter (✉)
Methodist Sports Medicine, Indiana University, Indianapolis, IN, USA

Indianapolis Colts, Indiana University, Purdue University, Indianapolis, IN, USA

Wabash College, Crawfordsville, IN, USA

Volunteer Clinical Faculty, Department of Orthopedics, Indiana University, Indianapolis, IN, USA
e-mail: dporter@methodistsports.com

K. Hurst · M. Walrod
Methodist Sports Medicine, Indiana University, Indianapolis, IN, USA
e-mail: kmhurst@iupui.edu; mwalrod@butler.edu

15.1 Introduction

Historically, the literature is sparse regarding ankle fractures in athletes despite ankle injuries accounting for 15–25% of all athletic injuries [1]. Ankle fractures account for 7–10% of all acute sports injury, a 0.11–0.19 rate of injury per 1000 [2, 3]. Although treatment algorithms for the general population are available, there are additional considerations in this population, mainly quick and effective return to play that minimizes disability. There has been a scarcity of investigations to determine the best care for athletes with an ankle fracture. Walsh and Hughston [4] in 1976 first reported on four athletes that required operative fixation after failed non-operative treatment for Weber C/deltoid (three athletes) and one athlete with a Weber B fibula fracture and deltoid ligament injury. Interestingly, the deltoid ligament was repaired with suture in all athletes with a Weber C/deltoid injury, but there was only fixation of the fibula and a syndesmosis screw in the other. All four athletes returned to athletic participation. Not until 2005 was the next small case series reported by Donley et al. [5] on three NFL players with pronation/external rotation injuries that underwent ORIF of the fibula with screw fixation of the syndesmosis. All returned to play the following NFL season. Together, Clanton and Porter [6] explored common foot and ankle injuries, including ankle fractures to help differentiate debilitating injuries from those that can initially present as sprains and strains. With a growing number of athletic injuries related to the foot and ankle, Jelinek et al. [1] expanded on the assessment and treatment of ankle fractures in the athletic population, focusing on the operative care of athletes. More recently, in 2008, Porter et al. [7] focused on postoperative functional outcome in athletes with ankle fractures: ORIF followed by early motion and weight-bearing allowed return-to-play at pre-injury level in 2–4 months with little pain or morbidity. Literature related to ankle injuries in athletes continued to advance as evidenced by Hsu, Lareau, and Anderson [8] reporting on outcomes of acute superficial deltoid avulsion repair during

G. A. J. Robertson, N. Maffulli (eds.), *Fractures in Sport*, https://doi.org/10.1007/978-3-030-72036-0_15

ankle fracture fixation in National Football League players, a treatment which had been highly controversial for decades.

In principle, we favor a more aggressive approach with ankle fractures in athletes. As early as the 1980's, there has been interest in early rigid fixation to allow early range-of-motion in the non-athlete [9]. Michelson [10] has proposed that ankle fracture classification stress stability versus instability rather than just fracture pattern. Unstable fractures do better with surgical fixation and inherently stable fractures can still be treated in many situations with non-operative treatment [1, 7]. Robertson et al. [3] also stressed that stable, nondisplaced fractures are best treated non-operatively [3]. It is critical to determine ligamentous integrity, fracture stability and joint surface congruity. Hunt and colleagues showed that even mild instability or syndesmotic injury leads to decreased contact area and increased joint contact forces in the ankle [11]. Subtle ligamentous laxity impacts injury prognosis and future athletic participation [11]. We will discuss techniques to assess occult instability as well as tips for obtaining and assessing joint congruity.

The Lauge-Hansen [12] and Weber [13] classifications (Fig. 15.1) provide guidance regarding the application of fixation hardware and techniques for fixation. They are also helpful in describing the injury and its likely mechanism, but are poor in determining stability, prognosis, and success of operative versus non operative treatment.

Initial research focused on the importance of anatomic reduction and surgical techniques to obtain and maintain reduction. With significant advances in bone and joint specific implants allowing reliable healing, soft tissue concerns have become more critical in optimizing outcomes. This is particularly important in athletes. One particular area of recent interest within the athletic population involves the deltoid ligament. Historically, there has been controversy regarding whether the lateral aspect or medial aspect of the ankle is more critical in providing stability and prognosis for recovery. Both sides are critical as subtle injuries on either side can result in rotational instability, pain and degenerative changes. Therefore, traditional and historical methods of evaluation can be inadequate in determining the appropriateness of operative versus non operative treatment. For instance, the study by Park [14], assessing gravity stress radiographs with "isolated", short oblique fibular fractures notes this gravity stress testing does not account for isolated

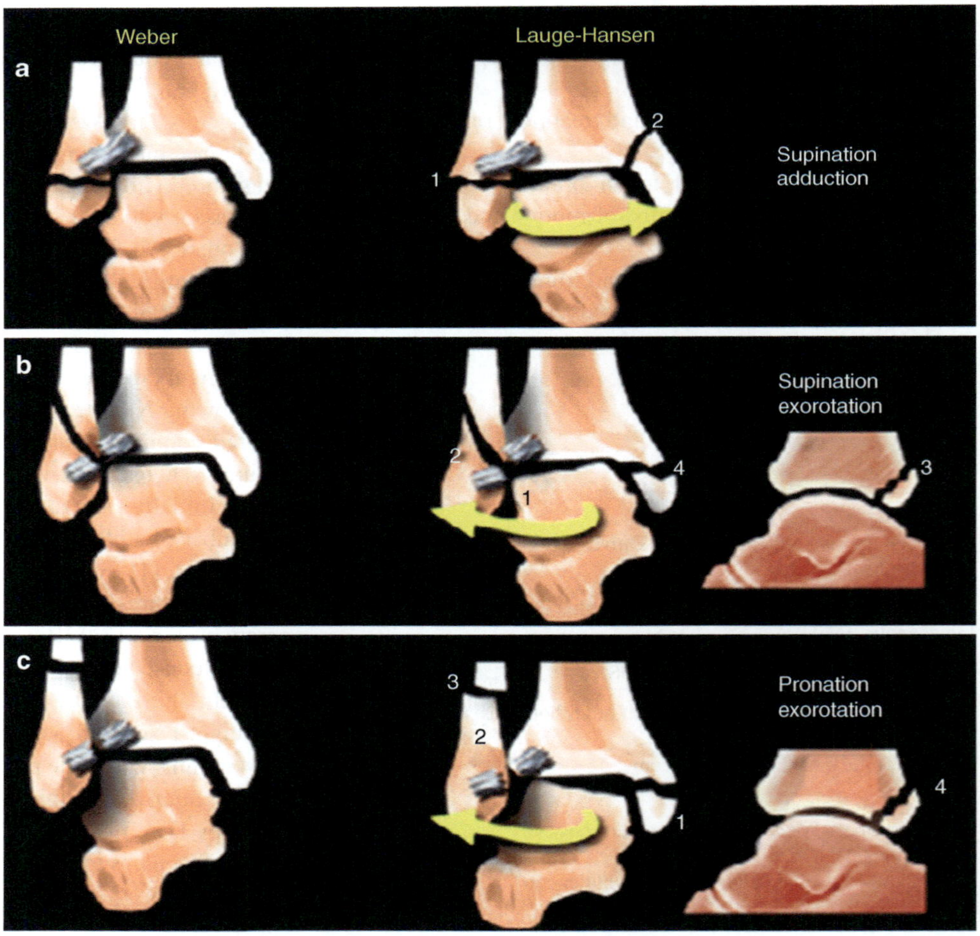

Fig. 15.1 Ankle fracture—Weber and Lauge-Hanson classification. Both Weber classification of distal fibular fractures and Lauge-Hansen of ankle fractures. (*Robin Smithuis* Radiology Department of the Riinland Hospital, Leiderdorp, The Netherlands, 2012-08-23)

anterior deltoid ligament injuries which can result in increased external rotation. This increased external rotation, despite the intact deep deltoid ligament, can be problematic for athletes long-term and it is more difficult to treat in the chronic setting than in the acute setting. Zhao and co-workers recently noted improved medial clear space (MCS) and an association of less mal-reduction of the ankle joint with open repair of the deltoid ligament at the time of fixation of the fracture compared to non-operative treatment of the deltoid with ankle fracture fixation [15]. However, only a small number of these patients were athletes [15]. We will focus on this assessment of the deltoid and its relationship to ankle fractures in athletes.

15.2 Chip Fractures with Ligament Rupture

Small avulsion chip fractures occur off the medial malleolus and the distal fibula. Traction avulsion fractures occur from ligament attachment. These injury patterns signify a ligamentous avulsion off the medial malleolus (deltoid ligament) or distal fibula (anterior talofibular ligament—ATFL) and need to be treated as ligament injuries rather than bone injuries. The small bony flecks can be subtle. Acute versus chronic avulsions is important to distinguish. An acute "fracture" has irregular, non-sclerotic borders and would not be present on prior images if available (Fig. 15.2a, b). Chronic ossicles are common and appear with rounded, sclerotic margins and are often visible on prior imaging when available.

15.2.1 Epidemiology

These small, acute chip avulsion fractures occur commonly with "ankle sprain" mechanism.

Medial malleolar chip fractures occur with eversion injuries causing tension on the deltoid (primarily the deep deltoid) and avulsing a small fleck of bone off the distal tip. It is important to recognize that a serious complete deltoid rupture can occur and must be treated aggressively (see isolated deltoid rupture below). Partial deltoid ligament rupture can also occur which portends a less concerning injury, but is not innocuous.

Distal fibula avulsions commonly occur with lateral ankle sprain mechanisms. This small chip fracture indicates a

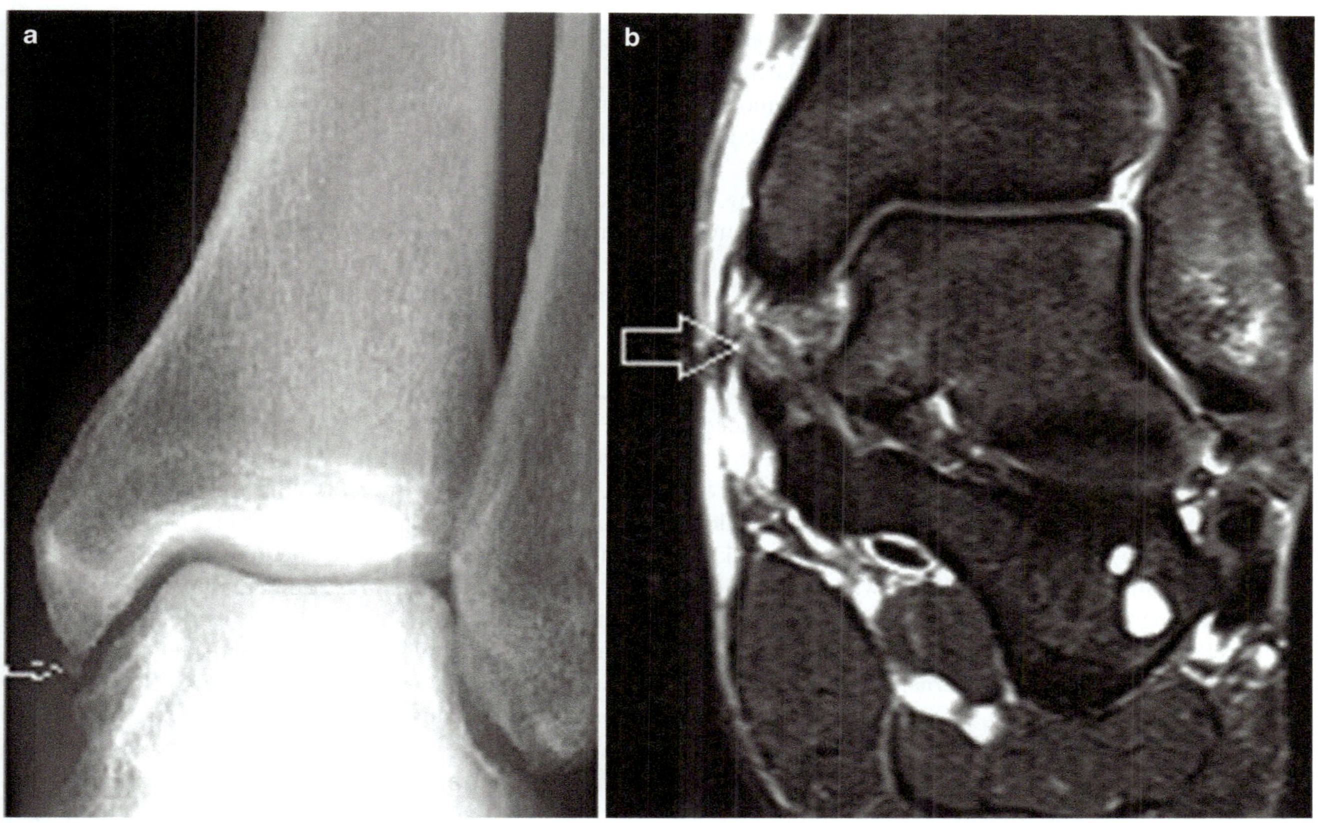

Fig. 15.2 (**a**, **b**) Anterior-posterior radiograph and coronal STIR Magnetic Resonance Imaging (MRI) left ankle demonstrating deltoid ligament rupture with chip fracture. (**a**) antero-posterior radiograph of left ankle denoting small avulsion fracture tip of the medial malleolus in an Olympic gymnast. (**b**) Coronal STIR MRI image of left ankle of the same athlete demonstrating actual complete, isolated deep deltoid ligament rupture. This avulsion "fracture" was treated for the deltoid ligament rupture, rather than the avulsion fracture. It is thus important to realize this acute tiny "fracture" was attached to a large avulsed ligament

Grade II or III lateral sprain. Despite the appearance of the avulsion being inferior and possibly in the CFL, the avulsion chip is most commonly at the origin of the ATFL.

15.2.2 Classification

There is no commonly used classification system for these chip fractures. As mentioned, the most important distinction to make is whether these bony fragments are acute fractures or chronic ossicles. Therefore, the classification would simply be acute versus chronic. The acute fracture will have sharp edges, and the donor site will match up to this corresponding chip fracture. Acute chip fractures will have swelling and ecchymosis, whereas chronic ossicles may have focal pain, but typically no ecchymoses and minimal swelling.

15.2.3 Diagnosis (History/Physical Examination/Imaging)

Diagnosis is centered around a precise history and careful examination. It is critical to determine the mechanism of injury. In particular, did the athlete have an inversion injury which can result in both medial (impaction) and lateral (distraction—ligament tear) pain, swelling and ecchymosis, or did the athlete have an eversion or external rotation component to the injury.

Medial malleolar chip fractures, in an acute setting, can occur from inversion sprains with medial impingement. More concerning are eversion and external rotation injuries with associated dorsiflexion which can present with small avulsion fractures that are actually significant deltoid ligament injuries (Fig. 15.3a–c). Careful examination of the athlete will reveal tenderness at the site of the chip fracture off the medial malleolus. If swelling, ecchymosis, and tenderness are present only over the medial aspect, and there is a history of an eversion and/or external rotation injury with dorsiflexion, a high-grade deltoid ligament injury should be suspected. In this setting, the lateral aspect of the ankle is typically nonpainful and not swollen. Swelling laterally or diffuse swelling and ecchymosis throughout the ankle will suggest either a high-grade lateral ankle sprain with medial impingement, or a significant external rotation and syndesmosis injury.

Distal fibular chip fractures present in a different manner. These injuries are typical of a lateral ankle sprain mechanism. Often athletes focus on fear, the level of pain, and recovery timeline. In other words, "when do I get better?" Discipline on the part of the examining healthcare provider is again important to solicit a detailed history of the mechanisms of injury. Demonstration with one's own foot and ankle may help athletes clarify the position of the foot in relationship to the ankle at the time of injury. A lateral Grade II or III ankle sprain will have significant lateral ecchymosis and swelling with tenderness over the lateral ligaments. With higher Grade II and III injuries, there is also some medial tenderness from impingement, but the level of swelling and ecchymosis is less than what is seen laterally.

Radiographic evaluation typically involves standing, weight-bearing three views (antero-posterior, lateral and oblique/mortise) of the ankle. Special attention should be directed at the alignment of the ankle joint including the medial clear space, the tibio-fibular interval and overlap, and any bony injury. To reiterate, avulsion fractures are often small and located at the tip of the medial malleolus, or the anterior tip of the fibula (Figs. 15.2a, b and 15.3a–c). Further advanced imaging is reserved for suspicious deltoid ligament ruptures and to evaluate high-grade lateral ankle sprains for evaluation of bone bruise and occult osteochondral lesions/fractures. Magnetic resonance imaging (MRI) is typically the most helpful test in this regard (Figs. 15.2a, b and 15.3a–c). Computed tomography (CT) can be used to identify small osteochondral lesions or extra-articular chip fractures which can be difficult to evaluate on MRI imaging.

15.2.4 Treatment

Significant lateral ankle sprains which result in distal fibular or medial malleolar chip fractures without medial-sided instability are typically treated as lateral ankle sprains [6]. Medial-sided "chip fractures" that appear chronic and rounded off can be treated symptomatically. Acute medial malleolar chip fractures that involved significant deltoid ligament injury are treated as discussed below in Sect. 15.3.

15.2.5 Complications

Complications related to these small fractures around the ankle are typically limited to insufficient diagnosis, or insufficient treatment. Insufficient diagnosis is related to a failure to recognize the ligamentous injury present with the initially underwhelming radiographic appearance of a small chip fracture. This results in insufficient treatment of a complete deltoid ligament injury medially or inadequate periods of immobilisation for Grade III lateral ankle sprains. Misdiagnosis, or under treatment, of isolated deltoid ligament injuries can have a devastating effect on the athlete. Outcomes after reconstruction for chronic isolated deltoid ligament injuries can be unpredictable [16]. Delayed treatment often results in chronic pain, residual instability and ultimately early arthritis and inability to return to sports. Appropriate early immobilisation and/or operative repair have both produced predictably good to excellent results [17].

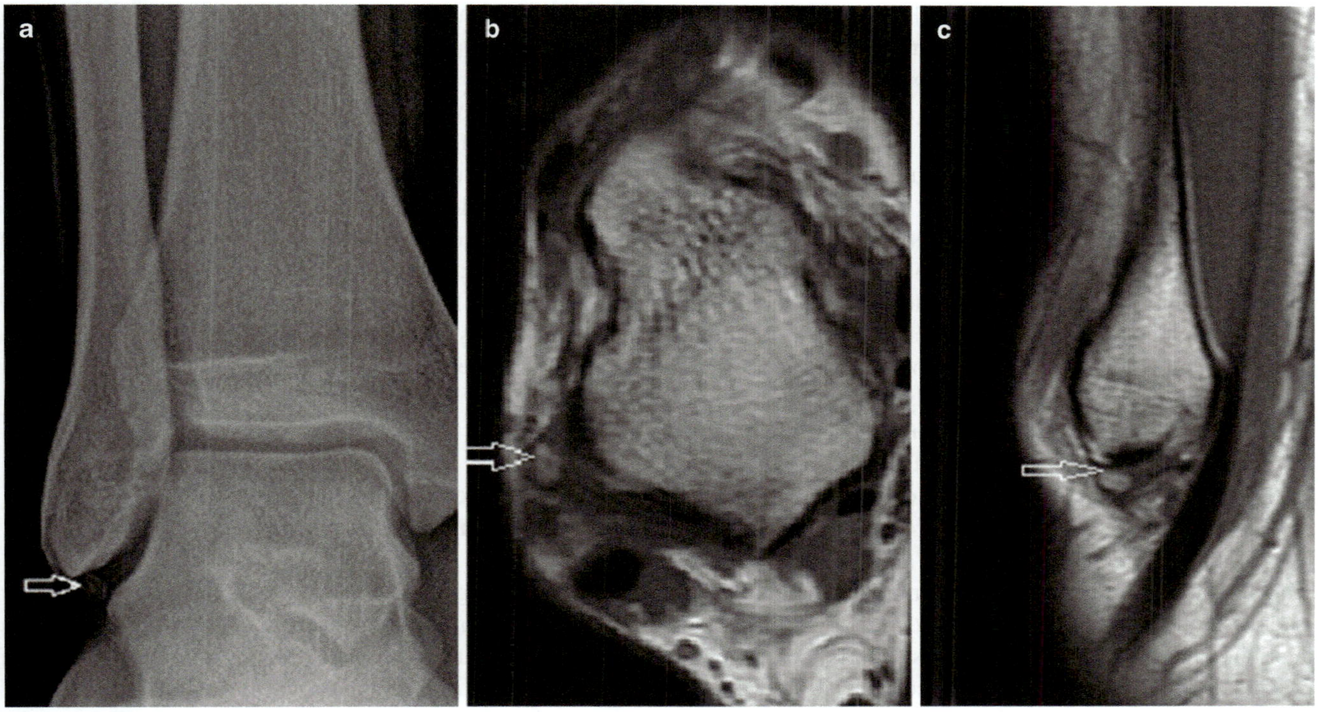

Fig. 15.3 (a–c) Plain radiographs and MRI of distal fibular avulsion fracture. (**a**) antero-posterior image of right ankle in Division 1 gymnast with distal fibular avulsion fracture (arrow). This can be confused with an acute fracture, but is actually an ossicle in the anterior talofibular ligament (ATFL) and will be treated more as a ligament injury than fracture. (**b**) Axial T1 MRI image of the right ankle showing an ossicle within the substance of the ATFL (arrow). (**c**) Sagittal T1 MRI image showing an ossicle within the substance of the ATFL ligament (arrow). Note the more anterior location at the ATFL attachment, well anterior to the peroneal tendons

15.2.6 Rehabilitation

Rehabilitation of acute medial malleolar chip fractures with a deltoid ligament injury follow the rehabilitation protocol of isolated deltoid ligament injuries. Chronic medial malleolar ossicles aggravated by an acute injury are typically treated symptomatically and return should be rapid (as quickly as 1–3 weeks). Grade II lateral ankle sprains with small chip fractures require a short period of immobilisation with a typical return to play between 3 and 5 weeks with a brace. Grade III lateral ankle sprains with associated small chip fractures should be treated similarly to an ankle dislocation and require 5–8 weeks for full recovery. An aggressive weight-bearing program with immobilisation and treatment at night to keep the ankle in dorsiflexion is critical [18]. Functional rehabilitation is effective for all lateral ankle sprains [19].

15.2.7 Preventative Measures

Preventative measures will focus on reducing the risk of recurrent ankle sprain. Therefore, since the small avulsion fractures are typically more ligament related, protocols that are geared toward proprioception and functional return to daily activity are most critical for prevention of re-injury [19]. Goals of rehabilitation should include full range of motion, full strength return, and return to normal proprioception.

15.3 Isolated Deltoid Ligament Ruptures

15.3.1 Epidemiology

The deltoid ligament is a complex (DLC) structure of the tibiotalar joint that is integral to overall medial ankle stability and specifically limits talar tilt, eversion and anterior and/or anteromedial translation [6]. The deltoid ligamentous complex [20] is divided into superficial and deep layer, with the superficial layer having four bands and the deep having two. The superficial layer crosses both the tibiotalar joint and the subtalar joint and is subdivided into two major components: the tibial-spring ligament (TSL) and the tibionavicular ligament (TNL) which constitute the *anterior deltoid*, and two additional bands—the superficial posterior tibiotalar ligament (SPTL) and the tibiocalcaneal ligament (TCL) which are superficial layers of the *deep deltoid*. The deep layer of the DLC crosses the ankle joint and consists of the primary deep posterior tibiotalar ligament (DPTL) and an additional band, the anterior deep tibiotalar ligament (ADTL) [21, 22]. The *anterior deltoid ligament* is responsible for controlling external rotation and the *deep deltoid ligament* controls principally eversion.

Isolated deltoid ligamentous injuries, or medial ankle sprains (MAS), occur less commonly than injuries to the lateral ligamentous structures, but they still account for 3–16% of ankle sprains. The mechanism of injury is a pronation or eversion trauma where the foot is externally rotated and the tibia is simultaneously internally rotated [6, 16]. Examples include running downstairs, landing on uneven surfaces, and dancing with the body simultaneously rotating in the opposite direction [16]. Injuries occur on a spectrum, ranging from sprains to complete rupture of the deltoid ligament. Isolated deltoid ligament injuries most commonly involve the superficial parts [23], while complete deltoid ligament tears, both superficial and deep parts, are almost always seen with lateral malleolar or bimalleolar fractures [16, 23]. A study of collegiate athletes found an equal predilection for laterality and gender [24]. Highest risk sports include men's basketball, rugby, lacrosse, and soccer as well as women's cheerleading, soccer, basketball, and volleyball. Our personal experience for isolated MAS has been in American Football and tumbling with cheer leading and gymnastics. MAS during American football typically occurs in a pile up or while landing from a jump. Tumbling involves an awkward landing, often when landing "short". Both scenarios involve the ankle dorsiflexed and the heel forced into isolated eversion, thus isolating the forces medially without external rotation.

Medial ankle instability can result from an acute injury to the deltoid ligament with a varied injury pattern [16]. It can also result from a chronic laxity due to various etiologies including residual instability from an ankle sprain, inefficiency of the posterior tibial tendon, or chronic overload [16]. Most medial ligament injuries are associated with concomitant injury to the lateral ligaments (AITFL), syndesmosis, or fibula [6, 23]. However, isolated injuries to the medial ankle do occur, accounting for less than 10% of all ankle sprains [6]. Though rarely isolated, it is important to diagnose these isolated injuries as return to sport with a completely disrupted DLC can lead to instability, delayed rehabilitation, and potentially long-term medial instability [23]. If the ankle has severe medial swelling and ecchymosis without lateral pain and a consistent mechanism of injury, an isolated tear must be suspected and thoroughly evaluated.

15.3.2 Classification

Classification of acute deltoid ligament injuries is based on the location and extent of the injury. Deltoid ligament injury can be graded on a scale of I–III. Grade I is an isolated deltoid ligament sprain with no instability [6]. Grade II involves partial tear and often involves significant anterior deltoid ligament injury with an intact deep deltoid. Grade III is a complete tear of the ligament [6]. Hintermann et al. [16] divided injuries to the anterior bundles of the deltoid ligament into three lesion types: Type I, proximal tear or avulsion of the deltoid ligament; Type II, intermediate tear of the deltoid ligament; Type III distal tear or avulsion of the deltoid and spring ligaments. In a series of 52 patients with medial ankle instability treated operatively, Type-I lesions were found to be the most common, comprising 71% compared to 10% for Type II, and 19% for Type III [25].

15.3.3 Diagnosis (History/Physical Examination/Imaging)

Acute deltoid ligament injuries occur from a pronation or eversion injury of the foot. Therefore, obtaining a clear and precise history of the patient's account of the mechanism of injury and specifically the position of the foot at the time of injury is helpful in determining the diagnosis. This can be difficult in practice, as patients often cannot remember the specific mechanism or have a history of multiple ankle sprains. Patients with an acute deltoid ligament injury will complain of anteromedial ankle pain, and often present with corresponding medial ecchymosis. Weight bearing may be impossible or significantly limited secondary to pain. Physical examination may include loading the ankle joint associated with instability [16]. Chronic injuries classically present with pain in the medial gutter which may be provoked by palpation of the anterior border of medial malleolus [16]. Excessive valgus and pronation of the affected foot while weightbearing indicate more diffuse medial ankle laxity [16]. Reliable clinical tests include varus and valgus tilt stress applied to the heel, as well as the anterior drawer test to be performed bilaterally [16]. Other essential examinations include the external rotation test and squeeze, which should be performed to rule out syndesmosis injury in all athletes [6].

Standard plain radiographs are recommended in acute trauma to rule out fractures. MRI may be used to evaluate the deltoid ligament complex; however, this modality is be less sensitive than arthroscopic assessment and may not be helpful in determining treatment, especially in the *anterior deltoid ligament* and in chronic laxity, which is difficult to visualize with MRI [16, 26, 27]. MRI can be helpful in assessing the cartilage and if there is associated chronic tendon involvement. Radiographic evidence of medial ankle sprains includes 2–3 mm widening of medial clear space, displaced lateral malleolus, syndesmosis disruption [6]. Isolated deltoid ligament injury may present with only a small medial malleolar chip fracture. This subtle finding has to be appreciated as a deltoid ligament injury in the right clinical setting (Fig. 15.2a, b). Weight-bearing radiographs are key, particularly when assessing chronic instability [16].

Although judicious use of MRI is recommended in the general population, in athletes with a suspected isolated deltoid ligament injury, an MRI is very helpful to confirm injury and distinguish the extent of the tear (Fig. 15.4a–c). Determining and distinguishing isolated anterior deltoid ligament injury from partial deep and anterior deltoid ligament and complete deep and anterior deltoid ligament tear is critical in athletes. Also, concomitant assessment of the syndesmosis and AITFL is critical to planning treatment. We do routinely use MRI scan in athletes since timing and missing a subtle injury can be so devastating. We then confirm instability with stress radiographs (Fig. 15.4b).

15.3.4 Treatment

Isolated deltoid ligament sprains can be successfully treated with a period of cast immobilisation and gradual return to pre-injury activity level. No randomized data has been published comparing non-operative treatment protocols for medial ankle sprains. However, accepted immobilisation is typically implemented for 6 weeks. We prefer operative repair if there are any loose bodies or significant cartilage injury that needs to be addressed and if the athlete is more comfortable with operative intervention. We reserve non-operative treatment for those patients with no cartilage or other associated ligament/tendon injury. We prefer 4 weeks of cast immobilisation followed by a custom short-articulated AFO (ShAFO—Fig. 15.19a) for 6–10 weeks, and, depending on field position and sport, we use the Short-articulating AFO for initial return to sports.

Operative treatment of complete deltoid ligament injuries is controversial. McCallum et al. [23] and Hsu [8] recommends arthroscopy for complete deltoid ligament injuries to assess the extent of the ligament injury and to treat intra-articular pathology. In-folding of the ruptured deltoid ligament is a common cause of persistent increased medial clear space, mal-reduction, and postoperative pain and instability [8, 23]. If identified, the deltoid ligament must be explored with the talus accurately reduced and ligament repaired [23]. In the acute setting, complete ruptures often involve the proximal deltoid ligament [16]. Surgical treatment includes reinsertion to the medial malleolus by suturing directly to the bone with or without bony anchor [16]. Furthermore, Clanton and Porter [6] recommended open repair with anatomic alignment of the medial clear space in the mortise could not be achieved.

Surgical repair of deltoid ligament tears in the acute setting has become more popular in association with other lateral sided injury e.g. unstable fibula fractures, and ankle fractures with syndesmotic injuries. Hsu recommended a more aggressive approach in Weber C fibula fracture in NFL players [8]. However, no studies exist currently regarding the optimal treatment for isolated complete deltoid ligament injuries in athletes. We tend to favor a more aggressive approach in professional athletes and Division I athletes after having good success with repair in ankle fracture. However, this is anecdotal and a personal preference.

Surgical treatment is dependent on the type of lesion, i.e. the location of the injury. Type I and III injuries may be

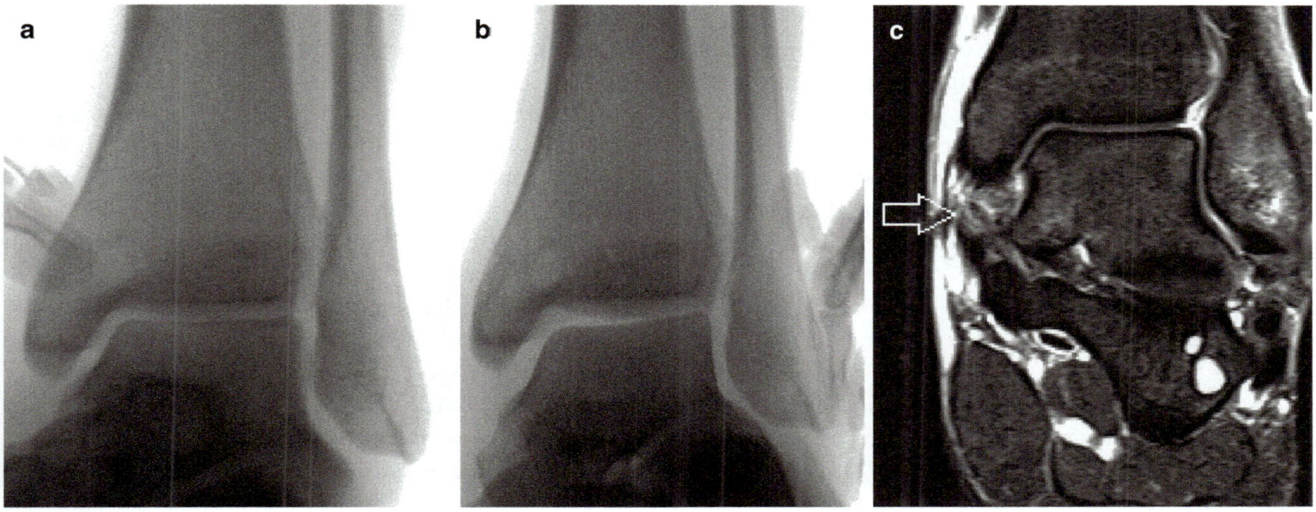

Fig. 15.4 (**a**) Anterior-posterior radiograph of left ankle in non-stressed position. Note normal appearing alignment, including normal medial clear space. (**b**) Stress antero-posterior Radiographs of the same left ankle noting mild talar tilt and increased widening in the medial clear space suggesting complete tear of the deltoid ligament. (**c**) Coronal STIR MRI scan of the left ankle confirming complete rupture of the deep deltoid ligament with normal appearing cartilage in the ankle

repaired with suture anchors or trans-osseous sutures to repair the avulsed tissue back to its anatomical origin or insertion. In Type-II lesions the ligament is typically hypertrophied and redundant. This tissue is divided and the deep part repaired to the malleolar tip as in Type I lesions. The portion originating at the medial malleolus is then brought down superficially and repaired to the navicular tuberosity using a second anchor. Finally, when ligament quality does not permit repair with anchors, autologous reconstruction with a free tendon graft should be considered. Careful attention must be paid to reconstruct the deltoid ligament in its anatomical position and not to overtighten the repair [28]. Hsu [8] recommended only reattachment of the *anterior deltoid ligament* to the medial malleolus with suture anchors, but this approach may not be adequate in acute, isolated, complete deltoid ligament ruptures. Repair of both the anterior and deep deltoid ligament is favored when there is a complete, isolated tear [1].

Chronic rupture of deep deltoid ligament often includes an extended tear of the superficial *anterior deltoid ligament* bundles of the deltoid ligament [16]. Importantly, reconstruction must account for the entire deltoid ligament [16]. Treatment of complete, chronic deltoid ligament ruptures are beyond the scope of this chapter.

15.3.5 Complications

The greatest challenge of this injury is chronic medial instability from incompetence of the deep deltoid ligament despite tendon augmentation [16]. To overcome this challenge, Hintermann favored a triple arthrodesis to achieve appropriate alignment and stability [16]. Despite providing excellent realignment, pain relief and stability, we have not seen athletes able to return to competitive sports after this procedure. This heightens the need for accurate and precise acute treatment. Chondral injury are another potential complications in the acute and chronic settings. Removal of loose chondral fragments and microfracture can be beneficial in the acute setting. Chronic deltoid ligament laxity must be prevented to avoid chronic chondral lesions and post-traumatic arthritis.

15.3.6 Rehabilitation

There is little literature available regarding return to sport and training following a deltoid ligament repair without fracture in athletes [23]. Hintermann et al. [16] recommends casting for 6 weeks postoperatively with a walker or stabilizing shoe to follow, along with initiation of physiotherapy. Rehabilitation includes active and passive range of motion and strengthening. Even with operative repair, we use 4 weeks of casting. ROM is initiated at 4 weeks, biking with the cast or boot can begin at 2–4 weeks. Progressive return to sports occurs after 3–4 months.

15.3.7 Preventative Measures

The two most common sports for isolated deltoid ligament rupture are gymnastics and American football. Prevention of injury in gymnastics is related to careful advancement within new skills and not over extending the abilities of young gymnasts. The injury is typically related to landing short and awkwardly on the involved, dorsiflexed ankle while the heel is in slight valgus. Young gymnasts who try to be overly aggressive with extending the routine often find themselves in compromised positions while landing.

American football presents a different set of circumstances. These players are in a compromised position while being tackled, within a pile up, or landing awkwardly while being flipped or after trying an acrobatic catch or maneuver. Educating athletes to avoid jumping over defenders is one way to prevent this significant ligamentous injury. There is data currently within the injury prevention segment of the National football league regarding the length of cleats and the giving away at the cleat field surface that may be involved in preventive measures also. That is, there is a certain amount of torque required to rupture this ligament, and shorter cleats may allow the foot to disengage from the surface before reaching this critical stress. This preventative approach is more studied and assessed within the syndesmosis and external rotation injuries.

15.4 Salter-Harris Growth Plate Fractures

15.4.1 Epidemiology

Pediatric ankle fractures are defined as tibia and fibula fractures distal to the diaphysis with open physes [29]. As the younger population increasingly participates in sporting activities, it is not uncommon to see unstable ankle injuries with open physes as this injury pattern typically occurs during sport or low-energy trauma [29]. Fifteen percent (15%) of all injuries in children involve the physis, and one 33.5% of all physeal injuries occurred during competitive sports with competitive sports having a higher rate than recreational sports [30]. Reportedly, ankle fractures account for 5% of all pediatric fractures and approximately 15% of physeal injuries [1, 29]. There is a greater incidence of ankle fractures in children with increased BMI, as well as those who partake in basketball, soccer, and football [29]. The growth plate is more susceptible to injury with direct blow or indirect trauma since the resistance of stress is up to 2–5× less at the epiphysis than surrounding bone and ligaments [31].

15.4.2 Classification

The Salter-Harris (SH) classification is commonly used to describe physeal injuries [1, 7, 29, 32]. This system groups physeal injuries into Types I–V. Salter-Harris Type I involves only the physis with minimal widening or translation [29]. Salter Harris Type II extends proximally from the physis into the metaphysis, while Type III extend from the physis into and through the epiphysis [7, 29]. Salter-Harris Type IV fractures extend from the physis to both distally to the epiphysis and proximally into the metaphysis [33, 34]. Lastly, Salter-Harris Type V is the rare fracture in which a crush injury occurs within the physis itself [29]. This Type V crush injury is the most susceptible to physeal injury because of the traumatic disruption within the whole growth plate, which can lead to growth arrest, resulting shortening and/or malalignment.

The Tilleaux and Triplane fractures are the more specific types of the Salter Harris fracture patterns seen in athletes. The Tilleaux fracture results from the pattern of distal tibia growth plate closure that starts centrally, progresses to medial closure leaving the anterolateral distal growth plate susceptible to "avulsion" supination and inversion injuries. The Tilleaux fracture is common in the young teen athlete ages 12–15. The Triplane fracture (Fig. 15.5a, b) is a specific SH-IV pattern with a posterior metaphyseal "Thurston-Holland" fragment, an axial intraphyseal component with a distal, sagittal oriented, intra-articular epiphyseal fracture. Displacement greater than 2–3 mm requires operative reduction and screw fixation (Fig. 15.6a–d). Also, SH-II of the distal tibia with displacement also requires anterior to posterior screw fixation to reduce the risk of growth plate premature closure. When a growth plate injury is displaced, there can be interposition of the thickened periosteum within the fracture, preventing closed reduction. In these patients, at surgery it is necessary to gently free the fracture ends of the periosteum, followed by accurate reduction and fixation with at least one screw (Fig. 15.7).

15.4.3 Diagnosis (History/Physical Examination/Imaging)

The history of the patient is important in distinguishing an ankle fracture from an ankle sprain. Presentation typically follows a twisting injury to the ankle with complaints of inability to bear weight, bony tenderness, swelling or deformity [29]. Physical examination should include assessing neurovascular compromise, ligamentous injury, as well as tenderness along bony anatomy. To assess syndesmosis, a squeeze test or a stress test can be performed [29]. Isolated syndesmosis disruption without fracture is rare in adolescents.

Ankle radiographs with three views are used to evaluate for fracture in each adolescent ankle injury with swelling,

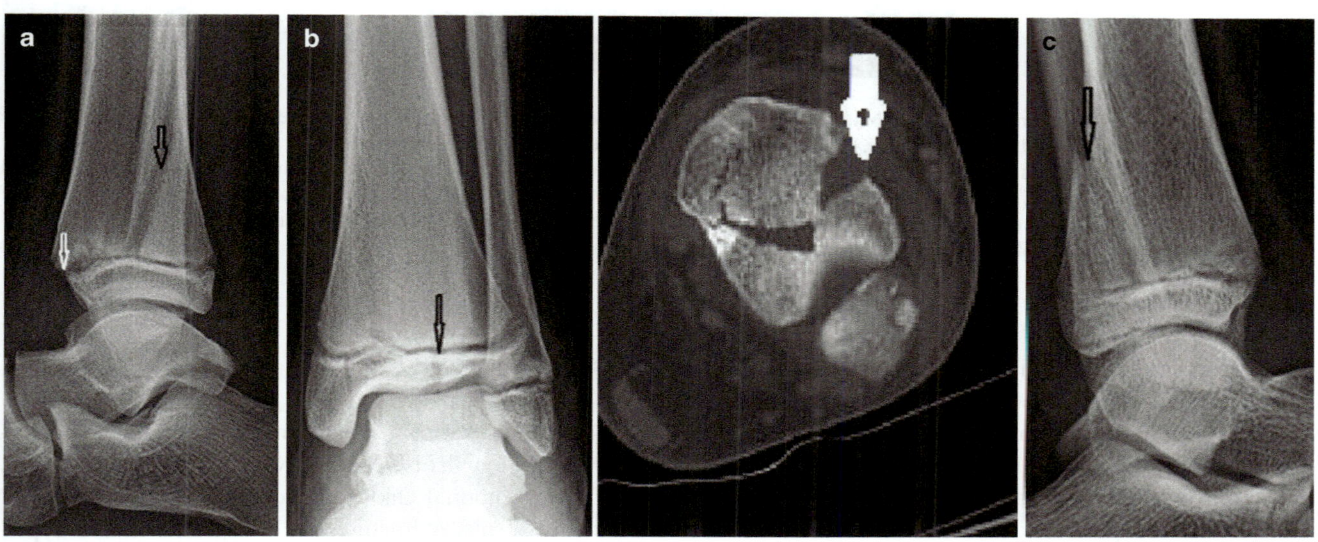

Fig. 15.5 (**a**) is lateral radiograph demonstrating displaced metaphyseal Salter-Harris II fracture of tibia in a 10-year-old female soccer goalie, Note the white arrow depicting the posterior displacement of the intact epiphysis on the metaphysis and the black arrow depicting the more proximal displaced tibia extending to the posterior cortex. (**b**) is an antero-posterior ankle image noting the subtle vertical fracture line (black arrow) in the distal tibial epiphysis of a 12-year-old female soccer player who fell awkwardly. Note the severe displacement of the distal tibial epiphysis with rotational malalignment but has intact distal tibial metaphysis thus a Salter-Harris III distal epiphyseal fracture. (**c**) A lateral radiographic image of a 16-year-old male football running back who had another player land on his ankle in a pile-up. Note the lateral image depicts the displaced tibial metaphysis fracture extending to the posterior-superior cortex, thus demonstrating a Salter-Harris II distal tibia fracture

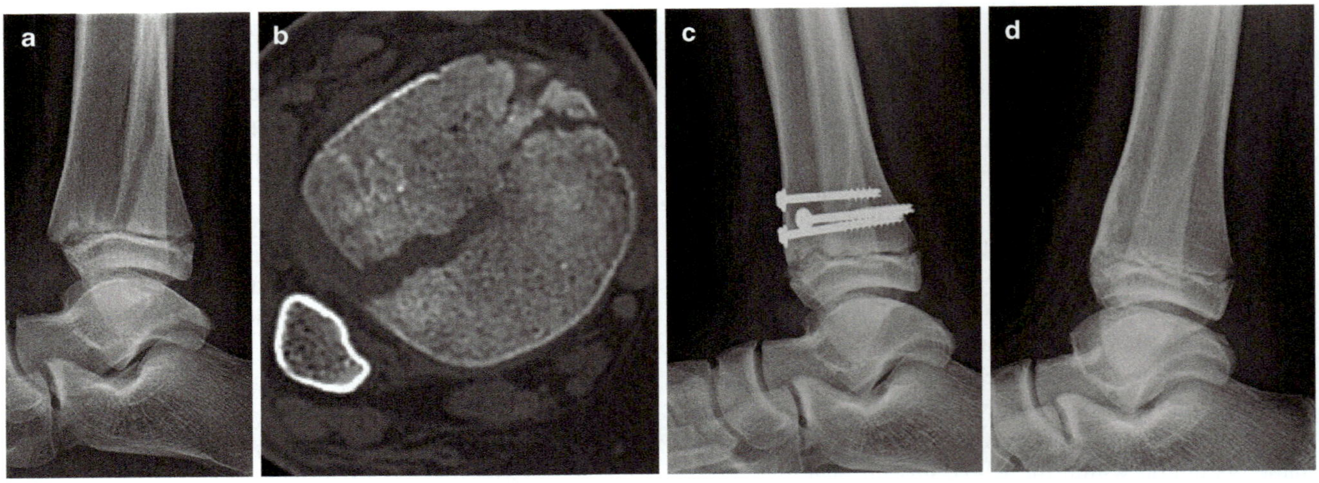

Fig. 15.6 (**a**) Lateral radiograph of 12-year-old soccer player with displaced Salter-Harris II (SH II) distal tibia fracture. Note that the distal epiphysis is posteriorly displaced showing malalignment of the distal growth plate. (**b**) Axial Computed axial tomogram of SH II fracture distal tibia with 4.5 mm of displacement. (**c**) Lateral image of distal tibia after Open Reduction Internal Fixation (ORIF) SH II distal tibia fracture with three, parallel, 4.0 mm screws with washers and anatomic reduction. (**d**) Anatomically reduced SH II distal tibia fracture after healing and removal hardware. Note open distal tibial growth plate despite growth fracture/injury

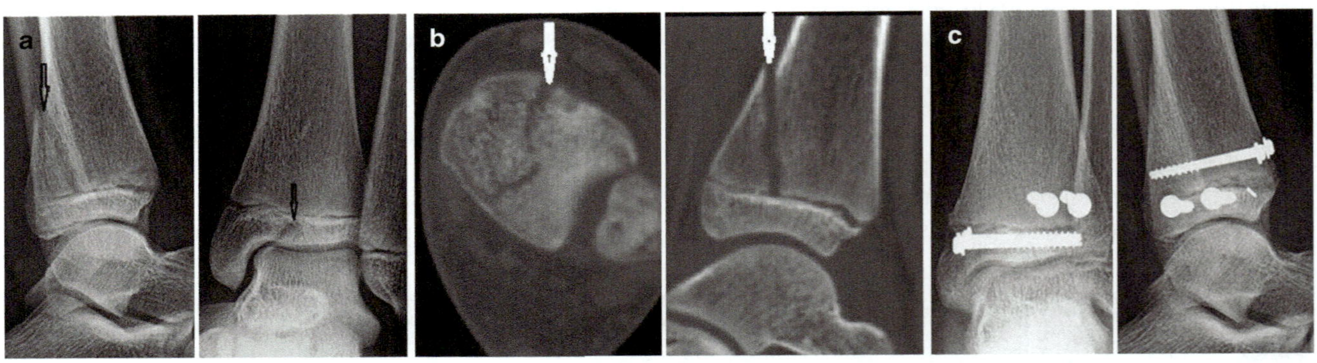

Fig. 15.7 (**a–c**) Triplane fracture of the distal tibia in 16-year-old High School running back. (**a**) Lateral and antero-posterior radiograph of left ankle suspicious for Salter-Harris IV (triplane) fracture distal tibia. Not suspected fracture tibial metaphysis and distal tibia epiphysis (black arrows) with possible intra-articular displacement. (**b**) Axial and sagittal CT image left tibia confirming displaced intra-articular epiphysis and displaced tibia metaphysis (white arrows). Associated fracture through growth plate itself accounts for the three planes of fracture. (**c**) antero-posterior and lateral left ankle showing anatomic reduction and rigid screw fixation triplane (SH IV) fracture. Note small broken tip of guide wire that can happen with these small cannulated screws/drills

ecchymosis and/or inability to bear weight. Evaluation should include assessment for physeal widening, which could indicate a Salter-Harris Type I [29]. A Salter-Harris Type II of the tibia is best seen on lateral radiographs [29]. Salter Harris II of the fibula can be seen on any of the three views. Other imaging modalities, including CT and MRI scanning, should be considered if an intra-articular fracture pattern is suspected on radiographs (SH III–IV) [29]. Conversely, stress radiographs, which are often key to diagnose instability in adults, are often not recommended in the pediatric population because of injury risk to the growth plate [29].

15.4.4 Treatment

The goals of treatment include minimizing angular deformity and leg length discrepancy, avoid osteoarthritis changes, and achieve normal ankle function [29]. Non-displaced or minimally displaced fractures, including Salter-Harris Type I and II can be treated with closed reduction (Type II) and casting [1, 29]. This author actually prefers boot immobilisation rather than casting if the patient and family are reliable [35]. Of note, multiple manipulation attempts should be avoided as it has been linked to greater risk of growth arrest and early closure of the physis [29].

Displaced Salter-Harris II–IV benefit from reduction, internal fixation, and anatomic restoration of the joint surface, as this is linked to lower rates of growth arrest [29]. Surgical intervention is also recommended with residual displacement after attempted closed reduction of greater than 2 mm [1]. Care should be taken to avoid crossing the physes with rigid screw fixation [1]. Porter et al. [7] reported on four athletes with Salter-Harris fractures, ranging from Type II to Type IV, treated surgically with three of the four athletes rating their ankles 100% on AAOS Ankle Module questionnaire postoperatively. The remaining athlete reported occasional swelling [7].

15.4.5 Complications

Complications associated with physeal injuries include growth arrest and joint problems. Salter-Harris I–II are associated with overall risk of premature closure of 2–67%, and Salter-Harris III–IV have an overall risk of 8–50% [29]. Other factors contributing to growth arrest include fracture type, greater displacement, and multiple manipulation attempts [29]. Other ankle joint problems include arthritis, stiffness, and pain [29]. Salter-Harris III–IV distal tibial fractures have a greater risk of post-traumatic arthritis, especially if angular deformity remains [29]. Reflex sympathetic dystrophy (RSD), or complex regional pain syndrome (CRPS), has also occurred about ankle injuries with a higher prevalence in young females compared to males [29]. A recent non-published pilot study presentation suggested via questionnaire data from Pediatric Orthopedic surgeons, that removable boot immobilisation had a lower complication rate for chronic pain, RSD/CRPS and stiffness [35].

In general, the risk of growth arrest (complete or partial) increases with SH grade. However, non-displaced fractures regardless of grade (except SH-V) have a low propensity of growth plate injury. Displaced SH fractures require reduction and fixation in athletes. Displacement by definition does not occur in SH-I lesions. If there is no bony injury and there is displacement through the physes, we would classify it as SH-V. We recommend following these more worrisome growth plate injuries until closure or 1–2 years for all displaced Salter Harris fractures.

15.4.6 Rehabilitation

Porter [7] has delineated most specifically a rehabilitation protocol for these fractures. There has been very little reported on growth plate fracture in the adolescent population. Porter [7] reported on four athletes with Salter-Harris fractures. There were three Salter-Harris III fractures of the distal tibia (one also had a SH III of the fibula) and one Salter Harris IV distal tibia fracture (with a SH II of the fibula). These authors recommended early weight bearing and early range-of-motion (ROM) with intermittent immobilisation if rigid fixation can be obtained. This more progressive rehabilitation counteracts the "cast disease" often noted with less progressive approaches [35]. That is, the severe atrophy and stiffness seen with non-weight bearing and prolonged rigid casting is negated with the intermittent immobilisation, early ROM and even weight bearing within 2–3 weeks of rigid fixation. Jelinek [1], reporting on the similar population, reiterated the need to remove any interposed periosteum to achieve anatomic reduction of the growth plate to reduce the risk of physeal injury. After this careful reduction and rigid fixation, they felt the more progressive approach to rehabilitation was safe [1].

15.4.7 Preventative Measures

Though injuries are an inevitable part of sports, there may be ways to avoid such incidents. Some prevention strategies include education and behavioral intervention, environmental interventions, and enforcement or legislative interventions [36]. Examples of such strategies include pre-season physical examinations, medical coverage at sporting events, proper coaching and officiating, suitable equipment and protective wear, and appropriate playing conditions [36]. As mentioned above, proper removal of the interposed periosteum with careful and non-traumatic reduction of the physes with rigid screw fixation of the fracture without violation of the physes is a technical point to always keep in mind to reduce the risk of growth plate injury. Youth sports have adopted weight restrictions and guidelines to decrease injuries. Interestingly, one study indicated there was no increased risk to a smaller player when there were no weight limits [37]. From this paper's perspective, it was interesting to note that ankle fracture was the most common "significant injury" during this football study season [37].

15.5 Unstable Syndesmosis/Maisonneuve Fracture

15.5.1 Epidemiology

External rotation ankle injuries can involve several different structures. These injuries that result in fractures are discussed below (Weber C/B with deltoid). Up to 23% of ankle fractures in the general population involves the distal tibial-fibular syndesmosis [37]. Maisonneuve fractures include a proximal fibula fracture with disruption of the syndesmosis and deltoid ligament. There is a continuum of ligament injury. Traditionally, the external rotation injury/syndesmosis ankle "fracture" or "sprain" is graded as stable (Grade I), occult unstable (Grade II) or unstable (Grade III). As there is a continuum of injury within Grade I and into Grade II, this needs further subclassification. This further delineation is critical to correct treatment approaches. Treatment of this injury has drawn a great deal of media attention because of high profile athletes.

These ER injuries can occur with contact, such as in American football (one player landing on outer aspect of the ankle causing ER and abduction) or non-contact, such as landing awkwardly from a jump or planting the foot and suffering the ER/Abduction injury.

Syndesmotic injuries, often referred to as high ankle sprains because they affect structures more proximal than the more commonly injured lateral ligaments, involve the ligamentous structures between the tibia and fibula. These are well described and include the anterior-inferior tibiofibular ligament (AITFL), interosseous ligament (IOL), interosseous membrane, posterior-inferior tibiofibular ligament (PITFL), and inferior transverse ligament [1, 6, 23, 38]. Syndesmotic injuries typically occur in high energy mechanisms and are more common in sports involving high speed collisions, uneven terrain, artificial turf, and high impact cutting or jumping. Examples include American football, soccer, rugby, skiing, or hockey. These injuries account for about 12% of all ankle sprains and occur when an external rotation force is applied to the foot in a dorsiflexed position [39]. This action forces the talus in between the tibia and fibula, causing the fibula to separate, externally rotate, and displace posteriorly [40]. This mechanism reliably produces injury first to the AITFL followed by medial injury to the deltoid ligament and propagation superiorly along the tibiofibular interval [41].

Unstable syndesmosis injuries occur when the membrane between the tibia and fibula is disrupted. It can occur in isolation or with fractures. The most common mechanism of injury is external rotation through the foot and ankle while the ankle is in dorsiflexion and the foot is pronated [23]. Syndesmosis injuries account for 1–18% of ankle sprains [23], but this likely underestimates the incidence of syndesmosis injuries as it is easily underdiagnosed or missed diagnosed [6, 23]. Additionally, there is a higher incidence of syndesmosis injury in high-impact sports such as skiing, ice hockey, and soccer [23].

Syndesmosis injuries can commonly occur with fractures, including Maisonneuve fractures [6]. It is most commonly associated with complete rupture of the deltoid ligament, AITFL, interosseous membrane, and proximal fibular fracture [6].

15.5.2 Classification

Syndesmotic injuries have previously been graded via radiographic images and clinical examination [23]. The West Point Ankle grading system is based on physical examination and is graded I–III. Grade I is a mild clinical sprain or tear to AITFL with no instability and no ecchymosis on exam. The radiographic findings are normal and by definition there is no complete tear of any of the ligaments. Grade II is a slight instability (moderate clinical findings) with a positive squeeze or external rotation test and a tear of AITFL with partial tear of interosseous ligament. These Grade II injuries have been associated with normal non-stressed radiographs of the ankle and lower leg. Grade III involves a definite instability with complete disruption of all the ligaments, with severe injury and radiographic gross instability [6, 23]. Traditionally, this system led to discrepancy and inconsistency on Grade II injuries being stable or unstable. This classification system lacks good differentiation between those that required surgery and those that could be treated non-operatively. To further address this confusion and as experience led to a developed understanding, Calder has updated their system. Calder and co-workers especially addressed the West Point Ankle grading system Grade II classification utilizing the "squeeze test" as an adjunct to the MRI findings, clinical examination and radiographs in 2016 [42]. Grade I remains a stable injury with no deltoid ligament injury, no pain with squeeze test and an intact deltoid. The Grade II has been separated in a IIA and IIB injury. Grade IIA injuries are still considered stable, present with an AITFL tear, some portion of interosseus ligament injury but a negative squeeze test. However, grade IIB injuries are unstable, present with an AITFL tear, interosseus injury of varying degree and either/or a positive pain at the ankle with squeeze test or deltoid ligament injury. A Grade III injury is unchanged, and is a frank instability with tear of the AITFL, interosseus ligament high grade tear and a complete deltoid ligament tear.

15.5.3 Diagnosis (History/Physical Examination/Imaging)

Visual evaluation is the first assessment and is important and insightful. Little to no swelling is seen with a true stable, Grade I injury with no ligament rupture. The presence of ecchymosis indicates some level of ligament tear and the degree and location of swelling is also telling. Swelling confined to the anterior medial ankle and anterolateral ankle would suggest injury to the AITFL and anterior deltoid ligament only. Tenderness should confirm the locations of injury. With unstable syndesmosis, even without fractures, severe swelling medially, laterally and half the way up the lower leg is observed and alerts the examiner to its severity. Athletes are hesitant to weigh bear with most of these syndesmosis injuries. However, with Grade I stable injuries, most athletes will bear weight after physical examination confirms that the ankle is stable. In more severe (Grade II and III) injuries, athletes will be unable to bear weight, even with encouragement, pointing the treating clinician to the increased severity of the injury.

Some special physical examination tests are utilized in the evaluation. Careful and gentle palpation is critical to assess which ligaments were injured, although the degree of injury (sprain versus rupture) will require advanced imaging. External rotation stress testing and the proximal "squeeze test" are both helpful in assessing distal stability. Wolf and Amendola described applying syndesmotic circumferential taping at the level of the distal syndesmosis for the Grade I–II differential [43]. Secure, firm taping that reduces pain with weight bearing suggests an unstable syndesmosis.

Pain is commonly diffuse and tenderness to palpation may extend proximally. This distance proximal to the ankle joint has been referred to as tenderness length and has been purported to correlate with return to sport [44]. Several provocative maneuvers aimed at assessing syndesmotic stability have been described including the squeeze, external rotation stress, Cotton, fibular translation, and the cross-leg tests. Physical examination should include external rotation test and squeeze test [6]. A positive squeeze test was predictive of a prolonged return to sport [23]. The external rotation test had the highest sensitivity with lowest interobserver error [23]. The squeeze test places a medial to lateral compressive force using both hands at the midpoint of the tibia/fibula. The external rotation stress test places an external force on the foot with the tibia stabilized. The Cotton test places a lateral translational force on the talus within the mortise, and, if positive, suggests associated deltoid ligament pathology with syndesmotic sprain. The fibular translation test places an anterior/posterior force on the fibula with the tibia stabilized. Increased pain or laxity relative to the contralateral limb indicates injury. Finally, the crossed leg test places the patient in a seated figure-of-4 position while gentle pressure is applied to the medial knee. Reproducible increased pain with all of these maneuvers indicates possible syndesmotic injury. One series comparing MRI and exam maneuvers found the squeeze test to be the most sensitive and specific, however the external rotation stress test is the only maneuver with high intra and inter-rater reliability [45, 46].

The history and physical examination along with appropriate work up to follow is critical in evaluation of patients with possible syndesmotic injury. Missed diagnoses can lead to marked impairment. Patients may report a mechanism consistent with syndesmotic injury such as a collision while the foot was planted and externally rotated, resulting in a forward fall that caused further dorsiflexion. Common symptoms reported during initial evaluation include inability to bear weight, pain during the push-off phase of gait, pain located along anterolateral ankle, swelling, and a giving way sensation [23]. Despite thorough examination, 25% of syndesmotic injuries are missed [23].

Imaging should include standard weight-bearing radiographs to assess fracture or diastasis [1, 6, 23]. A tibiofibular clear space greater than 6 mm, 1 cm above the plafond on antero-posterior and mortise views is suggestive of injury [6, 23]. Other suggestive evidence includes widening of the medial clear space which could indicate injury to the syndesmosis and deltoid ligament [23]. Other imaging modalities include CT, MRI, and sonography. CT scanning is useful in detecting small avulsion fractures and showing the relationship of the tibia and fibula, while MRI easily displays the structures comprising the syndesmosis [23]. MRI has high sensitivity and specificity along with ability to reveal nondisplaced fractures or bony edema [47]. Ankle arthroscopy can be useful for diagnosis and treatment with direct visualization and assessment of the syndesmosis/AITLF intraoperatively. Guyton and associates reported that a 3 mm increase in the syndesmosis noted arthroscopically correlated well with instability in a cadaveric model [48]. One common open technique is to use the Cotton test, when a towel clamp or bone clamp is used to place a direct lateral pulling stress on the fibula [33]. The test is positive for instability if there is translation greater than 1 mm [33].

Mal-reduction of the syndesmosis has been reported as high as 52% and the shape of the incisura has been postulated as a predisposing factor [49, 50]. Cheney, studying postoperative CT scans, reported that patients with a shallow incisura had a higher rate of anterior displacement, while those with a deeper incisura had more posterior malreduction and suffered more external rotation malalignment [50]. Temporary clamp fixation followed by screw fixation could inadvertently result in rigid anterior or posterior fibular malalignment [51].

Although these studies are not specific to the athlete, they highlight the potential malreduction and possible complications that can occur with syndesmosis treatment and fixation. Surgeon should be vigilant in assuring anatomic positioning of the fibula. Visual verification of the reduction in the anterior syndesmosis is helpful, and flexible fixation with suture buttons can aid in alignment in the anterior and posterior plane [52]. We favor a hybrid approach to fixation when there is a severely unstable Maisonneuve dislocation to counteract the vertical displacement that can still occur with suture button fixation in this particular injury pattern (Fig. 15.8a–d).

Warner et al. [53] later reported on follow-up evaluation of rotational ankle fractures that if the malalignment was only moderate in the incisura, that is ≤1.5 mm, the patients did well. Only when the syndesmotic reduction was more severe did the outcome appear to deteriorate [53]. Coetzee and Ebeling first described the TightRope fixation technique [54]. There have been several reports discussing its advantages, disadvantages, concern for "creep" (gradual loss of fixation due to stretching out of suture or loosening within the suture button interface), prominent suture knots, and yet optimization of syndesmotic reduction.

15.5.4 Treatment

Syndesmosis injuries with associated fracture warrant surgical repair. However, injuries without fracture are treated depending on the extent of the ligament injury [6]. For athletes, non-operative management, which includes a short period of non-weight bearing followed by aggressive rehabilitation, good results with an average return to sport of 13.4 weeks for stable injuries [23]. Clanton and Porter [6] recommended that stable sprains with negative routine and stress radiographs could be treated with conservative treatment with an estimated return to sport in 3 months from initiation of treatment.

If the athlete has negative routine radiographs, but diastasis on stress radiographs, operative management is recommended [6]. One study reported a group of professional athletes with Grade III syndesmotic injuries and divided them into two treatment groups: surgical stabilization versus conservative treatment with cast immobilisation. Though there was no significant difference in long-term performance between the two groups, the surgical group was able to return to play approximately 3 weeks faster than the conservative treatment group [23].

It is likely that the anatomic position and maintenance of reduction of the syndesmosis is the most important factor in outcome with these injuries [55]. Tornetta et al. [55] proposed that direct visual confirmation of the reduction at the level of the ankle joint is the most reliable technique [56, 57]. Intra-operative radiographic evaluation can be misleading. Others recommend post-operative CT imaging to confirm reduction, but mal-reduction would then require a second procedure. Syndesmosis screw removal after mild mal-reduction does appear to result in improved positioning and in some cases anatomic reduction. This may be especially true in the hybrid fixation technique mentioned above. Involvement of the syndesmosis resulted in a lower pain and function score compared to the other fracture patterns [7]. More recently, Litrenta reported mildly negative outcome if the syndesmosis was involved in operatively treated Weber B (SE4) fracture [58]. This study was not in athletes, but implies that disruption of the syndesmosis results in a more guarded outcome in all patients, athletes included [58].

Thus, to reiterate, if there is an unstable syndesmosis (with a Maisonneuve or no fracture), we recommend stabilization of the syndesmosis with two suture button TightRopes for dynamic stabilization [57, 59]. If there is a Maisonneuve fracture, and there is vertical instability of the fibula, we recommend a hybrid fixation of one syndesmosis screw (typically a 4.5 mm, with four cortices) and two suture button TightRopes (Fig. 15.8a–d). We undertake a direct repair of the deltoid ligament and we include the deep deltoid ligament repair [1, 8]. We use suture anchors as needed either in the medial malleolus (for anterior deltoid [8]) or the talus (for the deep deltoid). We will occasionally suggest 2–4 weeks of casting to support the deltoid ligament repair if needed.

A common question has always been whether and when screw(s) fixation used for syndesmosis fixation should be removed. There is still controversy regarding whether screws should be removed and if so, what is the optimal

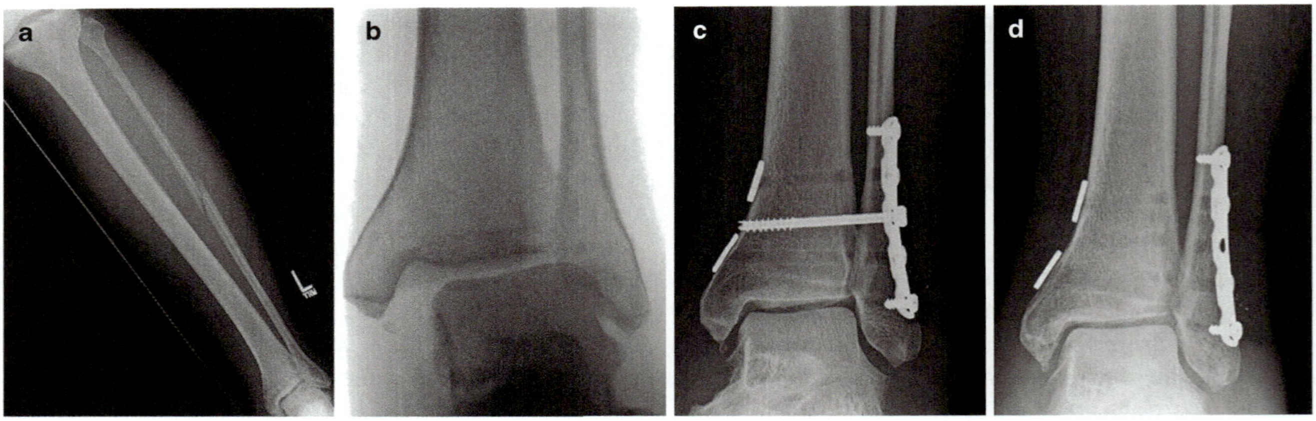

Fig. 15.8 (**a**) antero-posterior of tibia and fibula demonstrating mid-shaft fibula fracture which is not fixed at time of surgery so can result in vertical instability of fibula. (**b**) intra-operative external rotation and abduction stress image showing severe instability. (**c**) immediate post-operative antero-posterior image of left ankle showing hybrid syndesmosis fixation with two suture buttons and one syndesmosis screws. The suture buttons give syndesmosis medial-lateral stability and "center" the fibula on incisura and the rigid screw fixation supplies vertical stability of the fibula. (**d**) 2–3 month post-operative antero-posterior image of left ankle after single screw syndesmosis removal in office with excellent syndesmosis alignment

time of removal? Boyle and co-workers addressed this in the non-athletic population and reported no difference in overall ROM, AOFAS score, AAOS lower extremity score, radiographic alignment or arthritis in those patients with screw removal at 3 months and those without screw removal [60]. Van Heest and Lafferty noted that screw removal may allow for spontaneous correction of syndesmosis malreductions [57].

Another frequent question is whether the syndesmosis can be "overtightened" during fixation? Some have recommended dorsiflexion of the ankle while placing syndesmosis fixation. Tornetta noted in the cadaveric specimen that fixation in plantarflexion did not inhibit ankle dorsiflexion and thus argued against the possibility of excessive tightness [55]. Dynamic suture button fixation would be less apt to overtighten also. We have noted in some situations, screw fixation can apparently tighten the syndesmosis to the point of "distracting" the tibial-talar joint and have slightly loosened our screw to not "overtighten". We still err on the side of a real snug fit, visual inspection of the reduction and dynamic or hybrid fixation to optimize maintenance of reduction.

Maisonneuve fractures are treated similar to Grade III diastasis without fracture [8].

15.5.5 Complications

Involvement of the syndesmosis can cause prolonged dysfunction and delayed return to sport [23]. Missed and chronically unstable injuries can lead to osteoarthritis [23]. Malreduction of the fibula in the tibial incisura (often anterior translation) is a complication of fixation. Dynamic fixation results in a lower rate of malreduction and a lower reoperation rate [59]. Nerve and vessel injuries are rare, as is deep infection. Stiffness and pain result from delayed initiation of weight bearing and ROM exercised from prolonged cast immobilisation.

15.5.6 Rehabilitation

Recommended postoperative rehabilitation includes toe touch-weight bearing in a removable boot for 10–14 days [23]. Range of motion activities and partial weight bearing begins 2–4 weeks postoperatively [23]. Full weight bearing begins at 4 weeks after surgery and running or other high-impact activities are started around postoperative Week 8–12 [23]. We prefer intermittent immobilisation to allow ROM, desensitization and some cross training [7].

15.5.7 Preventative Measures

New data has recently been obtained with the expanding injury prevention arm of the National Football League. A great deal of mechanical shoe surface evaluation has been undertaken. The amount of torque required to produce a significant syndesmosis injury has been calculated and the only preventative measure to date that appears to have any impact on external rotation injuries is reducing the grasp between the shoe and field surface. This is obtained by altering the cleating pattern and the length of the cleats so that the shoe will give way from the turf interface with less total torque than that required to produce a significant ligamentous injury. Again, American football is the most common sport with this external rotation injury and this data shows some promise.

15.6 Isolated Weber A/B/C (Without Ligament Injury)

15.6.1 Epidemiology

Ankle fractures are common injuries, and the majority of ankle fractures are stable, isolated lateral malleolar injuries [33]. Criteria for the diagnosis of "isolated" lateral malleolar fracture includes radiographic evidence of fibular fracture without medial malleolar involvement, disruption of the mortise (widening of the medial clear space), medial tenderness, swelling or syndesmosis widening [33].

Weber A fibular fracture involves inversion and adduction of the ankle and hindfoot. This results in a varus tilt to the ankle causing a transverse avulsion fracture of the fibula at or slightly below the level of the ankle joint. This can be from a blow to the medial ankle with the foot firmly planted on the ground, or landing from a fall or jump with the heel in slight varus. This is a low-grade supination-adduction injury without medial-sided injury.

Weber B fibular fracture pattern occurs with supination abduction or supination and external rotation. This is the most common fibula fracture pattern in all sports. It involves the fracture initiating at the level of the ankle joint or slightly above the anterior inferior tibio-fibular ligament and then extending posteriorly and superiorly to different degrees depending on the position of the ankle. This injury can occur in a pile up in football, landing from a jump in any sport, landing on an uneven surface or even stepping often uneven curb.

Weber C fibula fracture patterns involves pronation and external rotation. This type of ankle fracture occurs commonly in American football resulting from another player landing on the outside of the involved athlete's ankle with the foot in slight pronation resulting in forced pronation external rotation. This mechanism does not result in an isolated Weber C fibular fracture. The Weber C fibular fracture by definition is a fracture line that initiates above the level of the ankle. It is typically a short oblique fracture with often some lateral comminution. For an isolated Weber C fibular fracture, it is more commonly just a direct blow to the lateral ankle without associated pronation or external rotation. This can cause a more transverse fracture and often is even further above the ankle than the pronation external rotation injury. Some athletes incur a "leg whip" in either American football or soccer and results in more of a fibular shaft fracture which is transverse. This isolated fracture can often be treated non operatively.

15.6.2 Classification

Ankle fractures are most commonly classified using Lauge-Hansen and Danis-Weber systems. Danis-Weber classification is made according to the location of the fibular fracture in relation to the syndesmosis, or the level of the tibial plafond [1, 61]. Type A falls below the plafond/ankle joint, Type B is at the level of the plafond/ankle joint, and Type C is above the tibial plafond [1, 61]. The higher the grade, or the more proximal the fracture on the fibula, the greater the risk of having concomitant syndesmosis injury, medial sided injury and greater instability [1]. Furthermore, lesions of the cartilage, especially on the talus, are associated with more proximal fibula injury [62]. Specifically, cartilaginous lesions increased in number and severity from Weber B to Weber C [62].

Harper performed a cadaveric study on the isolated Weber B distal fibular fracture and reported 25° of external rotation of the distal fibula and 20° of external rotation of the talus even with an "isolated" fibular fracture [63]. He also reported up to 1 mm of direct lateral talar shift even with this "isolated" injury [63]. He surmised this degree of rotation or lateral displacement resulted in incongruence at the tibial-talar joint which caused incongruence and potential long-term arthritis [63]. The deltoid ligament prevented talar eversion but did not prevent the initial 2–3 mm of lateral talar displacement. Magnusson reviewed 118 isolated fibular fractures with a mean follow-up of over 6 years and reported that 30% of patients reported some ankle discomfort and had some evidence of early arthritis on follow-up radiographs [64]. Cedel compared operatively reduced and internally stabilized isolated fibula fractures and reported superior results to Magnusson's report with this more aggressive approach [65]. Harper also concluded that operative intervention may be considered in the high-performance athlete [63].

Ramsey and Muller both reported that even 1 mm of lateral translation can result in significant decrease in tibiotalar joint surface area and thus must be taken in consideration, especially in athletes [66, 67]. Hunt and co-workers noted similar increases in joint pressure with small increases in displacement in the syndesmotic model [38]. This study by Hunt was specifically designed to examine the impact on athletic activity with a subtle ligament injury and displacement [38].

15.6.3 Diagnosis (History/Physical Examination/Imaging)

As mentioned above, isolated lateral malleolar fractures should not have medial tenderness or swelling on clinical examination. Radiographs are often sufficient to diagnose isolated Weber fractures, but it is imperative to be cognizant of radiographic pitfalls, including two-dimensional representation and lack of standardization for magnification [33]. CT scanning has been proven to better display anatomical alignment, though it is often not necessary [33].

Michelson assessed gravity stress radiographs of "isolated", short oblique fibular fractures and noted this gravity stress testing does not account for isolated anterior deltoid ligament injuries which can result in increased external rotation [68]. This increased external rotation despite the intact deep deltoid ligament can be problematic for athletes in the long-term, since it is much more difficult to treat in the chronic than in the acute setting. We will focus on this assessment of the deltoid ligament and its relationship to ankle fractures in athletes later in the chapter. Furthermore, Park noted that the position of the ankle was critical in assessing whether the deep deltoid ligament was intact, i.e. whether this fracture is truly "isolated" [14]. These authors implied that isolated tears of the anterior deltoid ligament was not as critical in assessment of medial stability, contrary to some more recent data from the NFL [8].

15.6.4 Treatment

The majority of isolated lateral malleolar fractures can be treated non-operatively with no long-term consequences [33]. Immobilisation should focus on protecting the ankle from further injury with the use of casting material for splinting, walking cast, boot immobilisation or high-top tennis shoe, which have all shown similar and acceptable results [33]. However, if there is displacement greater than or equal to 3 mm, reduction and fixation of the lateral malleolus may be recommended, especially in the athletic population to aid in a more rapid return to sport [1].

Sanders et al. [69] demonstrated that non-operative treatment of even seemingly "stable", "isolated" lateral malleolus fracture result in patients with greater medial clear space and also lower union rates. Thus, we caution non-operative treatment in these athletes and propose ORIF may be a more "conservative" approach.

For unstable Weber A fibula fractures, operative treatment is chosen. There are several options including a "hook" plate, small interfragmentary screws and tension band wiring. We do not recommend simple lateral neutralization plates since most Weber A fractures have inadequate fixation surface distal to the fracture. We prefer partially threaded, retrograde screw fixation (Fig. 15.9a–c). A direct lateral approach centered just at or distal to the fracture line allows tenaculum stabilization, removal of periosteum at the fracture site and adequate exposure to get a cannulated guide wire retrograde up the canal. A 4.5–5.5 screw typically fits well and gets good proximal purchase. The starting point is crucial and screw threads need to be past the fracture and purchase the distal diaphysis. We counter-sink the screw head to avoid painful hardware removal after healing.

For Weber B fibula fracture in athletes, we prefer an antiglide construct (Fig. 15.10a, b). The antiglide placement gives a true buttress effect and counteracts the posterior and superior displacement common in this pattern. A 1/3 tubular small fragment plate is commonly used, but we prefer a 2.4 mm LCDC plate with 2.7 mm screw in most athletes. The large (>250 lb) athlete we will still use a 3.5 mm 1/3 tubular plate with 3.5 screws. The 2.4 mm plate gives great strength and its width fits better in most athletic

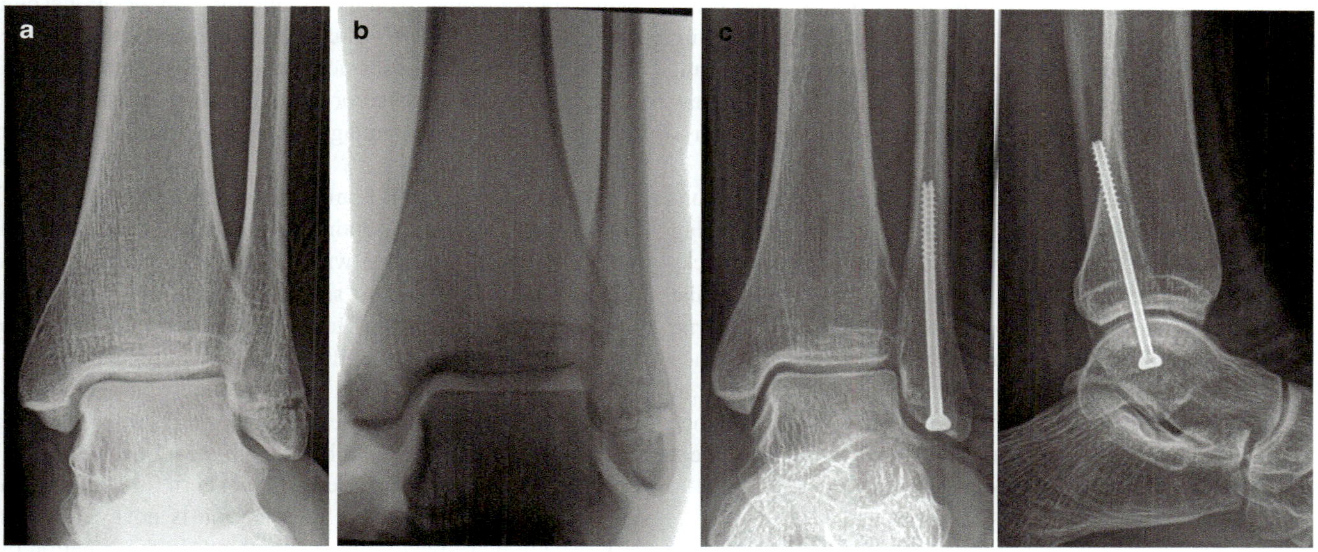

Fig. 15.9 (**a**) Anterior-posterior radiograph showing isolated, transverse distal fibula fracture just distal to the ankle joint (Weber A). (**b**) Varus talar tilt stress antero-posterior showing "opening up" of the distal fibula fracture denoting unstable Weber A fracture. (**c**) antero-posterior and lateral post-operative radiograph showing anatomic reduction and fixation with retrograde cannulated 4.5 mm screw

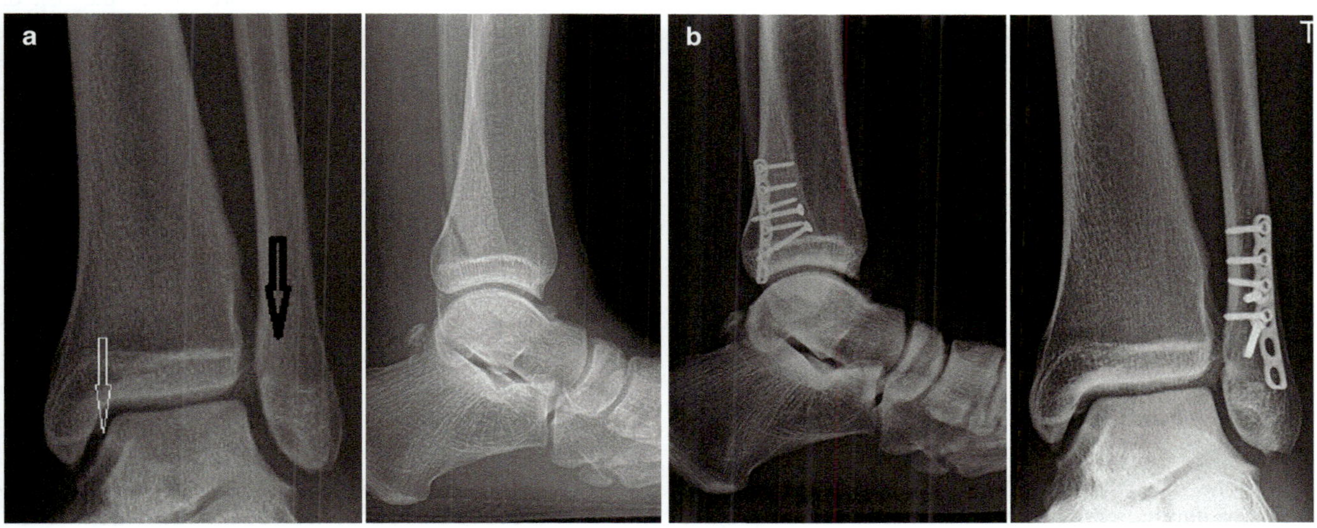

Fig. 15.10 (**a**) Pre-operative antero-posterior and lateral radiographs showing oblique distal fibula fracture (black arrow on antero-posterior image) consistent with Weber B fibula. Note that the fracture starts at the level of the ankle joint and extends proximally. The displacement is typically lateral, posterior and superior. There is no lateral displacement, but there is mild posterior and superior displacement. Note the medial clear space is normally aligned (white arrow). (**b**) Post-op antero-posterior and lateral radiographs of left ankle after distal fibular fixation with a 2.4 mm LCDC plate placed in a posterolateral anti-glide position to counter act posterior and superior displacement. (Note the incidental apophyseal nonunion seen on preop and post-operative lateral images)

frames. We caution against placing the plate too distal into the peroneal tendon sheath itself as this can irritate the tendon and require removal. Avoiding the last 1–2 holes in the plate still gives excellent buttress and avoids tendon irritation also. Otherwise, we have found rare need for removal of the antiglide plate. We use an anterior-posterior 2.7 lag screw first to stabilize the fracture and allow easy plate application.

For the true isolated Weber C fracture with operative fixation, we utilize a lateral side plate on the fibula. We get at least three holes above and below the fracture and use a locking 1/3 tubular plate in the true Weber C. The locking plate is thicker, but we do not use locking screw, but standard 3.5 mm screws. We attempt to get a 2.7 lag screw across any short oblique fracture but is not always possible.

For the large athlete with an isolated fibular shaft fracture a heavier LCDC plate (large 4.5 or small 3.5) with a lag screw if possible is utilized. We occasionally can use a locking small fragment 1/3 tubular plate as mentioned with the true isolated Weber C, but error on the larger plate. This true diaphyseal fracture can be a slow healer but requires patience since the large surrounding muscle belly supplies excellent cushioning for the larger plate and good vascular support. Care must be taken to avoid injury to the superficial peroneal nerve (SPN) with lateral exposure.

15.6.5 Complications

In one review, complications from surgical fixation of isolated lateral fractures included 1–3% risk of serious wound complication or infection and longer swelling times [33]. Conversely, there was found to be no adverse sequelae with nonoperative treatment [33]. Nonunions with chronic pain are the most preventable complications and typically fixation has a lower nonunion rate.

Hardware pain is always possible with fibular fixation, but is minimized with counter-sinking the retrograde screw, and a well-placed antiglide construct. Weber C hardware is often underneath a good muscle layer, so is less prominent.

15.6.6 Rehabilitation

Postoperative management typically consists of initial walking boot intermittent immobilisation followed by progressive weight bearing and ROM exercises [33]. Early mobilization has been proven safe in lateral malleolar fractures, however, there appears to be minimal benefit from early weight bearing or ROM in the first few weeks after surgery [33].

15.6.7 Preventative Measures

Preventative measures are focused around identifying stable versus unstable injuries. There are no studies indicating specific ability to prevent these traumatic injuries. However, mis-diagnosing and under diagnosis in these injuries can lead to nonunions and poor outcome.

The most critical aspect for the Weber A fibular fracture is whether the fracture is stable or unstable. The very nature of this fracture is one of inversion with supination. Near complete, spontaneous, anatomic reduction can occur despite periosteal interposition. Therefore, any distraction at the fracture site must raise suspicion for soft tissue interposition which can lead to delayed or nonunion if treated non operatively. Therefore, stress imaging may be required to prevent inadequate treatment.

The isolated Weber B fibular fracture has a long history of controversy regarding optimal treatment. True isolated Weber B fibular fractures with 2 mm or less displacement can be treated well in most situations, even in athletes, with non-operative treatment. However, we tend to be more aggressive with operative reduction and fixation, particularly in competitive athletes. Even small amounts of external rotation and shortening have been shown to result in chronic ankle pain particularly in high-level athletes. Despite no specific literature guidance, there is still concern for nonunion in elite athletes. The operative intervention is not without its risk. Anatomic re-positioning of the fibula and evaluation of the ankle and ligaments under anesthesia can be very helpful in confirming the extent of other associated injuries.

Isolated Weber C fibular fractures are most commonly from direct blow. The isolated fracture carries the risk of compartment syndrome because of the direct blow. Therefore, it is imperative that the evaluating clinician assess clearly for soft tissue injuries which could lead to an acute compartment syndrome. Also, operative intervention of these Weber C fibular fractures must include careful evaluation and protection of the superficial peroneal nerve. The superficial peroneal nerve will be in the operative field. The nerve courses in either the lateral or the anterior compartment and will cross the fibula at the area of the fracture and/or incision. In fact, a careful neurologic exam should be done to assess for neurapraxia or more severe nerve injury because of either fracture displacement or the lateral impaction which produced the fracture.

15.7 Isolated Medial Malleolar Fracture

15.7.1 Epidemiology

Isolated medial malleolar fractures occur by one of two mechanisms. The most common is a straight eversion injury such as landing awkwardly from a jump or stepping on an uneven surface, such as another players foot, with the lateral hindfoot causing eversion of the ankle. This type of mechanism results in an avulsion of the medial malleolus and oblique fracture at the joint then extending medial or inferomedial (Fig. 15.11a). The eversion mechanism often results in the periosteum of the medial ankle tearing proximal to the fracture and enveloping and interposing into the fracture as it spontaneously reduces. The periosteal interposition is one reason this fracture is operative. Also, this pattern of fracture is inherently unstable because of the natural pronation of the hind foot with normal gait ambulation and the deltoid ligament attachment.

The second mechanism is related to a prior early or occult medial malleolar stress fracture and is an isolated ankle inversion or adduction injury also from landing awkwardly or stepping on an uneven surface such as another players foot with the medial hindfoot. The prior occult or early stress fracture causes a stress-riser vertically in the medial malleolus and results in an acute on chronic vertical medial malleolar fracture (Fig. 15.12a, b).

15.7.2 Classification

Classification of medial malleolus do not have a true classification scheme. We just note the difference in acute avulsion chip fractures that was discussed above under deltoid avulsion and rupture. The other classification is just between an oblique avulsion fracture and verstical fractures (Lauge-Hansen supination adduction). Epidemiology and treatmenttcover these differences well.

15.7.3 Treatment

Both of these fracture patterns are unstable and require operative fixation and stabilization. With the avulsion fracture pattern, if the fracture is truly non-displaced, non-operative treatment can be successful. With the vertical fracture pattern, even "nondisplaced" fracture commonly requires fixation because of the commonly associated underlying stress pattern and influence on healing. Open treatment with extraction of the interposed periosteum is undertaken for the avulsion type pattern. Two screws are placed obliquely across the metaphysis and perpendicular to the avulsion fracture pattern (Fig. 15.11a, b). Repair of the periosteum can aid periosteal healing. Open approach is required for the treatment of the vertical pattern also. There is no periosteal interposition in this pattern of fracture. But the vertical pattern is not treated well with screw fixation only. We have seen several nonunions with oblique screw fixation only. We favor a distal tibial peri-articular plate with open placement of the distal transverse screws in the metaphysis but we often place the most proximal screw(s) percutaneous to minimize dissection. The distal screws are inserted with a cannulated drill to ensure that they are parallel to the distal tibial articular surface (Fig. 15.12a–c).

15.7.4 Complications

Complications include delayed healing nonunion, arthritis, stiffness and pain with inadequate treatment or rehabilitation, joint penetration and infection. Painful hardware and an inability to return to sports are also potential difficulties. It is

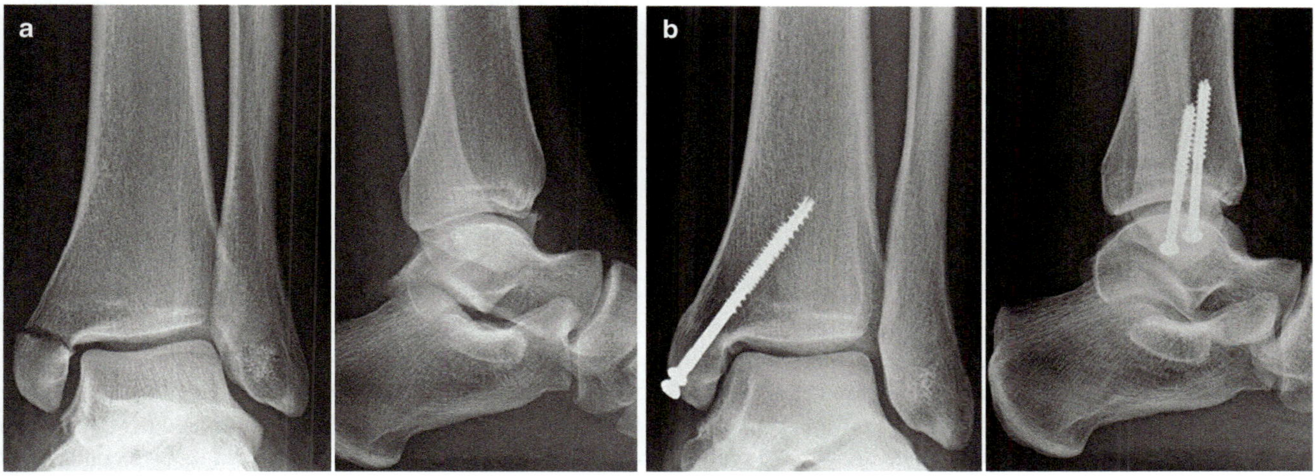

Fig. 15.11 (**a**) antero-posterior and lateral radiographs of left ankle of 17-year-old high school football player with sports injury and displaced, isolated medial malleolus fracture. (**b**) antero-posterior and lateral image of left ankle after operative fixation with two, 4.0 partially threaded lag screws obliquely across the medial malleolus fracture with anatomic reduction

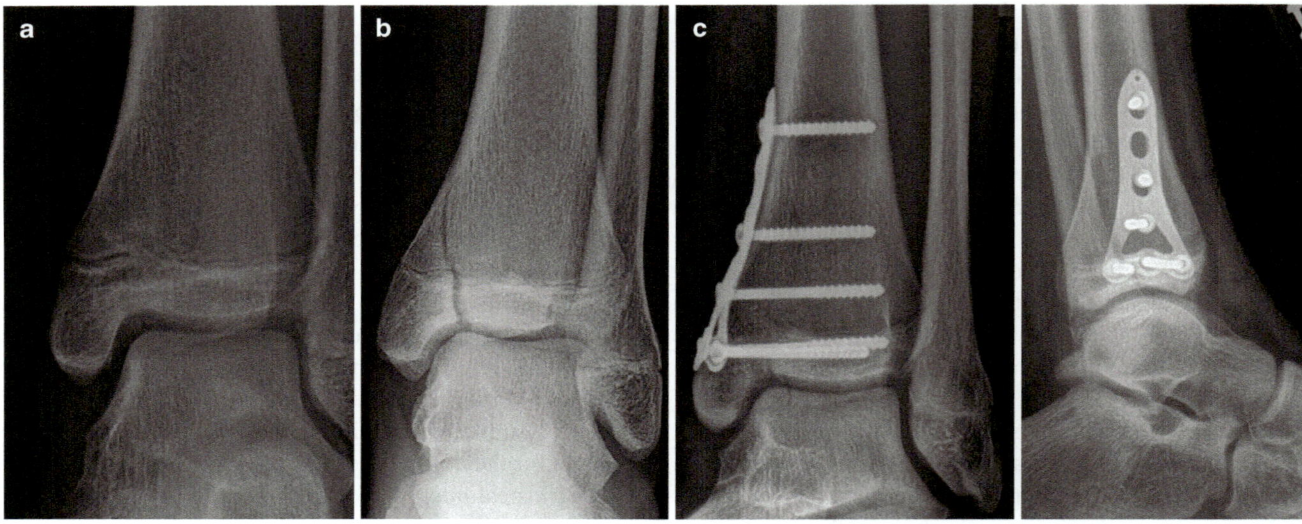

Fig. 15.12 (**a**) antero-posterior radiograph of left ankle with subtle, early medial malleolus fracture with vertical orientation consistent with early stress fracture in 15-year-old male basketball player. The fracture initially was not identified. (**b**) antero-posterior radiograph of same 15-year-old athlete 4 months later with acute on chronic vertical medial malleolus fracture with mild displacement. Now the fracture is easily identified and requires operative fixation. (**c**) antero-posterior and lateral images of same left ankle after ORIF of medial malleolus with medial plate and 4.0 screws with anatomic reduction. Distal most aspect of fracture identified still after reduction indicating the portion of the fracture that was likely the early stress fracture

critical to make the determination whether the isolated medial malleolus fracture is vertically oriented (Fig. 15.12a, b) and high risk for nonunion; or the oblique avulsion fracture (Fig. 15.11a) which is much more amenable to operative intervention and uncomplicated healing. Failure to appreciate the severity of the isolated vertical medial malleolus fracture leads to inadequate treatment, delayed union and often nonunion. The vertically oriented fracture is more commonly associated with the cavo-varus foot and significant anterior-medial ankle spurring and impingement.

15.7.5 Rehabilitation

Rehabilitation can be aggressive in both of these operative fixation fractures. However, immobilisation is still required for 4–6 weeks and especially, with the vertically oriented medial malleolar fractures, the risk for nonunion is high. We do a gradual weaning off the crutches over a 2–3-week period of time and initiate biking with a brace at 4–6 weeks if fixation allows [7]. We typically wean out of the boot into a stirrup type brace after 6 weeks in use of brace until there is complete healing shown on plain radiographs or CT scans. Sports participation without bracing usually requires 3–4 months. Return to sports is 8–12 weeks with the oblique avulsion fracture and 3–4 months with the vertically oriented fracture. Longer periods of immobilisation, non-weight bearing, and return to sports are required if there is any bone grafting, comminution, or impaction of the distal tibia weight-bearing surface.

15.7.6 Preventative Measures

Preventative measures, though ideal, are difficult to determine. We do recommend careful evaluation of anterior medial ankle pain in jumping and running athletes as often the vertically oriented fracture shows early development of stress reaction or stress fracture and early intervention can prevent fracturing and displacement (Fig. 15.12a, b). Oblique isolated medial malleolus fracture arise almost exclusively from acute traumatic injury and preventative measures are difficult to implement or define.

15.8 Bimalleolar Fracture (Medial/Lateral)

15.8.1 Epidemiology

The mechanism of injury must be kept in mind when assessing "bimalleolar" and "bimalleolar equivalent injuries". Underappreciation of this associated ligamentous instability can be devastating even if the "bimalleolar" or "equivalent" components are treated appropriately. Bimalleolar equivalent injuries are covered below. We will focus on the two true bimalleolar ankle fracture. Bimalleolar ankle fractures can occur in any sport, especially those that involve contact and jumping e.g. American football, soccer, gymnastics/tumbling/cheering, baseball/softball (hitting a base awkwardly or sliding into a player/bag).

The supination adduction type pattern is usually associated with landing from a jump or fall. In this mechanism, there is an impaction injury medially and a distraction injury laterally. The impaction injury medially results in a more vertically oriented medial malleolar fracture and there is often impaction of the medial tibial plafond which much be appreciated at the time of surgery. Laterally, with the supination adduction injury, there is a distraction injury which results either in a Weber A fibular fracture, or a Grade III lateral ankle sprain.

The eversion and external rotation mechanism for the bimalleolar injury results in an avulsion type oblique fracture of the medial malleolus and most commonly, a Weber B fibular fracture. A Weber C fibular fracture can also occur, but often that results in a trimalleolar ankle fracture with associated posterior malleolus fracture also. A bimalleolar equivalent injury has a similar mechanism as described with the bimalleolar fracture but with injury to the deltoid ligament. In this instance, the deltoid ligament presents a partial or complete tear in association with the same Weber B or Weber C fibular fracture with the medial malleolus spared.

15.8.2 Classification

The Lauge-Hansen classification (Fig. 15.13) allows to understand the mechanism of ankle fractures [33], and is based on the position of the foot and the direction of forces causing fracture at time of injury [61]. This produces classification by distinct injury pattern. The patterns include supination-adduction (SA), supination-external rotation (SER) pronation-adduction (PA), and pronation-external rotation (PER) [1]. The system is graded on severity and dislocation, ranging for Grade I being least severe to Grade IV being most severe [61]. The most common injury is supination-external rotation, which accounts for 85% of ankle fractures (Fig. 15.13) [33].

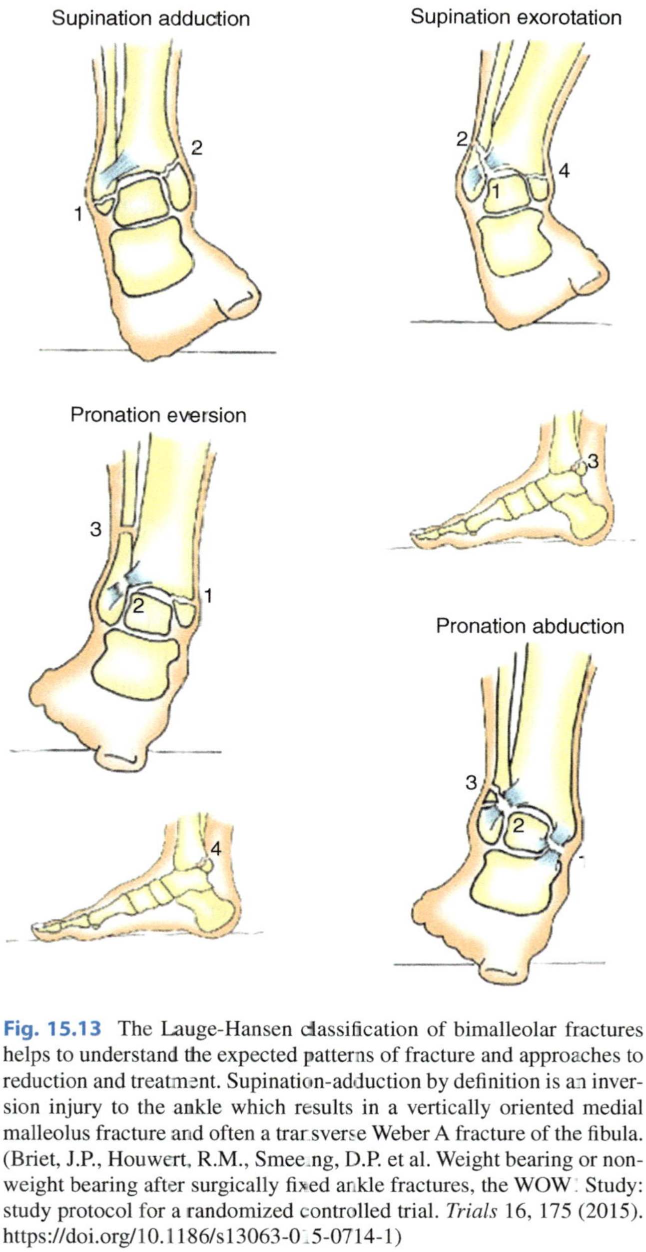

Fig. 15.13 The Lauge-Hansen classification of bimalleolar fractures helps to understand the expected patterns of fracture and approaches to reduction and treatment. Supination-adduction by definition is an inversion injury to the ankle which results in a vertically oriented medial malleolus fracture and often a transverse Weber A fracture of the fibula. (Briet, J.P., Houwert, R.M., Smeeing, D.P. et al. Weight bearing or non-weight bearing after surgically fixed ankle fractures, the WOW! Study: study protocol for a randomized controlled trial. *Trials* 16, 175 (2015). https://doi.org/10.1186/s13063-015-0714-1)

15.8.3 Diagnosis (History/Physical Examination/Imaging)

Athletes with a bimalleolar ankle fracture experience marked pain and have significant swelling and ecchymosis both medially and laterally. Athletes are reluctant to walk on the ankle because of the instability and pain. The skin can demonstrate mild to moderate swelling, all the way to severe fracture blistering depending on the level of displacement and the initial treatment. Care must be taken to be certain there is no skin disruption and an occult open fracture is not involved.

This fracture pattern occurs in all sports, especially those involving more high-energy injuries. That is, contact football, soccer, and both water and downhill skiing. A careful history is very helpful in understanding the mechanism of injury which will give the physician insights regarding evaluation of the plain radiographs. That is, was the injury more adduction or eversion-external rotation.

A history of an eversion, external rotation mechanism with an isolated Weber B fibular fracture must be carefully evaluated for possible bimalleolar equivalent injury. Although medial tenderness and swelling has not been associated with clear evidence of disruption of the deltoid, we have still found examination very helpful to decide whether further stress radiographs are needed. In the acute setting, a completely nontender and non-swollen medial aspect rules out a high-grade deltoid ligament injury or medial malleolus fracture. On the other hand, significant swelling, bruising and tenderness to deep palpation medially merits further workup to assess for deltoid ligament disruption or medial malleolus fracture. A high degree of suspicion must occur in this setting.

A history of a supination adduction injury points towards a medial tibial plafond impaction injury in association with a vertical medial malleolus fracture. Also, a medial-sided fracture with a normal fibula in this setting must be evaluated closely for a Grade III lateral ligament disruption. Of course, a vertical medial malleolus fracture with some impaction can also present with a Weber A fibular fracture.

Thus, a very thorough history and careful physical examination with the above nuances should be undertaken in a detailed manner on all athletes with suspicion of a bimalleolar fracture. A careful neurovascular examination is needed also to assess for subtle or overt neurologic injury and vascular compromise. Also, it should be kept in mind that there can be concomitant ankle fractures and significant midfoot injuries also. These can include cuboid impaction fractures, fifth metatarsal avulsion fractures, Lisfranc ligamentous injuries, and subtle fractures of the talus and calcaneus. We have seen missed anterior process fractures of the calcaneus, unidentified sustentaculum fractures of the calcaneus, and even talar neck fractures in these high energy complex fractures in athletes.

Standard three view weight-bearing, or simulated weight-bearing radiographs of the ankle are undertaken. For the very swollen and apprehensive athlete, simulated weight-bearing radiographs at least give much better clarification of alignment and fracture displacement than completely non-weightbearing and poorly rotated images. There is a low threshold for further imaging of the whole foot and hindfoot. Advanced imaging can be helpful to evaluate subtleties of the fracture, intra-articular chip fracture, osteochondral impaction or occult fracturing and to assess for bone bruising. Bone bruising that communicates with the articular surface and subchondral bone can imply more significant occult cartilage injury and can develop into an OCL. It is important to be clear regarding subtle and occult articular surface injury since these impact long term recovery and function. CT scanning is used to assess fragmentation, medial impaction and lateral loose fragments. MRI is particularly helpful to classify deep deltoid ligament injury, bone bruising and subtle cartilage injury. The MRI scan can also be helpful to make initial assessment of the AITFL and distal syndesmosis. We favor intra-operative arthroscopy and ankle-block or intra-operative stress imaging to make definitive assessments of the extent of subtle syndesmosis and anterior deltoid ligament disruption. Most professional athletes have an MRI for prognostic purposes. The cartilage and ligament assessment are also valuable for preoperative planning.

15.8.4 Treatment

Bimalleolar fractures are considered unstable and are almost exclusively treated operatively in athletes. Should the fracture result in dislocation or marked displacement, closed reduction and splinting allow the swelling to subside [33]. Post reduction imaging is necessary to confirm reduction and often to better define the fracture pattern. Jelinek and Porter [1] advocate surgical stabilization of both lateral and medial components in athletes with bimalleolar fractures or its equivalent. The lateral malleolus is stabilized first followed by reduction and stabilization of the medial malleolus [1, 33]. Despite this order of fixation, we often find opening medially first is helpful to remove loose fragments and interposed medial periosteum with definitive fixation delayed until after the lateral fixation. Lateral fixation reduces the talus under the tibia and supports medial reduction.

Preoperative planning and treatment involve optimizing the athlete both mentally and physically for surgery. Obtaining good pain control, clear and concise diagnosis with good communication to the *team of care givers* is crucial [70].

15.8.4.1 Hardware

For Weber B long oblique fibula fractures, we prefer an antiglide plate fixation if athlete present good quality bone and no comminution. We currently use a 2.7 anterior-posterior lag screw(s) and a 2.4 mm LCDC antiglide plate with 2.7 screws. For Weber C fibula fractures, we use a locking small fragment plate (but use non-locking screws in athletes with good bone stock) because it is thicker than the non-locking 1/3 tubular plate. These plates have contours/recess to allow suture button fixation of the syndesmosis that is often required with this type of fracture.

For the medial malleolus, we use either a 3.0 partially threaded lag screw for small anterior fragments and use one or two screws. For a typical oblique medial malleolus fracture, we use two, 4.0 screws. Cannulated screws medially allow placement in optimal radiographic position and cannulated drilling. A solid or cannulated screw can then be placed. For vertical medial malleolar fractures, we prefer a medial, distal tibial peri-articular plate with transverse lag screws placed after cannulated drilling. We place the plate subperiosteally, and can slide it under the periosteum proximally after exposing the fracture and reducing it anatomically. This is the same approach as mentioned in the isolated vertical fracture above. Arthroscopic evaluation and reduction with possible bone grafting or open reduction with bone grafting is occasionally needed for the medial impaction seen with supination-adduction injury pattern. Fixation in Weber A fracture with the supination-adduction pattern is the same as mentioned above *under isolated Weber A lateral malleolus* fracture with a retrograde screw (or other options as mentioned). We check the syndesmosis after final medial and lateral stabilization. Suture button fixation is applied as indicated.

15.8.5 Complications

Spare literature exists regarding the complications of bimalleolar ankle fractures in athletes. In fact, as mentioned, there is just sparse literature on true bimalleolar fractures in athletes in general. The obvious complications involve infection (<1–2%), nonunions (up to 5–10%), mal-reduction/malunions (most commonly in Weber C fibula fractures), nerve injury (both traumatic and iatrogenic). Stiffness and arthrofibrosis should not be underestimated or under appreciated. Arthritis is associated with initial cartilage injury (a case for arthroscopy at the time of fixation-see below) or with malunion/nonunions. Associated tendon interposition or injury can occur, but are not common. Hardware pain or loosening can occur after both medial or lateral fixation and with loosening from inadequate fixation. SPN injury can occur with any lateral approach to the ankle. Saphenous vein injury can be common with medial approaches (although the straight longitudinal approach lessens this risk). Early exposure and careful protection during the entire procedure is paramount.

15.8.6 Rehabilitation

The principles of rehabilitation are covered below. We favor anatomic rigid fixation that allows for early ROM and prudent early weigh bearing [7]. Initial wound healing is paramount to allow ROM and open chain activation of muscle and tendons with Theraband-type stimulation/strengthening. Aquatic and cross training can begin after wound healing and suture removal in many instances in athletes with good bone quality and rigid fixation. Vertical medial malleolar fractures and comminuted fractures in particular must be watched closely with a slower progression of weight bearing.

15.8.7 Preventative Measures

Prevention is principally a focus of pre-operative and post-operative prevention of complications. Preventive measures have not been delineated regarding the prevention of these severe traumatic injuries. Proper conditioning and counselling regarding sports techniques constitute a large part of prevention. Youth sports have adopted weight restrictions and guidelines to decrease injuries. Interestingly, one study indicated there was no increased risk to smaller players when there were no weight limits. From this chapter's perspective, it was interesting to note that ankle fracture was the most common "significant injury" during this football season study [37].

15.9 Bimalleolar Equivalent (Weber B/Weber C Fibula and Deltoid)

15.9.1 Epidemiology

Bimalleolar equivalent fractures include fibular fracture with damage to the deltoid ligament. The mechanism of injury is often due to a pronation-abducted force, which results in fibular fracture and damage to the medial ligaments [34] (Fig. 15.14). This disruption results in the talus externally rotating causing misalignment of the mortise [71]. It would be thought that the outcomes of bimalleolar and bimalleolar equivalent injuries would be similar. No study has compared these injuries in athletes, but, in the non-athletic population, the outcome is better in the bimalleolar equivalent [72].

15.9.2 Classification

Bimalleolar equivalent ankle fractures are typically classified by Lauge-Hasen and Danis-Weber systems discussed above. One of the most common ankle fractures is SER pattern with deltoid ligament rupture, or SER IV deltoid ligament variant, as it is suspected to account for 10% of all fractures involving the lateral malleolus [71].

15.9.3 Diagnosis (History/Physical Examination/Imaging) (Fig. 15.14)

Athletes with a bimalleolar equivalent ankle fracture experience marked pain and have significant swelling and ecchymosis and present similarly to the bimalleolar secetion. For sake of brevity, we will not duplicate what is well spelled out above. Since the equivalency is related to the deltoid disruption rather than a medial malleolar fracture, particular care must be taken to be certain there is no skin disruption and an occult open fracture is not involved. There is nearly uniform subluxation/dislocation with the deltoid rupture.

This fracture pattern occurs in all sports similar to the bimalleolar epidemiology. Contact football is a particularly common sport with another player landing on the lateral ankle causing the pronation/ER injury among others. A care-

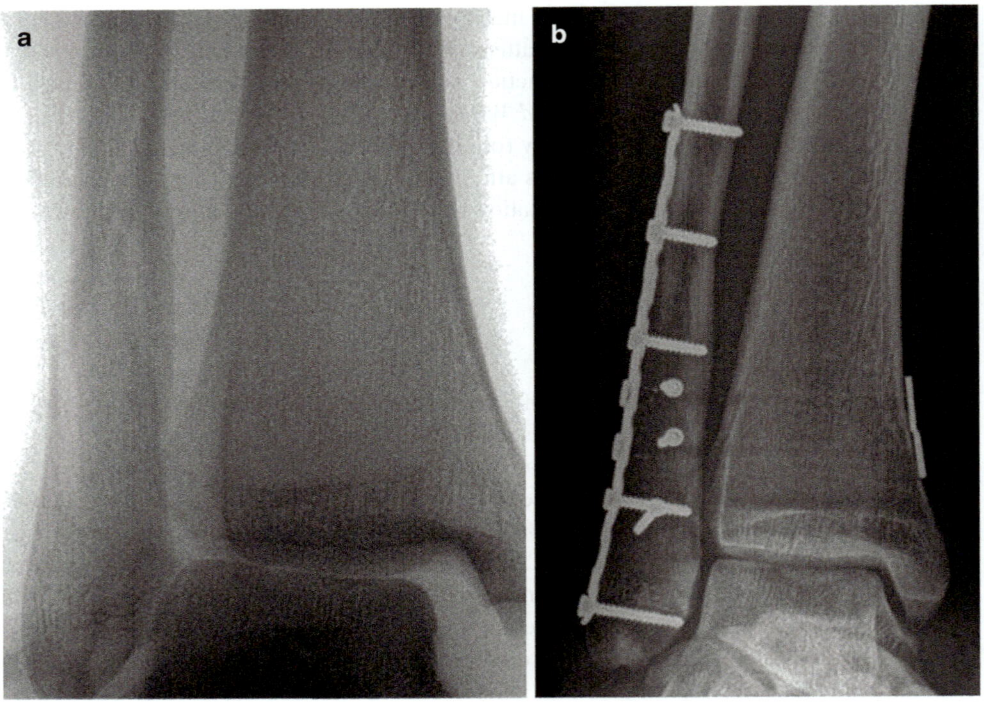

Fig. 15.14 (**a**, **b**) Weber B Fibula with deltoid. (**a**) Anterior-posterior radiograph of athlete with right ankle pain with Weber C variant of distal fibula fracture and distal syndesmosis disruption with wide medial clear space suggesting complete deltoid ligament rupture. (**b**) Post-operative antero-posterior image demonstrating lateral fibular plate, two antero-posterior lag screws. Note also two suture buttons for syndesmosis stabilization and resultant normal medial clear space after open deltoid ligament repair. Note the endo buttons on medial malleolus "snug" on bone below periosteum

ful history is very critical to understand the mechanism of injury By definition, a bimalleolar equivalent injury involves a deltoid rupture, so medial and lateral tenderness will be present. The rest of the exam and radiographic evaluation is similar to that noted above. Thus, a very thorough history and careful physical examination with the above nuances should be undertaken in a detailed manner on all athletes with suspicion of a bimalleolar equivalent injury.

Standard three view weight-bearing (or simulated weight bearing). Advanced imaging can be helpful to assess for communited fractures and to assess if there is any component of a pilon fracture or posterio malleolus fracture. MRI is particularly helpful to classify deep deltoid ligament injury, bone bruising and subtle cartilage injury and is routine in the elite athlete and judicous use if warranted in the less elite level player. We favor intra-operative arthroscopy and ankle-block or intraoperative stress imaging to make definitive assessments of the extent of subtle syndesmosis and anterior deltoid ligament disruption these images as delineated above re: bimalleolar injuries also.

15.9.4 Treatment

The treatment of bimalleolar equivalent fractures has been greatly debated. In earlier times, it was standard for surgeons to repair the ruptured deltoid ligament. The current trend from publications of the 1980s and 1990s is to not directly repair the deltoid ligament complex [71]. If there was proper anatomic alignment with ORIF, repair of the deltoid ligament was not necessary and the outcomes reported were satisfactory [73]. Lateral malleolar fixation with proper alignment of mortise did not warrant suture of the deltoid ligament, all patients returned to work, and 15 of the 19 patients who participated in sports were able to return without restriction [61]. Conversely, Jones and Nunley [74] compared the outcomes of bimalleolar equivalents treated with lateral malleolus ORIF with trans-syndesmotic fixation versus lateral malleolus ORIF with deltoid ligament repair. They found no significant difference between the two groups in functional outcomes or subjective questionnaires supporting deltoid ligament repair [74]. However, the patients in the ORIF with syndesmotic fixation group had to undergo an additional procedure to remove the implant. Another investigation looking at outcomes between bimalleolar equivalent fractures reported no difference in outcomes related to pain or activity between repaired deltoid ligaments and those left to heal non-operatively [34].

Of note, the referred publications did not mention the professional or competitive athletic population, which leaves the question does ORIF alone provide adequate function of the ankle during high performance situations without deltoid ligament repair. To address this question in this specific population, Hsu et al. [8] reported on 14 NFL players with a pronation-external rotation injury patterns who underwent ankle fracture fixation and syndesmotic fixation with open superficial deltoid ligament complex repair. They found that all players were able to return to running and cutting by 6 months postoperatively [8]. Overall, return to play the following season was 84%, though all players were medically cleared, and upon final follow-up, no players reported medial pain or instability [8]. Though this study is limited by the lack of subjective patient outcome measures and a control group for comparison, the authors recommend that, in athletes, repair of the deltoid ligament with ORIF should be considered.

Further studies recently favor more aggressive deltoid ligament repair in athletes with concomitant lateral bony injury [1, 7].

Hardware choices for the fibula fractures are the same as listed above under *Isolated Malleolar* and *Bimalleolar Fracture*.

15.9.5 Complications

The complications are the same as listed under bimalleolar fractures with a few additions and notes to make. The risk of chondral injury is higher in the deltoid ligament lateral sided injury with often more significant joint displacement and dislocation. Scuffing to frank chondral disruption to true osteochondral fracture occur with greater force of dislocation and greater degree of subluxation. Also, ligamentous laxity and rotational instability is always a concern with deltoid ligament disruption. Thus, our interest in anatomic deltoid ligament repair at the time of fracture fixation and our interest in arthroscopy with ankle fracture treatment is highlighted.

15.9.6 Rehabilitation

The 14 NFL players mentioned above underwent a standardized rehabilitation program following ORIF and deltoid ligament repair. This consisted of non-weight bearing in a splint for 2 weeks postoperatively, followed by non-weight bearing cast from 2 to 4 weeks to support the anterior deltoid ligament repair [8]. Transition to CAM boot took place at 4–6 weeks with the start of physical therapy occurring 6 weeks postoperatively [8]. Physical therapy consisted of ROM, stretching, and nonimpact strengthening exercises [8]. The athlete was weaned from CAM boot to lace-up ankle brace with weight bearing as tolerated from 6 to 12 weeks [8]. Gradual increase inactivity occurred from 12 to 16 weeks, with no running or jumping until after 16 weeks [8].

15.9.7 Preventative Measures

Preventative measures in our hands focus on preventing arthritis, cartilage deterioration, nonunions, arthrofibrosis and ligamentous laxity. These injuries are all traumatic and true prevention is illusive at best. Arthritis is most commonly a result of cartilage injury at the time of fracture/dislocation. Anatomic, rigid fixation significantly reduces the risk of nonunions, delayed unions and malunions. However, we still recommend consideration of external bone growth stimulator in the comminuted fibular shaft fractures. Orthobiologic can be considered in delayed unions and autogenous bone grafting is still preferred for nonunions and for some comminuted distal fibular fractures. Progressive rehabilitation, arthroscopy at the time of fixation and more aggressive deltoid ligament repair are means to reduce arthrofibrosis, inadvertent cartilage injury from loose fragments or untreated chondral injuries and long-term ligament laxity.

15.10 Trimalleolar Fracture

15.10.1 Epidemiology

Trimalleolar fractures, by definition, include all three malleoli: medial, lateral, and posterior. The posterior component is an avulsion or impaction fracture of the posterior plafond [74]. This type of fracture is relatively uncommon in the competitive athlete, and accounts for only 7% of all ankle fractures [75].

15.10.2 Classification

Malleoli fractures are classified based on the number of malleoli involved. Unimalleolar fracture include either the lateral, medial, or posterior malleolus, while bimalleolar contain two malleoli, and thus, trimalleolar consist of all three malleoli [75].

We prefer the Lauge-Hansen and Weber classification (Figs. 15.1 and 15.13) for the complex ankle fracture dislocation. Trimalleolar, like bimalleolar fractures, medially can involve either the deltoid ligament or the medial malleolus. On rare occasions, there can be both bony and ligamentous injury in the same athletic injury.

15.10.3 Diagnosis (History/Physical Examination/Imaging)

Please see bimalleolar and bimalleolar equivalent inury as the approach is similar. However, we obtain a CT scan on all triamalleolar ankle fratures to assess comminution and location and extent of the posterior malleolar fracture.

15.10.4 Treatment

Treatment of trimalleolar fractures involves operative fixation in athletes. In regards to the posterior malleolar fragment, small fragments reduce spontaneously with fibular

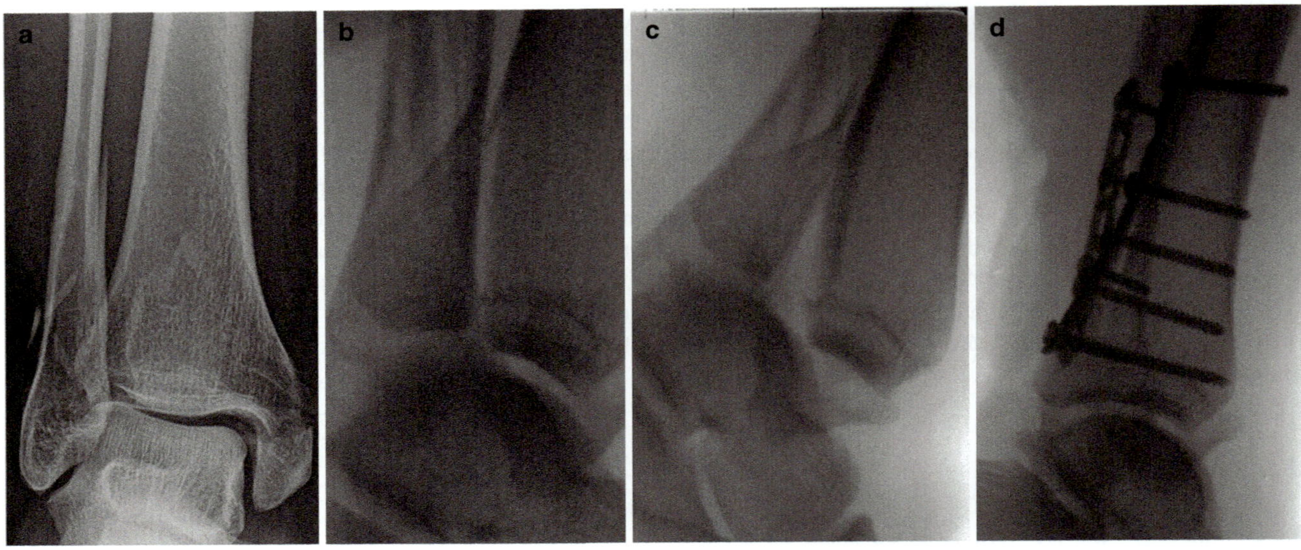

Fig. 15.15 (**a**) antero-posterior radiograph noting valgus tilt, comminuted fibula fracture, displaced medial malleolar avulsion fracture and suggestion of posterior malleolar fracture. (**b**) Lateral intra-operative image with anterior translation noting mild-moderate posterior malleolar displacement. (**c**) Lateral intra-operative image with posterior directed stress showing severe posterior instability necessitating posterior malleolar fixation. (**d**) Lateral intra-operative image showing anatomic reduction and fixation of the posterior malleolus fracture with posterior plate and fixation of the fibula with a posterior anti-glide plate applied through the same posterolateral incision, note medial malleolus fracture not address while in the prone position. Medial malleolus fixed was performed by placing the athlete in the supine position with arthroscopy performed at that time

fracture reduction due to the PITFL [33]. The need for separate reduction and fixation is determined preoperatively and/or intraoperatively [33]. However, in non-athletes, it is considered unstable if it includes >25–30% of the articular surface of the plafond and remains >2 mm displaced after lateral malleolar reduction [33]. We favor a more aggressive approach in athletes. Although this is not a common injury in competitive athletes, we do not accept any step-off posteriorly. Also, if the fragment involves more than 15–25% of the articular surface or if there is any posterior instability we prefer operative reduction and fixation (Fig. 15.15c).

Historically, little has been known about the functional outcomes of trimalleolar fractures in athletes. However, in the general population there has been poorer functional outcome scores, severe osteoarthritic changes, and residual symptoms depending on the posterior malleolar fragment size [75]. In retrospective case series, 47 patients with bimalleolar or trimalleolar fractures were analyzed. Twenty-six of the 47 patients complained of residual pain, 29 complained of stiffness, and 21 reported persistent ankle swelling despite majority of the patients reporting good to excellent results according to Olerud and Molander scores [75]. Of the 47 patients, 33 patients participated in sporting activities prior to injury. Nine of the 33 athletic patients returned to preinjury function and return to play, while 6 of the 33 were unable to participate in sporting activities at all [75]. Though the data referenced above accounts for both bimalleolar and trimalleolar fractures, the authors found no difference between the two groups in regards to functional outcomes or return to sport [75]. Similarly to the findings above, another investigation found that only 25% of patients returned to preinjury level of activity with no difference among the types of fractures, indicating the poor prognosis in this severe injury [75].

15.10.5 Current Approach to Posterior Malleolar Fractures

The management of large posterior malleolar fractures in association with bony injuries of the medial malleolus and fibula is somewhat controversial. Nondisplaced fractures in isolation can be treated non operatively. However, large fractures that involves significant portions of the articular surface and result in posterior instability, require operative fixation (Fig. 15.15a–d).

There is a recent trend to be more aggressive with posterior malleolar fractures for two reasons. The posterior malleolus typically involves the posterior tibio-fibular ligament (PITFL) which is a portion of the syndesmosis. Fixation of the posterior malleolus results in stabilization of the syndesmosis and can negate the need for further syndesmosis fixation. Secondly, improved techniques and improved hardware for the posterior malleolus, have resulted in improved stability and fixation. As surgeons have become more comfortable with this posterior approach, we have seen the advantage of being more aggressive with posterior fixation. And in all circumstances, when there is posterior instability associated with the posterior malleolar fracture, will believe posterior fixation is warranted and recommended in athletes. The amount of weight-bearing surface involvement to merit posterior fixation without obvious posterior instability, is a more difficult question to determine. We prefer a more aggressive approach with posterior fixation if there is any question or doubt. Somewhere between 15% and 30% of the weight-bearing surface has traditionally been the cut-off point for posterior fixation in the non-athlete. We tend to undertaken surgical fixation if there is 15% or greater articular surface involvement in athletes.

Fixation of the posterior malleolus is best approached with the patient in a prone position and we prefer a posterior lateral approach. We use the flexor hallucis-peroneal tendon interval. Often the posterior periosteum is not torn since it is a vertical shear force (impaction versus avulsion) with the ankle in equinus. Typically, we cut thru the periosteum to expose the fracture and insure anatomic reduction. We use either the 2.4 mm LCDC locking plate or more commonly, the 3.5 1/3 tubular plate. Both plates contour to the posterior tibia with screw fixation. Imaging is mandatory in the antero-posterior and lateral view to verify reduction and screw placement. We use 3.5 lag screws across the fractured portion of the malleolus and cannulated drilling can help with placement. Fixation of the fibula with an antiglide placement is accessible in this exposure. Rigid, anatomic fixation can be obtained with this approach. We turn the patient supine to fix the medial malleolus and perform arthroscopy at that time (Fig. 15.15a–d).

15.10.6 Complications

In addition to the outcomes mentioned above, another complication noted by Hong et al. [75] was a tri-malleolar fracture with a prominent screw requiring changes of screw under local anesthetic. Five patients also requested a follow-up procedure at least 1 year after surgery with evidence of union on radiograph for implant removal [75].

Furthermore, the authors reported on sporting activity in 33 athletes with either bimalleolar or tri-malleolar ankle fractures [75]. Only 9 of the 33 (27.3%) athletes were able to return to their preinjury level of sport with no difficulty and 6 of the 33 were not able to return to sports at all, highlighting the severe impact these more severe fractures can have on athletic participation.

Nonunions and malunion are certainly a known complication after trimalleolar ankle fractures. In the athletic population, this is still a significant complication. There is not enough literature to document the risk, but significant diaphyseal comminuted fractures of the fibula and comminuted medial malleolar fractures or ones with vertical orientation are at higher risk.

Posttraumatic arthritis of the ankle is a significant risk in these athletes. This is particularly true with associated subluxation or dislocations typically involved with these injuries. Arthroscopic assessment and treatment at the time of fracture reduction and fixation have in theory reduced the risk and identified the athletes with significant chondral injuries and osteochondral fractures at the time of injury. The advent of bone and joint specific hardware has significantly decreased the risk of malunion and nonunions. Therefore, chondral and osteochondral injuries in the ankle are some of the highest complication risk for return to preinjury sport activity.

Postoperative infections should be less than 1% in this population. Mild delayed wound healing or superficial epidermolysis can be common because of the significant soft tissue injury.

Stiffness, arthrofibrosis, and weakness are all complications that can be common after this fracture pattern.

15.10.7 Rehabilitation

The rehabilitation principles as delineated below should be incorporated into the preoperative and postoperative management. The ability to begin early range of motion, that is after the wounds have healed well, are an easy principle to apply even in these severe trimalleolar ankle fractures. Simple maneuvers such as toe curls and sitting toe raises as well as active assisted range of motion with towels and Thera-Band can be applied with discretion as early as 1–2 weeks' post-surgery. Weight-bearing status in these injuries will depend on the degree of weight-bearing surface disruption, stability chondral status. Unlike the non-athlete, the young athletic patient with good bone stock can have excellent stability with anatomic realignment with bone specific and location specific hardware. Therefore, weight-bearing status may be allowed sooner than the non-athletic population. There is interest in the trauma literature regarding being more progressive with weight-bearing post-surgical fixation also [76]. We apply those principles within the athletic population. With trimalleolar ankle fractures, the soft tissue injury is more concerning and the balance between range of motion and weight-bearing has to be obtained with prudent judgment and experience.

15.10.8 Preventative Measures

Preventative measures focus on eliminating or significantly reducing the postoperative complications. The improvement in hardware specificity around the ankle has significantly reduced the risk of nonunions and malunions. We favor low-profile bone and position specific hardware to reduce the risk of soft tissue compromise, stiffness and painful prominent hardware. Surgeon should be conversant with the different hardware options, as both titanium and stainless steel and dynamic fixation products around the distal syndesmosis allow to obtain anatomic reduction, rigid fixation, and dynamic stabilization. After rigid and anatomic fixation, early range of motion and early weight-bearing can be initiated thus reducing many of the historical complications. That is, stiffness, disuse atrophy, osteopenia, stress fractures with return to sports, and weakness.

Preoperative and postoperative management of soft tissue is critical in these injuries for prevention of catastrophic skin and soft tissue coverage. With trimalleolar ankle fractures, this awareness must be heightened. Judicious elevation, compression and cold therapy can be instrumental in optimizing the soft tissue envelope both preoperatively and in the immediate postoperative recovery. We prefer utilization of intermittent immobilisation with low-level compression and intermittent cold compression in the preoperative period (Cryocuff DJO Carlsbad, CA). We do not utilize extreme pressure or extreme cold therapy in the preoperative or immediate postoperative period. We get athletes as quickly as possible in intermittent and removable immobilisation device post-operatively such as a removable splint or more commonly a removable walking boot with a cold compression device within the boot that can be utilized throughout the day and even intermittently into the evening. This can have a significant impact on the timing required for optimal treatment and the post-operative swelling and pain. We have not found it necessary to utilize external fixation in the setting of this fracture. We prefer not to violate the soft tissue envelope prior to definitive surgical intervention to decrease the risk of infection. Postoperatively, we use cold compression therapy even more intermittently because of the "injury" produced by multiple incisions and arthroscopy. We do not allow devices such as GameReady® until the wounds have healed and are suitable for suture removal.

15.11 Pilon Fracture

15.11.1 Epidemiology

Pilon fractures are relatively rare in competitive athletes, and can be misinterpreted as less severe fractures. Pilon fractures are comminuted fracture of the distal tibia resulting from axial loading and producing injury to the distal tibial articular surface [7]. These fractures often occur in high-energy incidents [33]. This fracture is more common in motor vehicle accidents or a fall from heights. Therefore, pilon fractures in athletes will be associated with significant violence, and are prevalent in motor cross sports or high-speed skating or skiing. These injuries will more likely be treated by orthopedic surgeons specializing in trauma rather than sports.

15.11.2 Classification

Pilon fracture classification involves both soft tissue and bony classifications. The soft tissue classifications are based on the degree of skin and muscle injury as well as whether the fracture is open or closed. Detailed and careful evaluation of the soft tissue is crucial to determine the appropriate timing of surgical intervention to optimize soft tissue healing. The soft tissue envelope must be optimized before definitive surgery can be undertaken. These high energy injuries can require provisional external fixation prior to definitive internal fixation. After optimization of the soft tissues which can require up to 2–3 weeks, we prefer the below Table 15.1 listed bony classification system. This classification system primarily delineates severity of injury more so than actual fracture reduction or definitive fixation.

Fortunately, most Sports Medicine providers of athletic Pilon fractures involve types A1 and A2 as well as possibly types B1 and B2 fractures. Our report, in Foot and Ankle in International in which we reported on one Pilon fracture, involved a B1 type fracture and that athlete did well [7].

15.11.3 Diagnosis (History/Physical Examination/Imaging)

A pilon fracture should be suspected when the lateral plafond has a valgus alignment or obvious comminution of the distal tibial plafond [33]. Confirmation and delineation of the plafond alignment fracture pattern should be evaluated by CT [33].

Table 15.1 Pilon fracture classification system of J Ortho Trauma as presented *Medscape* May 20, 2019 Pilon Fractures Workup [77]

Type A—These fractures are extra-articular and subcategorized as simple (A1), comminuted (A2), or severely comminuted (A3)
Type B—These fractures involve only a portion of the articular surface and a single column; subcategories include pure split (B1), split with depression (B2), and depression with multiple fragments (B3)
Type C—These fractures involve the whole of the articular surface; they may be categorized as a simple split in the articular surface and the metaphysis (C1), an articular split that is simple with a metaphysis split that is multifragmentary (C2), or a fracture with multiple fragments of the articular surface and the metaphysis (C3)

15.11.4 Treatment

Surgical management of pilon fractures is complex, and using standard ankle fracture management concepts may result in an unstable valgus ankle [33]. Porter et al. [7] assessed functional outcomes in athletes with ankle fractures following ORIF. In this study, one athlete sustained a pilon fracture and was treated surgically by ORIF with low profile plates and screws as needed [7]. The athlete returned to activity in 8 weeks, and was competing at 16 weeks postoperatively with a subjective rating of the ankle at 80% relative to preinjury activity, with numbness and stiffness [7]. To our knowledge, no other reports on pilon fractures in athlete have been published.

15.11.5 Complications

Patients should be advised that the articular damage from the initial injury may lead to rapid joint degeneration [33]. Hinterman has linked the occurrence of intra-articular cartilage damage seen arthroscopically at time of ORIF of ankle fractures to long term poor outcomes [62]. The impaction nature of the pilon fracture puts the cartilage at particular increased risk! There is no study in athletes which has evaluated articular surface injury or long-term outcomes in athletes. The single patient reported by Porter [7] reported that the involved ankle was 80% of normal and, was noted to have the "lowest score on AAOS lower leg and foot and ankle module" compared to the other athletes with fractures. The athlete cited stiffness and numbness as the principal limiting factors.

15.11.6 Rehabilitation

A Rehabilitation program for pilon fractures was described by Porter et al. [7]. The athlete used a CryoCuff™ with a walking boot following surgery and was non-weightbearing initially for 4–6 weeks [7]. While early weight bearing was encouraged in the other fracture patterns after rigid fixation, because of the inherent articular surface and weightbearing surface injury with Pilon fractures weightbearing was delayed. However, the ankle was intermittently immobilized to allow early ROM for cartilage nutrition [7, 78]. Stationary biking in the walking boot was permitted once the athlete was weightbearing off crutches [7]. Over the course of several weeks, athletes are slowly weaned out of boot into a brace, and increase their activity [7]. Return to activity is started once athletes complete a sport-specific functional progression program, which include running without pain or discomfort [7]. In general, rehabilitation after this high impaction type injury with articular surface fracturing has to be more conservative. ROM exercises should be initiated as soon as they are safe, in the first 1–2 weeks following surgery. Sitting toe raises and active as well as, active assisted ROM can be very helpful in the chondral surface injuries. Once there is confirmed healing of the bony structures, then progression of activities can continue along the lines of other less severe fractures.

15.11.7 Preventative Measures

Preventative measures are centered around avoiding complications to treatment. It starts with detailed pre-operative planning. Control and management of preoperative swelling and the soft tissue trauma is paramount to preventing catastrophic outcomes. We utilize cold and gravity compression therapy (Boot with Cryocuff in boot), but wait on mechanical cold compression therapy (GameReady) until after complete wound healing and suture removal after definitive fixation to decrease risk of cold/compression injury.

15.12 Rehabilitation Principles

15.12.1 Goals/Principles

Rehabilitation involves preoperative planning, intraoperative assessment of bone quality the-cartilage condition-rigidity of fixation and post-operative treatment. Preoperative planning is crucial to optimize the soft tissues around the ankle and prepare and educate the athletes about their condition and plan for recovery. Communication is an important part also to those involved with the care of athletes, including the parents for the young athlete, the trainers and coaches for the collegiate athletes, and management, training staff, and agents at the professional level [70]. Significant orthopedic injuries to the ankle can produce a "death-like" experience for the athlete. Such fractures are emotionally crushing and anxiety provoking: "*... the psychological response to injury can trigger or unmask serious mental health issues such as depression, anxiety, disordered eating, and substance use or abuse*" [79]. Thus, educating athletes about the injury and helping athletes normalize their approach to a serious injury can be critical to the athletes' mental health. Awareness of what this injury might unmask mentally and socially are critical parts of rehabilitation also. Although there is controversy regarding the risk of pre-operative swelling on post-operative complications, we still favor giving time and attention to reducing edema and de-stressing the skin after serious acute injuries. We utilize cold and compression therapy (see below) similar to post-operative care to optimize timing and skin condition.

Intraoperative assessment is the foundation for postoperative rehabilitation decision-making. That is, the integrity of the articular surface, the rigidity of fixation and the presence or lack of comminution drives the decision-making of rehabilitation. With rigid fixation of ankle fractures and healthy athletes, early range of motion and early weight-bearing carries significant advantages [7]. Cartilage nutrition is clearly enhanced by early range-of-motion and limited weight-bearing. Wolf's law of bone healing plays a real role in optimizing the timing and functionality of fracture healing. We assess the quality of the bone as we place appropriate hardware. The rigidity of the fixation will be determined both by the hardware that can be used, as well as the amount of comminution. Optimizing the anatomic alignment and rotation with bone specific hardware can allow the surgeon to feel much more comfortable with early weight-bearing and certainly early range of motion. Though not specifically in athletes, recent confirmation of the benefits of early weight bearing and ROM have been supported in the trauma literature [79, 80]. Also, a recent article by Schubert et al. from Australia demonstrated improved early General Health Status as measured by the EuroQol SD visual analog scale with weight-bearing at 2 weeks versus 6 weeks' post-operative [81]. At 6 months, this benefit was maintained and was similar to the delayed weight bearing group.

Postoperative rehabilitation initially focuses on wound healing and edema control. After wound healing, more aggressive range of motion and weight-bearing is initiated. Barill and co-workers have outlined an extensive approach for rehabilitation after ankle fractures and Syndesmosis fixation [82–84]. We utilize their approach and the approach of Porter et al. [7]. Briefly, early ROM (2 weeks) can include sitting toe raises to initiate movement without significant forces across the joint. Desensitization massage is initiated in Weeks 1–2 since feet are highly susceptible to Complex Regional Pain Syndrome (CRPS). Stationary biking can be performed with the boot as early as 2–4 weeks in appropriate settings. Seated BAPS board, seated to standing double toe raises then to single toe raises are begun 2–6 weeks after surgery. Theraband strengthening can be initiated at 2–3 weeks in stable directions and 6 weeks in unstable directions. The athlete is begun on stationary bike program and then progresses to stairstepper/elliptical and then running. Each stage requires 30–40 min of exercise 3–4 days/week with a brace without discomfort. We use sports-specific functional progression to clear the athlete for sports performance and return-to-play. At the Division 1 and professional level, GPS monitoring of volume of activity tolerance and top speed return can be evaluated [83]. Skill return and position specific instincts are evaluated by position specific coaches, and/or trainers after release by the medical team.

15.12.2 Intermittent Immobilisation with Early Range-of-Motion (ROM) and Weight Bearing

We favor early ROM to decrease risk of arthrofibrosis, improve cartilage nutrition, and apply Wolf's law for soft tissue. Early weight bearing is favored and allowed when the fracture pattern and rigid fixation is adequate. We are never able to allow immediate weight bearing on Pilon fractures and joint surface injury requiring decompression and bone grafting, but always allow WBAT in the first 1–2 weeks for isolated, non-comminuted fibula fracture and isolated, non-comminuted rigidly fixed medial malleolus fracture. Bimalleolar and bimalleolar and bimalleolar equivalent fractures fall somewhere in between these patterns. Isolated syndesmosis fixation can support WBAT after 2–3 weeks but syndesmosis fixation in conjunction with ankle fracture fixation is dependent on the fracture itself.

15.12.3 Functional Recovery and Progression to Sports/Activity

We have discussed return to sport and functional recovery within each of the fracture types above. To be more detailed, this portion of the rehabilitation is critical to full return to pre-injury pattern and can be lost in some general fracture care rehabilitation. Athletes do not consider radiographic fracture healing with healed wounds with minimal swelling as the end point for recovery. Athletes are focused on full, uninhibited return to high-level performance as the goal of recovery. Thus, the functional, sports specific high intensity training needed after traditional rehabilitation is the final and distinctive piece to athletic recovery to an ankle fracture. Often, pre-surgical rehabilitation to prepare for optimization of post-surgical recovery and detailed post-surgery rehabilitation make a major difference following treatment of athletic ankle fractures [84]. Close collaborations between surgeons and rehabilitation specialists and coaches are beneficial to full return to performance, as these specialists continue the sports specific rehabilitation and conditioning for faster return to play. In practice, surgeons determine when an athlete is no longer restricted in rehabilitation and practice, but only trainers and coaches can fully evaluate when an athlete is truly cleared for return to play [82, 84].

15.13 Complications

15.13.1 Malunions and Nonunions

None of the sport-specific ankle fracture studies mention malunion or nonunion, but certainly this complication can occur. The lack of article with enough subjects and different fracture types likely leads to this more optimistic outcome. Comminuted Weber C fibula and comminuted, impacted medial malleolus fracture (mild pilon—Supination adduction) would intuitively have the highest rate for both malunions and non-unions.

15.13.2 Infection

Infection is a most dreaded complications and must be discussed with each athlete. Fortunately, with appropriate preventative measures it is uncommon. None of the articles mention rates of infection in athletes. In the general population, infection following open reduction and internal fixation of ankle fractures ranges from 1.44% to 8.6% [85, 86]. In our setting, we have not had an infection in an athlete with ankle fracture fixation and our infection rate in the general population is less than 1% in non-diabetic and non-comorbidity patients. We did report 2 of the 27 patients in our athletic ankle fracture study with suspected infection at time of syndesmosis hardware, but evaluation was negative for bacterial infection [7]. Hsu and Hong reported no deep infections and one superficial wound infection respectively. The wound infection resolved with oral antibiotics [8, 75].

15.13.3 Metal Allergy

Nickel is the most common metal allergy that impacts fracture care. Contact dermatitis to nickel has been reported to be 20% or higher [87]. There was speculation that the sensitivity was increasing because of trace Ni in technology products [87]. The sensitivity in women can be as high as 17–25% whereas in men is lower at 5%. Implant quality stainless steel used in orthopedic hardware is 13–15% Ni by weight [88]. There is no consensus on the rate of symptomatic reaction to nickel in implants placed under the skin, but there is clear reactivity reported and speculated. Nickel free stainless steel is currently under investigation [88]. Interestingly, there is a definite association between post-operative infection and implant sensitivity, but it is unclear whether there is a direct cause-effect relationship [89]. That is, was the increased sensitivity due to the infection or was the infection brought on by the increased sensitivity? Patch testing has been advocated as the most common method for preoperative evaluation if suspicion exist regarding metal allergy and Nickel is by far the most prevalent metal allergy (Fig. 15.16).

15.13.4 Cartilage Injury and Arthritis

Post traumatic arthritis is a potentially debilitating complication of ankle fractures. Post-traumatic arthritis can result from osteochondral and chondral injuries at the time of impaction with fracture dislocation (Fig. 15.16). Development of cartilage loss can also occur due to malreduction and malalignment, as well as, progression of cartilage injury due to cartilage impaction at the time of injury which was not visible radiographically or arthroscopically.

Post-traumatic arthritis has been identified traditionally by repeated plain radiographs over time with slow development of cartilage interval decrease and spurring. With the development of and more common use of arthroscopic eval-

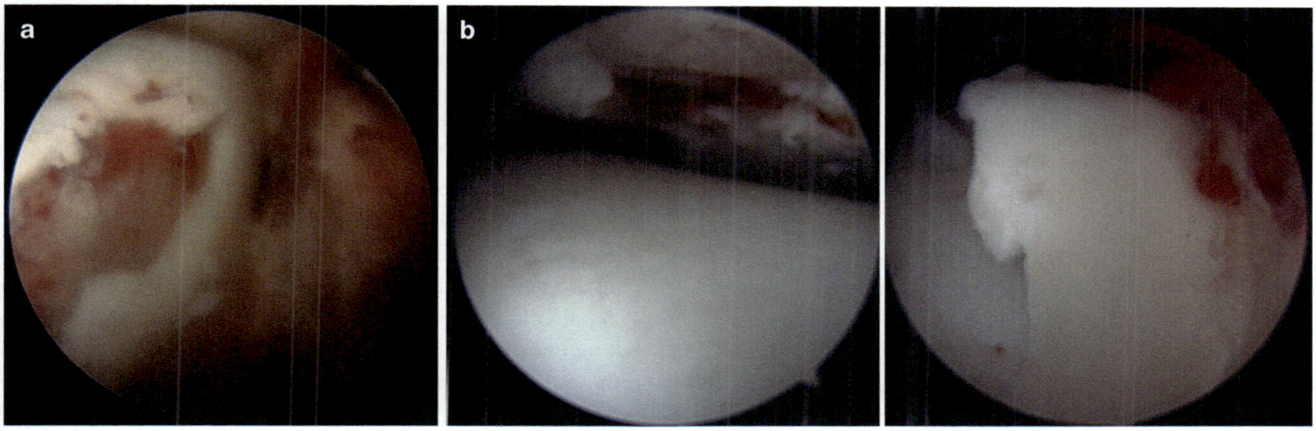

Fig. 15.16 (**a**, **b**) Arthroscopic images of chondral injury after deltoid ligament rupture. (**a**) Medial gutter talar dome injury with full thickness cartilage injury from eversion injury causing complete deltoid ligament rupture, mild syndesmosis injury with lateral impaction of fibula on lateral talus. Treated with debridement and microfracture but no change in weight bearing because of non-weightbearing surface and good short-term outcome. (<1 year). (**b**) Arthroscopic view of anterior distal tibial osteochondral lesion with large non-reparable chondral injury with minimal bony attachment. Required removal of loose cartilage, microfracture of distal tibia and non-weightbearing for 4 weeks. Good short term result with return to full activity in less than 1 year

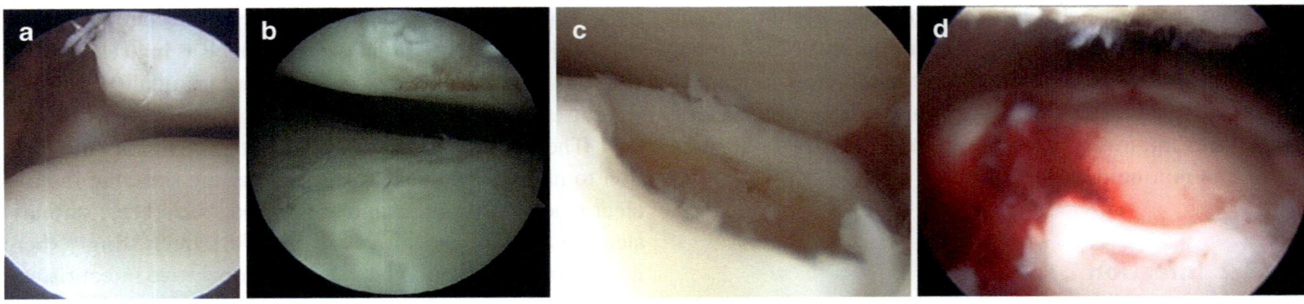

Fig. 15.17 (**a–d**) Arthroscopic appearance of ankle fractures with assessment of cartilage. (**a**) Arthroscopic view of normal tibial and talar cartilage in athlete with Isolated Weber B fibula fracture. Note debridement of Anterior Inferior Tibial Fibular Ligament (AITFL). (**b**) Arthroscopic view of central talar scuffing of the cartilage in an elite athlete with fracture dislocation of ankle. There is no exposed bone, so prognosis is still good if there is no occult full thickness chondral impaction injury. (**c**) Arthroscopic view after debridement of an osteochondral lesion of the lateral talar dome in an athlete with bimalleolar equivalent fracture dislocation. Note the microfracture puncture holes at the base of debrided lesion. (**d**) Arthroscopic view of pure chondral avulsion injury in a Division 1 athlete with a Weber C fibula fracture, and complete deltoid ligament rupture with dislocation. Note the bare subchondral bone and 1.5 cm chondral loss. This is a potentially poorer prognosis, and necessitated 4 weeks non-weightbearing with microfracture of the lesion

uation at the time of fracture reduction and fixation, the assessment of cartilage and osteochondral injury at the time of fixation has been better elucidated. As noted in Sect. 15.14, there is a high incidence of chondral and/or osteochondral injuries associated with ankle fractures in athletes. The incidence and degree of chondral and osteochondral injury increases with the severity of the fracture and is significantly elevated when there is subluxation or dislocation (Fig. 15.17). It is uncommon to see the same changes in isolated medial or lateral malleolar fractures.

As mentioned above, development of more joint and bone specific implants have significantly reduced the potential malreduction and nonunions associated with prior fractures in athletes. Not that long ago, severe fracture dislocation of the ankle was a career ending injury in athletes. However, more recent reports indicate a high rate of return can be achieved with proper fixation and attention to stabilization of associated ligamentous injuries. Thus, development of post-traumatic arthritis now is more commonly associated with the severity of cartilage injury at the time of the fracture and the degree of impaction and "silent" cartilage injury (Fig. 15.17).

15.14 Arthroscopy

Arthroscopy of the ankle is becoming more common. The first report of ankle arthroscopy was in 1939 by Tagaki from Japan, and Watanabe, in 1972, published the first series on ankle arthroscopy [90, 91]. Later, Plank in 1978 and Andrews in 1985 reported on arthroscopy and its usefulness in pathologic ankle conditions and the normal arthroscopic ankle anatomy [92, 93]. Hinterman reported a 79.2% incidence of chondral injuries in patients with ankle fractures and noted importance of assessing the cartilage [62]. The authors noted a higher incidence in the Weber C fractures than Weber B. Hinterman's study was not limited to athletes, but did note that the younger patients (<30) did have a higher rate of chondral injury. Aktas reported that 24 of 86 (28%) patients had a chondral injury and distal fibula fractures had the highest rate (14/20) [94]. Only 4 of the 86 fractures had a syndesmosis injury, indicating a less severe subluxation/injury pattern. His data included bimalleolar (4/27 chondral injury), trimalleolar (6/15 with chondral injury) and as noted, 14/20 distal fibular fractures. Ankle arthroscopy has become prevalent amongst sports orthopedist and foot and ankle specialists and is now considered common place. However, arthroscopic assessment and treatment associated with ankle fractures is a more recent development. Thordardson in 2001 reported on nine ankle fracture patients with 8/9 having chondral injuries [95]. The results were compared to ten patients with ankle fractures that did not have arthroscopy. Despite no short-term differences in outcome, the authors mention the advantage of arthroscopic assessment of chondral injuries with ankle fractures and the high incidence of chondral injury (89%). Ferkel's group, in 2002, reported a 63% incidence of chondral injury that could be treated at the time of surgery in 48 patients with ankle fractures [96]. There was also an increased incidence of chondral injuries with concurrent syndesmosis injury. Ono, in 2004, reported on 105 patients with a much lower chondral injury rate of 20% but mention the ability to shave off chondral irregularity and remove loose fragments as well as the ability to visualize reductions as clear advantages to arthroscopy with ankle fractures [86]. Ono did not report outcomes, however. Leontartis, in 2009, noted a higher incidence of chondral injury with more severe fracture [97]. The authors also concluded: "(there is) diagnostic value and better (assessment) for intra-articular fracture pattern and severity, (as well as better) visualization of reduction".

Despite these clear diagnostic advantages and the ability to treat the chondral surface changes at the time of fracture fixation, no study to date has shown statistical outcome improvements with arthroscopy [98, 99]. Fuchs reported no improvement in PROMIS scores with arthroscopy but noted no complications and the average operative time was increased by only 15 min [98]. Gonzalez also noted in a multi-study analysis that arthroscopically assisted surgery for fracture fixation was a valuable tool for assessing and treating chondral injuries, but that there was limited data to suggest an improved outcome [99]. The authors noted arthroscopy as a potentially excellent adjunct in fracture fixation but came short of recommending it as a routine.

This senior author began performing arthroscopy with ankle fracture fixation late in 2015. We have taken the view that prognostically and medical legally, there is enough advantage with such little risk, that arthroscopy is used to document and treat chondral injury. We have found the procedure relatively easy to perform and very helpful in treatment of chondral injuries and loose body removal. We often debride a torn AITFL to reduce post-operative scar. Some unpublished data has suggested that even the process of lavaging the ankle can be helpful for the cartilage long-term as it removes harmful blood factors that are "toxic" to cartilage. We have directed our rehabilitation based on the severity of the chondral injury or lack thereof. We prefer, as mentioned above, a more aggressive weight-bearing approach with rigid, anatomic fixation of fractures. If there is significant chondral injury with exposed bone, we alter this more immediate weight-bearing protocol. We have decided to perform concomitant arthroscopy prior to fixation in any athlete with an ankle fracture that resulted in either dislocation or subluxation. Therefore, arthroscopy is not routinely undertaken in isolated medial malleolus fractures or isolated Weber B fibular fractures. We highly recommend arthroscopy in more unstable fracture patterns which had some form of ankle joint displacement. Our personal experience has been that most all unstable and displaced ankle fractures have some form of chondral injury and it is best to evaluate, document, and treat as necessary the articular surface injury at the time of fracture fixation. Delayed treatment may result in more extensive degeneration.

The set-up of ankle arthroscopy requires some positioning preparation which allows gravity distraction of the ankle or soft tissue distractor to obtain adequate visualization. We have used a trauma triangle underneath the ipsilateral knee which allows gravity distraction of the ankle and excellent visualization with a minimal disruption of setup for ankle fracture fixation (Fig. 15.18a–c). We can still do an ankle block to help with intra-operative and postoperative pain control despite typically employing general anesthetic for non-isolated malleolar fractures. We use a sterile tourniquet on the distal calf which allows excellent hemostasis as well as giving slight reduction in the risk for postoperative deep venous thrombosis. We use standard anterior medial and anterior lateral portals. These portals have been adequate for us to visualize the articular surfaces. Because of the unstable nature of the fractured ankle, visualization can be obtained without external distractors (Fig. 15.18).

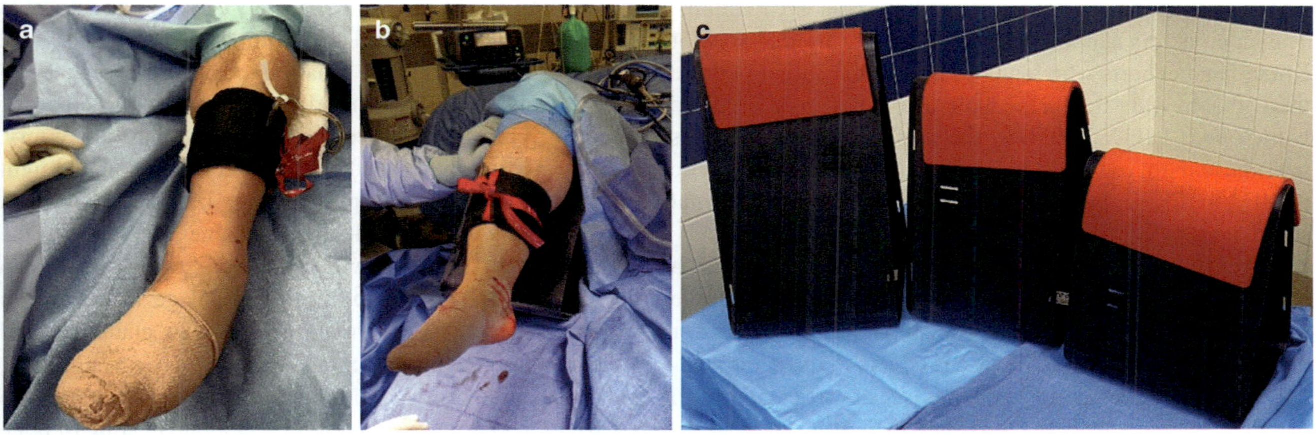

Fig. 15.18 (**a**–**c**) Arthroscopy set up for scope during Fracture treatment. (**a**) Head on view of athlete's draped left lower leg showing large towel-roll under left knee and calf tourniquet to allow arthroscopic access to the left ankle prior to definitive open fixation. (**b**) Similar set up during ankle fracture fixation with trauma triangle under left knee to take left foot/ankle off the operative bed and allow arthroscopy before fracture fixation. (**c**) Several different sized trauma triangles (11″, 14″, 16″) that can be used to allow arthroscopic access to ankle before fracture fixation. Size used will depend on size/height of athlete and length of lower leg. We typically use small (11″) and medium size (14″), unless a tall NBA player, then a 16″ may be needed

15.15 Future Developments/New Horizons

15.15.1 Orthobiologics

Orthobiologics are "biological products made from the variety of natural sources (human, animal, or microorganism) or the final products of advanced biotechnologies for medical applications (www.Fda.gov/aboutfda)" [100].

Schwartz recommends a modest metabolic workup of all athletes with an acute fracture including 25 Hydroxy-Vitamin D, parathyroid hormone, calcium and phosphorus [101]. We also favor aggressive evaluation and utilization of Vitamin D and calcium as metabolic factors in bone health and healing. Most authors recommend a serum level up to 40 ng/ml, a level similar to that recommended by Schwartz [101]. McCabe recommended supplementation even in the young athletic-aged athlete of 1000–2000 IU per day to maintain the serum level to at least 36–40 ng/mL [102]. In the face of true insufficiency or deficiency, most authors recommend between 10,000 IU a day to 50,000 IU a week until the level has reached the acceptable serum levels. Schwartz recommends Vitamin D supplementation, external bone stimulation, and further recommends consideration be given to augmenting with Teriparatide 20 mg subcutaneous daily until confirmed four quadrant healing on appropriate radiographic imaging [101].

External bone stimulation has become popular and recommended in nonunion fractures of the foot in athletes [103, 104]. No literature has specifically examined external bone stimulation use in athletes with acute ankle fractures. However, in the professional and elite college athlete, external bone stimulation is often used, especially in the troublesome fractures such as, comminuted fibular shaft, diaphyseal Weber C fractures, and vertical medial malleolar fractures. This approach is supported in the literature by the work of Kinami and cohorts who reported improved healing in acute tibia diaphyseal fractures with (Low Intensity Pulsed UltraSound) LIPUS [105]. In the professional setting, it is not unusual to use both the LIPUS and electromagnetic (CMF or PEMF-pulsed electromagnetic field) external stimulators.

Other forms of orthobiologics such as platelet rich plasma (PRP), stem cells, bone marrow aspirate concentrate (BMAC) have much of their application within delayed or nonunions also. The role of these products in the acute fracture are still in development. Schon et al. articulates well their current role in nonunions and their role in cartilage healing and repair [100].

15.15.2 Functional Bracing

Immobilisation is an important part of the post-operative and non-operative care of ankle fractures in athletes. Immobilisation takes different form at different times in the care and for different fracture types. As noted in each section above with each fracture type, there is little to do to prevent the initial fracture. However, we believe brace support after fracture fixation is helpful in preventing re-injury and supporting ligaments, fractures and muscle in the recovery phase. We take this approach intuitively and also because of the support we see in the literature with recovery from ankle fractures [106]. We use different braces depending on the fracture type and level of instability corrected. We always use a removable boot initially and then wean into a functional brace 2–6 weeks after initial fixation (Fig. 15.19a–c).

15.16 Conclusion

The treatment and care of athletes with ankle fractures is an exciting and evolving field. Recent advancements have resulted in improved prognosis with most treatment approaches allowing full return to even high level and professional sport. Open rigid internal fixation with low profile plates and screw fixation with appropriate use of dynamic fixation continues to be the gold standard. Augmentation with arthroscopy to assess and treat articular cartilage both optimizes treatment and guides rehabilitation as well as prognosis. We favor, and have outlined, a progressive rehabilitation approach that highlights intermittent immobilisation, where appropriate, to allow early ROM and early weight-bearing. Some ligament injuries, despite anatomic repair, require short periods of rigid casting or removable splinting until early soft tissue healing has occurred. Early ROM optimizes soft tissue rehabilitation. Early weight bearing is advantageous with rigid fixation, anatomic repair of ligament injury and limited or well treated cartilage injury. Cross training rehabilitation with aqua therapy and weight off-loading is a critical aspect of optimizing return to play. Cross training allows gradual establishment of stress to the repaired ankle. Bone growth stimulators, orthobiologics to augment healing and help "repair" cartilage injury are an exciting new area that should continue to challenge and enhance our treatment. Supplementation with nutrition, nutrients and hormonal/vitamin replacement continues to evolve as a means to enhance and accelerate healing of bone and soft tissue. A new area is the use of bone growth stimu-

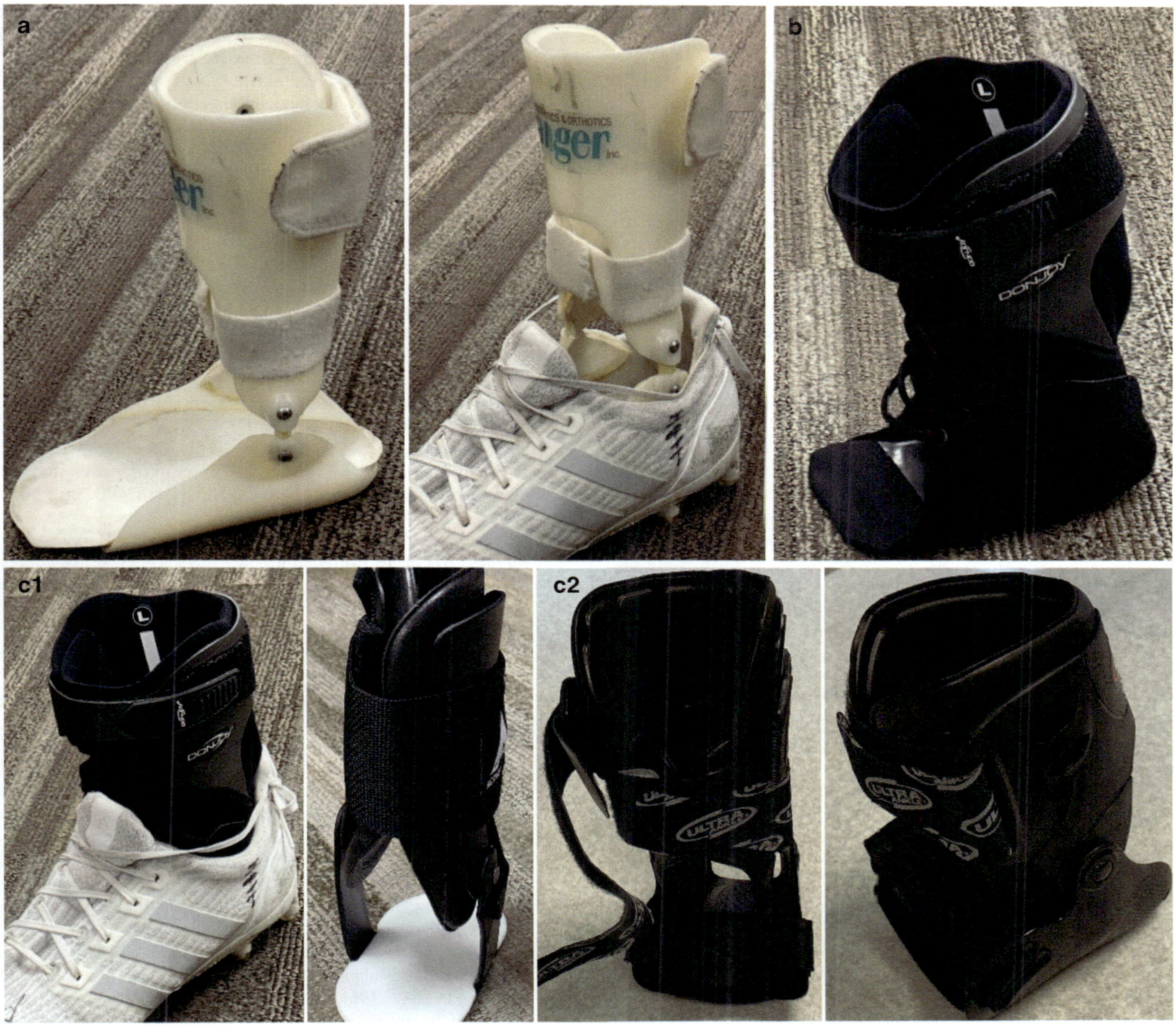

Fig. 15.19 (a–c) Functional braces for use after ankle fracture fixation in the athlete. (a) Short-articulating custom Ankle Foot Orthosis. Note the rubberized, mildly flexible hinge used to be more functional for the athlete. Note good fit in a football cleat allowing dorsiflexion-plantarflexion but resists external rotation. (b) Off-the-Shelf lace-up and stirrup combination in-shoe brace. This is good for most ankle fractures, but best for non-operatively treated High-Ankle sprains and post-surgical fixation that includes the deltoid and/or syndesmosis. (c1, c2) Two stirrup in-shoe braces used post-operatively. (c1) The pure stirrup brace is very low profile, preferred for return to full sport brace and after isolated lateral malleolus or medial malleolus fracture. (c2) This other brace has more of a foot-plate to help control external rotation and has an extension to be effective with more complicated post-surgical fracture. We often start with the extension in place (left brace) as the athlete comes out of the walking boot, then remove the upper extension for return to sport (right brace without extension for return to sports)

lants to help with delayed and nonunions that still occur despite optimal care and treatment. We look forward to new developments in the area of ankle fracture treatment to allow full return with minimal long- and short-term problems.

References

1. Jelinek A, Porter DA. Management of unstable ankle fractures and syndesmosis injuries in athletes. Foot Ankle Clin. 2009;14(2):277–98. https://doi.org/10.1016/j.fcl.2009.03.003.
2. Court-Brown CM, Wood AM, Aitken S. The epidemiology of acute sports-related fractures in adults. Injury. 2008;39:1365–72.
3. Robertson GAJ, Wood AM, Aitken SA, Court-Brown C. Epidemiology, management, and outcome of sport-related ankle fractures in a standard UK population. Foot Anke Int. 2014;35(11):1143–52.
4. Walsh WM, Hughston JC. Unstable ankle fractures in athletes. Am J Sports Med. 1976;4(4):173–83. https://doi.org/10.1177/036354657600400409.
5. Donley BG, Maschke S, Bergfled JA, et al. Pronation-external rotation ankle fractures in 3 professional football players. Am J Orthop. 2005;34:547–50.
6. Clanton TO, Porter DA. Primary care of foot and ankle injuries in the athlete. Clin Sports Med. 1997;16(3):435–66.
7. Porter DA, May BD, Berney T. Functional outcome after operative treatment for ankle fractures in young athletes: a retrospective case series. Foot Anke Int. 2008;29(9):887–94. https://doi.org/10.3113/fai.2008.0887.
8. Hsu AR, Lareau CR, Anderson RB. Repair of acute superficial deltoid complex avulsion during ankle fracture fixation in national football league players. Foot Anke Int. 2015;36(11):1272–8. https://doi.org/10.1177/1071100715593374.
9. Purvis GD. Displaced, unstable ankle fractures: classification, incidence, and management of a consecutive series. Clin Orthop Relat Res. 1982;165:91–8.
10. Michelson JD, Magid D, McHale K. Clinical utility of a stability-based ankle fracture classification system. J Orthop Trauma. 2007;21(5):207–315.
11. Hunt KJ, Goeb Y, Behn AW, Criswell B, Chou L. Ankle joint contact loads and displacement with progressive syndesmotic injury. Foot Anke Int. 2015;36(9):1095–103.
12. Lauge-Hansen N. Fractures of the ankle: III. Genetic roentgenologic diagnosis of fractures of the ankle. Am J Roentgenol Radium Therapy, Nucl Med. 1954;71:456–71.
13. Danis R. Les fractures malleolaires. In: Danis R, editor. Theorie et Pratique de l'Osteosynthese. Paris: Masson; 1949. p. 133–65.
14. Park SS, Kubiak EN, Egol KA, Kummer F, Koval KJ. Stress radiographs after ankle fracture. The effect of ankle position and deltoid ligament status on medial clear space measurements. J Orthop Trauma. 2006;20(1):11–8.
15. Zhao HM, Zhang F, Wen X, Li Y, Hao DJ, Liang ZJ. Surgical treatment of ankle fracture with or without deltoid ligament repair: a comparative study. BMC Musculoskelet Disord. 2017;18:543–9. https://doi.org/10.1186/s12891-017-1907-4.
16. Hintermann B, Knupp M, Pagenstert GI. Deltoid ligament injuries: diagnosis and management. Foot Ankle Clin. 2006;11(3):625–37. https://doi.org/10.1016/j.fcl.2006.08.001.
17. Kerkhoffs GM, Rowe BH, Assendelft WJ, Kelly KD, Struijs PA, van Dijk CN. Immobilisation for acute ankle sprain: a systematic review. Arch Orthop Trauma Surg. 2001;121:462–71.
18. Smith RW, Reischl SF. Treatment of ankle sprains in young athletes. Am J Sports Med. 1986;14(6):465–71.
19. Arnold BL, Wright CJ, Ross SE. Functional ankle instability and health-related quality of life. J Athl Train. 2011;46(6):634–41. https://doi.org/10.4085/1062-6050-46.6.634.
20. Campbell KJ, Michalski MP, Wilson KJ, et al. The ligament anatomy of the deltoid complex of the ankle: a qualitative and quantitative anatomical study. J Bone Jt Surg Am. 2014;96(8):e62. https://doi.org/10.2106/jbjs.m00870.
21. Milner CE, Soames RW. The medial collateral ligaments of the human ankle joint: anatomical variations. Foot Ankle Int. 1998;19(5):289–92. https://doi.org/10.1177/107110079801900504.
22. Yammine K. The morphology and prevalence of the deltoid complex ligament of the ankle: a meta-analysis of cadaveric studies. Foot Ankle Spec. 2017;10(1):55–62. https://doi.org/10.1177/1938640016675409.
23. McCollum GA, Michel P, Van Den Bekerom J, Kerkhoffs GMMJ, Calder JDF, Dijk CNV. Syndesmosis and deltoid ligament injuries in the athlete. Knee Surg Sports Traumatol Arthrosc. 2012;21(6):1328–37. https://doi.org/10.1007/s00167-012-2205-1.
24. Waterman BR, Belmont PJ, Cameron KL, DeBerardino TM, Owens BD. Epidemiology of ankle sprain at the United States Military Academy. Am J Sports Med. 2010;38(4):797–803. https://doi.org/10.1177/0363546509350757.
25. Hintermann B, Valderrabano V, Boss A, Trouillier HH, Dick W. Medial ankle instability: an exploratory, prospective study of fifty-two cases. Am J Sports Med. 2004;32(1):183–90. https://doi.org/10.1177/0095399703258789.
26. Hermans JJ, Wentink N, Beumer A, Hop WC, Heijboer MP, Moonen AF, et al. Correlation between radiological assessment of acute ankle fractures and syndesmotic injury on MRI. Skelet Radiol. 2012;41(7):787–801. https://doi.org/10.1007/s00256-011-1284-2.
27. Nortunen S, Lepojarvi S, Savola O, Niinimaki J, Ohtonen P, Flinkkila T, et al. Stability assessment of the ankle mortise in supination-external rotation-type ankle fractures: lack of additional diagnostic value of MRI. J Bone Joint Surg Am. 2014;96(22):1855–62. https://doi.org/10.2106/JBJS.M.01533.
28. Lötscher P, Lang TH, Zwicky L, et al. Osteoligamentous injuries of the medial ankle joint. Eur J Trauma Emerg Surg. 2015;41:615–21. https://doi.org/10.1007/s00068-015-0548-2.
29. Su AW, Larson AN. Pediatric ankle fractures: concepts and treatment principles. Foot Ankle Clin. 2015;20(4):705–19. https://doi.org/10.1016/j.fcl.2015.07.004.
30. Peterson HA, Madhok R, Benson JT, Ilstrup DM, Melton LJ. Physeal fractures. Part I. Epidemiology in Olmsted County, Minnesota, 1979–1988. J Pediatr Orthop. 1994;14:423–30.
31. Larson RL, McMahan RO. The epiphyses and the childhood athlete. JAMA. 1966;196(7):607–12. https://doi.org/10.1001/jama.1966.0310020004hsu.
32. Salter RB, Harris WR. Injuries involving the epiphyseal plate. J Bone Joint Surg Am. 1963;45:587–622.
33. Michelson JD. Ankle fractures resulting from rotational injuries. J Am Acad Orthop Surg. 2003;11(6):403–12. https://doi.org/10.5435/00124635-200311000-00004.
34. Stromsoe K, Hoqevold H, Skjeldal S, Alho A. The repair of a ruptured deltoid ligament is not necessary in ankle fractures. J Bone Jt Surg Br. 1995;77-B(6):920–1. https://doi.org/10.1302/0301-620x.77b6.7593106.
35. Beck J, et al. ePaper 281. Presented at American Academy of Orthopaedic Surgeons Annual Meeting, March 24–28; 2020.
36. Adirim TA, Cheng TL. Overview of injuries in the young athlete. Sports Med. 2003;33(1):75–81.
37. Stuart MJ, Morrey MA, Smith AM, Meis JK, Ortiguera CJ. Injuries in youth football: a prospective observational cohort analysis among players aged 9 to 13 years. Mayo Clin Proc. 2002;77(4):317–22.
38. Hunt KJ, et al. High ankle sprains and syndesmotic injuries in athletes. J Am Acad Orthop Surg. 2015;23(11):661. Gale OneFile: Health and Medicine, https://link-gale-com.proxy.ulib.uits.iu.edu/apps/doc/A436439962/HRCA?u=iulib_iupui&sid=HRCA&xid=b0c64b16.

39. Waterman BR, Belmont PJ Jr, Cameron KL, Svoboda SJ, Alitz CJ, Owens BD. Risk factors for syndesmotic and medial ankle sprain: role of sex, sport, and level of competition. Am J Sports Med. 2011;39(5):992–8.
40. Haraguchi N, Armiger RS. A new interpretation of the mechanism of ankle fracture. J Bone Joint Surg Am. 2009;91(4):821–9.
41. Wei F, Villwock MR, Meyer EG, Powell JW, Haut RC. A biomechanical investigation of ankle injury under excessive external foot rotation in the human cadaver. J Biomech Eng. 2010;132(9):091001.
42. Calder JD, Bamford R, Petrie A, McCollum GA. Stable versus unstable grade II high ankle sprains: a prospective study predicting the need for surgical stabilization and time to return to sports. Arthroscopy. 2016;32(4):634–42.
43. Wolf BR, Amendola A. Syndesmosis injuries in the athlete: when and how to operate. Curr Opin Orthop. 2002;13(2):151–4.
44. Sikka RS, Fetzer GB, Sugarman E, et al. Correlating MRI findings with disability in syndesmotic sprains of NFL players. Foot Ankle Int. 2012;33(5):371–8.
45. de Cesar PC, Avila EM, de Abreu MR. Comparison of magnetic resonance imaging to physical examination for syndesmotic injury after lateral ankle sprain. Foot Ankle Int. 2011;32(12):1110–4.
46. Sman AD, Hiller CE, Refshauge KM. Diagnostic accuracy of clinical tests for diagnosis of ankle syndesmosis injury: a systematic review. Br J Sports Med. 2013;47(10):620–8.
47. Takao M, Ochi M, Oae K, Naito K, Uchio Y. Diagnosis of a tear of the tibiofibular syndesmosis: the role of arthroscopy of the ankle. J Bone Joint Surg (Br). 2003;85(3):324–9.
48. Guyton GP, DeFontes K III, Barr CR, Parks G, Camire LM. Arthroscopic correlates of subtle syndesmotic injury. Foot Anke Int. 2017;38(5):502–6.
49. Gardner MJ, Demetrakopoulos D, Briggs SM, Helfet DL, Lorich DJ. Malreduction of the tibiofibular syndesmosis in ankle fractures. Foot Anke Int. 2006;27(10):688–92.
50. Cheney SM, Sprague-Hughes AG, McAndrew CM, Ricci WM, Gardner MJ. Incisura morphology as a risk factor syndesmotic malreduction. Foot Anke Int. 2016;37(7):748–54.
51. Miller AN, Barei DP, Iaquinto JM, Ledoux WR, Beingessner DM. Iatrogenic syndesmosis malreduction via clamp and screw placement. J Orthop Trauma. 2013;27(2):100–6.
52. Miller AN, Carroll EA, Parker RJ, Boraiah S, Helfet DL, Lorich DJ. Direct visualization for syndesmotic stabilization in ankle fractures. Foot Anke Int. 2009;30(5):419–26.
53. Warner SJ, Fabricant PD, Garner MR, Schottel PC, Helfet DL, Lorich DG. The measurement and clinical importance of syndesmotic reduction after operative fixation of rotational ankle fractures. J Bone Joint Surg Am. 2015;97(23):1935–44. https://doi.org/10.2106/JBJS.O.00016.
54. Coetzee CJ, Ebeling P. Treatment of syndesmosis disruption TightRope fixation. Tech FAS. 2008;7(3):196–202. https://doi.org/10.1097/BTF.0b013e3181757476.
55. Tornetta P, Spoo JE, Reynolds FA, Lee C. Overtightening of the ankle syndesmosis: is it really possible? JBJS. 2001;83(A):489–92.
56. Tornetta P, Yakavonis M, Veltre D, Shah A. Reducing the syndesmosis under direct vision: where should I look? J Orthop Trauma. 2019;33(9):450–4.
57. Van Heest TJ, Lafferty PM. Current concepts review: injuries to the ankle syndesmosis. J Bone Joint Surg. 2014;96:603–13.
58. Litrena J, Saper D, Tornetta P, Phieffer L, Jones CJ, Mullis BH, et al. Does syndesmotic injury have a negative effect on functional outcome? A multicenter prospective evaluation. J Orthop Trauma. 2015;29(9):410–3.
59. Grassi A, Samuelson K, D'Hooghe PD, Romagnoli M, Mosca M, Zaffagnini S, Amendola A. Dynamic stabilization of syndesmosis injuries reduce complications and reoperations as compared to screw fixation. Am J Sports Med. 2019;20(10):1–14.
60. Boyle MJ, Gao R, Frampton CM, Coleman B. Removal of the syndesmotic screw after the surgical treatment of a fracture of the ankle in adult patients does not affect one-year outcomes: a randomized controlled trial. J Bone Joint Surg. 2014;96-B(12):1699–705. https://doi.org/10.1302/0301-620X.96B12.34258.
61. Zeegers AV, Werken CVD. Rupture of the deltoid ligament in ankle fractures: should it be repaired? Injury. 1989;20(1):39–41. https://doi.org/10.1016/0020-1383(89)90043-0.
62. Hintermann B, Regazzoni P, Lampert C, Stutz G, Gächter A. Arthroscopic findings in acute fractures of the ankle. J Bone Jt Surg Br. 2000;82-B(3):345–51. https://doi.org/10.1302/0301-620x.82b3.0820345.
63. Harper MC. An anatomic study of the short oblique fracture of the distal fibula and ankle stability. Foot Anke Int. 1983;4(1):23–9.
64. Magnusson R. On the late results in non-operated cases of malleolar fracture. I. Fractures by external rotation. Acta Chir Scan (Suppl). 1944;84:1.
65. Cedel CA. Supination-outward rotation injuries of the ankle: a clinical and roentgenological study with special reference to the operative treatment. Acta Orthop Scand. 1967;38(Suppl 110):1.
66. Ramsey PL, Hamilton W. Changes in tibiotalar area of contact caused by lateral talar shift. J Bone Joint Surg. 1976;58A:356–7.
67. Muller ME, Allgower M, Willenegger H. Technique of internal fixation of fractures. New York, NY: Springer; 1965. p. 543–8.
68. Michelson JD, Varner KE, Checcone M. Diagnosing deltoid injury in ankle fractures. The gravity stress view. Clin Orthop Relat Res. 2001;(387):178–82.
69. Sanders DW, Tieszer C, Corbett B. Canadian Orthopedic Trauma Society. Operative versus nonoperative treatment of unstable lateral malleolar fractures: a randomized multicenter trial. J Orthop Trauma. 2012;26(3):129–34. https://doi.org/10.1097/BOT.0b013e3182460837.
70. Porter DA. The team in the care of the athlete. In: Porter DA, Schon LS, editors. *Baxter's*, The foot and ankle in sports. 3rd ed. Philadelphia, PA: Elsevier Press; 2020.
71. Brockwell J, Yeung Y, Griffith JF. Stress fractures of the foot and ankle. Sports Med Arthrosc Rev. 2009;17(3):149–59. https://doi.org/10.1097/jsa.0b013e3181b1272.
72. Tejwani NC, Mclaurin TM, Walsh M, Bhadsavle S, Egol KA, Koval KJ. Are outcomes of bimalleolar fractures poorer than those of lateral malleolar fractures with medial ligamentous injury? J Bone Jt Surg Am. 2007;89(7):1438–41. https://doi.org/10.2106/00004623-200707000-00005.
73. Bluman EM. Deltoid ligament injuries in ankle fractures: should I leave it or fix it? Foot Anke Int. 2012;33(3):236–8. https://doi.org/10.3113/fai.2012.0236.
74. Jones CR, Nunley JA. Deltoid ligament repair versus syndesmotic fixation in bimalleolar equivalent ankle fractures. J Orthop Trauma. 2015;29(5):245–9. https://doi.org/10.1097/bot.0000000000000220.
75. Hong CC, Roy SP, Nashi N, Tan KJ. Functional outcome and limitation of sporting activities after bimalleolar and trimalleolar ankle fractures. Foot Anke Int. 2013;34(6):805–10. https://doi.org/10.1177/1071100712472490.F.
76. Dehghan N, McKee MD, Jenkinson RJ, et al. Early weightbearing and range of motion versus non-weightbearing and immobilization after open reduction and internal fixation of unstable ankle fractures: a randomized controlled trial. J Orthop Trauma. 2016;30(7):345–52.
77. Marsh JL, Slongo TF, Agel J, Broderick JS, Creevey W, DeCoster TA, et al. Fracture and dislocation classification compendium - 2007: Orthopedic Trauma Association classification, database and outcomes committee. J Orthop Trauma. 2007;21(10 Suppl):S1–133.

78. Salter RB, Simmonds D, Malcolm BW, Rumble EJ, MacMichael D, Clements N, et al. The biological effect of continuous passive motion on the healing of full thickness defects in articular cartilage. J Bone Joint Surg. 1980;62A:1232.
79. Putukian M. How being injured affects mental health. In: NCAA mind, body and sport: understanding and supporting student-athlete mental wellness. Indianapolis, IN: National Collegiate Athletic Association; 2014.
80. Simanski CJP, Maegele MG, Lefering R, et al. Functional treatment and early weightbearing after an ankle fracture: a prospective study. J Orthop Trauma. 2006;20(2):108–14. https://doi.org/10.1097/01.bot.0000197701.96954.8c.
81. Schubert J, Kimber C, Denk K, Cho M, Doornber JN, Jaarsma RL, Jaarsma RL. Effect on overall health status with weightbearing at 2 weeks vs 6 week after open reduction and internal fixation of ankle fractures. Foot Ankle Int. 2020;41(6):658–65.
82. Barill E, Porter DA. Principles of rehabilitation for the foot and ankle. In: Porter DA, Schon LS, editors. Baxter's the foot and ankle in sports. Philadelphia, PA: Mosby; 2007. p. 607–9.
83. Waldrop NE, Smith KS. Rehabilitation of specific foot and ankle issues. In: Porter DA, Schon LS, editors. Baxter's, the foot and ankle in sports. Philadelphia, PA: Elsevier; 2020.
84. Barill E, Carroll D, Porter DA. Principles of rehabilitation for the foot and ankle. In: Porter DA, Schon LS, editors. Baxter's the foot and ankle in sports. Philadelphia, PA: Elsevier; 2020. p. 572–4.
85. Mak KH, Chang KM, Leung PC. Ankle fracture treated with the AO principle-an experience with 116 cases. Injury. 1985;16(4):265–72.
86. Ono A, Nishikawa S, Nagao A, Irie T, Sasaki M, Kouno T. Arthroscopically assisted treatment of ankle fractures: arthroscopic findings and surgical outcomes. Arthroscopy. 2004;20:627–31.
87. Dador D. 20 percent of people in US allergic to nickel, health experts say. In: Healthy Living KABC, Los Angeles, CA, March 16; 2016.
88. Disegi JA. Eschback L Stainless steel in bone surgery. Injury. 2000;31(Suppl 4):D2–6.
89. Heirholzer S, Hierholzer G. Allergy to metal following osteosynthesis. Uncallchirurgie. 1982;8(6):347–52.
90. Takagi K. The arthroscope: the second report. J Jpn Orthop Assn. 1939;14:441.
91. Watanabe M. Development of the Selfoc-arthroscope. J Jpn Orthop Assoc. 1972;46:154.
92. Plank E. Die Arthroskopie des oberen Sprunggelenkes. Helfe zur Unfallheilkunde. 1978;131:245.
93. Andrews JR, Previte WJ, Carson WG. Arthroscopy of the ankle: technique and normal anatomy. Foot Ankle. 1985;6:29.
94. Aktas S, Kocaoglu B, Gereli A, Nalbantodlu U, Guven O. Incidence of chondral lesions of talar dome in ankle fracture types. Foot Ankle Int. 2008;29(3):287–92.
95. Thordardson DB, Bains R, Shepherd LE. The role of ankle arthroscopy on the surgical management of ankle fractures. Foot Anke Int. 2001;22:123–5.
96. Loren G, Ferkel R. Arthroscopic assessment of occult intra-articular injury in acute ankle fractures. Arthroscopy. 2002;18(4):412–21.
97. Leontartius N, Hinojosa L, Panchbhavi VK. Arthroscopically detected intra-articular lesions associated with acute ankle fractures. J Bone Jt Surg Am. 2009;91:333–9.
98. Fuchs DJ, Ho BS, LaBelle MW, Kelikian AS. Effect of arthroscopic evaluation of acute ankle fractures on PROMIS intermediate-term functional outcomes. Foot Ankle Int. 2016;37(1):51–7.
99. Gonzalez TA, Macaulay AA, Ehrlichman LK, Drummond R, Mittal V, DiGiovanni CW. Arthroscopically assisted versus standard open reduction and internal fixation techniques for the acute ankle fracture. Foot Ankle Int. 2016;37(5):554–62.
100. Schon LS, Karli D, Anderson RB, Gould H, Zhang Z. Orthobiologics in foot and ankle applications. In: Porter DA, Schon LS, editors. *Baxter's* the foot and ankle in sports. Philadelphia, PA: Elsevier Press Kerkhoff; 2020.
101. Schwartz EN, Edmondson CP. Medical and metabolic considerations in athletes with stress fracture. In: Porter DA, Schon LS, editors. *Baxter's*, the foot and ankle in sports. 3rd ed. Philadelphia, PA: Elsevier Press; 2020.
102. McCabe MP, Smyth MP, Richardson DR. Current concept review: vitamin D and stress fractures. Foot Anke Int. 2012;33(6):526–33.
103. Lareau CR, Anderson RB. Jones fractures. Pathophysiology and treatment. J Bone Jt Surg Rev. 2015;3(7):1–8.
104. Porter DA. Fifth metatarsal jones fractures in the athlete: a review. Foot Anke Int. 2018;39(2):250–8. https://doi.org/10.1177/1071100717741856.
105. Kinami Y, Noda T, Ozaki T. Efficacy of low-intensity pulsed ultrasound treatment for surgically managed fresh diaphyseal fractures of the lower extremity: multi-center retrospective cohort study. J Orthop Sci. 2013;18(3):410–8.
106. Vuurberg G, Hoorntje A, Wink LM, et al. Diagnosis, treatment and prevention of ankle sprains: update of an evidence-based clinical guideline. Br J Sports Med. 2018;52:956.

16 Acute Fractures in Sport: Foot

Karan A. Patel, Sean M. Richards, Jonathan Day, and Mark C. Drakos

Learning Objectives

- Understand mechanisms of acute foot fractures in sports
- Describe in detail operative and non-operative indications and management for acute foot fractures in athletes.
- Generally understand return-to-play time frame for acute foot fractures

16.1 Fifth Metatarsal Fractures

16.1.1 Background

Metatarsal fractures account for a substantial portion of foot injuries. Namely, approximately 35% of all foot fractures are metatarsal fractures [1]. Fifth metatarsal fractures, the most common type of metatarsal fracture, are common in the athletic population, and are often a source of pain, disability, and loss of playing time [2–4]. Fractures of the base of the fifth metatarsal likely result from the pull by the peroneus brevis or tertius and plantar fascia during a plantar flexion and inversion injury [5–7]. Fractures located in the more diaphyseal portion likely occur secondary to a large adduction moment on the forefoot with the ankle in plantar flexion [5–7]. It is critical that these injuries are not missed in patients presenting with a potential ankle sprain, as the mechanisms can be similar.

Since the first description of these fractures, there has been much interest in their management given their propensity to poor healing depending on the location of the fracture. The fifth metatarsal has three main sources of blood supply: nutrient artery, periosteal arteries, and the metaphyseal perforators. A watershed area exists between the nutrient artery and metaphyseal perforators, and this corresponds to the area of clinical concern for healing at the metaphyseal-diaphyseal junction [8–10] (Fig. 16.1). Prompt diagnosis and proper classification are crucial for successful treatment.

16.1.2 Classification

Sir Robert Jones was the first to define these fractures in 1902, coining the term "Jones fracture" [11]. Since the term was first coined, there has been ambiguity and lack of standardized application of the term "Jones" fracture. These injuries can be classified by location as described by Lawrence and Botte [5] and Dameron [6, 12]. Zone 1 fractures, also called "Pseudo-jones" fractures, are tuberosity avulsion fractures, with or without involvement of the tarsometatarsal joint. Zone 2 fractures, which some would classify as Jones fractures, involve fractures of the metaphysis-diaphysis junction extending into the fourth–fifth intermetatarsal facet [13]. Lastly, Zone 3 fractures are proximal diaphyseal stress fractures [14]. While Zone 1 fractures are very common and usually easily treatable, Zones 2 and 3 fractures are quite susceptible to both delayed union and non-union, making them more difficult to treat [13]. As previously discussed, these areas are prone to delayed union and non-union because of the unique blood supply of the fifth metatarsal. Zones 2 and 3 fractures occur in the watershed region between the metaphyseal artery and the nutrient artery (Fig. 16.1). There is no consistency on the classification of a Jones fracture, with some authors advocating for a combination of Zones 2 and 3 fracture, and others only using one of these groups [15] (Fig. 16.2).

16.1.3 Diagnosis

Patients who suffer acute fifth metatarsal fractures present with typical fracture symptoms, complaining of difficulty

K. A. Patel (✉)
Hospital for Special Surgery, New York, NY, USA

Mayo Clinic Arizona, Phoenix, AZ, USA
e-mail: Patel.karan@mayo.edu

S. M. Richards · J. Day · M. C. Drakos (✉)
Hospital for Special Surgery, New York, NY, USA
e-mail: dayj@hss.edu; drakosm@hss.edu

G. A. J. Robertson, N. Maffulli (eds.), *Fractures in Sport*, https://doi.org/10.1007/978-3-030-72036-0_16

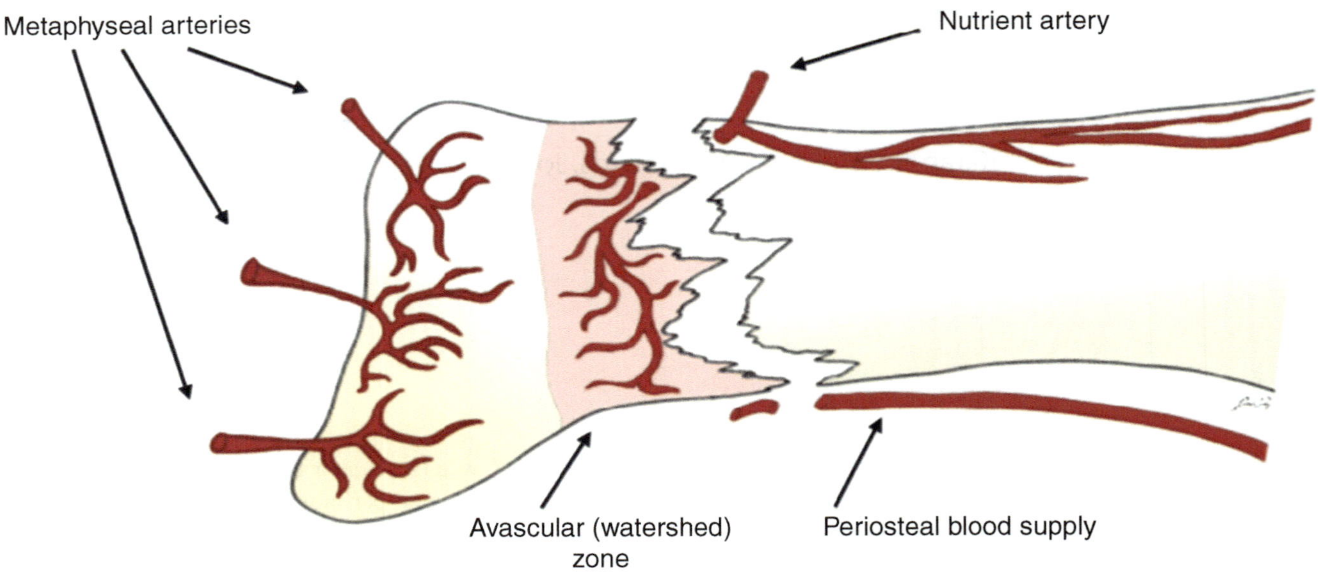

Fig. 16.1 Depiction of the blood supply of the fifth metatarsal base

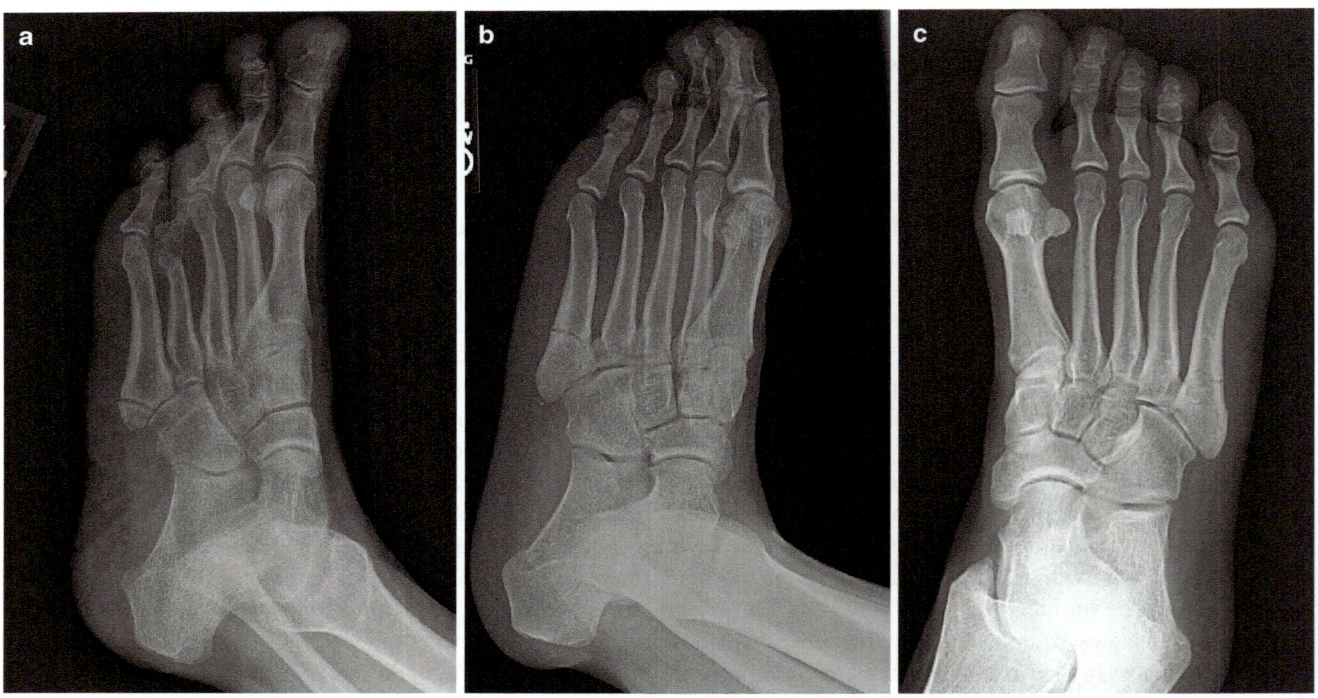

Fig. 16.2 Typical location for a Zone 1 fracture (**a**), Typical location for a Zone 2 fracture extending into the fourth–fifth metatarsal articulation (**b**), Typical location for a Zone 3 fracture. It is in the proximal diaphysis just distal to the fourth–fifth articulation (**c**)

walking or weight bearing. The lateral aspect of their foot is edematous, painful and tender on palpation, and there may be ecchymosis [16]. Another subset of patients will present with an insidious onset of pain over the lateral border of the foot, complicated by an acute injury or progression of pain. When examining these patients, it is crucial to evaluate both the distal fibula and lateral ligamentous structures as well. It is also critical to evaluate foot alignment, as this can factor into healing potential. Patients with cavovarus foot alignment are more susceptible to fifth metatarsal fractures, as well as delayed union or refractures of these injuries. In addition, athletes with forefoot adductus are also at increased risk

[17]. Plain radiographs display radiolucency proximal to the metaphyseal-diaphyseal junction, with fractures generally occurring perpendicular to the long axis of the fifth metatarsal [18]. Radiographs are generally sufficient in distinguishing between acute fractures or acute fractures on previous underlying chronic changes, but, when pain persists without typical radiographic findings, CT can be utilized to further evaluate them [19].

16.1.4 Management

The management of these fractures depends on several factors, including patient age, activity level, and health, as well as fracture location. The most paramount factor is fracture location.

16.1.4.1 Nonoperative Management

Zone 1 fractures typically respond well to non-operative management, with a non-union rate of only 0.5% following a period of protected weight bearing in a hard soled shoe or boot [20]. These patients can return to sport in a graduated fashion once they are pain free. Management of fractures in Zone 2 or 3 more often depends on patient factors. In recreational athletes or sedentary patients, nonweightbearing in a cast or boot for a period of 6–8 weeks can provide healing rates of up to 98%, with a subset of patients who will have a delayed union [20]. Considering the risk of non-union in this region, these patients should be followed clinically and radiographically to ensure healing prior to return to sport: this typically occurs in 12–14 weeks.

16.1.4.2 Operative Management

When treating elite or competitive athletes who sustained fifth metatarsal fractures in Zone 2 or 3, nonoperative management is often not a viable option. Specifically, when managed nonoperatively, acute fractures have a union rate of 76% [15], with an alarmingly high refracture risk of 33% [21]. However, intramedullary screw fixation, the most common technique, more typically yields promising outcomes with a union rate of 96% and return to sport between 4 and 18 weeks [15] (Fig. 16.3). Intramedullary screw fixation can be performed with or without an autologous bone graft. Specifically, athletes with non-unions and refractures after undergoing screw fixation without bone grafting who subsequently undergo screw fixation with bone graft are able to return to their previous level of activity relatively quickly, and exhibit strong clinical and radiographic signs of cortical healing [22]. Generally, surgery is only contraindicated in patients with vascular compromise, neuropathy, or local infection in the foot [13].

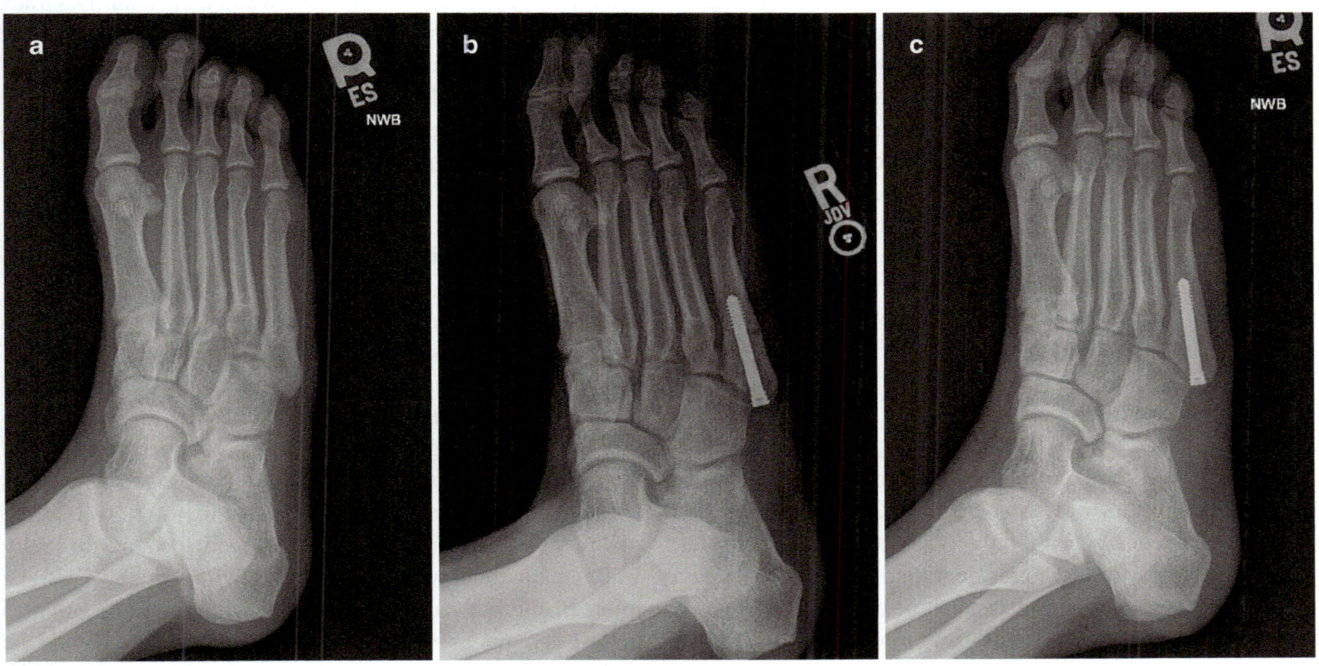

Fig. 16.3 Fracture in Zone 2 (Jones fracture) (**a**). Acute post-operative fixation of the fracture in Zone 2 with a single partially threaded compression screw (**b**), Healed Zone 2 fracture approximately 8 weeks post-operatively (**c**)

16.1.5 Complications

In general, complications arising from acute fifth metatarsal fractures include delayed union, nonunion, and refracture [13]. All of these can be addressed with surgical procedures. For tuberosity avulsion fractures exhibiting nonunions (Zone 1), excision or fixation of the avulsed fragment can be employed to resolve the nonunion, depending on fracture length, with repair of the peroneus brevis as needed [23]. In athletes, Jones fractures (Zone 2) that exhibit nonunion or refracture after conservative treatment are typically managed by intramedullary screw fixation with a large screw and autologous bone grafting [22]. There are many intra-and post-operative complications of screw fixation, including wound infection, impingement by the prominent screw head on the cuboid, peroneus brevis tendon damage, and peroneal and sural nerve injury [13].

16.1.6 Rehabilitation

Following intramedullary screw fixation, the patient should be kept non-weightbearing in a splint and immobilized in a short leg splint for 2 weeks [24]. Once sutures have been removed, the patient can begin progressive weightbearing in a short-leg walking cast or boot for 4–6 weeks [19]. Only after the fracture site is minimally tender, radiographs exhibit bridging trabeculation, and there is no pain on weightbearing can the patient begin wearing a running shoe and return to sport [24]. The time frame of return to competition is highly debated, and most advocate a 9–12 weeks time frame, with advanced imaging (CT) that indicates complete healing at the fracture site. It is important to consider the patient's overall alignment prior to return to sport. If the patient exhibits significant pes cavus, a full length orthotic recessed for the first metatarsal can be used if the deformity is flexible. In theory, this will reduce the stresses placed on the lateral aspect of the foot [19].

16.2 Lisfranc Injuries

16.2.1 Background

Lisfranc injuries are increasingly common injuries in athletes. Although they only account for 0.2% of fractures and have an incidence rate of only 1/55,000 people per year, Lisfranc injuries are more prevalent than epidemiologic data would indicate, as they are frequently undiagnosed. Males are approximately two to four times more susceptible to suffer these injuries. Moreover, Lisfranc injuries occur most frequently to males in their 20s, but are seen across all age groups. Given the growing prevalence of high-performance training, the incidence of Lisfranc fracture-dislocations in athletes is increasing [25, 26]. In non-athletes, Lisfranc injuries typically occur secondary to high-energy injuries, such as a motor vehicle accident. However, in the athletic population these injuries are generally attributed to low-energy indirect forces, commonly involving axial load and plantarflexion, resulting in midfoot sprains [27, 28].

16.2.2 Classification

There are a several ways of classifying Lisfranc injuries based on many factors. Generally, they can be categorized as Type A, B, or C injuries. Type A injuries are defined by total displacement of every metatarsal bone or incongruity of the entire Lisfranc joint complex. Type B injuries involve at least one metatarsal displacement and partial incongruity of the Lisfranc joint complex. Finally, Type C injuries occur when the medial and lateral metatarsals are displaced in opposite directions, a phenomenon known as divergent displacement (Fig. 16.4). Lisfranc fracture-dislocations can also be classified simply based on whether the metatarsals are dislocated on the same side (homolateral) or opposite side (divergent) [25] (Fig. 16.4). Moreover, Lisfranc fracture-dislocations can be defined by degree of displacement. Grade I injuries involve essentially no displacement, Grade II are defined by dislocations of half the bone shaft, and Grade III involve total shaft displacement [29]. Sprains of the Lisfranc ligament can also be categorized by grade. Grade I sprains elicit mild joint pain with minimal edema and no instability, Grade II sprains involve increased joint pain and edema, and Grade III sprains are characterized by complete ligamentous disruption and possibly fracture-dislocation [30]. While these classification and grading schemes are descriptive, unfortunately none of them guide treatment and prognosis.

16.2.3 Diagnosis

Lisfranc injuries are commonly misdiagnosed, perhaps as frequently as 20% of the time [31]. This is a consequence of the subtleties in presentation, requiring a high clinical suspicion. For this reason, it is critical to consider the mechanism of injury, including foot position, direction of force, and degree of energy involved [27]. At presentation, patients complain of diffuse pain of the midfoot region as well as the inability to bear weight. In particular, patients have difficulty walking on their toes because of loading of the Lisfranc joint. If midfoot pain and difficulty with push-off activities persist for more than 5 days, a Lisfranc injury should be highly considered. Additionally, a Lisfranc injury should be suspected and evaluated in any patient with midfoot pain and plantar ecchymosis. When examining patients with suspected Lisfranc injuries, palpation should begin distally and

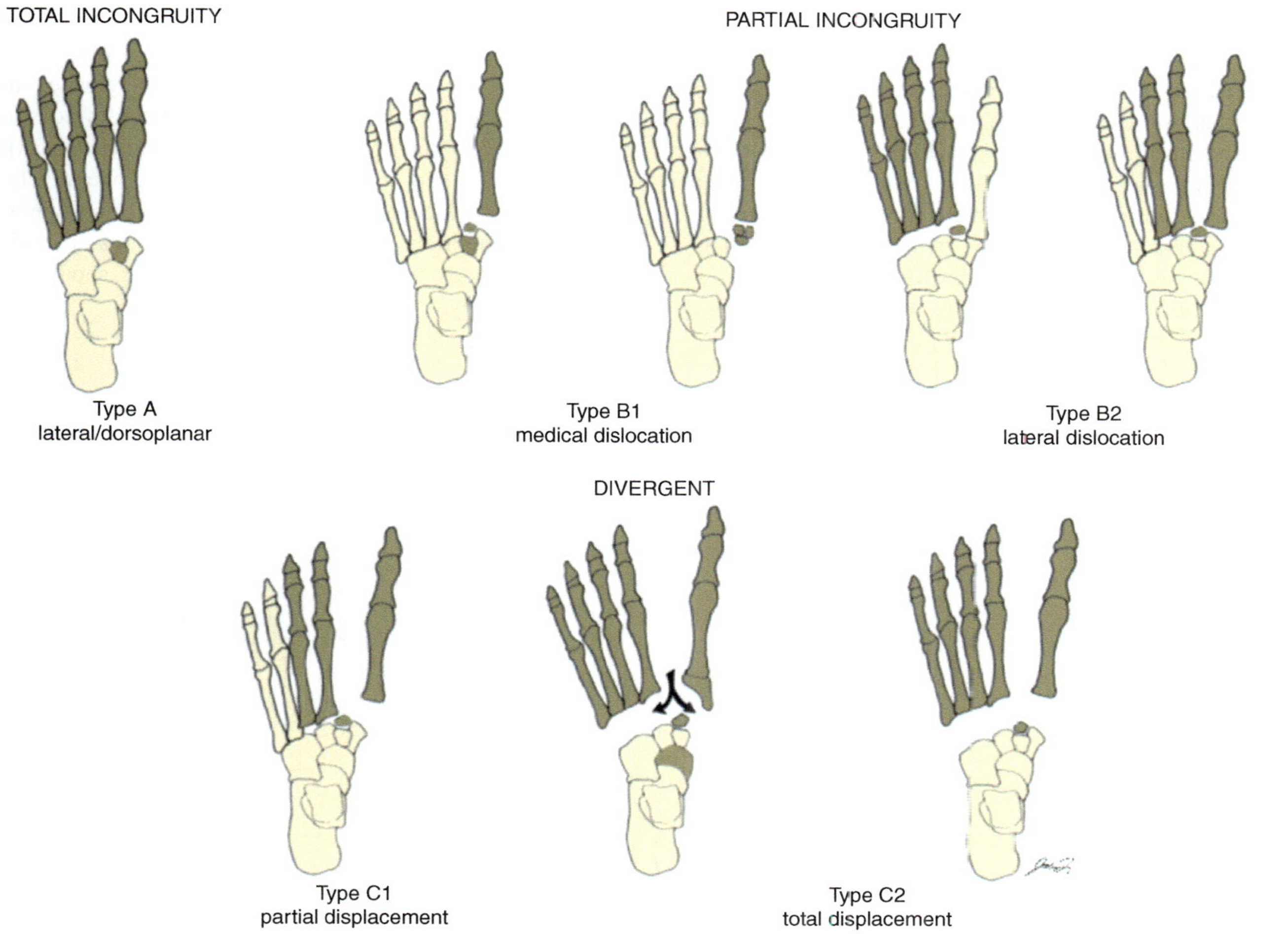

Fig. 16.4 Classification of Lisfranc injuries based on direction and amount of displacement

continue proximally to each tarsometatarsal joint. Midfoot pain on palpation, specifically at the tarsometatarsal joints, plantar ecchymosis, and significant edema are all highly suggestive of a Lisfranc injury [25, 30]. An instability test can also be performed. The forefoot should be dorsiflexed with the other hand palpating the tarsometatarsal joints. An evidence of dorsal subluxation suggests instability.

After midfoot injuries, initial radiographs should include weightbearing anteroposterior, lateral, and internal oblique views [32]. If a Lisfranc injury is suspected, weightbearing imaging of both the injured and uninjured foot on the same film for comparison should be employed to rule out diastasis or small displacements [33]. On weightbearing radiographs, tarsometatarsal joint dislocation can be demonstrated by loss of in-line arrangement of both the lateral margin of the first metatarsal base and the medial margin of the second metatarsal base with the lateral edge of the first cuneiform and the medial edge of the second cuneiform, respectively, as well as the presence of tiny avulsed fragments [30, 34, 35]. Generally, there are five critical radiographic signs indicating the presence of midfoot mobility, which greatly assist in the diagnosis of Lisfranc injuries. Examples of these are shown in Table 16.1. If weight bearing imaging cannot be performed because of pain, an injection of local anesthetic can be considered into the Lisfranc joint to allow for weight bearing. Another option is to perform a stress exam, with forced forefoot abduction during an anteroposterior radiograph, or forced first ray plantar flexion during a lateral radiograph. Moreover, CT scans may also be employed in the diagnosis of Lisfranc injuries, as they are instrumental in detecting minor displacements [25, 35].

16.2.4 Management

Lisfranc injuries can be managed either nonoperatively or operatively depending on anatomical stability and degree of displacement.

16.2.4.1 Nonoperative Management

Anatomically stable, nondisplaced Grade I injuries can be managed conservatively by having the patient wear a non-weightbearing cast or CAM boot for 4–6 weeks or until complete resolution of symptoms [30, 32]. The patient may then commence weightbearing activities, engage in range of motion exercises, and begin wearing a regular shoe [27]. If the patient does experience persistent pain, reimaging should be performed to rule out more serious injuries or joint instability [32]. Otherwise, minor Lisfranc injuries generally allow prompt return to sport and minimal long-term residual problems with nonoperative management [37]. Recently, a systematic review by Robertson et al. demonstrated 100% return rates at an average of 9 weeks in patients with 2–5 mm of diastasis of the Lisfranc joint [38]. Conventionally, these injuries are often treated operatively, however, this evidence indicates some success non-operatively. It is important to follow these patients, as any evidence of midfoot collapse or further diastasis should be treated surgically.

Table 16.1 Displays examples the critical radiographic signs indicative of midfoot instability as well as the radiographic views on which these can be seen

Critical radiographic sign	View	Example
1. Discontinuity of line drawn from medial base of second metatarsal to medial side of middle cuneiform	Weight bearing Anteroposterior	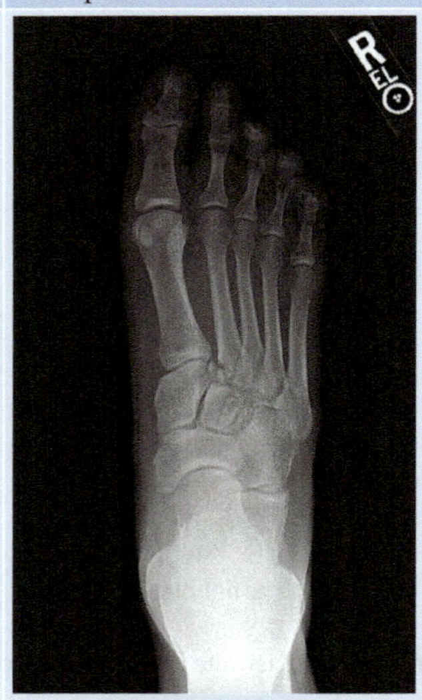
2. Widening of distance between first and second digit	Weight bearing Anteroposterior	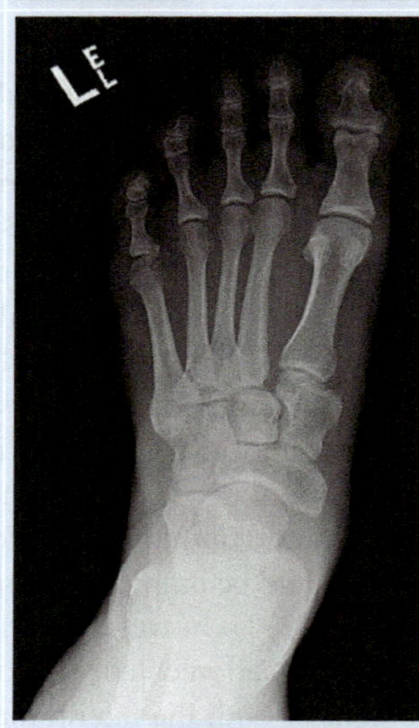
3. Dorsal displacement of proximal base of first or second metatarsal	Weight bearing Lateral	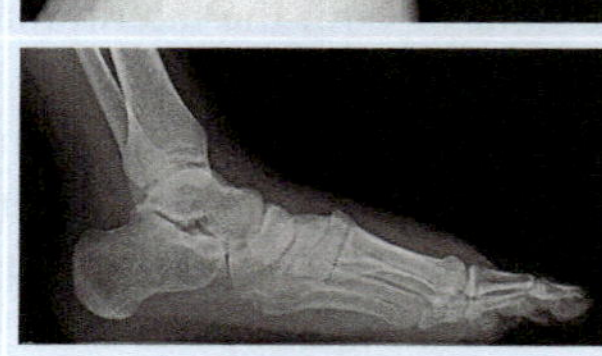

Table 16.1 (continued)

Critical radiographic sign	View	Example
4. Medial side of fourth metatarsal base does not align with medial side of cuboid	Weight bearing Oblique	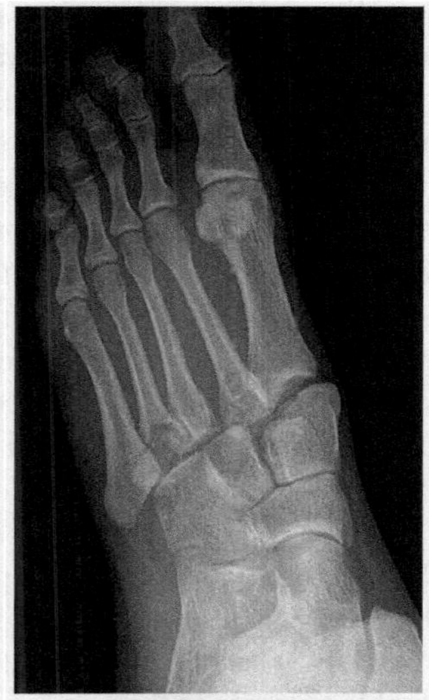
5. Disruption of medial column line	Weight bearing Oblique	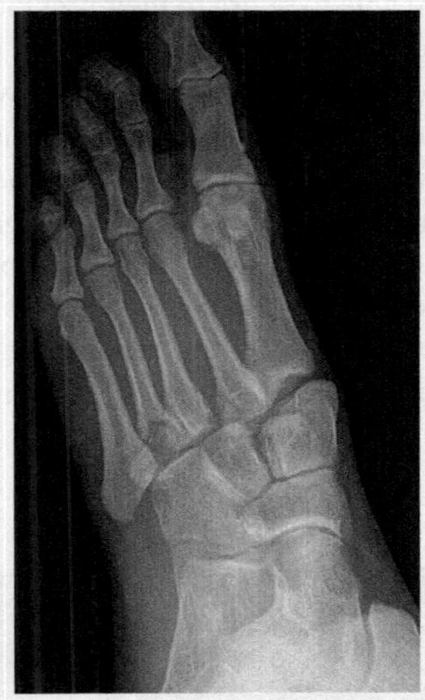
6. Stress Examination	Forced Forefoot Abduction, Anteroposterior	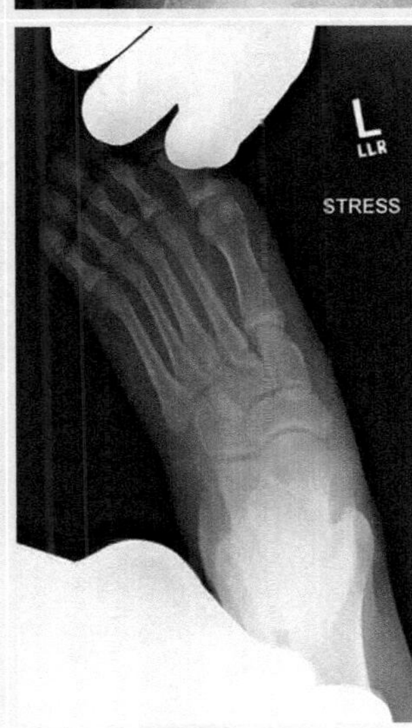

16.2.4.2 Operative Management

There is some controversy regarding which Lisfranc injuries should be managed operatively. Many investigators believe a displacement of greater than 2 mm warrants surgical intervention, especially in athletes [30, 39, 40]. Surgery should be performed as soon as possible after edema has resolved, generally 1–2 weeks following injury. If the fracture-dislocation is amenable to intraoperative reduction under fluoroscopy, percutaneous fixation may be attempted. However, if closed reduction is not possible, open reduction and internal fixation (ORIF) with transarticular screw placement or bridge plate fixation is the gold standard, as it ensures sufficient stabilization of the joint [25, 32] (Figs. 16.5 and 16.6). Recently, primary arthrodesis, which acts by requiring only limited loss of motion and function of the involved medial and middle column joints, has become a more popular option in Lisfranc injuries [27]. One study suggests arthrodesis may be superior to ORIF alone. Namely, 92% of patients treated with primary arthrodesis were able to return to their previous level of activity, compared to 65% of patients treated with only ORIF [41]. The long term consequences of fusion following injuries has not been reported yet. The current recommendation is to base the choice of operative management on the quality of the articular cartilage. In those patients with significant damage to the articular cartilage, arthrodesis should be considered, as well as in patients with purely ligamentous damage. There are no long-term follow-up studies comparing arthrodesis and ORIF. Therefore, ORIF is preferred over arthrodesis in the young, athletic population.

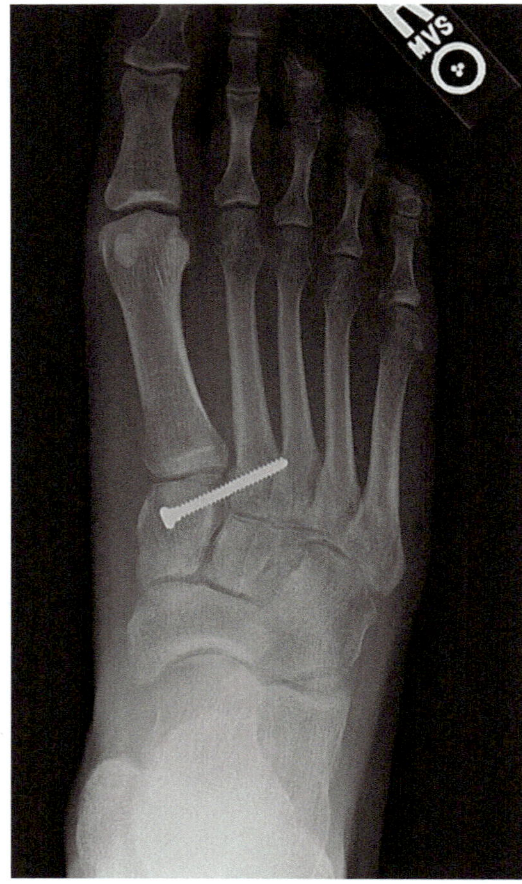

Fig. 16.6 Operative treatment of a Lisfranc injury with transarticular Lisfranc screw

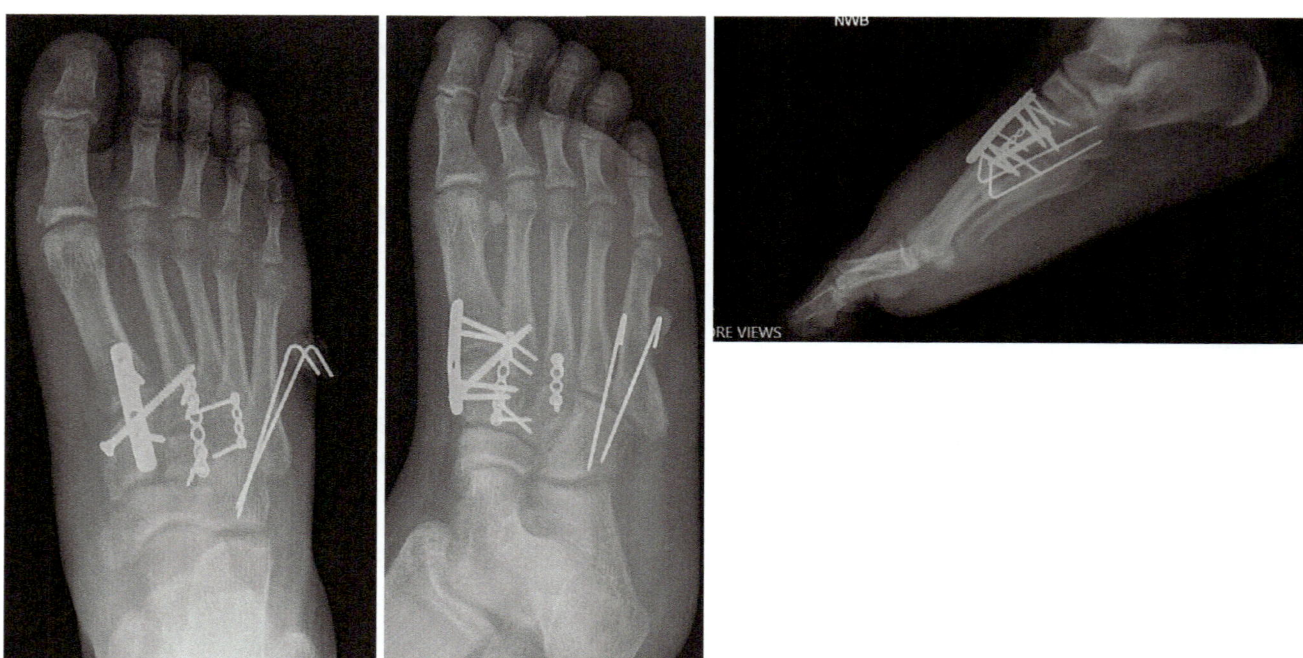

Fig. 16.5 Operative treatment of Lisfranc injury using a bridge plate technique

The method of fixation for these injuries is highly debated. The gold standard is typically a trans-articular screw that traverses from the medial cuneiform to the second metatarsal base with the addition of a plate-screw construct between the first metatarsal and the medial cuneiform.

16.2.5 Complications

The most common complication of Lisfranc injuries is the development of post-traumatic osteoarthritis. Damage to articular surfaces, insufficient reduction, or a combination of the two can contribute to midfoot osteoarthritis. Symptoms include pain, edema, difficulty weightbearing, and gradual deformity. If pain and limited mobility persist for 6 months after nonoperative treatment, surgery should be strongly considered [30, 32, 42]. In patients undergoing fusion, there is also a risk of nonunion.

Hardware removal in athletes is typically undertaken at approximately 16 weeks postoperatively [43]. Removal of hardware should facilitate restoration of joint mobility and avoid hardware failure complications. Following hardware removal in people with an elevated body mass index and the elderly population, loss of reduction can occur. Loss of reduction can also occur if ORIF is performed for purely ligamentous injuries, as there is no reliable method to evaluate the integrity of the healing Lisfranc ligament. For this reason, fusion is considered in patients with a pure ligamentous injury.

16.2.6 Rehabilitation

After undergoing ORIF, patients should be kept nonweightbearing for approximately 8–12 weeks. Healing is generally assessed through radiographs at the sixth postoperative week. Full weightbearing high impact activities should not be attempted until the trans-articular screw has been removed, approximately 4–5 months after surgery. Following screw removal, the patient may begin to wear a protective shoe with an orthosis [30, 44].

Although several factors dictate when athletes may return to sport following a Lisfranc injury, severity of injury may offer the most accurate prognosis. One particular study found that athletes with Grade I and II injuries returned to sport in 11–18 weeks and 12–20 weeks, respectively, with excellent outcomes, while athletes who sustained Grade III injuries generally returned to sport significantly later [28]. The unfortunate reality is that recovery from surgically managed Lisfranc injuries can be lengthy. In one study evaluating return to play for professional football players who sustained Lisfranc injuries, 90% of the athletes were able to return to sport at their pre-injury level of activity, but at a median of 11.1 months after injury [45]. Nevertheless, undergoing operative treatment for Lisfranc injuries may be worthwhile for athletes despite the extended rehabilitation period. Nonoperative management may lead to permanent disability, including midfoot degenerative arthritis [46], which may plague athletes for the remainder of their careers.

16.3 Navicular Fractures

16.3.1 Background

The tarsal navicular is a C-shaped bone that articulates with the three cuneiforms distally, the talus proximally, and the cuboid laterally [47]. Proximally, the talonavicular joint is a highly mobile joint that articulates with the subtalar joint to form the coxa pedis, which affects the mobility of the entire foot. Overall, the navicular plays a crucial role in upholding the medial longitudinal arch of the foot, and is closely associated with hindfoot motion and efficient locomotion [48, 49]. As such, navicular fractures can be highly problematic, though rare in sports. They more commonly occur from high energy trauma such as motor vehicle collisions.

Navicular fractures can occur secondary to acute traumatic injury or chronic stress, with stress fractures being much more common. Specifically, navicular stress fractures comprise as much as one-third of total stress fractures [50]. Moreover, navicular fractures occur most commonly in the younger and athletic populations, with basketball and football being the more common sports [51]. Depending on fracture type, acute navicular fractures following trauma can be either low-energy or high-energy injuries, with most of the latter occurring secondary to motor vehicle collisions. Lower energy injuries are typically an exacerbation of an underlying chronic stress injury. Other causes of acute navicular fractures include falls and blunt injuries [47, 52].

16.3.2 Classification

Acute navicular fractures can be broadly categorized into three types: avulsion, tuberosity, and body fractures [53]. Avulsion fractures are low-energy injuries that present on the dorsal lip or medial surface of the bone, accounting for approximately 50% of navicular fractures. Tuberosity fractures occur secondary to an acute eversion or valgus injury to the hindfoot, which causes traction of the posterior tibial tendon or spring ligament complex [47, 53, 54]. Injuries in athletes tend to be the avulsion or tuberosity type (Fig. 16.7), although the largest category is navicular stress fractures. Sangeorzan et al. further classified acute navicular body fractures based on direction of fracture line, direction of forefoot and midfoot displacement, and pattern of joint

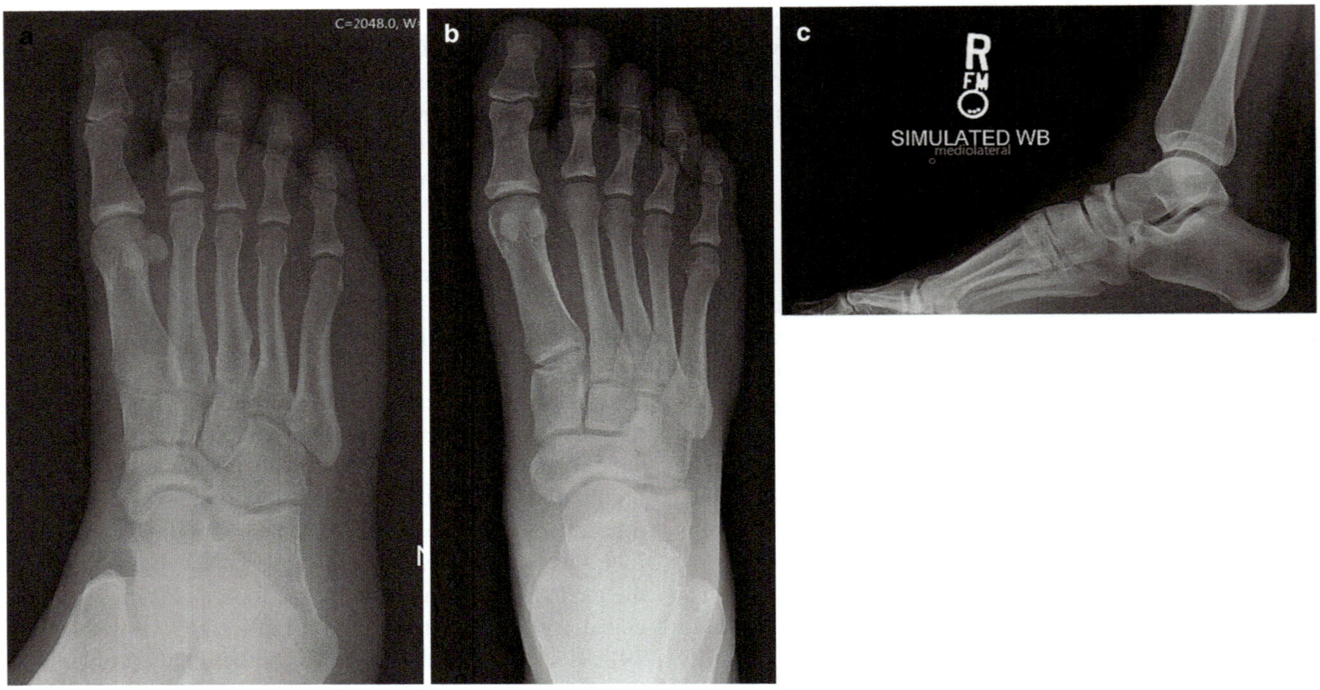

Fig. 16.7 (a–c) Acute navicular avulsion fracture

disruption. Type 1 injuries are those in which the fracture line is in the coronal plane with no associated angulation of the forefoot. Type 2 injuries occur when the fracture line is dorsolateral to plantarmedial, and there is associated medial displacement of both the major fragment and forefoot. Lastly, Type 3 injuries are comminuted fractures in the sagittal plane of navicular body with lateral displacement of the forefoot [47, 55]. As acute navicular fractures may vary in severity, proper classification at the time of diagnosis is crucial when planning management.

16.3.3 Diagnosis

Intuitively, acute navicular fractures present differently based on fracture type. Patients with avulsion fractures typically complain of midfoot pain which is exacerbated by push-off activities. When patients suffer fractures of the body of the navicular, however, they have difficulty weight-bearing, and present with considerable edema of the dorsal and medial portions of the midfoot. On examination, acute navicular fractures often elicit midfoot point tenderness and occasionally gross deformity. When patients present with navicular stress fractures, the symptoms can often be vague, leading to delayed diagnosis in many patients. In any athlete with vague, chronic ankle pain, navicular stress fracture should be high on the differential diagnosis.

Non-weightbearing anteroposterior, lateral, and oblique radiographs are generally employed to diagnose acute navicular fractures. Additionally, weight-bearing and stress radiographs can be helpful in identifying ligamentous injuries in patients with minor injuries and some avulsion fractures. If a tuberosity fracture is suspected, an external oblique radiograph should be used, as this view best visualizes these injuries. CT should always be performed in diagnosing navicular fractures as they help delineate complex fracture patterns of high-energy injuries, determine talonavicular joint involvement, assist in operative planning, and produce three-dimensional reconstructions of the navicular [47, 48]. Advanced imaging (both CT and MRI) can be helpful in the diagnosis of navicular stress fractures.

16.3.4 Management

Management of acute navicular fractures depends both on fracture type and degree of displacement.

16.3.4.1 Nonoperative Management

Most acute navicular fractures are amenable to nonoperative management. Generally, small avulsion fractures, tuberosity fractures with less than 2–3 mm of displacement, and non-displaced navicular body fractures do not warrant surgical intervention. However, there are other factors to consider, including the condition of the soft tissue of the foot, the presence of additional foot injuries, and medical comorbidities. Athletes sustaining minor navicular fractures can expect a prompt return to sport after injury, following 6 weeks in a weight-bearing short leg cast and an additional 4–6 weeks in a walking boot to prevent further displacement [47, 49]. Non-operative management can also be employed for navicular stress fractures according to Torg, though recently there has been a shift to early operative management [56, 57].

16.3.4.2 Operative Management

Most avulsion and tuberosity fractures of the navicular can be managed nonoperatively. However, the majority of displaced navicular body fractures should be surgically managed. Surgery is also indicated for intra-articular fractures with greater than 1 mm of incongruity and fractures associated with subluxation, instability, or dislocation of the naviculocuneiform or talonavicular joints. Open reduction and internal fixation (ORIF) is the recommended surgical approach in most patients, although external fixation can also be attempted in patients with comminuted fractures and a poor surrounding soft-tissue envelope [47, 48] (Fig. 16.8). The goals of ORIF are to anatomically reduce the talonavicular joint, restore medial column length, and reestablish rigid fixation, facilitating improved range of motion [49]. Additionally, mini-fragment plate fixation has been used for complex Types 2 and 3 injuries [50]. Evans et al. performed ORIF with mini-fragment plate fixation on 24 patients with good results: all fractures united, with no loss of reduction in any fracture [58]. In addition, patients with navicular stress fractures can be treated operatively, with the most common fixation method with two screws from lateral to medial, plus or minus autologous bone grafting [57].

16.3.5 Complications

Two common complications arising from acute navicular fractures are nonunion and osteonecrosis, which can lead to posttraumatic collapse of the navicular resulting in foot deformity [50]. Mild non-unions are amenable to nonoperative management with a stiff orthotic supporting the medial midfoot [59], while more serious non-unions require revision ORIF with autologous bone grafting. Osteonecrosis is a more serious complication which often results in marked deformity. Insufficient blood supply to the navicular and the stripping of soft-tissue during surgery can both contribute to developing osteonecrosis. Talonavicular fusion can be employed to reduce pain and rectify length and alignment irregularities arising from osteonecrosis [47, 50].

16.3.6 Rehabilitation

After undergoing ORIF for an acute navicular fracture, the foot should be kept non-weightbearing in a splint for 2 weeks until suture removal; at that point, the patient may begin ankle, forefoot, and hindfoot range of motion exercises.

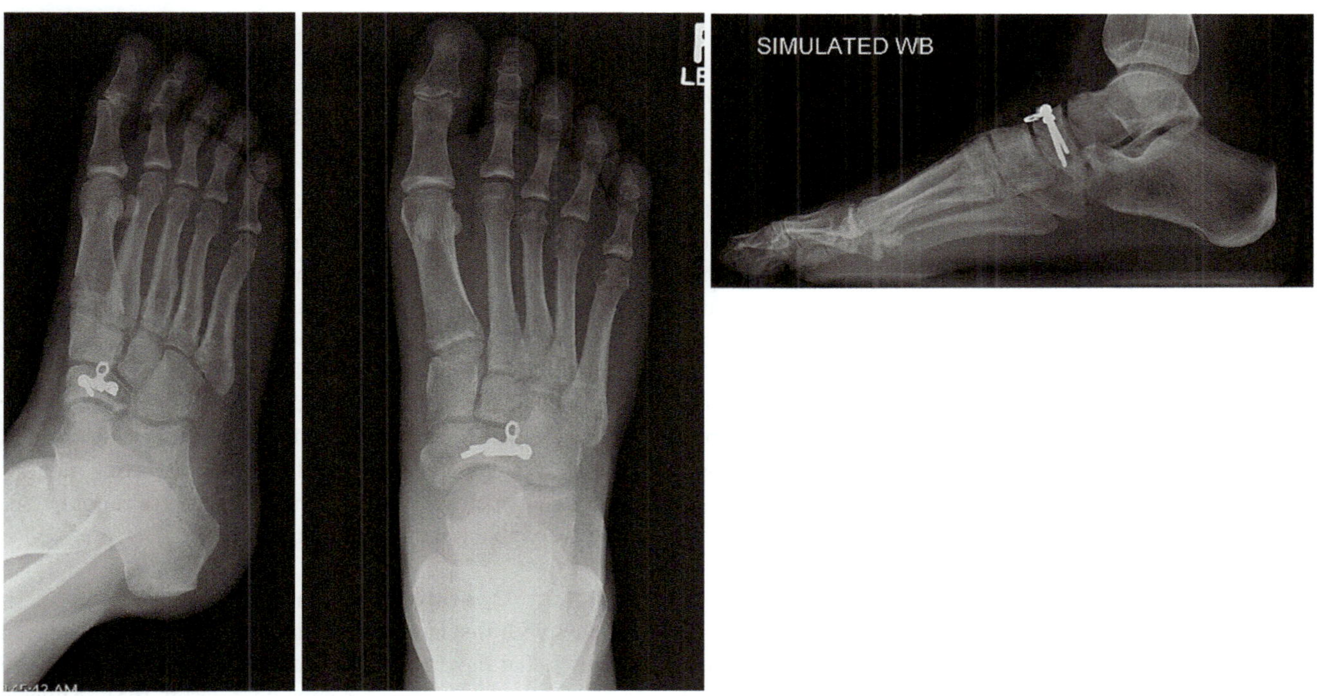

Fig. 16.8 Fixation of an acute navicular avulsion fracture

After approximately 6 weeks, partial weightbearing can be attempted. Radiographs should be repeated throughout the rehabilitation period to assess fracture healing [49]. Athletes typically return to sport between 4 and 6 months after surgery [57]. While management of acute navicular fractures can be challenging since acute fractures are managed quite differently than stress fractures, a thorough understanding of the mechanism of injury and a prompt, accurate diagnosis can effectively guide treatment. In any patient with a stress fracture, follow up with CT scan should be used to evaluate union.

16.4 Sesamoid Fractures

16.4.1 Background

Sesamoid fractures can be painful, debilitating, and often difficult to identify. Considering the many different types of sesamoid injuries, it can be challenging to accurately diagnose these fractures. Acute sesamoid fractures only account for 10% of sesamoid injuries, while sesamoiditis and stress fractures account for 40% and 30% of sesamoid injuries, respectively [60]. Other common sesamoid injuries include osteochondritis, osteoarthritis, and bursitis [61]. Overall, sesamoid injuries represent approximately 9% of foot and ankle injuries [62], and sesamoid fractures are most frequently seen in female dancers, runners, and gymnasts [63]. Acute sesamoid fractures usually occur secondary to severe hyperextension or abduction of the hallux [64].

16.4.2 Classification

The two sesamoid bones, the tibial (medial) and fibular (lateral) sesamoids, articulate at the hallucal metatarsophalangeal joint with the metatarsal bone [61]. In some people, two or more ossification centers may fail to coalesce, leading to a 'bipartite sesamoid' [65]. Unfortunately, bipartite sesamoids can be difficult to distinguish from acute sesamoid fractures, as they are present in up to 35% of the population. Tibial sesamoids are bipartite 10 times more frequently than the fibular sesamoids [66]. Therefore, the presence of multiple fragments in the fibular sesamoid following trauma should be considered as an acute sesamoid fracture until proven otherwise.

16.4.3 Diagnosis

Patients with acute sesamoid fractures generally complain of acute pain secondary to forced hyper-dorsiflexion of first metatarsophalangeal joint. The pain is generally located on the plantar aspect of the foot, directly over the injured sesamoid [64]. Examination may reveal point tenderness on palpation, significant edema, ecchymosis, and diminished range of motion of the hallux [67]. Certain criteria have been devised to help distinguish acute sesamoid fractures from bipartite sesamoids. Namely, acute sesamoid fractures present with irregular or unequal separation of the affected sesamoid, callus formation as evidence of attempted healing seen on radiographs, the absence of similar findings in the unaffected foot, and gross or microscopic evidence of fracture appreciated during surgical intervention [68]. As bipartite sesamoids are present bilaterally in up to 85% of patients, the absence of similar findings in the uninjured foot is a strong indication that a sesamoid fracture has occurred. Additionally, a sharp-edged, irregular contour seen on radiograph should raises suspicion for an acute sesamoid fracture instead of a bipartite sesamoid, as the latter generally displays a smoother border on radiograph. Moreover, in an acute fracture, the size of the fragments combined should relatively approximate the size of the other sesamoid. If the combination of fragments appears larger, bipartite sesamoid can be considered. Advanced imaging (MRI) can be helpful in delineating a difference as well. Lastly, CT scans are helpful in the diagnosis of acute sesamoid fractures, since they better delineate sharp-edged contours that may represent fractures [65, 66]. An injury can occur through a previous synchondrosis of a bipartite sesamoids: this is evident by increased signal on T2 sequences at the synchondrosis in patients with pain in this region.

16.4.4 Management

Acute sesamoid fractures may be managed nonoperatively or operatively depending on degree of displacement.

16.4.4.1 Nonoperative Management

Nondisplaced acute sesamoid fractures are generally amenable to nonoperative management. There is some discrepancy regarding which nonoperative management regimen is the most effective for a prompt recovery. A 6- to 8-week period of non-weightbearing and immobilisation is generally recommended [69]. However, others recommend casting for 3–4 weeks followed by having the patient wear a firm-soled shoe with padding [70]. Regardless of the approach, nonoperative management of nondisplaced acute sesamoid fractures is a viable treatment strategy.

16.4.4.2 Operative Treatment

Patients with displaced sesamoid fractures or nondisplaced fractures that have not healed after prolonged nonoperative treatment should obtain orthopedic referral [65]. Athletes should also be given strong consideration for early referral. In the past, excision of either the affected sesamoid or both sesamoids was the standard surgical treatment. However, complications arising from excising the sesamoids have led to the advent of other techniques [61, 65]. Percutaneous screw fixation with autologous bone grafting is a reliable option to manage sesamoid fractures unresponsive to conservative treatment [71] (Fig. 16.9). One study evaluated the results of percutaneous screw fixation on nine patients, each of whom reported significant post-operative pain relief [72]. When considering excision of the fractured sesamoid, it is crucial to preserve the attachment of the flexor hallicus brevis to prevent deformity of the great toe. This can be accomplished by fixation of the soft tissue complex to the base of the proximal phalanx or performing an all soft tissue repair (Fig. 16.10).

16.4.5 Complications

Unfortunately, many complications are associated with acute sesamoid injuries. Following excision of both sesamoids, patients may develop an intrinsic minus/claw deformity of the hallux. Moreover, excision of only the fibular sesamoid may increase the likelihood of developing hallux varus, while hallux valgus may be exacerbated by excision of only the tibial sesamoid. Chronic post-operative pain secondary to nerve damage during surgery is another possible complication. Fortunately, these complications can be avoided with knowledge of foot anatomy and scrutiny in assessing both the indications and contraindications for each specific procedure and selecting the optimal strategy [65, 66].

16.4.6 Rehabilitation

Post-operative protocol following surgical fixation of acute sesamoid fractures depends on the surgical approach employed. Athletes who undergo bone grafting of non-unions, for instance, are kept immobilized in a short-leg cast for 3–4 weeks. Subsequently, patients wear a short-leg walking cast or boot for 8 weeks, while active exercises and gentle passive range-of-motion exercises are performed as tolerated. Radiographs and potentially CT scans are employed at 10–12 weeks to confirm union with return to sport to follow if the patient is pain-free [67]. Return to sport varies in a case-by-case basis, but some athletes who undergo percutaneous screw fixation resume full activities as early as 3 months post-op [72].

16.5 First and Central Metatarsal Fractures

16.5.1 Background

Metatarsal fractures are extremely common injuries in both athletes and non-athletes, accounting for approximately 35% of foot fractures. They also comprise 5–6% of all skeletal injuries, yielding an incidence rate of approximately 6.7/10,000. As detailed in Sect. 16.1, fifth metatarsal fractures are the most common metatarsal fracture. While first metatarsal fractures are least common and generally present fewer complications, central metatarsal fractures (those that occur in the second through fourth digits) present a unique

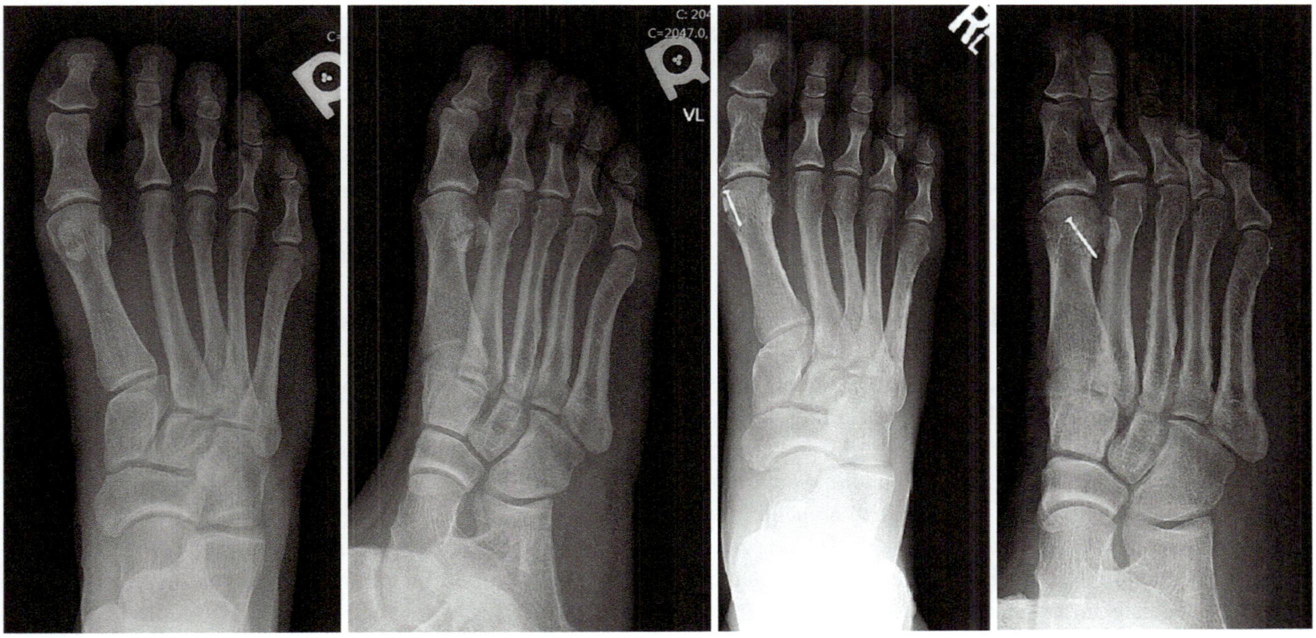

Fig. 16.9 Fixation of a tibial sesamoid fracture with a screw

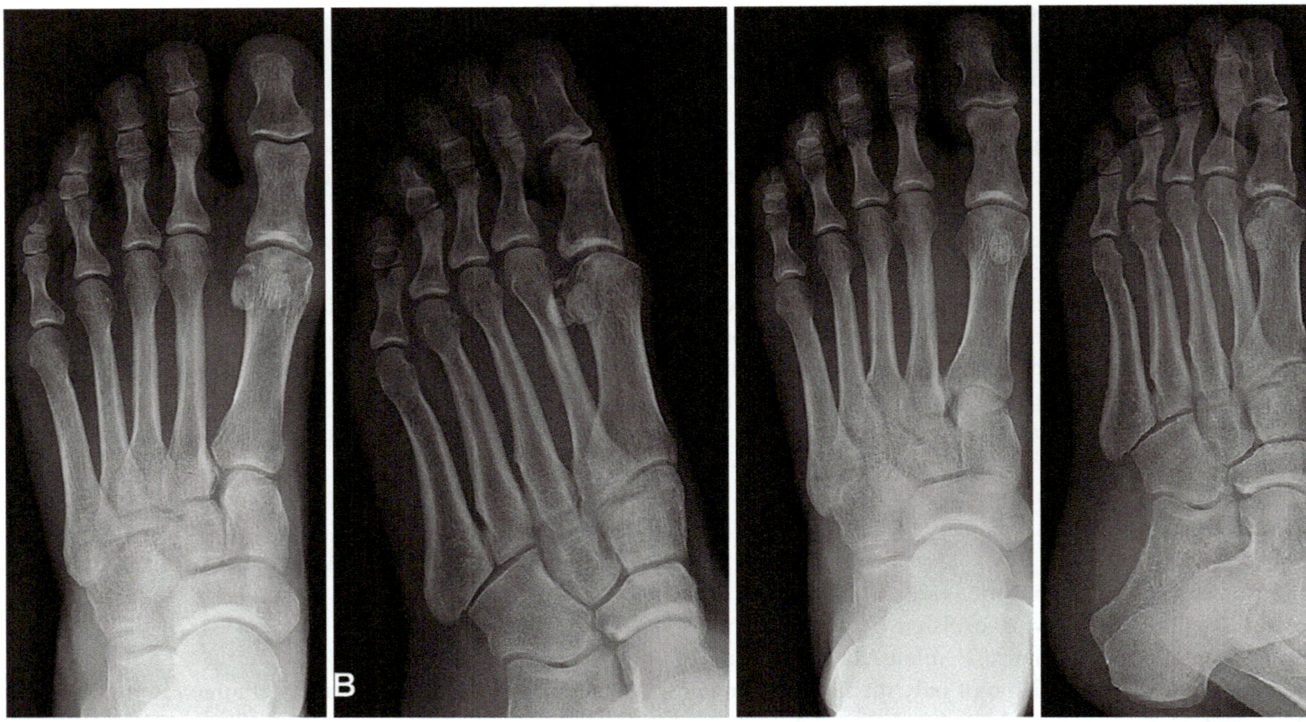

Fig. 16.10 Excision of sesamoid following fracture

problem as there is a high likelihood of contiguous fracture in a neighboring metatarsal. In fact, approximately 60% of cases involving third metatarsal fractures are associated with either second or fourth metatarsal fractures [73].

Although first through fourth metatarsal fractures are less prominent than fifth metatarsal fractures, these fractures require distinct attention as they can be associated with involvement of the Lisfranc ligament complex, which is responsible for keeping the metatarsals in place and anchored to the rest of the body as well as preserving the arch of the foot. Unfortunately, a fracture of the first through fourth metatarsals with an associated Lisfranc injury can lead to long-term disability without early detection [74].

16.5.2 Classification and Diagnosis

In general, first and central metatarsal fractures can be classified based on anatomical location, including proximal, metaphyseal, diaphyseal, cervical (neck), and cephalic (head) fractures. Additionally, it is crucial to rule out Lisfranc joint involvement if a patient presents with an acute first or central proximal metaphyseal fracture [75]. As always, proper classification of acute first and central metatarsal fractures is essential, as factors such as fracture location, fracture pattern, degree of displacement, and stability of the fracture dictate the treatment decision [1]. Standard radiographs of the foot allow to diagnose these injuries. Displacement of these fractures is often times prevented as the metatarsals are held together by the intermetatarsal ligaments.

16.5.3 Management

As in acute fifth metatarsal fractures, management of first and central metatarsal fractures depends on a variety of factors.

16.5.3.1 Nonoperative Management

In general, nondisplaced and minimally displaced (less than 3 mm) first and central metatarsal fractures can be effectively managed nonoperatively in both athletes and non-athletes. Initial management involves posterior splint immobilisation, use of crutches, and avoiding weight-bearing activities. Moreover, patients should be advised to apply ice regularly, keep the foot elevated, and use pain medications as needed [1, 76]. Return to play can be expected between 6 and 12 weeks.

16.5.3.2 Operative Management

There are several clinical indications for surgery after sustaining an acute metatarsal fracture. For central metatarsal fractures, surgery is indicated if there is an open fracture, a fracture dislocation, multiple metatarsal fractures, intra-articular fractures, greater than 3 mm of displacement, more than 10° angulation in the dorsoplantar plane, or 50% dorsal displacement. It is important to assess the metatarsals in the sagittal plan, as extensive displacement can lead to transfer metatarsalgia. As the first metatarsal is crucial for weight bearing and arch support, a surgical consultation is warranted if there is any displacement or angulation [76].

As was the case for acute fifth metatarsal fractures, central metatarsal fractures can be managed with intramedullary screw fixation with either antegrade or retrograde Kirschner wires, or "K-wires," which reduce the risk of injury to neighboring soft tissue. Another treatment option is open reduction and plate fixation, which decreases the possibility of pin site complications and metatarsophalangeal stiffness, both of which can occur following K-wire insertion [1]. Similarly, first metatarsal fractures can be effectively managed by K-wire insertion or plate osteosynthesis depending on whether or not the fracture can be managed by closed reduction [1, 77].

16.5.4 Complications

Most complications of acute first and central metatarsal fractures can be avoided with prompt treatment. Unfortunately, fractures of the first metatarsal base and metatarsophalangeal joint are often associated with unrecognized ligament damage. Further, fractures of the metatarsophalangeal joint and sesamoid complex often result in joint instability and dislocations [78]. Metatarsalgia resulting from malunion is especially common with first metatarsal fractures, but can also be associated with central metatarsal fractures. Additional complications of central metatarsal fractures include arterial injury, neurologic injury (specifically to the medial dorsal cutaneous superficial peroneal nerve branch and deep peroneal nerve in second metatarsal fractures), and osteomyelitis [74, 78].

16.5.5 Rehabilitation

Immediately after diagnosis, patients should be instructed to avoid weight bearing activities and to keep leg immobilized in a posterior splint. Radiographs should then be utilized 1 week after injury to confirm fracture stability and if stable, the patient may begin wearing a short leg walking cast. Once callus formation is seen on radiography and the patient has no residual point tenderness, which usually occurs at approximately 6 weeks following injury, the patient can discontinue immobilisation. Lastly, the patient should commence calf stretching/strengthening and ankle range-of-motion exercises before he/she returns to sport [74, 76].

16.6 Phalanx Fractures

16.6.1 Background

Phalanx fractures are seen in athletes of all age groups and levels of participation. Studies suggest phalanx fractures of the hallux are most common, accounting for 38–56% of phalanx fractures [79, 80]. Unfortunately, serious fractures to the hallux can often be misconstrued as a mild injury, such as toe stubbing with minimal soft tissue disruption, and can lead to severe dysfunction and long term pain without proper diagnosis [81]. For this reason, a high index of suspicion in the primary care setting is necessary.

16.6.2 Classification

Phalanx fractures can be simply classified based on anatomical position (e.g. proximal, middle, or distal phalanx fractures). Certain phalanges are more susceptible to fracture than others. Namely, fractures of the distal phalanx of the hallux are more common than fractures of the proximal phalanx of the hallux [81]. Diagnosis is made through standard radiographs and clinical suspicion.

16.6.3 Treatment

16.6.3.1 Nonoperative Management

Fortunately, the vast majority of acute phalanx fractures in athletes may be managed conservatively with a quick return to sport [82]. Nondisplaced fractures are generally managed by splinting the affected toe by employing the buddy taping technique, wherein the affected toe is taped to an adjacent toe for support. Similarly, displaced fractures of the lesser toes may be managed conservatively in most cases. However, the bone fragments must be manipulated into anatomical position, whereby the physician holds the tip of the toe and applies longitudinal traction under local anesthesia [83]. The patients can return to sport as their symptoms allow.

16.6.3.2 Operative Management

While phalanx fractures of the lesser toes rarely warrant surgical intervention, surgery is indicated in hallucal phalanx fractures in which there is greater than 2 mm of displacement, the fracture is open, or if there is a displaced physeal injury following an attempted closed reduction [80]. Open reduction and internal fixation is a reliable technique for traumatic phalanx fractures of the hallux using a dorsomedial incision [84].

16.6.4 Rehabilitation

In general, acute phalanx fractures are managed conservatively with the exception of severe hallucal phalanx fractures [80, 84]. Most commonly, the buddy taping technique is used until point tenderness resolves, usually after 3–4 weeks. Ice and elevation are recommended for the first few days after injury as well. Once splinting has been discontinued, the patient may begin gentle range-of-motion exercises. Radiographs should be taken weekly for 2 to 3 weeks in potentially unstable or intra-articular fractures of the hallux to survey fracture position, and they should be repeated once treatment is complete to confirm adequate healing [83]. Athletes can return to sport as their pain allows, especially if the injury is stable.

16.7 Talar Fractures

16.7.1 Background

Talar fractures are relatively uncommon, comprising between 3% and 6% of foot fractures [85]. They are more frequent in males than females; one study reports that as high as 72% of talar fractures are seen in men. Interestingly, there is no specific age group predisposed to sustaining talar fractures [86]. In the athletic population, lateral process talar fractures are most frequently seen. These injuries are generally associated with a high-energy, acute mechanism of injury, including snowboarding injuries, falls from heights, direct trauma, and football and rugby injuries [87]. Lateral process talar fractures are being recognized and diagnosed more frequently, thus increasing the annual incidence rate of these injuries [88]. Athletes also often present with acute osteochondral lesions of the talus.

16.7.2 Diagnosis

Unfortunately, up to 50% of lateral process talar fractures are missed due to similarity in presentation to ankle sprains [89]. Patients generally complain of acute localized tenderness, edema, and painful range of motion. On examination, there may be a hematoma close to the tip of the lateral malleolus [87, 88, 90]. These signs and symptoms, coupled with a history of high-energy trauma, should raise high suspicion for a lateral process talar fracture. Pain lasting longer than 6 weeks following an acute ankle sprain should be investigated further. Radiographic investigations should include lateral, anteroposterior, and mortise views. Specifically, a lateral radiograph with ankle dorsiflexion and inversion enables clear visualization of the fracture fragment [88, 91]. However, CT scans are considered the gold standard in the diagnosis of fractures of the lateral process of the talus, as they better delineate the degree of bony injury [92]. If there is concern for an acute osteochondral fractures of the talus, MRI can be helpful to assess location and displacement of these lesions. The amount of bony involvement will often times determine the method of treatment. Various of osteochondral lesions exist, Fig. 16.11 demonstrates a lateral inverted fracture of the talus (LIFT lesion).

16.7.3 Treatment

16.7.3.1 Nonoperative Management

In general, nondisplaced lateral process talar fractures and fractures with less than 2 mm of displacement may be managed conservatively. The leg is immobilized in a short-leg cast and kept partial weightbearing for approximately 6 weeks [93]. However, some authors believe that Type I fractures warrant operative treatment, as up to 38% of patients with Type I fractures experience bothersome symptoms when managed conservatively [94].

16.7.3.2 Operative Management

Typically, extra-articular lateral process talar fractures may be managed conservatively. However, lateral process talar fractures involving the articular surface should be managed operatively. The subtalar and ankle joint do not tolerate step-off and incongruity well. Some of less displaced intra-articular fractures are amenable to arthroscopic excision [95]. However, fractures with a single, large displaced fragment as well as comminuted fractures should be managed by either arthroscopic screw fixation or open reduction and internal fixation [87, 88, 93]. Additionally, large comminuted fragments should be excised rather than internally fixed. Regardless of the degree of displacement, prompt treatment of lateral process talar fractures is instrumental in obtaining the optimal result [96]. In patients with displaced, acute osteochondral lesions, excision versus repair should be considered, depending on the extent of involvement of the bone.

16.7.4 Rehabilitation

Immediately following ORIF, patients are recommended bed rest and elevation for 2–3 days. Subsequently, the ankle is immobilized in a walking boot, and patients are kept partial weightbearing for 6 weeks. Afterwards, full weightbearing is permitted. Return-to-sport time can vary significantly depending on the extent of injury. In 16 snowboarders who underwent ORIF of fractures of the lateral process of the talus, the average recovery time was 27 weeks. Despite the

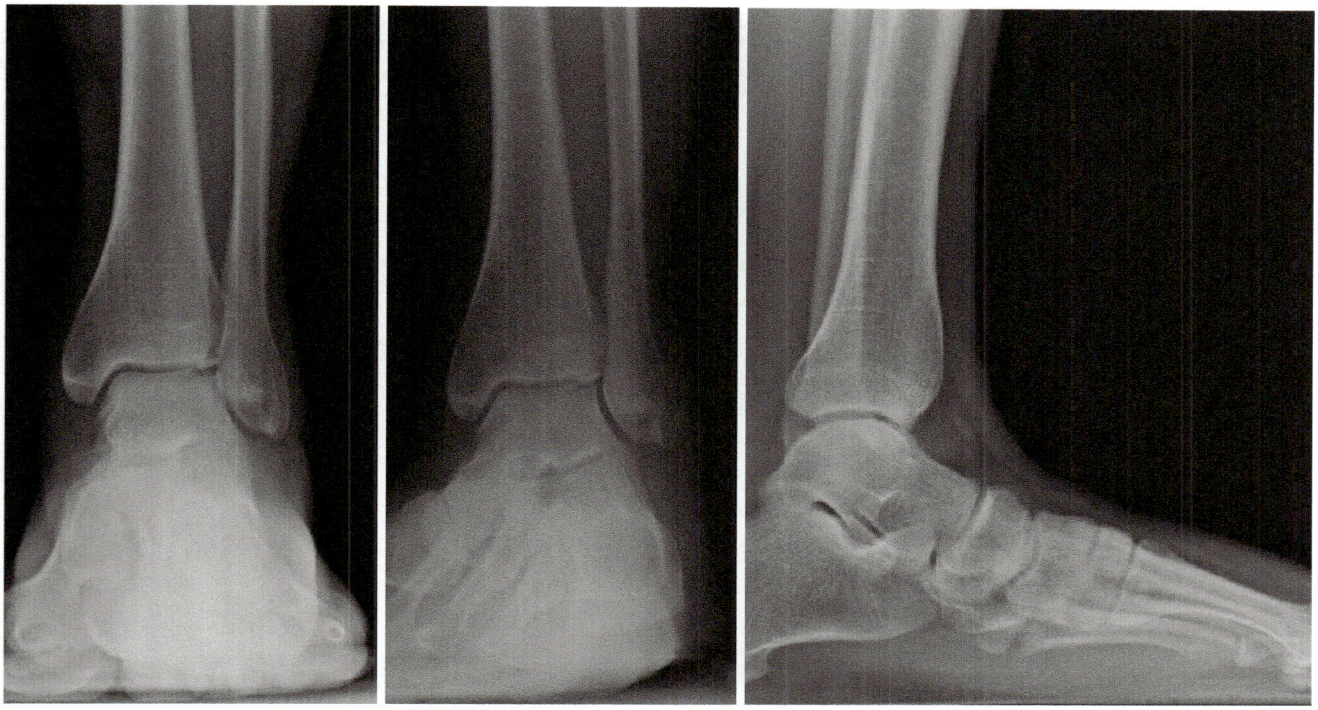

Fig. 16.11 Radiographs demonstrated a lateral inverted osteochondral lesion of the talus (LIFT lesion)

extended recovery time in some patients, most of the athletes were able to return to their previous level activity following operative management [90].

16.8 Calcaneal Fractures

16.8.1 Background

Acute calcaneal fractures are uncommon but potentially devastating. The annual incidence rate of these fractures is approximately 11.5/100,000, with the majority seen in males aged 20–29. Fortunately, most acute calcaneal fractures are isolated injuries, but some may be associated with lower limb or spinal injuries [97]. In the athletic population, anterior process calcaneal fractures are particularly common. Unfortunately, they are often misdiagnosed because of their similarity in presentation to ankle sprains [98]. An anterior process fracture is commonly caused by extreme tension on the bifurcate ligament during inversion and plantar flexion, which results in an avulsion fracture [99, 100].

16.8.2 Diagnosis

After sustaining an anterior process calcaneal fracture, the patient will generally complain of an aching pain about the anterior and lateral ankle, exacerbated on weightbearing. On examination, significant edema and ecchymosis on the lateral calcaneal aspect is often appreciated in addition to anterior talocalcaneal tenderness on palpation [98, 99, 101]. Radiographic evaluation should include anteroposterior, lateral, and mortise views. Oblique radiograph of the foot can also help in diagnosis (Fig. 16.12). However, MRI is instrumental in the diagnosis of anterior process calcaneal fractures, as it can better demonstrate tendon or ligamentous injuries and facilitate detection of nondisplaced fractures [98, 102].

16.8.3 Management

16.8.3.1 Nonoperative Management

Fortunately, the vast majority of anterior process fractures may be managed nonoperatively. For nondisplaced or minimally displaced fractures, the injured foot is placed in a boot and can be made partial weight bearing. After 6 weeks, the patient may begin participating in progressive weightbearing activities and range-of-motion exercises as tolerated [101, 103]. Most patients who proceed with conservative management for anterior process fractures report positive functional outcomes [104].

16.8.3.2 Operative Management

While most anterior process calcaneal fractures are amenable to nonoperative management, displaced fractures may be at a

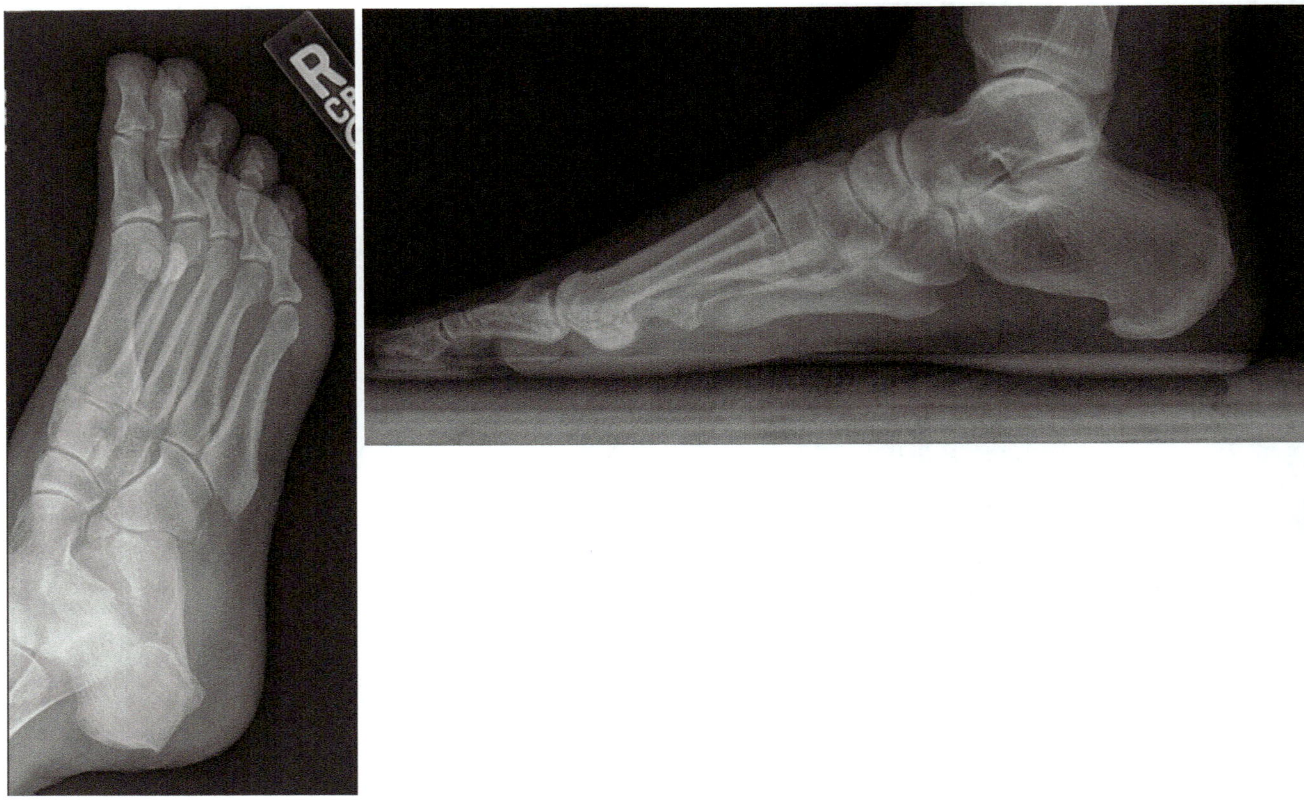

Fig. 16.12 Radiographs demonstrating anterior process of the calcaneus fracture

higher risk for non-union [101, 105]. Open reduction and internal fixation (ORIF) is the preferred surgical approach for large dislocated fractures, and should also be considered when patients experience persistent pain or symptomatic non-union after conservative management [104]. Patients who undergo ORIF of fractures of the anterior process of the calcaneus generally experience good results. In a study of 18 patients who underwent ORIF of fractures of the anterior process of the calcaneus, most reported satisfactory outcomes, were asymptomatic at an average time of 8 weeks, and were able to resume full activities at an average time of 4.3 months [106]. Excision, even of large fragments, can be considered, as the anterior process of the calcaneus contributes little to stability.

16.8.4 Rehabilitation

Postoperatively, patients are advised to begin gentle subtalar range-of-motion exercises as soon as the wound heals and patient can tolerate them, usually at 7–10 days. Suture removal generally occurs at 3 weeks post-op, after which gentle strengthening exercises of foot and ankle muscles may be attempted. When union has been confirmed on radiograph, the patient may begin partial weightbearing, which generally occurs 8–10 weeks postoperatively. Finally, gradual full weightbearing is resumed over a period of 4–6 weeks [106].

Acknowledgement Oliver B. Hansen (Figure prep and manuscript editing), Stephanie K. Eble (Figure prep and manuscript editing)

Funding None

Review

Questions

1. What is the optimal treatment for a Zone 2 fifth metatarsal fracture in a 65-year old sedentary individual?
   (a) Open Reduction internal fixation with a plantar based plate
   (b) Open reduction internal fixation with a single partially threaded screw
   (c) Open reduction internal fixation with a single partially threaded screw with autograft bone
   (d) Non-weight bearing in a cast or boot for a period of 6 weeks

2. What is the typical mechanism for a Lisfranc fracture?
   (a) Plantar flexion, axial force, forefoot abduction
   (b) Dorsiflexion, axial force, forefoot abduction
   (c) Plantar flexion, axial force, forefoot adduction
   (d) Dorsiflexion and inversion
3. What is a complication following treatment of a medial (tibial) sesamoid fracture by excision?
   (a) Hallux Varus
   (b) Hallux Valgus
   (c) Hallux Rigidus
   (d) Curly Toe deformity
4. True or False: The sesamoids are encased inside of the flexor hallucis longus tendon
5. If there is clinical concern for Lisfranc injury, which of the following should be obtained initially?
   (a) MRI
   (b) CT scan
   (c) Weight bearing CT scan
   (d) Non-weight bearing radiographs
   (e) Weight bearing radiographs

Answers

1. D—While this fracture is at a higher risk for non-union, in elderly or more sedentary patients, non-weight bearing in a cast is the indicated treatment.
2. A—Typically mechanism involves axial force and forefoot abduction of a hyper plantar flexed foot
3. B—If the soft tissues are not repaired properly, pull by the fibular sesamoid can cause the patient to develop a hallux valgus deformity
4. False—They are incased inside of the flexor hallucis brevis tendon
5. E—initial evaluation of a Lisfranc injury should include weight bearing radiographs (one should also include the contralateral foot in the same plate in order to properly evaluate the Lisfranc joint)

References

1. Sarpong NO, Swindell HW, Trupia EP, Vosseller JT. Metatarsal fractures. Foot Ankle Orthop. 2018;3:2473011418775094.
2. Lareau CR, Hsu AR, Anderson RB. Return to play in national football league players after operative jones fracture treatment. Foot Ankle Int. 2016;37:8–16.
3. Kaplan LD, Jost PW, Honkamp N, Norwig J, West R, Bradley JP. Incidence and variance of foot and ankle injuries in elite college football players. Am J Orthop. 2011;40:40–4.
4. Bigsby E, Halliday R, Middleton RG, Case R, Harries W. Functional outcome of fifth metatarsal fractures. Injury. 2014;45:2009–12.
5. Lawrence SJ, Botte MJ. Jones' fractures and related fractures of the proximal fifth metatarsal. Foot Ankle. 1993;14:358–65.
6. Dameron TB. Fractures of the proximal fifth metatarsal: selecting the best treatment option. J Am Acad Orthop Surg. 1995;3:110–4.
7. Chuckpaiwong B, Queen RM, Easley ME, Nunley JA. Distinguishing Jones and proximal diaphyseal fractures of the fifth metatarsal. Clin Orthop Relat Res. 2008;466:1966–70.
8. McKeon KE, Johnson JE, McCormick JJ, Klein SE. The intraosseous and extraosseous vascular supply of the fifth metatarsal: implications for fifth metatarsal osteotomy. Foot Ankle Int. 2013;34:117–23.
9. Smith JW, Arnoczky SP, Hersh A. The intraosseous blood supply of the fifth metatarsal: implications for proximal fracture healing. Foot Ankle. 1992;13:143–52.
10. Shereff MJ, Yang QM, Kummer FJ, Frey CC, Greenidge N. Vascular anatomy of the fifth metatarsal. Foot Ankle. 1991;11:350–3.
11. Jones R. I. Fracture of the base of the fifth metatarsal bone by indirect violence. Ann Surg. 1902;35:697–700.2.
12. Dameron TB. Fractures and anatomical variations of the proximal portion of the fifth metatarsal. J Bone Joint Surg Am. 1975;57:788–92.
13. Cheung CN, Lui TH. Proximal fifth metatarsal fractures: anatomy, classification, treatment and complications. Arch Trauma Res. 2016;5:e33298. https://doi.org/10.5812/atr.33298.
14. Bowes J, Buckley R. Fifth metatarsal fractures and current treatment. World J Orthop. 2016;7:793–800.
15. Roche AJ, Calder JDF. Treatment and return to sport following a Jones fracture of the fifth metatarsal: a systematic review. Knee Surg Sports Traumatol Arthrosc. 2013;21:1307–15.
16. Zwitser EW, Breederveld RS. Fractures of the fifth metatarsal; diagnosis and treatment. Injury. 2010;41:555–62.
17. Karnovsky SC, Rosenbaum AJ, DeSandis B, Johnson C, Murphy CI, Warren RF, Taylor SA, Drakos MC. Radiographic analysis of national football league players' fifth metatarsal morphology relationship to proximal fifth metatarsal fracture risk. Foot Ankle Int. 2019;40:318–22.
18. Strayer SM, Reece SG, Petrizzi MJ. Fractures of the proximal fifth metatarsal. AFP. 1999;59:2516.
19. Lareau CR, Anderson RB. Jones fractures: pathophysiology and treatment. J Bone Jt Surg Rev. 2015;3:01874474-201503070-00004. https://doi.org/10.2106/JBJS.RVW.N.00100.
20. Konkel KF, Menger AG, Retzlaff SA. Nonoperative treatment of fifth metatarsal fractures in an orthopaedic suburban private multispeciality practice. Foot Ankle Int. 2005;26:704–7.
21. Zelko RR, Torg JS, Rachun A. Proximal diaphyseal fractures of the fifth metatarsal--treatment of the fractures and their complications in athletes. Am J Sports Med 1979;7:95–101.
22. Hunt KJ, Anderson RB. Treatment of Jones fracture nonunions and refractures in the elite athlete: outcomes of intramedullary screw fixation with bone grafting. Am J Sports Med. 2011;39:1948–54.
23. Ritchie JD, Shaver JC, Anderson RB, Lawrence SJ, Mair SD. Excision of symptomatic nonunions of proximal fifth metatarsal avulsion fractures in elite athletes. Am J Sports Med. 2011;39:2466–9.
24. Sakellariou VI, Kyriakopoulos S, Sofianos IP, Papagelopoulos PJ. Fractures of the Proximal Part of the 5th Metatarsal. J Trauma Treat. 2014;3:1–4.
25. Kalia V, Fishman EK, Carrino JA, Fayad LM. Epidemiology, imaging, and treatment of Lisfranc fracture-dislocations revisited. Skelet Radiol. 2012;41:129–36.
26. Buchanan BK, Donnally CJ III. Lisfranc dislocation. Treasure Island, FL: StatPearls; 2019.
27. Clare MP. Lisfranc injuries. Curr Rev Musculoskelet Med. 2017;10:81–5.

28. Nunley JA, Vertullo CJ. Classification, investigation, and management of midfoot sprains: lisfranc injuries in the athlete. Am J Sports Med. 2002;30:871–8.
29. Leenen LP, van der Werken C. Fracture-dislocations of the tarsometatarsal joint, a combined anatomical and computed tomographic study. Injury. 1992;23:51–5.
30. Burroughs KE, Reimer CD, Fields KB. Lisfranc injury of the foot: a commonly missed diagnosis. AFP. 1998;58:118.
31. Goossens M, De Stoop N. Lisfranc's fracture-dislocations: etiology, radiology, and results of treatment. A review of 20 cases. Clin Orthop Relat Res. 1983:154–62.
32. Llopis E, Carrascoso J, Iriarte I, Serrano MP, Cerezal L. Lisfranc injury imaging and surgical management. Semin Musculoskelet Radiol. 2016;20:139–53.
33. Hatem SF. Imaging of lisfranc injury and midfoot sprain. Radiol Clin N Am. 2008;46:1045–60, vi.
34. Vuori JP, Aro HT. Lisfranc joint injuries: trauma mechanisms and associated injuries. J Trauma. 1993;35:40–5.
35. Myerson M. The diagnosis and treatment of injuries to the Lisfranc joint complex. Orthop Clin North Am. 1989;20:655–64.
36. Ho V, Hawkes N, Flemming D. Subtle lisfranc injury: low energy midfoot sprain. Mil Med. 2007;172:6.
37. Meyer SA, Callaghan JJ, Albright JP, Crowley ET, Powell JW. Midfoot sprains in collegiate football players. Am J Sports Med. 1994;22:392–401.
38. Robertson GAJ, Ang KK, Maffulli N, Keenan G, Wood AM. Return to sport following lisfranc injuries: a systematic review and meta-analysis. Foot Ankle Surg. 2019;25:654–64.
39. Mantas JP, Burks RT. Lisfranc injuries in the athlete. Clin Sports Med. 1994;13:719–30.
40. Trevino SG, Kodros S. Controversies in tarsometatarsal injuries. Orthop Clin North Am. 1995;26:229–38.
41. Ly TV, Coetzee JC. Treatment of primarily ligamentous Lisfranc joint injuries: primary arthrodesis compared with open reduction and internal fixation. A prospective, randomized study. J Bone Joint Surg Am. 2006;88:514–20.
42. Arntz CT, Veith RG, Hansen ST. Fractures and fracture-dislocations of the tarsometatarsal joint. J Bone Joint Surg Am. 1988;70:173–81.
43. Deol RS, Roche A, Calder JDF. Return to training and playing after acute lisfranc injuries in elite professional soccer and rugby players. Am J Sports Med. 2016;44:166–70.
44. Lorenz DS, Beauchamp C. Functional progression and return to sport criteria for a high school football player following surgery for a lisfranc injury. Int J Sports Phys Ther. 2013;8:162–71.
45. McHale KJ, Rozell JC, Milby AH, Carey JL, Sennett BJ. Outcomes of lisfranc injuries in the national football league. Am J Sports Med. 2016;44:1810–7.
46. Desmond EA, Chou LB. Current concepts review: lisfranc injuries. Foot Ankle Int. 2006;27:653–60.
47. Rosenbaum AJ, Uhl RL, Dipreta JA. Acute fractures of the tarsal navicular. Orthopedics. 2014;37:541–6.
48. Cronier P, Frin J-M, Steiger V, Bigorre N, Talha A. Internal fixation of complex fractures of the tarsal navicular with locking plates. A report of 10 cases. Orthop Traumatol Surg Res. 2013;99:S241–9.
49. Al-Ashhab MEA. Treatment for displaced navicular body fractures. Egypt Orthop J. 2015;50:63.
50. Ramadorai MUE, Beuchel MW, Sangeorzan BJ. Fractures and dislocations of the tarsal navicular. J Am Acad Orthop Surg. 2016;24:379–89.
51. Khan KM, Brukner PD, Kearney C, Fuller PJ, Bradshaw CJ, Kiss ZS. Tarsal navicular stress fracture in athletes. Sports Med. 1994;17:65–76.
52. Richter M, Wippermann B, Krettek C, Schratt HE, Hufner T, Therman H. Fractures and fracture dislocations of the midfoot: occurrence, causes and long-term results. Foot Ankle Int. 2001;22:392–8.
53. Eichenholtz SN, Levine DB. Fractures of the tarsal navicular bone. Clin Orthop Relat Res. 1964;34:142–57.
54. Pinney SJ, Sangeorzan BJ. Fractures of the tarsal bones. Orthop Clin North Am. 2001;32:21–33.
55. Sangeorzan BJ, Benirschke SK, Mosca V, Mayo KA, Hansen ST. Displaced intra-articular fractures of the tarsal navicular. J Bone Joint Surg Am. 1989;71:1504–10.
56. Torg JS, Moyer J, Gaughan JP, Boden BP. Management of tarsal navicular stress fractures: conservative versus surgical treatment: a meta-analysis. Am J Sports Med. 2010;38:1048–53.
57. Saxena A, Behan SA, Valerio DL, Frosch DL. Navicular stress fracture outcomes in athletes: analysis of 62 injuries. J Foot Ankle Surg. 2017;56:943–8.
58. Evans J, Beingessner DM, Agel J, Benirschke SK. Minifragment plate fixation of high-energy navicular body fractures. Foot Ankle Int. 2011;32:S485–92.
59. Penner MJ. Late reconstruction after navicular fracture. Foot Ankle Clin. 2006;11:105–19, ix.
60. McBryde AM, Anderson RB. Sesamoid foot problems in the athlete. Clin Sports Med. 1988;7:51–60.
61. Sims AL, Kurup HV. Painful sesamoid of the great toe. World J Orthop. 2014;5:146–50.
62. Julsrud ME. Osteonecrosis of the tibial and fibular sesamoids in an aerobics instructor. J Foot Ankle Surg. 1997;36:31–5.
63. Stein CJ, Sugimoto D, Slick NR, Lanois CJ, Dahlberg BW, Zwicker RL, Micheli LJ. Hallux sesamoid fractures in young athletes. Phys Sportsmed. 2019;47:441–7.
64. Imerci A, Aydoğan NH, Gemci C, Topsakal FE. Fracture of the fibular sesamoid bone of the metatarsophalangeal joint of the big toe. J Clin Anal Med. 2018;9:147. https://doi.org/10.4328/jcam.5200.
65. Dedmond BT, Cory JW, McBryde AJ. The hallucal sesamoid complex. J Am Acad Orthop Surg. 2006;14:745.
66. Jahss MH. The sesamoids of the hallux. Clin Orthop Relat Res. 1981:88–97.
67. Richardson EG. Hallucal sesamoid pain: causes and surgical treatment. J Am Acad Orthop Surg. 1999;7:270–8.
68. Brown TI. Avulsion fracture of the fibular sesamoid in association with dorsal dislocation of the metatarsophalangeal joint of the hallux: report of a case and review of the literature. Clin Orthop Relat Res. 1980:229–31.
69. Leventen EO. Sesamoid disorders and treatment. An update. Clin Orthop Relat Res. 1991:236–40.
70. Scranton PE, Rutkowski R. Anatomic variations in the first ray: Part II. Disorders of the sesamoids. Clin Orthop Relat Res. 1980:256–64.
71. Anderson RB, McBryde AM. Autogenous bone grafting of hallux sesamoid nonunions. Foot Ankle Int. 1997;18:293–6.
72. Blundell CM, Nicholson P, Blackney MW. Percutaneous screw fixation for fractures of the sesamoid bones of the hallux. J Bone Joint Surg (Br). 2002;84:1138–41.
73. Petrisor BA, Ekrol I, Court-Brown C. The epidemiology of metatarsal fractures. Foot Ankle Int. 2006;27:172–4.
74. Hatch RL, Alsobrook J, Clugston JR. Diagnosis and management of metatarsal fractures. AFP. 2007;76:817–26.
75. Point-counterpoint: central metatarsal fractures: cut or cast? In: Podiatry Today. https://www.podiatrytoday.com/point-counterpoint-central-metatarsal-fractures-cut-or-cast. Accessed 2 Sep 2019.
76. Bica D, Sprouse RA, Armen J. Diagnosis and management of common foot fractures. AFP. 2016;93:183–91.
77. Rammelt S, Heineck J, Zwipp H. Metatarsal fractures. Injury. 2004;35:77–86.

78. Adelaar RS. Complications of forefoot and midfoot fractures. Clin Orthop Relat Res. 2001;(391):26.
79. Van Vliet-Koppert ST, Cakir H, Van Lieshout EMM, De Vries MR, Van Der Elst M, Schepers T. Demographics and functional outcome of toe fractures. J Foot Ankle Surg. 2011;50:307–10.
80. Eves TB, Oddy MJ. Do broken toes need follow-up in the fracture clinic? J Foot Ankle Surg. 2016;55:488–91.
81. York PJ, Wydra FB, Hunt KJ. Injuries to the great toe. Curr Rev Musculoskelet Med. 2017;10:104–12.
82. Churchill RS, Donley BG. Managing injuries of the great toe. Phys Sportsmed. 1998;26:29–39.
83. Hatch RL, Hacking S. Evaluation and management of toe fractures. Am Fam Physician. 2003;68:2413–8.
84. Nishikawa DRC, Duarte FA, de Cesar NC, Monteiro AC, Albino RB, Fonseca FCP. Internal fixation of displaced intra-articular fractures of the hallux through a dorsomedial approach: a technical tip. Foot Ankle Spec. 2018;11:77–81.
85. Melenevsky Y, Mackey RA, Abrahams RB, Thomson NB. Talar fractures and dislocations: a radiologist's guide to timely diagnosis and classification. RadioGraphics. 2015;35:765–79.
86. Dale JD, Ha AS, Chew FS. Update on talar fracture patterns: a large level I trauma center study. AJR Am J Roentgenol. 2013;201:1087–92.
87. Boack D-H, Manegold S. Peripheral talar fractures. Injury. 2004;35(Suppl 2):SB23–35.
88. Majeed H, McBride DJ. Talar process fractures. EFORT Open Rev. 2018;3:85–92.
89. Mills HJ, Horne G. Fractures of the lateral process of the talus. Aust N Z J Surg. 1987;57:643–6.
90. von Knoch F, Reckord U, von Knoch M, Sommer C. Fracture of the lateral process of the talus in snowboarders. J Bone Jt Surg Br. 2007;89-B:772–7.
91. Bladin C, McCrory P. Snowboarding injuries. An overview. Sports Med. 1995;19:358–64.
92. Whitby EH, Barrington NA. Fractures of the lateral process of the talus--the value of lateral tomography. Br J Radiol. 1995;68:583–6.
93. McCrory P, Bladin C. Fractures of the lateral process of the talus: a clinical review. "Snowboarder's ankle". Clin J Sport Med. 1996;6:124–8.
94. Perera A, Baker JF, Lui DF, Stephens MM. The management and outcome of lateral process fracture of the talus. Foot Ankle Surg. 2010;16:15–20.
95. Veazey BL, Heckman JD, Galindo MJ, McGanity PL. Excision of ununited fractures of the posterior process of the talus: a treatment for chronic posterior ankle pain. Foot Ankle. 1992;13:453–7.
96. Heckman JD, McLean MR. Fractures of the lateral process of the talus. Clin Orthop Relat Res. 1985:108–13.
97. Mitchell MJ, McKinley JC, Robinson CM. The epidemiology of calcaneal fractures. Foot (Edinb). 2009;19:197–200.
98. Graham P. Anterior process fracture of the calcaneus: a case report and discussion. Orthop Nurs. 2016;35:45.
99. Renfrew DL, El-Khoury GY. Anterior process fractures of the calcaneus. Skelet Radiol. 1985;14:121–5.
100. Yu SM, Yu JS. Calcaneal avulsion fractures: an often forgotten diagnosis. Am J Roentgenol. 2015;205:1061–7.
101. Sessa P, Mascarello M. Isolated "nutcracker" fracture of the anterior calcaneal process: do we need a more comprehensive classification for this injury spectrum? A case report. Orthop Surg. 2018;3:3.
102. Robbins MI, Wilson MG, Sella EJ. MR imaging of anterosuperior calcaneal process fractures. Am J Roentgenol. 1999;172:475–9.
103. Fadl SA, Ramzan MM, Sandstrom CK. Core curriculum illustration: anterior process fracture of the calcaneus. Emerg Radiol. 2018;25:205–7.
104. Massen FK, Baumbach SF, Böcker W, Kammerlander C, Herterich V, Polzer H. [Fractures of the anterior process of the calcaneus-frequently overlooked injuries following ankle sprains]. Unfallchirurg. 2018;121:730–8
105. Berkowitz MJ, Kim DH. Process and tubercle fractures of the hindfoot. J Am Acad Orthop Surg. 2005;13:492–502.
106. Mostafa MF, El-Adl G, Hassanin EY, Abdellatif M-S. Surgical treatment of displaced intra-articular calcaneal fracture using a single small lateral approach. Strat Trauma Limb Reconstr. 2010;5:87–95.

Part IV

Acute Fractures in Sport: Spine and Pelvis

Acute Fractures in Sport: Cervical Spine

17

Andrew Platt, Arjang Ahmadpour, and Julian E. Bailes

Learning Objectives

- Describe different classification systems for cervical spine fractures and spinal cord injuries
- Understand different treatment modalities for upper and subaxial cervical spine fractures
- Understand differences between neurogenic shock and spinal shock in terms of treatment options and clinical implications
- Describe preventative measures to prevent spinal cord injury in athletes
- Describe the proper way to identify athletes with presentations concerning for cervical spine injuries and how to evacuate them from the field of play

Although acute cervical spine injuries in sport are rare, physicians caring for athletes in all sports types must maintain a thorough knowledge of the treatment principles of cervical spine injuries in order to potentially prevent otherwise devastating neurological outcomes. Historically, the sports with the greatest risk for vertebral column injuries and spinal cord injury (SCI) are American football, ice hockey, wrestling, diving, skiing, snowboarding, rugby, cheerleading, and baseball [1, 2]. Regional popularity of sports influences the mechanism of injury. In the United States, gymnastics, wrestling, and American football are the most common sports types in which cervical spine injuries occur [3, 4]. In Canada, ice hockey is the sport with the highest incidence of cervical spine injuries [5]. Rugby is the leading cause of cervical spine injuries in Europe [4, 6].

Despite dramatic improvements in safety regulations since the 1970s, cervical spine injuries remain the most common injury type to the axial skeleton in American football players. Less than 1.0% of cervical spine injuries result in SCI or cervical spine fracture [4, 7]. Although the overall incidence of SCIs in American football is rare, the higher popularity of the sport results in a higher overall prevalence [8–10]. An estimated 1.8 million athletes participate in American football per year. Approximately 1.5 million of these participants are in high school, 75,000 are college athletes, and 2000 play at the professional level [10, 11].

This chapter will include a concise description of the epidemiology, contemporary management principles, predicted outcome and preventative measures of sport-related acute fractures of the upper cervical and subaxial cervical spine as well as an examination of sports-related spinal cord injury.

17.1 Upper Cervical Spine Fractures

Upper cervical spine injuries include injuries to the occipital condyles, C1 and C2 vertebrae and ligaments of the cranio-cervical junction.

17.1.1 Epidemiology

Injuries to the upper cervical spine can range from stable fractures to severe fracture dislocations. Overall, upper cervical spine injuries in athletes are rare and occur in only 4.6% of the cervical spine injuries of American football players [4, 12]. Spinal cord injuries in the upper cervical spine can result in quadriplegia, respiratory failure, or sudden death, especially in the setting of atlanto-occipital dislocation (AOD) [13–15]. The stability of the upper cervical spine is mainly due to the strong ligamentous structures and osseous anatomy that forms the occipital condyles, atlas, and axis. The incidence of occipital condyle fractures (OCFs) ranges from 4.0% to 19.0% of all cervical spine injuries [16]. Traumatic atlanto-occipital dislocation (AOD) is associated with a high incidence of neurological morbid-

A. Platt · A. Ahmadpour
Section of Neurosurgery, University of Chicago, Chicago, IL, USA
e-mail: andrew.platt@uchospitals.edu; Arjang.Ahmadpour@uchospitals.edu

J. E. Bailes (✉)
Department of Neurosurgery, NorthShore University HealthSystem, Evanston, IL, USA
e-mail: JBailes@northshore.org

G. A. J. Robertson, N. Maffulli (eds.), *Fractures in Sport*, https://doi.org/10.1007/978-3-030-72036-0_17

ity and mortality [17–22]. Twenty percent to 30% of all cervical spine injury-related deaths are the result of AOD [23, 24]. C1 fractures account for 3.0–13.0% of all cervical spinal injuries [25, 26]. Forty percent to 44% of C1 fractures are associated with fractures of C2 [25]. C2 fractures account for 18.0% of all cervical spine traumatic injuries with odontoid fractures being the most common fracture type in athletes [27–33]. Odontoid process fractures represent approximately 60.0% of C2 fractures. A neurological deficit is seen with 8.5% of C2 fractures, and mortality is associated with 2.4% [34]. Traumatic spondylolisthesis of C2, also known as a hangman's fracture, is due to a bilateral fracture of the C2 pars interarticularis. These injuries account for 4.0–7.0% of all cervical spine fractures and 20.0–22.0% of all C2 fractures [35].

Extreme sports are also a common cause of cervical spine injuries. Sharma et al. identified 78,355 cervical spine injuries in extreme sports between 2000 and 2011 [36]. Motocross and skateboarding composed the largest number of severe head and neck injuries. Cervical spine fractures sustained during motocross accounted for 27.6% of all reported neck fractures in the extreme sports group [36]. Surfing also has a fair amount of cervical spine injuries and carries a 38 times greater risk of suffering a cervical spine fracture than skateboarding [36].

17.1.2 Classification

Various classification systems have been created to aid in management of upper cervical spine injuries. The AO spine classification (*Arbeitsgemeinschaft für Osteosynthesefragen* German for "Association for the Study of Internal Fixation") system separates the upper cervical spine into three sections, the occipital condyle and craniocervical junction, the C1 ring and C1–2 joint, and C2 and the C2–3 joint (Table 17.1) [13, 37]. Injuries are further classified as Type A (bony injury only), Type B (tension band/ligamentous injury), and Type C (translation injuries with specifically translation of the vertebral bodies). Type A injuries are stable and include isolated condyle fractures. The stability of Type B injuries depends on injury specifics whereas Type C injuries are unstable. Modifiers and neurologic status are further applied to the classification system [13, 37, 38].

In regards to occipital condyle fractures, Anderson and Montesano, the most frequently used classification type, classified occipital condyle fractures into three classes (Table 17.2) [39]. Type I occipital condyle fractures occur secondary to axial loading of the skull onto C1 and result in a comminuted fracture of the condyle without significant displacement. Type II occipital condyle fractures result secondary to a direct blow to the skull and are an extension of a fracture of the skull base. Type I and II fractures are usually stable secondary to an intact tectorial and contralateral alar ligament. In the case of a Type II condylar fracture, usually both alar ligaments are intact. Type III occipital condyle fractures can result from rotation, lateral bending, or a combination and lead to an avulsion fracture of the occipital condyle fracture by the alar ligament. Type III fractures are the most concerning and require further testing and evaluation to determine stability [39]. Tuli et al. published a second classification system (Table 17.3) of occipital condyle fractures with a greater emphasis on displacement of the fragments and how that relates to stability [40].

There are several classifications systems to address atlanto-occipital dislocation. The Traynelis classification groups (Table 17.4) traumatic occipitocervical dislocation based on the direction of displacement [18].

Type I involves anterior displacement of the occiput with respect to the atlas. Type II is primarily a longitudinal distraction. Type III atlanto-occipital dislocation results when there is posterior displacement of the occiput on the atlas [18]. The Harborview classification (Table 17.5) includes the

Table 17.1 AO Spine International Upper Cervical Spine fracture classification system

Type	Injury
I: Occipital condyle and craniocervical junction	
IA	Isolated bony injury (condyle)
IB	Non-displaced ligamentous injury (craniocervical)
IC	Any injury with displacement on spinal imaging
II: C1 ring and C1–C2 joint	
IIA	Isolated bony only (arch)
IIB	Ligamentous injury (transverse atlantal ligament)
IIC	Atlantoaxial instability/Translation in any plane
III: C2 and C2–C3 joint	
IIIA	Bony injury only without ligamentous, tension band, disc injury
IIIB	Tension band/Ligamentous injury with or without bony injury
IIIC	Any injury that leads to vertebral body translation in any directional plane

Table 17.2 Anderson and Montesano occipital condyle fracture classification

Type	Description of fracture
I[a]	Non displaced comminuted fracture
IIA[a]	Fracture through skull base extending to condyle
IIB[b]	Fracture through skull base extending to condyle
III[b]	Avulsion fracture of ipsilateral condyle by alar ligament

[a]Stable
[b]Unstable

Table 17.3 Tuli et al. occipital condyle fracture classification

Type	Description of fracture
I	Non-displaced fracture
II	Displaced fracture
IIA	No ligamentous instability
IIB	Ligamentous instability

degree of displacement to classify the level of instability. A Stage 1 injury is defined as a stable minimally or nondisplaced craniocervical injury, and includes unilateral alar ligament avulsion. A Stage 2 injury represents a partially or completely reduced injury which fails a traction test. A Stage 3 injury denotes a highly unstable injury defined by gross craniocervical malalignment [41].

There are three main classification systems for atlas fractures [30, 42, 43]. The Jefferson classification (Table 17.6), classifies fractures as involving the anterior arch, posterior arch, burst fractures, lateral mass fractures, and lateral mass plus posterior arch fractures. The Jefferson classification was originally unnumbered however has been modified and now includes the following classes: Type 1 (an isolated fracture through the anterior or posterior arch), Type 2 (a four part burst fracture through both the anterior and posterior arch), and Type 3 (a lateral mass fracture) [43]. To make matters more confusing, the eponymous "Jefferson Fracture" refers to the type 2 fracture, which is a burst fracture of the atlas. "Jefferson Fractures" are usually secondary to axial loading injuries. The Landells classification follows the same numbering as the modified Jefferson fracture classification. The Gehweiler classification (Table 17.7) classifies atlas fractures into five subtypes. Type I fractures are isolated fractures through the anterior arch. Type II fractures include the posterior arch and are usually bilateral. Type III fractures are bilateral fractures of the posterior arch with an associated unilateral or bilateral anterior arch fracture, synonymous with a "Jefferson Fracture" or type 2 fracture. Type III fractures are felt to be more unstable in the setting of transverse atlantal ligament (TAL) disruption and are referred to as type IIIb fractures. Type IV fractures are lateral mass fractures. Type V are isolated fractures of the transverse process [30, 43]. Any injury to C1 requires evaluation of the traverse atlantal ligament as it is required for C1 stability. The Dickman classification assesses TAL integrity. A central TAL rupture is classified as a Type I injury whereas a bony avulsion of the transverse ligament from the lateral mass is a Type II injury [43].

Axis fractures are classified by two main classification systems, one for fractures of the odontoid and a second for fractures of the pars. The classification system for odontoid fractures was defined by Anderson and D'Alonzo (Table 17.8). Type I odontoid fractures are the rarest and involve an isolated odontoid tip fracture. Type II fractures are the most common and involves the base of the odontoid process tip. Type IIA fractures include a comminuted fracture associated with a Type II fracture. Type IIA fractures account for approximately 5.0% of odontoid fractures. One third of all odontoid fractures are Type III fractures. Type III fractures involve a fracture that extends through the C2 vertebral body [27–29]. In regards to C2 pars fractures (hangman's fractures) the Levine-Edwards modification of the Effendi (Table 17.9) classification system is the most used classification system, and classifies fractures based on the mechanism of injury. Type I fractures are the only fractures to result from a predominantly extension mediated injury and are usually stable. Type II fractures result from a combined extension

Table 17.4 Traynelis atlanto-occipital dislocation classification

AOD type	Description of dislocation
I	Anterior displacement of the occiput with respect to the atlas
II	Longitudinal distraction with separation of the occiput from the atlas
III	Posterior displacement of the occiput on the atlas

AOD atlanto-occipital dislocation

Table 17.5 Harborview classification of craniocervical injuries

Stage	Description of injury
1	MRI evidence of injury to craniocervical osseoligamentous stabilizers; craniocervical alignment within 2 mm of normal; distraction of ≤2 mm on provocative traction radiography
2	MRI evidence of injury to craniocervical osseoligamentous stabilizers; craniocervical alignment within 2 mm of normal; distraction of >2 mm on provocative traction radiography.
3	Craniocervical malalignment of >2 mm on static radiography

Table 17.6 Jefferson classification of atlas fractures

Type	Description of fracture
I	An isolated fracture through the anterior or posterior arch.
II	A four-part burst fracture through both the anterior and posterior arch
III	A lateral mass fracture

Table 17.7 Gehweiler classification of atlas fractures

Type	Description of fracture
I	Isolated fractures through the anterior arch
II	Fractures include the posterior arch and are usually bilateral
IIIA[a]	Bilateral fractures of the posterior arch with an associated unilateral or bilateral anterior arch fracture
IIIB[b]	Bilateral fractures of the posterior arch with an associated unilateral or bilateral anterior arch fracture with disruption of the traverse atlantal ligament
IV	Lateral mass fractures
V	Isolated fractures of the transverse process

[a]Stable
[b]Unstable

Table 17.8 Anderson and D'Alonzo classification of odontoid fractures

Type	Description of fracture
I	Isolated odontoid tip fracture
II	Fracture through the base of the dens
IIA	Comminuted fracture associated with a Type II fracture
III	Fracture extends through the C2 vertebral body

Table 17.9 Levine and Edwards classification of *hangman fractures of C2*[a]

Type	Description of fracture
I	Fracture with <3 mm antero-posterior deviation without angular deviation
II[b]	Fracture with >3 mm antero-posterior deviation with significant angular deviation and disruption of the posterior longitudinal ligament
IIA[b]	Fracture line is horizontal with significant angular deviation without anterior translation
III[b]	Type II fracture with bilateral C2–3 facet joint dislocation

[a]Also referred to as traumatic spondylolisthesis of the axis
[b]Unstable fractures

and flexion injury, whereas Type IIa and Type III fractures result from a predominantly flexion mediated injury. Type II, IIa, and III fractures are unstable secondary to involvement of the C2–3 disc and anterior/posterior longitudinal ligament [35, 44].

17.1.3 Diagnosis (History/Physical Exam/Radiological Investigations)

Please see Sect. 17.3.3 for a discussion of on-field management, evacuation, and initial evaluation of athletes with concern for spinal injury. Many academic Level I trauma centers have individualized cervical spine clearance protocols. Not all patients require radiologic investigations. If there is low concern for a spinal injury, and the athlete is awake, neurologically non-altered, asymptomatic, without neck pain or tenderness, with a normal neurologic examination, and a lack of distracting injuries, the patient can be cleared of cervical spinal precautions without a radiologic evaluation if they are able to complete functional range of motion (flexion, extension, lateral rotation, lateral bending) [45–47]. It is our practice to always get at least cervical spine X-Rays in pediatric patients.

In awake, symptomatic patients, the imaging modality of choice for identification of a cervical spine fractures is a high definition computed tomography (CT) scan [45–47]. CT measures density and is the best imaging modality for identifying osseous injuries. American football helmets and shoulder pads have been shown to interfere with adequate imaging of the cervical spine, particularly at the cervicothoracic junction and should be removed prior to scanning [11]. The process of removing equipment is complicated and requires multiple clinicians to both remove equipment and hold strict spinal precautions in a specific and coordinated way avoiding any malalignment or manipulation of the head and neck [46]. If there is concern for ligamentous or soft tissue injury, acute disc herniation, or epidural hematoma, magnetic resonance imaging (MRI) is also ascertained. If there is evidence of ligamentous injury by MRI, and it is unclear whether a patient is unstable, flexion/extension X-Rays can be ascertained: however, these should not be done in an obtunded patient [45]. Patients with fractures involving a foramen transversarium or any significant displacement should also have a CT-Angiogram or MR-Angiogram to assess the vertebral arteries and for preoperative planning.

17.1.4 Treatment

In the upper cervical spine, since there are multiple types of fractures and injuries, the treatment of choice is usually predicated by the location and degree of injury. Treatment of upper cervical fractures can be divided into three main categories, collar placement, halo placement, and operative fixation and fusion. Operative fixation and fusion is almost always carried out in a posterior fashion. Placement of an anterior odontoid screw is possible in patients with Type II dens fractures however is uncommonly performed in athletes. Indications for halo vest placement include C1 Jefferson (burst) fractures, Type II hangman's fractures, Type II and III odontoid fractures, C2 comminuted fractures, and combinations of C1 and C2 fractures [48].

Nearly all occipital condyle fractures, without associated ligamentous injury, can be managed without internal fixation [15]. A recent review of occipital condyle fractures recommended getting magnetic resonance imaging (MRI) to assess the integrity of the craniocervical ligaments [49]. They further recommended external cervical immobilisation for all types of OCFs with consideration of halo vest placement with bilateral OCF's patients with associated atlanto-occipital ligamentous disruption should be treated with occipitocervical fusion or halo placement [49].

For treatment of atlanto-occipital dissociation, according to the Harborview classification, stage 1 injuries can be managed non-operatively whereas stage 2 and 3 injuries require internal fixation [41]. Historically, we do not place patients with concern for AOD in traction, nor do we rely on orthoses for cervical stabilization. We favor halo placement only as a temporary intervention until occipital-cervical fixation can be carried out. Bellabarba et al. in a case series of 17 patients with AOD performed operative fixation on all patients [41]. Of 13 patients with incomplete spinal cord injury preoperatively, 85.0% improved by at least one ASIA grade [41].

The treatment of atlas fractures is controversial. Kandziora et al. recommend cervical spine immobilisation with a soft collar for 6 weeks for Gehweiler Types 1, 2, and 5 [43]. For Gehweiler type 3a fractures without TAL injury, they recommend rigid collar immobilisation. For type 3b fractures with Dickman Type II TAL injuries Kandziora et al. recommend direct osteosynthesis of the atlas or halo placement for 6–12 weeks. For type 3b fractures with a Dickman Type I TAL injury they recommend C1–2 fusion [43].

Odontoid fractures, Type I and III, are typically treated with rigid external immobilisation. There is a 97.0% fusion rate in a halo vest for Type III fractures. Type II odontoid fractures are associated with a nonunion rate of up to 40.0% when treated with external immobilisation alone. Type II fractures with less than 5 mm of dens displacement are appropriate candidates for stabilization with a halo. The rate of failure associated with external immobilisation alone for Type II fractures with more than 5 mm of dens displacement is greater than 86.0%; these fractures should be addressed surgically [27–33]. In a recent systematic review of patients with C2 pars fractures (hangman's fractures), Murphy et al. showed the most commonly used method of nonsurgical treatment was the halo vest (15.7%), followed by Minerva jacket and hard collar (8.2%) [35]. The remaining patients were treated surgically. The authors found the chance of non-union to be lower in surgically treated patients without a difference in the mortality rate [35].

17.1.5 Complications

The incidence of complications with halo vest treatment varies widely in the literature, ranging from 11.0% to 92.0% (mostly in 30.0–50.0% range), with the majority classified as "minor" complications [48]. A review by Lee et al. found that pin loosening, pin site infection, and spinal instability were the most common complications related to halo vest immobilisation and found that pin site infection significantly correlated to pin penetration of the cranial outer table [48]. Advanced age is classically felt to be a contraindication to halo placement, however, data supporting this is inconclusive and contradictory [48, 50–53]. In a case-control study of patients with Type II dens fractures after halo placement, Lennarson et al. found that age more than 50 years was a highly significant risk factor for failure of halo immobilisation and that the risk of failure of halo immobilisation is 21 times higher in patients aged 50 years or more [26].

In regards to C2 pars fractures treated with nonsurgical intervention, Murphy et al. in a systematic review found no difference in union rate, mortality rate, treatment failure, or complications between patients treated with a rigid cervical orthosis versus a halo vest [35]. In regards to surgical intervention they also found no difference in union rate, mortality rate, treatment failure, or complications between ACDF, posterior fusion, and combined anterior-posterior fusion [35].

17.1.6 Rehabilitation

Please see Sect. 17.3.6 for a discussion of rehabilitation in patients with spinal cord injuries.

17.1.7 Preventative Measures

Please see Sect. 17.3.7 for a discussion of preventative measures in sport to prevent cervical spine injury.

17.2 Subaxial Cervical Spine Fractures

17.2.1 Epidemiology

The subaxial spine includes levels C3–C7. The C3 vertebra is an uncommon location for an isolated injury and accounts for less than 1.0% of all cervical spine injuries. Isolated C3 fractures may be relatively protected from injury because it is situated between the two more vulnerable areas of the C1–C2 complex and C5–C6 complex [27, 32, 54]. The most common level of cervical vertebral fracture is C5 and the most common level of subluxation injury is the C5–C6 interspace [27, 54]. Vertebral body fractures are the most common type of injury to occur in the subaxial cervical spine and when associated with subluxation result in high incidence of spinal cord injury [31, 55, 56]. Facet dislocations account for approximately 10.0% of all subaxial cervical spine fractures, which can be unilateral or bilateral [57]. Bilateral facet dislocations have a nearly 100% incidence of neurological injury, and those with unilateral facet dislocations have an incidence of 80.0% of neurological injury [31].

17.2.2 Classification

One of the first classifications systems for subaxial cervical spine fractures is the Allen and Ferguson classification which stratifies fractures by the mechanism of injury into six categories: compression-flexion, vertical compression, distraction-flexion, compression-extension, distraction-extension and lateral flexion [57, 58]. Facet dislocations are classified as distraction-flexion injuries.

Two more recent classification systems for subaxial cervical spine fractures are the AO Spine subaxial classification system (Table 17.10), and the Sub-axial Injury Classification (SLIC) and Severity Scale (Table 17.11). The AO Spine subaxial classification system classifies injuries into three main classes Type A (compression injuries), Type B (tension band injuries), and Type C (translation injuries) [59, 60]. Type A

Table 17.10 AO Spine subaxial cervical spine injury classification

Type	Injury
Type A: Compression injuries with integrity of the posterior tension band	
Without posterior wall involvement	
A0	Minor injury (fracture of the spinous or transverse process)
A1	Compression fracture involving a single endplate
A2	Split (or pincer) type fracture involving both endplates
Posterior wall involvement (Burst fractures)	
A3	Burst fracture of a single endplate
A4	Fracture of both endplates
Type B: Anterior or posterior tension band injury	
B1	Transosseous disruption of posterior tension band
B2	Ligamentous disruption of posterior tension band; with or without osseous involvement
B3	Disruption of the anterior tension band with an intact posterior tension band
Type C: Displacement/translational injury	
C	Displacement of the cranial and caudal portions of the spinal column in any plane
Type F: Facet joint complex injury	
F1	Non-displaced facet fracture (fracture fragment <1 cm)
F2	Facet fracture with potential for instability
F3	Floating lateral mass
F4	Pathologic subluxation or perched/dislocated facet

Table 17.11 The Sub-axial Injury Classification (SLIC) and severity scale

Sub-axial injury classification scale	Points
Morphology	
No abnormality	0
Compression	1
Burst	2
Distraction	3
Rotation/Translation	4
Disco-ligamentous complex (DLC)	
Intact	0
Indeterminate	1
Disrupted	2
Neurological status	0
Intact	0
Root injury	1
Complete cord injury	2
Incomplete cord injury	3
Continuous cord compression with neurological deficit	+1

injuries are further classified according to the amount of the vertebral body involvement with the most severe fracture being a complete burst (A4) [60]. A separate category Type F, is used to describe injuries isolated to the facet. As with the upper cervical spine classification system, injury modifiers and neurologic status are further applied to the final classification [60]. The Sub-axial Injury Classification (SLIC) and Severity Scale grades injuries according to fracture morphology, status of the disco-ligamentous complex, and neurologic status [61]. The scoring system is used to suggest surgical vs. non-surgical treatment with a score of 5 or greater being the cutoff for surgical management [61]. Clay Shoveler's fractures are avulsion fractures of the spinous processes of the cervical spine caused by hyperflexion. They are named for the workers who would sustain stress injuries from the overhead rotational forces required to throw clay with a long shovel out of a clay pit. These fractures are usually stable and do not require further intervention as long as other occult fractures are ruled out [62].

17.2.3 Diagnosis (History/Physical Exam/Radiological Investigations)

Please see Sect. 17.3.3 for a discussion of on-field management, evacuation, and initial evaluation of athletes with concern for spinal injury, and Sect. 17.1.3 for a discussion on radiologic investigations that should be performed in athletes with concern for cervical spine injuries.

With injuries in the subaxial cervical spine, clinicians should also be cognizant about recognizing patients with ankylosed spines. Persons with ankylosing spondylitis or diffuse idiopathic skeletal hyperostosis can suffer catastrophic neurologic injuries from spinal injuries caused by low-energy trauma that may be missed in the initial emergency evaluation [47]. Although less common in young patients who are typically involved in athletics, patients with ankylosed spines require advanced imaging evaluation including CT or MRI prior to clearance [47].

17.2.4 Treatment

In the subaxial cervical spine, the treatment of choice is usually predicated by the type of injury. Treatment of subaxial cervical fractures can be divided into three main categories, reduction, operative fixation and fusion and collar placement. Halo placement is less common in subaxial injuries than in the upper cervical spine.

For treatment of facet dislocations, intervention is carried out in two stages: first reduction, which can be performed closed with traction or surgically, and second internal fixation, both of which can be performed by an anterior or posterior approach (Fig. 17.1) [57]. Timing of closed reduction and whether or not to get a MRI prior to reduction is controversial [47, 57]. Studies have shown that early reduction is more likely to successfully reduce the patient and may be associated with improved neurologic outcomes [63, 64]. As previously mentioned, a MRI is helpful if there is concern for ligamentous or soft tissue injury, acute disc herniation, or epidural hematoma. Obtaining a MRI may take a significant amount of time to coordinate and requires increased mobilization of the patient into and out of the scanner that could

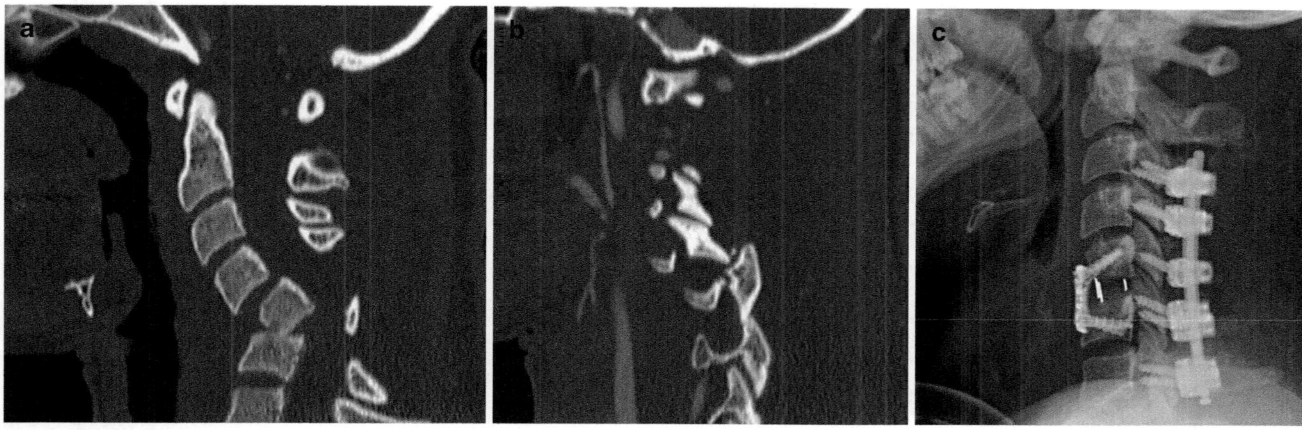

Fig. 17.1 (**a, b**) Preoperative sagittal Computerized Tomography (CT) image of a patient with a traumatic three column cervical spine injury. (**c**) Post-operative lateral cervical spine X-ray. The patient underwent initial traction for reduction, then a staged anterior cervical discectomy and fusion, followed by a posterior cervical decompressive laminectomy and instrumented fusion

potentially be avoided. The reasoning for a MRI prior to reduction is that a large disc herniation may injure the spinal cord during reduction if it is carried out prior to decompression. Some experts have recommended a MRI prior to reduction unless a patient has a near complete neurologic injury while others prefer immediate closed reduction prior to a MRI in any patient who is awake and alert [65, 66].

In terms of choosing an anterior or posterior approach each approach has advantages and disadvantages. The anterior approach which includes an anterior discectomy and fusion (Fig. 17.2) or anterior corpectomy and fusion has advantages of being able to directly decompress a disc extrusion and not needing to flip a patient with an unstable spine from supine to prone position. The posterior approach has the advantage of being able to directly address the facet dislocation as the facet is easily exposed. A recent meta-analysis of two randomized controlled trials, although hindered by limited and poor quality of evidence, found no significant difference in long-term neurological status, pain or patient-reported quality of life between the anterior and posterior approach [57, 67, 68].

Burst fractures of the subaxial spine can be associated with retropulsion of disc or osseous materials into the spinal cord however can be treated surgically or with collar immobilisation depending on neurologic status, integrity of the posterior ligamentous complex, and other factors [4, 61]. Athletes who sustain burst fractures and are treated with collar immobilisation should be closely watched for development of a kyphotic deformity, especially in athletes who sustain C7 burst fractures [4]. Flexion tear drop injuries, flexion-compression injuries in which the posterior tension band is disrupted and there is simultaneous compression and fracture of the vertebral body, present with a high likelihood of spinal cord injury and almost always require surgical stabilization [4, 9]. Injuries to the anterior tension band (distraction-extension injuries) are more rare in athletes than flexion-mediated injuries, however, can present with significant neurologic injury and almost always require surgical intervention, especially if there is a translational component [4].

17.2.5 Complications

In regards to athletes undergoing anterior cervical fusion, Maroon et al. reported that among 15 patients, 13 (86.7%) returned to play at an average time of 6 months (range 2–12 months) [69]. Of all patients undergoing anterior cervical discectomy and fusion, morbidity rates range from 13.2% to 19.3% with dysphagia (1.7–9.5%) and postoperative hematoma (0.4–5.6%) being the most common [70]. The pseudoarthrosis rate after anterior cervical discectomy and fusion is largely dependent on the number of levels fused. The reoperation rate after ACDF is 11.1% [70]. In a recent systematic review of patients undergoing posterior cervical decompression and fusion, Youssef et al. reported 98.3% of patients had successful fusion whereas 1.1% of patients required revision and 9.0% of patients had complications or adverse events (with axial pain, C5 nerve palsy, transient neurologic worsening and wound infection most commonly) [71].

17.2.6 Rehabilitation

Please see Sect. 17.3.6 for a discussion of rehabilitation in patients with spinal cord injuries. In regards to athletes undergoing anterior cervical fusion; Maroon et al. reported advancing patients with progressive ambulation and light exercise within the first week. They reported increasing lower extremity exercise (stationary bike, treadmill, elliptical machine) as well as light weights in the second week,

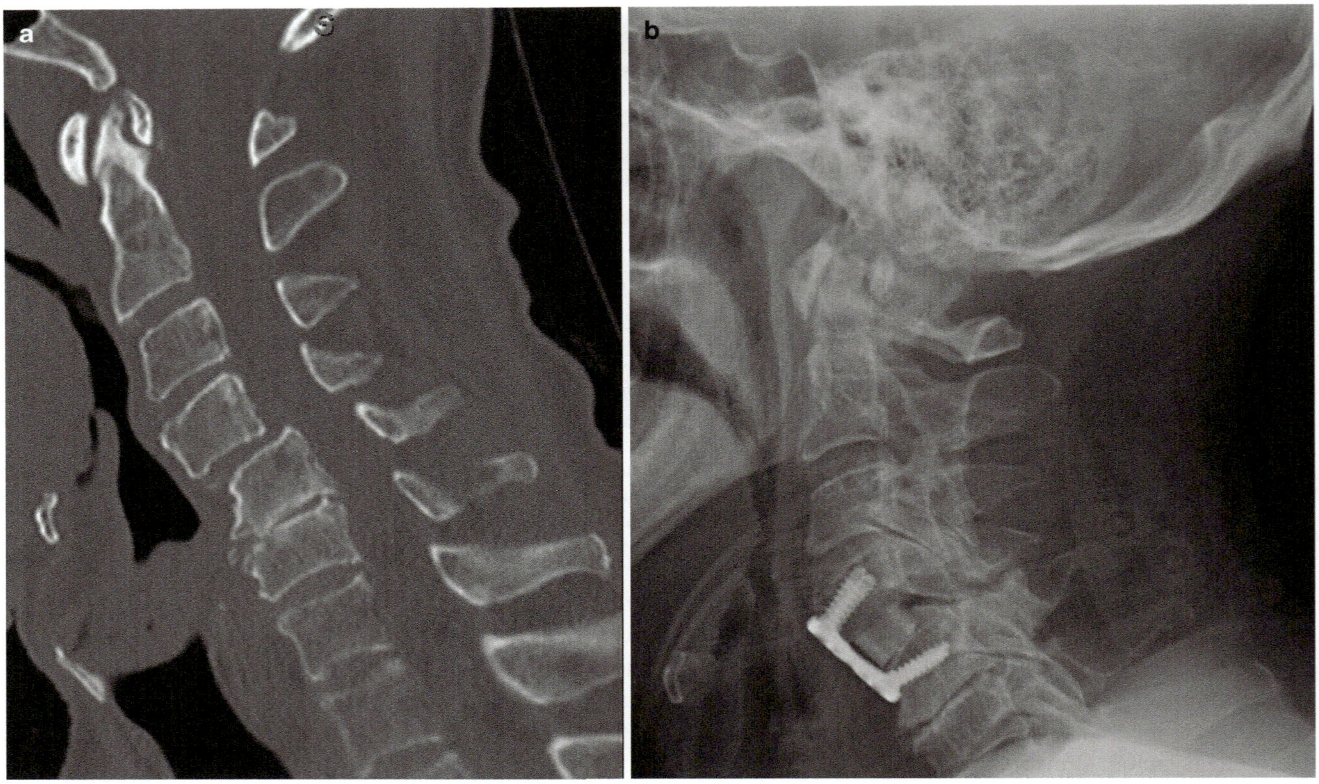

Fig. 17.2 A patient with a grade 2, C4–C5 cervical spondylolisthesis. (**a**) before and (**b**) after a C4–C5 anterior cervical discectomy and fusion

followed by progressive weight training with a focus on flexibility and endurance in the third week. During the fourth week postoperatively, they reported advancing athletes to full aerobic exercise and weight training at 50.0% of their preoperative capability [69]. Maroon et al. further reported allowing athletes to return to light contact drills with full return of neurologic function and demonstration of arthrodesis and return to full contact after multi-disciplinary (surgeon, athlete, trainer, etc.) approval [69].

Studies have evaluated return to play after athletes have undergone cervical fusion. Although the fusions were mostly performed for cervical spondylosis (degeneration) and not after fractures, the implications are important. Maroon et al. evaluated 15 professional athletes who had undergone a 1-level fusion in the subaxial spine from an anterior approach. Athletes were cleared for return to play after a normal neurological examination and radiographic appearance of early fusion. All patients in the study were cleared for return to play; 13/15 players returned at on average 6 months (range 2–12 months) [69]. Mai et al. published a retrospective case series of 101 professional athletes who had undergone anterior fusion, posterior fusion, and cervical total disc replacement. They found that patients undergoing posterior fusion had a significantly higher rate of return to play and shorter time to return after surgery, however, had a higher rate of index level reoperation than patients undergoing ACDF [72].

17.2.7 Preventative Measures

Please see Sect. 17.3.7 for a discussion of preventative measures in sport to prevent cervical spine injury.

17.3 Spinal Cord Injury

17.3.1 Epidemiology

Spinal cord injuries (SCI) in athletes are rare; 2.4% of hospitalizations caused by sports injuries are related to SCI [4, 73]. Despite increased protective measures for athletes in the modern era, 8.7–9.2% of all SCIs sustained in the United States are acquired during athletic activity [2, 4]. Hyperflexion injury is the most common cause of serious cervical injuries [74–77]. Although American football is associated with a higher number of catastrophic neck injuries, Canadian ice hockey players suffer spinal cord injuries at three times the annual incidence of American football players [10, 11, 78].

Cantu et al. analyzed catastrophic spine injuries in American football from 1977 to 2001 and found that 223 football players sustained a catastrophic cervical spine injury with incomplete or no recovery [8]. These injuries occurred in 183 high school athletes, 29 college athletes, and seven professional athletes, with resultant incidence rates for catastrophic spine injury per 100,000 participants over the past 25 years of 0.52 in high school, 1.55 in college, and 14 in professional football [8, 9]. In a study evaluating severe injuries in NCAA sports, head and neck injuries account for 11.2% of all injuries [79].

17.3.2 Classification

Cervical spinal cord trauma may result in a variety of clinical syndromes depending on the type and severity of the impact and bony displacement as well as the subsequent secondary insults such as hemorrhage, ischemia, and edema [80]. Complete spinal cord injury, as the name implies, results in a complete loss of function below the level of injury, these injuries are rarely reversible. Central cord syndrome includes an incomplete loss of motor function with a greater impact on the upper extremities compared with the lower extremities. This condition is thought to be the result of hemorrhagic and/or ischemic injury to the corticospinal tracts related to their somatotopic arrangement [80]. Fibers of cervical nerves that innervate the upper extremities are arranged more medially than those innervating the lower extremities and are more susceptible to ischemic phenomenon. American Football players can present with a mild form of central cord syndrome called "Burning Hands Syndrome" [81]. Central cord syndrome carries a good prognosis in terms of recovering at least some function after injury. In some cases, total functional recovery is experienced [80].

Anterior spinal cord syndrome describes an injury that occurs to the anterior two thirds of the spinal cord in the region supplied by the anterior spinal artery [80]. The neurologic deficit consists of a complete loss of all motor function below the level of injury, with loss of sensation conveyed by the spinothalamic tracts (STT) (pain and temperature) [80]. Upper and lower extremity function is more equally affected than in central cord syndrome as is sphincteric and sexual dysfunction. Dorsal column-medial lemniscus (DC-ML) tracts which convey proprioception, light touch, and vibration may be preserved. Brown-Sequard syndrome consists of a spinal cord hemisection and includes ipsilateral motor loss below the lesion, ipsilateral sensory loss (DC-ML) and contralateral STT loss. Posterior spinal cord syndromes are rare, and can cause isolated sensory deficits.

The most common classification system used for spinal cord injuries is the American Spine Injury Association (ASIA) impairment scale (AIS) which grades spinal cord injuries using the International Standards for Neurological Classification of Spinal Cord Injury (ISNCSCI) worksheet.

Patients in whom no motor or sensory function is preserved in the lowest sacral segments (S4–S5) are deemed to be AIS A. Patients with sensory sparing in the lowest sacral segments with no motor function are AIS B. Patients with preserved motor function below the neurologic level, with the majority of myotomes having a muscle grade of 2 or less, are AIS C, whereas those with a muscle grade of 3 or more in half or more of muscle groups are AIS D. Patients with normal motor and sensory function are considered to be AIS E [47, 82, 83]. The athlete must be assessed for spinal shock prior to being graded for the level of spinal cord injury. Spinal shock is distinct from neurogenic shock, and is defined as the temporary physiologic state of the acutely traumatized spinal cord, manifested by the transient absence of reflexive function distal to spinal cord injury [47]. Patients cannot be actively graded for their degree of spinal cord injury until spinal shocks resolves which can be between 24 and 48 h after injury. The end of spinal shock is normally is signaled by the return of the bulbocavernosus reflex.

Bailes et al. [3] classified cervical spine injuries in athletes into three categories. Type 1 injuries result in neurologic injury and preclude patients from returning to contact play. Type 2 injuries consist of transient neurological deficits without radiological abnormalities and do not prohibit further participation in contact sports unless they become repetitive. Type 3 injuries are those that cause a radiological abnormality however no neurologic injury [3, 84].

The importance of accurately grading degree of spinal cord injury at initial assessment is that it highly predicts ability for neurologic recovery. Fisher et al. followed the neurologic outcomes of 70 patients with spinal injury. After an unobstructed neurologic examination following the return of the bulbocavernosus reflex, these patients were confirmed to have complete spinal cord injuries (AIS A). Two years post injury, none of the 70 patient recovered distal lower extremity motor function [85]. Incomplete spinal cord injuries carries a significantly better prognosis. Roughly half of patients with AIS B injuries will regain enough lower extremity strength to become ambulatory whereas approximately three quarters of patients with AIS C injuries will become ambulatory and virtually all patients who are graded AIS D will regain their pre-injury lower extremity strength and become ambulatory [47, 86].

Burners/stingers are fairly common injuries in athletes and are characterized by self-resolving sudden pain and paresthesia in a single extremity that often is non-dermatomal [4]. They are felt to be related to stretch injury of the upper trunk of the brachial plexus, foraminal compression of exiting cervical nerve roots, or direct supraclavicular trauma [4, 46]. Athletes who feel burners/stingers should be evaluated with a full neurologic workup and may be limited from return to play after multiple episodes [4]. Most importantly, athletes with burners/stingers should have transient cervical cord neuropraxia ruled out prior to return to play. Repetitive brachial plexus or cervical root injuries can lead to permanent neurologic deficits and force retirement for athletes.

Athletes with transient spinal cord injury (TSCI) most commonly present with quadriplegia with sensory deficits which resolve within 15–30 min or may last up to 48 h prior to resolution [87]. In a study of ten patients presenting after TSCI, Bailes et al. found evidence of spinal stenosis at three or more levels in all patients. Spinal stenosis, especially in the sagittal dimension, can cause an increased risk of SCI due to less available space to accommodate excursions of the spinal cord after elongation, compression, or momentary impingement [87].

17.3.3 Diagnosis (History/Physical Exam/ Radiological Investigations)

The first moments after a spinal injury are pivotal. If there is any concern for a spinal or cranial injury to an athlete all play must be immediately stopped so that the concerning player can be assessed. With aquatic sports such as swimming, diving, or water polo the player must be carefully removed from the pool with careful attention to maintenance of cervical spine precautions and immobilisation [88]. During the on-field primary assessment, if a player is found to be unresponsive, the Emergency Medical Services (EMS) should be contacted while a simultaneous assessment of respiratory/ cardiac function occurs following Basic Life Support (BLS) guidelines [46]. With upper spinal cord injury involving C3–5 there is concern for diaphragmatic dysfunction which may necessitate bag valve mask ventilation or intubation by qualified personnel. Strict cervical spine precautions must be maintained at all times and a jaw thrust can be used to open the airway. Once the primary survey is complete a secondary survey including a brief neurologic exam should take place. Any athlete that is unconscious, has a neurologic deficit, or is complaining of neurologic symptomatology such as neck pain, numbness/tingling/weakness in arms or legs should be treated as if he or she has a cervical spine fracture, stabilized and transported for further testing and diagnosis [80].

Prior to movement of the player off the field the athlete should be properly secured to a rigid spine board in such a way that the spine is immobilized, and the airway is accessible [89]. If necessary, this involves multiple people "log-rolling" the patient with maintenance of strict spinal precautions. All athletic gear including helmets and pads should be left on. If the athlete is wearing a facemask this should be disconnected from the helmet to allow access to the airway. When the patient is being cared for by experienced medical professionals who can hold the cervical spine steady, the helmet may be gently removed, and the pads cut off and removed while maintaining strict spinal precautions. A cervical collar can be placed or if obstructed from helmet or athletic gear foam blocks or sandbags can be placed on each side of the head with tape or elastic straps to then secure the head, blocks, and backboard in place [4, 46, 80].

Once the athlete arrives in the emergency department the primary and secondary survey are again repeated. The patient should be assessed by the Glasgow Coma Scale (GCS) and with a cranial nerve, musculoskeletal, sensory, and rectal exam. With maintenance of strict spine precautions the entire spine should be palpated for tenderness, "step-offs" or any other abnormalities [46]. If the patient is deemed to be stable for imaging by the emergency room physician or trauma surgeon, a computed tomography scan of the cervical spine is the initial imaging modality of choice if there is concern for a cervical spinal injury. CT of the thoracic or lumbar spine should be done if there is concern for injury to those areas. If there is any concern for a spinal cord injury or any abnormality on neurologic examination or imaging, a spine consultation (neurosurgery or orthopedic spine surgery) should be immediately placed.

Once the spinal consultant arrives to examine the patient a repeat focused neurologic and musculoskeletal examination takes place. This includes a reassessment of GCS, cranial nerve function, and a musculoskeletal examination. A rectal examination must be performed to test for perianal sensation, rectal tone (both passive and voluntary), and bulbocavernosus reflex. A patient without a bulbocavernosus reflex may be in spinal shock. In order to accurately grade a patient as AIS A, a patient must be out of spinal shock, and active rectal tone must be absent.

17.3.4 Treatment

The principles of treatment of spinal cord injury include decompression/stabilization, and prevention of secondary injury. For decompression/stabilization please see Sects. 17.1.4 and 17.2.4. Several strategies have been previously tried to minimize secondary injury including blood pressure augmentation, therapeutic hypothermia, anti-inflammatory medications including steroids, and agents to promote plasticity and axonal regeneration; however many have failed to be effective or are still purely investigational [90].

In terms of blood pressure augmentation, guidelines of the American Association of Neurological Surgeons/ Congress of Neurological Surgeons (AANS/CNS) Joint Section on Spine and Peripheral Nerves advise correcting hypotension and maintaining a mean arterial pressure (MAP) goal of 85–90 mmHg for 7 days post injury [90–92]. The data for blood pressure augmentation is mainly from retrospective case series without comparative groups [90]. In a systematic review of the literature, Saadeh et al. identified only one comparative study that showed a benefit of keeping MAP >85 at all times for 5 days after injury [90, 93]. A difficulty of maintaining MAP >85 in athletes presenting after cervical spine injuries is that patients may present in neurogenic shock a syndrome of hypotension and bradycardia secondary to loss of sympathetic tone to vasculature. Fluids can be used to replace losses however the treatment for neurogenic shock is vasopressors. Previously the recommendation for patients in neurogenic shock has been to give dopamine or norepinephrine due to both alpha and beta adrenergic effect [46, 90].

Timing of surgical intervention after cervical spinal cord injury is another controversial topic. In a multicenter, prospective, cohort study, the Surgical Timing in Acute Spinal Cord Injury Study (STASCIS) compared patients undergoing decompression prior to and after 24 h, and found patient undergoing early decompression had significantly improved neurologic outcome, defined as at least a 2 grade AIS improvement at 6 months follow-up [94]. The most recent spinal cord injury guidelines from the AANS/CNS, however, reported that since methodological flaws downgraded the study from Class II to III evidence, it is unhelpful for establishing quality and certainty in the case of acute surgical intervention in spinal cord injury [91]. A recommendation regarding the use of systemic hypothermia was also left out of the most recent guidelines due to insufficient evidence [91]. The most controversial intervention in spinal cord injury is without a doubt the use of steroids which is now not recommended [91].

17.3.5 Complications

Management of acute spinal cord injury is complicated by broad pathophysiologic derangements in nearly every organ system [95, 96]. Neurologic complications of spinal cord injury include neuropathic pain, spasticity, and mood/adjustment disorders [95]. In terms of cardiovascular complications, patients with spinal cord injuries can present with neurogenic shock necessitating vasopressor treatment for several days. In addition to frequent vital and laboratory checks, echocardiography and pulmonary catheter placement may aid treatment [96]. Within 3–5 days of injury, patients may also develop severe cardiac arrhythmias such as bradycardia, supraventricular tachycardia, or ventricular tachycardia. Estimates of cardiac arrest following cervical spinal cord injuries are as high as 15.0% [96]. More chronically, patients may develop orthostatic hypotension and autonomic dysreflexia. Pulmonary complications include a compromised cough/stiff chest wall, atelectasis, risk of aspiration and pneumonia [95]. Gastrointestinal and genitourinary complications include constipation (decreased gut motility), bladder spasticity, detrusor-sphincter dyssnergia, urinary retention, urinary tract infections, and erectile dysfunctions [95]. Patients are at high risk of development of pressure ulcers both acutely from immobilisation and use of a backboard and chronically secondary to restricted movement [47, 89, 95]. Thromboembolic complications are prevalent after spinal cord injury with an incidence as high as 81–100%, with the most significant risk occurring between 72 h and 2 weeks following injury [95, 96]. Patients may benefit from early usage of mechanical and chemical thromboprophylaxis or placement of inferior vena cava filters.

17.3.6 Rehabilitation

Patients with spinal cord injuries should be discharged to inpatient rehabilitation centers as soon as they are medically fit for transfer. If available, inpatient rehabilitation centers that specialize in recovery of patients with spinal cord injuries should be sought out. Acute inpatient rehabilitation in spinal cord injury focuses mainly on development of functional compensatory changes so that patients may be safely discharged back to the community [95]. There is little evidence to provide guidelines on specific treatment approaches for specific patient profiles in rehabilitation of spinal cord injury patients [95].

In terms of rehabilitation in patients specifically with central cord syndromes, Tow et al. reported in 73 spinal cord injured patients with central cord syndrome that patients after inpatient rehabilitation showed significant improvements in the admission/discharge ASIA motor scores and Modified Barthel Index (MBI) scores and reported that 92.0.0 of patients were continent of bladder on discharge compared to 64.4% on admission [97]. They further reported that factors associated with a better functional outcome were higher admission MBI scores, absence of spasticity and younger age [97].

It is unclear if it is safe to let patients with transient neurologic deficits with radiographic evidence of cervical stenosis return to contact play [87]. Kepler et al. proposed nine absolute contraindications to participation in intense athletic activity after cervical spine fracture: occipital-cervical arthrodesis, atlantoaxial instability, Spear Tackler's Spine, residual subaxial spine instability, substantial sagittal malalignment, narrowing of the spinal canal as a result of retropulsed fragments, residual neurologic deficits, loss of cervical spine range of motion, and arthrodesis of three or more disk levels [4, 98].

17.3.7 Preventative Measures

When looking at sports injuries, it is important to consider the annual incidence of spinal cord injuries over time.

Comparing the trends in SCIs between sports types and controlling for the number of participants in each type, will better demonstrate how well the governing organizations of each sports type are doing at improving safety measures. This applies at the high school, collegiate, or professional level. Torg and colleagues were instrumental in reducing the rate of quadriplegia as a result of cervical injury after they showed tackling another player using the top of the head (termed "spearing") was the major source of permanent cervical quadriplegia in players [2, 99]. The National Collegiate Athletic Association Football Rules Committee and high school American football governing bodies banned headfirst contact in January 1976 [9]. This rule change had a profound effect on reducing the incidence of spinal cord injury related to American football. Overall, the rate of catastrophic cervical injuries dropped 80.0% from 1976 to 1987 [2, 74]. At the high school level, the rate of cervical spine injuries from 1976 to 1987 decreased 70.0%, from 7.72 per 100,000 to 2.31 per 100,000 [9, 99]. In 1976, the rate of permanent quadriplegia per year was 2.24 per 100,000 participants in high school American football and 10.66 per 100,000 participants in college American football. This rate decreased to 0.38 per 100,000 and 0 per 100,000 by 1984 [9, 10, 99].

The evolution of safety regulations in high-speed motor sports, further demonstrates the impact that athlete centered protective measures can have on safeguarding cervical spine injury. Fatal craniovertebral junction (CVJ) injuries were the most common cause of death in high-speed motor sports prior to 2001 [100]. From 1990 to 2002, 204 drivers died at motor sports events [100]. Shear and loading forces sustained by the neck during collisions can be three times the magnitude needed to cause catastrophic injury. The Head and Neck Support (HANS) device was created by biomechanical engineer Robert Hubbard and race car driver Jim Downing in 1990 and allows for an 80.0% reduction in flexion-distraction force on the head and neck compared with controls and a reduction in neck tension to less than 225 pounds [100]. After the death of NASCAR legend Dale Earnhardt in 2001 due to severe cranial-vertebral joint injury resulting from high force flexion-distraction, NASCAR mandated the use of the HANS device beginning in 2001.

Review

Questions

1. What are the differences between neurogenic and spinal shock in terms of treatment options and clinical implications?
2. If there is concern for a cervical spine injury, how should athletes with shoulder pads and helmets be secured prior to movement off the field of play?

Answers

1. Neurogenic shock is a type of shock that can occur in spinal cord injury causing bradycardia and hypotension secondary to loss of sympathetic tone to vasculature. It is important to identify neurogenic shock quickly and to treat with pressors, classically dopamine or norepinephrine. Spinal shock is distinct from neurogenic shock, and is defined as the temporary physiologic state of the acutely traumatized spinal cord, manifested by the transient absence of reflexive function distal to spinal cord injury.
2. If the athlete is wearing a facemask this should be disconnected from the helmet to allow access to the airway. A cervical collar can be placed or if obstructed from helmet or athletic gear foam blocks or sandbags can be placed on each side of the head with tape or elastic straps to then secure the head, blocks, and backboard in place.

References

1. Boden BP, Prior C. Catastrophic spine injuries in sports. Curr Sports Med Rep. 2005;4(1):45–9.
2. Boden BP, Jarvis CG. Spinal injuries in sports. Phys Med Rehabil Clin N Am. 2009;20(1):55–68, vii.
3. Bailes JE, Hadley MN, Quigley MR, Sonntag VK, Cerullo LJ. Management of athletic injuries of the cervical spine and spinal cord. Neurosurgery. 1991;29(4):491–7.
4. Schroeder GD, Vaccaro AR. Cervical spine injuries in the athlete. J Am Acad Orthop Surg. 2016;24(9):e122–33.
5. Tator CH, Provvidenza C, Cassidy JD. Spinal injuries in Canadian ice hockey: an update to 2005. Clin J Sport Med. 2009;19(6):451–6.
6. Andrews J, Jones A, Davies PR, Howes J, Ahuja S. Is return to professional rugby union likely after anterior cervical spinal surgery? J Bone Joint Surg (Br). 2008;90(5):619–21.
7. Mall NA, Buchowski J, Zebala L, Brophy RH, Wright RW, Matava MJ. Spine and axial skeleton injuries in the National Football League. Am J Sports Med. 2012;40(8):1755–61.
8. Cantu RC, Li YM, Abdulhamid M, Chin LS. Return to play after cervical spine injury in sports. Curr Sports Med Rep. 2013;12(1):14–7.
9. Banerjee R, Palumbo MA, Fadale PD. Catastrophic cervical spine injuries in the collision sport athlete, Part 1: Epidemiology, functional anatomy, and diagnosis. Am J Sports Med. 2004;32(4):1077–87.
10. Frederick O, Mueller RCC. Catastrophic sports injury research twenty-sixth annual report fall 1982 - SPRING 2008. Chapel Hill, NC: National Centre for Catastrophic Sports Injury Research; 2008.
11. Banerjee R, Palumbo MA, Fadale PD. Catastrophic cervical spine injuries in the collision sport athlete, part 2: principles of emergency care. Am J Sports Med. 2004;32(7):1760–4.
12. Boden BP, Tacchetti RL, Cantu RC, Knowles SB, Mueller FO. Catastrophic cervical spine injuries in high school and college football players. Am J Sports Med. 2006;34(8):1223–32.
13. Maeda FL, Formentin C, de Andrade EJ, Rodrigues PAS, Goyal DKC, Shroeder GD, et al. Reliability of the new AOSpine classification system for upper cervical traumatic injuries. Neurosurgery. 2019;83:E271.
14. Joaquim AF, Ghizoni E, Tedeschi H, Yacoub AR, Brodke DS, Vaccaro AR, et al. Upper cervical injuries: clinical results

using a new treatment algorithm. J Craniovertebr Junct Spine. 2015;6(1):16–20.
15. Joaquim AF, Ghizoni E, Tedeschi H, Lawrence B, Brodke DS, Vaccaro AR, et al. Upper cervical injuries - a rational approach to guide surgical management. J Spinal Cord Med. 2014;37(2):139–51.
16. Ryan MD, Henderson JJ. The epidemiology of fractures and fracture-dislocations of the cervical spine. Injury. 1992;23(1):38–40.
17. Bools JC, Rose BS. Traumatic atlantooccipital dislocation: two cases with survival. AJNR Am J Neuroradiol. 1986;7(5):901–4.
18. Traynelis VC, Marano GD, Dunker RO, Kaufman HH. Traumatic atlanto-occipital dislocation. Case report. J Neurosurg. 1986;65(6):863–70.
19. Dickman CA, Papadopoulos SM, Sonntag VK, Spetzler RF, Rekate HL, Drabier J. Traumatic occipitoatlantal dislocations. J Spinal Disord. 1993;6(4):300–13.
20. Nischal K, Chumas P, Sparrow O. Prolonged survival after atlanto-occipital dislocation: two case reports and review. Br J Neurosurg. 1993;7(6):677–82.
21. Kaufman RA, Dunbar JS, Botsford JA, McLaurin RL. Traumatic longitudinal atlanto-occipital distraction injuries in children. AJNR Am J Neuroradiol. 1982;3(4):415–9.
22. Noble ER, Smoker WR. The forgotten condyle: the appearance, morphology, and classification of occipital condyle fractures. AJNR Am J Neuroradiol. 1996;17(3):507–13.
23. Leone A, Cerase A, Colosimo C, Lauro L, Puca A, Marano P. Occipital condylar fractures: a review. Radiology. 2000;216(3):635–44.
24. Legros B, Fournier P, Chiaroni P, Ritz O, Fusciardi J. Basal fracture of the skull and lower (IX, X, XI, XII) cranial nerves palsy: four case reports including two fractures of the occipital condyle--a literature review. J Trauma. 2000;48(2):342–8.
25. Greene KA, Dickman CA, Marciano FF, Drabier JB, Hadley MN, Sonntag VK. Acute axis fractures. Analysis of management and outcome in 340 consecutive cases. Spine. 1997;22(16):1843–52.
26. Lennarson PJ, Mostafavi H, Traynelis VC, Walters BC. Management of type II dens fractures: a case-control study. Spine. 2000;25(10):1234–7.
27. Sonntag VK, Hadley MN. Nonoperative management of cervical spine injuries. Clin Neurosurg. 1988;34:630–49.
28. Reiss SJ, Raque GH Jr, Shields CB, Garretson HD. Cervical spine fractures with major associated trauma. Neurosurgery. 1986;18(3):327–30.
29. Hadley MN, Zabramski JM, Browner CM, Rekate H, Sonntag VK. Pediatric spinal trauma. Review of 122 cases of spinal cord and vertebral column injuries. J Neurosurg. 1988;68(1):18–24.
30. Gehweiler JA Jr, Clark WM, Schaaf RE, Powers B, Miller MD. Cervical spine trauma: the common combined conditions. Radiology. 1979;130(1):77–86.
31. Ross SE, Schwab CW, David ET, Delong WG, Born CT. Clearing the cervical spine: initial radiologic evaluation. J Trauma. 1987;27(9):1055–60.
32. Gleizes V, Jacquot FP, Signoret F, Feron JM. Combined injuries in the upper cervical spine: clinical and epidemiological data over a 14-year period. Eur Spine J. 2000;9(5):386–92.
33. Coyne TJ, Fehlings MG, Wallace MC, Bernstein M, Tator CH. C1-C2 posterior cervical fusion: long-term evaluation of results and efficacy. Neurosurgery. 1995;37(4):688–92; discussion 92–3.
34. Guiot B, Fessler RG. Complex atlantoaxial fractures. J Neurosurg. 1999;91(2 Suppl):139–43.
35. Murphy H, Schroeder GD, Shi WJ, Kepler CK, Kurd MF, Fleischman AN, et al. Management of Hangman's fractures: a systematic review. J Orthop Trauma. 2017;31(Suppl 4):S90–s5.
36. Sharma VK, Rango J, Connaughton AJ, Lombardo DJ, Sabesan VJ. The current state of head and neck injuries in extreme sports. Orthop J Sports Med. 2015;3(1):2325967114564358.
37. Vaccaro A. AOSpine knowledge forum traumu. In: AOSpine upper cervical classification system; 2018.
38. Divi SN, Schroeder GD, Oner FC, Kandziora F, Schnake KJ, Dvorak MF, et al. AOSpine-Spine trauma classification system: the value of modifiers: a narrative review with commentary on evolving descriptive principles. Global Spine J. 2019;9(1 Suppl):77s–88s.
39. Anderson PA, Montesano PX. Morphology and treatment of occipital condyle fractures. Spine. 1988;13(7):731–6.
40. Tuli S, Tator CH, Fehlings MG, Mackay M. Occipital condyle fractures. Neurosurgery. 1997;41(2):368–76; discussion 76–7.
41. Bellabarba C, Mirza SK, West GA, Mann FA, Dailey AT, Newell DW, et al. Diagnosis and treatment of craniocervical dislocation in a series of 17 consecutive survivors during an 8-year period. J Neurosurg Spine. 2006;4(6):429–40.
42. Kandziora F, Scholz M, Pingel A, Schleicher P, Yildiz U, Kluger P, et al. Treatment of atlas fractures: recommendations of the spine section of the German Society for Orthopaedics and Trauma (DGOU). Global Spine J. 2018;8(2_suppl):5S–11S.
43. Kandziora F, Chapman JR, Vaccaro AR, Schroeder GD, Scholz M. Atlas fractures and atlas osteosynthesis: a comprehensive narrative review. J Orthop Trauma. 2017;31(Suppl 4):S81–s9.
44. Levine AM, Edwards CC. The management of traumatic spondylolisthesis of the axis. J Bone Joint Surg Am. 1985;67(2):217–26.
45. Ryken TC, Hadley MN, Walters BC, Aarabi B, Dhall SS, Gelb DE, et al. Radiographic assessment. Neurosurgery. 2013;72(Suppl 2):54–72.
46. Sindelar B, Bailes JE. Neurosurgical emergencies in sport. Neurol Clin. 2017;35(3):451–72.
47. Schouten R, Albert T, Kwon BK. The spine-injured patient: initial assessment and emergency treatment. J Am Acad Orthop Surg. 2012;20(6):336–46.
48. Lee D, Adeoye AL, Dahdaleh NS. Indications and complications of crown halo vest placement: a review. J Clin Neurosci. 2017;40:27–33.
49. Theodore N, Aarabi B, Dhall SS, Gelb DE, Hurlbert RJ, Rozzelle CJ, et al. Occipital condyle fractures. Neurosurgery. 2013;72(Suppl 2):106–13.
50. Boakye M, Arrigo RT, Kalanithi PS, Chen YR. Impact of age, injury severity score, and medical comorbidities on early complications after fusion and halo-vest immobilization for C2 fractures in older adults: a propensity score matched retrospective cohort study. Spine. 2012;37(10):854–9.
51. van Middendorp JJ, Slooff WB, Nellestein WR, Oner FC. Incidence of and risk factors for complications associated with halo-vest immobilization: a prospective, descriptive cohort study of 239 patients. J Bone Joint Surg Am. 2009;91(1):71–9.
52. Bransford RJ, Stevens DW, Uyeji S, Bellabarba C, Chapman JR. Halo vest treatment of cervical spine injuries: a success and survivorship analysis. Spine. 2009;34(15):1561–6.
53. Horn EM, Theodore N, Feiz-Erfan I, Lekovic GP, Dickman CA, Sonntag VK. Complications of halo fixation in the elderly. J Neurosurg Spine. 2006;5(1):46–9.
54. Bohlman HH. Acute fractures and dislocations of the cervical spine. An analysis of three hundred hospitalized patients and review of the literature. J Bone Joint Surg Am. 1979;61(8):1119–42.
55. Mesard L, Carmody A, Mannarino E, Ruge D. Survival after spinal cord trauma. A life table analysis. Arch Neurol. 1978;35(2):78–83.
56. Hadley MN, Dickman CA, Browner CM, Sonntag VK. Acute axis fractures: a review of 229 cases. J Neurosurg. 1989;71(5 Pt 1):642–7.

57. Del Curto D, Tamaoki MJ, Martins DE, Puertas EB, Belloti JC. Surgical approaches for cervical spine facet dislocations in adults. Cochrane Database Syst Rev. 2014;(10):Cd008129.
58. Allen BL Jr, Ferguson RL, Lehmann TR, O'Brien RP. A mechanistic classification of closed, indirect fractures and dislocations of the lower cervical spine. Spine. 1982;7(1):1–27.
59. Schnake KJ, Schroeder GD, Vaccaro AR, Oner C. AOSpine classification systems (subaxial, thoracolumbar). J Orthop Trauma. 2017;31(Suppl 4):S14–s23.
60. Vaccaro AR, Koerner JD, Radcliff KE, Oner FC, Reinhold M, Schnake KJ, et al. AOSpine subaxial cervical spine injury classification system. Eur Spine J. 2016;25(7):2173–84.
61. Vaccaro AR, Hulbert RJ, Patel AA, Fisher C, Dvorak M, Lehman RA Jr, et al. The subaxial cervical spine injury classification system: a novel approach to recognize the importance of morphology, neurology, and integrity of the disco-ligamentous complex. Spine. 2007;32(21):2365–74.
62. Olivier EC, Muller E, Janse van Rensburg DC. Clay-shoveler fracture in a paddler: a case report. Clin J Sport Med. 2016;26(3):e69–70.
63. Lee AS, MacLean JC, Newton DA. Rapid traction for reduction of cervical spine dislocations. J Bone Joint Surg (Br). 1994;76(3):352–6.
64. Kahn A, Leggon R, Lindsey RW. Cervical facet dislocation: management following delayed diagnosis. Orthopedics. 1998;21(10):1089–91.
65. Hart RA. Cervical facet dislocation: when is magnetic resonance imaging indicated? Spine. 2002;27(1):116–7.
66. Vaccaro AR, Nachwalter RS. Is magnetic resonance imaging indicated before reduction of a unilateral cervical facet dislocation? Spine. 2002;27(1):117–8.
67. Kwon BK, Fisher CG, Boyd MC, Cobb J, Jebson H, Noonan V, et al. A prospective randomized controlled trial of anterior compared with posterior stabilization for unilateral facet injuries of the cervical spine. J Neurosurg Spine. 2007;7(1):1–12.
68. Brodke DS, Anderson PA, Newell DW, Grady MS, Chapman JR. Comparison of anterior and posterior approaches in cervical spinal cord injuries. J Spinal Disord Tech. 2003;16(3):229–35.
69. Maroon JC, Bost JW, Petraglia AL, Lepere DB, Norwig J, Amann C, et al. Outcomes after anterior cervical discectomy and fusion in professional athletes. Neurosurgery. 2013;73(1):103–12; discussion 12.
70. Epstein NE. A review of complication rates for Anterior Cervical Diskectomy and Fusion (ACDF). Surg Neurol Int. 2019;10:100.
71. Youssef JA, Heiner AD, Montgomery JR, Tender GC, Lorio MP, Morreale JM, et al. Outcomes of posterior cervical fusion and decompression: a systematic review and meta-analysis. Spine J. 2019;19(10):1714–29.
72. Mai HT, Chun DS, Schneider AD, Hecht AC, Maroon JC, Hsu WK. The difference in clinical outcomes after anterior cervical fusion, disk replacement, and foraminotomy in professional athletes. Clin Spine Surg. 2018;31(1):E80–e4.
73. Nalliah RP, Anderson IM, Lee MK, Rampa S, Allareddy V, Allareddy V. Epidemiology of hospital-based emergency department visits due to sports injuries. Pediatr Emerg Care. 2014;30(8):511–5.
74. Torg JS, Guille JT, Jaffe S. Injuries to the cervical spine in American football players. J Bone Joint Surg Am. 2002;84(1):112–22.
75. Melvin WJ, Dunlop HW, Hetherington RF, Kerr JW. The role of the faceguard in the production of flexion injuries to the cervical spine in football. Can Med Assoc J. 1965;93(21):1110–7.
76. Ciccone R, Richman RM. The mechanism of injury and the distribution of 3000 fractures and dislocations caused by parachute jumping. J Bone Joint Surg Am. 1948;30(1):77–97.
77. Tator CH, Edmonds VE. National survey of spinal injuries in hockey players. Can Med Assoc J. 1984;130(7):875–80.
78. Tator CH, Carson JD, Edmonds VE. Spinal injuries in ice hockey. Clin Sports Med. 1998;17(1):183–94.
79. Chung AS, Makovicka JL, Hassebrock JD, Patel KA, Tummala SV, Deckey DG, et al. Epidemiology of cervical injuries in NCAA football players. Spine. 2019;44(12):848–54.
80. Bailes JE, Petschauer M, Guskiewicz KM, Marano G. Management of cervical spine injuries in athletes. J Athl Train. 2007;42(1):126–34.
81. Maroon JC. 'Burning hands' in football spinal cord injuries. JAMA. 1977;238(19):2049.
82. Kirshblum S, Waring W III. Updates for the international standards for neurological classification of spinal cord injury. Phys Med Rehabil Clin N Am. 2014;25(3):505–17, vii.
83. Schuld C, Franz S, Bruggemann K, Heutehaus L, Weidner N, Kirshblum SC, et al. International standards for neurological classification of spinal cord injury: impact of the revised worksheet (revision 02/13) on classification performance. J Spinal Cord Med. 2016;39(5):504–12.
84. Maroon JC, Bailes JE. Athletes with cervical spine injury. Spine. 1996;21(19):2294–9.
85. Fisher CG, Noonan VK, Smith DE, Wing PC, Dvorak MF, Kwon BK. Motor recovery, functional status, and health-related quality of life in patients with complete spinal cord injuries. Spine. 2005;30(19):2200–7.
86. Waters RL, Adkins RH, Yakura JS, Sie I. Motor and sensory recovery following incomplete tetraplegia. Arch Phys Med Rehabil. 1994;75(3):306–11.
87. Bailes JE. Experience with cervical stenosis and temporary paralysis in athletes. J Neurosurg Spine. 2005;2(1):11–6.
88. Bailes JE, Herman JM, Quigley MR, Cerullo LJ, Meyer PR Jr. Diving injuries of the cervical spine. Surg Neurol. 1990;34(3):155–8.
89. White CC, Domeier RM, Millin MG. EMS spinal precautions and the use of the long backboard - resource document to the position statement of the National Association of EMS Physicians and the American College of Surgeons Committee on Trauma. Prehosp Emerg Care. 2014;18(2):306–14.
90. Saadeh YS, Smith BW, Joseph JR, Jaffer SY, Buckingham MJ, Oppenlander ME, et al. The impact of blood pressure management after spinal cord injury: a systematic review of the literature. Neurosurg Focus. 2017;43(5):E20.
91. Walters BC, Hadley MN, Hurlbert RJ, Aarabi B, Dhall SS, Gelb DE, et al. Guidelines for the management of acute cervical spine and spinal cord injuries: 2013 update. Neurosurgery. 2013;60(CN_suppl_1):82–91.
92. Ryken TC, Hurlbert RJ, Hadley MN, Aarabi B, Dhall SS, Gelb DE, et al. The acute cardiopulmonary management of patients with cervical spinal cord injuries. Neurosurgery. 2013;72(Suppl 2):84–92.
93. Dakson A, Brandman D, Thibault-Halman G, Christie SD. Optimization of the mean arterial pressure and timing of surgical decompression in traumatic spinal cord injury: a retrospective study. Spinal Cord. 2017;55(11):1033–8.
94. Fehlings MG, Vaccaro A, Wilson JR, Singh AW, Cadotte D, Harrop JS, et al. Early versus delayed decompression for traumatic cervical spinal cord injury: results of the Surgical Timing

in Acute Spinal Cord Injury Study (STASCIS). PLoS One. 2012;7(2):e32037.
95. Stampas A, Tansey KE. Spinal cord injury medicine and rehabilitation. Semin Neurol. 2014;34(5):524–33.
96. Evans LT, Lollis SS, Ball PA. Management of acute spinal cord injury in the neurocritical care unit. Neurosurg Clin N Am. 2013;24(3):339–47.
97. Tow AM, Kong KH. Central cord syndrome: functional outcome after rehabilitation. Spinal Cord. 1998;36(3):156–60.
98. Kepler CK, Vaccaro AR. Injuries and abnormalities of the cervical spine and return to play criteria. Clin Sports Med. 2012;31(3):499–508.
99. Torg JS, Vegso JJ, O'Neill MJ, Sennett B. The epidemiologic, pathologic, biomechanical, and cinematographic analysis of football-induced cervical spine trauma. Am J Sports Med. 1990;18(1):50–7.
100. Kaul A, Abbas A, Smith G, Manjila S, Pace J, Steinmetz M. A revolution in preventing fatal craniovertebral junction injuries: lessons learned from the Head and Neck Support device in professional auto racing. J Neurosurg Spine. 2016;25(6):756–61.

Acute Fractures in Sport: Thoraco-Lumbar Spine

18

Chelsea J. Hendow, Harvey E. Smith, Jose A. Canseco, Parthik D. Patel, and Alexander R. Vaccaro

Learning Objectives

- Detail the prevalence of and risk factors for acute thoracolumbar fractures in athletes
- Describe the classification schemes for thoracolumbar fractures and their utility
- Understand how to diagnose and evaluate acute thoracolumbar fractures
- Determine appropriate treatment for athletes with acute thoracolumbar fractures
- Identify the factors considered in determining return-to-play and prevention of acute thoracolumbar fractures

18.1 Epidemiology

Although literature case reports of thoracic (T1–T10) spine fractures in football exist, these injuries are rarely seen in sports, a likely consequence of the stability afforded by the ribs in the thoracic spine [1]. Keene et al. evaluated all back pain injuries in collegiate athletes over a 10 year period, and found a thoracolumbar fracture prevalence of 7% with 59% of these secondary to an acute injury [2]. Eighty percent of all thoracolumbar spine fractures occurred in practice, followed by 14% in preseason conditioning, and 6% in competition. The injuries were thoracic (T1–T10) in 14% of cases, thoracolumbar (T11–L1) in 5%, and lumbar (L2–L5) in 81%. Of 17 sports examined, football and gymnastics showed the highest prevalence rates at 17 and 11 injuries per 100 participants, respectively; badminton, the next highest sport, had an 8% prevalence [2].

Collision sports, such as football, involve purposely colliding with other athletes or inanimate objects, and convey greater risks to the player overall. A biomechanical study of Division I collegiate football players hitting a blocking sled showed that the magnitude of the forces through the L4/L5 motion segment in these athletes exceeded those found in previous fatigue studies necessary to cause lumbar disk and pars interarticularis injuries, such as burst fractures and spondylolysis [3].

Despite collisions being inadvertent, infrequent, or even nonexistent in limited contact or noncontact sports, such as skateboarding and weightlifting, serious injuries may still occur [4]. Sports with significant axial loading, such as weightlifting, may incur mild anterior thoracolumbar compression fractures, as the vertebral body lacks horizontal trabeculations [5]. Significant spine fractures causing instability in noncontact sports are uncommon, except in high speed sports such as auto racing and skiing [5]. Extreme sports, such as mountain biking and airborne winter sports, are increasingly popular, and these athletes are particularly vulnerable to thoracolumbar fractures. One study of helicopter rescues of extreme athletes described a 56% rate of thoracolumbar fractures with the highest percentage of these injuries, i.e. 68%, among paragliders [6]. Airborne sports, such as paragliding or base jumping, have a particularly high rate of spine fractures, representing nearly half of all injuries requiring hospitalization in this population. Over 90% of these spine fractures are compression fractures in the thoracic and lumbar spine [7]. Similarly, the increased popularity of motocross has resulted in an increase in spine fractures, the majority of which are thoracolumbar burst fractures in male patients [8]. In equestrian sports, spine fractures account for between 3% and 7% of injuries [9, 10]. Siebenga et al. reviewed 13 years of horse-related spine injuries, and found these patients to be at particular risk for thoracolumbar fractures, with 78% of spine fractures occurring from T11 to L2 [11].

C. J. Hendow (✉) · H. E. Smith
Department of Orthopaedic Surgery, University of Pennsylvania, Philadelphia, PA, USA
e-mail: chelsea.hendow@pennmedicine.upenn.edu; Harvey.smith@uphs.upenn.edu

J. A. Canseco · P. D. Patel · A. R. Vaccaro
Department of Orthopaedic Surgery, Rothman Institute, Thomas Jefferson University Hospital, Philadelphia, PA, USA
e-mail: Jose.canseco@rothmanortho.com; Parthik.patel@rothmanortho.com; alex.vaccaro@rothmanortho.com

G. A. J. Robertson, N. Maffulli (eds.), *Fractures in Sport*, https://doi.org/10.1007/978-3-030-72036-0_18

The epidemiology of acute thoracolumbar fractures may be expected to vary seasonally given the timing of recreational sports. In coastal cities, trauma centers see a surge in cases in the warmer months [12]. Winter sports, such as alpine skiing, snowboarding, snowmobiling, and tobogganing, often involve high speeds, and are examples of noncontact sports with considerable risk of spinal injuries in the case of a bad fall. Spine trauma represents between 1% and 17% of injuries in skiers and snowboarders [13]. In a review of thoracolumbar fractures in winter sports, Keene et al. found that they account for up to 14% of snowmobile injuries, 5% of Alpine skiing injuries, and 8% of freestyle skiing injuries [14]. Retrospective reviews by trauma centers in the regions of major ski resorts demonstrate that thoracic and lumbar fractures account for the vast majority of spine fractures among alpine skiers and snowboarders, and their incidence is increasing [15]. The mechanism of injury resulting in thoracolumbar fractures in skiers tends to involve a high-speed fall or collision, whereas spine fractures in snowboarders involve jumping and a younger patient population than down hill skiers [16, 17]. There is mixed evidence regarding the comparative risk of spinal injuries and injury severity between snowboarders and skiers, but mechanisms involving a collision tend to result in the most severe injuries [15, 18]. Transverse process, vertebral body compression, and burst fractures are the most common fracture types seen in these patient populations [16, 17, 19].

Isthmic spondylolysis generally refers to a chronic stress fracture of the pars interarticularis due to repetitive loading. These fractures may occur acutely depending on the degree of trauma. In a computed tomography study evaluating 40 young athletes with low back pain and positive bone scans, 40% had acute pars fractures [20]. The prevalence of spondylolysis in the general population is between 3% and 6% [21–23]. While the prevalence is not higher in athletes overall, some types of athletes are particularly at risk, including football players, gymnasts, divers, wrestlers, throwing athletes, dancers, and rowers [5, 24–26]. Pars defects typically occur in young athletes at L5 secondary to repetitive hyperextension and axial loading maneuvers often performed by offensive and defensive football linemen and gymnasts [5]. Torsion against resistance is another important mechanism responsible for the high incidence of spondylolysis among elite athletes [24]. Additionally, pedicle stress fractures are associated with contralateral spondylolysis, although they may occur alone or involve both sides [27–29].

18.2 Classification

There are several classification systems that may be applied to thoracolumbar fractures. Many of these systems focus on characterizing an injury based on stability as a major determinant of operative treatment. It was originally thought that injury to the posterior column alone, comprised of the posterior elements and posterior ligamentous complex, would be sufficient to produce spinal instability [30]. Subsequent studies cast doubt on this assertion, indicating that injury to the posterior ligamentous complex alone does not produce instability, and that an intact posterior ligamentous complex may not protect against deformity in nonoperatively treated fractures [31, 32].

In response, Denis conceptualized the three-column spine model in 1983, dividing spinal segments into three parts: anterior, posterior, and middle column [33] (Fig. 18.1). Denis was first to characterize the middle column, comprised of the posterior longitudinal ligament, the posterior annulus fibrosus, and the posterior vertebral body. When the middle column is disrupted in addition to the posterior ligamentous complex, flexion instability may result. After retrospectively

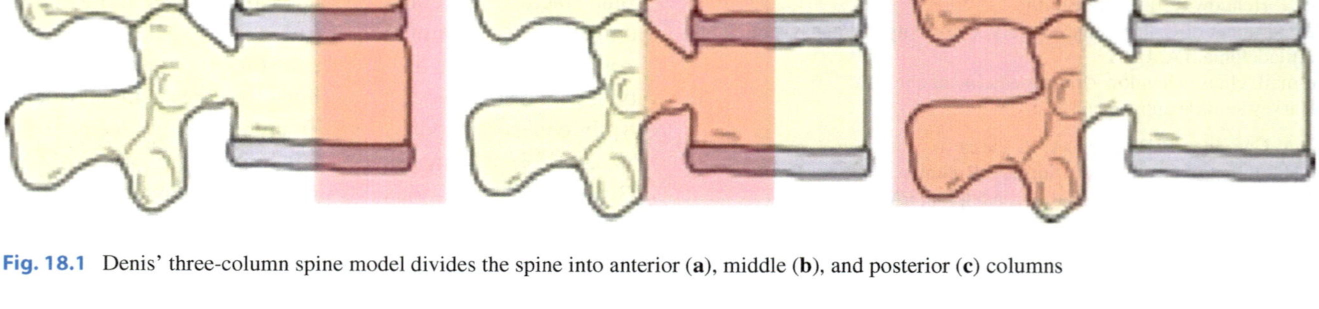

Fig. 18.1 Denis' three-column spine model divides the spine into anterior (**a**), middle (**b**), and posterior (**c**) columns

reviewing 412 thoracolumbar injuries from a single institution, Denis divided injuries into major and minor, then subdivided them by anatomic type and mechanism. Minor fractures are isolated injuries to part of one column, and do not lead to spinal instability. Major spinal injuries were divided into compression fractures, burst fractures, seatbelt-type injuries, and fracture dislocations, which were then subdivided by mechanism. Compression fractures are failures of the anterior column with an intact middle column, resulting from anterior or lateral flexion-compression mechanisms. Burst fractures, in contrast, result from compression by an axial load, with failure of the anterior and middle columns. In seatbelt-type injuries, the posterior and middle columns fail under tension caused by flexion. Finally, all three columns fail in fracture-dislocation injuries, with varied underlying mechanisms. These types are associated with increasing severity of neurological injury and instability, but do not explicitly guide management or predict outcomes [33]. The simple categories allow for interobserver reliability and ease of communication, but may not be inclusive of all fractures observed. Denis may have over-emphasized the role of the middle column in stability, and further research has demonstrated that Holdsworth's original two-column model may be more biomechanically relevant [34].

The AO (Magerl) classification scheme attempts to systematically classify fractures by broad mechanism of injury into:

- Type A: Compression (Fig. 18.2)
- Type B: Distraction (Fig. 18.3)
- Type C: Rotational (Fig. 18.4)

Instability and neurological injury increase across these types, which are in turn subdivided into over 30 subtypes. This system is comprehensive, accounting for morphologic details such as osseous versus ligamentous injuries, direction of displacement, and orientation of fracture [38]. However, it is less reproducible than the Denis classification without producing any advance in prognostic indication [39].

Multiple classification systems have been developed to offer clear indications for specific types of operative treatment. McCormack et al.'s load sharing classification (LSC) assigns points for degree of vertebral body injury, displacement, and need for kyphotic deformity correction as a means of not only describing an injury, but also of predicting success with operative fixation. By identifying fractures at risk for instrumentation failure in cases with isolated short-segment transpedicular constructs, a numerical score >6 should suggests that an anterior reconstruction with a strut graft would improve long term construct success [40]. Dai and Jin found the load sharing classification to have almost perfect inter- and intra-observer reliability [41]; Elzinga et al. analyzed reliability with respect to recommendation categories and found that the LSC has only fair reliability with respect to its recommendation for anterior or posterior stabilization [42].

Additional classification systems focus on relevance to treatment, such as McAfee's classification, which combines morphology and mechanism of injury to delineate six injury types:

- Wedge-compression fracture
- Stable burst fracture
- Unstable burst fracture
- Chance fracture
- Flexion-distraction injury
- Translational injury.

According to this classification system, injuries without failure of the middle column do not require operative fixation, with the exception of multi-level wedge-compression fractures with progressive deformity and neurological deficits. Furthermore, the classification provides recommendations for methods of operative fixation as indicated by mechanism of injury: if the middle column failed in distraction, compressive fixation strategies are indicated; if the middle column failed in compression, compressive fixation strategies are contraindicated [43].

In an effort to synthesize an overall assessment of spinal instability in a reliable classification scheme, Vaccaro et al. developed the Thoracolumbar Injury Severity Scale and Score (TLISS) [44]. This system assigns points assessing mechanism of injury, neurological status, and integrity of the posterior ligamentous complex in an effort to guide clinical decision-making, with 3 or less points indicating nonoperative treatment, and surgical intervention indicated with 5 or more points (Table 18.1).

The TLISS classification was revised to the Thoracolumbar Injury Classification and Severity Score (TLICS), replacing the mechanism of injury with fracture morphology [45]. The morphological categories, in ascending point value, include: compression fractures, burst fractures, translational/rotational injuries, and distraction injuries. Though the injury morphology was thought to be a more objective criterion than the mechanism of injury, the TLISS interrater reliability was still found to be superior [45]. Nevertheless, the TLICS has since been clinically validated, with high inter- and intra-rater reliability [46]. Furthermore, Joaquim et al. demonstrated the reliability of the scoring system in its recommendation for surgical intervention in 65 consecutive patients. None of the patients experienced worsening neurological function, and only two patients originally treated nonoperatively eventually necessitated operative treatment from axial back pain and focal kyphosis [47]. The two classification schemes are simple, comprehensive, reliable, and useful as a treatment algorithm and communication tool between providers.

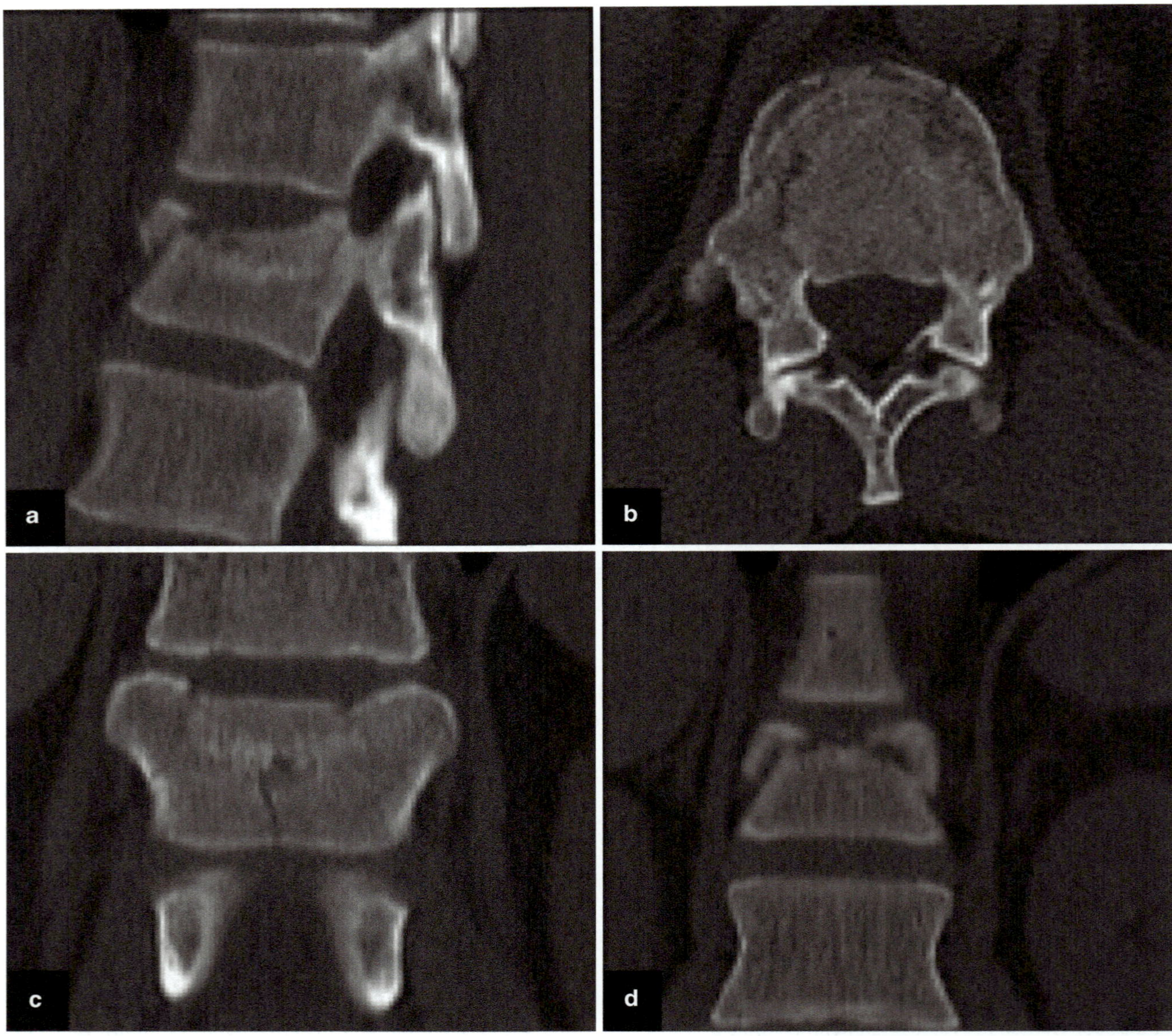

Fig. 18.2 Sagittal (**a**), axial (**b**), and coronal (**c-d**) CT images demonstrating AO Magerl type A thoracolumbar compression fracture. (Copyright © 2009 Schmidt et al.; licensee BioMed Central Ltd., with permission [35])

Recently the TLICS score has evolved into the AOSpine Thoracolumbar Spine Injury Classification System (TL AOSIS) in an attempt to produce a globally accepted system that would settle the widespread controversies with regards to classification of thoracolumbar trauma, particularly those in neurologically intact patients with burst fractures. This classification system similarly separates fractures by morphologic subtypes, then assigns points for severity of injury, neurologic status, and PLC integrity. It takes into consideration variations of burst fracture morphology, such as single verse both endplates failure. Recommendations are based on the input of over 500 international spine surgeons, and the classification is both valid and reliable [48].

18.3 Diagnosis

18.3.1 History

Clinicians should be alert to athletes with significant back pain or decreased range of motion after an acute axial load or severe violent flexion injury. Patients often complain of persistent midline back pain with a history of a suspicious mechanism of injury. Particularly in athletes, images or video of the injury are often available, and their review reveals pertinent details, such as energy and direction of the injury, which alert the clinician to the possibility of a thoracolumbar injury.

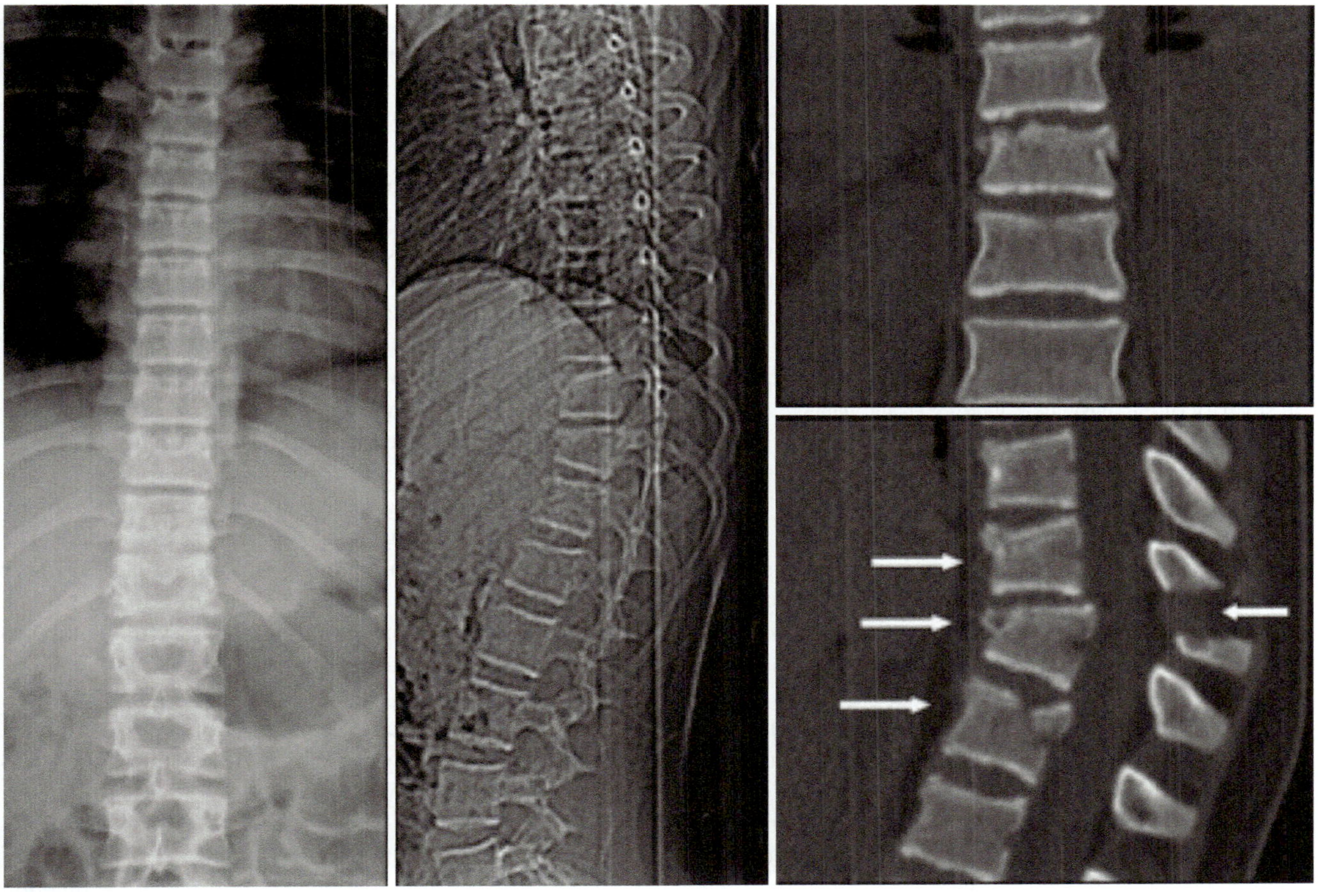

Fig. 18.3 AP and lateral radiographs, and sagittal and coronal CT scan demonstrating AO Magerl Type B distraction thoracolumbar fracture. (Copyright © 2011 Springer-Verlag, with permission [36])

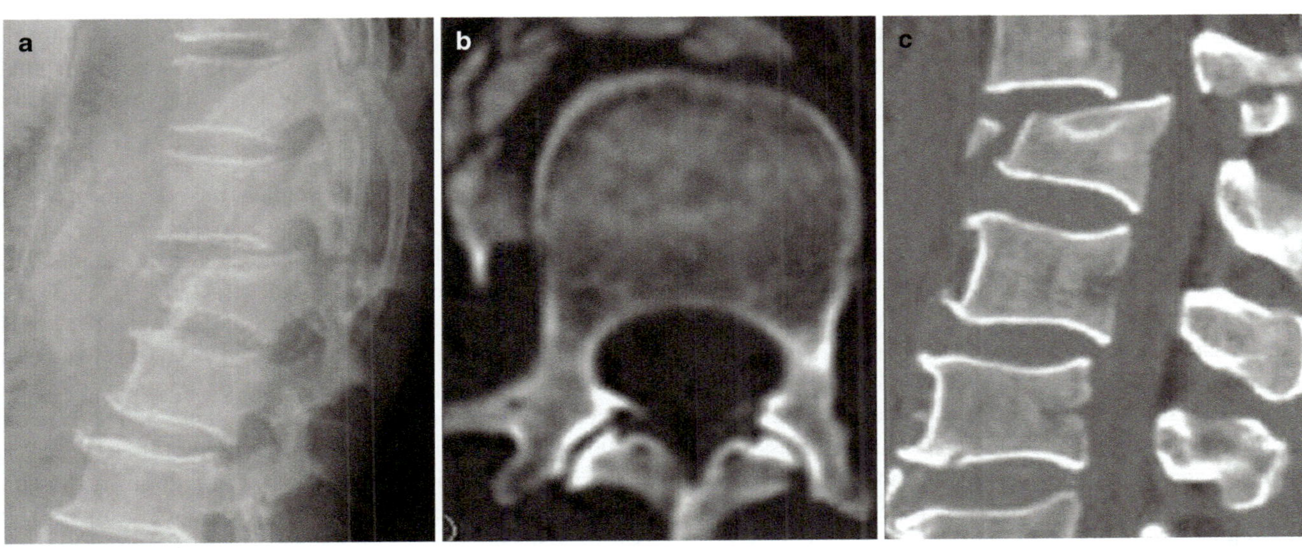

Fig. 18.4 Lateral radiograph (**a**), axial CT scan (**b**), and sagittal CT scan (**c**) demonstrate AO Magerl Type C rotational thoracolumbar injury. (Copyright © 2007 The Korean Neurosurgical Society, with permission [37])

Table 18.1 Thoracolumbar injury severity score

Mechanism of injury	Compression	1 point
	Burst fracture or lateral angulation	1 additional point
	Translational or rotational injury	3 points
	Distraction injury	4 points
Posterior ligamentous complex (PLC)	Intact	0 points
	Indeterminate status	2 points
	Disrupted	3 points
Neurological status	Intact	0 points
	Nerve root, complete spinal cord, or complete conus medullaris injury	2 points
	Incomplete spinal cord or conus medullaris injury, or cauda equina syndrome	3 points

Patients with any neurologic symptoms should receive a thorough evaluation, but subtle neurologic findings may go undetected without a careful history, including genitourinary dysfunction. Denis found that a subset of patients with major thoracolumbar fractures who were neurologically intact on presentation endorsed less than 1 h of paresthesias or weakness at the time of injury [33]. In Keene et al.'s series of 14 consecutive patients with thoracolumbar fractures and normal neurologic exams, 5 patients experienced urologic dysfunction [14]. Postvoid residual should be documented in the acute period if there are any concerns for urologic dysfunction; even if examined at a later date, a history of retention may be revealing and warrant further urological examination. Thoracic spine fractures in particular may be difficult to diagnose due to poorly localizing symptoms. As such, a high index of suspicion must be utilized in injuries involving axial compression on a flexed thoracic spine [1].

18.3.2 Physical Examination

Initial on-field evaluation should follow a systematic approach with the goal of identifying serious injuries. A rapid and standardized approach should be used to evaluate the patient. In patients in whom a thoracolumbar fracture is suspected, cervical precautions should be observed until the entire spine has been evaluated given the high prevalence of noncontiguous spine injuries [16, 19, 49]. A brief history with respect to mechanism of injury, loss of consciousness, and significant complaints is obtained before an assessment of mental status and intact voluntary motion of all extremities. Any injured patient should then be transported for an in-depth exam off-site, with the location of that exam determined by severity of injury. Specifically regarding thoracolumbar spine injuries, only those patients with minor muscular strains that do not impair performance should be allowed to return to play if determined safe by a trained clinician [50]. While there are no accepted guidelines for thoracolumbar spine clearance, there is evidence that a clinical examination alone is not sufficient to rule out fracture, particularly in high energy mechanisms such as those experienced by collision athletes [51]. Physicians should have a low threshold for a comprehensive evaluation and treatment in a hospital-setting that includes advanced imaging prior to considering return-to-play status.

A complete in-depth off-site examination should include observation and palpation of the posterior spine for midline tenderness or step-off. A careful neurologic examination should be performed, with deficits fully characterized using the American Spinal Injury Association classification [52]. Comparable standardized, comprehensive exams are acceptable, though the ASIA exam facilitates interprovider communication and aids in directing clinical decision making by clearly categorizing injuries as complete or incomplete. The exam comprises grading strength of key muscles in upper and lower extremities, and testing sensation to light touch and pinprick in all dermatomal distributions, in addition to assessing sacral sensation and rectal tone. Sensation and strength determine the neurological level of injury (NLI), defined as the most caudal segment of the cord with intact sensation and antigravity strength. A letter is then assigned to indicate the severity injury where:

- Grade A is complete
- Grade B is sensory incomplete, with no motor function but with preserved sacral sensation
- Grade C is motor incomplete, with preserved voluntary rectal tone
- Grade D is motor incomplete, with preservation of key muscle functions below the neurological level of injury
- Grade E is assigned to patients who sustained a spinal cord injury but at the time of exam are neurologically normal.

Patients without a spinal cord injury are not graded. Serial neurological examinations are critical to the care of a patient with a thoracolumbar injury, and a change in examination may direct further treatment.

Several tests have been proposed to detect lumbar instability. Passive lumbar extension, where a positive sign involves low back pain when the legs of a prone patient are passively extended, has a sensitivity of 84% and specificity of 90%, with excellent intra-rater reliability [53] (Fig. 18.5). Signs such as the instability catch sign, painful catch sign, and apprehension sign are specific but not sensitive [53]. Keene et al. advocates a prone instability test, where pain on ventral pressure over the affected vertebrae is relieved with contraction of the paraspinous musculature [14]. These findings may be subtle indications of a spinal injury requiring further radiographic evaluation [14].

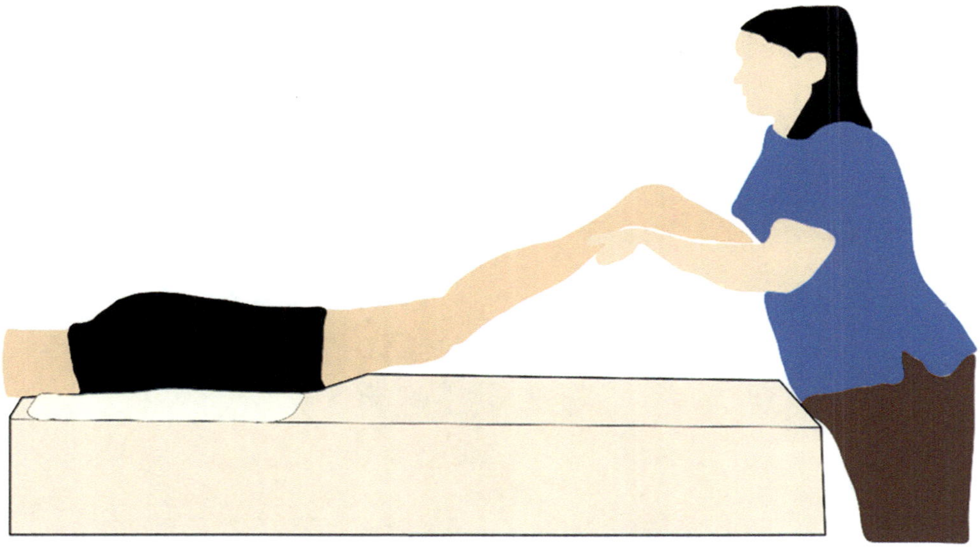

Fig. 18.5 The passive lumbar extension test is one way to determine lumbar injury on physical examination

18.3.3 Imaging Investigations

Appropriate and quality imaging studies are central to accurate diagnosis and complete evaluation of acute thoracolumbar fractures. The goals of imaging are to identify the level of any bony or soft tissue injury, classify the injury, and thereby determine the patient's predicted clinical course including treatment and return-to-play. Although advanced imaging is increasingly the first diagnostic study performed in the setting of trauma, antero-posterior and lateral radiographs maintain their utility in rapid, convenient diagnosis and longitudinal assessment of injuries to the thoracolumbar spine [54] (Fig. 18.6). Dynamic flexion and extension views in a patient without a spinal cord injury are used to evaluate stability, while an oblique view may identify a pars defect. The interspinous gap change at the concerning level can be compared to adjacent levels during flexion and extension, and an abnormal interspinous diastasis is 82% sensitive and 61% specific for instability on flexion-extension radiographs [56].

Computed tomography (CT) has an important role in both identifying and further characterizing acute thoracolumbar injuries due to its improved resolution, three-dimensional nature, and speed. A CT scan involves a high dose of radiation, and as such exposure should be minimized particularly in the young athlete [57, 58]. CT is recommended in the initial evaluation of a patient with a radiograph-proven thoracolumbar fracture, or as the first imaging modality in the presence of a spinal cord injury or a suspected thoracolumbar fracture. In high energy blunt trauma patients, as it often occurs in sports trauma, thoracolumbar spine clearance may require CT scanning [51]. One prospective observational study demonstrated that using physical examination alone was inadequate to detect significant thoracolumbar fractures, and advocated for CT imaging in any injury involving high-energy mechanisms or in elderly patients, in addition to those with positive physical exam findings or those who are unexaminable [51]. Furthermore, serial CT scans are useful in following bony union in conjunction with adjunct studies such as radiographs, although this is often discouraged because of the amount of radiation exposure one would experience [59].

While bony elements are best-defined on CT scans, MRI is a useful adjunct in the trauma setting. Edema on MRI is highly sensitive for subtle fractures and superior visualization of soft tissues allows for diagnosis of ligamentous and discogenic injuries and evaluation of the neural elements. In particular, 30–40% of distraction injuries are initially misdiagnosed [60, 61]. In one study, 29% of flexion distraction injuries in which the posterior disruption is primarily ligamentous cannot be detected on plain radiographs or CT scan [62]. Though local kyphosis, a reduced vertebral body height, and increased interspinous distance are indicative of posterior column injury [61, 63, 64], MRI has a high sensitivity for detecting PLC injuries [65] (Fig. 18.7). Comparisons with intraoperative findings have yielded sensitivity between 79% and 100%. Specificity may be as low as 53%, though agreement between MRI and intraoperative findings improves in more severe injuries [65, 67]. Caution should be exercised to avoid over-diagnosis and treatment based on MRI findings alone, yet MRI represents an important adjunct in the diagnosis of suspected ligamentous injuries.

Bony edema of the pars interarticularis on MRI is a non-specific finding indicating a stress response. Single-photon emission computed tomography (SPECT) may be used to differentiate an acute stress fracture from a chronic spondylolysis [68].

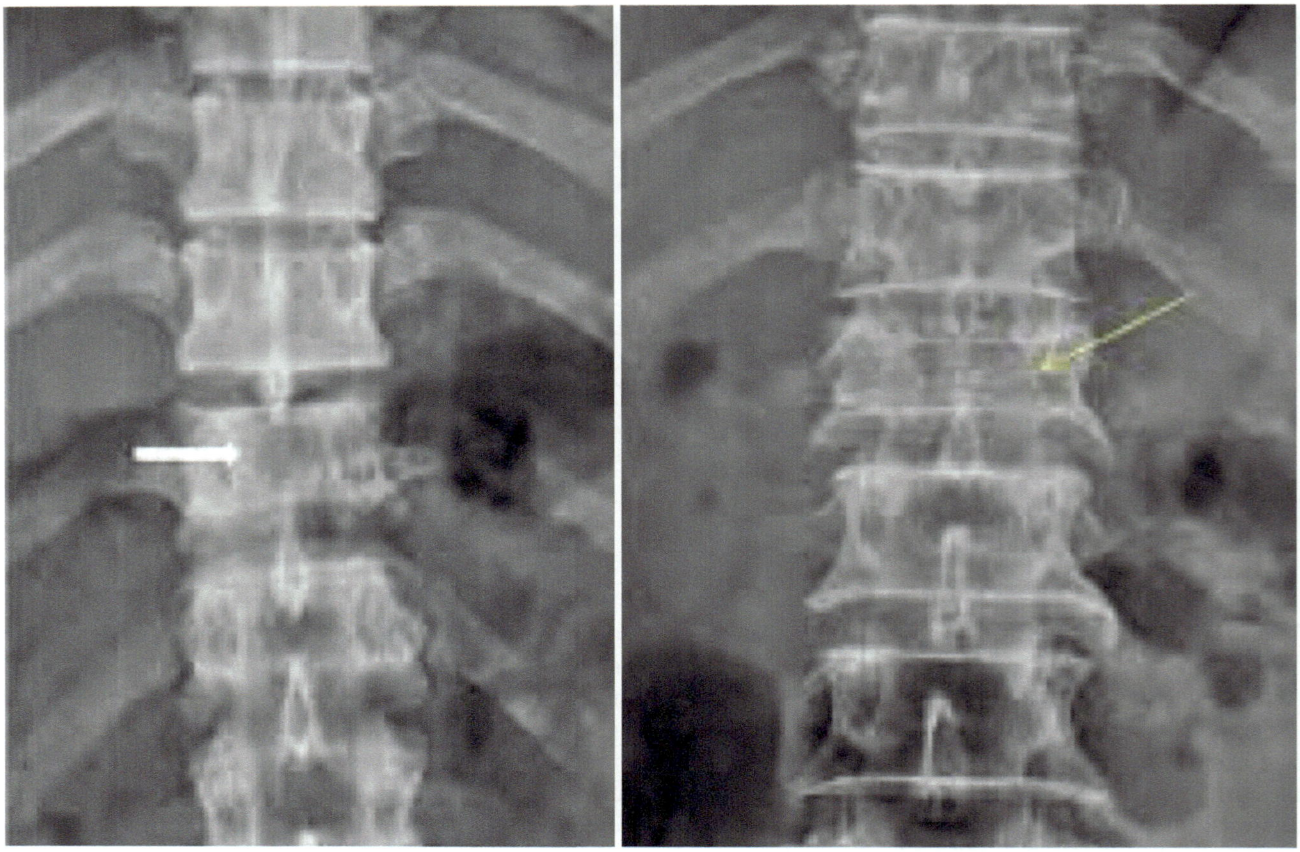

Fig. 18.6 AP radiographs demonstrating interspinous diastasis (arrows) in a distraction thoracolumbar injury. (Copyright © 2016, Rights Managed by Georg Thieme Verlag KG Stuttgart, New York, with permission [55])

Given the high energy resulting in acute thoracolumbar fractures, patients should be evaluated for related injuries including those to the abdominal organs.

18.4 Management

More recent classification schemes, such as the TLISS and TLICS, are designed to guide clinical decision making. Assessment of the mechanical and neurological stability of a fracture pattern is key. When possible, the goals of the athlete should be taken into account in choosing the timing and strategy of management. Furthermore, consideration should be given to the extremes of patient physical size often encountered both when planning for bracing and for any operative intervention or relevant instrumentation [69].

18.4.1 Conservative Management

Nonoperative management typically consists of immobilisation in an external brace. Depending on the device, motion can be limited to varying degrees, but no device eliminates motion of the lumbar spine [70]. Hyperextension braces resist flexion without significantly impacting rotational or lateral bending forces, while a custom thoracolumbosacral orthosis (TLSO) reduces motion in multiple planes. To reduce motion at the L5/S1 junction, a leg cuff is required, while a cervical extension is required to brace T7 and above [71]. These extensions may prove impractical or intolerable for patients, and thus are often foregone in favor of activity limitations and careful observation or operative stabilization.

Bracing is reasonable for most compression fractures, as these are by nature stable fractures [72]. It may also be indicated for stable burst fractures without neurological injury, or those with complete spinal cord injuries as a part of comfort care [72].

The treatment of neurologically intact patients with thoracolumbar burst fractures is controversial. Multiple studies have shown long-term favorable outcomes of nonoperative treatment in neurologically intact stable burst fracture, i.e. those with an intact posterior column [73, 74]. Cantor et al. advocated bracing with early ambulation for this group, showing satisfactory results in a series of stable burst fractures [75]. Wood et al. performed a prospective randomized

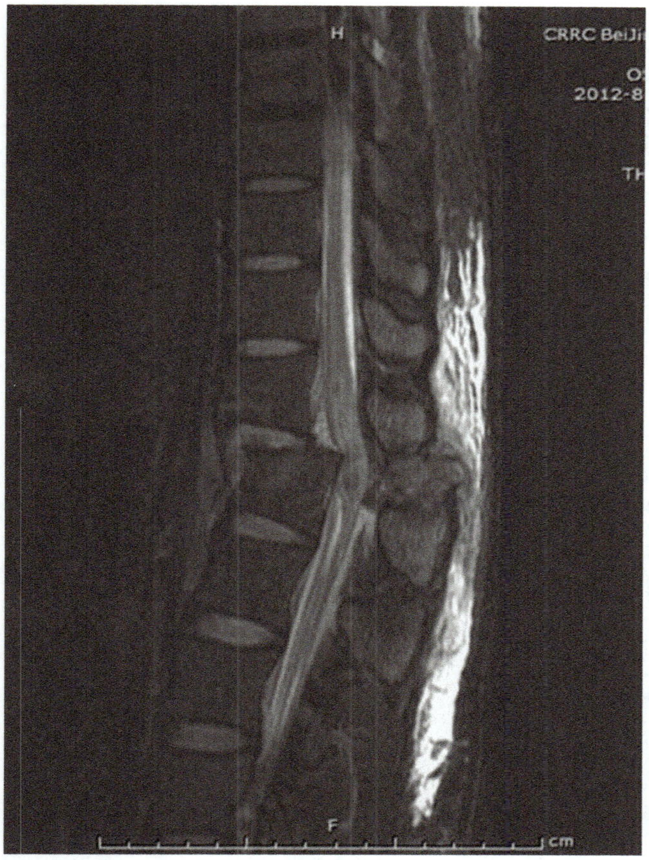

Fig. 18.7 Sagittal T2-weighted fat-suppressed MRI demonstrates distraction thoracolumbar injury with PLC injury. (Copyright © 2015 Wolters Kluwer Health, Inc. All rights reserved, with permission [66])

study of operative versus nonoperative treatment in these patients, and long-term results demonstrate no difference in kyphotic deformity but superior functional scores in those treated nonoperatively [76]. Bracing for 10–12 weeks may be trialed, and nonoperatively treated patients should be followed with serial standing radiographs [77].

18.4.2 Surgical Treatment

Operative treatment is intended to convey immediate stability, correct deformity, and decompress neural elements [78]. Indications for operative intervention are therefore based on avoiding negative outcomes associated with prolonged immobilisation in nonoperative treatment, minimizing neural impingement to optimize clinical outcomes, and preventing pain and neurologic dysfunction associated with mechanical instability [78]. Classifications systems such as the LSC and TLISS focus on PLC injury and neurological deficit, and are designed to assist the provider in identifying patients who would benefit from operative intervention.

A prospective randomized study of AO type A thoracolumbar fractures suggested that operative treatment of compression fractures may be superior [79]. After a mean 4.3 years follow-up, those patients treated operatively with short-segment transpedicular arthrodesis demonstrated significantly less local kyphosis and superior functional outcomes. Furthermore, a significantly larger number of operatively treated patients were able to return to work, at an average of 6.7 months, compared to 13.8 months in the nonoperatively treated group. Particularly in athletes, for whom an expeditious recovery and return to activity is desirable, operative treatment should be considered especially if return to play is considered [79].

The posterior surgical approach to the thoracolumbar spine provides low-morbidity access to reduce, decompress, and stabilize an injured spine. It is possible to address significant causes of neural compression in a traumatic setting, including epidural hematomas and traumatic dural tears. Any decompressive technique is combined with an instrumented arthrodesis to avoid further destabilizing a fractured spine.

A posterior instrumented fusion can re-establish the posterior tension band of the spine, and as such is widely applied. Unstable burst fractures that are neurologically intact or are neurologically compromised with only a moderate degree of canal stenosis may benefit from a posterior spinal fusion [80]. By distracting through the injured segment, ligamentotaxis may be utilized to reduce retropulsed bony fragments and expand the spinal canal [81] (Fig. 18.8). This is most efficacious when completed in the acute period and in cases with less than 67% canal compromise, as these patients are most likely to have bony elements in continuity with their original soft tissue structures [83, 84]. A meta-analysis compared the results of treatment of burst fractures using a posterior approach to those of anterior approach: despite superior decompression and canal remodeling in burst fractures treated with anterior approaches, clinical outcomes are not superior to those treated with a posterior approach. Rather, the anterior approach had greater blood loss, longer operative times, and higher associated costs [85].

Flexion-distraction injuries and fracture-dislocations may also be addressed with posterior instrumented arthrodesis. Other posterolateral techniques have been described and may be utilized based on the specific needs of the patient. Transpedicular short-segment fixation, extending one level above and below the level of injury, are advocated as a motion-preserving, low-morbidity surgical option for relatively stable fractures requiring operative treatment [86]. The posterior approach and transpedicular short-segment fixation must be used judiciously, as McCormack et al. have demonstrated higher rates of failure when used improperly, such as in fracture patterns with significant comminution or displacement [87]. There is controversy regarding whether to

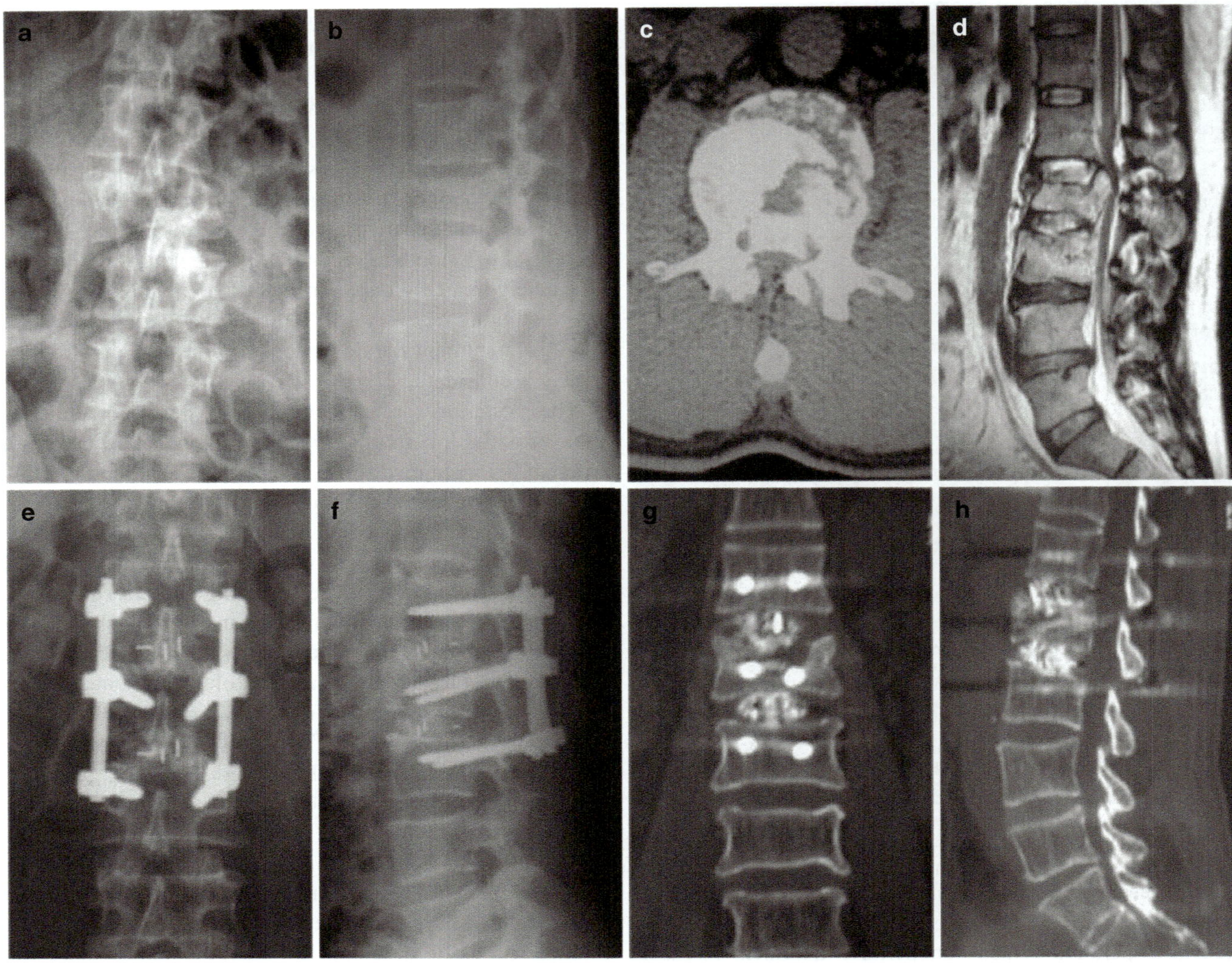

Fig. 18.8 AP and lateral radiographs (**a**, **b**), axial CT scan (**c**), and sagittal MRI (**d**) of the thoracolumbar spine demonstrate AO Magerl type A burst fracture with significant retropulsion and canal stenosis. AP and lateral radiographs (**e**, **f**) and axial and sagittal CT scan (**g**, **h**) are postoperative images of the same injury after short-segment transpedicular fixation, in addition to interbody instrumented fusion. (Copyright © 2014 Wang et al.; licensee BioMed Central Ltd, with permission [82])

instrument the fracture level. Biomechanical analysis indicates that a short-segment fusion with inclusion of screws at the fracture level increases the stiffness of the construct to a level comparable with circumferential fusion for unstable burst fractures [86]. Inclusion of the fracture level does increase operative times and blood loss with mixed clinical outcomes, though there is evidence that patients without screws at the fracture level are at a higher risk for worsening kyphosis and failure than those with screws at the fracture level. This risk is more pronounced for patients with more unstable injuries, such as AO Magerl Type C injuries [86].

These more unstable fractures may require long-segment fixation, with extension of the arthrodesis two levels above and below the level of injury [88]. Long-segment fixation may be ideal in severely unstable fractures requiring a stiffer construct, or in fracture patterns precluding transpedicular instrumentation at the level of fracture, such as severe burst fractures requiring removal of a pedicle for adequate canal decompression [86]. Some authors advocate transpedicular decompression with a posterior-only fixation approach, allowing direct decompression and anterior column reconstruction without the morbidity of an anterior approach, particularly in high-energy injuries which may have concurrent visceral injuries [89, 90].

An anterior approach affords superior access to decompress retropulsed bone fragments from the posterior vertebral body into the spinal canal, and as such is indicated in patients with incomplete spinal cord injuries and significant spinal canal stenosis [80, 91]. In those patients in whom an anterior procedure is indicated, multiple studies have shown favorable short- and long-term outcomes [85, 92–95]. Kaneda et al. analyzed 150 consecutive thoracolumbar burst fractures with neurological deficits treated with anterior decompression and instrumented fusion, and found that more than 90% went on to solid fusion, improved neurologically, and eventually returned to work [94].

A circumferential approach may be indicated in patients with significant anterior and posterior instability, severely comminuted fractures, or poor bone quality, in whom isolated anterior or posterior stabilization would not be adequate. McCormack et al.'s load sharing classification was in part designed to identify candidates for circumferential fixation, those patients with significant instability owing to destruction of the anterior column [40]. A prospective case series with 1-year follow-up of 74 patients who underwent circumferential fusion as indicated by the load sharing classification's guidelines demonstrated lasting regional deformity correction in addition to satisfactory functional clinical outcomes [96]. In the aforementioned study, the anterior procedure was staged an average of 15 days with the goal of avoiding the morbidity of the acute peritraumatic period, though some advocate for simultaneous circumferential approaches to maximize immediate stability and optimize the potential for fracture reduction [96]. However, a systematic review comparing circumferential to posterior approaches for thoracolumbar burst fractures demonstrated no clinically significant difference in radiographic or functional outcomes. The same study found strong evidence that a circumferential approach results in longer operative times, greater blood loss, and higher costs [97]. This approach should be used judiciously, and reserved for those patients with marked instability in addition to incomplete neurological injury requiring decompression of anterior elements [98].

Finally, minimally invasive approaches play an increasing role in the approach to surgical treatment of thoracolumbar fractures. Endoscopic or thoracoscopic treatment of thoracolumbar fractures has a role in specific fracture patterns. Complications of thoracoscopic surgery are similar to those of anterior thoracic surgery, including pleural effusions, pneumothorax, intercostal neuralgia, and brachial plexopathy. Further, patients with restricted cardiopulmonary function or severe medical comorbidities are not appropriate candidates. However, for the young, healthy athlete, these approaches may provide for a cosmetically pleasing and muscle-preserving method of surgical stabilization [99].

18.5 Complications

Chronic back pain is a common yet unelucidated long-term complication of thoracolumbar injuries. Despite a widespread belief that kyphotic deformity is responsible for long-term axial back pain [100], studies have not substantiated this connection [101–103]. Rather, the importance of soft-tissue injury, specifically injuries to the disco-vertebral complex and posterior facet joints, is emerging as a possible causative factor of long-term back pain and kyphosis after thoracolumbar injuries [65].

Injuries requiring an arthrodesis warrant a discussion with the athlete regarding future potential for adjacent segment disease. The risk is specific to the length and stiffness of the construct, and thus the patient. Thoracolumbar trauma may require only limited arthrodesis of one to two levels, resulting in more normal spinal motion and less stress concentration in adjacent motion segments. Yet even single level fusions is associated with accelerated disc degeneration that may be further accelerated with continued athletic participation [104]. With an increased force translated across adjacent segments, athletes should carefully consider any return to contact sports.

18.6 Rehabilitation

In patients with spinal instability with low back pain without neurological deficit, rehabilitation involves strengthening of the paraspinal musculature [14].

Return to activity guidelines for the elite athlete after any injury must be tailored to the specific sport, and often include a task-specific evaluation. Most protocols involve 10–12 weeks of immobilisation for nonoperative treatment, with progressive activity reintroduction. Minor fractures without instability such as transverse process, spinous process, and facet fractures can resume play when asymptomatic during full range of motion, and during activities consistent with their sport [5]. Neurologic status, coronal and sagittal alignment, range of motion, and pain in specific sports related activities are all assessed in order to determine timing of return-to-play. Residual deficits in any of these categories may be an indication for continued rehabilitation without return to play after a trial of nonoperative treatment, or of an inadequate construct in those patients who have already undergone surgical stabilization.

In cases requiring instrumented arthrodesis, practice patterns vary widely depending on many of the same factors considered in nonoperatively treated patients. Patients may be allowed to resume full activities once a solid fusion is attained, typically after 6–12 months. A recent systematic review demonstrated that return-to-play after thoracolumbar surgery most often occurs at 6 months for noncontact sports and at greater than 12 months for contact sports, if at all [105]. Physical rehabilitation during the period of activity restriction focuses on maintaining muscle tone and lower extremity strength, with restrictions on truncal rotation and bending. Fusion may be monitored with serial imaging and clinical exams.

Considerations for return to play after thoracolumbar trauma requiring surgery include the potentially catastrophic consequences of reinjury as well as known potential for adjacent segment disease [106]. Participation in sports at the same level may not be an option. In operatively-treated spine fractures in snowboarders, the majority of which were thoracolumbar, none returned to play any sports even though some patients recovered neurologic function [107]. However, multiple case reports of athletes returning to competition after thoracolumbar arthrodesis exist with uncomplicated follow-up at 4 years postoperatively [106, 108]. After percutaneous pedicle screw fixation for thoracolumbar fractures, 93% of pediatric patients are eventually able to return to their previous level of activity [105]. Competitive weightlifters may need their activity restricted indefinitely to prevent worsening of previous compression fractures [5].

18.7 Preventative Measures

Sports that present a risk for spine fractures need to be recognized as such, with the help of epidemiological data and public education. The foci of preventative measures are twofold: training and equipment. The high-risk nature of high-speed and collision sports make these relevant targets for prevention, particularly given the known risks of inexperience and intoxication in snow, equestrian, and airborne sports [7, 10, 18].

In snow sports, lessons with an emphasis on hill etiquette and safe, collision-free skiing and snowboarding may be encouraged or required. Education may focus on minimizing risk factors, such as fatigue, alcohol consumption, high speeds, technically challenging tricks, and listening to music [18]. Development and maintenance of trails and terrain parks may minimize injuries by designing trails with ample opportunity for rest, obstacle demarcation, and space for instruction of safe jumping and landing techniques [18]. Appropriate, well-fitting equipment such as helmets reduce the risk of serious head injury and are now required in competitions [18] (Fig. 18.9a). Spine protectors are controversial, and their use is currently not supported by evidence. While they may protect the thoracolumbar spine, there are theoretical concerns that rigidity may predispose the cervical spine to injury [18]. Further investigation into the benefits of spine/rib protectors is required before making formal recommendations (Fig. 18.9b).

Horse riders are more frequently injured with young and inexperienced horses, and leisure riders are more likely to be seriously injured than pupils or contest riders [10]. An awareness of the increased risk in these circumstances may allow the rider to proceed with an appropriate level of caution. In one review, nearly half of horse-related deaths occurred outdoors without a trainer. Furthermore, thoracic trauma occurred most frequently when a horse rolled over. These data suggest that inexperienced riders should train indoors with a trainer. Finally, avoiding slippery ground conditions may aid in preventing a horse from rolling [10].

In football, linemen frequently assume two different positions that expose them to increased forces through their lumbosacral spines. The typical starting position is a three- or four-point stance in which the lumbar spine is markedly flexed and the cervical spine is extended, causing loss of lumbar lordosis and narrowing of anterior disc spaces, a position known to put increased stress on the pars interarticularis. From this position they drive forward and upward, extending the lumbosacral spine as they collide with the opposing players. This motion places a shearing force on the apophyseal joints, theoretically resulting in high stresses on the pars and an increased rate of spondylolysis [109]. Good coaching and practice techniques may prevent injuries in at-risk athletes.

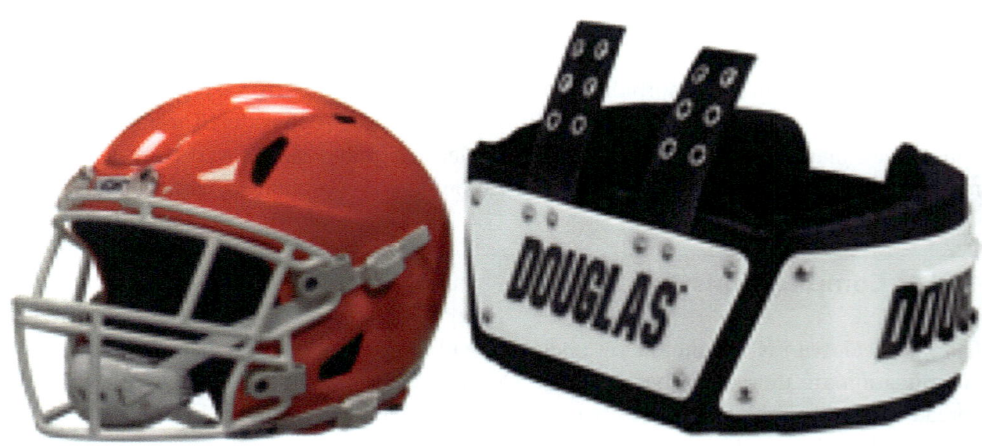

Fig. 18.9 Protective equipment including a helmet (**a**) and a spine/rib protector (**b**) may play a role in spine injuries in sports. (Images courtesy of Light Helmets™ and Douglas Pads and Sports, Inc., with permission)

Clinical Pearls

- Acute thoracolumbar fractures in sport may occur in contact or noncontact sports, and represent high energy injuries
- The most common acute thoracolumbar fractures in athletes are transverse process, compression, and burst fractures.
- A comprehensive history and physical exam with complete characterization of any neurologic deficits is key.
- Spinal instability and neurologic deficits are surgical indications, and classification systems such as the TLIC and TLISS system both identify these indications and also are intended to be used as a treatment algorithm.
- Rehabilitation and return to sport considerations are predicated on radiographic healing and task-specific assessments. Athletes should understand the risks of returning to full participation.
- Education, both to promote awareness of risk and training for safe competition, is integral to prevention.

Review

Questions

1. A 24 year-old male snowboarder sustains an injury while performing a jump. Which of the following is the most likely injury?
   (a) Odontoid fracture
   (b) Thoracolumbar compression fracture
   (c) Thoracolumbar flexion distraction injury
   (d) Sacral fracture
2. On examination, the patient has no motor function of his lower extremities, with intact voluntary anal contraction. What is this patient's ASIA Impairment Scale classification?
   (a) ASIA A
   (b) ASIA B
   (c) ASIA C
   (d) ASIA D
3. The patient is found to have an unstable thoracolumbar burst fracture, without evidence of posterior ligamentous complex injury. How many points would be assigned using the Thoracolumbar Injury Severity Score, and what is the corresponding recommended course of action based on this classification system?
   (a) 4 points; indeterminate
   (b) 5 points; indeterminate
   (c) 4 points; nonoperative management
   (d) 5 points; operative management

Answers

1. The answer is (B) thoracolumbar compression fracture. Thoracic and lumbar fractures account for the majority of spine fractures among skiers and snowboarders, and are increasing. The mechanism of injury resulting in thoracolumbar fractures in skiers tends to involve a fall or collision, whereas spine fractures in snowboarders involve jumping and a younger patient population. Transverse process, anterior compression. and burst fractures are the most common fracture types.
2. The answer is (C) ASIA C. With no lower extremity motor function, the patient is either classified as complete, sensory incomplete, or motor incomplete. With intact motor function at the most caudal sacral segments, this patient is classified as motor incomplete.
3. The answer is (D) 5 points; operative management. Using the TLISS, the patient is assigned one point for a compression type mechanism, and an additional point for a burst fracture. An incomplete spinal cord injury earns 3 points, and zero points are assigned for an intact PLC, for a total of five points. Patients with 3 or less points can likely be managed nonoperatively, and those with five or more would likely benefit from operative intervention.

References

1. Elattrache N, Fadale PD, Fu FH. Thoracic spine fracture in a football player: a case report. Am J Sports Med. 1993;21(1):157–60.
2. Keene JS, Albert MJ, Springer SL, Drummond DS, Clancy WG. Back injuries in college athletes. J Spinal Disord. 1989;2:190–5.
3. Gatt CJ, Hosea TM, Palumbo RC, Zawadsky JP. Impact loading of the lumbar spine during football blocking. Am J Sports Med. 1993;25(3):317–21. http://journals.sagepub.com.libproxy2.usc.edu/doi/pdf/10.1177/036354659702500308.
4. Rice SG. Medical conditions affecting sports participation. Pediatrics. 2008;121(4):841–8.
5. Dunn IF, Proctor MR, Day AL. Lumbar spine injuries in athletes. Neurosurg Focus. 2006;21(E4):1–5.
6. Gosteli G, Yersin B, Mabire C, Pasquier M, Albrecht R, Carron PN. Retrospective analysis of 616 air-rescue trauma cases related to the practice of extreme sports. Injury. 2016;47(7):1414–20.
7. Hasler RM, Hüttner HE, Keel MJB, Durrer B, Zimmermann H, Exadaktylos AK, et al. Spinal and pelvic injuries in airborne sports: a retrospective analysis from a major Swiss trauma centre. Injury. 2012;43(4):440–5.
8. Singh R, Bhalla A, Ockendon M, Hay S. Spinal motocross injuries in the United Kingdom. Orthop J Sport Med. 2018;6(1):1–5.
9. Buckley SM, Chalmers DJ, Langley JD. Injuries due to falls from horses. Aust J Public Health. 1993;17(3):269–71.
10. Ingemarson H, Grevsten S, Thoren L. Lethal horse-riding injuries. J Trauma. 1989;29(1):25–30.

11. Siebenga J, Segers MJM, Elzinga M, Bakker FC, Haarman HJTM, Patka P. Spine fractures caused by horse riding. Eur Spine J. 2006;15:465–71.
12. Kane I, Ong A, Radcliff KE, Austin LS, Maltenfort M, Tjoumakaris F. Epidemiology of aquatic and recreational water sport injuries: a case-control analysis. Orthopedics. 2015;38(9):e813–8.
13. Owens BD, Nacca C, Harris AP, Feller RJ. Comprehensive review of skiing and snowboarding injuries. J Am Acad Orthop Surg. 2018;26(1):e1–10.
14. Keene JS. Thoracolumbar fractures in winter sports. Clin Orthop Relat Res. 1987:39–49.
15. Weber CD, Horst K, Lefering R, Hofman M, Dienstknecht T, Pape HC. Major trauma in winter sports: an international trauma database analysis. Eur J Trauma Emerg Surg. 2016;42(6):741–7.
16. Franz T, Hasler RM, Benneker L, Zimmermann H, Siebenrock KA, Exadaktylos AK. Severe spinal injuries in alpine skiing and snowboarding: a 6-year review of a tertiary trauma centre for the Bernese Abs ski resorts, Switzerland. Br J Sports Med. 2008;42(1):55–8.
17. Yamakawa H, Murase S, Sakai H, Iwama T, Katada M, Niikawa S, et al. Spinal injuries in snowboarders: risk of jumping as an integral part of snowboarding. J Trauma Inj Infect Crit Care. 2001;50(6):1101–5.
18. Bigdon SF, Gewiess J, Hoppe S, Exadaktylos AK, Benneker LM, Fairhurst PG, et al. Spinal injury in alpine winter sports: a review. Scand J Trauma Resusc Emerg Med. 2019;27(1):1–11.
19. Floyd T. Alpine skiing, snowboarding, and spinal trauma. Arch Orthop Trauma Surg. 2001;121(8):433–6.
20. Congeni J, McCulloch J, Swanson K. Lumbar spondylolysis a study of natural progression in athletes. Am J Sports Med. 1997;25(2):248–53.
21. Roche MB, Rowe GG. The incidence of separate neural arch and coincident bone variations: a survey of 4,200 skeletons. Anat Rec. 1951;109:233.
22. Amato M, Totty WG, Gilula LA. Spondylolysis of the lumbar spine: demonstration of defects and laminal fragmentation. Radiology. 1984;153(3 I):627–9.
23. Fredrickson B, Baker D, McHolick W, Yuan H, Lubicky JP. The natural history of spondylolysis. Surgery. 1984;66(5):699.
24. Soler T, Calderon C. The prevalence of spondylolysis in the Spanish elite athlete. / Frequence de la spondylolyse chez des athletes espagnols de haut niveau. Am J Sports Med. 2000;28(1):57–62. http://articles.sirc.ca/search.cfm?id=S-163857%5Cn.
25. Rossi F, Dragoni S. Lumbar spondylolysis, occurrence in competitive athletes: updated achievements in a series of 390 cases. J Sports Med Phys Fitn. 1990;30(4):450–2.
26. Gottschlich LM, Young CC. Spine injuries in dancers. Curr Sports Med Rep. 2011;10(1):40–4.
27. Amari R, Sakai T, Katoh S, Sairyo K, Higashino K, Tachibana K, et al. Fresh stress fractures of lumbar pedicles in an adolescent male ballet dancer: case report and literature review. Arch Orthop Trauma Surg. 2009;129(3):397–401.
28. Ireland ML, Micheli LJ. Bilateral stress fracture of the lumbar pedicles in a ballet dancer. A case report. J Bone Jt Surg Am. 1987;69(1):140–2.
29. Parvataneni HK, Nicholas SJ, McCance SE. Bilateral pedicle stress fractures in a female athlete. Spine (Phila Pa 1976). 2004;29(2):E19–21.
30. Holdsworth F. Fractures, dislocations, and fracture-dislocations of the spine. J Bone Jt Surg. 1970;52-A(8):1534–51.
31. Purcell GA, Markolf KL, Dawson EG. Twelfth thoracic-first lumbar vertebral mechanical stability of fractures after harrington-rod instrumentation. J Bone Jt Surg. 1981;63-A(1):71–8.
32. Alanay A, Yazici M, Acaroglu E, Turhan E, Cila A, Surat A. Course of nonsurgical management of burst fractures with intact posterior ligamentous complex: an MRI study. Spine (Phila Pa 1976). 2004;29(21):2425–31.
33. Denis F. The three column spine and its significance in the classification of acute thoracolumbar spinal injuries. Spine (Phila Pa 1976). 1983;8(8):817–31.
34. James KS, Wenger KH, Schlegel JD, Dunn HK. Biomechanical evaluation of the stability of thoracolumbar burst fractures. Spine. 1994;19:1731–40.
35. Schmidt OI, Gahr RH, Gosse A, Heyde CE. ATLS® and damage control in spine trauma. World J Emerg Surg. 2009;4(1):1–11.
36. Pizones J, Izquierdo E, Álvarez P, Sánchez-Mariscal F, Zúñiga L, Chimeno P, et al. Impact of magnetic resonance imaging on decision making for thoracolumbar traumatic fracture diagnosis and treatment. Eur Spine J. 2011;20(Suppl 3):390–6.
37. Shin T-S, Kim H-W, Park K-S, Kim J-M, Jung C-K. Short-segment pedicle instrumentation of thoracolumbar burst-compression fractures; short term follow-up results. J Korean Neurosurg Soc. 2007;42(4):265.
38. Magerl F, Aebi M, Gertzbein SD, Harms J, Nazarian S. A comprehensive classification of thoracic and lumbar injuries. Eur Spine J. 1994;3(4):184–201. http://link.springer.com/10.1007/BF02221591.
39. Oner F, Ramos L, Simmermacher R, Kingma P, Diekerhof C, Dhert W, et al. Classification of thoracic and lumbar spine fractures: problems of reproducibility: a study of 53 patients using CT and MRI. Eur Spine J. 2002;11(3):235–45.
40. McCormack T, Karaikovic E, Gaines RW. The load sharing classification of spine fractures. Spine (Phila Pa 1976). 1994;19(15):1741–4. http://www.ncbi.nlm.nih.gov/pubmed/7973969.
41. Dai LY, Jin WJ. Interobserver and intraobserver reliability in the load sharing classification of the assessment of thoracolumbar burst fractures. Spine (Phila Pa 1976). 2005;30(3):354–8.
42. Elzinga M, Segers M, Siebenga J, Heilbron E, De Lange-De Klerk ESM, Bakker F. Inter- and intraobserver agreement on the load sharing classification of thoracolumbar spine fractures. Injury. 2012;43(4):416–22.
43. McAfee P, Yuan H, Fredrickson B. The value of computed tomography in thoracolumbar fractures. J Bone Jt Surg. 1983;65A(4):461–73. http://citeseerx.ist.psu.edu/viewdoc/download?doi=10.1.1.132.9115&rep=rep1&type=pdf.
44. Vaccaro AR, Zeiller SC, Hulbert RJ, Anderson PA, Harris M, Hedlund R, et al. The thoracolumbar injury severity score: a proposed treatment algorithm. J Spinal Disord Tech. 2005;18(3):209–15. http://www.ncbi.nlm.nih.gov/pubmed/15905761.
45. Vaccaro AR, Lehman RA, Hurlbert RJ, Anderson PA, Harris M, Hedlund R, et al. A new classification of thoracolumbar injuries. Spine (Phila Pa 1976). 2005;30(20):2325–33.
46. Magnusson E, Spina N, Fernando ND. Classifications in brief: the thoracolumbar injury classification. Clin Orthop Relat Res. 2018;476(1):160–6.
47. Joaquim AF, Ghizoni E, Tedeschi H, Batista UC, Patel AA. Clinical results of patients with thoracolumbar spine trauma treated according to the Thoracolumbar Injury Classification and Severity Score: Clinical article. J Neurosurg Spine. 2014;20(5):562–7.
48. Schroeder GD, Harrop JS, Vaccaro AR. Thoracolumbar trauma classification. Neurosurg Clin N Am. 2017;28(1):23–9. https://doi.org/10.1016/j.nec.2016.07.007.
49. Vaccaro AR, An HS, Lin S, Sun S, Balderston RA, Cotler JM. Noncontiguous injuries of the spine. J Spinal Disord. 1992;5(3):320–9.
50. Khan N, Husain S, Haak M. Thoracolumbar injuries in the athlete. Sports Med Arthrosc. 2008;16(1):16–25.
51. Inaba K, Nosanov L, Menaker J, Bosarge P, Williams L, Turay D, et al. Prospective derivation of a clinical decision rule for thoracolumbar spine evaluation after blunt trauma: an American

Association for the Surgery of Trauma Multi-Institutional Trials Group Study. J Trauma Acute Care Surg. 2015;78(3):459–67.
52. Kirshblum SC, Waring W, Biering-Sorensen F, Burns SP, Johansen M, Schmidt-Read M, et al. Reference for the 2011 revision of the international standards for neurological classification of spinal cord injury. J Spinal Cord Med. 2011;34(6):547–54.
53. Kasai Y, Morishita K, Kawakita E, Kondo T, Uchida A. A new evaluation method for lumbar spinal instability: passive lumbar extension test. Phys Ther. 2006;86(12):1661–7.
54. Antevil JL, Sise MJ, Sack DI, Kidder B, Hopper A, Brown CVR. Spiral computed tomography for the initial evaluation of spine trauma: a new standard of care? J Trauma Inj Infect Crit Care. 2006;61(2):382–7.
55. Anissipour AK, Belding J, Bellabarba C, Bevevino AJ, Bransford RJ, Brodke DS, et al. AO spine masters series: thoracolumbar spine trauma, AO spine masters series, vol. 6. Stuttgart: Georg Thieme Verlag; 2016. http://www.thieme-connect.de/products/ebooks/book/10.1055/b-006-149770.
56. Ahn K, Jhun HJ. New physical examination tests for lumbar spondylolisthesis and instability: low midline sill sign and interspinous gap change during lumbar flexion-extension motion Orthopedics and biomechanics. BMC Musculoskelet Disord. 2015;16(1):1–6.
57. Miglioretti DL, Johnson E, Williams A, Greenlee RT, Weinmann S, Solberg LI, et al. The use of computed tomography in pediatrics and the associated radiation exposure and estimated cancer risk. JAMA Pediatr. 2013;167(8):700–7.
58. Pearce MS, Salotti JA, Little MP, McHugh K, Lee C, Kim KP, et al. Radiation exposure from CT scans in childhood and subsequent risk of leukaemia and brain tumours: a retrospective cohort study. Lancet. 2012;380(9840):499–505. https://doi.org/10.1016/S0140-6736(12)60815-0.
59. Carreon LY, Glassman SD, Djurasovic M. Reliability and agreement between fine-cut CT scans and plain radiography in the evaluation of posterolateral fusions. Spine J. 2007;7(1):39–43.
60. Leferink V, Veldhuis E, Zimmerman K, Ten Vergert E, Ten Duis H. Classificational problems in ligamentary distraction type vertebral fractures: 30% of all B-type fractures are initially unrecognised. Eur Spine J. 2002;11(3):246–50.
61. Hartmann F, Nusselt T, Mattyasovszky S, Maier G, Rommens PM, Gercek E. Misdiagnosis of thoracolumbar posterior ligamentous complex injuries and use of radiographic parameter correlations to improve detection accuracy. Asian Spine J. 2019;13(1):29–34.
62. Schnake KJ, von Scotti F, Haas NP, Kandziora F. Typ-B-Distraktionsverletzungen der thorakolumbalen WirbelsäuleType B injuries of the thoracolumbar spine. Unfallchirurg. 2008;111(12):977–84.
63. Hiyama A, Watanabe M, Katoh H, Sato M, Nagai T, Mochida J. Relationships between posterior ligamentous complex injury and radiographic parameters in patients with thoracolumbar burst fractures. Injury. 2015;46(2):392–8. https://doi.org/10.1016/j.injury.2014.10.047.
64. Rajasekaran S, Maheswaran A, Aiyer SN, Kanna R, Dumpa SR, Shetty AP. Prediction of posterior ligamentous complex injury in thoracolumbar fractures using non-MRI imaging techniques. Int Orthop. 2016;40(6):1075–81. https://doi.org/10.1007/s00264-016-3151-1.
65. Vaccaro AR, Rihn JA, Saravanja D, Anderson DG, Hilibrand AS, Albert TJ, et al. Injury of the posterior ligamentous complex of the thoracolumbar spine: a prospective evaluation of the diagnostic accuracy of magnetic resonance imaging. Spine (Phila Pa 1976). 2009;34(23):841–7.
66. Li X, Zhang J, Tang H, Lu Z, Liu S, Chen S, et al. Comparison between posterior short-segment instrumentation combined with lateral-approach interbody fusion and traditional wide-open anterior-posterior surgery for the treatment of thoracolumbar fractures. Medicine (Baltimore). 2015;94(44):e1946.
67. Rihn JA, Yang N, Fisher C, Saravanja D, Smith H, Morrison WB, et al. Using magnetic resonance imaging to accurately assess injury to the posterior ligamentous complex of the spine: a prospective comparison of the surgeon and radiologist. J Neurosurg Spine. 2011;12(4):391–6.
68. Leone A, Cianfoni A, Cerase A, Magarelli N, Bonomo L. Lumbar spondylolysis: a review. Skelet Radiol. 2011;40(6):683–700.
69. DeCoster TA, Stevens MA, Albright JP. Sports fractures. Iowa Orthop J. 1994;14:81–4.
70. Miller RA, Hardcastle P, Renwick SE. Lower spinal mobility and external immobilization in the normal and pathologic condition. Orthop Rev. 1992;21(6):753–7.
71. Vander KD, Abad G, Basford JR, Maus TP, Yaszemski MJ, Kaufman KR. Lumbar spine stabilization with a thoracolumbosacral orthosis: evaluation with video fluoroscopy. Spine (Phila Pa 1976). 2004;29(1):100–4.
72. Shen W-J, Shen Y-S. Nonsurgical treatment of three-column thoracolumbar junction burst fractures without neurologic deficit. Spine (Phila Pa 1976). 1999;24(4):412–5.
73. Moller A, Hasserius R, Redlund-Johnell I, Ohlin A, Karlsson MK. Nonoperatively treated burst fractures of the thoracic and lumbar spine in adults: a 23- to 41-year follow-up. Spine J. 2007;7(6):701–7.
74. Aligizakis A, Katonis P, Stergiopoulos K, Galanakis I, Karabekios S, Hadjipavlou A. Functional outcome of burst fractures of the thoracolumbar spine managed non-operatively, with early ambulation, evaluated using the load sharing classification. Acta Orthop Belg. 2002;68(3):279–87.
75. Cantor JB, Lebwohl NH, Garvey T, Eismont FJ. Nonoperative management of stable thoracolumbar burst fractures with early ambulation and bracing. Spine (Phila Pa 1976). 1993;18(8):971–6.
76. Wood KB, Buttermann GR, Phukan R, Harrod CC, Mehbod A, Shannon B, et al. Operative compared with nonoperative treatment of a thoracolumbar burst fracture without neurological deficit: a prospective randomized study with follow-up at sixteen to twenty-Two years. J Bone Jt Surg Am. 2015;97(1):3–9.
77. Gnanenthiran SR, Adie S, Harris IA. Nonoperative versus operative treatment for thoracolumbar burst fractures without neurologic deficit: a meta-analysis Clin Orthop Relat Res. 2012;470(2):567–77.
78. Kepler CK, Vaccaro AR. Thoracolumbar spine fractures and dislocations. In: Court-Brown CM, Heckman JD, McQueen MM, Ricci WM, Tornetta P, editors. Rockwood and Green's fractures in adults. 8th ed. Philadelphia, PA: Lippincott Williams & Wilkins; 2015. p. 1757–93.
79. Siebenga J, Leferink VJM, Segers MJM, Elzinga MJ, Bakker FC, Haarman HJTM, et al. Treatment of traumatic thoracolumbar spine fractures: a multicenter prospective randomized study of operative versus nonsurgical treatment. Spine (Phila Pa 1976). 2006;31(25):2881–90.
80. Esses S, Botsford D, Kostuik J. Evaluation of Surgical Treatment for Burst Fractures. Spine (Phila Pa 1976). 1990;15(7):667–73.
81. Anderson PA, Crutcher J, King H, Montano P. Spinal canal decompression in thoracolumbar burst fractures treated with posterior distraction rods. J Orthop Trauma 1989;3(2):160–1.
82. Wang L, Li J, Wang H, Yang Q, Lv D, Zhang W, et al. Posterior short segment pedicle screw fixation and TLIF for the treatment of unstable thoracolumbar/lumbar fracture. BMC Musculoskelet Disord. 2014;15(1):1–11.
83. Gertzbein SD. Scoliosis Research Society: multicenter spine fracture study. Spine (Phila Pa 1976). 1992;17(5):528–40.
84. Harrington R, Budorick T, Hoyt J, Anderson P, Tencer A. Biomechanics of indirect reduction of bone retropulsed into the spinal canal in vertebral fracture. Spine (Phila Pa 1976). 1993;18(6):692–9.

85. Xu GJ, Li ZJ, Ma JX, Zhang T, Fu X, Ma XL. Anterior versus posterior approach for treatment of thoracolumbar burst fractures: a meta-analysis. Eur Spine J. 2013;22(10):2176–83.
86. Joaquim AF, Maslak JP, Patel AA. Spinal reconstruction techniques for traumatic spinal injuries: a systematic review of biomechanical studies. Glob Spine J. 2019;9(3):338–47.
87. McLain RF, Sparling E, Benson D. Early failure of short-segment pedicle instrumentation for thoracolumbar fractures. A preliminary report. J Bone Joint Surg Am. 1993;75:162.
88. Razak M, Mahmud M, Mokhtar SA, Omar A. Thoracolumbar fracture--dislocation results of surgical treatment. Med J Malaysia. 2000;55(Suppl C):14–7. http://www.ncbi.nlm.nih.gov/pubmed/11200038.
89. Jo DJ, Kim KT, Kim SM, Lee SH, Cho MG, Seo EM. Single-stage posterior subtotal corpectomy and circumferential reconstruction for the treatment of unstable thoracolumbar burst fractures. J Korean Neurosurg Soc. 2016;59(2):122–8.
90. Agrawal M, Garg M, Kumar A, Singh PK, Satyarthee GD, Agrawal D, et al. Management of pediatric posttraumatic thoracolumbar vertebral body burst fractures by use of single-stage posterior transpedicular approach. World Neurosurg. 2018;117:e22–33. https://doi.org/10.1016/j.wneu.2018.05.088.
91. Schnee CL, Ansell LV. Selection criteria and outcome of operative approaches for thoracolumbar burst fractures with and without neurological deficit. J Neurosurg. 2009;86(1):48–55.
92. Dai LY, Jiang LS, Jiang SD. Anterior-only stabilization using plating with bone structural autograft versus titanium mesh cages for two- or three-column thoracolumbar burst fractures: a prospective randomized study. Spine (Phila Pa 1976). 2009;34(14):1429–35.
93. Sasso RC, Best NM, Reilly TM, McGuire RA. Anterior-only stabilization of three-column thoracolumbar injuries. J Spinal Disord Tech. 2005;18(Suppl):S7–14. http://www.ncbi.nlm.nih.gov/pubmed/15699808.
94. Kaneda K, Taneichi H, Abumi K, Hashimoto T, Satoh S, Fujiya M. Anterior decompression and stabilization with the Kaneda device for thoracolumbar burst fractures associated with neurological deficits. J Bone Jt Surg Am. 1997;79(1):69–83.
95. Wood KB, Bohn D, Mehbod A. Anterior versus posterior treatment of stable thoracolumbar burst fractures without neurologic deficit: a prospective, randomized study. J Spinal Disord Tech. 2005;18(SUPPL. 1):15–23.
96. Ould-Slimane M, Damade C, Lonjon G, Gilibert A, Cochereau J, Gauthé R, et al. Instrumented circumferential fusion in two stages for instable lumbar fracture: long-term results of a series of 74 patients on sagittal balance and functional outcomes. World Neurosurg. 2017;103:303–9.
97. Oprel P, Tuinebreijer WE, Patka P, den Hartog D. Combined anterior-posterior surgery versus posterior surgery for thoracolumbar burst fractures: a systematic review of the literature. Open Orthop J. 2010;4(1):93–100.
98. Kepler CK, Vroome C, Goldfarb M, Nyirjesy S, Millhouse P, Lonjon G, et al. Variation in the management of thoracolumbar trauma and postoperative infection. J Spinal Disord Tech. 2015;28(4):E212–8.
99. Wood KB, Li W, Lebl DS, Ploumis A. Management of thoracolumbar spine fractures. Spine J. 2014;14(1):145–64. https://doi.org/10.1016/j.spinee.2012.10.041.
100. Folman Y, Gepstein R. Late outcome of nonoperative management of thoracolumbar vertebral wedge fractures. J Orthop Trauma. 2003;17(3):190–2.
101. Gertzbein S, Crowe P, Fazl M, Schwartz M, Rowed D. Canal clearance in burst fractures using the AO internal fixator. Spine (Phila Pa 1976). 1992;17(5):558–60.
102. Weinstein JN, Collalto P, Lehmann TR. Thoracolumbar "burst" fractures treated conservatively: a long-term follow-up. Spine. 1988;13:33–8.
103. Wall BA, Moskowitz A, Whitaker MC, Jones TL, Stuckey RM, Carr-Maben CL, et al. Functional outcomes of thoracolumbar junction spine fractures. Kansas J Med. 2017;10(2):30–4. http://www.ncbi.nlm.nih.gov/pubmed/29472964.
104. Quinnell RC, Stockdale HR. Some experimental observations of the influence of a single lumbar floating fusion on the remaining lumbar spine. Spine (Phila Pa 1976). 1981;6(3):263–7.
105. Sellyn GE, Hale AT, Tang AR, Waters A, Shannon CN, Bonfield CM. Pediatric thoracolumbar spine surgery and return to athletics: a systematic review. J Neurosurg Pediatr. 2019:1–11.
106. Micheli LJ. Sports following spinal surgery in the young athlete. Clin Orthop Relat Res. 1985;198:152–7.
107. Masuda T, Miyamoto K, Wakahara K, Matsumoto K, Hioki A, Shimokawa T, et al. Clinical outcomes of surgical treatments for traumatic spinal injuries due to snowboarding. Asian Spine J. 2015;9(1):90–8.
108. Gotfryd AO, Franzin FJ, Hartl R. Thoracolumbar Chance fracture during a professional female soccer game: case report. Einstein (Sao Paulo). 2016;14(1):67–70.
109. Ferguson RJ, Mcmaster JH, Stanitski CL. Low back pain in college football linemen. Am J Sports Med. 1974;2(2):63–9.

Acute Fractures in Sport: Pelvis and Acetabulum

19

Nikolaos Patsiogiannis and Peter V. Giannoudis

19.1 General Considerations

19.1.1 Epidemiology

Injuries to the hip and pelvis account for approximately 5–6% of all injuries sustained in adult athletes and about 10–24% in the paediatric athletes [1, 2]. A particular group of athletes such as ballet dancers, runners and soccer players have a higher incidence of this kind of injuries 43.8%, 2–11% and 5.4–13% respectively [1]. Noteworthy, these injuries are also very common in high impact sports such as American football, hockey, cycling and equestrianism [3].

19.1.2 Differential Diagnosis

The aetiology of hip and pelvic symptoms varies in relation to different age groups.

In the *paediatric population*, the musculoskeletal system is still immature, and hip and pelvic pain can be caused by one or more of the following pathologies [3]:

- Skeletal (hip dislocations, physeal, non-physeal, apophyseal avulsions, stress and pathologic fractures)
- Soft tissue (muscular/musculotendinous strains, injury to the apophyseal insertion site, soft-tissue contusion)
- Non-traumatic (slipped capital femoral epiphysis, Leg-Calve-Perthes disease, DDH, septic arthritis)
- Referred pain from structures in the torso, viscera, lumbar spine, genitalia

In *adults*, hip and pelvic pain could be related to a number of clinical entities, including [3]:

- Trauma to the bony structures of the femur, acetabulum and pelvis (hip dislocations, fractures of the femur, pelvis or acetabulum, stress fractures)
- Soft tissue injuries (Contusions, musculotendinous strains, hamstrings injuries, adductors/abductor injuries)
- Non-traumatic (AVN, myositis ossificans, Greater Trochanteric Pain Syndrome—GTPS, Snapping Hip-Coxa Saltans, bursitis, meralgia paresthetica, osteitis pubis, piriformis syndrome, labral tears, ischiofemoral impingement, Fig. 19.1)
- Referred pain from structures in the torso, viscera, lumbar spine/sacroiliac joints, genitalia, hernias
- Early degenerative disease

19.1.3 Signs and Symptoms

Each injury may present with a different history of trauma mechanism (contact or non-contact). The athlete can refer an audible pop or snap (avulsion injuries). Ability to finish the athletic activity-game can direct towards the diagnosis, as severe injuries can present with inability to weight bear (hip fracture-dislocations, acetabular fractures).

Athlete usually reports pain and weakness. A complete physical examination of the spine, pelvis and hip is required, including a full neurological assessment.

N. Patsiogiannis
Department of Trauma and Orthopaedics, Leeds General Infirmary, Leeds, UK
e-mail: nikolaos.patsiogiannis@nhs.net

P. V. Giannoudis (✉)
Academic Department of Trauma and Orthopaedics, School of Medicine, Leeds General Infirmary, University of Leeds, Leeds, UK

NIHR Leeds Biomedical Research Centre, Chapel Allerton Hospital, Leeds, UK
e-mail: p.giannoudis@leeds.ac.uk

G. A. J. Robertson, N. Maffulli (eds.), *Fractures in Sport*, https://doi.org/10.1007/978-3-030-72036-0_19

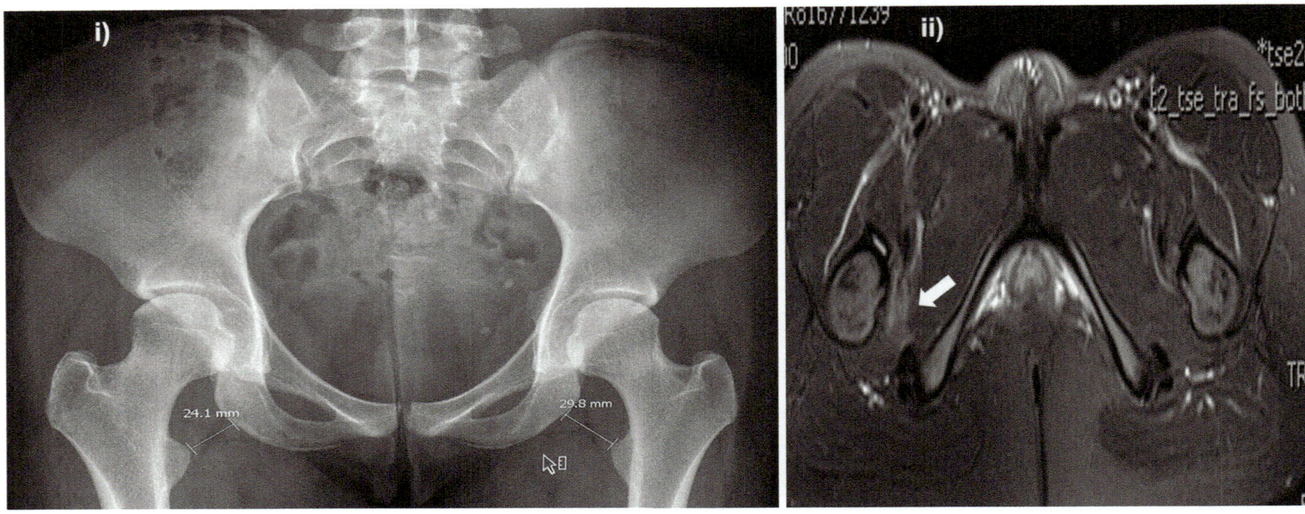

Fig. 19.1 Antero-posterior pelvic radiograph in a 18 year old ballet dancer presenting with right hip pain. (i) Antero-posterior radiograph showing the presence of right sided ischiofemoral impingement; (ii) MRI T2 slice axial cut showing soft tissue oedema (arrow)

19.2 Apophyseal Injuries: Avulsions of the Pelvis

19.2.1 Anatomy

There are a few bony prominences (apophyses) around the pelvis where muscles originate from. The sartorius and tensor fascia lata muscles originate from the anterior superior iliac spine (ASIS). The hip adductors originate from the body of the pubis, the hamstrings from the ischial tuberosity (IT), and the direct head of the rectus femoris from the anterior inferior iliac spine (AIIS) (Fig. 19.2).

An avulsion fracture represents a type of bony injury that occurs when the growth plate of an apophysis is injured from a sudden tensile force applied through a forceful, normally eccentric, contraction of the attaching musculotendinous unit without external trauma. These injuries can either be acute or chronic. They are usually IT, AIIS and ASIS avulsions but iliac crest, greater and lesser trochanter avulsions have also been reported.

19.2.2 Epidemiology

The prevalence of these injuries is higher in adolescents [4], with a strong male preponderance. In children and adolescents, the growth plate is weaker than the attaching musculotendinous structure until its fusion at the time of skeletal maturation. This is the reason why the apophysis growth plate is susceptible to injuries when the attaching musculotendinous unit is contracted.

Most of these fractures occur during the eccentric phase of a sporting activity from the higher forces produced by this modality of muscular contractions [4]. These injuries can also occur at other locations, such as the spinous process or the lesser tuberosity, but they are more common around the hip and the pelvis as the apophyses there appear and fuse later compared to other areas [5].

The body of literature surrounding avulsion fractures is largely comprised of case reports and case series. Rossi and Dragoni in an Italian Sports clinic retrospectively studied 1238 pelvic radiographs taken over 22 years in competitive athletes with an age range of 11–35 years, and compared the findings to focal traumatic symptoms [6]. They found 203 avulsion fractures of the pelvic apophyses.

In more than half of the cases (n = 109), the ischial tuberosity (IT) was affected followed by the anterior inferior iliac spine (AIIS) in 45 cases and the anterior superior iliac spine (ASIS), in 39 cases. They also reported seven cases of avulsion of the superior corner of the pubic symphysis (SCPS) and three cases of iliac crest (IC) avulsion. Soccer and gymnastics were the sports with the highest number of avulsion fractures. More rarely, these injuries also involved the lesser or, the greater trochanter [6].

19.2.3 Symptoms and Signs

In acute injuries, patients usually describe an eccentric load to the muscle-tendon unit. The athlete will experience sudden pain which might be associated with a pop/snap referred to the involved apophysis in the skeletally immature individual.

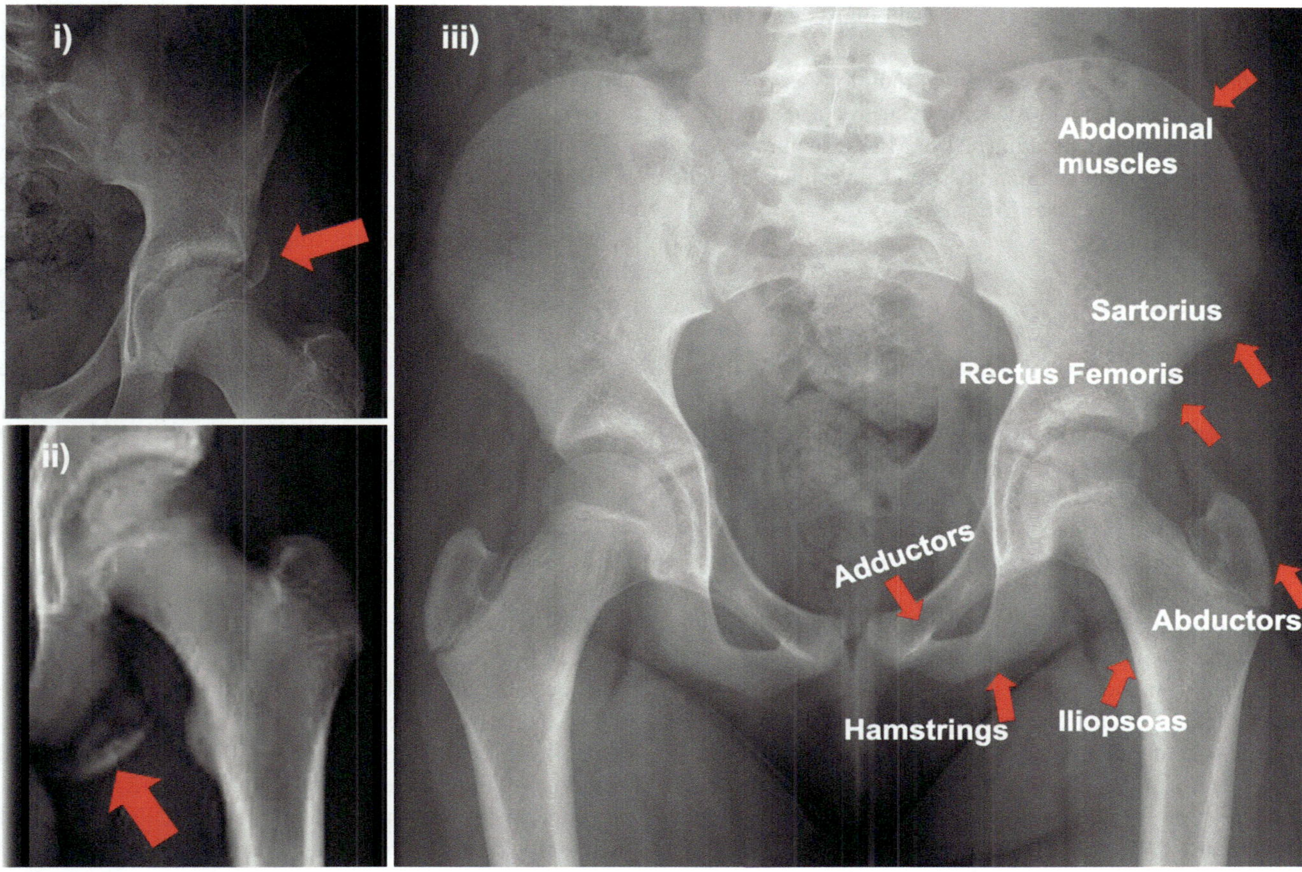

Fig. 19.2 (i) Antero-posterior left hip radiograph showing avulsion injury of the anterior inferior iliac spine. (ii) Antero-posterior radiograph left hip showing avulsion fracture of ischium. (iii) Bony prominences (apophyses) around the pelvis where muscles originate from and are associated with apophyseal injuries

Regarding the mechanism, this is relevant to the site of the injury as below:

- Ischial tuberosity (IT) avulsion fractures usually result from sudden forceful flexion of the hip joint when the knee is extended, and the hamstrings are powerfully contracted [7]. Avulsions of the ischial tuberosity are often related to sports such as soccer, waterskiing, track and field, and other competitive sports [8].
- Avulsions of the AIIS occur due to a forceful hip hyperextension and knee flexion and are also referred as sprinter's fractures because they primarily occur in sports such as American football, rugby, and soccer during the kicking phase [5].
- ASIS avulsions may occur from eccentric hip and knee extension.

All these injuries may result in bruising, pain, swelling and tenderness on palpation. Pain will be reproduced with stretching of the involved musculotendinous unit. Weakness may also be present in relation with the attached muscle group (hamstrings weakness for IT avulsions, hip flexion for ASIS/AIIS avulsions, adductor for pubic symphysis avulsions). Finally, in severe injuries or in the early acute phase, athlete may walk with a limp.

19.2.4 Imaging

Radiographs usually will reveal a displaced fracture in skeletally immature individuals, but they can also be missed because of the location and small size of the fragments. In adults, the equivalent is usually a soft tissue injury not apparent on radiographs.

Given their rarity, these injuries can regularly be missed on initial presentation, causing chronic problems (pain, neurological symptoms). In chronic cases, excessive bone formation can occur, and other pathologies such as bone tumours are regularly suspected by radiologists less familiar with the condition.

In most acute cases, conventional radiology is enough to formulate a correct diagnosis. However, in chronic, unclear cases or in the adult population, CT or MRI scan may become necessary to confirm the diagnosis and investigate/exclude other non-traumatic causes [5].

19.2.5 Treatment

Most of these injuries are treated conservatively with bed rest, ice, NSAIDS and initially a period of non or protected weight-bearing with crutches. A gradual stretching regimen can be initiated with pain as a guide. When pain resolves, strengthening physiotherapy can be initiated until full ROM and muscle strength are restored. Return to sport is advised only when strength is 90% of the contralateral side to avoid further injury.

Complications following conservative treatment include heterotopic ossification and non-union. The non-union risk is significantly higher for IT avulsions with displacement greater than 1.5 cm. "Hamstring syndrome" can develop from shortening and fibrosis at the origin of the muscle which can trap the sciatic nerve and lead to chronic pain, inability to sit for long periods of time, and reduced athletic performance [9].

There is no consensus regarding surgical treatment in this type of injuries, especially in the adult population.

In injuries with significant acute displacement greater than 1.5–2 cm, particularly around the IT, surgical fixation can be considered [10].

Ferlic et al. treated 13 patients with IT avulsion fractures with a median age of 15 years: in patients with displacement greater than 15 mm, conservative treatment yields excellent results, and early operative intervention should be considered in physically active patients with such displacement [10].

Pogliacomi et al., regarding anterior iliac spine fractures (AIIS, ASIS), suggested surgical treatment for injuries with displacement and fragment size greater than 2 cm [11].

A recent systematical review with meta-analysis comparing avulsion fractures with a displacement of greater than 1.5 cm in adults found significantly better outcomes in the operatively treated group; delay of return to sport was also noted to be shorter after surgery [12].

Surgical treatment might also be considered for patients who failed to respond to conservative management, developed complications (painful non-unions) and in high demand athletes: consideration should be given to the professional status of the athlete, and the need for a rapid rehabilitation program and a prompt return to their professional career.

19.2.6 Prognosis

The prognosis of such injuries is generally good, and full recovery and return to sports can be expected. IT avulsions and hamstrings injuries can though take more time to recover.

Uzun et al. reported nine patients with avulsion fractures of the AIIS who sought treatment after conservative management at a mean of 3 months after the initial injury. All the clinical results were rated as excellent. At final follow-up, no patients reported pain, evidence of impingement, limitation of motion or restriction of sports activity [13].

Overall, both conservative and operative methods provide excellent outcomes in most patients. However, surgery may result in shorter recovery time and is preferable in athletes with greater displacements and high professional demands [9].

19.3 Acetabular Fractures

19.3.1 Anatomy

In the acetabulum, the head of the femur meets the concave side of the pelvis to form the hip joint. The acetabulum is formed by three different bones: the ilium, the ischium, and the pubis. All three bones are referred together as the innominate bone, and join at the tri-radiate cartilage. Final fusion of the innominate bone occurs in the late teens period.

The acetabulum has an anterior and a posterior wall, a roof, and is floored by the quadrilateral plate (Fig. 19.3, i). The acetabulum is supported by two columns of bone. On the lateral view, the innominate bone resembles the Greek letter lambda "λ", with the longer limb forming the anterior column, and the shorter forming the posterior column (Fig. 19.3, ii, iii).

The shorter **posterior column** is comprised of the quadrilateral surface, the posterior half of the acetabulum, the ischium and the sciatic notches.

The **anterior column** is comprised of the anterior ilium (iliac crest, iliac spines), the anterior wall and dome, the iliopectineal eminence, and the lateral superior pubic ramus.

19.3.2 Epidemiology

Acetabular fractures follow a bimodal distribution. In patients older than 60 years, the most common mechanism of injury is a fall, as opposed to high energy injuries (motor vehicle accidents) in younger patients [14]. This is consistent with the fact that the elderly patients more commonly present with an acetabular fracture as an isolated injury.

From data available from the UK after the enactment of mandatory seatbelt legislation in 1983, the overall incidence

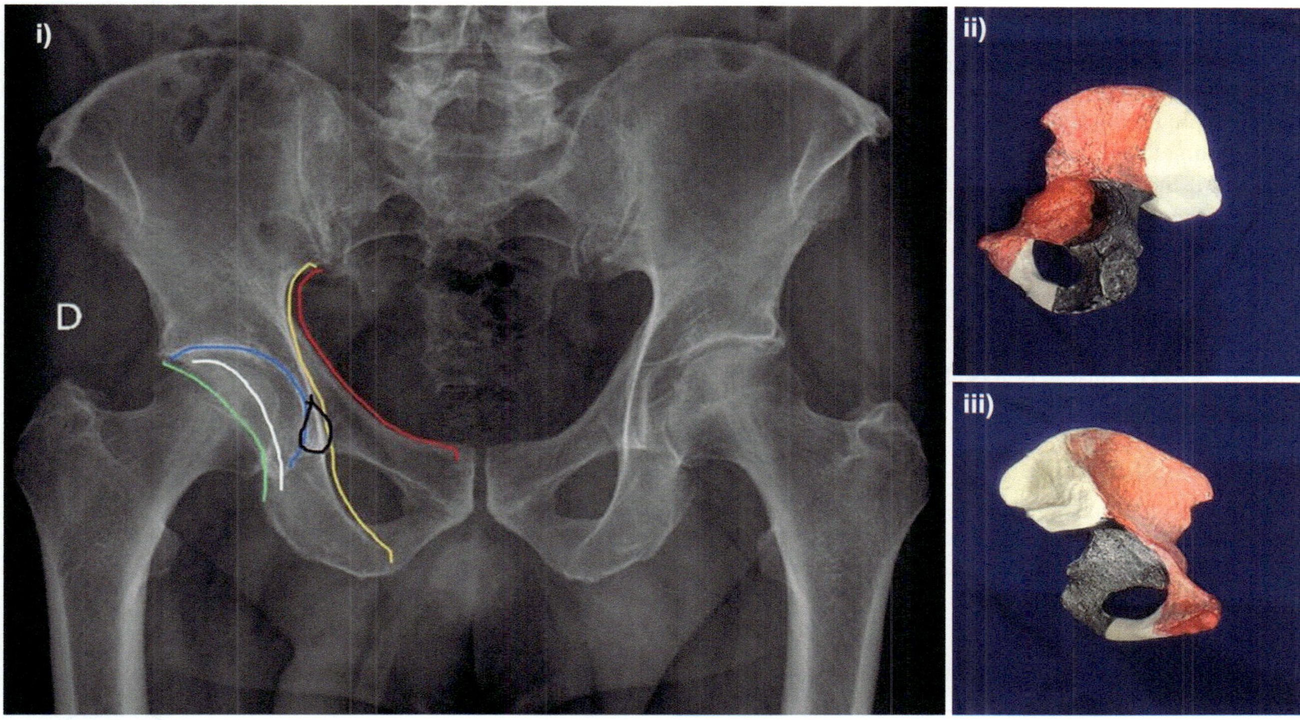

Fig. 19.3 (i) Antero-posterior view of the pelvis. Colour lines represent the following: Red: iliopectineal line. Yellow: ilioischial line. Green: Posterior wall. White: Anterior wall. Blue: dome of the acetabulum. Black: Radiographic teardrop. (ii) Obturator oblique view; (iii) Iliac oblique view: Plastic hemipelvis bone model demonstrating the two-column concept as described by Judet-Letournel. Red colour: anterior column Black colour: posterior column

of this fractures was approximately 3 patients/100,000/year, and has remained stable since [15].

Although acetabular fractures are common in the general population, they rarely occur in athletes, and only few case series and case reports have been documented. Good et al. reported two cases of acetabular fractures following rugby tackles, both requiring fixation [16]. Morrissey et al. managed four closed, isolated acetabular fractures in skeletally immature patients (13–16 year old) three of which were in conjunction with hip dislocations [17]. Stilger et al. reported a posterior wall fracture in an intercollegiate American football player, which was judged unstable under anaesthesia and underwent fixation [18]. Williams et al. evaluated the incidence and MRI appearance of acetabular (fatigue) fractures in military endurance athletes and recruits. Of 178 17–45 year old trainees with a history of activity-related hip pain which were evaluated with MRI and bone scan, 12 demonstrated acetabular stress fractures [19]. Acetabular fractures have also been reported following a game of squash [20] and during competitive cycling [21, 22].

19.3.3 Signs and Symptoms

A fractured acetabulum will be almost always painful. The pain is worsened with movement and weight-bearing, but it may be still possible to put some weight on the affected extremity. Patients will usually report hip pain on examination and also complain of diffuse pain around the groin and thigh. If any nerve damage co-exists, patients may exhibit weakness, numbness or a tingling sensation down the leg. A full neurological examination is always mandatory if these injuries are suspected.

As these fractures are usually high energy traumatic events, especially in the athletic population, other associated injuries may need to be assessed and managed first (lower extremity, spine, head, chest, abdominal and genitourinary injuries). The advanced trauma life support (ATLS) protocol should always be followed. The presence of a hip dislocation, a femoral neck fracture or sciatic nerve palsy should always be excluded. The overlying skin should be assessed for a Morel-Lavallee degloving lesion which might predispose to wound complications (high rate of S. Epidermidis colonisation) [23].

19.3.4 Imaging

Conventional anteroposterior pelvic radiographs with the addition of Judet (obturator and iliac oblique) views are usually recommended. Inlet/outlet pelvic views can also be requested if there are concerns for pelvic ring involvement, and sometimes fluoroscopic evaluation under anaesthesia might be useful to assess posterior wall stability.

Currently, the gold standard is a pelvic CT scan which provides more details regarding the fracture configuration and helps with decision making and operating planning if required. A 3D reconstruction is also beneficial.

19.3.5 Classification

Judet and Letournel classified these injuries to five elementary and five associated patterns as follows (Figs. 19.4 and 19.5) [24–26].

19.3.6 Treatment

Acetabular fractures are intra-articular fractures, and there is a low threshold for surgical treatment, especially in the presence of displacement aiming to avoid the most common long-term complication, post-traumatic arthritis. Over the past 50 years, their treatment has shifted from conservative to operative. Nevertheless, conservative treatment can provide a good outcome, and some patient-related factors are important for decision making. Indications for nonoperative treatment include:

- Contraindication to surgery: high operative risk patients (elderly patients, multiple comorbidities)
- Severe injuries to the skin and soft tissues (Morel-Lavallee)
- Morbidly obese patients
- Late presentation (greater than 3 weeks)
- Undisplaced/minimally displaced fractures (less than 2 mm)

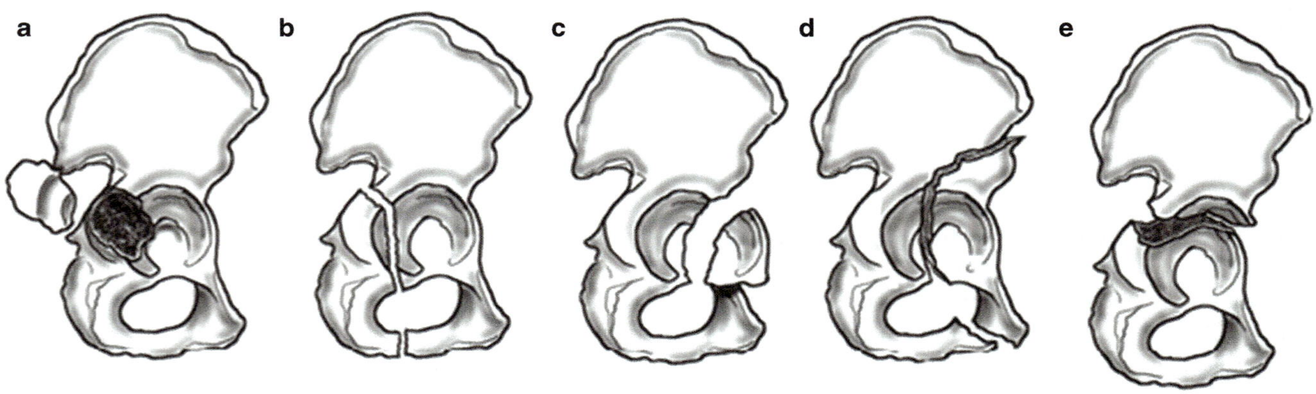

Fig. 19.4 The five elementary acetabulum fracture patterns: **Type A** posterior wall fracture (PW), **Type B** posterior column fracture (PC), **Type C** anterior wall fracture (AW), **Type D** anterior column fracture (AC), **Type E** transverse fracture (TV)

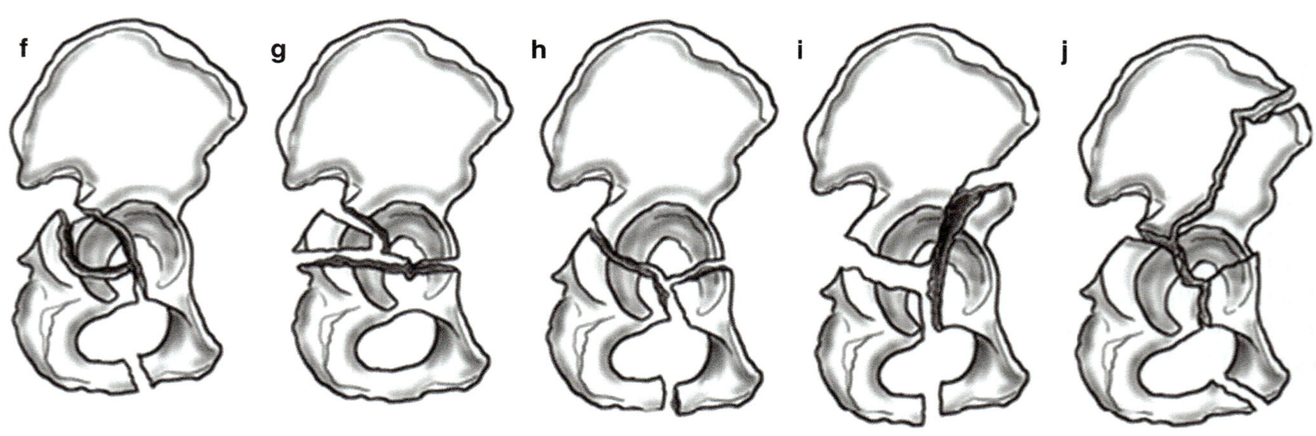

Fig. 19.5 The five associated acetabulum fracture patterns: **Type F** posterior column and posterior wall fracture (PC/W), **Type G** transverse posterior wall fracture (TV/PW), **Type H** T-shaped fracture, **Type I** anterior column and posterior hemitransverse fracture (AC/PHTV), **Type J** both column fracture (ABC)

- Displacement with congruency of the femoral head with the acetabular roof on antero-posterior and Judet views and a minimum of 50% of the posterior wall is intact on all CT cuts [24, 27].
- Congruent both column fracture patterns without significant displacement
- Comminuted fractures in the presence of severely osteopenic/osteoporotic, precluding optimal fixation following fracture reduction.

Indications of operative treatment are presented below:

- *Requirement for emergency fixation* [23, 28]*:*
  - Irreducible hip dislocation
  - Recurrent hip dislocation following reduction despite traction
  - Progressive sciatic nerve palsy following reduction
  - Associated vascular injuries requiring repair
  - Open fractures
- *Indications for acetabular fixation:*
  - Incongruent hip joint from incarcerated fragments/intra-articular loose bodies.
  - Ipsilateral femoral neck fracture
  - Marginal posterior wall impaction.
  - Unstable fracture (e.g. fracture involving more than 40–50% of the posterior wall compared to the contralateral side)

    When less than 40–50% is involved, fluoroscopic evaluation under anesthesia (EUA) is recommended to assess the stability of the hip
- Displacement of the acetabular roof greater than 2 mm
- Less than 3 weeks from the injury

Treatment strategy can be summarised as follows:

- *Nonoperative:*
  - Non-weight bearing (NWB) mobilisation on the affected side or protected weight bearing (PWB) for about 6–8 weeks based on the fracture characteristics. Lowest joint reactive forces are seen with toe-touch weight-bearing.
  - Thromboprophylaxis is required to avoid deep vein thrombosis (DVT)
  - Subsequent progression to full weight-bearing after 6–8 weeks.
  - Physiotherapy
  - Close clinical and radiographical follow up
  - Once union is demonstrated, and the patient is pain-free, they can initiate light training and gradually build up activity levels.
- *Operative:*

  When surgery is required, it is better to take place 3–5 days following the injury. This period will allow optimisation of the patient status and help decrease excessive intraoperative bleeding. At 10 days, the fragments are difficult to manipulate, and the worsts outcomes are reported if treatment delays more than 3 weeks. The choice of approach is dictated by the fracture characteristics and displacement, but also on personal preferences and experience of the surgeons (Figs. 19.6a–c and 19.7).

The existing options of approaches to fixing these injuries are as follows:

- **Kocher Langenbeck**: provides access to the posterior acetabular elements (posterior wall and posterior column, most transverse and T-shaped).
- **Ilioinguinal**: provides access to anterior elements (anterior wall and anterior column, both column fracture, posterior hemitransverse).
- **Extended Iliofemoral**: provides extensive exposure of anterior and posterior elements. This is the only approach which allows direct visualisation of both columns (some transverse fractures and T types, some both column fractures)
- **Modified Stoppa**: provides access to the anterior elements with improved exposure of the quadrilateral surface and the posterior column.

Lately, several mini-open and percutaneous techniques have been developed that allow the surgeon to avoid extensile approaches and their morbidity [24].

19.3.7 Complications

- Post-traumatic arthritis is by far the most common, occurring in approximately 20% of the patients [29].
- Heterotopic ossification.
- AVN (avascular necrosis of the femoral head).
- Deep vein thrombosis and pulmonary embolism.
- Neurovascular injuries (sciatic nerve palsy).
- Infection.
- Intraarticular hardware placement.

19.3.8 Prognosis

Overall outcomes are related to the fracture pattern and the possible complications. Kheir et al. have reported results of patients who had surgical treatment for isolated acetabular or pelvis injuries and were able to return to their previous sporting activities. Despite the severity of acetabular and pelvic rim fractures, most patients resumed a satisfactory level of sports activity. The worst prognosis lies with fractures of both column and posterior wall acetabular [30]. Stilger et al. [18] reported a return to full athletic activities in a patient treated with ORIF for an unstable posterior wall acetabular fracture. Cerynik et al. [22] in a case series reported full return to competition 8 weeks after the original injury of a cyclist with an undisplaced acetabular fracture treated conservatively. Patel et al. [20], in a case report of a minimally displaced both column fracture following a game of squash, reported that, although the patient regained pain-free movements of the hip, he did not return to squash.

19.4 Pelvic Ring Injuries

19.4.1 Anatomy

The pelvic ring is formed by the two innominate bones and the sacrum. The ilium, ischium and pubic bones fuse at the triradiate cartilage to become the innominate bones. Strong ligaments stabilise the pelvis. Anteriorly, the symphyseal ligaments resist mostly external rotation. The sacrospinous and sacrotuberous ligaments of the pelvis floor resist shear and flexion forces and the posterior complex around the sacroiliac joints resist forces in multiple directions (anterior-posterior displacement, cephalad-caudal displacement and rotation). The posterior sacroiliac complex (anterior sacroiliac ligament, posterior sacroiliac ligament and interosseous sacroiliac ligament) is the strongest ligamentous structure in the human body and the most important for pelvic stability.

The pelvic ring is composed of three joints. The hip joint, which is a ball and socket joint, the sacroiliac joints posteriorly, and the pubic symphysis anteriorly.

19.4.2 Epidemiology

Fractures of the pelvic ring, though are rare, have been reported in athletes involved in high impact sport, including cyclists, motorcyclists and horse riders. O'Farrell et al. published a case series of nine pelvic injuries caused by horse riding accidents. Five of them were "open book" type

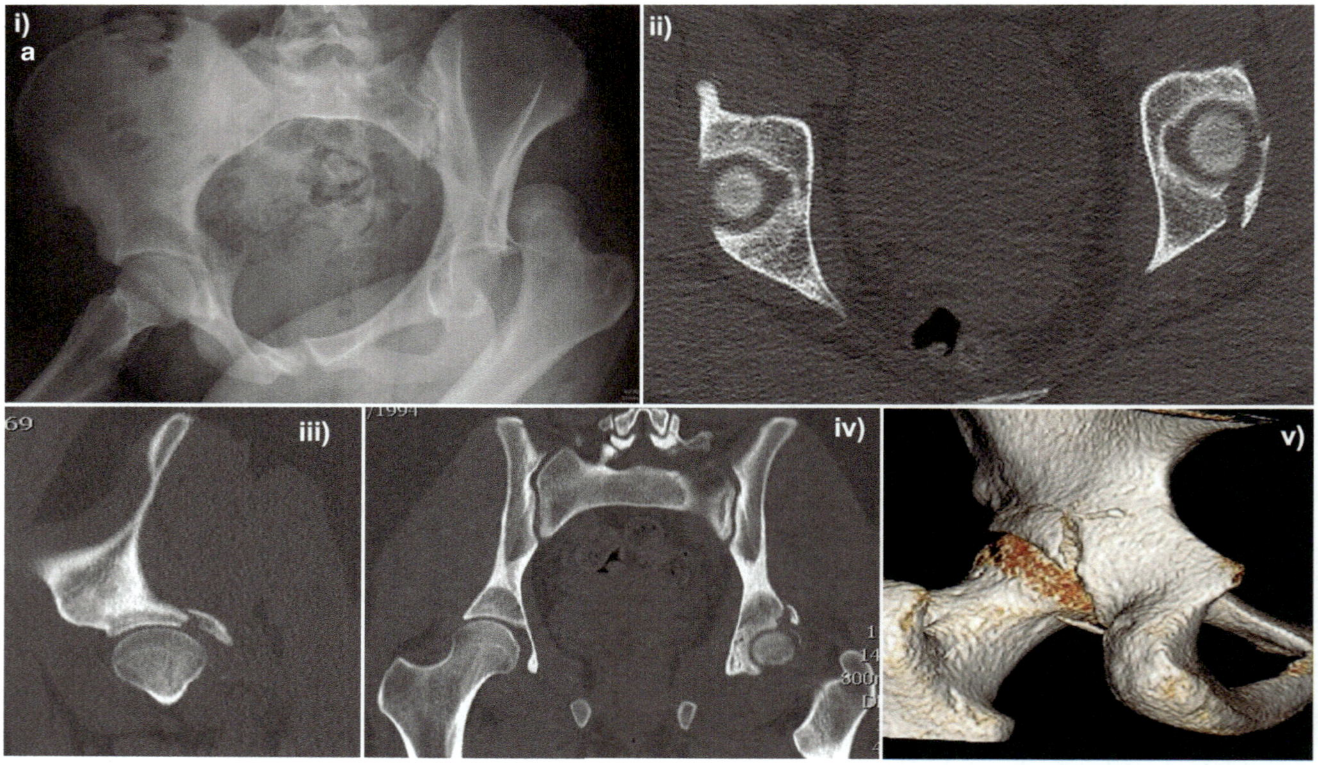

Fig. 19.6 (**a**) (i) Antero-posterior radiograph in a 18 year old female American footballer who sustained a left hip fracture dislocation following a tackle. (ii) CT slice axial cut; (iii) CT slice sagittal cut; (iv) CT slice coronal cut; (v) 3D model left hip showing fracture of the posterior wall. (**b**) (i) intraoperative images of the left hip, which was approached using a Kocher-Langebeck incision showing a labral tear (white arrow); (ii) Labral tear was repaired with a mitek suture (white arrow); (iii) Antero-posterior and (iv) Obturator oblique fluoroscopic images showing stabilisation of the posterior wall fragment with screws and a buttressing 3.5 mm plate. (**c**) (i, ii) Post-operative CT showing safe placement of the metal work. (iii) AP; (iv) Obturator oblique; (v) Iliac oblique radiographs 2 years after injury showing a congruent hip joint with no evidence of AVN or poste-traumatic arthritis

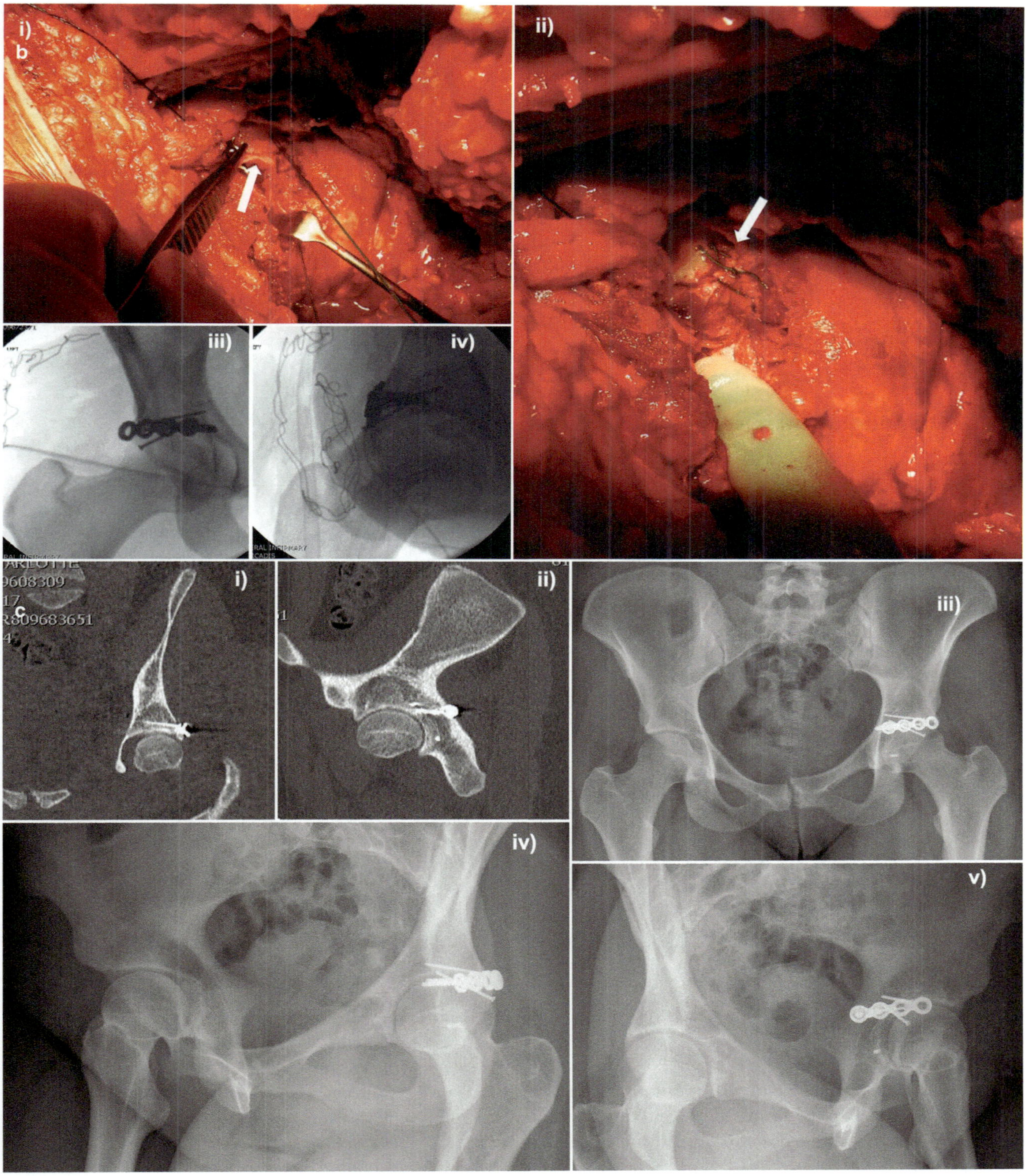

Fig. 19.6 (continued)

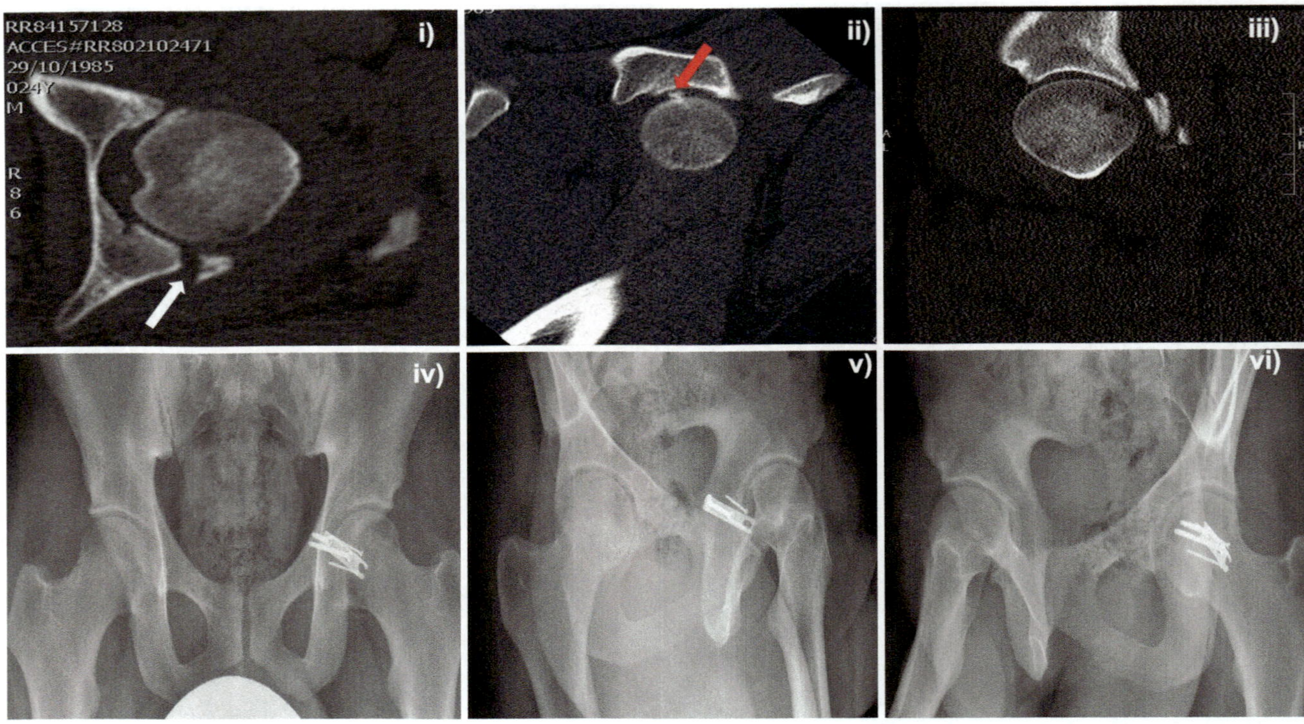

Fig. 19.7 (i–iii) CT pelvic cuts in a 28 year old professional rugby player who sustained a fracture dislocation of his left hip during a match. The hip was reduced at the accident and Emergency Department. In slice (ii) an incarcerated bone fragment is shown. (iv) Using a Kocher Langebeck approach, the left hip was exposed, the floating fragment was removed and the fracture was stabilised with screws and a spring plate. (iv) AP; (v) Iliac oblique; and (vi) obturator oblique radiograph taken 2 years after fixation

injuries, and two were fractures of the ilium without pelvic ring disruption [31]. Flynn et al. have also reported two cases of pelvic ring injuries treated conservatively while horse riding [32] while Mulhal et al. [33] described three cases of pubic symphysis diastasis on horse riders treated operatively. Service et al. [34] have retrospectively investigated the rate of urethral trauma and pubic symphysis diastasis in saddle horn injuries compared to pelvic fractures from other mechanisms. Saddle horn injuries had a higher rate of lower genitourinary injuries, and pubic symphysis diastasis was higher in these patients.

19.4.3 Classification

Tile, in 1988, classified pelvic ring injuries into A, B, and C types, based on the degree of instability and more specifically on the integrity of the posterior sacroiliac ligamentous complex [24].

A. **Stable injuries**.
   The sacroiliac complex is intact.
   A1: Avulsion fractures of the innominate bone (not involving the ring).
   A2: Stable iliac wing or stable minimally displaced ring fractures.
   A3: Transverse fractures of the sacrum or the coccyx
B. **Partially stable** (Rotationally unstable but vertically stable).
   They are caused by rotational forces.
   Partial disruption of the posterior sacroiliac complex exists.
   B1: 'open book' (external rotation).
   B2: lateral compression injury (internal rotation).
   B3: lateral compression, contralateral, or bucket-handle-type injury.
C. **Rotationally and vertically unstable**.
   These fractures have complete disruption of the posterior sacroiliac ligamentous complex, with the pelvic ring being completely disrupted at two or more places (Fig. 19.8).
   C1: unilateral
   C2: bilateral
   C3: involving acetabular fractures

The most widely used classification today is that of Young and Burgess, introduced in 1990. This classification system is useful to guide treatment based on the mechanism of the injury. It classifies pelvic fractures by the vector of applied force

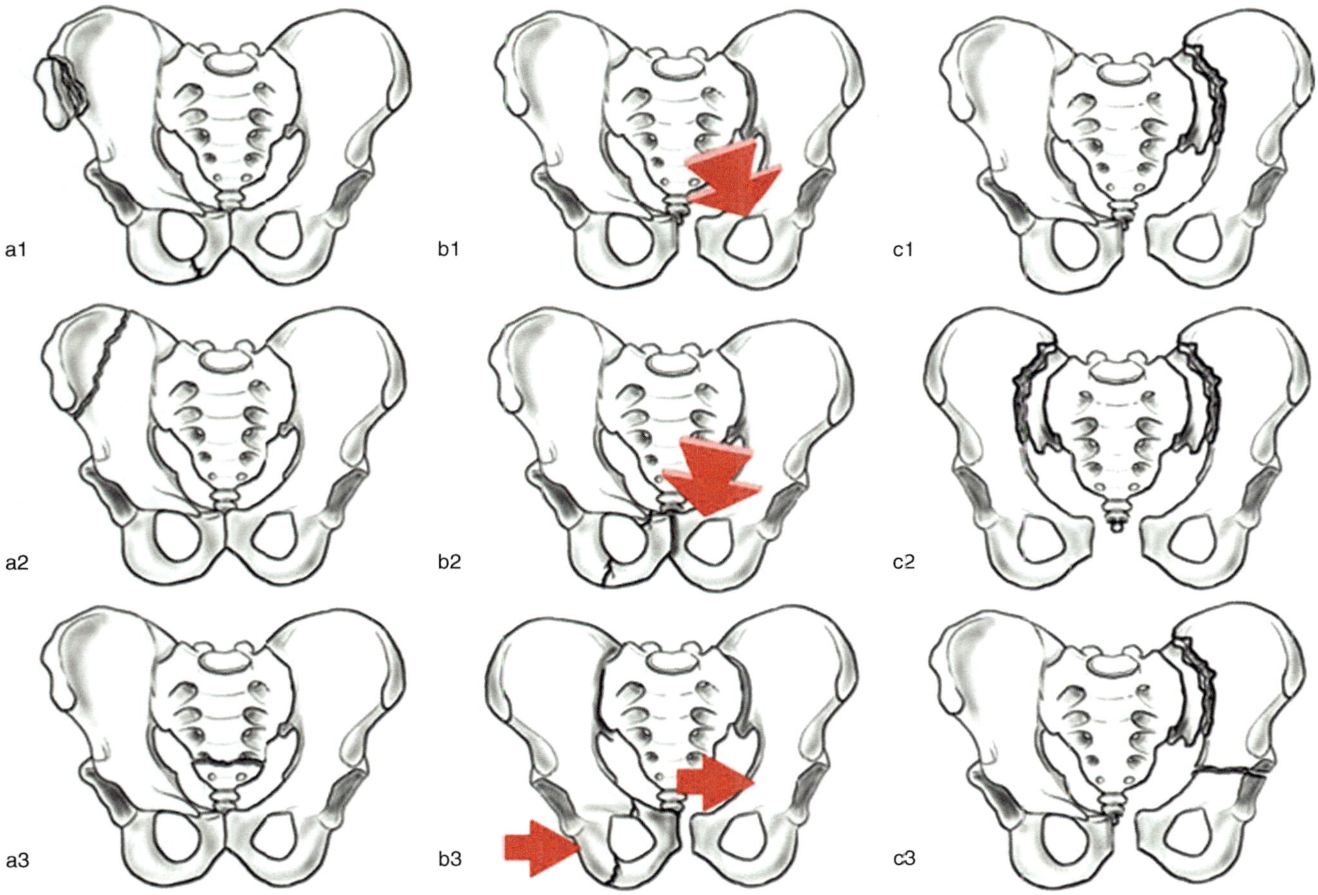

Fig. 19.8 The Tile classification: **Type A1** avulsion fracture; **Type A2** stable iliac wing or rami fracture; **Type A3** transverse sacral-coccyx fractures; **Type B1** open book anteroposterior compression fracture; **Type B2** ipsilateral lateral compression injury; **Type B3** contralateral compression injury; **Type C1** unilateral disruption with rotational and vertical pelvic ring instability; **Type C2** bilateral disruption with rotational and vertical pelvic ring instability; **Type C3** rotational and vertical pelvic ring instability with acetabular fracture

- anteroposterior compression (APC)
- lateral compression (LC)
- vertical shear (VS)

APC and LC fractures are sub-divided into Types I, II and III with increasing degrees of severity (Figs. 19.9, 19.10, and 19.11).

Vertical Shear Injuries

These injuries are completely unstable (rotationally and vertically) (Fig. 19.12).

Some injuries may result from a more complex force vector and can involve a combination of the above fractures.

19.4.4 Assessment

Pelvic ring trauma is a severe injury which requires immediate evaluation and resuscitation, as it carries a high mortality rate, with haemorrhage being the overall major cause of death. A multidisciplinary team approach that will involve general surgeons, orthopaedic surgeons and urologists is advised.

The ATLS protocol should always be followed. As part of the initial treatment, a pelvic binder is usually applied, but in unstable injuries, external fixation may also be acutely used. In the haemodynamically unstable individual, urgent angio-embolisation may also be required.

Following initial resuscitation, a full neurological examination is mandatory to rule out lumbosacral plexus injuries, including a rectal examination to evaluate anal tone and perianal sensation. Urogenital examination might reveal haematuria which is more common in males, and vaginal/rectal examination is mandatory to rule out open fractures. In male patients, a retrograde urethrogram to exclude urethral injury is usually necessary before catheterisation of the bladder. This is not required all times in female patients, as in females the urethra is shorter. Following catheterisation, a cystogram is obtained. Other common associated injuries also need to be excluded (chest and spinal injury, long bone fractures).

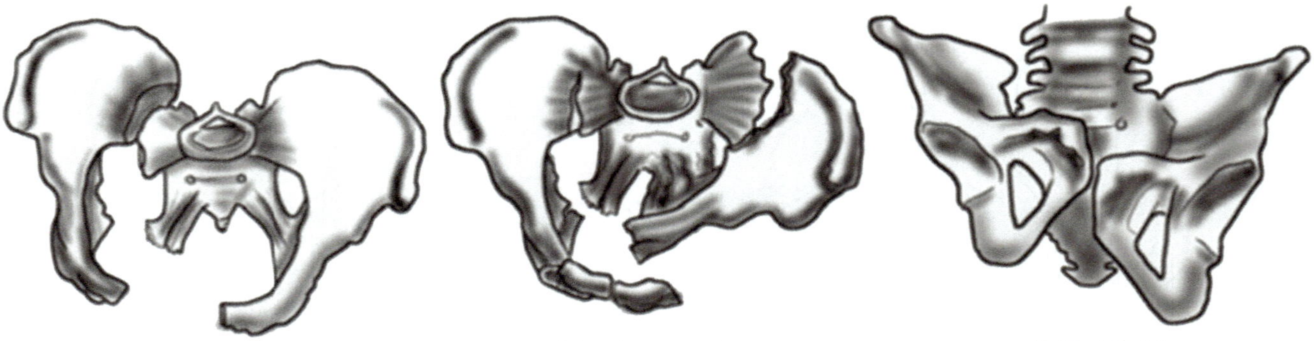

Fig. 19.9 The three basic types according to the vector of causative forces as defined at the Young and Burgess classification system

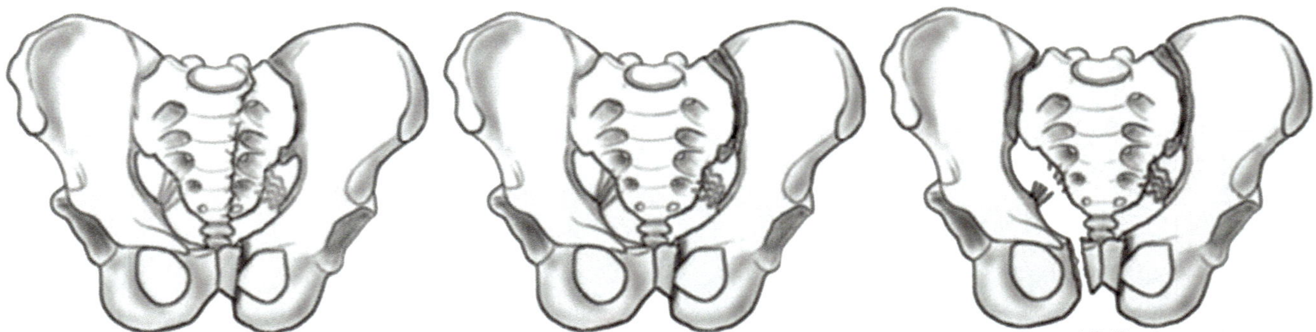

Fig. 19.10 Lateral Compression (LC) fractures: **LC-I** horizontal-oblique fractures of the rami with crush fracture of the sacrum; **LC-II** horizontal-oblique fractures of the rami with iliac wing fracture and/or sacroiliac joint separation; **LC-III** as per Type I and II with external rotation of the contralateral side and bilateral posterior instability

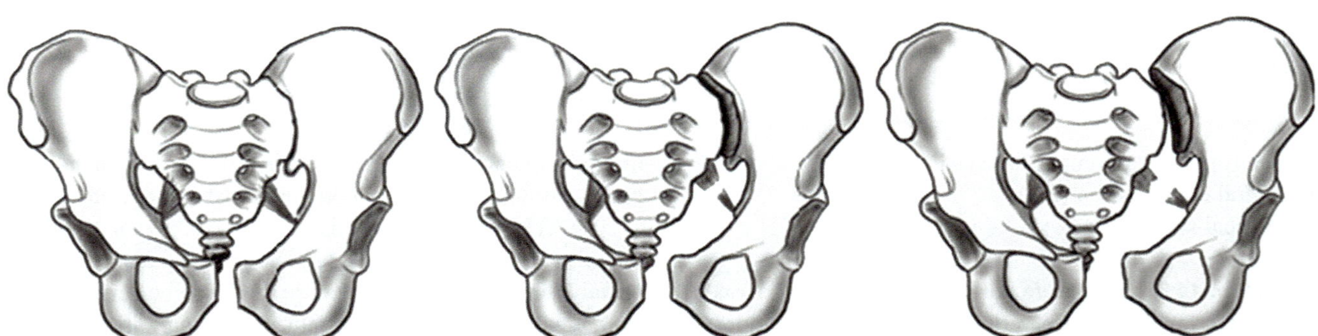

Fig. 19.11 Antero-Posterior Compression (APC) fractures: **APC-I** diastasis of the symphysis without posterior disruption; **APC II** >2.5 cm of diastasis of the symphysis with disruption of the sacrospinous sacrotuberous and anterior sacroiliac ligaments (open book); **APC-III** complete disruption of the symphysis and the posterior sacroiliac ligamentous complex

19.4.5 Imaging

Standard radiographs such as anteroposterior view of the pelvis (part of ATLS protocol), including inlet and outlet views, are recommended. CT scan is a routine part of the investigation that will provide sufficient information and better characterisation of the injuries and will help to guide treatment.

19.4.6 Treatment

19.4.6.1 Nonoperative

Conservative management with either bed rest, a non-weight bearing period or weight-bearing as tolerated is suggested for stable pelvic ring injuries.

These are:

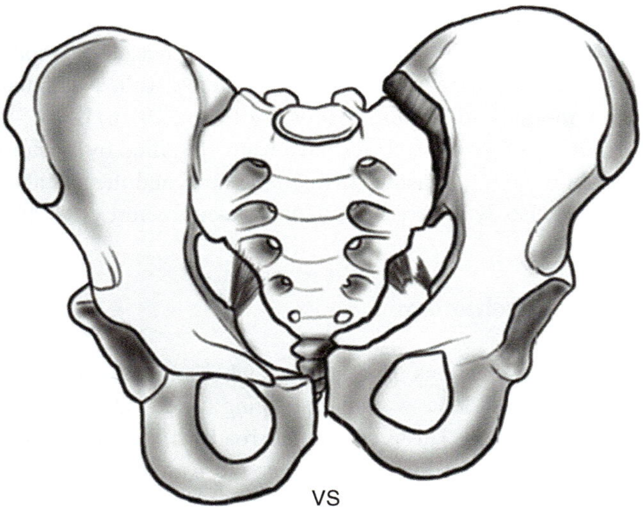

Fig. 19.12 The **Vertical Shear** type of injury with an unstable pelvic ring and vertical displacement of the hemipelvis

- Stable pelvic injuries (LC1, APC1)
- Vast majority of Tile type A fractures
- Isolated pubic rami fractures

However, not all LC1 injuries are stable. Tosounidis et al. reported that, when there is a complete sacral fracture posteriorly on the coronal and axial CT scan images, operative stabilisation is indicated, given the presence of persistent painful stimuli and rotational instability of the pelvic ring (Fig. 19.13) [33].

Similarly, API injuries can be associated with a degree of chronic instability and pain when the ligaments fail to heal. In this scenario, pubic symphysis fusion is recommended (Fig. 19.14).

19.4.6.2 Operative

Pelvic injuries requiring surgical treatment include:

- Pelvic ring injuries with more than 2.5 cm of pubic diastasis.
- Displacement of the SI joint of more than 1 cm.
- Sacral fractures with more than 1 cm displacement or neurological deficit.
- Open fractures.
- Most of Tile Type C injuries.

Operative treatment includes options of either anterior, posterior or both anterior and posterior fixation. Anteriorly, an external fixator can be used; ORIF with screws and plates or, alternatively, percutaneous fixation. Posteriorly, ORIF can be achieved either through an anterior or posterior approach. Close percutaneous fixation can be achieved with sacroiliac screws.

Some studies examined surgeons' variability in the management of pelvic ring injuries; although there is a consensus towards nonoperative management for Tile type A injuries (95.3%) and operative for the unstable Type C (80.7%), the treatment modality of Type B fractures varies between surgeons (nonoperative 36.6% vs. 63.4%) [35].

19.4.7 Complications

- Urogenital injuries (more common in males)
- Neurological injuries.
- Deep vein thrombosis.
- Chronic pelvic instability (in conservatively treated injuries)

19.4.8 Prognosis

The outcome is related to the fracture pattern and the possible complications. Mulhall et al. [33] reported that all three patients treated surgically were able to participate in all their activities, but only one had returned to horse riding at 1 year follow up.

Flynn et al. [32] reported on two patients, both receiving conservative treatment; one was able to continue horse-riding without difficulties.

19.5 Traumatic Hip Dislocations

19.5.1 Anatomy

The hip joint is a ball and socket synovial joint, with the femoral head being the ball while the acetabulum forms the socket. It is an inherently stable joint because of its bony anatomy, thick fibrous capsule, joint labrum and ligaments, all of which providing significant stability. These ligaments (iliofemoral and pubofemoral ligament anteriorly and the ischiofemoral ligament posteriorly) form the hip capsule and attach to the femoral neck. The ligamentous teres is another ligament which is located entirely within the joint itself from the inferior aspect of the femoral head to the acetabulum at the cotyloid fossa.

The blood supply to the femoral head has been well studied. An extracapsular vascular ring is formed at the base of the femoral neck. The major contributor is the medial femoral circumflex (branch of the profunda femoris) with some contribution to the anterior and inferior head from the lateral femoral circumflex artery. There is also some contribution from the inferior gluteal artery. A small vascular supply also travels directly to the head through the ligamentum teres artery, which originates from the obturator artery [36].

19.5.2 Epidemiology

Traumatic hip dislocations are rare during sporting activities, as they are mostly associated with high energy trauma and motor vehicle accidents. However, early recognition and appropriate treatment are of paramount importance as these dislocations can lead to significant complications. The true incidence of these injuries in athletes is unclear. Most of the cases reported occur during high energy sports such as American football, rugby, skiing and cycling [37–41]. Isolated cases in basketball, soccer and during gymnastic vault have also been reported [42–44].

19.5.3 Classification

Traumatic hip dislocations can be divided into two groups, namely anterior and posterior, with the posterior being by far the most common (80–90%). This is also the case for dislocations that are related to sports injuries. They can be simple or complex with fracture of the acetabulum or proximal femur.

Posterior hip dislocations have been classified by Thompson and Epstein based on the presence, topography and severity of associated fractures (posterior wall, acetabular and femoral head fractures) (Figs. 19.15 and 19.16) [24, 45].

Anterior hip dislocations have been classified by Epstein based on the relationship between the head and the acetabulum and also by the presence of associated fractures [24, 46].

19.5.4 Mechanism

Posterior dislocations usually occur when a force is directed against a flexed knee with the hip being flexed, adducted and internally rotated. This is common in road traffic accidents and in field sports when the athlete's knee is driven into the ground during a tackle. Anterior dislocations result from abduction and external rotation of the hip in splits-type injury [38].

19.5.5 Assessment

Following injury, athletes experience acute pain, with deformity and inability to bear weight in the acute setting, the

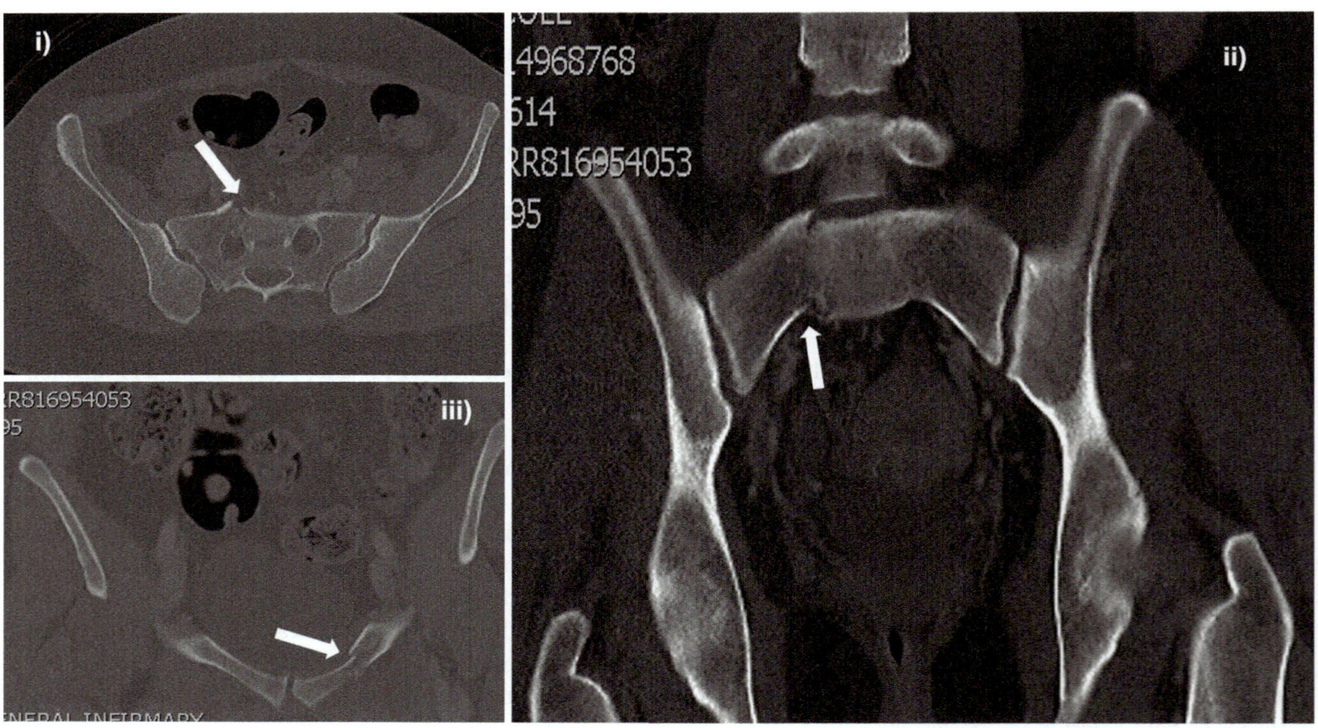

Fig. 19.13 A 23 year of age fell whilst horse riding sustaining a pelvic ring injury. (**a**) (i–iii) CT scan pelvic cuts (axial and coronal) showing a complete right sacral wing fracture and a left pubic rami fracture. (**b**) Fluoroscopic images during fixation of the LC1 unstable pelvic fracture. (i) Sacral lateral view for identification of the safe corridor for insertion of a cannulated 7.2 mm partially threaded screw into the body of S1. (ii) Antero-posterior view showing safe placement of the guide wire in the middle of the sacral ala. (iii) Inlet view showing advancement of the screw beyond the fracture level for compression. (iv) Outlet view showing safe screw placement above the Sacral 1 foramina (dotted white lines). (v) Guide wire insertion and reaming to left superior pubic ramus for fracture fixation. (**c**) (i) AP; (ii) Inlet; (iii) Outlet pelvic views at 2 years follow up showing osseous fracture healing

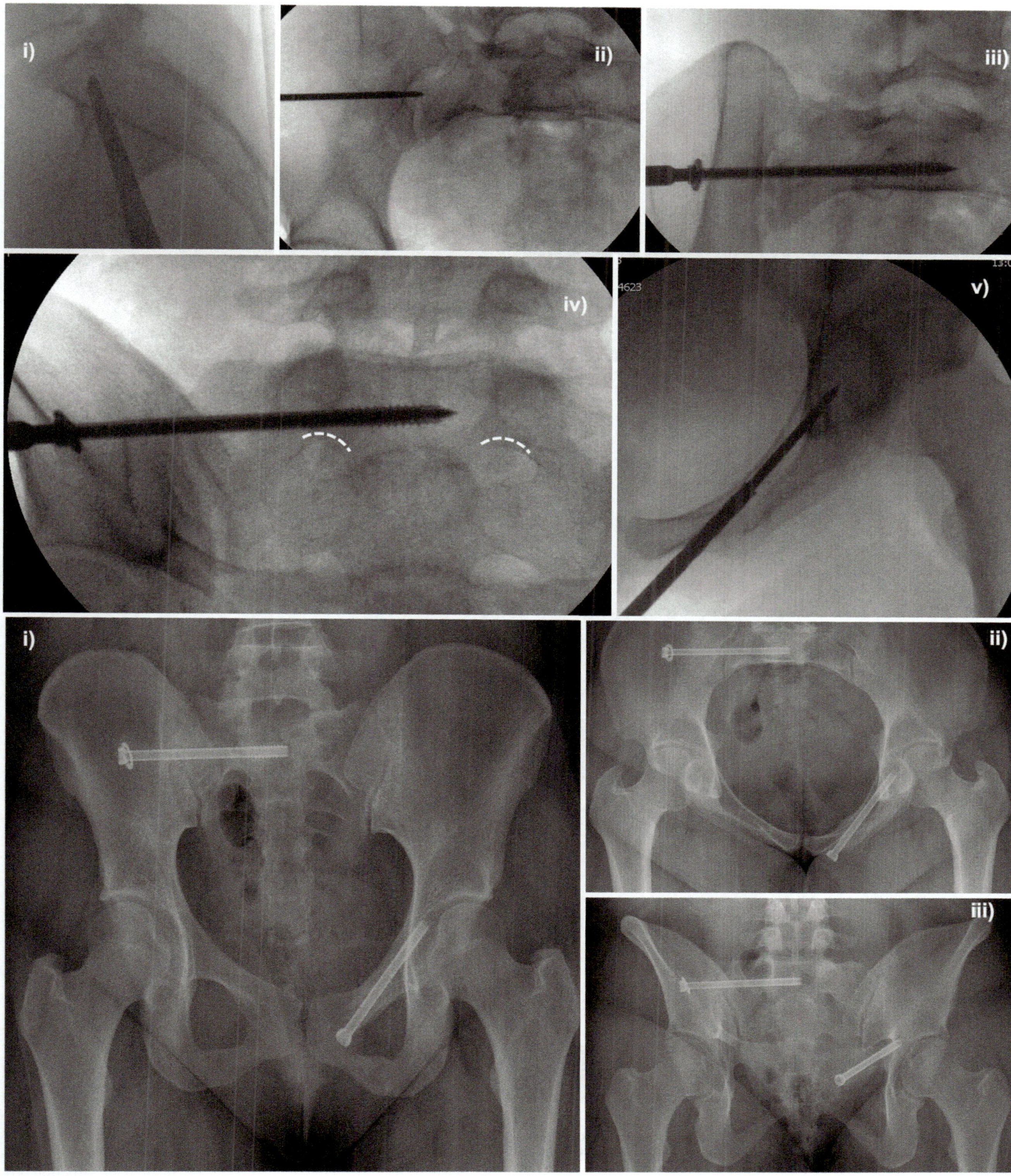

Fig. 19.13 (continued)

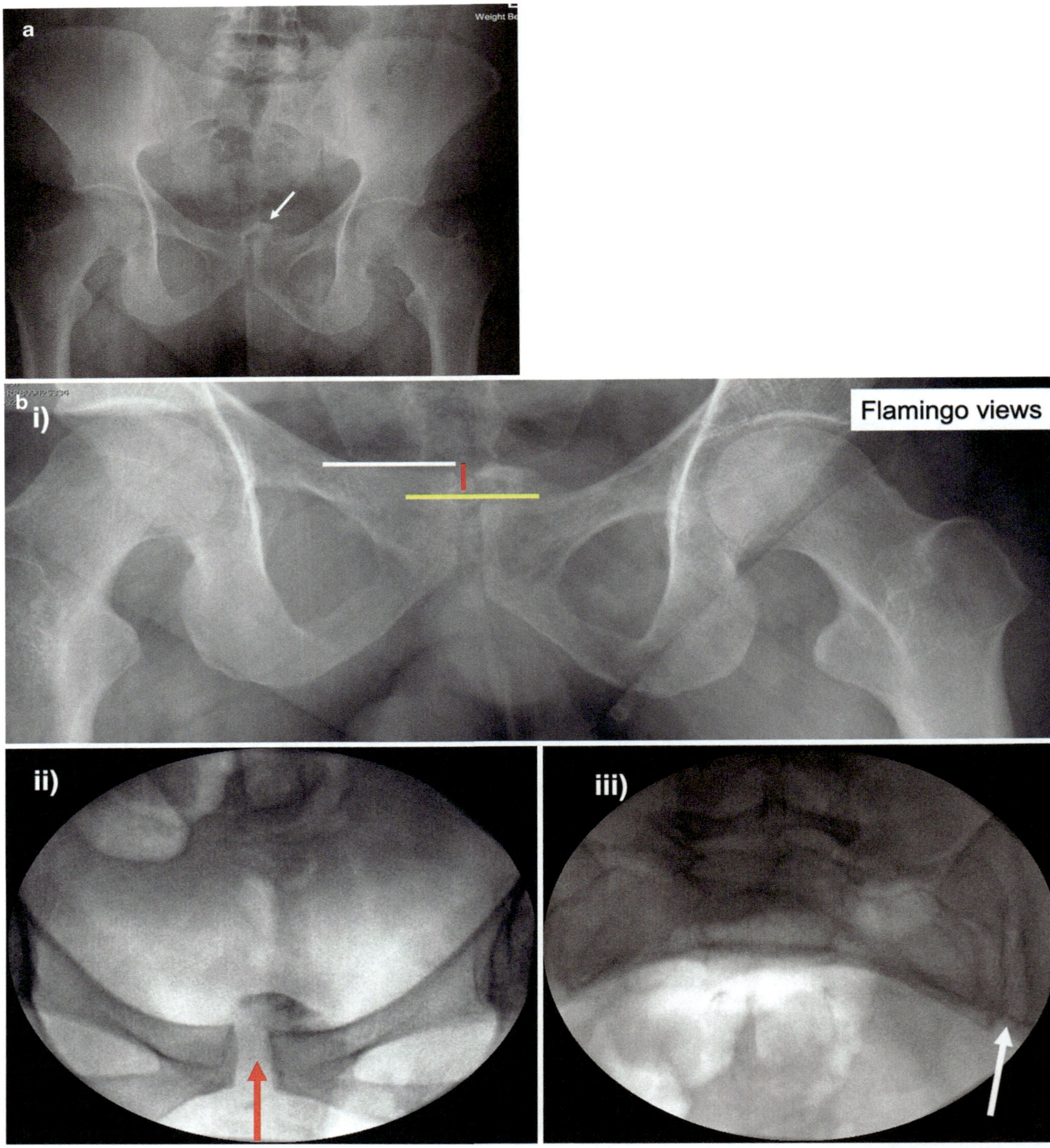

Fig. 19.14 (a) Antero-posterior radiograph of a 29-year-old professional racing motorcyclist who sustained a pelvic injury API 18 months previously. He was referred with chronic pain and inability to ride. Radiograph demonstrated ossification over the pubic symphysis (white arrow). (b) (i) Flamingo (stork) views revealed pelvic instability. (ii) Operative intervention was undertaken – Fluoroscopic stress views in theatre revealed opening of the pubic symphysis (red arrow); (iii) and opening of left SI joint (White arrow). (c) Intraoperative picture demonstrating pubis symphysis (white arrow) and the pubic rami (green arrows) which have been prepared with an osteotome to accept a tricortical T-shape graft from the iliac crest for the fusion reconstruction procedure. (d) Intraoperative pictures showing (i) Tricortical graft harvested from iliac crest (ii, iii) T-shape tricortical graft prior to implantation in the pubis symphysis. (iv) Stabilisation of the pubic symphysis with a 3.5 mm plate. (e) Antero-posterior pelvic radiograph at 12 months follow up showing fusion of the pubic symphysis

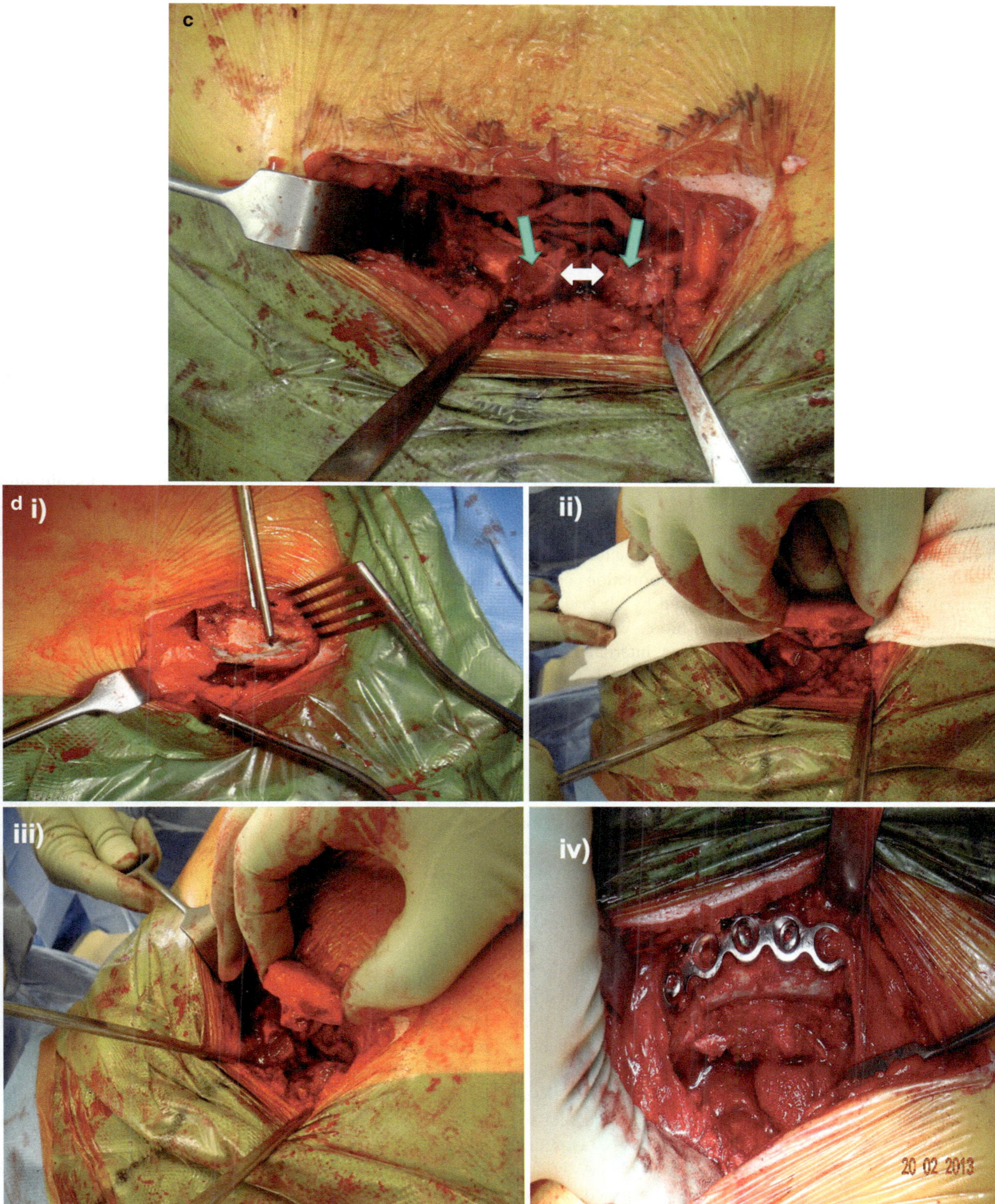

Fig. 19.14 (continued)

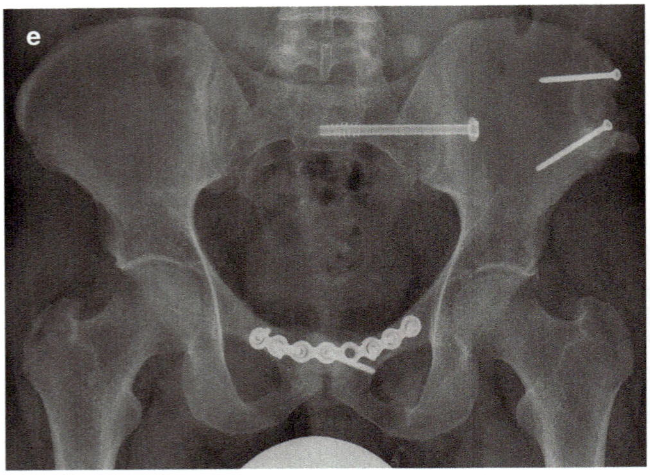

Fig. 19.14 (continued)

injury might be identifiable as the athlete with a dislocated hip usually prefers a 'fetal' position with the dislocated hip facing up [38]. Palpation of the area will reveal tenderness around the hip joint and muscles. The ATLS protocol should always be part of the approach to the patient, including a full neurovascular examination. Further information can be obtained if a hip dislocation is suspected by observing the position of the injured extremity. The more common posterior dislocations will present with a flexed, internally rotated and adducted hip; in an anterior dislocation the hip will be extended, externally rotated and abducted.

19.5.6 Imaging

Antero-posterior radiographs of the pelvis and a cross-table lateral of the affected hip are initially obtained, and they will help to differentiate between anterior and posterior dislocation and to rule out a fracture of the proximal femur prior to any reduction attempt. Following reduction, another antero-posterior view must be obtained together with additional views (inlet/outlet, Judet) if required.

Post reduction CT scan is essential for all traumatic hip dislocations to rule out persistent incongruency and to identify associated fractures or the presence of loose fragments.

MRI can also provide useful information about the cartilage and the labrum, and can rule out surrounding soft tissue injuries, evaluate the key muscles around the hip joint for avulsion type injuries and recognise early AVN (avascular necrosis) [38]. Poggi et al., attempting to predict AVN, followed up 14 patients for 24 months. They proposed an algorithm for the early recognition of osteonecrosis following posterior hip dislocation [44]. An MRI scan at 4–6 weeks looking for abnormal marrow signal on the T1 and T2 images has been recommended. If the scan reveals normal marrow signal, no further imaging is needed. In the case of abnormal signal, a further MRI at 3 months was advised. If the changes initially observed (at 4–6 weeks) persist or worsen, a diagnosis of AVN can be made. If the second scan reveals normal signal or considerable improvement, the initial changes were considered transient and probably not indicative of osteonecrosis. Patients with no head bone marrow changes at 4–6 weeks had a low risk of AVN [47].

19.5.7 Management

Early closed reduction is essential and should be provided within 6 h to avoid complications such as avascular necrosis of the femoral head or sciatic nerve injury. The only contraindication to early closed reduction is an ipsilateral femoral neck fracture. Reduction can be performed under sedation, spinal or general anaesthesia. If the dislocation cannot be reduced, bony fragments may be incarcerated in the hip joint or significant soft tissue damage may be present. In that situation, the surgeon should proceed with open reduction with fixation of the associated fractures primarily or in a later stage.

A simple on the field reduction technique has been described at an NFL Physician's Society meeting. This requires that the player lies supine and relaxed with the hip supported and flexed at 90°. The physician should place his bent knee under the injured leg and apply traction in line with the femur. The hip should be maintained in an internally rotated position. The femoral head will be felt reducing back once the musculature fully relaxes. If successful reduction has not been achieved over several minutes, the player should be placed on a backboard and to the emergency room for radiological investigation (Xrays). It is essential that the reduction should not be forced to prevent further injuries, and that anterior hip dislocations should not be addressed on the field because they are far more challenging to reduce [38, 48].

Several reduction techniques have been described by Allis et al. [49], Stimson et al. [50] and Bigelow, though the last which requires forced rotational movements of the hip is not recommended given the increased risk of femoral neck fractures [38]. Usually, any attempt of reduction will require sedation, but occasionally general anaesthesia might be needed. In all cases, the surgeon must be prepared for an open reduction in the situation of a nonreducible injury. For open reduction of posterior hip dislocations, a posterior approach is used (Kocher-Langenbeck) and an anterior approach (Smith-Petersen) for anterior dislocations. At the same session, associated fractures or other injuries (e.g. labral injuries) should be addressed.

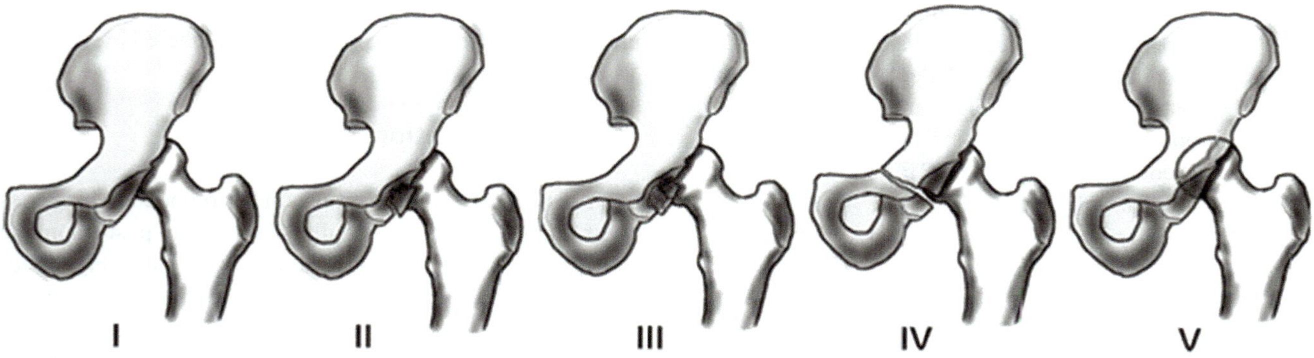

Fig. 19.15 The five types of the Thompson-Epstein classification system: **Type I** simple dislocation with or without a minor posterior wall fragment; **Type II** dislocation with single large posterior wall fragment; **Type III** dislocation with comminuted fragments of the posterior acetabular wall; **Type IV** dislocation with fracture of the acetabular roof/floor; **Type V** dislocation with fracture of the femoral head

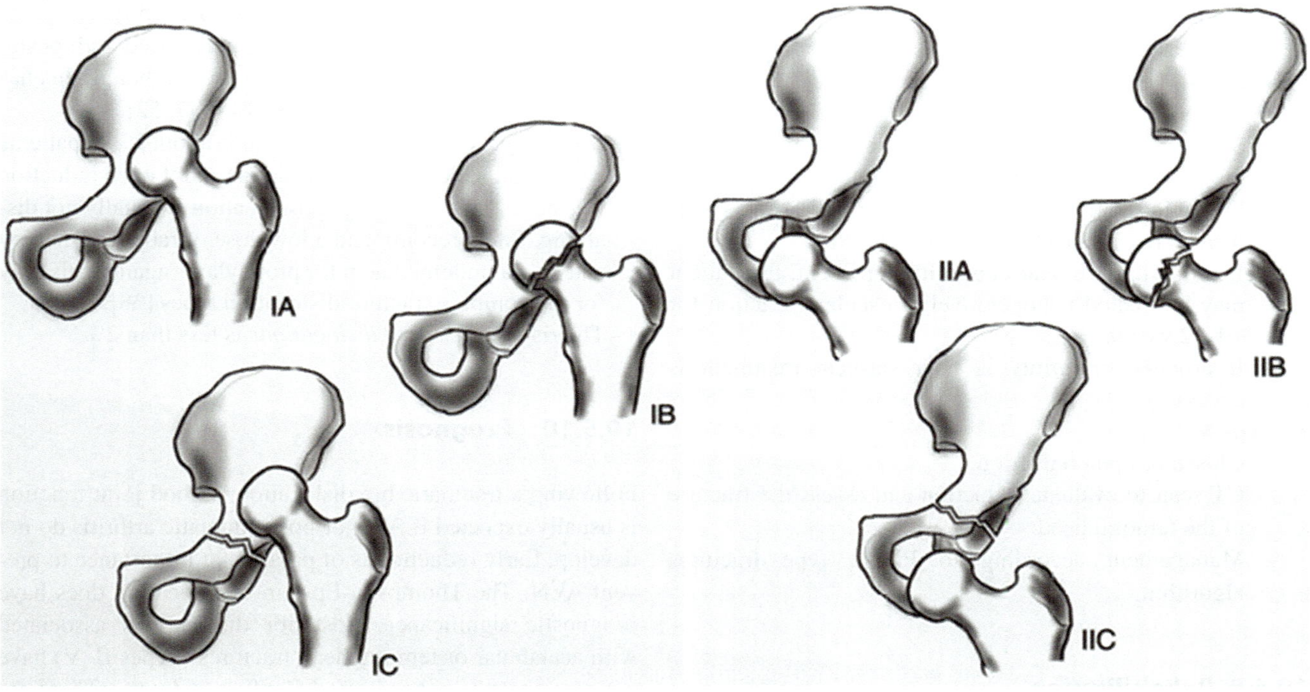

Fig. 19.16 The six types/subtypes of anterior hip fracture-dislocations according to the Epstein classification: **Type IA** superior dislocation without associated fractures; **Type IB** superior dislocation with fracture or impaction of the femoral head; **Type IC** superior dislocation with associated fracture of the acetabulum; **Type IIA** inferior dislocation without fractures; **Type IIB** inferior dislocation with fracture or impaction of the femoral head; **Type IIC** inferior dislocation with associated fracture of the acetabulum [24]

A simple treatment algorithm based on the Thompson–Epstein classification can be as follows [24]:

- **Type I**
  - Urgent closed reduction.
  - Post reduction CT scan to evaluate joint congruency and identify associated fractures femoral head/acetabulum or loose intraarticular bodies.
  - Early ROM exercises avoiding hip flexion, adduction and internal rotation.
  - Partial weight-bearing (PWB) for 4–6 weeks.
  - Full weight-bearing (FWB) 6 weeks after the injury.
- **Type II**
  - Closed or open reduction.
  - Evaluation under anaesthesia (EUA) of the stability of the reduction (posterior wall fracture).

  - CT scan for reduction evaluation and assessment of the posterior wall acetabular fracture.
  - If the reduction is stable and depending on the size of the posterior wall fragment, the injury may be treated non-operatively.
  - If the reduction is unstable ORIF of the posterior wall fracture is usually required.
  - Mobilisation protocol will be as per Type I.
- **Type III**
  - Closed or open reduction.
  - Evaluation under anaesthesia (EUA) of the stability of the reduction (posterior wall comminution).
  - CT scan for reduction evaluation and assessment of the posterior wall comminution.
  - Reduction in most cases is unstable because of fracture's comminution, so ORIF of the posterior wall fracture is usually required.
  - Mobilisation protocol will be as per Type I.
- **Type IV**
  - Closed or open reduction.
  - Skeletal traction may be necessary to improve and maintain the reduction.
  - Following satisfactory reduction, a CT scan is performed to evaluate the acetabular fracture.
  - If satisfying articular congruity is present, the patient may be treated nonoperatively in skeletal traction for 10–12 weeks.
  - If articular congruity is poor surgical treatment is necessary.
- **Type V**
  - Closed or open reduction.
  - CT scan to evaluate reduction and assess the fracture of the femoral head.
  - Management according to Pipkin type fractures algorithm.

19.5.8 Rehabilitation

Early, active and aggressive rehabilitation has been proposed [51]. There is no increased risk of AVN for patients allowed to early weight bear [52, 53]. Post-reduction/post-fixation prolonged and strict immobilisation may lead to intra-articular adhesions and arthritis. It should be avoided where possible, especially for more stable injuries (Type I posterior hip dislocations) [24].

Athletes should proceed throughout a protocol aiming at managing pain, improving ROM, stretching and strengthening the surrounding muscles. They can return to high-level activities once there is symmetrical lower limb function (strength, dexterity).

An early MRI is considered by some important to evidence femoral head ischemia. It should be taken at around 1–2 weeks following the injury. If evidence of femoral head ischaemia is present, the rehabilitation protocol can be altered [38].

19.5.9 Complications

- *Post-traumatic arthritis*. Epstein has reported in his series of 426 hip dislocations of all types a 23% of post-traumatic arthritis. This percentage though is probably higher for the complex fracture-dislocation type injuries. The initial injury to the articular cartilage is the critical factor.
- *AVN 5–40%*, time from dislocation to reduction plays an important role (ideally within 6 h of the injury and certainly within 24 h). Hougaard et al. in a series of 100 patients reported AVN rates of 4.8% for those patients which had reduction within 6 h; hips reduced later than 6 h developed AVN in 52.9% of the cases [54].
- *Sciatic nerve injuries* are commonly reported with posterior dislocations in 5–10% of the cases, although this has been reported higher by some (20%) [37, 52].
- *Heterotopic ossification* may occur in about 2% of patients who sustained complex dislocations and if open reduction was necessary. Heterotopic ossification is usually not disabling. Some recommend a low dose of radiation therapy and or oral indomethacin for prophylaxis against this only for the complex fracture-dislocation types [38].
- The risk of *recurrent dislocations* is less than 2%.

19.5.10 Prognosis

Following a traumatic hip dislocation, a good joint function is usually expected if AVN or post-traumatic arthritis do not develop. Early reduction is of paramount importance to prevent AVN. The Thompson-Epstein classification does have prognostic significance. Posterior dislocations associated with acetabular or femoral head fractures (Types II–V) have a worse prognosis than Type I.Conflict of InterestThere are no conflicts of interest.

References

1. Boyd KT, Peirce NS, Batt ME. Common hip injuries in sport. Sports Med. 1997;24(4):273–88.
2. Lloyd-Smith R, et al. A survey of overuse and traumatic hip and pelvic injuries in athletes. Phys Sportsmed. 1985;13(10):131–41.
3. Scopp JM, Moorman CT III. Acute athletic trauma to the hip and pelvis. Orthop Clin North Am. 2002;33(3):555–63.
4. Porr J, Lucaciu C, Birkett S. Avulsion fractures of the pelvis - a qualitative systematic review of the literature. J Can Chiropr Assoc. 2011;55(4):247–55.
5. Singer G, et al. Diagnosis and treatment of apophyseal injuries of the pelvis in adolescents. Semin Musculoskelet Radiol. 2014;18(5):498–504.

6. Rossi F, Dragoni S. Acute avulsion fractures of the pelvis in adolescent competitive athletes: prevalence, location and sports distribution of 203 cases collected. Skelet Radiol. 2001;30(3):127–31.
7. Bolgla LA, et al. Hip pain in a high school football player: a case report. J Athl Train. 2001;36(1):81–4.
8. Kujala UM, et al. Ischial tuberosity apophysitis and avulsion among athletes. Int J Sports Med. 1997;18(2):149–55.
9. Calderazzi F, et al. Apophyseal avulsion fractures of the pelvis. A review. Acta Biomed. 2018;89(4):470–6.
10. Ferlic PW, et al. Treatment for ischial tuberosity avulsion fractures in adolescent athletes. Knee Surg Sports Traumatol Arthrosc. 2014;22(4):893–7.
11. Pogliacomi F, Calderazzi F, Paterlini M, Pompili M, Ceccarelli F. Anterior iliac spine fractures in the adolescent athletes: surgical or conservative treatment? Med Sport. 2013;66(2):231–40.
12. Eberbach H, et al. Operative versus conservative treatment of apophyseal avulsion fractures of the pelvis in the adolescents: a systematical review with meta-analysis of clinical outcome and return to sports. BMC Musculoskelet Disord. 2017;18(1):162.
13. Uzun M, Alpan B, Ozger H. Avulsion fractures involving the straight and reflected heads of the rectus femoris. Hip Int. 2014;24(2):206–9.
14. Ferguson TA, et al. Fractures of the acetabulum in patients aged 60 years and older: an epidemiological and radiological study. J Bone Joint Surg (Br). 2010;92(2):250–7.
15. Laird A, Keating JF. Acetabular fractures: a 16-year prospective epidemiological study. J Bone Joint Surg (Br). 2005;87(7):969–73.
16. Good DW, et al. Acetabular fractures following rugby tackles: a case series. J Med Case Rep. 2011;5:505.
17. Morrissey DI, Good D, Leonard M. Acetabular fractures in skeletally immature rugby players. BMJ Case Rep. 2016;2016:bcr2015211637.
18. Stilger VG, Alt JM, Hubbard DF. Traumatic acetabular fracture in an intercollegiate football player: a case report. J Athl Train. 2000;35(1):103–7.
19. Williams TR, et al. Acetabular stress fractures in military endurance athletes and recruits: incidence and MRI and scintigraphic findings. Skelet Radiol. 2002;31(5):277–81.
20. Patel ND, Trehan RK. Acute isolated acetabular fracture following a game of squash: a case report. J Med Case Rep. 2007;1:156.
21. Bass A, Lovell ME. Two cases of acetabular fractures sustained during competitive cycling. Br J Sports Med. 1995;29(3):205–6.
22. Cerynik DL, et al. Pelvic fractures in professional cyclists: a report of 3 cases. Sports Health. 2009;1(3):265–70.
23. Giannoudis PV, Pape H-C. Practical procedures in orthopaedic trauma surgery. Cambridge: Cambridge University Press; 2014.
24. Lasanianos NGK, Kanakaris NK, Giannoudis PV. Trauma and orthopaedic classifications. London: Springer; 2016.
25. Judet R, et al. [Fractures of the acetabulum. Classification and guiding rules for open reduction]. Arch Orthop. 1968;31(3):119–58.
26. Judet R, Judet J, Letournel E. Fractures of the acetabulum: classification and surgical approaches for open reduction. Preliminary report. J Bone Joint Surg Am. 1964;46:1615–46.
27. Tornetta P III. Non-operative management of acetabular fractures. The use of dynamic stress views. J Bone Joint Surg (Br). 1999;81(1):67–70.
28. Court-Brown CM, Rockwood CA, Green DP. Rockwood and Green's fractures in adults. Philadelphia, PA: Wolters Kluwer; 2015.
29. Giannoudis PV, et al. Operative treatment of displaced fractures of the acetabulum. A meta-analysis. J Bone Joint Surg (Br). 2005;87(1):2–9.
30. Kheir E, et al. Return to sport after fixation of pelvic and acetabular fractures. Injury Extra. 2007;38:153.
31. O'Farrell DA, et al. Major pelvic injuries in equestrian sports. Br J Sports Med. 1997;31(3):249–51.
32. Flynn M. Disruption of symphysis pubis while horse riding: a report of two cases. Injury. 1973;4(4):357–9.
33. Mulhall KJ, et al. Diastasis of the pubic symphysis peculiar to horse riders: modern aspects of pelvic pommel injuries. Br J Sports Med. 2002;36(1):74–5.
34. Service, C.A, et al. Urethral trauma following pelvic fracture from horseback saddle horn injury versus other mechanisms of pelvic trauma. Urology. 2019;124:260–3.
35. Furey AJ, et al. Surgeon variability in the treatment of pelvic ring injuries. Orthopedics. 2010;33(10):714.
36. Gautier E, et al. Anatomy of the medial femoral circumflex artery and its surgical implications. J Bone Joint Surg (Br). 2000;82(5):679–83.
37. Mohanty K, Gupta SK, Langston A. Posterior dislocation of hip in adolescents attributable to casual rugby. J Accid Emerg Med. 2000;17(6):429.
38. Pallia CS, Scott RE, Chao DJ. Traumatic hip dislocation in athletes. Curr Sports Med Rep. 2002;1(6):338–45.
39. Sherry E. Hip dislocations from skiing. Med J Aust. 1987;146(4):227–8.
40. Venkatachalam S, Heidari N, Greer T. Traumatic fracture-dislocation of the hip following rugby tackle: a case report. Sports Med Arthrosc Rehabil Ther Technol. 2009;1:28.
41. Giannoudis PV, et al. Posterior fracture-dislocation of the hip in sports. Eur J Trauma. 2003;29(6):399–402.
42. Bakalakos M, et al. Posterior hip dislocation in a non-professional football player: a case report and review of the literature. Eur J Orthop Surg Traumatol. 2019;29(1):231–4.
43. Mitchell JC, et al. A rare fracture-dislocation of the hip in a gymnast and review of the literature. Br J Sports Med. 1999;33(4):283–4.
44. Tennent TD, Chambler AF, Rossouw DJ. Posterior dislocation of the hip while playing basketball. Br J Sports Med. 1998;32(4):342–3.
45. Thompson VP, Epstein HC. Traumatic dislocation of the hip; a survey of two hundred and four cases covering a period of twenty-one years. J Bone Joint Surg Am. 1951;33A(3):746.
46. Epstein HC, Wiss DA. Traumatic anterior dislocation of the hip. Orthopedics. 1985;8(1):130, 132–4.
47. Poggi JJ, et al. Changes on magnetic resonance images after traumatic hip dislocation. Clin Orthop Relat Res. 1995;319:249–59.
48. Collins J, Trulock S, Chao DJ. Field management and rehabilitation of an acute posterior hip dislocation in a professional football player. Prof Footb Athlet Train. 2001;19:1–3.
49. Allis OH. An inquiry into the difficulties encountered in the reduction of dislocations of the hip. Philadelphia, PA: Doran; 1896.
50. Stimson LA. A treatise on fractures. Philadelphia, PA: H.C. Lea's son & co.; 1883.
51. Stewart MJ, Milford LW. Fracture-dislocation of the hip; an end-result study. J Bone Joint Surg Am. 1954;36A(2):315–42.
52. Amihood S. Posterior dislocation of the hip. Clinical observations and review of literature. S Afr Med J. 1974;48(24):1029–32.
53. Brav EA. Traumatic dislocation of the hip: army experience and results over a twelve-year period. JBJS. 1962;44(6):1115.
54. Hougaard K, Thomsen PB. Traumatic posterior dislocation of the hip--prognostic factors influencing the incidence of avascular necrosis of the femoral head. Arch Orthop Trauma Surg. 1986;106(1):32–5.

Part V

Stress Fractures in Sport: Upper Limb

Stress Fractures in Sport: Shoulder

20

Alex C. DiBartola, Gregory L. Cvetanovich, and Timothy L. Miller

Learning Objectives

- Understand the difference between stress fractures and traumatic fractures
- Recognize imaging findings for shoulder girdle stress fractures
- Recognize common youth athlete stress response locations
- Describe the unique areas about the shoulder girdle where stress fractures occur in adult athletes
- Understand treatment modalities for shoulder girdle stress fractures

20.1 Epidemiology and Background

Stress injuries to bone are a continuum of structural failure from simple bone marrow edema (stress reaction) to a small microcrack with minor cortical disruption to a complete fracture with or without displacement to nonunion. Stress fractures predominantly occur in the lower extremities secondary to the repetitive impact loading [1–3]. Stress fractures about the shoulder girdle are much less common but still can be debilitating for athletes [1–4]. Large series of rib and upper extremity stress fractures demonstrate the following categories of activities that put athletes at risk of sustaining and upper extremity bony stress injury [5, 6].

- weight lifting
- upper extremity weight bearing
- throwing
- axial rotation
- rowing

Throwing and/or swinging motions are the two most common inciting activities that result in stress fractures of the shoulder girdle [6]. Stress fractures of the ribs are common among rowers. However, overhead throwers are more likely to present with stress fractures about the elbow. Weightlifters demonstrate the greatest anatomical variability for location of injury, with injuries occurring as far proximal as the sternum and as far distal as the scaphoid.

As awareness of overuse injuries of the thorax and shoulder girdle increases, so has the rate of diagnosis of stress fractures of the ribs and upper extremities [6]. A thorough history and physical examination along with appropriate imaging is essential to diagnosis. Nonoperative and operative treatment recommendations are made based on location, injury classification, and causative activity.

General guiding principles for shoulder gridle stress fractures are as follows:

- Strain is generated by the rotational torque of swinging or throwing.
- Tensile and compressive forces result from muscle contraction [7].
- Repetitive axial loading can produce microtrauma to bone.
- Key risk factors for stress fractures are:
  - pre-participation conditioning
  - volume (frequency, duration, and intensity) of the causative activity [8]
  - abnormal bony alignment
  - muscular imbalance
  - improper technique/biomechanics
  - poor blood supply to bone [9]

A. C. DiBartola
Department of Orthopaedic Surgery, The Ohio State University, Columbus, OH, USA
e-mail: Alex.DiBartola@osumc.edu

G. L. Cvetanovich · T. L. Miller (✉)
Department of Orthopaedic Surgery, The Ohio State University, Columbus, OH, USA

Department of Sports Medicine, The Ohio State University, Columbus, OH, USA
e-mail: Gregory.Cvetanovich@osumc.edu; Timothy.miller@osumc.edu

G. A. J. Robertson, N. Maffulli (eds.), *Fractures in Sport*, https://doi.org/10.1007/978-3-030-72036-0_20

20.2 Classification

Understanding the continuum of severity for stress fractures in general is imperative to ultimately treat an athlete with this injury. Grading of the cortical failure is used to describe the injury stage, determine prognosis, and communicate treatment options [10]. The continuum throughout which stress fractures occur include:

- simple bone-marrow edema (stress reaction)
- small unicortical disruptions
- complete fractures with or without displacement
- nonunion (malunion of stress fractures is rare)

The management of bony stress injuries should be based on:

- fracture location
- severity grade of stress injury or fracture
- healing potential of the bone

A classification system developed by Kaeding and Miller is shown below and is based on CT, MRI, bone scan, X-ray, in conjunction with patient clinical history [11].

- Grade I: *no* pain *with* imaging evidence of stress fracture without discernable fracture line
- Grade II: pain *with* imaging evidence of stress fracture without discernable fracture line
- Grade III: pain *with* imaging evidence of a non-displaced fracture line
- Grade IV: pain *with* displaced fracture (>2 mm of displacement)
- Grade V: pain *with* non-union

20.3 Diagnosis

20.3.1 History

Clinical history coupled with the clinician's high degree of suspicion for stress injuries about the bone is critical to the diagnosis of stress fractures about the shoulder. Below are important components or risk factors that may be obtained during clinical interview [4, 9, 12]:

- Atraumatic shoulder or chest wall discomfort associated with repetitive activity must raise suspicion for possible stress fracture.
- Repetitive resisted scapular retraction and humeral torsion may place athletes at risk (e.g., pitcher, javelin).
- Upper extremity repetitive weightbearing is a risk factor (e.g., cheerleading, gymnastics).
- Patients often may not recall specific injury or trauma.
- Symptom onset is most often insidious.
- Concomitant or isolated soft tissue overuse injuries must be diagnosed more easily.
- Pain is initially present only during the inciting activity early in the development of a stress fracture.

20.3.2 Physical Examination

The physical examination performed for suspected shoulder girdle stress fractures should begin with general evaluation of the following nearby anatomy first, as pathology about other areas may in fact be more common than shoulder girdle stress fractures:

- Neck/cervical spine
- Chest
- Heart
- Lungs
- Costal cartilage

A focused exam of the shoulder must include the following:

- inspection
- palpation for tenderness
- assessment of active and passive range of motion
- comprehensive strength testing of the shoulder girdle musculature
- neurovascular exam

20.4 Diagnostic Imaging Modalities

20.4.1 Radiographs

Plain radiographs are usually unremarkable early in the course of stress fractures in general and in shoulder girdle stress fractures in particular. The following points are key to remember when using radiographs to make the diagnosis of shoulder girdle stress fractures:

- Over two-thirds of initial radiographs are negative.
- Half will be positive approximately 3 weeks after symptom onset once healing begins [13].
- Evidence of bony healing allows for eventual diagnosis.
- Signs of healing (cortical thickening and bone edema) are subtle and easily overlooked [13, 14].
- Radiographs may be inconclusive with advanced imaging being required.
- MRI or bone scan may be necessary to make a diagnosis.
  - MRI has superior specificity (>85%) compared to bone scan

20.4.2 Computed Tomography (CT)

Advanced imaging may be useful when the diagnosis of a stress fracture is indeterminate based on plain radiographs [9].

- CT can delineate complete fractures versus incomplete fractures.
- CT has a high radiation dose and is not as commonly used as MRI.
- CT is useful for demonstrating evidence of healing or demonstrating nonunions (Figs. 20.1b and 20.3b).

20.4.3 Bone Scan

Bone scan or bone scintigraphy may be up to 100% sensitive for stress fractuers (Figs. 20.1, 20.2, 20.3, and 20.4) [14]. Bone scintigraphy allows early diagnosis of stress injuries and can diagnose bony stress injuries at multiple sites simultaneously. Uptake on bone scan often requires 12–18 months to normalize, lagging behind the resolution of clinical symptoms, making them less useful helpful for guiding return to activity and/or sports participation.

20.4.4 Magnetic Resonance Imaging

Magnetic resonance imaging (MRI) is the most sensitive and specific imaging study available for stress fracture diagnosis [15, 16]. Key points regarding using MRI to evaluate stress fractures include [9, 16]:

- MRI may detect injuries earlier than bone scan.
- MRI may be able to detect stress injuries up to 2 weeks prior to bone scans

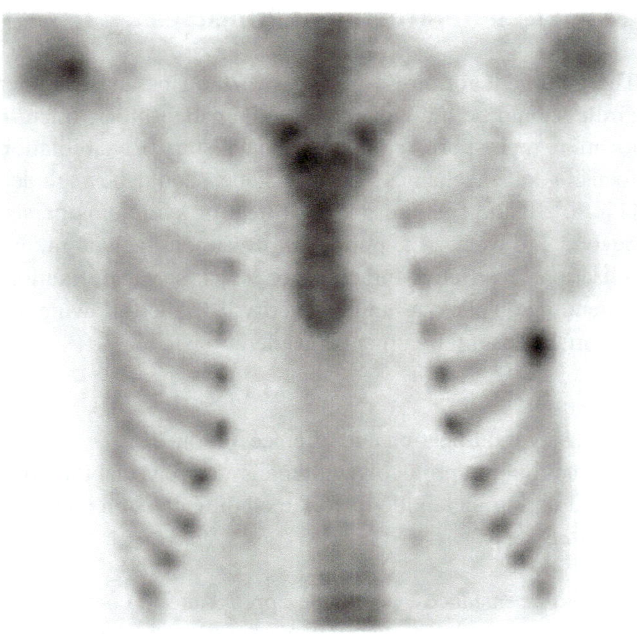

Fig. 20.1 Bone Scan demonstrating stress fracture of the left mid seventh rib

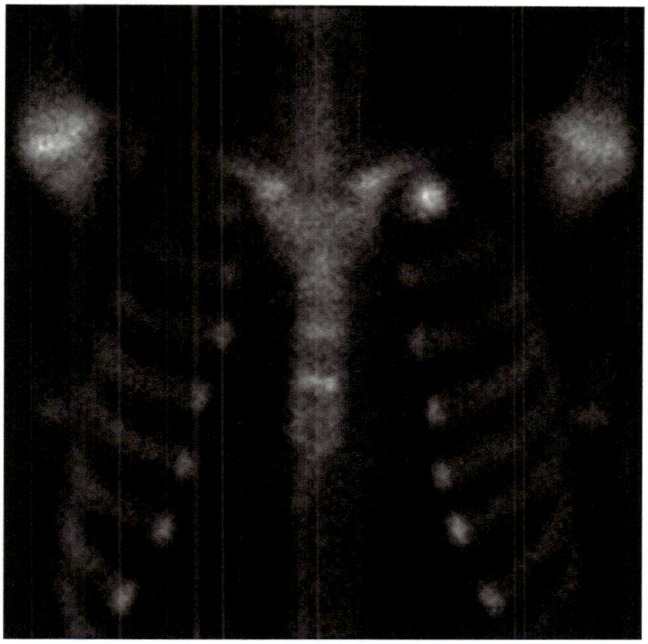

Fig. 20.2 Bone Scan images demonstrating left first rib stress fracture in a collegiate gymnast

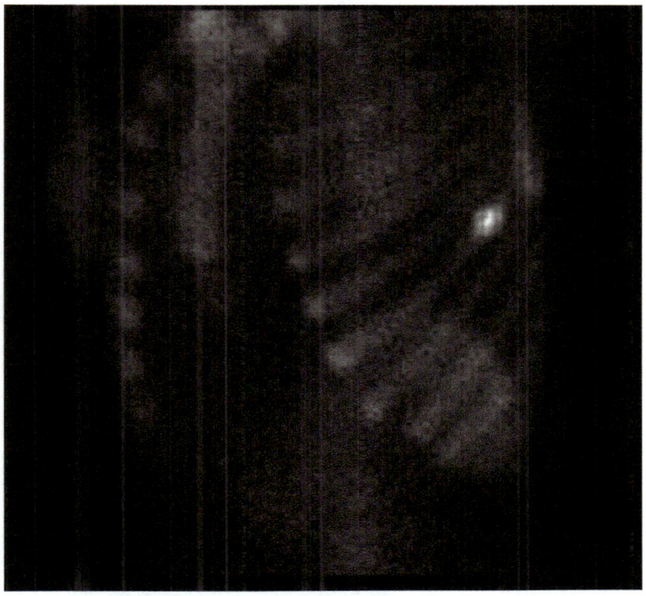

Fig. 20.3 Bone Scan demonstrating stress fracture of the left mid eighth rib

- T2 sequences demonstrate a band of low signal corresponding to a fracture line.
- Surrounding high signal intensity on T2 sequences represents marrow edema (Figs. 20.5 and 20.6)

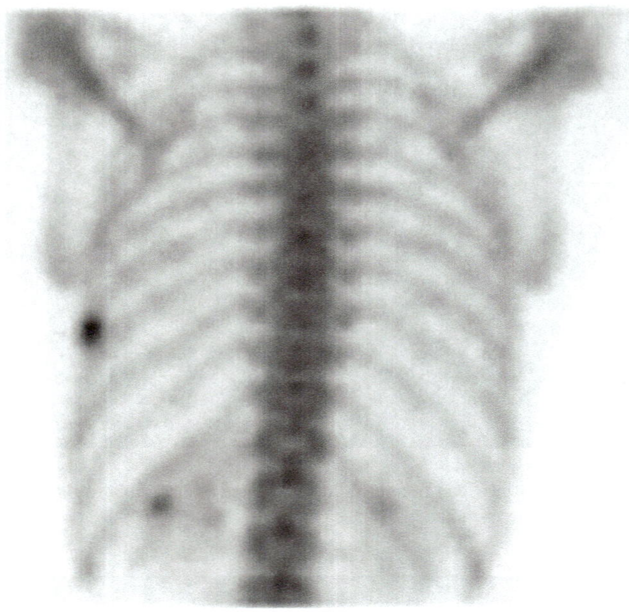

Fig. 20.4 Bone Scans of right sided seventh rib stress fracture

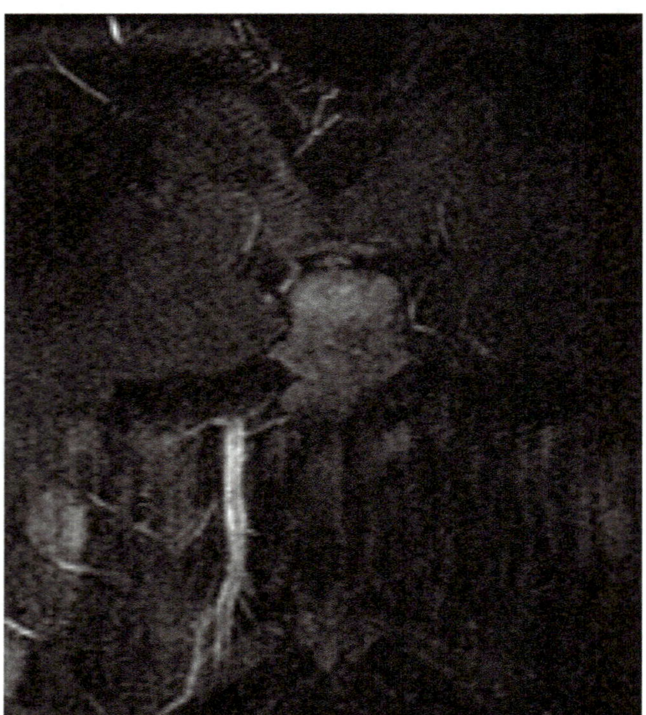

Fig. 20.5 T2 coronal MRI cut demonstrating stress fracture of the mid sternum in a competitive weight lifter

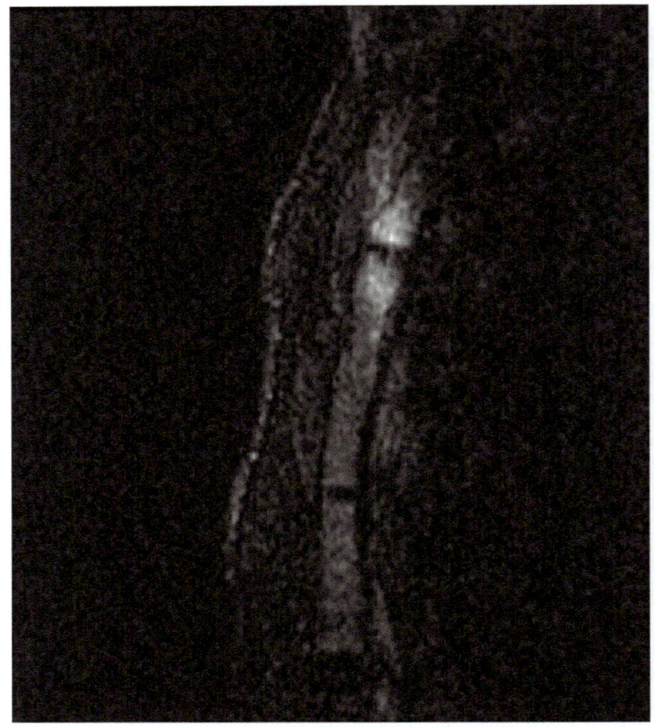

Fig. 20.6 T2 sagittal MRI cut demonstrating stress fracture of the mid sternum in a competitive weight lifter

- Soft tissue data obtained with MRI may also be diagnostically valuable.

20.5 General Treatment Principles

The treatment for stress fractures of the ribs and shoulder girdle should be individualized to the patient, their fracture location, their sport, and their clinical history. Rehabilitation focusing on mechanics and technique should be included [17–20]. If the fracture does not heal or symptoms persist beyond 4–6 weeks, the options for treatment include immobilisation, restrictive bracing, or even surgical fixation, depending on site and injury severity [9]. The following are important general treatment considerations:

- rest
- activity modification and often cessation
- rehabilitation protocols with integrated physical therapy
- addressing metabolic factors including calcium and vitamin D

In some instances, it may be appropriate to continue but decrease the causative activity in the presence of a stress fracture. This decision must be made in conjunction with the athlete. The activity may be continued with pain as a guide, however, close follow-up of these patients is necessary to ensure compliance with activity restrictions and to prevent fracture progression to a higher-grade.

Among all treatment plans, the goals of treatment are symptomatic relief and to decrease the repetitive stress at the fracture site, thus restoring the balance between bony damage and repair [8, 9]. Regardless of the treatment plan, should pain persist or intensify despite activity modification alone, treatment must be advanced to include complete rest, immobilisation or possibly surgical stabilization [9].

20.5.1 Return to Sport (RTS)

Return to sport decision making following a stress fracture must be multifactorial. Critical to RTS is an understanding of the risk of injury progression by the physician, athlete, coaches, trainers, and family. All patients, particularly those with stress fractures at sites with poor healing potential, must understand the risks of commencing a RTS treatment plan, too early. However, treatment plans must be tailored to athletic and personal goals. Athletes near the end of a competitive season may desire to be healed from their injury prior to returning training or competition. For these individuals, the treatment plan should include strict rest and activity modification to a pain-free level. Mid-season athletes with low-risk stress fractures may desire to finish the season and pursue treatment at a later time. General return to sport criteria include the following:

- pain free
- >90% strength compared to the uninjured limb
- healed fracture or resolution of stress response
- nontender to palpation at the injury site
- continued implementation alterations to technique and/or mechanics
- continued nutritional, calcium, and vitamin D supplementation

20.6 Prevention

Prevention of shoulder girdle stress fractures is preferred. This begins with a pre-participation physical examination where an evaluation of risk should occur. Below are important considerations regarding prevention:

- Determine if a history of stress fractures exists.
- Correct menstrual irregularities.
- Evaluate and correct poor nutritional status.
- Calcium and vitamin D supplementation is recommended.
- Optimize general nutrition.
- Consider video analysis with appropriate muscular strengthening.
- Use proper equipment.
- Make technique alterations as appropriated to the causative activity.

20.7 Sternum

20.7.1 Epidemiology

Please refer to the above general epidemiology and background section. Activities which result in repetitive contraction of the pectoralis, triceps, or rectus abdominis muscles may result in stress fractures of the sternum.

20.7.2 Classification

There is no specific classification system for sternal stress fractures. Fractures are classified based on anatomic location and aforementioned grade.

20.7.3 Diagnosis

Stress fractures of the sternum are typically diagnosed on radiographs, CT scan, technetium bone scan, or MRI. The presenting history is typically that of dull to progressively sharp anterior chest pain. Stress fractures of the sternum have been described in the following sporting activities [21–25]:

- military training
- weight lifting
- golf
- cycling
- wrestling
- core exercises

20.7.4 Treatment

Relative rest from the causative activity often leads to resolution of symptoms within 6–10 weeks. Sternal stress fractures rarely require further treatment.

20.7.5 Complications

Complications are rare but include nonunion and delayed union.

20.7.6 Rehabilitation

Rehabilitation from sternal stress fractures generally includes rest from the causal activity followed by a gradual return to play program with physical therapy.

20.7.7 Preventative Measures

Please refer to the general prevention section above.

20.8 Scapula

20.8.1 Epidemiology

The scapula has a complex array of muscle attachments and corresponding bone stress patterns [4, 6, 9]. Depending on the specific patient's motion, stress concentration occurs at a variety of locations in the scapula. Stress fractures of the scapula are uncommon, though they have been well-documented in athletes [4, 9, 26–28]. Those participating in the following sports are at greatest risk [4, 9, 26–28]:

- gymnastics
- baseball pitching
- golf
- football
- jogger carrying weights
- professional football player
- trap shooting
- intensive shoulder rehabilitation programs

Figure 20.7 demonstrates a scapular spine stress fracture in a high school football quarterback. In addition, stress fractures can occur about the coracoid, acromion (Figs. 20.8 and 20.9), scapular spine, and scapular body [9, 17, 26]. Furthermore, stress fractures may also occur about acromion process after total shoulder arthroplasty and may be a source of post-operative pain (Fig. 20.10).

20.8.2 Classification

There is no specific classification system for scapula stress fractures. Fractures are classified based on anatomic location and aforementioned grade.

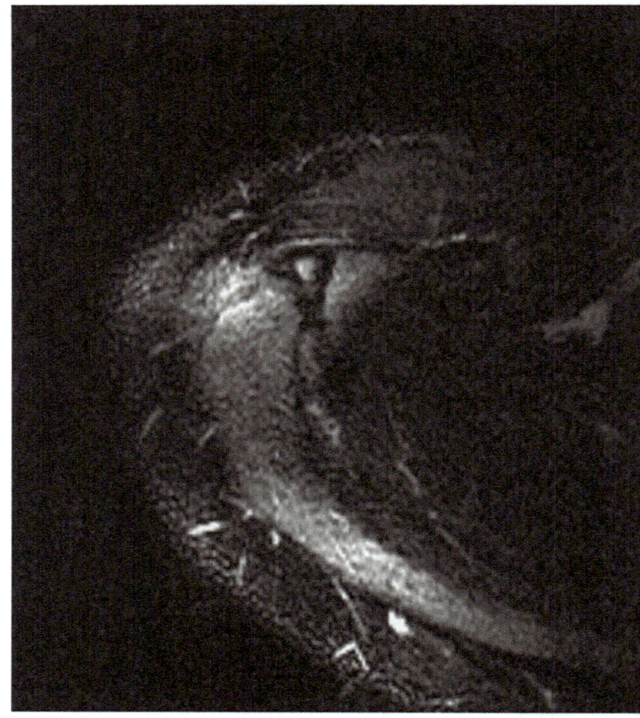

Fig. 20.7 Axial cut T2 MRI of the right shoulder of a high school quarterback demonstrating a stress reaction of the scapular spine

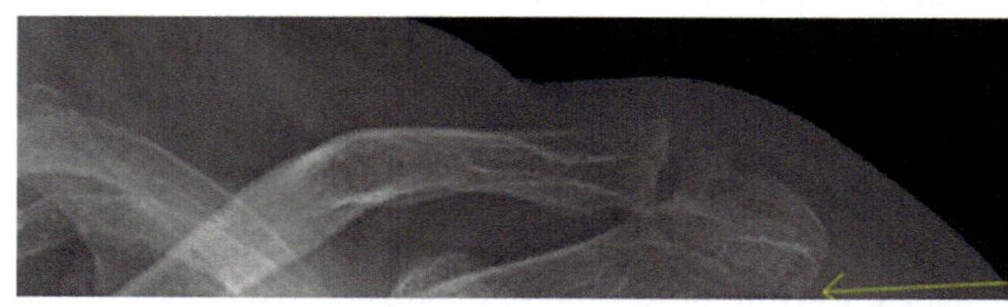

Fig. 20.8 T2 Axial MRI demonstrating Grade 2 stress fracture of the medial scapular spine in the dominant right shoulder of a high school quarterback (unstable os acromiale also present)

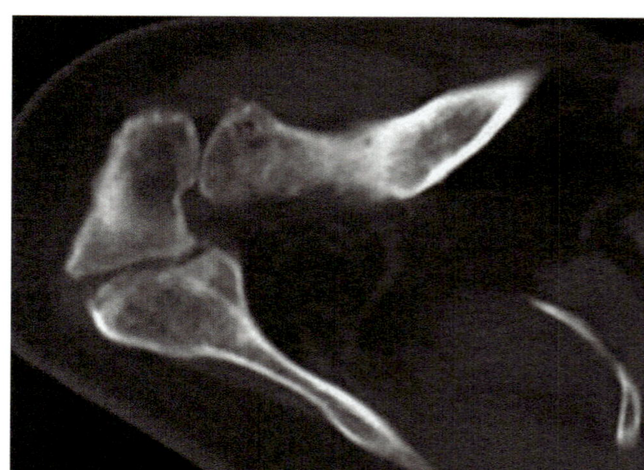

Fig. 20.9 Axial CT demonstrating a right sided acromion stress fracture

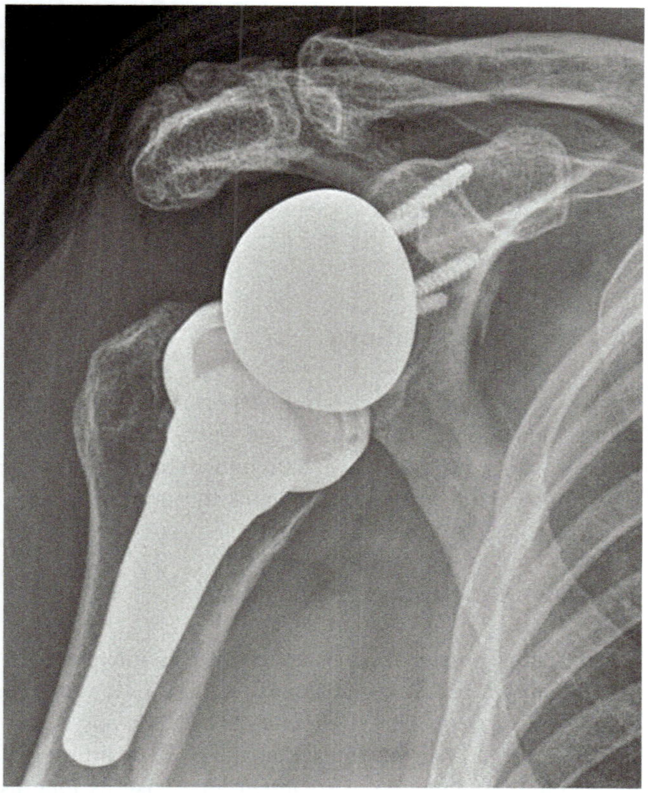

Fig. 20.10 Radiograph demonstrating a right sided acromion stress fracture after total shoulder arthroplasty

20.8.3 Diagnosis

Stress fractures of the scapula are typically diagnosed on CT scan, technetium bone scan, or MRI.

20.8.4 Treatment

Relative rest from the causative activity often leads to resolution of symptoms within 6–10 weeks. Scapular stress fractures rarely require further treatment.

20.8.5 Complications

Complications are rare but include nonunion and delayed union.

20.8.6 Rehabilitation

Rehabilitation from scapula stress fractures generally includes rest from the causal activity followed by a gradual return to play program with physical therapy.

20.8.7 Preventative Measures

Please refer to the general prevention section above.

20.9 Clavicle

20.9.1 Epidemiology

There are numerous muscular attachments to the clavicle, with multiple resultant force vectors. Abnormal shear and rotational forces can develop across the clavicle if there is an imbalance in muscular contraction between the pectoralis major, deltoid, and sternocleidomastoid muscles [4]. Athletes at risk of clavicle stress fractures include the following sporting activities [4, 5, 29]:

- rowing
- diving
- javelin
- weightlifting
- gymnastics
- baseball

20.9.2 Classification

There is no specific classification system for clavicle stress fractures. Fractures are classified based on anatomic location and aforementioned grade.

20.9.3 Diagnosis

Seyahi et al. [29] described a patient with a clavicular stress fracture presenting as atypical arm pain radiating throughout the upper extremity and hemithorax, further highlighting the importance of a high degree of suspicion and a thorough clinical exam.

20.9.4 Treatment

Relative rest from the causative activity often leads to resolution of symptoms within 6–10 weeks. Clavicular stress fractures rarely require further treatment.

20.9.5 Complications

Complications are rare but include nonunion and delayed union.

20.9.6 Rehabilitation

Rehabilitation from clavicle stress fractures generally includes rest from the causal activity followed by a gradual return to play program with physical therapy. Activity modification, postural training, and scapulothoracic stabilization exercises reliably yield symptom resolution [4, 29].

20.9.7 Preventative Measures

Please refer to the general prevention section above.

20.10 Proximal Humerus

20.10.1 Epidemiology

Poor conditioning and fatigue of the shoulder girdle musculature allows for increased rotational strain at the cortical surface of the proximal humerus. Bending forces generated by the deltoid and pectoralis major muscles is thought to contribute to transversely oriented stress fractures in weight lifters [30]. Stress fractures of the proximal humerus occur most commonly in the following sporting activities [31–34]:

- baseball
- throwers
- overhead activities
- weight lifting
- tennis

20.10.2 Classification

There is no specific classification system for proximal humerus stress fractures. Fractures are classified based on anatomic location and aforementioned grade.

20.10.3 Diagnosis

Stress fractures of the proximal humerus are typically diagnosed on radiographs, technetium bone scan, or MRI.

20.10.4 Treatment

In general, if the fracture is incomplete or non-displaced, proximal humeral stress fractures may be treated nonoperatively in a sling or functional brace until the athlete is pain free with activities of daily living or radiographic healing is evident. In addition to cessation of activity and rest, physical therapy for analgesia control, stretching, and deltoid and rotator cuff strengthening exercises may also be incorporated for treatment of proximal humerus stress fractures [18]. If there is fracture displacement, open reduction and internal fixation may be necessary to ensure timely healing and return to play.

20.10.5 Complications

Complications with nonoperative management are rare but include nonunion, delayed union and fracture displacement. Patients who require operative fixation will be subject to the standard complications associated with this procedure.

20.10.6 Rehabilitation

Rehabilitation from proximal humerus stress fractures generally includes rest from the causal activity followed by a gradual return to play program with physical therapy. A progressive return to throwing program and close monitoring of pitch counts is imperative. Treatment may take as long as 12 months for athletes to become asymptomatic [9].

20.10.7 Preventative Measures

Please refer to the general prevention section above.

20.11 Little League Shoulder

20.11.1 Epidemiology

Little League Shoulder is an epiphysiolysis of the proximal humerus secondary to repetitive microtrauma and rotational torque sustained during overhead activity that occurs exclusively in younger patients with open proximal humeral physes [35, 36]. The proximal humeral physis fuses between approximately 14 and 17 years of age among females and between 16 and 18 years among males [36–38]. In general, little league shoulder injuries are found among pitchers between the ages of 11–14, just prior to physeal fusion. The following factors contribute to the development of Little League shoulder:

- excessive throwing
- poor throwing technique
- muscular imbalance

20.11.2 Classification

There exist two published classification systems for little league shoulder stress fractures. That by Kanematsu, Y. et al. determines grade based on radiographic findings [39]. An older system determines grade based on epiphyseal displacement [40].

- Grade I: Widening of the epiphyseal plate in the lateral area only
- Grade II: Widening in all areas of the epiphyseal plate and metaphyseal demineralization
- Grade III: Slipped epiphysis

20.11.3 Diagnosis

Clinical history often includes diffuse shoulder pain predominately during throwing, often following an increase in the throwing frequency or intensity [41–43]. The following physical exam findings are common:

- weakness with resisted abduction and internal rotation
- tenderness at the proximal and lateral humerus
- swelling over the proximal and lateral shoulder

Little leaguer shoulder is typically diagnosed on radiographs, technetium bone scan, or MRI. Radiographs will reveal widening of the proximal humeral physis (Fig. 20.11). Plain radiographs may display fragmentation or demineralization of the metaphysis, cyst formation, physeal fragmentation or widening, or periosteal reaction [41–44]. MRI of the shoulder is required when the diagnosis is unclear (Fig. 20.12).

20.11.4 Treatment

The following treatment considerations are specific to management of proximal humeral stress fractures in adolescents [43]:

- rest from throwing for 6–12 weeks
- a progressive throwing program
- alterations to the athlete's throwing techniques and biomechanics
- monitoring of pitch counts

20.11.5 Complications

Complications are rare but include nonunion and delayed union.

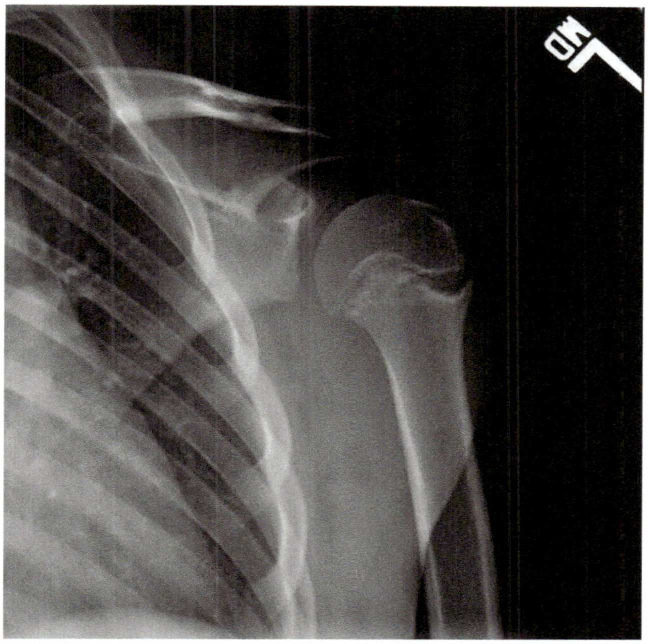

Fig. 20.11 Radiograph showing lateral widening at the proximal humeral physis

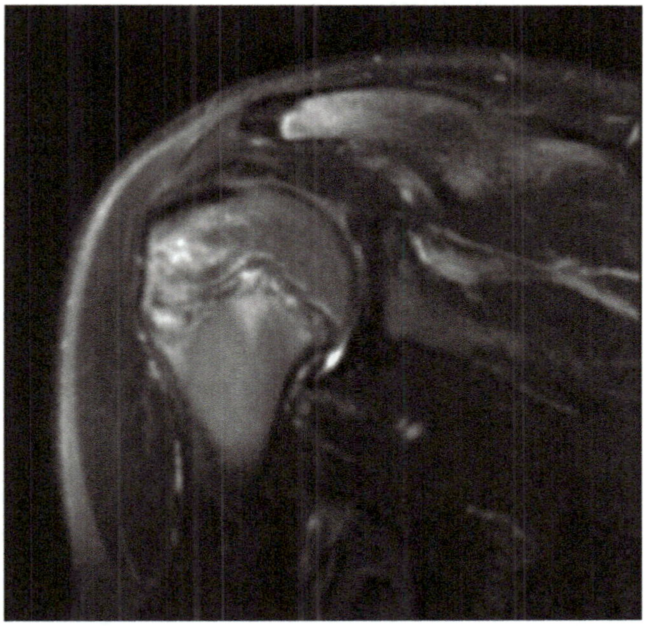

Fig. 20.12 Coronal T2 MRI image demonstrating periphyseal stress fracture of the proximal humerus

20.11.6 Rehabilitation

Rehabilitation includes rest from the causal activity followed by a gradual return to play program with physical therapy. A progressive return to throwing program and close monitoring of pitch counts is imperative.

20.11.7 Preventative Measures

Please refer to the general prevention section above.

20.12 Humeral Diaphysis

20.12.1 Epidemiology

Stress fractures of the humeral diaphysis are exceedingly rare when compared to those of the proximal humerus. The deltoid and pectoralis major muscles exert stress across the humeral diaphysis in weight lifters [30–34].

20.12.2 Classification

There is no specific classification system for humeral diaphyseal stress fractures, though fractures may be classified based on anatomic location and aforementioned grading system.

20.12.3 Diagnosis

Stress fractures of the humeral diaphysis may be diagnosed on radiographs, technetium bone scan, or MRI.

20.12.4 Treatment

Humeral diaphyseal stress fractures are routinely treated nonoperatively in a sling or functional brace until the athlete is pain free. The athlete should be followed-up with serial radiographs until healing is confirmed. Similarly to proximal humerus stress fracture treatment, cessation of activity and rest, physical therapy, stretching, and deltoid and rotator cuff strengthening exercise are imperative [18].

20.12.5 Complications

Complications are rare but include nonunion, delayed union and fracture displacement. If significant, fracture displacement may warrant open reduction and internal fixation of the fracture.

20.12.6 Rehabilitation

Rehabilitation from humeral diaphyseal stress fractures generally includes rest from the causal activity followed by a gradual return to play program with physical therapy.

20.12.7 Preventative Measures

Please refer to the general prevention section above.

20.13 Rib Stress Fractures

20.13.1 Epidemiology

Rib stress fractures must be considered when evaluating athletes with vague shoulder pain after repetitive activities as these injuries are well described and are frequently missed. Tensile muscular forces (rather than axial compressive forces) are predominantly responsible for rib stress fractures, as ribs are non-weight-bearing bones [7]. The most common sites of fracture include the anterolateral first rib (Fig. 20.13), the posterolateral fourth through ninth ribs, and the posterolateral upper ribs [9, 12]. Rib stress fractures are almost always reported on the throwing or dominant limb [45]. Patients with first-rib stress fractures present with insidious onset of dull, vague pain in the anterior cervical triangle and mid-clavicular region, with occasional radiation to the sternum and pectoral region [12]. Repetitive strain on the torso contributes to middle- and lower-rib stress fractures (Figs. 20.14 and 20.15) [5, 6, 19, 46–48]. The following sporting activities are at risk for rib stress fractures [4, 6, 49–52]:

- discus
- rowing
- rugby

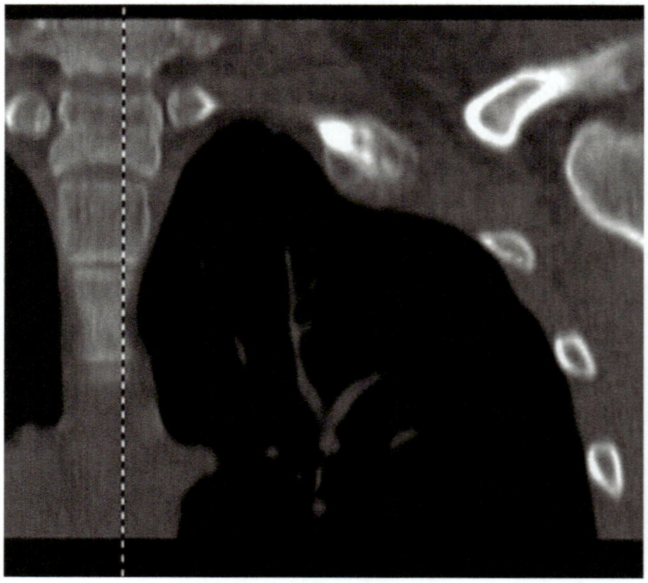

Fig. 20.13 CT scan demonstrating left first rib stress fracture in a male collegiate gymnast with abundant callus formation

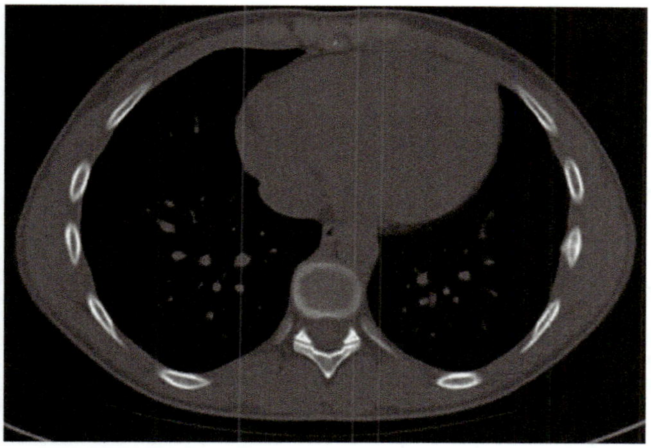

Fig. 20.14 CT scan demonstrating stress fracture of the left mid seventh rib with callus formation

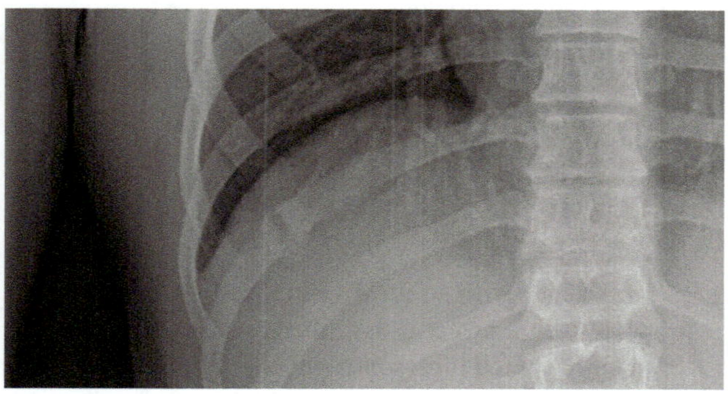

Fig. 20.15 Chest radiographs demonstrating nonunion (Grade 5) of the right tenth rib stress fracture in a male collegiate rower

- golf
- weightlifting
- volleyball
- gymnastics
- judo
- tennis
- table tennis
- baseball
- basketball
- lacrosse
- soccer
- javelin
- backpacking
- wind surfing

20.13.2 Classification

There is no specific classification system for rib stress fractures. Fractures are classified based on anatomic location and aforementioned grade.

20.13.3 Diagnosis

Importantly, when reviewing elite rowers throughout their entire career, they have been found to suffer a first rib stress fracture rate of 8–9% [53]. This highlights the importance of sport-specific diagnostic acumen. A recent review by Funakoshi et al. [54, 55] demonstrated that the most common presenting symptoms for athletes with first rib stress fractures included posterior shoulder or upper thoracic back pain. Cervical spine imaging may more accurately identify first rib stress fractures when compared to shoulder radiographs [54]. Prisk et al. [56] described the "trapezius squeeze test" for the diagnosis of first rib stress fractures. This test involves applying pressure to the anterior aspect of the trapezius muscle, causing involuntary contraction of the muscle and eliciting rib pain (Fig. 20.16). This test was found to be reliable for diagnosing first rib stress fractures on physical examination in five cases of stress fractures in ballet dancers [9, 56].

20.13.4 Treatment

Treatment of rib stress fractures includes the following [57]:

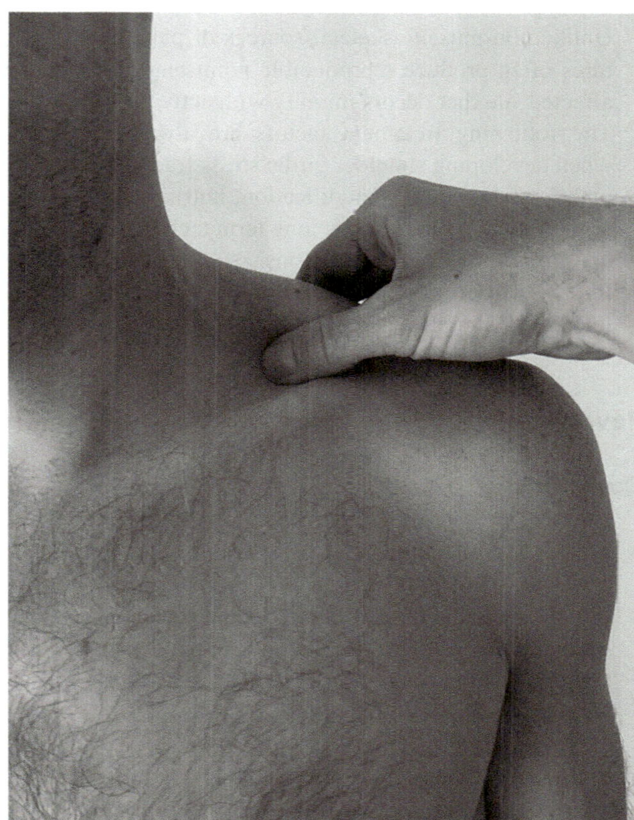

Fig. 20.16 Trapezius squeeze or pinch test

- physical therapy
- rest until deep breathing is pain free
- gradual return to sport

20.13.5 Complications

Complications are rare but include nonunion and delayed union.

20.13.6 Rehabilitation

Rehabilitation includes rest from the causal activity followed by a gradual return to play program with physical therapy.

20.13.7 Preventative Measures

Please refer to the general prevention section above.

Clinical Pearls

- A high sense of clinical suspicion is required to accurately diagnose a shoulder girdle stress fracture given the multitude of other differential diagnoses in an athlete to consider.
- Unlike non-musculoskeletal sources of pain, stress fractures often produce reproducible point tenderness at the affected site that occurs initially with activity.
- The following treatment factors are always important when developing shoulder girdle stress fracture treatment plans: rest or activity modification, nutritional optimization, gradual return to play, long term technique or shoulder girdle mechanical alterations.
- Return to sport timing must be individualized to the athlete, sport, symptom duration, and season remaining.

Review

Questions

1. A 23 year old male high performing collegiate rower presents with a 3 week history of left chest wall discomfort. He has no trouble breathing and denies any recent trauma. Which of the following physical exam tests or signs has been shown to have high sensitivity for evaluation of first rib stress fractures?
   (a) Loss of internal range of motion
   (b) Pain with resisted arm forward elevation
   (c) Pain with trapezius squeeze test
   (d) Pain with shoulder external rotation
   (e) Reduction in shoulder girdle range of motion
2. Which of the following choices corresponds to the common time-period when proximal humeral physeal stress injuries occur?
   (a) 5–8 years old
   (b) 7–10 years old
   (c) 11–14 years old
   (d) 13–16 years old
   (e) 15–18 years old
3. A 28 year-old female professional power lifter presents with a multiple month history of recurrent activity-related left shoulder pain. She notes this pain usually occurs during repetitive lifting sessions of greater than 30 repetitions. On physical examination, she has point tenderness over the scapular spine. Her radiographs do not demonstrate any abnormalities. Which of the following choices demonstrates the next best step in treatment?
   (a) Continued activity as tolerated
   (b) MRI of left shoulder
   (c) Repeat radiographs in 2 weeks
   (d) Surgical stabilization
   (e) Whole body bone scan

Answers

1. Choice C: The rib stress fractures section describes the trapezius squeeze test as described by Prisk et al. This test has demonstrated high sensitivity for first rib stress fractures. Rowers are at particularly high risk for rib stress injuries in general due to the high tensile loads placed on ribs during repetitive rowing activity.
2. Choice C: In general the proximal humeral physis fuses between approximately 14 and 17 years of age among females and between 16 and 18 years among males. As such, league shoulder injuries are commonly found among pitchers between the ages of 11–14, just prior to physeal fusion.
3. Choice B: The athlete likely has a stress fracture of the shoulder girdle; likely of her scapula given her physical exam and clinical history. An MRI would yield the most useful data to diagnose a shoulder girdle stress fracture. A bone scan is not as specific *and* sensitive as an MRI.

References

1. Matheson GO, et al. Stress fractures in athletes. A study of 320 cases. Am J Sports Med. 1987;15:46–58. https://doi.org/10.1177/036354658701500107.
2. Fredericson M, Jennings F, Beaulieu C, Matheson GO. Stress fractures in athletes. Top Magn Reson Imaging. 2006;17:309–25. https://doi.org/10.1097/RMR.0b013e3180421c8c.
3. Brukner P. Stress fractures of the upper limb. Sports Med. 1998;26:415–24. https://doi.org/10.2165/00007256-199826060-00004.

4. Jones GL. Upper extremity stress fractures. Clin Sports Med. 2006;25:159–74. https://doi.org/10.1016/j.csm.2005.08.008, xi.
5. Sinha A, Kaeding C, Wadley G. Upper extremity stress fractures in athletes: clinical features of 44 cases. Clin J Sport Med. 1999;4:199–202.
6. Miller TL, Kaeding CC. Upper-extremity stress fractures: distribution and causative activities in 70 patients. Orthopedics. 2012;35:789–93. https://doi.org/10.3928/01477447-20120822-09.
7. Vinther A, et al. Exercise-induced rib stress fractures: potential risk factors related to thoracic muscle co-contraction and movement pattern. Scand J Med Sci Sports. 2006;16:188–96. https://doi.org/10.1111/j.1600-0838.2005.00473.x.
8. Kaeding CC, Spindler KP, Amendola A. Management of troublesome stress fractures. Instr Course Lect. 2004;53:455–69.
9. Miller TL, Harris JD, Kaeding CC. Stress fractures of the ribs and upper extremities: causation, evaluation, and management. Sports Med. 2013;43:665–74. https://doi.org/10.1007/s40279-013-0048-7.
10. Miller T, Kaeding CC, Flanigan D. The classification systems of stress fractures: a systematic review. Phys Sportsmed. 2011;39:93–100. https://doi.org/10.3810/psm.2011.02.1866.
11. Kaeding CC, Miller T. The comprehensive description of stress fractures: a new classification system. J Bone Joint Surg Am. 2013;95:1214–20. https://doi.org/10.2106/JBJS.L.00890.
12. McDonnell LK, Hume PA, Nolte V. Rib stress fractures among rowers: definition, epidemiology, mechanisms, risk factors and effectiveness of injury prevention strategies. Sports Med. 2011;41:883–901. https://doi.org/10.2165/11593170-000000000-00000.
13. Banks KP, et al. Overuse injuries of the upper extremity in the competitive athlete: magnetic resonance imaging findings associated with repetitive trauma. Curr Probl Diagn Radiol. 2005;34:127–42. https://doi.org/10.1067/j.cpradiol.2005.04.001.
14. Anderson MW. Imaging of upper extremity stress fractures in the athlete. Clin Sports Med. 2006;25:489–504, vii. https://doi.org/10.1016/j.csm.2006.02.006.
15. Kiuru MJ, Pihlajamäki HK, Perkiö JP, Ahovuo JA. Dynamic contrast-enhanced MR imaging in symptomatic bone stress of the pelvis and the lower extremity. Acta Radiol. 2001;42:277–85.
16. Ishibashi Y, et al. Comparison of scintigraphy and magnetic resonance imaging for stress injuries of bone. Clin J Sport Med. 2002;12:79–84.
17. Bugbee S. Rib stress fracture in a golfer. Curr Sports Med Rep. 2010;9:40–2. https://doi.org/10.1249/JSR.0b013e3181cb12df.
18. Godoy IRB, Malavolta EA, Lundberg JS, da Silva JJ, Skaf A. Humeral stress fracture in a female CrossFit athlete: a case report. BMC Musculoskelet Disord. 2019;20:150. https://doi.org/10.1186/s12891-019-2532-1.
19. Dragoni S, Giombini A, Di Cesare A, Ripani M, Magliani G. Stress fractures of the ribs in elite competitive rowers: a report of nine cases. Skelet Radiol. 2007;36:951–4. https://doi.org/10.1007/s00256-007-0350-2.
20. Lord M, Ha K, Song K. Am J Sports Med. 1996;1:118–22.
21. Keating TM. Stress fracture of the sternum in a wrestler. Am J Sports Med. 1987;15:92–3. https://doi.org/10.1177/036354658701500115.
22. Hill PF, Chatterji S, DeMello WF, Gibbons JR. Stress fracture of the sternum: an unusual injury? Injury. 1997;28:359–61.
23. Barbaix EJ. Stress fracture of the sternum in a golf player. Int J Sports Med. 1996;17:303–4. https://doi.org/10.1055/s-2007-972851.
24. Lee J, Fields KB. Sternal stress fracture in a middle-aged woman. BMJ Case Rep. 2017;2017:bcr2016218203. https://doi.org/10.1136/bcr-2016-218203.
25. Robertson K, Kristensen O, Vejen L. Br J Sports Med. 1996;30:176–7.
26. Herickhoff PK, Keyurapan E, Fayad LM, Silberstein CE, McFarland EG. Scapular stress fracture in a professional baseball player: a case report and review of the literature. Am J Sports Med. 2007;35:1193–6. https://doi.org/10.1177/0363546506298278.
27. Hall RJ, Calvert PT. Stress fracture of the acromion: an unusual mechanism and review of the literature. J Bone Joint Surg (Br). 1995;77:153–4.
28. Boyer DW. Trapshooter's shoulder: stress fracture of the coracoid process. Case report. J Bone Joint Surg Am. 1975;57:862.
29. Seyahi A, Atalar AC, Demirhan M. [An unusual cause of shoulder pain: stress fracture of the clavicle]. Acta Orthop Traumatol Turc. 2009;43:264–6, https://doi.org/10.3944/AOTT.2009.264.
30. Jones G. AOSSM sports medicine update. 2009.
31. Evans PA, Farnell RD, Moalypour S, McKeever JA. Thrower's fracture: a comparison of two presentations of a rare fracture. J Accid Emerg Med. 1995;12:222–4. https://doi.org/10.1136/emj.12.3.222.
32. Polu KR, et al. Stress fracture of the humerus in a collegiate baseball pitcher. A case report. Am J Sports Med. 1999;27:813–6. https://doi.org/10.1177/03635465990270062201.
33. Joseph TA, Zehr RJ. Spontaneous humeral shaft fracture in a weight lifter. Orthopedics. 2000;23:603–5.
34. Horwitz BR, DiStefano V. Stress fracture of the humerus in a weight lifter. Orthopedics. 1995;18:185–7.
35. Chen FS, Diaz VA, Loebenberg M, Rosen JE. Shoulder and elbow injuries in the skeletally immature athlete. J Am Acad Orthop Surg. 2005;13:172–85.
36. Wu M, Fallon R, Heyworth BE. Overuse injuries in the pediatric population. Sports Med Arthrosc Rev. 2016;24:150–8. https://doi.org/10.1097/JSA.0000000000000129.
37. Webb L, Mooney J, Swiontkowski M. Skeletal trauma in children. Philadelphia, PA: WB Saunders; 1998.
38. Stanitski C, DeLee J, Drez D. Pediatric and adolescent sports medicine. Philadelphia, PA: WB Saunders; 1998.
39. Kanematsu Y, et al. Epidemiology of shoulder injuries in young baseball players and grading of radiologic findings of Little Leaguer's shoulder. J Med Invest. 2015;62:123–5. https://doi.org/10.2152/jmi.62.123.
40. Neer CS, Horwitz BS. Fractures of the proximal humeral epiphysial plate. Clin Orthop Relat Res. 1965;41:24–31.
41. Carson WG, Gasser SI. Little leaguer's shoulder. A report of 23 cases. Am J Sports Med. 1998;26:575–80. https://doi.org/10.1177/03635465980260041901.
42. Ireland ML, Andrews JR. Shoulder and elbow injuries in the young athlete. Clin Sports Med. 1988;7:473–94.
43. Kocher M, Walter PM, Micheli LJ. Upper extremity injuries in the pediatric athlete. Sports Med. 2000;30:117–35.
44. Popkin CA, Posada A, Clifford PD. Little leaguer's shoulder. Clin Imaging. 2006;30:365–7. https://doi.org/10.1016/j.clinimag.2006.02.005.
45. Coris EE, Higgins HW. First rib stress fractures in throwing athletes. Am J Sports Med. 2005;33:1400–4. https://doi.org/10.1177/0363546505275349.
46. Holden DL, Jackson DW. Stress fracture of the ribs in female rowers. Am J Sports Med. 1985;13:342–8. https://doi.org/10.1177/036354658501300509.
47. Lee AD. Golf-related stress fractures: a structured review of the literature. J Can Chiropr Assoc. 2009;53:290–9.
48. Gerrie BJ, Harris JD, Lintner DM, McCulloch PC. Lower thoracic rib stress fractures in baseball pitchers. Phys Sportsmed. 2016;44:93–6. https://doi.org/10.1080/00913847.2015.1116363.
49. Chaudhury S, Hobart SJ, Rodeo SA. Bilateral first rib stress fractures in a female swimmer: a case report. J Shoulder Elb Surg. 2012;21:e6–10. https://doi.org/10.1016/j.jse.2011.08.048.
50. Eng J, Westcott J, Better N. Stress fracture of the first rib in a weightlifter. Clin Nucl Med. 2008;33:371–3. https://doi.org/10.1097/RLU.0b013e31816a78c8.
51. Evans GM, Bhogal G. Unusual cause of thoracic wall pain in a kayaker: a case report. Clin J Sport Med. 2018;28:e85–6. https://doi.org/10.1097/JSM.0000000000000453.

52. Low S, Kern M, Atanda A. First-rib stress fracture in two adolescent swimmers: a case report. J Sports Sci. 2016;34:1266–70. https://doi.org/10.1080/02640414.2015.1108452.
53. D'Ailly PN, Sluiter JK, Kuijer PP. Rib stress fractures among rowers: a systematic review on return to sports, risk factors and prevention. J Sports Med Phys Fitn. 2016;56:744–53.
54. Funakoshi T, et al. First-rib stress fracture in overhead throwing athletes. J Bone Joint Surg Am. 2019;101:896–903. https://doi.org/10.2106/JBJS.18.01375.
55. Kawashima K, et al. Stress fractures of the first rib related to swinging of a baseball bat: two case reports. Clin J Sport Med. 2016;26:e108–10. https://doi.org/10.1097/JSM.0000000000000278.
56. Prisk VR, Hamilton WG. Stress fracture of the first rib in weight-trained dancers. Am J Sports Med. 2008;36:2444–7. https://doi.org/10.1177/0363546508326710.
57. Vinther A, Thornton JS. Management of rib pain in rowers: emerging issues. Br J Sports Med. 2016;50:141–2. https://doi.org/10.1136/bjsports-2014-094168.

Stress Fractures in Sport: Elbow

21

Robert A. Jack II and Christopher C. Dodson

21.1 Stress Fractures Around the Elbow: General Principles

21.1.1 Epidemiology

Early reports revealed that 17% of young baseball players will experience elbow pain in their dominant elbow [1]. More recent data from 2013 showed that this percentage has increased to 30% in adolescent baseball players [2]. Most of the data surrounding elbow injuries in athletes is in regards to injuries to the ulnar collateral ligament (UCL). In adolescents aged 15–19 years old the incidence of ulnar collateral ligament reconstruction (UCLR) has been reported as 6.3 per 1000 [3]. Over the last 15 years there has been a greater than 300% increase in UCLR and is projected to continue to increase over the next 5–10 years [3]. One can postulate that the increase in UCLR may also indicate an overall increase in elbow injuries as a whole.

Early sport specialization is thought to be the culprit for the recent increase in elbow injuries and elbow surgeries in the young throwing athlete population. Early sport specialization is defined as an athlete less than 12 years old playing in a single sport for at least 8 months per year [4, 5]. This has been shown to have a detrimental effect on athletes, increasing overall overuse injuries which are dependent on the athletes sport [6, 7]. In throwing athletes, specifically, there is a reported increase in overall arm injuries and missed games due to injury [8].

Unfortunately, even with the large body of evidence showing the detriments of specializing early, parents and coaches remain in the dark. A recent study showed that parents and the athletes themselves are often not aware of their status as a specialized athlete [8]. A 2018 survey-based study revealed that over half of little league coaches do not keep pitch counts per recommendations of the American Sports Medicine Institute or the 2006 US Baseball Medical and Safety Advisory Committee, and were not aware of risk factors for overuse injury of the upper extremity [9]. The early addition of off-speed pitches such as a curveball or slider to a pitcher's repertoire continues to be debated as a contributing factor to elbow injury [10]. However, most will agree that early introduction of off-speed pitches in an athlete who has poor or undeveloped biomechanics probably predisposes that athlete to upper extremity injury.

The effect of overuse in adolescent athletes is not restricted to adolescence. The risk of injury as a professional baseball player is higher for athletes who had early sports specialization, with the average age of specialization being 9 years in one study of professional baseball players [5]. These professional athletes have also been shown to have an increased number of upper extremity injuries and missed games as a professional [11].

Stress fractures about the elbow are rare in athletes. Most commonly, the soft tissue structures around the elbow are injured including the medial ulnar collateral ligament, flexor-pronator muscle-tendon complex, common extensor muscle-tendon complex, and the ulnar nerve [12]. Bony or cartilage injuries can occur as well which may include osteochondritis dissecans, valgus extension overload, or apophyseal stress injuries in the pediatric population most commonly at the medial epicondyle [12].

The athlete's sport absolutely plays a role in the type of stress fracture they may incur. Stress fractures around the elbow are typically seen with throwing athletes [13]. Throwers may also experience stress fractures of the ribs, while track and field, ballet, and tennis athletes are more prone to tibial shaft stress fractures, and basketball athletes more prone to tibial shaft or metatarsal stress fractures [13]. A systematic review of stress fractures about the elbow in throwing athletes reported 88.5% of athletes participated in baseball, 7.7% in javelin, 1.9% in American football and softball [14].

R. A. Jack II (✉)
Houston Methodist Orthopedics and Sports Medicine, Houston, TX, USA

C. C. Dodson
Rothman Institute, Philadelphia, PA, USA

G. A. J. Robertson, N. Maffulli (eds.), *Fractures in Sport*, https://doi.org/10.1007/978-3-030-72036-0_21

The age of athletes who are diagnosed with a stress fracture ranges from 13 to 29 years old with the average being 20 years old [13, 14]. The majority of stress fractures are reported at the olecranon with a small minority at the proximal ulna or distal humerus [14–17]. Most commonly, athletes, who have a stress related injury, participate at the high recreational or competitive level of play [13].

21.1.2 Classification

The three main locations of stress fracture about the elbow reported in the literature are the olecranon, proximal ulna, and distal humerus. A recent case series also described a radial head stress reaction in gymnasts [18]. The large majority of stress fractures of the elbow are at the olecranon [13, 14]. Due to the rarity of these injuries, a consistent and widely used classification system for each individual injury does not exist.

Furushima et al. described a classification system for olecranon stress fractures in baseball players [19]. The five types of stress injuries to the olecranon described are physeal, classic, transitional, sclerotic, and distal [19]. The type of stress fracture is directly related to the age of the athlete: physeal (14.1 years old), classic (18.6 years old), transitional (16.9 years old), sclerotic (18 years old), and distal 19.6 years old). Each type is then subdivided into four stages based on severity. In stage 1 the epiphyseal plate on the contralateral side is closed incompletely and in stage 2 the epiphyseal plate on the contralateral side is completely closed [19]. In stage 3 there is epiphyseal plate dehiscence visible at the articular surface [19]. Finally, in stage 4 there is complete dehiscence of the epiphyseal plate from the articular surface to the dorsal olecranon [19]. Treatment is then dictated based on type and severity which will be covered later in this chapter.

21.1.3 Diagnosis

Elbow injuries can be complicated to diagnose based on history and physical exam alone. Diagnosing stress fractures around the elbow becomes even more challenging. Ultimately the physician likely will need to rule out other more common pathology prior to the diagnosis of a stress fracture.

21.1.3.1 History

Athletes will present with pain around the elbow and potentially a decreased level of play. The patient may describe decreased performance on the field associated with hampered elbow function. The physician should inquire about the timing and location of the pain. Specifically, to determine if pain extends beyond the sport and is an issue while at rest or with activities of daily living. Additional factors to explore are symptom duration, potential mechanism of injury, prior injuries, and associated symptoms [20–22]. Changes in workout intensity or diet, team advancement including expanded roles, and position changes may offer insight [23].

Timing may be the most critical indicator for throwing athletes. Acuity of the pain should be documented as throwers may have an acute event where a "pop" is heard or felt, or more chronic symptoms may be described for patients with a stress fracture. For throwing athletes, change in velocity, ball control, stamina, and perceived arm strength can be helpful as well. Timing within the athlete's season can also provide insight into the injury. In overhead athletes, flexor pronator strains may be more commonly seen in the early season due to inadequate conditioning, whereas a stress fracture may appear after 4–8 weeks of training [24]. Patients with mechanical symptoms are less likely to have a stress related problem.

Injury history and dietary history should be explored and can assist in the context of the diagnosis. For female athletes, inquiring about changes in menstrual cycle can provide a context for explanation of the injury. Specific history related to the shoulder or hips can also provide clues for diagnosis. An example would be a throwing athlete with prior posterior shoulder pain and a diagnosis of glenohumeral internal rotation deficit (GIRD) who underwent physical therapy. This may be indicative of an athlete with detrimental biomechanics during throwing or perhaps is actively changing their biomechanics during throwing which may have led to an elbow injury.

The six phases of throwing include wind-up, stride, cocking, acceleration, deceleration, and follow-through [21]. These phases are imperative to understand for physicians treating throwing athletes. Determining the point during the throwing motion that pain occurs or the point during the throwing motion pain began initially is essential [21]. In patients with UCL injury, 85% will feel pain during the acceleration phase of throwing and 25% will experience pain during the deceleration phase [25]. The late cocking or early acceleration phases will typically put strain on the medial elbow, while pain during the deceleration phase may signify posterior elbow pathology [20, 22, 26, 27].

Pitch type that exacerbates pain is a useful portion of the history. Different pitches, which are somewhat player specific, may predispose a player to injury at different locations about the elbow. An athlete sustaining an injury while throwing a fastball is likely attempting to throw as hard as possible thus putting the most strain on the medial elbow in the late cocking and early acceleration phase of throwing. By contrast, many pitchers will describe "snapping off" a curveball which is often a forced extension of the elbow prior to and at release of the baseball. An injury during this pitch may indicate posterior elbow pathology including olecranon stress fracture.

Early sports specialization has been linked to increased numbers of elbow injuries [28]. The physician treating these athletes should inquire about the athlete's year-round throwing routine including excessive pitch counts and provide guidance based upon current literature. Many high-school athletes are preparing for the next level and may be throwing in multiple showcases, tryouts, and matches, all at the same time. This amount of throwing, with the potential maximized effort to increase velocity, can put undue strain on the elbow with subsequent injury.

Physicians should be familiar with diagnosing UCL injury, flexor pronator strain, triceps tendon strain, cubital tunnel syndrome, and valgus extension overload. Occasionally these concomitant injuries may require a different non-operative course or potentially additional surgical procedures. Careful attention should be given to athlete's additional symptoms including instability, mechanical symptoms, numbness, paresthesias, and perceived weakness in order to diagnose and treat these concurrent issues.

21.1.3.2 Physical Exam

For overhead athletes, a complete elbow, shoulder, and hip exam should be completed on each patient, including contralateral assessment to evaluate side to side differences. As with other exams of the musculoskeletal system, the physician should begin with inspection and range of motion testing followed by palpation and special tests used to elucidate specific pathology of concern. For special testing it is imperative to clarify if pain mimics the symptomatology that brought the patient for the visit or if it is something "new" or potentially incidental. It is helpful to also get a general assessment of the patient's kinetic chain strength and coordination, by performance of a single leg squat or a single leg stance with controlled trunk rotation.

During the initial inspection stage, the physician should evaluate the skin and soft tissue envelope for signs of acute injury including ecchymoses, swelling, abnormal muscle contour, muscle quality including atrophy or hypertrophy, and the presence of prior surgical or accidental scars [29]. The carrying angle of the elbow should be measured which is defined as the angle between the humerus and the forearm with the elbow in extension and forearm in full supination. The normal carrying angle in the general population is typically 11–13° of valgus which may be slightly higher in women [30]. This angle may also be higher in throwers, often upwards of 15°. There are a few theories behind this including the "muscle theory" which is described as the increased strength in the brachioradialis and extensor carpi radialis longus of throwing athletes resulting in a greater radial deviation in full extension [29]. There is also a theory that the repetitive stress on the elbow joint may lead to increased laxity or adaptive changes through development, thus resulting in a larger carrying angle [23, 29].

Range of motion of the elbow, forearm, and shoulder should be measured both actively and passively. The normal range of motion of the elbow should be from full extension or slight hyperextension to 140° of flexion. Commonly in throwing athletes loss of elbow extension is found up to 20° which may be pathologic or developmental [23]. Forearm pronation and supination normally measure 75° and 85° respectfully [29]. Endpoints in passive range of motion should be evaluated with a solid endpoint in flexion potentially indicating an osteophyte in the coronoid fossa and a solid endpoint in extension potentially indicating an osteophyte in the olecranon fossa [23]. If mechanical symptoms are experienced during the exam, close attention should be given to the timing of the symptoms as it will aid in diagnosis.

Palpation should begin away from the site of discomfort. Laterally the structures palpated should include the radial head, capitellum, "soft spot" posterior to radiocapitellar joint, lateral epicondyle, and extensor wad. Posteriorly the triceps insertion, olecranon process, and soft spots corresponding to the medial and lateral gutters should be palpated. Anteriorly the distal biceps tendon, brachioradialis, and pronator teres should be palpated.

For patients with medial elbow pain the palpated structures should begin with the bony prominence of the medial epicondyle. With medial epicondylitis there is typically tenderness associated with palpating the anteromedial facet where the pronator teres and flexor carpi radialis originate [29]. The UCL should be palpated along its course from the inferior medial epicondyle to the sublime tubercle of the proximal ulna. This is best achieved in 50–70° of flexion where the flexor pronator muscles are shifted slightly anteriorly [23]. The ulnar nerve can be palpated in the cubital tunnel proximal to the medial epicondyle, posterior to the medial epicondyle, and distally. Attention should be given to whether the nerve subluxes anteriorly with the elbow taken from extension to flexion. Careful percussion of the nerve may elucidate a positive Tinel sign with radiating symptoms into the small finger.

Active resisted testing of the flexor pronator muscle mass should be performed to determine the extent of injury to these structures. This is done by resisting wrist flexion with the elbow in full extension. Resisted forearm pronation should also be tested with the elbow both in full extension and flexed to 90°. Negative tests with these maneuvers shift the examiner away from flexor pronator pathology to an injury to the UCL. Both ipsilateral and contralateral palmaris longus tendons should be assessed for their presence and quality, by having the patient flex the wrist and oppose the thumb to the small finger. The incidence of congenital absence of this tendon varies, but in some geographic populations, this can be as high as 64% [31].

There are a few special tests for evaluating the medial elbow in throwing athletes. [12, 20] To evaluate the anterior band of the UCL, various valgus stress testing maneuvers are described. For a valgus stress test of the elbow, the patient can be upright or supine. Valgus stress is given with the elbow at 15–20° of flexion in order to unlock the olecranon from the olecranon fossa [32]. The orientation of the forearm during this test is contentious: initially this was described to be in full supination; however, forearm pronation during this maneuver will prevent subtle posterolateral instability, from mimicking medial laxity [32, 33]. Medially based pain or instability during this maneuver should be considered a positive test.

The milking maneuver is another test used to evaluate valgus instability [12, 20]. The patient is in a seated position with the shoulder in 90° of abduction and the elbow at 90° of flexion. The examiner will apply a valgus stress by pulling the patient's thumb. Reproduction of medially-based pain or instability indicates a positive test. Alternatively, the moving valgus test can be performed in the same position or with the patient supine. The examiner will then slowly extend the elbow from 90° to 20° of flexion while applying valgus stress. Reproduced pain or instability at any point along this arc indicates a positive test.

The valgus extension overload test can be performed to evaluate posteromedial pain due to presence of a posteromedial osteophyte or olecranon fossa overgrowth [20]. The examiner will stabilize the humerus with one hand with the other hand will pronate the forearm and apply a valgus force while maximally extending the elbow [23]. A positive test is when the maneuver provokes pain posteromedially.

The bounce test can be used to elucidate pain over the olecranon. The examiner will hold the shoulder in slight forward flexion, with the elbow also in slight flexion. The examiner will then "bounce" the elbow by passively extending the patient's elbow to full extension. Pain reproduced posteriorly should raise concern for an olecranon or distal humerus stress fracture.

21.1.3.3 Imaging

Standard radiographs including the anteroposterior, lateral, and oblique views should be obtained for all patients with elbow pain. Often these radiographs will be negative for patients with a stress fracture. A lucency or sclerotic area in the proximal olecranon can indicate an olecranon stress fracture.(Fig. 21.1) Radiographs should be reviewed for the presence of olecranon osteophytes, calcification within the UCL, capitellar osteochondral injury, and loose bodies [12]. If particularly interested in posteromedial olecranon osteophytes, an oblique axial view can be taken with the elbow in 110° of flexion [26]. In patients where the discomfort is primarily more distal in the forearm, dedicated AP and lateral forearm radiographs should be obtained to evaluate for evidence of radial or ulnar diaphyseal stress fracture.

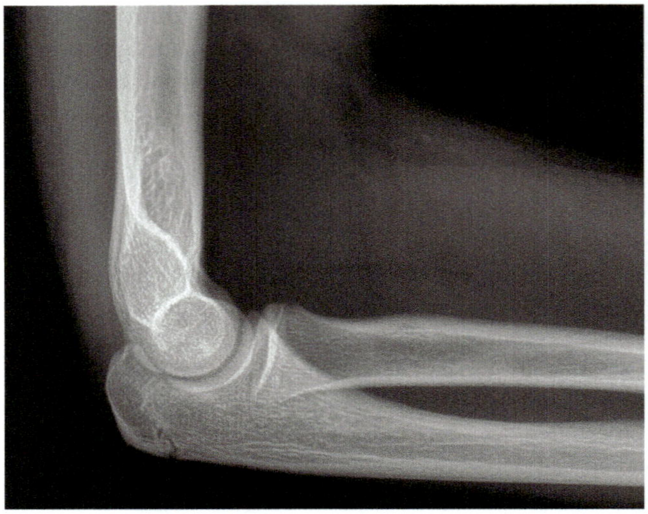

Fig. 21.1 Lateral elbow radiograph demonstrating an olecranon stress fracture at the previous physeal closure site

Magnetic resonance imaging (MRI) can be obtained for patients with a high clinical suspicion of stress fracture. Alternatively, a computed tomography (CT) scan or bone scan can be utilized. An MRI would be best for evaluating soft tissue structures if a concomitant or alternative injury was suspected such as a distal triceps tear. Additionally, an MRI would be preferable over CT scan for evaluating a less severe "stress reaction" or edema within the bone without an overt fracture line.

21.1.4 Treatment

According to Smith et al. most (76.9%) of stress fractures in throwing athletes undergo operative intervention [14]. However, this number may underrepresent straight forward nonoperative cases that are not presented in the literature. The mean duration of symptoms before diagnosis is reported as 2.8 months for successful nonoperative treatment and 6.7 months for operative treatment [14, 16, 34]. This emphasizes the need for definitive diagnosis in this challenging patient population and to move forward with advanced imaging in patients who are not improving with nonoperative measures. There are no reported studies in the literature of a stress fracture of the proximal ulna or distal humerus requiring operative management.

21.1.4.1 Nonoperative

In most cases without a completed stress fracture, 8–12 weeks of nonoperative treatment is pursued. Most authors recommend an initial 4–6 week period of rest and avoidance of activities that may apply a valgus stress to the elbow [16, 34]. A custom hinged elbow brace is an option at this timeframe as well. Schickendantz et al. suggest setting the elbow brace with full flexion to 20° short of full extension for the first 2–4 weeks with gradual increasing range of motion thereafter [15]. The next 2–6 weeks after injury should focus on motion and subsequently strengthening with weaning from the brace if applied [15, 23]. The physician should also identify other predisposing factors that may exist including GIRD, poor core strength or coordination, and kinetic chain weakness. During this period of relative rest and subsequent building of a strengthening program, kinetic chain coordination and shoulder health maintenance should not be overlooked. The physician should also send the athlete to an endocrinologist or nonoperative sports medicine physician to be evaluated for endocrine or hormonal abnormalities. This step is essential to correct an underlying medical reason for a stress fracture which may precipitate a recurrence if untreated. A bone growth stimulator may also be used to facilitate healing.

Assuming the athlete remains pain free without point tenderness over the stress fracture with the first 6–8 weeks of rehabilitation, introduction of plyometrics and sports specific exercises can begin. For throwers, an interval throwing program should be utilized [24]. A hitting progression program should also be used for baseball athletes who are primarily position players. A physician may choose to begin a hitting progression program prior to a throwing program as hitting is thought to have less force across the elbow. Once the athlete has progressed through these programs and is pain free, return to sport is recommended.

21.1.4.2 Operative

Operative management is indicated for patients who have failed nonoperative management, or those who have a stress fracture that is one of the following types: physeal (stage 3 or 4), classic, transitional, or distal [19]. Operative treatment is not typically recommended for sclerotic stress fractures [19].

Postoperatively the patient is placed in a posterior based splint for 7–10 days. Encouragement should be given for finger range of motion and light hand grasping exercises. After the initial splinting period, the wound is evaluated and sutures are removed if necessary. The patient is then placed optionally into a hinged elbow brace with progressive advancement of motion over the next 2–4 weeks until full range of motion is achieved. If a brace is used, the patient may wean from the brace at 4 weeks postoperatively. Encouragement should be given to focus on entire kinetic chain optimization as it relates to their sport including scapular posturing, low back and core strengthening, lower extremity strengthening, and overall flexibility and coordination. An interval throwing and hitting program should be utilized in the throwing athlete beginning between weeks 8 and 12 postoperatively. Once the athlete has progressed through these programs and is pain free, return to sport is recommended.

21.1.4.3 Symptom Resolution

In nonoperatively treated patients, symptoms resolved in an average of 20 weeks after beginning treatment [14]. In operatively treated patients, symptoms resolved 16 weeks after operative treatment [14]. The time to radiographic union is reported at 29.6 weeks on average in nonoperatively treated patients and 14.3 weeks on average in operatively treated patients [14] (Figs. 21.2 and 21.3). According to Smith et al., all patients treated nonoperatively had full symptom resolution and 97.5% of operatively treated patients had full symptom relief with one patient reporting continued elbow pain [14, 35].

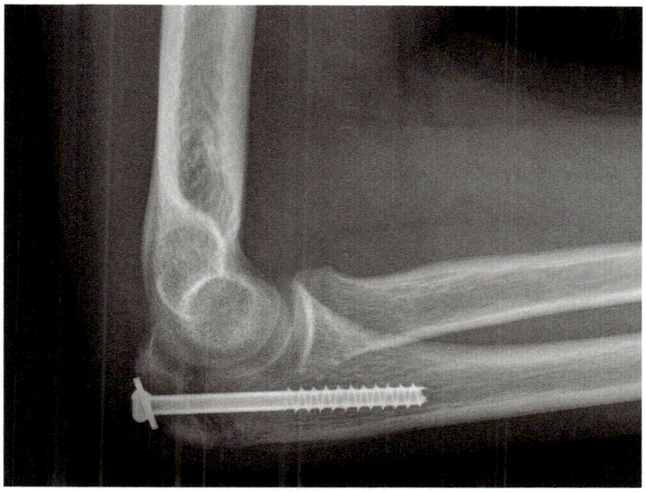

Fig. 21.2 Four-week postoperative lateral elbow radiograph of an olecranon stress fracture treated with a partially threaded cannulated screw and washer construct demonstrating initial increased lucency at the fracture site

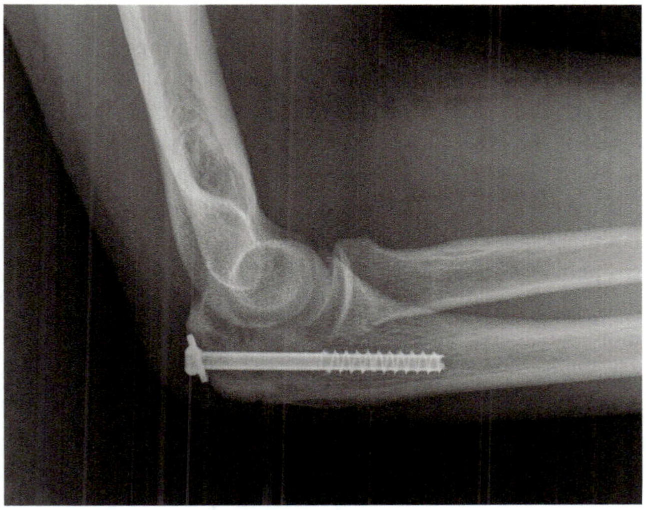

Fig. 21.3 Twenty-week postoperative lateral elbow radiograph of an olecranon stress fracture treated with a partially threaded cannulated screw and washer construct demonstrating bony healing of fracture site

21.1.4.4 Return to Sport

The overall reported return to sport rate for stress fractures around the elbow in throwing athletes is 96.2% [14]. Of the patients who did not return to sport, one was lost to follow-up after nonoperative management and one did not return due to unresolved pain after operative treatment with cannulated screws [14, 15, 35]. The average return to sport time for nonoperatively treated patients was 16 weeks and for operatively treated patients was 25.7 weeks [14]. All nonoperatively treated patients returned to their pre-injury level of sport and 95% of operatively treated patients returned to their pre-injury level of sport or higher [14].

21.1.5 Complications

Nonoperatively treated stress fractures need to be followed closely in the clinic setting with specific attention to pain profiles and radiographic changes. Patient's who eventually move towards operative management will experience fracture displacement, persistent nonunion, or continued elbow pain [36–39]. These patients have been reported to go through 20 weeks of nonoperative management before electing for surgery [37–40].

21.1.6 Rehabilitation

Nonoperative and operative regimens for early rehabilitation are described in the above sections. Sports specific rehabilitation should be coordinated for each patient. However, given that most of these patients are throwing athletes, the rehabilitation program for throwers is outlined here. Wilk et al. have described a four phase rehabilitation program for throwers [41]. The goal of Phase 1 is to maximize the effects of immobilisation, reestablish nonpainful range of motion, decrease pain and inflammation, and slow muscle atrophy [41]. Patients will begin to work on range of motion exercises of the elbow and shoulder in this phase and will last until week 4. Phase 2 begins once preoperative range of motion is achieved and consists primarily of reestablishing neuromuscular control of the elbow and improving muscle strength and endurance [41]. This phase allows for the beginning of Thrower's Ten exercises [42]. Phase 3 consists of more advanced strengthening and includes the Advanced Thrower's Ten to be performed over weeks 10–16 postoperatively [42]. The final phase is Phase 4 that lasts from week 16 to return to play and focuses on sports specific activities included interval programs [41].

The patient will ultimately return to sport when full range of motion is restored and is pain free. Additional criteria may include completing a rehabilitation protocol, interval throwing or hitting programs, and strength testing. Commonly the return to play decision is based on these factors as well as time from surgery.

21.1.7 Preventative Measures

Elbow injuries in the young throwing population are on the rise, likely due to early sport specialization. The current best preventative measures for all shoulder and elbow overuse injuries include following current recommendations regarding sports specialization and pitch counts for throwing athletes. Young athletes should be encouraged to pursue alternative sports in their offseason if a period of rest is not desired. It has been clearly shown that greater than 9 months of continued overhead play in these young athletes are not only detrimental acutely, but can continue to have an effect into their eventual professional career. Education of the parents of adolescents who participate in high risk sports for overuse injuries can have a significant impact on decreasing their child's likelihood to have an injury [43].

For those involved in on-field sports medicine and injury prevention, emphasis on a good diet should be continued. Adequate levels of Vitamin D and calcium in these athletes should be assured. The treating physician should be familiar with the Female Athlete Triad and make appropriate referrals for these patients as well as any patient with a stress fracture as there may be a metabolic reason for injury at the forefront.

Proper preseason conditioning is also essential. Overhead throwing athletes should be encouraged to participate in an interval throwing and hitting program at the beginning of each season, in addition to their strength, flexibility, and cardiovascular training. Acknowledgement of symptoms early on and avoidance of activities that produce symptoms should be a part of an athletes training regimen.

Additional details regarding the site-specific stress fractures around the elbow are provided below.

21.1.8 Distal Humerus

21.1.8.1 Epidemiology

There are multiple case reports of humeral stress fractures in the literature [17, 44, 45]. However, the incidence of these fractures is unknown.

21.1.8.2 Classification

There is no specific classification system for stress fractures of the distal humerus.

21.1.8.3 Diagnosis

The anterior to posterior squeeze and medial to lateral squeeze tests of the distal humerus have been described to aid in the diagnosis [46].

21.1.8.4 Treatment

The large majority of these fractures are treated in the nonoperative fashion. A completed stress fracture may be treated surgically by open reduction and internal fixation with plate and screw construct dependent on the orientation of the fracture.

21.1.8.5 Complications

Fractures that have been treated operatively with plate and screw construct should be monitored for a proximal stress shielding response to the humerus proximally resulting in a new humerus fracture at the level of the plate.

21.1.8.6 Rehabilitation

Please refer to the General Principles section.

21.1.8.7 Preventative Measures

Please refer to the General Principles section.

21.1.9 Little League Elbow

21.1.9.1 Epidemiology

Little Leaguer's elbow is often used as a broad term describing multiple pathologies about the elbow in an adolescent overhead athlete. It has been reported that 20–40% of school aged pitchers are affected [28, 47]. The spectrum of the disease may include delayed or accelerated growth of the medial epicondyle, traction apophysitis of the medial epicondyle, medial epicondylitis, osteochondritis of the capitellum, hypertrophy of the ulna, osteochondral injury to the radial head, and olecranon apophysitis with delayed physeal closure [48]. The purpose of this section is to discuss medial epicondyle apophysitis.

21.1.9.2 Classification

Medial epicondyle injuries have been classified based on patient age, fragment size, and ulnar collateral ligament integrity with the most common morphology of the epicondyle represented as small fragmentation [49, 50]. More recent work has been done to further classify these injuries based on medial epicondyle morphology. There are four types of medial epicondyle appearance: normal, irregular, hypertrophic, and fragmented [51]. In younger patients aged 11–12 the most common abnormal appearance is fragmented or irregular [51]. The most commonly encountered type in a patient older than 16 is hypertrophic [51]. Sixty-eight percent of athletes with abnormal appearance of their medial epicondyle reported concomitant elbow pain [51].

21.1.9.3 Diagnosis

Please refer to the General Principles section.

21.1.9.4 Treatment

The medial epicondyle injuries can be treated nonoperatively. However, in patients who have continued pain after trial of nonoperative treatment or displacement of the medial epicondyle, open reduction and internal fixation may be required. (Fig. 21.4).

21.1.9.5 Complications

Please refer to the General Principles section.

21.1.9.6 Rehabilitation

Please refer to the General Principles section.

21.1.9.7 Preventative Measures

Please refer to the General Principles section.

21.1.10 Radial Head

21.1.10.1 Epidemiology

There is one case series in the literature describing three young gymnasts with open physes sustaining Type IV Salter

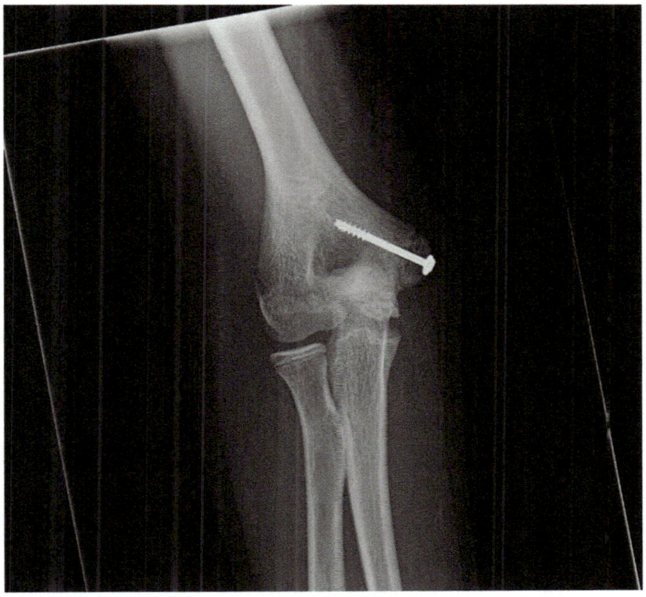

Fig. 21.4 Twelve-week postoperative radiograph of medial epicondyle apophysitis treated with a partially threaded cannulated screw and washer construct

Harris stress fractures of the radial head [18]. The high repetitive loads that gymnasts sustain place them at risk for these injuries. The average age of these patients was 11.7 years old and were all female [18].

21.1.10.2 Classification

There is no specific classification system for stress fractures of the radial head.

21.1.10.3 Diagnosis

Please refer to the General Principles section.

21.1.10.4 Treatment

The majority of radial head stress fractures can be treated nonoperatively. However in the only reported case series, one patient required open reduction and internal fixation after a period of nonoperative management which resulted in persistent nonunion [18].

21.1.10.5 Complications

Please refer to the General Principles section.

21.1.10.6 Rehabilitation

Please refer to the General Principles section.

21.1.10.7 Preventative Measures

Please refer to the General Principles section.

21.1.11 Olecranon

21.1.11.1 Epidemiology

The most common stress fracture about the elbow is the olecranon stress fracture reported to comprise between 58% and 98% of stress fractures in this location [13, 14]. In throwers, the most common stress fracture is the olecranon stress fracture [14]. The mechanism of injury is postulated to be similar to that of valgus extension overload [52]. Repetitive abutment of the medial olecranon in the olecranon fossa combined with forceful contraction of the triceps during deceleration is thought to play the primary role in this injury [52]. This may also be exacerbated by pitch selection as many pitchers will describe "snapping off" a curveball which is often a forced extension of the elbow prior to and at release of the baseball.

21.1.11.2 Classification

Stress fractures of the olecranon can be stratified using the classification system by Furushima et al. [19] This has been described above.

21.1.11.3 Diagnosis

Please refer to the General Principles section.

21.1.11.4 Treatment

Nonoperative

Please refer to the General Principles section.

Operative

Many techniques have been utilized for operative management including open reduction and internal fixation (ORIF) with cannulated screws, tension band wiring with Kirschner wires, bone grafting, fracture site drilling, and excision of the olecranon tip [35–40, 53–56].

Seventy-eight percent of studies have reported using ORIF with cannulated screws [14]. In this case the surgeon may use a single large (6.5 or 7.3 mm) partially threaded cannulated screw [23].(Fig. 21.5) The patient will be placed in the supine position with a hand table or two arm boards. The arm may either be draped over the patient's chest or maximally internally rotated at the shoulder to gain access to the posterior arm. A single, longitudinally based incision is made over the olecranon and distal triceps. A longitudinal split through the triceps tendon is recommended to insert the

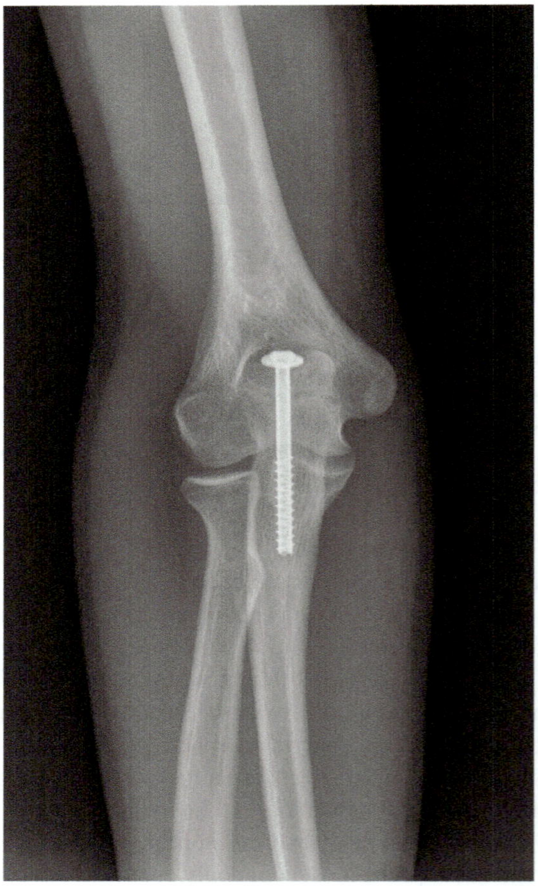

Fig. 21.5 Twenty-week postoperative anterior-posterior radiograph of an olecranon stress fracture treated with a partially threaded cannulated screw and washer construct

screw. Intraoperative radiographs are used to ensure appropriate placement of screw. The wound would then be irrigated and closed in a layered fashion. A secondary procedure for removal of the screw is explored if the screw is symptomatic and radiographic and clinical union has been achieved.

21.1.11.5 Complications

The overall reported complication rate after operative management of olecranon stress fractures is 17.3% [14]. Of the complications, 89% were related to symptomatic hardware which required reoperation [14]. In two (25%) of those patients, a deep infection was encountered which necessitated 6 weeks of intravenous vancomycin following irrigation and debridement with removal of hardware [35]. The last reported complication was related to the ulnar nerve and the patient ultimately underwent neurolysis of the ulnar nerve in the cubital tunnel [41]. In cases of revision surgery as reported by Smith et al., all primary procedures used tension band wiring with Kirschner wires which were subsequently removed and the fracture was then treated with ORIF and a screw [14].

21.1.11.6 Rehabilitation

Please refer to the General Principles section.

21.1.11.7 Preventative Measures

Please refer to the General Principles section.

21.1.12 Proximal Ulna

21.1.12.1 Epidemiology

The epidemiology of proximal ulna stress fractures is unknown. There are a few cases reported in the literature in throwing athletes [15, 16]. In all cases, the stress fracture was found at the posteromedial aspect of the proximal ulna [15, 16].

21.1.12.2 Classification

There is no specific classification system for stress fractures of the proximal ulna.

21.1.12.3 Diagnosis

Schickendantz et al. described the unreliable nature of plain radiographs with no stress fractures appearing on plain radiographs in seven cases [15]. The recommended imaging modality for diagnosing proximal ulna stress fractures is MRI [15].

21.1.12.4 Treatment

These injuries are predominantly treated nonoperatively. There are no reported cases of proximal ulna stress fractures being treated operatively.

21.1.12.5 Complications

Please refer to the General Principles section.

21.1.12.6 Rehabilitation

Please refer to the General Principles section.

21.1.12.7 Preventative Measures

Please refer to the General Principles section.

21.1.13 Radial Diaphysis

21.1.13.1 Epidemiology

The incidence of radial diaphyseal stress fractures is unknown. There are two reports of stress fracture in the literature in a baseball pitcher and kettlebell lifter [57, 58]. The proposed mechanism of injury is repetitive use of the supinator in the case of the baseball pitcher and repetitive overload of the radius in the kettlebell lifter [57, 58].

21.1.13.2 Classification

There is no specific classification system for stress fractures of the radial diaphysis.

21.1.13.3 Diagnosis

Please refer to the General Principles section.

21.1.13.4 Treatment

These injuries are predominantly treated nonoperatively. There are no reported cases of radial diaphyseal stress fracture being treated operatively.

21.1.13.5 Complications

Please refer to the General Principles section.

21.1.13.6 Rehabilitation

Please refer to the General Principles section.

21.1.13.7 Preventative Measures

Please refer to the General Principles section.

21.1.14 Ulnar Diaphysis

21.1.14.1 Epidemiology

The incidence of these injuries is unknown, however, there are multiple case reports in the literature regarding stress fractures of the ulna [59–66]. Most frequently, these are reported in the athletic population including softball pitchers, dancers, and a bowler [59–62, 64]. There are also reports of bilateral stress fractures in a weightlifter and military trainee [65, 66]. The proposed mechanism for injury is repetitive forearm rotation or increase load requirement in the case of a patient who was on crutches [63].

21.1.14.2 Classification

There is no specific classification system for stress fractures of the ulna diaphysis.

21.1.14.3 Diagnosis

Please refer to the General Principles section.

21.1.14.4 Treatment

Incomplete fractures of the ulna diaphysis can be treated successfully with nonoperative management, by activity modification, relative rest and return to activity. However, a completed stress fracture of the ulna should be treated with open reduction and internal fixation, using a plate and screw construct.

21.1.14.5 Complications

Please refer to the General Principles section.

21.1.14.6 Rehabilitation

Please refer to the General Principles section.

21.1.14.7 Preventative Measures

Please refer to the General Principles section.

References

1. Gugenheim JJ, Stanley RF, Woods GW, Tullos HS. Little league survey: the Houston study. Am J Sports Med. 1976. https://doi.org/10.1177/036354657600400501.
2. Matsuura T, Suzue N, Kashiwaguchi S, Arisawa K, Yasui N. Elbow injuries in youth baseball players without prior elbow pain: a 1-year prospective study. Orthop J Sport Med. 2013; https://doi.org/10.1177/2325967113509948.
3. Mahure SA, Mollon B, Shamah SD, Kwon YW, Rokito AS. Disproportionate trends in ulnar collateral ligament reconstruction: projections through 2025 and a literature review. J Shoulder Elb Surg. 2016; https://doi.org/10.1016/j.jse.2016.02.036.
4. Popkin CA, Bayomy AF, Ahmad CS. Early sport specialization. J Am Acad Orthop Surg. 2019; https://doi.org/10.5435/jaaos-d-18-00187.
5. Wilhelm A, Choi C, Deitch J. Early sport specialization: effectiveness and risk of injury in professional baseball players. Orthop J Sport Med. 2017; https://doi.org/10.1177/2325967117728922.
6. Fabricant PD, Lakomkin N, Sugimoto D, Tepolt FA, Stracciolini A, Kocher MS. Youth sports specialization and musculoskeletal injury: a systematic review of the literature. Phys Sportsmed. 2016; https://doi.org/10.1080/00913847.2016.1177476.
7. Post EG, Trigsted SM, Riekena JW, Hetzel S, McGuine TA, Brooks MA, Bell DR. The association of sport specialization and training volume with injury history in youth athletes. Am J Sports Med. 2017; https://doi.org/10.1177/0363546517690848.
8. Arnold A. Patterns of participation and performance in youth baseball players. Diss Abstr Int Sect B Sci Eng. 2018;
9. Knapik DM, Continenza SM, Hoffman K, Gilmore A. Youth baseball coach awareness of pitch count guidelines and overuse throwing injuries remains deficient. J Pediatr Orthop. 2018; https://doi.org/10.1097/BPO.0000000000001244.
10. Lyman S, Fleisig GS, Andrews JR, Osinski ED. Effect of pitch type, pitch count, and pitching mechanics on risk of elbow and shoulder pain in youth baseball pitchers. Am J Sports Med. 2002; https://doi.org/10.1177/03635465020300040201.
11. Confino JE, Irvine JN, Ahmad CS, Lynch TS. Early sports specialization is associated with increased upper extremity injuries and fewer games played in major league baseball players. Orthop J Sport Med. 2019; https://doi.org/10.1177/2325967119s00399.
12. Cain EL, Dugas JR, Wolf RS, Andrews JR. Elbow injuries in throwing athletes: a current concepts review. Am J Sports Med. 2003; https://doi.org/10.1177/03635465030310042601.
13. Iwamoto J, Takeda T. Stress fractures in athletes: review of 196 cases. J Orthop Sci. 2003; https://doi.org/10.1007/s10776-002-0632-5.
14. Smith SR, Patel NK, White AE, Hadley CJ, Dodson CC. Stress fractures of the elbow in the throwing athlete: a systematic review. Orthop J Sport Med. 2018; https://doi.org/10.1177/2325967118799262.
15. Schickendantz MS, Ho CP, Koh J. Stress injury of the proximal ulna in professional baseball players. Am J Sports Med. 2002; https://doi.org/10.1177/03635465020300051801.
16. Mamanee P, Neira C, Martire JR, McFarland EG. Stress lesion of the proximal medial ulna in a throwing athlete. A case report. Am J Sports Med. 2000; https://doi.org/10.1177/03635465000280022101.
17. Alpert J, Flannery R, Epstein R, Monaco R, Prendergast N. Humeral stress edema: an injury in overhead athletes quarterback with humeral "shin" splints-a case report. Clin J Sport Med. 2014; https://doi.org/10.1097/JSM.0000000000000036.
18. Santelli J, McCambridge TM, Valasek AE, Standiford K. Proximal radial head fractures in young gymnasts: a case series of newly described overuse injuries. Clin J Sport Med. 2019; https://doi.org/10.1097/JSM.0000000000000498.
19. Furushima K, Itoh Y, Iwabu S, Yamamoto Y, Koga R, Shimizu M. Classification of olecranon stress fractures in baseball players. Am J Sports Med. 2014; https://doi.org/10.1177/0363546514528099.
20. Cain EL, Dugas JR. History and examination of the thrower's elbow. Clin Sports Med. 2004; https://doi.org/10.1016/j.csm.2004.04.008.
21. Fleisig GS, Andrews JR, Dillman CJ, Escamilla RF. Kinetics of baseball pitching with implications about injury mechanisms. Am J Sports Med. 1995; https://doi.org/10.1177/036354659502300218.
22. McCall BR, Cain EL. Diagnosis, treatment, and rehabilitation of the thrower's elbow. Curr Sports Med Rep. 2005; https://doi.org/10.1097/01.CSMR.0000306218.40799.a0.
23. Kuremsky MA, Cain EL, Dugas JR, Andrews JR. Chapter 064: Elbow throwing injuries. DeLee, Drez, Miller's Orthop Sport Med. 2017. https://doi.org/10.1016/B978-1-4557-4376-6.00068-8.
24. Azar FM, Andrews JR, Wilk KE, Groh D. Operative treatment of ulnar collateral ligament injuries of the elbow in athletes/Traitement chirurgical des lesions du ligament lateral interne du coude chez les athletes. Am J Sports Med. 2000;
25. Conway JE, Jobe FW, Glousman RE, Pink M. Medial instability of the elbow in throwing athletes. Treatment by repair or reconstruction of the ulnar collateral ligament. J Bone Jt Surg Ser A. 1992; https://doi.org/10.2106/00004623-199274010-00009.
26. Wilson FD, Andrews JR, Blackburn TA, McCluskey G. Valgus extension overload in the pitching elbow. Am J Sports Med. 1983; https://doi.org/10.1177/036354658301100206.
27. Miller CD, Savoie FH. Valgus extension injuries of the elbow in the throwing athlete. J Am Acad Orthop Surg. 1994; https://doi.org/10.5435/00124635-199409000-00004.
28. Lyman S, Fleisig GS, Waterbor JW, Funkhouser EM, Pulley L, Andrews JR, Osinki ED, Roseman JM. Longitudinal study of elbow and shoulder pain in youth baseball pitchers. Med Sci Sports Exerc. 2001; https://doi.org/10.1097/00005768-200111000-00002.
29. Kuremsky MA, Lyle Cain E, JRD y JRA. Ch 057: Elbow anatomy and biomechanics. DeLee, Drez, Miller's Orthop Sport Med. 2017. https://doi.org/10.1016/B978-1-4557-4376-6.00061-5.

30. Beals RK. The normal carrying angle of the elbow. A radiographic study of 422 patients. Clin Orthop Relat Res. 1976; https://doi.org/10.1097/00003086-197609000-00029.
31. Ioannis D, Anastasios K, Konstantinos N, Lazaros K, Georgios N. Palmaris Longus muscle's prevalence in different nations and interesting anatomical variations: review of the literature. J Clin Med Res. 2015; https://doi.org/10.14740/jocmr2243w.
32. Norwood LA, Shook JA, Andrews JR. Acute medial elbow ruptures. Am J Sports Med. 1981; https://doi.org/10.1177/036354658100900103.
33. O'Driscoll SW, Bell DF, Morrey BF. Posterolateral rotatory instability of the elbow. J Bone Jt Surg Ser A. 1991; https://doi.org/10.12790/ahm.2018.23.2.69.
34. Nuber GW, Diment MT. Olecranon stress fractures in throwers: a report of two cases and a review of the literature. Clin Orthop Relat Res. 1992; https://doi.org/10.1097/00003086-199205000-00009.
35. Paci JM, Dugas JR, Guy JA, Cain EL, Fleisig GS, Hurst C, Wilk KE, Andrews JR. Cannulated screw fixation of refractory olecranon stress fractures with and without associated injuries allows a return to baseball. Am J Sports Med. 2013; https://doi.org/10.1177/0363546512469089.
36. Fujioka H, Tsunemi K, Takagi Y, Tanaka J. Treatment of stress fracture of the olecranon in throwing athletes with internal fixation through a small incision. Sport Med Arthrosc Rehabil Ther Technol. 2012; https://doi.org/10.1186/1758-2555-4-49.
37. Kvidera DJ, Pedegana LR. Stress fracture of the olecranon: report of two cases and review of literature. Orthop Rev. 1983;
38. Nakaji N, Fujioka H, Tanaka J, Sugimoto K, Yoshiya S, Fujita K, Kurosaka M. Stress fracture of the olecranon in an adult baseball player. Knee Surg Sport Traumatol Arthrosc. 2006; https://doi.org/10.1007/s00167-005-0622-0.
39. Suzuki K, Minami A, Suenaga N, Kondoh M. Oblique stress fracture of the olecranon in baseball pitchers. J Shoulder Elb Surg. 1997; https://doi.org/10.1016/S1058-2746(97)80004-3.
40. Rettig AC, Wurth TR, Mieling P. Nonunion of olecranon stress fractures in adolescent baseball pitchers: a case series of 5 athletes. Am J Sports Med. 2006; https://doi.org/10.1177/0363546505281802.
41. Wilk KE, Reinold MM, Andrews JR. Rehabilitation of the thrower's elbow. Clin Sports Med. 2004; https://doi.org/10.1016/j.csm.2004.06.006.
42. Wilk KE, Yenchak AJ, Arrigo CA, Andrews JR. The advanced throwers ten exercise program: a new exercise series for enhanced dynamic shoulder control in the overhead throwing athlete. Phys Sportsmed. 2011; https://doi.org/10.3810/psm.2011.11.1943.
43. Zabawa L, Alland JA. Association between parental understanding of pitch smart guidelines and youth baseball player injuries. Orthop J Sport Med. 2019; https://doi.org/10.1177/2325967119846314.
44. Godoy IRB, Malavolta EA, Lundberg JS, Da Silva JJ, Skaf A. Humeral stress fracture in a female CrossFit athlete: a case report. BMC Musculoskelet Disord. 2019; https://doi.org/10.1186/s12891-019-2532-1.
45. Zaremski JL, Wright TW, Herman DC. Humeral stress fracture with median nerve injury in a baseball player: a case report and discussion. Curr Sports Med Rep. 2018; https://doi.org/10.1249/JSR.0000000000000489.
46. Zaremski JL, Herman DC. Humeral stress fractures in overhead athletes: pearls for recognition, diagnosis, and management. Curr Sports Med Rep. 2016; https://doi.org/10.1249/JSR.0000000000000309.
47. Fleisig GS, Andrews JR. Prevention of elbow injuries in youth baseball pitchers. Sports Health. 2012; https://doi.org/10.1177/1941738112454828.
48. Bradley JP, Austin LS, Tjoumakaris FP. Ch 134: Elbow injuries in pediatric and adolescent athletes. Delee Drez's Orthop Sport Med. 2015. https://doi.org/10.1016/B978-1-4557-4376-6.00132-3.
49. Woods GW, Tullos HS. Elbow instability and medial epicondyle fractures. Am J Sports Med. 1977; https://doi.org/10.1177/036354657700500105.
50. Rudzki JR, Paletta GA. Juvenile and adolescent elbow injuries in sports. Clin Sports Med. 2004; https://doi.org/10.1016/j.csm.2004.05.001.
51. Otoshi K, Kikuchi S, Kato K, Sato R, Igari T, Kaga T, Konno S. Age-specific prevalence and clinical characteristics of humeral medial epicondyle apophysitis and osteochondritis dissecans: ultrasonographic assessment of 4249 players. Orthop J Sport Med. 2017; https://doi.org/10.1177/2325967117707703.
52. Ahmad CS, ElAttrache NS. Valgus extension overload syndrome and stress injury of the olecranon. Clin Sports Med. 2004; https://doi.org/10.1016/j.csm.2004.04.013.
53. Hulkko A, Orava S, Nikula P. Stress fractures of the olecranon in javelin throwers. Int J Sports Med. 1986; https://doi.org/10.1055/s-2008-1025760.
54. Imade S, Matsuura Y, Nishi H, Uchio Y. Olecranon stress fracture in an adult baseball pitcher: a case report. Curr Orthop Pract. 2011; https://doi.org/10.1097/BCO.0b013e31822140fc.
55. Pavlov H, Torg JS, Jacobs B, Vigorita V. Nonunion of olecranon epiphysis: two cases in adolescent baseball pitchers. Am J Roentgenol. 1981; https://doi.org/10.2214/ajr.136.4.819.
56. Torg JS, Moyer RA. Non union of a stress fracture through the olecranon epiphyseal plate observed in an adolescent baseball pitcher. A case report. J Bone Jt Surg Ser A. 1977; https://doi.org/10.2106/00004623-197759020-00026.
57. Gross C, Reese ME. Radial stress fracture in a kettlebell competitor: a case report. PM R. 2016.
58. Meijer KA, Fury MS, Ennis H, Grau L, Baraga M, Jose J, Andrews JR, Kaplan L. Radial shaft stress fracture in a major league pitcher. Am J Orthop (Belle Mead NJ). 2017;
59. Chen YH, Kuo CL, Lin LC, Wang SJ, Lee CH. Stress fracture of the ulna in a break-dancer. J Sports Sci Med. 2008;
60. Wiltfong RE, Carruthers KH, Popp JE. Completed ulnar shaft stress fracture in a fast-pitch softball pitcher. Orthopedics. 2017; https://doi.org/10.3928/01477447-20161108-01.
61. Bigosinski K, Palmer T, Weber K, Evola J. Ulnar shaft stress fracture in a high school softball pitcher. Sports Health. 2010; https://doi.org/10.1177/1941738109357300.
62. Hsu MC, Lue KH, Lin ZI, Lu KH. Stress fracture at the junction of the middle and distal third of the ulnar diaphysis in a spinner bowler: a case report and a review of the literature. Knee Surg Sport Traumatol Arthrosc. 2005; https://doi.org/10.1007/s00167-004-0560-2.
63. Venkatanarasimha N, Kamath S, Kambouroglou G, Ostlere SJ. Proximal ulna stress fracture and stress reaction of the proximal radius associated with the use of crutches: a case report and literature review. J Orthop Traumatol. 2009; https://doi.org/10.1007/s10195-009-0057-3.
64. Tornese D, Curci D, Nardo A, Cuccia A, Pozzi G. Stress fracture of the ulna in an elite ice dancer. J Sports Sci Med. 2014;
65. Lin HH, Chang WH, Huang TF, Hung SC, Ma HL, Liu CL. Bilateral stress fractures of the ulna in a young adolescent. J Pediatr Orthop Part B. 2012; https://doi.org/10.1097/BPB.0b013e328354db2f.
66. Steunebrink M, De Winter D, Tol JL. Bilateral stress fracture of the ulna in an adult weightlifter: a case report. Acta Orthop Belg. 2008;

Stress Fractures in Sport: Wrist

22

Joseph Shung and William Geissler

22.1 Introduction

Wrist and hand injuries constitute 3–9% of all injuries sustained in sport participation. Fractures of the wrist were once thought to be insignificant injuries with minimal morbidity [1]. However, clinical research has shown that delayed treatment of carpal fractures can irreversibly alter wrist biomechanics and adversely affect athletic performance. Carpal stress fractures in particular are often misdiagnosed for overuse injuries due to the lack of a traumatic event. Prompt recognition and appropriate treatment of carpal stress fractures are critical to minimize time away from sport and to avoid the complications of fracture nonunion.

When discussing stress fractures, it is important to differentiate between fatigue stress fractures and insufficiency stress fractures. Fatigue stress fractures are caused by increased force on biomechanically normal bone while insufficiency fractures are the result of normal load applied to abnormally weak bone. Among athletes, fatigue fractures occur far more frequently than insufficiency fractures. However in female athletes with low body mass and a history of stress fractures, the clinician should maintain a high index of suspicion for female athletic triad and osteoporosis. Fatigue fractures occur when applied stress approaches the upper limit of the elastic deformity range on the stress-strain curve. Although the stress level remains well below the magnitude required for catastrophic failure, the area of bone most vulnerable to stress sustains microscopic fractures. Normally, microfractures are repaired in a precisely balanced equilibrium between osteoblasts and osteoclasts. Bone healing, however, lags behind bone reabsorption by a period of several weeks [2]. If excessive stress is applied repetitively without providing sufficient time for bone healing, the microfractures persist and begin to coalesce. Elevated osteoclast activity also increases bone porosity which further weakens the bone [2]. If this cycle is not interrupted, a lucent fracture line develops and propagates through the entire cortex.

Several mechanisms are thought to play a role in the development of upper extremity stress fractures. Upper extremity weight bearing, seen in gymnastics and platform diving, increases the risk of upper extremity stress fractures especially distal to the elbow [3]. Muscle hypertrophy from intense training can outpace the rate of bone development, leading to stress fractures at the point of muscle insertion. Muscle fatigue has also been shown to be major factor in the development of stress fractures. Muscle contractions help shield the bone from stress by countering external forces. When muscles become fatigued, bones and ligaments are exposed to significantly greater stress which increases the risk of fracture development [4, 5].

Factors that contribute to fatigue fracture formation can be divided into two broad categories—extrinsic and intrinsic factors. Extrinsic factors include the nature of the sport, equipment, the field surface, and the training regimen. Intrinsic factors are related to the athletes themselves. Gender, age, ethnicity, fitness level, and anatomic proportions all contribute to a particular athlete's risk of developing fatigue fractures. Clinicians must also not overlook signs and symptoms of female athletic triad which can expose the athlete to significantly higher risk of insufficiency stress fractures [6, 7].

Overall, approximately 90% of athletic fatigue fractures occur in the lower extremities [8]. Anderson et al. reviewed the most common upper extremity fatigue fractures and noted that, with the exception of the scaphoid, stress fractures of carpal bones are exceedingly rare [4]. Sinha et al. surveyed approximated 50 physicians and trainers to estimate the prevalence of upper extremity stress fractures. The athletes were broadly classified by predominant upper extremity motion into weight lifters (power lifters, American football), upper extremity weight-bearers (gymnasts, divers, cheerleaders), throwers (pitchers, javelin throwers, soccer goalkeepers), and swingers (golf, tennis). Although distal

J. Shung (✉) · W. Geissler
Department of Orthopedic Surgery, University of Mississippi Medical Center, Jackson, MS, USA

G. A. J. Robertson, N. Maffulli (eds.), *Fractures in Sport*, https://doi.org/10.1007/978-3-030-72036-0_22

radius physeal stress injuries were excluded in the study, stress fractures involving the wrist represented less than 16% of the 44 stress fractures reported and consisted exclusively of fractures involving the scaphoid. They concluded that upper extremity stress fractures followed certain patterns corresponding to the predominant upper extremity motions utilized in each sport [3].

22.2 Imaging

Plain radiographs are known to be a poor screening tool for diagnosing stress fractures. Radiographs have a sensitivity of about 15% for detecting fractures at the time of presentation and only 50% of stress fractures can be seen on plain radiographs over time [9, 10]. The earliest radiographic sign is a subtle intracortical lucency or "grey cortex" that represents early bone reabsorption. The fracture becomes more apparent as periosteal and endosteal bone formation develops around the site of injury. Late findings of complete intracortical fractures or displaced fractures are often visible on plain radiographs.

CT scans have poor sensitivity for detecting stress fractures during the early stages of injury. However, the freedom to reformat orthogonal images along the fracture line make CT scan invaluable for mapping fracture morphology and monitoring fracture healing [11].

MRI scans are highly sensitive (100%) and specific (85%) for detecting early stress fractures and have the added advantage of providing a comprehensive assessment of the surrounding soft tissue structures [7]. Early signs consist of bone marrow edema and periosteal fluid accumulation, best seen on T2 fat saturation and STIR sequences. Fractures lines appear hypointense on MRI and are best seen on T1 and T2 sequences [7]. All MRI findings, however, should be correlated to the athlete's clinical presentation since asymptomatic areas of bone marrow edema can be indistinguishable from stress reaction [12].

Arendt et al., attempted to classify stress fractures using differences in signal intensity across various MRI sequences. She classified grade 0 as normal MRI and radiographic findings. Grade 1 was defined as increased signal intensity on STIR sequences only. Grade 2 involved increased signal intensity on both STIR and T2 sequences. Grade 3 involved increased signal intensity on STIR, T2, and T1 sequences, as well as early evidence of periosteal reactions. Finally, grade 4 was defined as clear cortical fracture lines visible on radiographic imaging [13]. From her clinical experience, she noted that Grade 1 and 2 injuries had more predictable and rapid recoveries compared to higher grade lesions. She labeled lower grade injuries "stress phenomenon" and permitted athletes with lower grade injuries to return to play more aggressively, using pain or discomfort as a central guide to modifying activity [14, 15]. Higher grade injuries, on the other hand, required prolonged restriction from play until radiographs revealed osseous healing. In contrast to lower extremity stress fractures, upper extremity stress injuries do not prevent the athlete from participating in most aerobic exercises. However, weightbearing and forceful use of the upper extremity should be limited to activities that do not cause abnormal discomfort.

While increased MRI signal intensity combined with clinical tenderness strongly suggests stress reaction, the clinician must as least consider infection and malignancy in the differential diagnosis. Infections often cause bone marrow edema that can closely resemble stress reaction. Osseous malignancies, especially bone marrow malignancies including lymphoma, leukemia, and multiple myeloma; exhibit bone hemorrhage and edema which can also mimic osseous injury. Bone bruising is another condition that can be mistaken for stress injury. Bone bruises are usually associated with direct trauma and located close to the articular surface [16]. Bone bruising on MRI demonstrates evidence of bone marrow hemorrhage and edema without involvement of the cortex, but signal changes can persist for up to 6 months [17].

Prior to the wide-spread use of MRI, bone scan was the primary imaging modality for detecting stress fractures. The advantage of radionuclide imaging is the ability to screen the entire body for increased osteoblastic activity. However, higher radiation exposure, longer image acquisition time, and lack of image resolution make bone scan inferior to MRI for diagnosing stress fractures in the majority of patients.

22.3 Scaphoid

Scaphoid fractures constitute 60–70% of all carpal injuries. A large percentage of the scaphoid surface is covered by articular cartilage with the exception of the dorsal ridge where it receives its major blood supply. The vessels perfuse the scaphoid in a retrograde manner and any interruption of the blood supply places the proximal pole at increased risk for avascular necrosis. Acute fractures of the scaphoid are usually caused by falling onto an outstretched hand with the wrist dorsiflexed greater than 90° [1]. Similarly, stress fractures of the scaphoid have been attributed to repetitive, forceful dorsiflexion of the wrist [18]. Dorsiflexion of the wrist shifts load transmission to the scaphoid facet of the radius and tightens the volar radiocarpal ligaments, causing the scaphoid to slide volarly within the facet [19]. The proximal pole of the scaphoid remains securely anchored to the volar radiocarpal ligaments, leaving the scaphoid waist exposed to the bending moments exerted across the wrist [20]. Forces that are insufficient to cause acute fracture in normal bone but are applied repeatedly, can lead to stress fractures across the scaphoid waist over time [21]. All cases of scaphoid stress fractures reported in the literature to date have occurred at the scaphoid waist [18, 20, 22–34]. Repetitive motion not only generates a cyclical loading pattern on the scaphoid, it also leads to muscle fatigue. High level athletes, in particular, have a tendency to push themselves beyond the limits of muscular endurance. Without the dynamic support of the surrounding musculature, the scaphoid is exposed to increased loading forces that accelerate the progression towards fracture [35, 36].

22.3.1 Epidemiology

Stress fractures of the scaphoid are the most commonly reported carpal stress fracture and have been observed across numerous athletic disciplines including shot put, gymnastics, tennis, badminton, platform diving, cricket, and soccer (goalkeeper) [18, 20, 22–34]. Certain movements, such as the high backhand volley in tennis, require forceful dorsiflexion of the wrist and places particular strain across the scaphoid [22, 37]. Platform divers exert incredible amounts of force across their wrists as they spring off the platform from a hyperextended, handstand position. The impact of the hyperextended wrist against the water upon entry places further stress across the scaphoid [31]. Gymnasts in particular are prone to wrist injuries, and 80–90% of those injuries can be attributed to overuse rather than acute accidents [38]. Skeletally immature athletes are particularly vulnerable to stress fractures of the scaphoid. Of the fractures reported in the literature, 19 of 22 occurred in high level athletes between the ages of 13 and 19 years old [18, 20, 22–34]. Youth athletes are starting to compete at earlier ages and at higher levels and than ever before [18, 39, 40]. Unfortunately, the immature skeleton is mechanically weak around the physes and the under-developed musculature is often inadequate to protect against stress injury [21].

22.3.2 Classification

Stress fractures of the scaphoid are uncommon injuries and no classification system pertaining specifically to scaphoid stress fractures has been developed. However, they share certain radiographic similarities to scaphoid nonunions. Geissler and Slade classified scaphoid nonunions into six classes [41]. Class one is defined as scaphoid fractures with a 4–12 week delay in presentation for treatment. Class two is defined as fibrous union with no cystic or sclerotic changes at the fracture margins. Class three is defined as minimal sclerosis and less than 1 mm of bone reabsorption at the nonunion interface. Class four is defined as cystic formation and sclerosis with less than 5 mm of bone resorption at the nonunion interface and no visible deformity of the fracture on the lateral radiograph. Class five is defined as over 5 mm of bone resorption at the nonunion interface with deformity and/or pseudoarthrosis of the fracture site. Class six is defined as radiocarpal or midcarpal arthritis secondary to scaphoid nonunion advance collapse. Scaphoid stress fractures may be diagnosed at any stage of nonunion progression. However, scaphoid stress fractures may have greater healing potential and appear to be more amenable to treatment with immobilisation than true scaphoid nonunions [26–32].

22.3.3 Diagnosis (History/Physical Exam/ Radiological Investigations)

The clinical presentation of scaphoid stress fractures is subtle and easily mistaken for other common pathologies. The clinical history resembles that of most overuse injuries with activity-related wrist pain and the absence of traumatic injury. The athlete may recall persistent, mild symptoms that started several months ago and have gradually progressed. A history of prolonged, repetitive wrist activity, perhaps from extended practice sessions or sequential competitive events, should alert the practitioner to the possibility of a stress fracture [22]. Unlike acute scaphoid fractures, the clinical presentation of scaphoid stress fractures can closely mimic tendonitis [30]. Physical exam may reveal tenderness to palpation over the snuff box associated with mild swelling. Watson's test may be positive in the affected wrist [30, 34]. Tenderness at the limits of wrist dorsiflexion and decreased dorsiflexion arc of motion compared to the contralateral side are also suggestive of scaphoid pathology [22]. Multiple case reports noted tenderness with Finkelstein's maneuver, and some athletes underwent prolonged treatment for de Quervain's tenosynovitis prior to being diagnosed with a scaphoid stress fracture [18, 26]. Symptoms can progress to the point where training becomes impossible, placing the athlete's career in jeopardy [31].

To add to the complexity, initial radiographs are often negative, and delayed diagnosis for up to 2 years have been reported [18]. Occasionally, delayed radiographs may reveal a nondisplaced fracture or subtle increase in bone density at the waist of the scaphoid [18, 22] (Fig. 22.1). Cases have been reported where routine evaluation of the contralateral wrist for pre-operative planning revealed asymptomatic stress fracture of the contralateral scaphoid. Bilateral cases may be seen more commonly in sports that stress both wrists equally, such as gymnastics, platform diving, and goal keeping [18, 30, 31, 34]. CT scans often reveal sclerosis and cystic changes at the fracture site suggesting a chronic process consistent with stress fracture [22]. MRI scan of the wrist demonstrates edema surrounding the fracture site, with low signal intensity on T1 images and iso-intensity to high intensity on T2 images (Fig. 22.2).

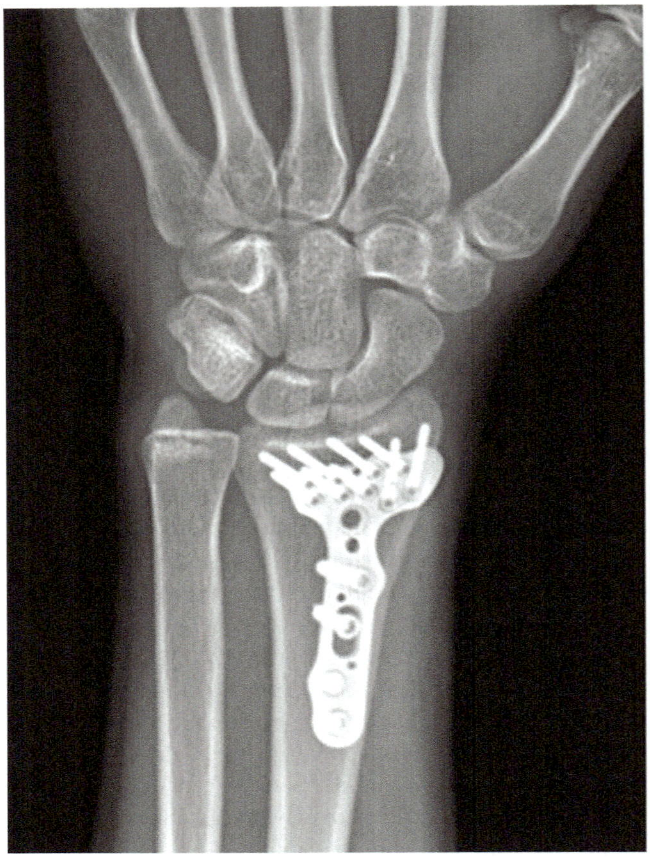

Fig. 22.1 PA radiograph of a 21 year old college second baseman who presented with activity-related wrist pain following a hyperextension injury to his wrist. He is approximately 2 years out from previous open reduction internal fixation of a distal radius fracture

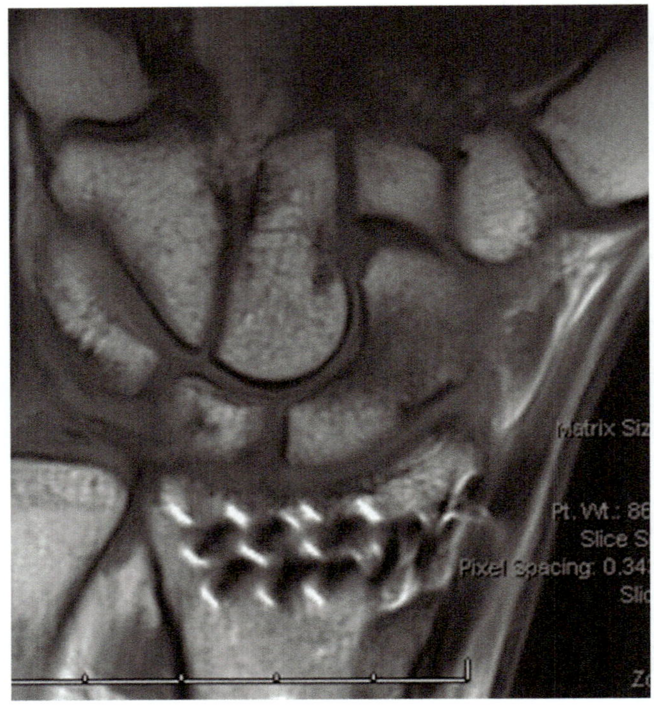

Fig. 22.2 MRI evaluation to the wrist shows increased signal at the waist of the scaphoid consistent with a stress fracture. The patient was acutely symptomatic and desired to return to play as soon as possible. Conservative versus operative management was discussed, and the decision was made to proceed with operative management, with the goal of early return to athletic competition

22.3.4 Treatment

A discussion should be had with the patient concerning the options of conservative versus surgical management. Cast immobilisation, though effective, is not benign and can lead to muscle atrophy and joint stiffness. An athlete may potentially lose their position or scholarship if the injury occurred mid-season. Athletes under stringent time constraints may benefit from early surgical management and accelerated rehabilitation. Fractures with sclerotic and cystic changes suggesting chronic nonunion may also be more effectively managed with internal fixation [31]. Surgical management allows the athlete to avoid joint stiffness, muscle atrophy, and osteopenia from prolonged immobilisation. Studies have also shown that internal fixation of scaphoid fractures shortens the time to osseous union [42, 43]. Of the 22 scaphoid stress fractures reported in the literature, nine were treated successfully with headless compression screws, inserted through percutaneous dorsal and open volar approaches [26–32]. Iliac crest bone graft was also added on occasion to enhance bone healing potential [30, 31].

The author's preferred technique for scaphoid fixation is to use wrist arthroscopy to allow for direct visualization of the fracture site, assess for any concomitant intraarticular pathology, and minimize morbidity. The hand is suspended in a traction tower (Acumed, Hillsboro, Oregon) with the wrist at 30° of flexion. The forearm support bar, which usually braces against the volar aspect of the forearm, is repositioned along the dorsal aspect of the forearm to facilitate fluoroscopic imaging later in the procedure (Fig. 22.3). The standard 3–4 and 6R portals are established and an arthroscopic survey is performed to identify any concomitant radiocarpal joint pathology. The scope is then inserted into the 6R portal and a 14 G needle is inserted into the 3–4 portal to established the guidewire starting point on the proximal pole of the scaphoid (Fig. 22.4). The ideal starting point is located at the junction of the scapholunate interosseous ligament with the proximal pole of the scaphoid along its middle third. The proximal pole of the scaphoid is impaled with the needle and the traction tower is flexed forward at its base to allow for fluoroscopic assessment of the start point location (Figs. 22.5 and 22.6). Keeping the 14 G needle firmly in place, a 0.045-in. guide wire is inserted through the needle and aimed towards the volar base of the first metacarpal. Fluoroscopic imaging should be used to monitor guide wire insertion and verify the

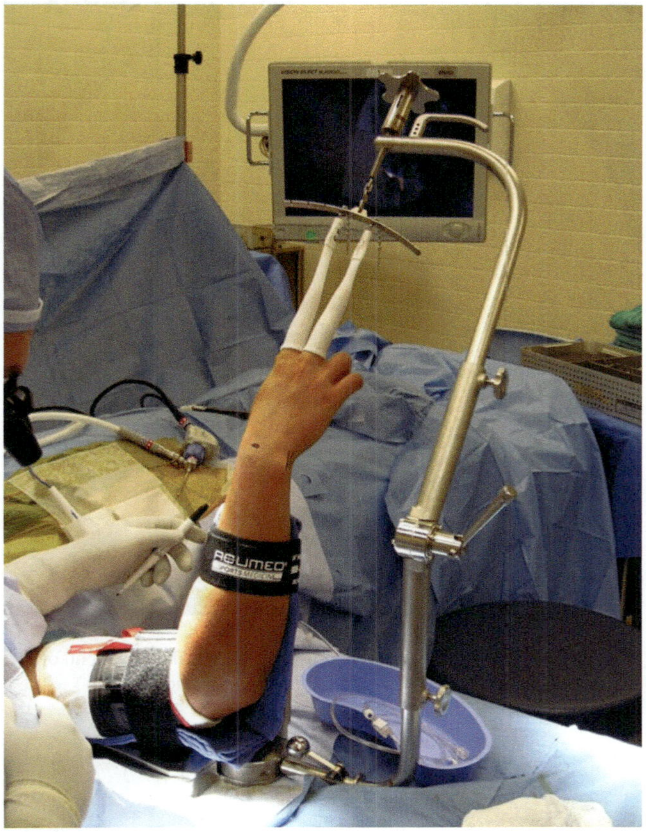

Fig. 22.3 The patient underwent arthroscopic fixation to his scaphoid fracture. The wrist was suspended with 10 pounds of traction in the Acumed traction tower (Hillsboro, Oregon). This tower is designed to accommodate fluoroscopy, in order to obtain an anatomic reduction to the scaphoid fracture with minimal surgical dissection

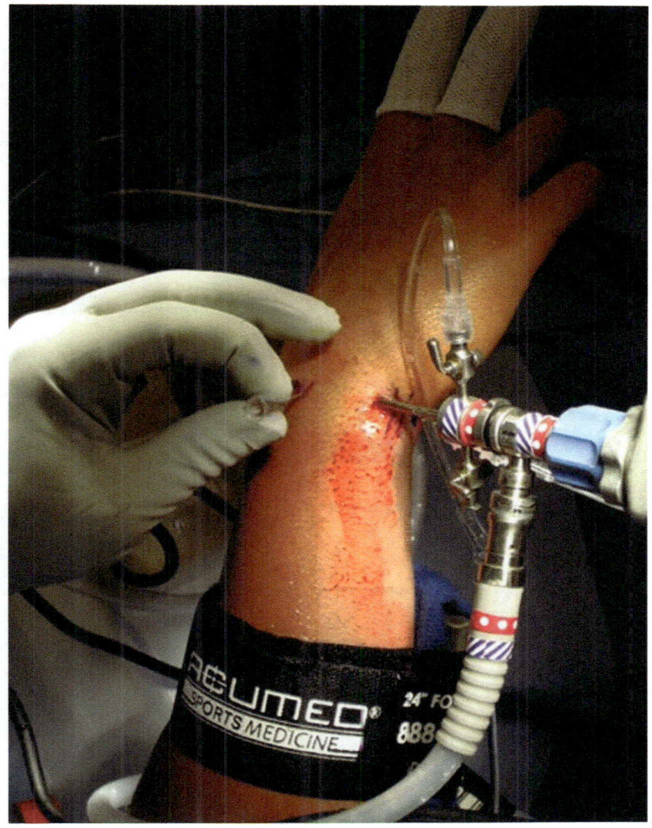

Fig. 22.4 With the arthroscope in the 6R portal, a 14 G needle is brought into the 3/4 portal, and the junction of the scapholunate interosseous ligament is palpated to the proximal pole of the scaphoid

final guidewire position. For nondisplaced fractures, the guidewire should be measured prior to penetration of the volar cortex to obtain the most accurate measurement possible. The measured length should be reduced by 4 mm to ensure that the screw is completely buried within the articular surfaces. It is important to advance the guidewire out the volar aspect of the wrist before reaming, for easy access to the guidewire in case it bends or breaks during reaming or screw insertion (Fig. 22.7). The scaphoid is then reamed under fluoroscopic control to minimize bending of the guidewire. The appropriately-sized screw is then inserted in an antegrade manner. The screw position and fracture reduction are checked under fluoroscopy (Fig. 22.8). Following screw insertion, it is important to place the arthroscope back into the radiocarpal space to ensure that the headless screw is fully inserted into the scaphoid (Fig. 22.9). The primary advantages of the arthroscopic assisted percutaneous technique include direct visualization of the reduction, precise placement of the starting point, assessment of additional intra-articular pathology, and avoiding wrist hyperflexion which can further displace the fracture [41].

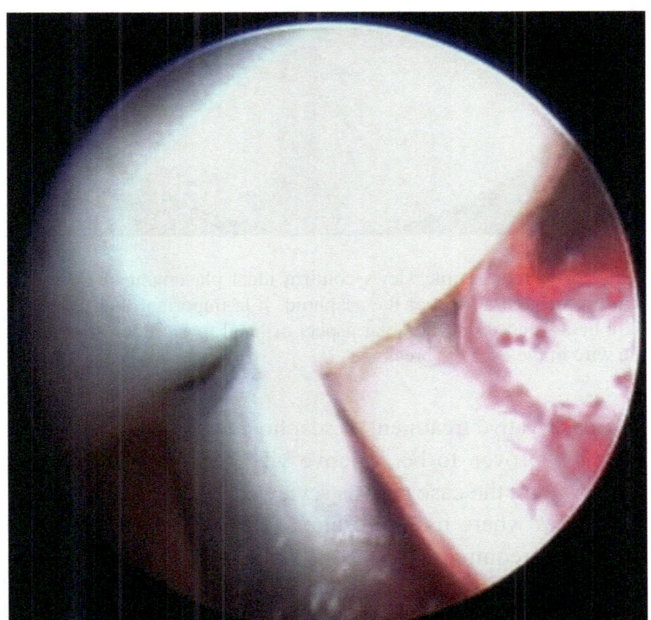

Fig. 22.5 Arthroscopic view with the arthroscope in the 6R portal as the 14 G needle is impacted into the proximal pole of the scaphoid just radial to junction of the interosseous ligament

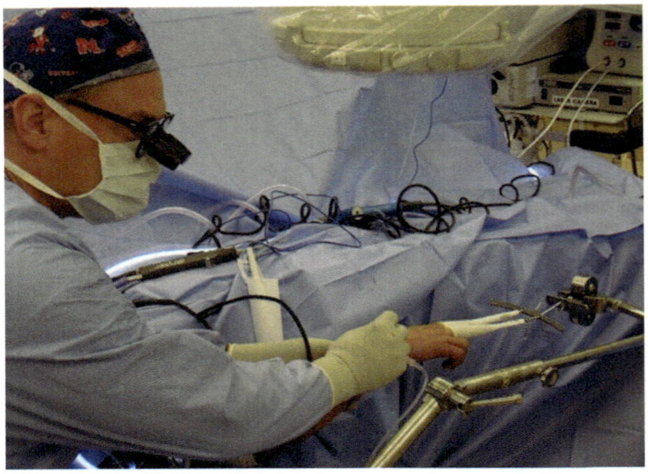

Fig. 22.6 The tower is flexed forward to confirm the ideal starting point under fluoroscopy

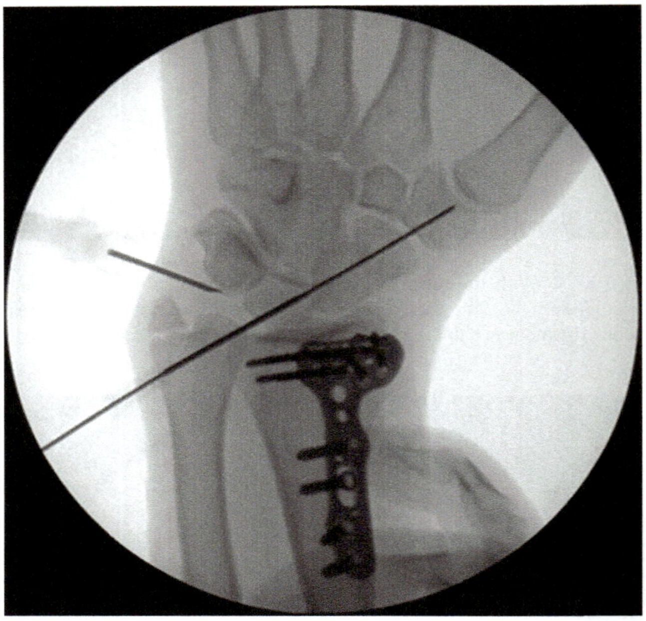

Fig. 22.7 Fluoroscopic views confirm ideal placement of the guide wire to the central axis of the scaphoid. It is important that the guide wire be advanced out the volar aspect of hand to facilitate removal of the wire in the event of breakage

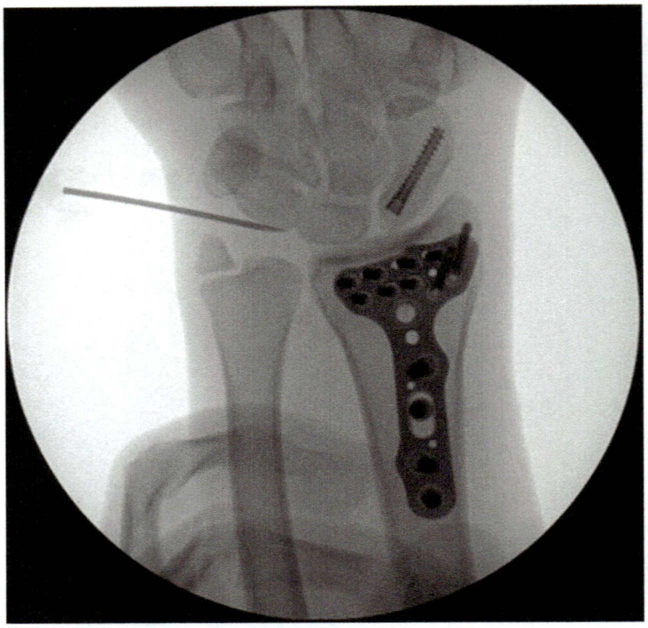

Fig. 22.8 Fluoroscopic view confirming an ideal placement of the screw across the stress fracture in the postero-anterior view

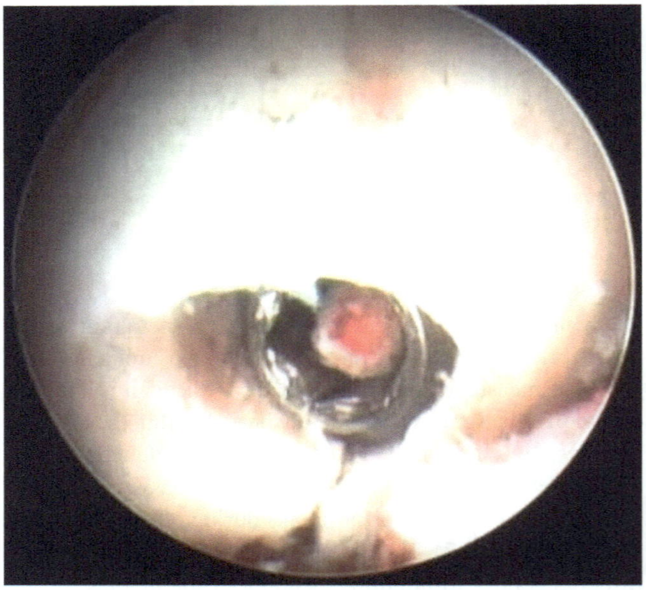

Fig. 22.9 Arthroscopic view confirming that the headless screw has been inserted deep to the articular surface of the scaphoid. Fluoroscopic evaluation is not a reliable method of confirming sufficient screw insertion. One does not want to leave the screw prominent as it could potentially damage the articular cartilage of the scaphoid facet of the distal radius

Conservative treatment of scaphoid stress fractures, however, has proven to be effective when applied consistently [22]. Among the case reports reviewed, there were only two incidences where immobilisation failed to achieve osseous union and required surgical intervention [28, 32]. Multiple treatment protocols have been described to successfully treat scaphoid stress fractures. Matskin et al. preferred a long arm thumb spica cast for 8 weeks, followed by a short arm splint for 4 weeks. His patient returned to gymnastic in 6 months and had full wrist range of motion without pain at 1 year [20]. Kohyama et al. started with 4 weeks immobilisation in a thumb spica short arm cast followed by 8 weeks of bracing. The athlete was encouraged to progress to active wrist range of motion exercises while in the brace. Gradual return to tennis practice was initiated at 3 months once fracture union was confirmed on CT scan [22]. Kohring et al. reported the case of an incomplete scaphoid stress fracture in a shot-putter, which was treated with a removable thumb spica brace for 6 weeks. During her treatment, she was restricted from shot-putting and weight training but allowed to continue discus throwing, which did not cause her pain. The athlete was released to full sport participation at 6 weeks and reported full wrist function without pain at 3 years [33]. In contrast, Yamagiwa et al. reported a similar case of a nondisplaced scaphoid stress fracture in a gymnast, which was treated with 2 months of immobilisation in a removal wrist brace. The athlete's symptoms persisted and radiographs revealed fracture displacement which warranted surgical fixation [28]. When treating scaphoid stress fractures conservatively, it is advisable that the athlete refrain from all activities that generate wrist pain and that the fracture is carefully monitored with serial radiographs to detect late fracture displacement.

22.3.5 Complications

As mentioned previously, cast immobilisation can lead to muscle atrophy and joint stiffness. If the injury occurred mid-season, prolonged restriction from training can lead to loss of position or scholarship. Athletes under stringent time constraints may benefit from early surgical management and accelerated rehabilitation. No complications have been reported following surgical fixation of scaphoid stress fractures. However, the spectrum of possible complications is likely identical to those seen following surgical fixation of acute scaphoid fractures, as discussed in the relevant chapter.

22.3.6 Rehabilitation

The protocol for rehabilitation following treatment of scaphoid stress fractures is identical to what would be used for rehabilitation of acute scaphoid fractures.

22.3.7 Preventative Measures

Stress fractures of the scaphoid are difficult to prevent, especially in high-level athletes. Individualized training and gradual progression of training volume may help prevent over stressing of the osseous structures. The key to preventing a protracted and difficult recovery is early detection of injury and immediate cessation of activity. Open communication between the coaching staff and the physician is critical to curb the cycle of injury as soon as possible. Athletes and trainers should be educated on the sentinel symptoms and on the importance of strict compliance with treatment protocols.

22.4 Lunate

22.4.1 Epidemiology

The lunate is a well-protected carpal bone cradled tightly between the lunate facet of the radius and the head of the capitate. Stress fractures of the lunate in athletes are seen almost exclusively among tennis players. Overuse is the most common cause of wrist injury especially among elite players [44].

22.4.2 Classification

To the authors' knowledge, no classification system has been proposed for stress fractures of the lunate.

22.4.3 Diagnosis (History/Physical Exam/ Radiological Investigations)

Maquirrian and Ghisi reported the largest series of lunate stress fractures consisting of five cases over a period of 2 years [45]. The players presented with dorsal wrist pain that worsened with activity and improved with rest. No history of trauma could be identified, but the players reported severe discomfort with hyperextension of the wrist during weight training and when performing a forehand stroke. Physical exam revealed symmetric active wrist range of motion and symmetric grip strength. However, passive hyperextension of the wrist and direct palpation over the lunate with the wrist in flexion generated exquisite tenderness. Less than half the patients also reported minor ulnar-sided wrist pain. Plain radiographs demonstrated no abnormality, but MRI revealed bone marrow edema on all sequences, localized to the distal facet of the lunate. Gadolinium enhanced studies revealed increased uptake in the lunate which helped differentiate the injury from avascular necrosis. After 6 weeks of semi-rigid wrist immobilisation, the players were gradually reconditioned and allowed to return to practice by 8 weeks. Complete resolution of all symptoms was achieved by 14 weeks. Final follow-up at 6 months confirmed no recurrence of symptoms and no residual wrist stiffness. Control MRI scans documented resolving bone edema at 6 months and resolution of marrow signal at 12 months.

The considerable differential diagnosis of dorsal wrist pain in athletes makes isolating the correct diagnosis quite challenging. Occult dorsal ganglion cysts are the most common cause of dorsal wrist pain, and typically present with point tenderness on palpation of the scapholunate joint [44]. Kienbock's disease, another common cause of dorsal wrist pain, is the most frequent condition associated with abnormal signal intensity in the lunate on MRI scan [46]. Wrist stiffness on physical exam and lack of enhancement with gadolinium imaging can help differentiate between Kienbock's disease and stress fractures of the lunate [45]. Ulnar impingement syndrome and interosseous ganglion cysts are additional pathologies that can present with isolated, signal intensity in the lunate [45]. The pattern of increased signal intensity within the distal aspect of the lunate, however, remains a unique finding highly associated with lunate stress fractures.

22.4.4 Treatment

The treatment protocol described in the series reported by Maquirrian and Ghisi consisted of 6 weeks of semi-rigid wrist immobilisation [45]. The players were then gradually reconditioned and allowed to return to practice by 8 weeks. Complete resolution of all symptoms was achieved by 14 weeks. Final follow-up at 6 months confirmed no recurrence of symptoms and no residual wrist stiffness. Control MRI scans documented resolving bone edema at 6 months and resolution of marrow signal at 12 months [45].

22.4.5 Complications

To the authors' knowledge, no complications from the treatment of lunate stress fractures have been reported in the literature. Recurrence of stress fracture is a potential complication if training resumes without preventative precautions.

22.4.6 Rehabilitation

Once symptoms have completely resolved, training may resume starting with the elements that cause the least discomfort and at significantly reduced volumes of repetition. Training intensity may be gradually increased over a period of several weeks. Weekly re-evaluations should help coaches and physicians determine if rehabilitation is progressing appropriately or if adjustments should be made.

22.4.7 Preventative Measures

Prevention of lunate stress fractures in tennis players requires a thorough review of the training regimen, stroke biomechanics, and predisposing risk factors. Elliot et al. estimated that approximately 20% of the final racquet velocity is contributed by the wrist [47]. The terminal position of the wrist during the forehand stroke is typically hyperextension and ulnar deviation. Not surprisingly, all the players in Maquirrian's series reported referred pain in the wrist when hitting a forehand stroke. Switching from a "Western" style grip to the "Eastern" style has been shown to decrease elbow flexion, forearm supination, wrist extension, and ulnar deviation, while minimizing the load exerted across the wrist joint [48]. In addition, ensuring proper grip mechanics during weight training can also help minimize injury from improper technique.

22.5 Triquetrum

22.5.1 Epidemiology

The triquetrum is the second most commonly fractured carpal bone, accounting for 3–4% of all carpal bone injuries [49, 50]. Among athletes, isolated triquetrum injuries are primarily caused by avulsion of the dorsal ligaments off the triquetrum, and impingement of the triquetrum on the ulnar styloid [1]. To the authors' knowledge, a stress fracture of the triquetrum has been reported only once in the literature.

22.5.2 Classification

To the authors' knowledge, no classification system has been proposed for stress fractures of the triquetrum.

22.5.3 Diagnosis (History/Physical Exam/Radiological Investigations)

Lohman et al. reported on a single case of triquetral stress reaction in a 17 year old break dancer [51]. Break dancing, while not a conventional sport, requires the performers to support their entire body weight on their wrists while performing complex acrobatic maneuvers. Injuries to the upper extremities are common and range from humeral shaft fractures to thumb ulnar collateral ligament avulsions [52, 53]. The patient in the case initially presented with right wrist pain of several months duration. He reported no history of injury and did not participate in any sport besides break dancing. Physical exam revealed non-specific diffuse hand tenderness with no evidence of tendonitis or wrist instability. X-ray of the wrist revealed no osseous abnormality, but focal edema within the triquetrum was identified on MRI, best seen on the T2 fat saturation coronal images. No other areas of tendonitis, ligament injury, or carpal edema were visualized on the scan.

22.5.4 Treatment

The break dancer in Lohman's case report was treated with complete rest from all break dancing activities. The patient's symptoms resolved completely within a few months [51].

22.5.5 Complications

Recurrence of stress fracture is a potential complication if activity is resumed too early with excessive intensity. In Lohman's case, the patient resumed break dancing as soon as he was symptom free and experienced immediate recurrence of right wrist pain. Follow-up MRI of the right wrist, performed 6 months after the initial scan, reveal recurrence of edema within the triquetrum, as well as additional signs of edema within the lunate and capitate bones [51].

22.5.6 Rehabilitation

Once symptoms have completely resolved, training may resume starting with the elements that cause the least discomfort and at significantly reduced volumes of repetition. Training intensity may be gradually increased over a period of several weeks. Weekly re-evaluations should help coaches and physicians determine if rehabilitation is progressing appropriately or if adjustments should be made.

22.5.7 Preventative Measures

Stress fractures of the triquetrum are difficult to prevent, especially in high-level athletes. Individualized training and gradual progression of training volume may help prevent over stressing of the osseous structures. The key to preventing a protracted and difficult recovery is early detection of injury and immediate cessation of activity. Open communication between the coaching staff and the physician is critical to curb the cycle of injury as soon as possible. Athletes and trainers should be educated on the sentinel symptoms and on the importance of strict compliance with treatment protocols.

22.6 Hook of the Hamate

The hook of the hamate protrudes from the base of the hamate body to form the hypothenar eminence. Structures that attach to the hook of the hamate include the flexor digiti minimi, opponens digiti minimi, pisohamate ligament, and the ulnar aspect of the transverse carpal ligament. The strategic location of the hook also allows it to serve as a pulley for the fourth and fifth finger flexor profundus tendons, and excision of the hook is associated with loss of up to 15% of finger flexion strength [54].

22.6.1 Epidemiology

Hamate fractures account for 2–4% of all carpal bone fractures [1]. Traumatic hook of the hamate injuries are usually seen in racquet sports, where direct compression of the handle against the hypothenar eminence results in acute fracture [1]. Stress fractures of the hook of the hamate can be caused by the repetitive impact of a racquet handle against the hook of the hamate [55]. However, the vast majority of hook of the hamate stress fractures involve sports that require intense gripping. Climbing athletes support the entire weight of their body on the arms, hands, and fingertips. The tension generated by the flexor tendons of the small and ring finger pressing against the radial aspect of the hook of the hamate, can lead to stress fracture over time [54, 56]. Ulnar deviation of the wrist further exacerbates the stress placed across the hook of the hamate, as demonstrated in the side under-cling grip used by climbers [56]. As a result, an increasing number of elite climbers with ulnar wrist pain have been diagnosed with stress fractures of the hook of the hamate [57]. Underwater rugby and polo players must also grip intensely with the outstretched arm for prolonged periods of time. In order to place spin on the ball as it is thrown, water polo players employ techniques to snap the ball from the wrist with maximal force. As the wrist is brought into extreme ulnar deviation prior to ball release, the tightly tensioned flexor tendons exert pressure on the hook of the hamate in the same manner seen in climbers Prolonged gripping of the ball with the outstretched hand can also exert significant strain through the hook of the hamate, by the direct pull of the hypothenar muscles [58, 59].

22.6.2 Classification

Hamate fractures can be primarily divided into fractures of the hook (Milch Type 1) and fractures of the hamate body (Milch Type 2). Fractures of the hook of the hamate can be further subdivided into fractures involving avulsion of the tip (Type 1), fractures through the middle (Type 2), and fractures at the base of the hook (Type 3) [60].

22.6.3 Diagnosis (History/Physical Exam/ Radiological Investigations)

Symptomatic athletes typically present with mild ulnar sided wrist pain at rest, and significant exacerbation of pain with certain gripping techniques. Typically, the symptoms have persisted for several months but without a history of direct trauma. Work-up by other trainers and clinicians often reveal no specific injury or diagnosis. Physical exam reveals loss of grip strength compared to the contralateral side, which is associated with hypothenar wrist pain. Tenderness around the pisiform may also be present which may mimic the symptoms of pisohamate arthritis. Injections into the hypothenar region may alleviate symptoms, but weakness and pain with motion often persist [61]. It is important when examining the patient to test excursion of the flexor tendons to ensure that they are not entrapped within the fracture site. Wright et al. described a pathognomic exam maneuver for hook of the hamate fractures which involved flexing the ulnar digits against resistance with the wrist in flexion and ulnar deviation, resulting in pain localized to the hypothenar eminence. Absence of pain when the maneuver is repeated with the wrist in extension and radial deviation helps to confirm the diagnosis [62]. Other potential causes of ulnar wrist pain in climbers should also be considered and investigated. Bouldering athletes, in particular, are at risk of direct impact fractures to the carpal bones since they are vulnerable to frequent falls [57]. Older climbers may be at risk for degenerative arthritis and cyst formation within the carpal bones [63, 64].

A history of chronic ulnar sided wrist pain with normal radiographic findings warrants evaluation by MRI or CT to evaluate for subtle osseous injury. MRI of the affected wrist may reveal bone edema and inflammation of the surrounding tissues. On occasion, MRI may demonstrate an isolated fluid collection at the insertional of the flexor retinaculum which may indicate a “ligamentopathy” rather than fracture [57]. Overuse bone marrow edema in the hands of climbers has also been described, and must be carefully differentiated from stress fracture by clinical exam [63]. The osseous structure can be further evaluated with high density CT to delineate subtle fracture lines [61]. Positioning the hands in a “praying position” allows for efficient comparison between the two wrists, and has a reported accuracy of 97.2% for diagnosing fractures of the hamate [65].

22.6.4 Treatment

Conservative management of hook of the hamate stress fractures consist of cast immobilisation for 6 weeks. This is followed by gradual return to training and climbing activities. Athletes with persistent pain following 6–8 weeks of immobilisation should be offered surgical intervention [57]. While some authors have recommended open reduction and internal fixation, the prognosis is guarded owing to the small size of the fragments and limited blood supply [66, 67]. Most studies have shown no functional deficit following excision, with earlier return to athletic activities [68, 69]. Excision of the hamate hook is performed through a volar approach by releasing Guyon’s canal. Careful dissection and retraction of the ulnar nerve is necessary, since the motor branch is in direct contact with the base of the hamate and can be easily injured. The base of the hamate is quite deep and the dissection can be tedious. The fractured edges are smoothed off and the periosteum closed to prevent irritation to the ulnar nerve. Inspection of the small and ring finger flexor tendons should be performed intraoperatively to assess for partial rupture. Athletes should be withheld from play for 4 weeks, after which they may resume without restriction. Full recovery of grip strength and wrist motion should be expected by 3 months [61].

Lutter et al. published one of the largest retrospective series on hook of the hamate stress fractures in climbers. The ten fracture cases were all Milch type 1, and evenly distributed among the three hook fracture subtypes. Conservative therapy was successful in seven of the ten patients. Bony union after 6 weeks of cast immobilisation was verified by computed tomography. All seven athletes returned to their pre-injury level of activity after an average recovery period of 8.2 weeks. Of the ten fracture cases, three athletes required surgical excision of the hook of the hamate. Two patients demonstrated persistent nonunion after cast immobilisation, and one patient had a concomitant volar ganglion cyst of the annular pulley. The primary advantage of managing hook of the hamate fractures conservatively is that the pulley mechanism for the small and ring finger flexor tendons remains intact. Grip strength is more likely to be preserved by retaining the hook of the hamate in contrast to excision [57]. Nonetheless, many authors advocate excision of the hook of the hamate in the setting of fracture [60, 70]. At final follow-up, all patients resumed their previous level of sport with complete resolution of symptoms.

22.6.5 Complications

To the authors’ knowledge, no long term complications from the treatment of hamate stress fracture have been reported in the literature. In fractures managed with immobilisation, recurrence of stress fracture is a potential complication, if activity resumes without preventative precautions. Potential complications from hook of the hamate excision include damage to the ulnar nerve motor branch and minor loss of grip strength [1, 57].

22.6.6 Rehabilitation

Once symptoms have completely resolved, training may resume starting with the elements that cause the least discomfort and at significantly reduced volumes of repetition.

Training intensity may be gradually increased over a period of several weeks. Weekly re-evaluations should help coaches and physicians determine if rehabilitation is progressing appropriately or if adjustments should be made.

22.6.7 Preventative Measures

Stress fractures of the hook of hamate are difficult to prevent, especially in high-level athletes. Individualized training and gradual progression of training volume may help prevent over stressing of the osseous structures. The key to preventing a protracted and difficult recovery is early detection of injury and immediate cessation of activity. Open communication between the coaching staff and the physician is critical to curb the cycle of injury as soon as possible. Athletes and trainers should be educated on the sentinel symptoms and on the importance of strict compliance with treatment protocols.

22.7 Capitate

22.7.1 Epidemiology

Capitate fractures comprise 1–2% of all carpal fractures and are usually associated with other carpal pathology, especially fractures of the scaphoid. Isolated capitate fractures are rare and account for only 0.3% of carpal injuries [71]. As the most central bone of the wrist, the capitate is shielded from excessive stress by an osseous wall of carpal structures, and stabilized by a network of intracarpal ligaments [72]. When capitate fractures do occur, injuries to adjacent bones and carpal ligaments are highly probable, as seen in perilunate and scaphoid fractures [73]. The capitate serves a central role in the kinematic behavior of the wrist joint. The axes of rotation for flexion-extension, as well as radio-ulnar deviation of the wrist, pass through the head of the capitate [74]. As a result, the capitate is vulnerable to stress fracture from repetitive activity of the wrist [75]. The capitate head is supplied in a retrograde manner by vessels entering the volar and dorsal aspects of the capitate body. In a study by Gelberman, 67% of the capitate heads received blood supply from both the dorsal and volar vessels, while 33% of the capitate heads received blood supply solely from the volar vessels. Avulsion of the vessels during traumatic fracture of the capitate may place the capitate head at risk for avascular necrosis [76]. While traumatic fractures of the capitate are usually associated with high energy mechanisms such as motor vehicle collisions and falls onto an extended wrist, the mechanism of capitate stress fractures is thought to involve repetitive low energy forces over an extended period of time [73]. Athletes that perform repetitive motions of the wrist, such as gymnasts and color guards, are at highest risk for this type of injury.

The vast majority of published reports on capitate stress fractures involve skeletally immature wrists [75]. Decreased cortical thickness, high physical activity, underdeveloped chondro-osseous junctions, and immature muscular development may contribute to the increases susceptibility of the skeletally immature wrist to capitate stress fractures [77]. According to a radiographic review of pediatric carpal stress fractures by Oestreich et al., capitate stress fractures were the most common carpal stress fracture followed by scaphoid and lunate fractures. However, the author noted that the carpal stress fractures documented in his study were often preceded by a period of cast immobilisation for a contiguous long bone fracture. The author concluded that the stress fractures resulted from aggressive overuse of the upper extremity while the carpal bones were still osteopenic from prolonged immobilisation of the injured extremity [75]. Case reports of capitate stress fractures in adults, on the other hand, are extremely rare, with only three cases reported over a 50 year span [78–80].

22.7.2 Classification

To the authors' knowledge, no classification system has been proposed for stress fractures of the capitate.

22.7.3 Diagnosis (History/Physical Exam/Radiological Investigations)

Vizkelety and Wouters described the earliest case involving a dock worker back in 1972 [79]. Allen et al. reported the case of a 42 year old gym teacher who presented with 4 months of bilateral wrist pain and night time paresthesias, as well as stiffness to his left wrist. He was diagnosed clinically with bilateral carpal tunnel syndrome. However, routine X-ray at the time also revealed a well-established capitate fracture nonunion within the distal third of the capitate body. The patient denied any history of injury to the wrist. An MRI was performed which demonstrated no evidence of avascular necrosis to the capitate head. The nonunion was managed with benign neglect and the patient's neuropathic symptoms resolved following bilateral carpal tunnel decompression [80]. Cho et al. reported the case of a 20 year old soldier who served in the honor guard. He reported persistent pain in his right wrist which developed gradually without any history of injury. Since his symptoms had persisted for over 5 months, CT scan of the wrist was performed, which revealed a fracture line through the subchondral bone adjacent to the midcarpal joint. Evaluation by MRI identified depression of the articular surface associated with bone marrow edema and small degenerative osteophytes. The volar capito-hamate ligament also demonstrated increased signal intensity consistent with injury. Wrist arthroscopy was used to visually inspect the articular surface and to debride the surrounding degenerative tissue. The fracture bed was perforated with a small drill bit to stimulate vascular ingrowth and accelerate fracture healing. The patient was able to resume his former activity at 2 months post-operation [78].

Traumatic capitate fractures are typically easy to identify on plain radiographs [81]. However, nondisplaced traumatic fractures and stress fractures of the capitate are often missed on plain X-ray and can go undiagnosed for prolonged periods of time (Figs. 22.10 and 22.11). Complications that can result from delayed treatment of nondisplaced capitate stress fractures include arthritis, nonunion, and avascular necrosis of the capitate head [82]. The risk of developing arthritis from non-displaced fractures of the capitate is unknown. Avascular necrosis from non-displaced capitate fractures has been reported but remains a rarely seen complication. A case of capitate head avascular necrosis in the setting of capitate stress fracture has never been reported.

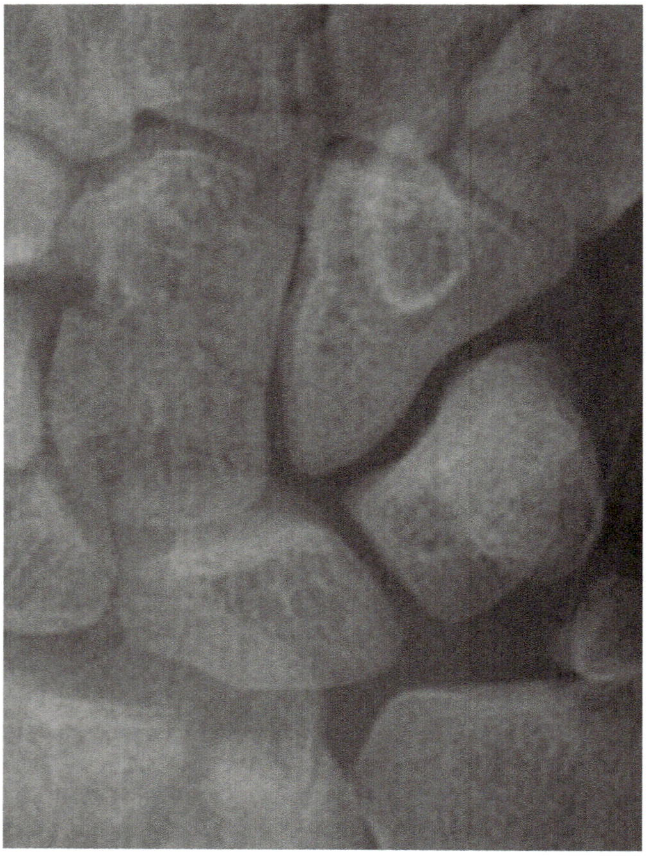

Fig. 22.10 Radiographic view of a subtle non-displaced fracture to the capitate. The patient was a 20 year old football player at a major college, and complained of approximately 2–3 months of dorsal wrist pain. The patient presented for treatment after a hyperextension injury associated with sudden increased pain and swelling to the wrist

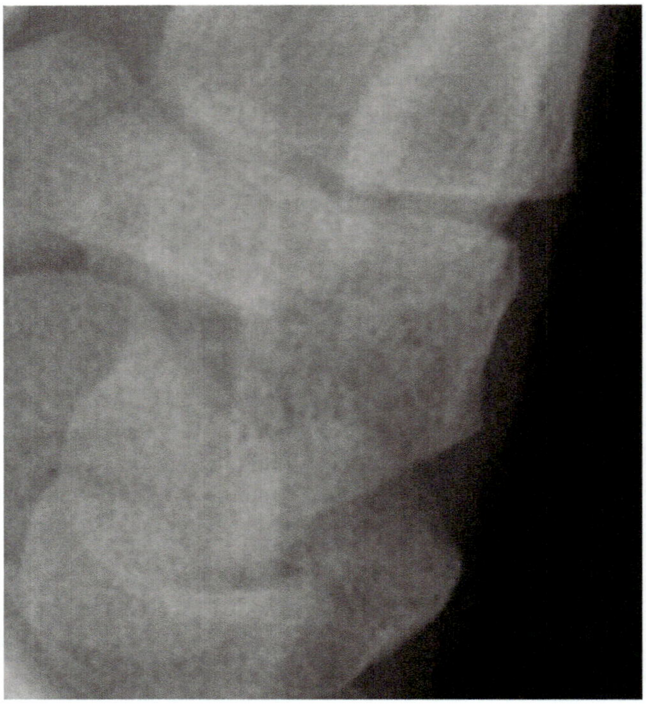

Fig. 22.11 Lateral view of a subtle non-displaced fracture across the waist of the capitate

22.7.4 Treatment

Treatment for nondisplaced capitate fractures usually consists of 6 weeks of immobilisation in a short arm cast which leads to clinical union and resolution of symptoms in most cases [81]. Displaced fractures require anatomic reduction to increase the rate of union and prevent complications. Fixation with compression screws can significantly decrease the athlete's time to return to competition [1] (Fig. 22.12). The incision is made between the third and fourth dorsal compartments in line with the radial border of the long finger. Palmar flexion of the wrist exposes the capitate head for placement of one or two cannulated compression screws, from a proximal to distal orientation [1]. When treating chronic nonunions, it is important to re-establish carpal height, in order to maintain normal carpal kinematics. Corticocancellous interposition bone grafts can be used to restore carpal height and prevent instability [1].

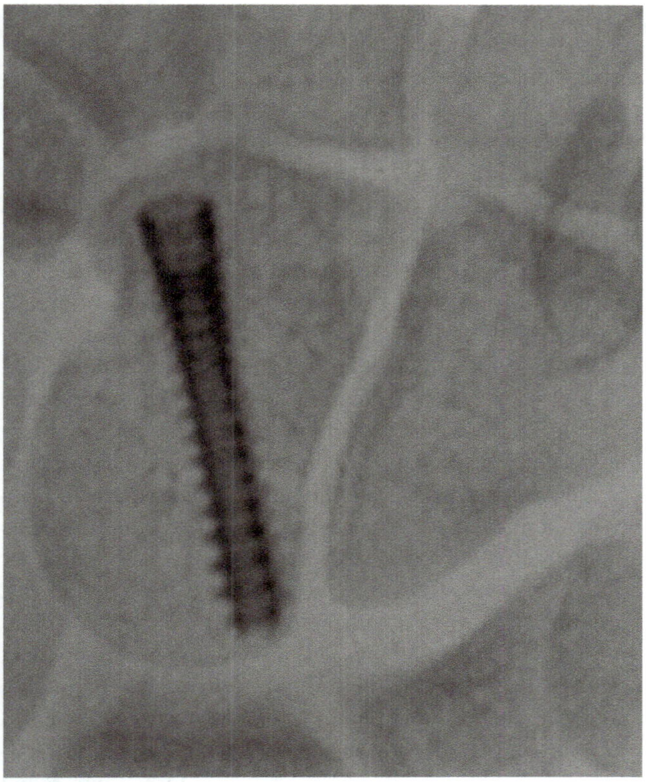

Fig. 22.12 The patient was offered non-operative versus operative management. The patient desired surgical stabilization for early return to sport. Percutaneous guidewire was placed between the webspace of the index and long metacarpals across the capitate, and a headless compression screw was inserted. The patient experienced almost immediate pain relief and returned to athletic competition within 1 week

22.7.5 Complications

To the authors' knowledge, no complications from the treatment of capitate stress fracture have been reported in the literature. Recurrence of stress fracture is a potential complication if training resumes without preventative precautions.

22.7.6 Rehabilitation

Once symptoms have completely resolved, training may resume starting with the elements that cause the least discomfort and at significantly reduced volumes of repetition. Training intensity may be gradually increased over a period of several weeks. Weekly re-evaluations should help coaches and physicians determine if rehabilitation is progressing appropriately or if adjustments should be made.

22.7.7 Preventative Measures

Stress fractures of the capitate are difficult to prevent, especially in high-level athletes. Individualized training and gradual progression of training volume may help prevent over stressing of the osseous structures. The key to preventing a protracted and difficult recovery is early detection of injury and immediate cessation of activity. Open communication between the coaching staff and the physician is critical to curb the cycle of injury as soon as possible. Athletes and trainers should be educated on the sentinel symptoms and on the importance of strict compliance with treatment protocols.

22.8 Distal Radius

22.8.1 Epidemiology

Stress injuries to the distal radius occur most often through the physes of adolescent athletes. Distal radius physeal stress fractures were first described by Read in 1981. He documented wrist pain in three adolescent female gymnasts, who had radiographic findings concerning for stress fracture adjacent to the physes. Achieving proficiency in gymnastics requires countless hours of repetition, often starting at a young age. Studies have shown that gymnasts between the ages of 10 and 14 years old, across both genders, are at higher risk of developing activity-related wrist pain [83]. The most vulnerable period for injury to the physis coincides with the peak of the growth spurt [84]. Biomechanical studies have demonstrated that the growing physis is especially vulnerable to shear stress and exhibits reduced fracture resistance [85]. In contrast, stress fractures of the mature distal radius, to the authors' knowledge, have been reported only a handful times in the literature [86–88].

22.8.2 Classification

To the authors' knowledge, no classification system has been proposed for stress fractures of the distal radius.

22.8.3 Diagnosis (History/Physical Exam/Radiological Investigations)

The clinical presentation begins with mild symptoms after a few hours of exercise which gradually worsens as the training progresses. Ice usually provides relief during the early stages but becomes ineffective over time [89]. Physical exam reveals symptoms with forced dorsiflexion of the wrist and tenderness to palpation over the distal radial epiphysis. Minimal swelling may be observed over the dorsal aspect of the wrist at the level of the physis. Read observed that the rotational torque exerted on the fulcrum wrist during vaulting was the likely mechanism of injury [90]. The sport of gymnastics routinely utilizes the upper extremities to support forces equal to several times the body weight during events such as vaulting, floor exercise, balance beam, and pommel horse [91, 92]. Any activity that requires forced dorsiflexion of the wrist may cause severe exacerbation of symptoms [89].

Athletes with activity related wrist pain should first be evaluated with standard radiographs to look for evidence of physeal stress reaction and to document ulnar variance. The classic radiographic findings of distal radial stress reaction were first described by Roy et al., and include widening of the physis radially and volarly, cystic irregularities of the metaphyseal margin, "beak effect" along the radial aspect of the physis, and haziness within the normally radiolucent area of the physis [89]. The pathophysiology of physeal widening is likely related to disruption of the metaphyseal blood supply adjacent to the physis. Decreased vascular ingrowth delays maturation of the zone of calcification and extends the productive life of the chondrocytes, leading to an increase in total cartilage volume [93]. However, not all cases of distal radial physeal stress reaction present with obvious radiographic findings, and advanced imaging may be necessary to accurately elucidate the diagnosis [89]. MRI scan will reveal increased signal intensity on T2 and STIR sequences localized to the distal radial physis [94].

In his series of 21 cases, Roy et al. observed that positive radiographic changes correlated to a difficult and prolonged recovery [89]. Among the ten cases in his series with radiographic changes, five gymnasts required 6 months to recover while another three athletes took 3 months. Athletes with identical clinical findings but normal wrist radiographs were able to return to gymnastic after 4 weeks of rest and rehabilitation. The cause for delayed healing in distal radius physeal injuries remains unclear. Delayed healing has not been observed in proximal humeral and medial epicondylar physeal injuries despite similar radiographic findings [95, 96].

To the authors' knowledge, stress fractures of the mature distal radius have been reported only a handful times in the literature. Loosli et al. described the earliest case involving a 25 year old female tennis player in 1987. The athlete complained of wrist pain in her dominant extremity which progressed from pain during play to pain with daily activities. She did not recall any traumatic injury, but her symptoms did not improve despite taking a month break from tennis. Her physical exam was significant for diffuse tenderness over the dorsal distal radius radiating into the second and third metacarpal bases. Dorsiflexion of the wrist and active extension of the thumb exacerbated her symptoms. X-ray of the affected wrist were normal. However, a Technetium 99m scan revealed increased uptake within the distal radius, consistent with a stress fracture. The patient was placed into a cast for 3 weeks, followed by splint immobilisation. At 8 weeks, the patient was able to hit without pain, and she returned to competition at 3 months from the time of immobilisation [86]. Hashiguchi et al. reported the case of a 16 year old judo athlete who presented with a 2 month history of gradual right wrist pain, without an inciting traumatic incident. Physical exam identified pain with wrist dorsiflexion and on direct palpation of the radial styloid. X-ray clearly revealed a small radial styloid bone fragment separated from the radial metaphysis by an osteosclerotic fracture line. The clinical presentation and radiographic appearance were consistent with stress fracture. The athlete was treated with cast immobilisation for 1 month, followed by 2 months of bracing. X-ray at 3 months revealed bony union and the patient reported complete resolution of symptoms. Following another month of rehabilitation, the patient was allowed to return to judo competition. However, at 5 months post-presentation, the patient's right wrist was forced into radial deviation during competition and his symptoms immediately recurred. Radiographs revealed refracture of the radial styloid with clear displacement through the former fracture site. MRI scan of the wrist revealed increased signal intensity on T2 sequences. Arthroscopic examination revealed complete discontinuity of the radial articular facet and free mobility of the styloid fragment. The treating surgeons decided to excise the fracture fragment in an effort to return the athlete to competition as soon as possible. Fibers of the radioscaphocapitate ligament which were attached to the fragment were immediately repaired to the remnant ligament. Post-operatively, the patient was placed into a cast for 3 weeks, followed by accelerated rehabilitation for another 5 weeks. The athlete was allowed to return to judo practice at 8 weeks post-operatively, and resumed competitive judo 1 month later. At 1 year, the athlete remained symptom free with normal wrist range of motion and no evidence of carpal instability [87]. Fujioka et al. reported a similar case involving an 18 year old gymnast. The athlete complained of pain in both wrists when performing hand stands and push-ups. Radiographs identified chronic fractures of bilateral radial styloids, and MRI scans revealed stress reactions in the scaphoid bones of both wrists. The radial styloid fragments were excised simultaneously and both wrists were immobilized in casts for 4 weeks. The athlete was able to resume gymnastic training at 2 months post-operatively. Final follow-up at 2 years documented no recurrence of symptoms and no evidence of wrist instability [88].

22.8.4 Treatment

Initial treatment of distal radius stress reactions should involve immediate cessation of all compression loading to the distal radial physis for a minimum of 6 weeks. Bracing may be indicated if symptoms persist even during non-athletic activities. The athlete's training regimen should be thoroughly evaluated, and recent changes in equipment or training practice should be carefully reviewed to determine if they may have contributed to the injury. Each training element should be correlated to a grade of wrist discomfort and the total number of repetitions of each training element in the athlete's current regimen should be carefully documented [97].

From the cases reported in the literature, stress fractures of the mature distal radius can occur by a variety of mechanisms include weight lifting, weight bearing, and repetitive impact. Forced radial deviation with the wrist in extension is likely to place the most stress across the radial styloid, from the direct impaction of the scaphoid against the radial articular facet [87]. Forced ulnar deviation can also exert stress across the radial styloid from the pull of the radioscaphocapitate ligament [87]. The options of conservative versus surgical treatment should be carefully discussed with the patient. Although cast immobilisation may be effective, long absence from sport and wrist stiffness from prolong immobilisation can adversely impact an athlete's career. The choice between radial styloid fragment excision versus osteosynthesis depends on the size of the fracture fragment. Nakamura et al. demonstrated that a radial stylectomy over 6 mm increased carpal translation, and recommended resection of no more than 3–4 mm from the tip of the styloid [98]. Excision of small radial styloid fragments with ligament repair, as necessary, has been shown to be an effective operation to return the athlete to sport expeditiously [87]. Fracture fragments over 6 mm in size are best managed by osteosynthesis.

The author's preferred method for osteosynthesis of radial styloid fractures is arthroscopic screw fixation. Direct visualization of the articular surface through the arthroscope improves the accuracy of the articular reduction, particularly fragment rotation, which is difficult to assess fluoroscopically. It also permits evaluation of concomitant TFCC and intercarpal ligament injuries. The standard 3–4, 6-U, and 6-R portals are first established for arthroscopic assessment of the radiocarpal joint. It is helpful to thoroughly lavage the joint, to clear out fracture debris and hematoma. Fluid is pumped through the 6-U inflow portal and out a canula at the 3–4 portal, until visualization improves. A shaver may be inserted through the 6-R portal to clear debris or trim the TFCC if necessary. The radial styloid fragment is best visualized with the arthroscope in the 6-R portal, particularly for rotation. The scaphoid articular facet is examined, which may demonstrate step-off of the articular surface and mobility of the radial styloid fragment. Two 0.045-in. guide wires are inserted into the radial styloid under fluoroscopic guidance, and used as joysticks to maneuver the fragment (Fig. 22.13). If necessary, a blunt trochar, inserted through the 3–4 portal, can be used to assist with mobilization and elevation of the fracture fragment (Fig. 22.14). Once ana-

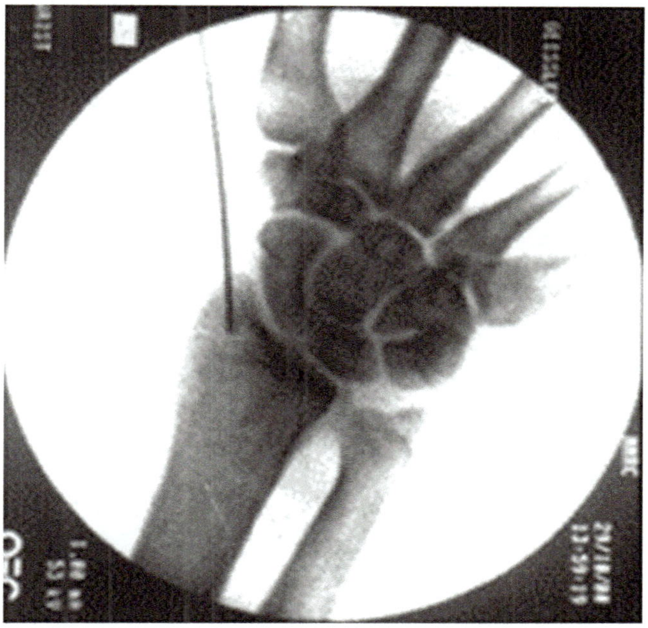

Fig. 22.13 PA fluoroscopic view of a non-displaced fracture of the radial styloid in a major college soccer player, following a hyperextension injury. The patient had a history of multiple falls associated with radial styloid wrist pain

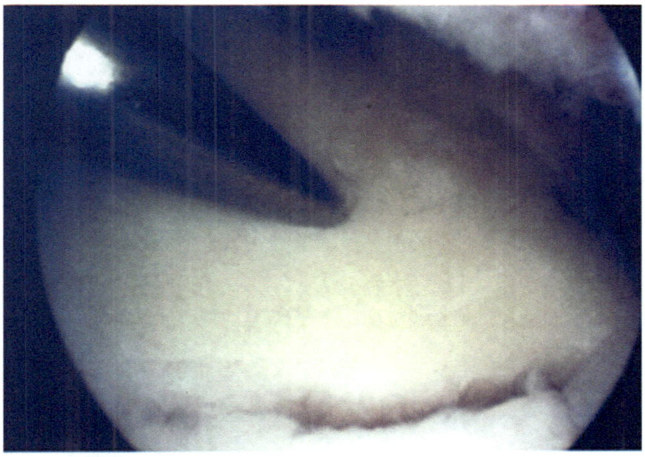

Fig. 22.14 Arthroscopic evaluation was recommended to evaluate the reduction of the fracture and to evaluate for scapho-lunate interosseous ligament injury. The best view to judge rotation of a radial styloid fragment is to place the scope in the 6R and look across the articular surface to access rotation. The guide wire was then placed in the radial styloid fragment to act as a joystick. A trocar, placed in 3/4 portal, can be used to help manipulate the fragment for an anatomic reduction

tomic reduction has been verified arthroscopically, the k-wires are advanced across the fracture and the more central k-wire is selected for screw placement (Fig. 22.15). The appropriately sized screw is inserted over the guidewire, while the other k-wire counters malrotation. A second headless screw may then be placed depending on the fracture pattern (Fig. 22.16). Compression of the fracture gap is verified arthroscopically, and the screw position is evaluated fluoroscopically. The primary advantages of this technique over fluoroscopic percutaneous fixation are direct visualization of the fracture reduction and concomitant evaluation of intraarticular structures [99].

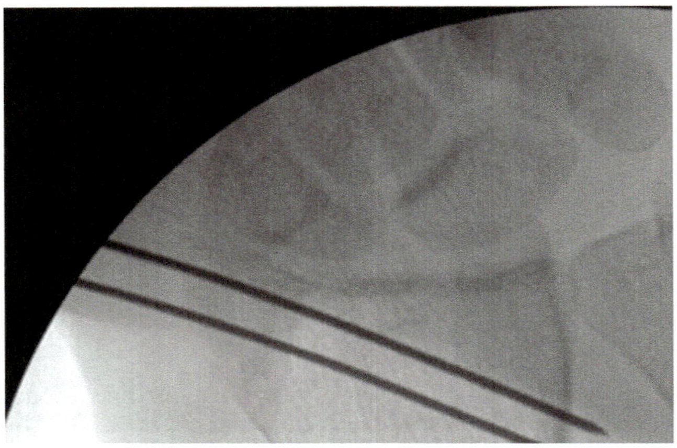

Fig. 22.15 Under oscillation, two guidewires were placed across the fracture site, under fluoroscopic and arthroscopic guidance

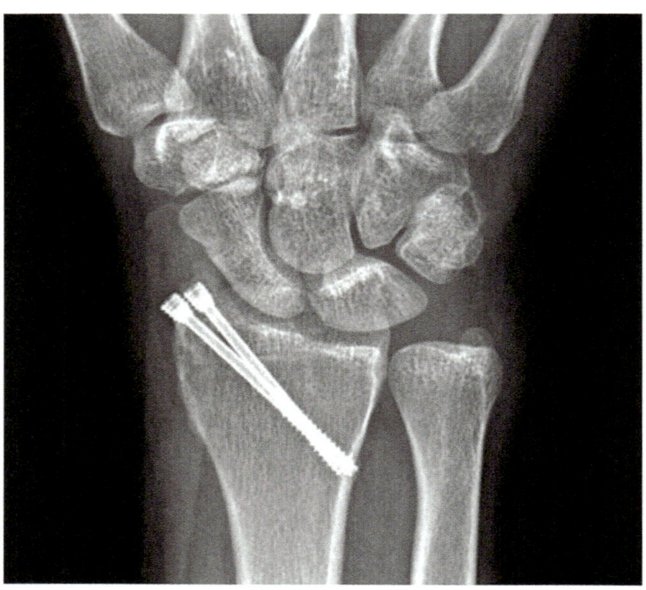

Fig. 22.16 Through a cannula, two percutaneous headless screws were placed to stabilize the radial styloid fragment. The patient was allowed to return to sport within one week in a playing cast

22.8.5 Complications

Distal radial physeal stress reactions typically resolve after appropriate treatment and leave no permanent deformity. In rare cases, physeal stress reactions have been shown to stunt radial growth, leading to positive ulnar variance [100]. Premature closure of the radial physis, relative to the ulnar physis, has also been documented using serial radiographs [101, 102]. Partial growth arrest of the radial physis is another potential sequelae of radial physeal stress reaction [103, 104].

No complications have been reported following excision of radial styloid fragments in the treatment of distal radius stress fractures. However, inadvertent injury to the radioscaphocapitate ligament can result in radiocarpal instability [98].

22.8.6 Rehabilitation

Once symptoms have completely resolved, training may resume starting with the element that caused least discomfort. The volume of repetitions should be reduced to 75% of pre-injury levels and gradually increased over a period of several weeks. Weekly re-evaluations should help coaches and physicians determine if rehabilitation is progressing appropriately or if adjustments should be made [97].

22.8.7 Preventative Measures

Prevention of distal radial stress reactions remain an active area of research and multiple strategies have been proposed to reduce the incidence of these wrist injuries. Individualized training and gradual progression of training volume, especially during the growth spurt period, may help prevent the distal radial physis from being over stressed. The key to preventing a protracted and difficult recovery is early detection of injury and immediate cessation from all weightbearing activities. Open communication between the coaching staff and the physician is critical to curb the cycle of injury as soon as possible. Athletes and trainers should be educated on the sentinel symptoms and on the importance of strict compliance with treatment protocols.

22.9 Distal Ulna

22.9.1 Epidemiology

Stress fractures of the ulna are usually observed along the ulnar diaphysis where muscular attachments can stress the bone excessively with repetitive activity [105]. In contrast, stress fractures of the distal ulna have only been reported a few times in the literature and are thought to be related to repetitive loading at the wrist [106].

22.9.2 Classification

To the authors' knowledge, no classification system has been proposed for stress fractures of the distal ulna. Hauck et al. classified ulnar styloid nonunions as Type 1 if the nonunion was associated with a stable distal radio-ulnar joint, and Type 2 if the nonunion was associated with subluxation of the distal radio-ulnar joint [107].

22.9.3 Diagnosis (History/Physical Exam/ Radiological Investigations)

Bell et al. reported the case of a 19 years old male competitive tennis player who complained of pain just proximal to the ulnar styloid of his non-dominant hand [106]. The patient reported activity-related wrist pain especially when performing his two-handed backhand swing. He had been previously treated for ECU tendonitis with ice, NSAIDs, and physical therapy, but noted little improvement. Physical exam revealed tenderness to palpation around an area approximately 3–4 cm proximal to the ulnar styloid, with no associated soft tissue swelling. The symptoms were exacerbated by dorsiflexion as well as supination and pronation. X-ray demonstrated a discrete periosteal reaction along the dorsal aspect of the distal ulna, with normal radiographic appearance of the cortex and medullary canal. Given the patient's history of activity-related wrist pain and physical exam findings consistent with stress fracture, the patient was encouraged to adopt a single-hand backhand technique while the injured wrist was immobilized in an extension blocking splint. After 4 weeks, the patient returned to his previous style of play with complete resolution of symptoms. Subsequent X-ray revealed increased callus formation surrounding the distal ulna. The authors observed that the two-hand backhand technique required the player to bring the non-dominant wrist into a position terminal hyperextension just prior to ball impact. Repetitive wrist hyperextension under load was thought to transmit stress through the ulno-carpal joint and into the distal ulna, resulting in a stress reaction.

To the authors' knowledge, a stress fracture of the ulnar styloid has only been reported once in the literature. Itadara et al. reported the case of a 15 years old kendo player (Japanese fencing) who complained of pain in his non-dominant wrist whenever he swung his "shinai" (bamboo sword) [108]. The high-level athlete denied any history of trauma, and localized the pain to the ulnar styloid of his left wrist. The symptoms had been present for 6 months and had not improved with conservative treatment. Physical exam revealed severe tenderness with direct palpation of the ulnar styloid, and a positive ulno-carpal impaction test where axial load was applied with the wrist in terminal ulnar deviation, while the forearm was brought through passive range of supination and pronation. X-ray revealed a radiolucent line through the tip of the ulnar styloid, bordered by sclerotic changes. Further imaging with wrist arthrography and MRI revealed no injury to the triangular fibrocartilage ligament complex. Since the fracture did not extend into the fovea and the athlete's symptoms did not improve with conservative management, excision of the fracture fragment was performed through a dorsal approach. The fragment was found to be loosely attached with fibrous tissue, and the triangular fibrocartilage complex (TFCC) was observed to be intact. At 9 months, the athlete had returned to his sport with complete resolution of symptoms. The authors concluded that repeated ulnar deviation of the wrist caused impaction of the triquetrum against the ulnar styloid, leading to fracture. Ulnar styloid impaction syndrome is a well-described cause of ulnar-sided wrist pain, especially in patients with proportionally prominent ulnar styloids [109]. However, the progression of ulnar styloid impaction syndrome to stress fracture of the ulnar styloid had never been previously reported. The decision to perform ulnar styloid excision was contingent upon stablity of the TFCC. The authors noted that instability of the TFCC would have been an indication for fracture osteosynthesis rather than fragment excision.

22.9.4 Treatment

Given the uncommon occurrence of distal ulna stress fractures, clinical information regarding treatment of distal ulnar stress fractures is limited to the case reports discussed in the previous section.

22.9.5 Complications

To the authors' knowledge, no complications from the treatment of distal ulna stress fracture have been reported in the literature. Recurrence of stress fracture is a potential complication if training resumes without preventative precautions. Inadvertent injury to the TFCC insertion during ulnar styloid excision can lead to distal radio-ulnar joint instability [107].

22.9.6 Rehabilitation

Once symptoms have completely resolved, training may resume starting with the elements that cause the least discomfort and at significantly reduced volumes of repetition.

Training intensity may be gradually increased over a period of several weeks. Weekly re-evaluations should help coaches and physicians determine if rehabilitation is progressing appropriately or if adjustments should be made.

22.9.7 Preventative Measures

Stress fractures of the distal ulna are difficult to prevent, especially in high-level athletes. Individualized training and gradual progression of training volume may help prevent over stressing of the osseous structures. The key to preventing a protracted and difficult recovery is early detection of injury and immediate cessation of activity. Open communication between the coaching staff and the physician is critical to curb the cycle of injury as soon as possible. Athletes and trainers should be educated on the sentinel symptoms and on the importance of strict compliance with treatment protocols.

22.10 Conclusion

Stress fractures of the wrist in athletes are rare injuries which could be easily misdiagnosed. Delayed treatment could severely impair the athlete's performance and negatively impact their athletic career. Prompt diagnosis with radiographic and advanced imaging is critical to prevent fracture nonunion and early-onset osteoarthritis. When managed appropriately, the vast majority of stress fractures heal without complication. When treating fractures of the scaphoid, capitate, hook of the hamate, radial styloid, and ulnar styloid, early operative intervention may be favored over conservative management to accelerate the athlete's return to sport.

References

1. Geissler WB. Carpal fractures in athletes. Clin Sports Med. 2001;20(1):167–88.
2. Frost HM. Some ABC's of skeletal pathophysiology. V. Microdamage physiology. Calcif Tissue Int. 1991;49:229–31.
3. Sinha AK, Kaeding CC, Wadley GM. Upper extremity stress fractures in athletes: clinical features of 44 cases. Clin J Sport Med. 1999;9:199–202.
4. Anderson MW. Imaging of upper extremity stress fractures in the athlete. Clin Sports Med. 2006;25(3):489–504.
5. Yoshikawa T, Mori S, Santiesteban AJ, et al. The effects of muscle fatigue on bone strain. J Exp Biol. 1994;188:217–33.
6. Boden BP, Osbahr DC, Jimenez C. Low-risk stress fractures. Am J Sports Med. 2001;29(1):100–11.
7. Matcuk GR, Mahanty SR, Skalski MR, Patel DB, White EA, Gottsegen CJ. Stress fractures: pathophysiology, clinical presentation, imaging features, and treatment options. Emerg Radiol. 2016;23(4):365–75.
8. Matheson GO, Clement DB, McKenzie DC, et al. Stress fractures in athletes: a study of 320 cases. Am J Sports Med. 1987;15:46–58.
9. Lord MJ, Ha KI, Song KS. Stress fractures of the ribs in golfers. Am J Sports Med. 1996;24:118–22.
10. Connolly LP, Connolly SA. Rib stress fractures. Clin Nucl Med. 2004;29:614–6.
11. Matsumoto T, Fujita K, Fujioka H, et al. Stress fracture of the first rib in a soccer player: a rare etiology of shoulder pain. J Shoulder Elb Surg. 2003;12:197–9.
12. Taimela S, Kujala UM, Orava S. Two consecutive rib stress fractures in a female competitive swimmer. Clin J Sport Med. 1995;5:254–7.
13. Arendt EA, Clohisy DR. Stress injuries of bone. In: Nicholas JA, Hershman EB, editors. The lower extremity and spine. 2nd ed. St. Louis: Mosby; 1995. p. 65.
14. Chisin R, Milgrom C, Stein M, et al. Clinical significance of nonfocal scintigraphic findings in suspected tibial stress fractures. Clin Orthop. 1987;220:200–5.
15. Kelsay JL, Behall KM, Prather TS. Effects of fiber from fruits and vegetables on metabolic responses of human subjects 11: calcium, magnesium, iron and silicon balances. Am J Clin Nutr. 1979;32:1876–80.
16. Griffiths HJ, Priest DR, Rector BE, et al. Bone bruises: their aetiology and importance. Imaging. 1995;7:286–90.
17. Arendt EA, Griffiths HJ. The use of MR imaging in the assessment and clinical management of stress reactions of bone in high-performance athletes. Clin Sports Med. 1997;16(2):291–306.
18. Hanks GA, Kalenak A, Bowman LS, Sebastianelli WJ. Stress fractures of the carpal scaphoid: a report of four cases. J Bone Joint Surg Am. 1989;71:938–41.
19. Majima M, Horii E, Matsui H, Hirata H, Genda E. Load transmission through the wrist in the extended position. J Hand Surg Am. 2008;33:182–8.
20. Matzkin E, Singer DI. Scaphoid stress fracture in a 13-year-old gymnast: a case report. J Hand Surg. 2000;25:710–3.
21. Coady CM, Micheli LJ. Stress fractures in the pediatric athlete. Clin Sports Med. 1997;16:225–36.
22. Kohyama S, Kanamori A, Tanaka T, Hara Y, Yamazaki M. Stress fracture of the scaphoid in an elite junior tennis player: a case report and review of the literature. J Med Case Rep. 2016;10(1):8.
23. Manzione M, Pizzutillo PD. Stress fracture of the scaphoid waist: a case report. Am J Sports Med. 1981;9:268–9.
24. Engel A, Feldner-Busztin H. Bilateral stress fracture of the scaphoid: a case report. Arch Orthop Trauma Surg. 1991;110:314–5.
25. Inagaki H, Inoue G. Stress fracture of the scaphoid combined with the distal radial epiphysiolysis. Br J Sports Med. 1997;31:256–7.
26. Hosey RG, Hauk JM, Boland MR. Scaphoid stress fracture: an unusual cause of wrist pain in a competitive diver. Orthopedics. 2006;29:503–5.
27. Rethnam U, Yesupalan RSU, Kumar TM. Non union of scaphoid fracture in a cricketer – possibility of a stress fracture: a case report. J Med Case Rep. 2007;1:37. https://doi.org/10.1186/1752-1947-1-37.
28. Yamagiwa T, Fujioka H, Okuno H, Tomatsuri M, Tsunemi K, Tanaka J, et al. Surgical treatment of stress fracture of the scaphoid of an adolescent gymnast. J Sports Sci Med. 2009;8:702–4.
29. Nakamoto JC, Saito M, Medina G, Schor B. Scaphoid stress fracture in high-level gymnast: a case report. Case Rep Orthop. 2011;2011:492407. https://doi.org/10.1155/2011/492407.
30. Pidemunt G, Torres-Claramunt R, Ginés A, de Zabala S, Cebamanos J. Bilateral stress fracture of the carpal scaphoid: report in a child and review of the literature. Clin J Sport Med. 2012;22:511–3.
31. Haflah NH, Nor NF, Abdullah S, Sapuan J. Bilateral scaphoid stress fracture in a platform diver presenting with unilateral symptoms. Singap Med J. 2014;55(10):e159.

32. Brutus JP, Chahidi N. Could this unusual scaphoid fracture occurring in a badminton player be a stress fracture? Chir Main. 2004;23(1):52–4.
33. Kohring JM, Curtiss HM, Tyser AR. A scaphoid stress fracture in a female collegiate-level shot-putter and review of the literature. Case Rep Orthop. 2016;2016
34. Saglam F, Gulabi D, Baysal Ö, Bekler HI, Tasdemir Z, Elmali N. Chronic wrist pain in a goalkeeper; bilateral scaphoid stress fracture: a case report. Int J Surg Case Rep. 2015;7:20–2.
35. Baker J, Frankel VH, Burstein A. Fatigue fractures: biomechanical considerations. J Bone Jt Surg. 1972;54-A:1345–6.
36. Weiker GG. Hand and wrist problems in the gymnast. Clin Sports Med. 1992;11:189–202.
37. Chow JW, Knudson DV, Tillman MD, Andrew DPS. Pre- and post-impact muscle activation in the tennis volley: effects of ball speed, ball size and side of the body. Br J Sports Med. 2007;41:754–9.
38. Dobyns JH, Gabel GT. Gymnast's wrist. Hand Clin. 1990;6:493–505.
39. Gabel GT. Gymnastic wrist injuries. Clin Sports Med. 1998;17:611–21.
40. Markiewitz AD, Andrish JT. Hand and wrist injuries in the preadolescent and adolescent athlete. Clin Sports Med. 1992;11:203–25.
41. Geissler WB, Adams JE, Bindra RR, Lanzinger WD, Slutsky DJ. Scaphoid fractures: what's hot, what's not. JBJS. 2012;94(2):169–81.
42. Arora R, Gschwentner M, Krappinger D, Lutz M, Blauth M, Gabl M. Fixation of nondisplaced scaphoid fractures: making treatment cost effective. Prospective controlled trial. Arch Orthop Trauma Surg. 2007;127(1):39–46.
43. Rettig AC, Kollias SC. Internal fixation of acute stable scaphoid fractures in the athlete. Am J Sports Med. 1996;24:182–6. Epub 2006 Sept 27
44. Rettig AC. Wrist problems in the tennis players. Med Sci Sports Exerc. 1994;10:1207–12.
45. Maquirriain J, Ghisi JP. Stress injury of the lunate in tennis players: a case series and related biomechanical considerations. Br J Sports Med. 2007;41(11):812.
46. Schmitt R, Christopoulos G, Kalb K, et al. Differential diagnosis of the signal-compromised lunate in MRI [abstract, in German]. Rofo. 2005;177:358–66.
47. Elliot B, Takahashi K, Noffal G. The influence of grip position on upper limb contribution to racket head velocity in a tennis forehand. J Appl Biomech. 1997;13:182–96.
48. Knudson DV. Factors affecting force loading on the hand in the tennis forehand. J Sports Med Phys Fitness. 1991;31:527–31.
49. Bartone NF, Bums JF. Fractures of the triquetnun. J Bone Joint Surg. 1956;38:353–6.
50. Bryan RS, Dobyns JH. Fractures of the carpal bones other than the lunate and navicular. Clin Orthop. 1980;14:107–11.
51. Lohman M, Kivisaari L, Partio EK. Stress reaction in the carpal bones caused by breakdancing. Emerg Radiol. 2003;10(2):102–4.
52. Hansen GR. Breaks and other bad breaks for breakers. JAMA. 1985;253:2047.
53. Winslet MC, Clarke NM, Mulligan PJ. Breakdancer's thumb—partial rupture of the ulnar collateral ligament with a fracture of the proximal phalanx of the thumb. Injury. 1986;17:201–2.
54. Demirkan F, Calandruccio JH, DiAngelo D. Biomechanical evaluation of flexor tendon function after hamate hook excision. J Hand Surg Am. 2003;28(1):138–43.
55. Guha AR, Marynissen H. Stress fracture of the hook of the hamate. Br J Sports Med. 2002;36(3):224–5.
56. Bayer T, Schweizer A. Stress fracture of the hook of the hamate as a result of intensive climbing. J Hand Surg Eur. 2009;34:276–7.
57. Lutter C, Schweizer A, Hochholzer T, Bayer T, Schöffl V. Pulling harder than the hamate tolerates: evaluation of hamate injuries in rock climbing and bouldering. Wilderness Environ Med. 2016;27(4):492–9.
58. Scheufler O, Kamusella P, Tadda L, Radmer S, Russo SG, Andresen R. High incidence of hamate hook fractures in underwater rugby players: diagnostic and therapeutic implications. Hand Surg. 2013;18(3):357–63.
59. Bishop AT, Beckenbaugh RD. Fracture of the hamate hook. J Hand Surg Am. 1988;13(1):135–9.
60. Xiong G, Dai L, Zheng W, Sun Y, Tian G. Clinical classification and treatment strategy of hamate hook fracture. J Huazhong Univ Sci Technol Med Sci. 2010;30:762–6.
61. Ueda H, Hama S, Yasuda M, Minato K, Miyashita M, Shin K. Stress fracture of the hamate hook in a water polo player. Case Rep Orthop. 2019;2019
62. Wright TW, Moser MW, Sahajpal DT. Hook of hamate pull test. J Hand Surg Am. 2010;35:1887–9.
63. Hochholzer TBT, Straub G, Schöffl V. Overuse bone marrow edema of the hands in sport climbers. Sport Orthop Traumatol. 2013;29:219–24.
64. Schoffl VR, Schoffl I. Finger pain in rock climbers: reaching the right differential diagnosis and therapy. J Sports Med Phys Fitness. 2007;47:70–8.
65. Egawa M, Asai T. Fractures of the hook of the hamate: report of six cases and the suitability of computerised tomography. J Hand Surg. 1983;8:393.
66. Failla JM. Hook of the hamate vascularity: vulnerability to osteonecrosis and nonunion. J Hand Surg. 1993;18A:1075–9.
67. Watson HK, Rodgers WD. Nonunion of the hook of the hamate. An argument for bone grafting the nonunion. J Hand Surg. 1989;14:486–90.
68. Bishop AT, Bechenbaugh RD. Fractures of the hamate hook. J Hand Surg. 1988;13A:135–9.
69. Futami T, Aoki H, Tsukamoto Y. Fractures of the hook of the hamate in eight athletes: eight cases followed for six years. Acta Orthop Scand. 1993;64:469–71.
70. Hirano K, Inoue G. Classification and treatment of hamate fractures. Hand Surg. 2005;10:151–7
71. Rand JA, Linscheid RL, Dobyns JH. Capitate fractures: a long-term follow-up. Clin Orthop. 1982;165:209–16.
72. Kaewlai R, Avery LL, Asrani AV, Abujudeh HH, Sacknoff R, Novelline RA. Multidetector CT of carpal injuries: anatomy, fractures, and fracture-dislocations. Radiographics. 2008;28: 1771–84.
73. Vigler M, Aviles A, Lee SK. Carpal fractures excluding the scaphoid. Hand Clin. 2006;22:501–16. abstract vii
74. Moojen TM, Snel JG, Ritt MJ, Venema HW, Kauer JM, Bos KE. In vivo analysis of carpal kinematics and comparative review of the literature. J Hand Surg Am. 2003;28:81–7.
75. Oestreich AE, Bhojwani N. Stress fractures of ankle and wrist in childhood: nature and frequency. Pediatr Radiol. 2010;40:1387–9.
76. Gelberman RH, Gross MS. The vascularity of the wrist: identification of arterial patterns at risk. Clin Orthop. 1986;202:40–9.
77. Jaimes C, Jimenez M, Shabshin N, Laor T, Jaramillo D. Taking the stress out of evaluating stress injuries in children. Radiographics. 2012;32:537–55.
78. Cho HJ, Hong KT, Kang CH, Ahn KS, Kim Y, Hwang ST. Stress fracture of the capitate. Investig Magn Reson Imaging. 2018;22(2):135–9.
79. Vizkelety T, Wouters HW. Stress fracture of the capitate. Arch Chir Neerl. 1972;24:47–57.
80. Allen H, Gibbon WW, Evans RJ. Stress fracture of the capitate. J Accid Emerg Med. 1994;11:59–60.
81. Calandruccio JH, Duncan SF. Isolated nondisplaced capitate waist fracture diagnosed by magnetic resonance imaging. J Hand Surg Am. 1999;24(4):856–9.
82. Hindman BW, Kulik WJ, Lee G, Avolio RE. Occult fractures of the carpals and metacarpals: demonstration by CT. AJR Am J Roentgenol. 1989;153:529–32.

83. DiFiori JP, Puffer JC, Mandelbaum BR, Mar S. Factors associated with wrist pain in the young gymnast. Am J Sports Med. 1996;24:9–14.
84. Carter SR, Aldridge MJ. Stress injury of the distal radial growth plate. J Bone Joint Surg Br. 1988;70-B:834–6.
85. Flachsmann R, Broom ND, Hardy AE, Moltschaniwskyj G. Why is the adolescent joint particularly susceptible to osteochondral shear fracture? Clin Orthop Relat Res. 2000;381:212–21.
86. Loosli AR, Leslie M. Stress fractures of the distal radius: a case report. Am J Sports Med. 1991;19:523–4.
87. Hashiguchi H, Iwashita S, Ohkubo A, Sawaizumi T, Takai S. Stress fracture of the radial styloid process in a judo player: a case report. J Nippon Med Sch. 2015;82(2):109–12.
88. Fujioka H, Tsunemi K, Tanaka J. Bilateral stress fractures of the radial styloid process in a gymnast. J Hand Surg Eur. 2010;35:243–4.
89. Roy S, Caine D, Singer KM. Stress changes of the distal radial epiphysis in young gymnasts: a report of twenty-one cases and a review of the literature. Am J Sports Med. 1985;13(5):301–8.
90. Read MT. Stress fractures of the distal radius in adolescent gymnasts. Br J Sports Med. 1981;15(4):272–6.
91. Koh TJ, Grabiner MD, Weiker GG. Technique and ground reaction forces in the back handspring. Am J Sports Med. 1992;20:61–6.
92. Markoff JL, Shapiro MS, Mandelbaum BR, Teurling L. Wrist loading patterns during pommel horse exercises. J Biomech. 1990;23:1001–11.
93. Jaramillo D, Laor T, Zaleske DJ. Indirect trauma to the growth plate: results of MR imaging after epiphyseal and metaphyseal injury in rabbits. Radiology. 1993;187:171–8.
94. Kwon SW, Hong SJ, Nho JH, Moon SI, Jung KJ. Physeal fracture in the wrist and hand due to stress injury in a child climber: a case report. Medicine. 2018;97(34)
95. Cahill BR. Little league shoulder: lesions of the proximal humeral epiphyseal plate. J Sports Med. 1974;2(3):150–3.
96. Grana WA, Rashkin A. Pitcher's elbow in adolescents. Am J Sports Med. 1980;8(5):333–6.
97. DiFiori JP, Caine DJ, Malina RM. Wrist pain, distal radial physeal injury, and ulnar variance in the young gymnast. Am J Sports Med. 2006;34(5):840–9.
98. Nakamura T, Cooney WP III, Lui WH, Haugstvedt JR, Zhao KD, Berglund L, An KN. Radial styloidectomy: a biomechanical study on stability of the wrist joint. J Hand Surg Am. 2001;26(1):85–93.
99. Geissler WB, Freeland AE. Arthroscopically assisted reduction of intraarticular distal radial fractures. Clin Orthop Relat Res. 1996;327:125–34.
100. Caine D, Knutzen K, Howe W, et al. A three-year epidemiological study of injuries affecting young female gymnasts. Phys Ther Sport. 2003;4:10–23.
101. Albanese SA, Palmer AK, Kerr DR, Carpenter CS, Lisi D, Levinsohn EM. Wrist pain and distal growth plate closure of the radius in gymnasts. J Pediatr Orthop. 1989;9:23–8.
102. Bak K, Boeckstyns M. Epiphysiodesis for bilateral irregular closure of the distal radial physis in a gymnast. Scand J Med Sci Sports. 1997;7:363–6.
103. Brooks TJ. Madelung deformity in a collegiate gymnast: a case report. J Athl Train. 2001;36:170–3.
104. Vender MI, Watson HK. Acquired Madelung-like deformity in a gymnast. J Hand Surg Am. 1988;13:19–21.
105. Jones GL. Upper extremity stress fractures. Clin Sports Med. 2006;25(1):159–74.
106. Bell RH, Hawkins RJ. Stress fracture of the distal ulna. A case report. Clin Orthop Relat Res. 1986;209:169–71.
107. Hauck RM, Skahen J III, Palmer AK. Classification and treatment of ulnar styloid nonunion. J Hand Surg Am. 1996;21(3):418–22.
108. Itadera E, Ichikawa N, Hashizume H, Inoue H. Stress fracture of the ulnar styloid process in kendo player—a case report. Hand Surg. 2001;6(01):109–11.
109. Topper SM, Wood MB, Ruby LK. Ulnar styloid impaction syndrome. J Hand Surg. 1997;22(4):699–704.

23 Stress Fractures in Sport: Hand

Paul H. C. Stirling and Christopher W. Oliver

Learning Objectives

- To describe the epidemiology of stress fractures of the metacarpals and finger phalanges in sport.
- To understand contemporary management principles for these injuries.
- To appreciate the outcomes following these injuries.
- To identify preventative measures to avoid these injuries in athletes.

23.1 Stress Fractures of the Metacarpals

23.1.1 Epidemiology

Stress fractures occur when the balance between bone resorption and new bone deposition is disrupted. In athletes this results from repetitive loading. Sports-related stress fractures of the upper extremity are far less common than those affecting the lower limb [1].

Metacarpal stress fractures are extremely rare injuries: they are thought to account for only 0.3–1.4% of all stress fractures in adults [1, 2]. In the past 30 years, 19 cases of metacarpal stress fractures have been reported, which occurred in 17 athletes [3–13]. These reports are summarized in Table 23.1 and Fig. 23.1.

The typical patient is an adolescent female tennis player. Based on currently reported cases the average age at presentation is 17 years (range 13–27 years; standard deviation 3 years). 12 patients were female (70%). 13 cases were related to racquet sports (11 tennis players, 1 badminton player, and 1 soft tennis player). One case each occurred in a rower, a softball pitcher, and a golfer. There was a single case of a military recruit who developed a metacarpal stress fracture following knuckle (military) press-ups. The second metacarpal was the most commonly injured (76%). Two cases (12%) occurred in the fourth metacarpal, and one case each occurred in the third and fifth metacarpals (6% each). All cases related to gripping occurred in the second metacarpal, apart from one case of a third metacarpal stress fracture. The vast majority of cases in racquet sports players occurred following a change from the Eastern to the Western grip [8, 9, 11]. Although this is recognised as a potential aetiological cause, the exact pathophysiology of this is not well-understood [13].

23.1.2 Classification

Conventional fracture classification systems aim to allow communication between specialists, facilitate research, and guide management. Due to the rarity of metacarpal stress fractures no specific classification system has been described. Traumatic metacarpal fractures are classified as head, neck, shaft, or base fractures according to their anatomical location [14], and this is also easily applicable to stress fractures. Stress fractures in other anatomical sites have been described as occurring on the tension side or compression side of the bone, depending on the position of the fracture in relation to the deforming force [15]; this nomenclature can also be applied to stress fractures of the metacarpal.

The most commonly reported site for metacarpal stress fractures is the metacarpal base (Fig. 23.1). Review of imaging from studies reporting fractures of the metacarpal base revealed the cortical breach to occur at the junction of the proximal third and distal two thirds of the shaft. These proximal shaft fractures occurred in 16 patients [4, 5, 7–9, 11–13]. Other fracture locations included one case of a fracture of the head [3], one of the neck [6], and a single intra-articular fracture of the true base [10]. All cases occurred on the compression side of the metacarpal: for racquet sports and the golfer, this was the ulnar side (14 cases), while the rower and military press up case occurred on the radial side.

P. H. C. Stirling (✉) · C. W. Oliver
Department of Trauma and Orthopaedic Surgery, Royal Infirmary of Edinburgh, Edinburgh, UK
e-mail: cwoliver@btopenworld.com

G. A. J. Robertson, N. Maffulli (eds.), *Fractures in Sport*, https://doi.org/10.1007/978-3-030-72036-0_23

Table 23.1 Summary of published reports of metacarpal stress fractures

Study	Number of cases	Sex	Age	Finger	Location	Side	Sport	Treatment	RTP (weeks)	Notes
Balius et al. [13]	9	6F 1M	15–17	Index (6) Middle (2) Ring (1)	Proximal shaft	Ulnar	Tennis	Cessation and physiotherapy	7–16	6 Western or Semi-Western grips, 1 Eastern grip
Muramatsu and Kuriyama [7]	1	F	13	Index	Proximal shaft	Ulnar	Soft tennis	Physiotherapy and grip change	6	Western grip
Bespalchuk et al. [11]	1	F	15	Index	Proximal shaft	Ulnar	Tennis	Cessation and grip change	12	Western grip
Rolison and Smoot [4]	1	M	19	Index	Proximal shaft	Ulnar	Golf	Cessation and splint	16	Returned with modified grip
Duarte et al. [5]	1	M	27	Index	Proximal shaft	Ulnar	Tennis	Cast, grip change	8	Eastern grip
Fukuda et al. [12]	1	F	15	Index	Proximal shaft	Ulnar	Badminton	Cessation	5	Western grip
Busche et al. [10]	1	M	19	Ring	Intraarticular base	Radial	Knuckle press-ups	Cast	4	Concomitant hamate stress fracture
Parsons et al. [6]	1	F	18	Ring	Neck	Radial	Rowing	Cessation	16	–
Jowett and Brukner [3]	1	F	18	Little	Head	–	Softball pitching	Cessation	6	–
Waninger and Lombardo [9]	1	F	14	Index	Proximal shaft	Ulnar	Tennis	Cessation and grip change	6	Precipitated by change from Eastern to Western grip
Murakami [8]	1	M	16	Index	Proximal shaft	Ulnar	Tennis	Cessation and grip change	6	–

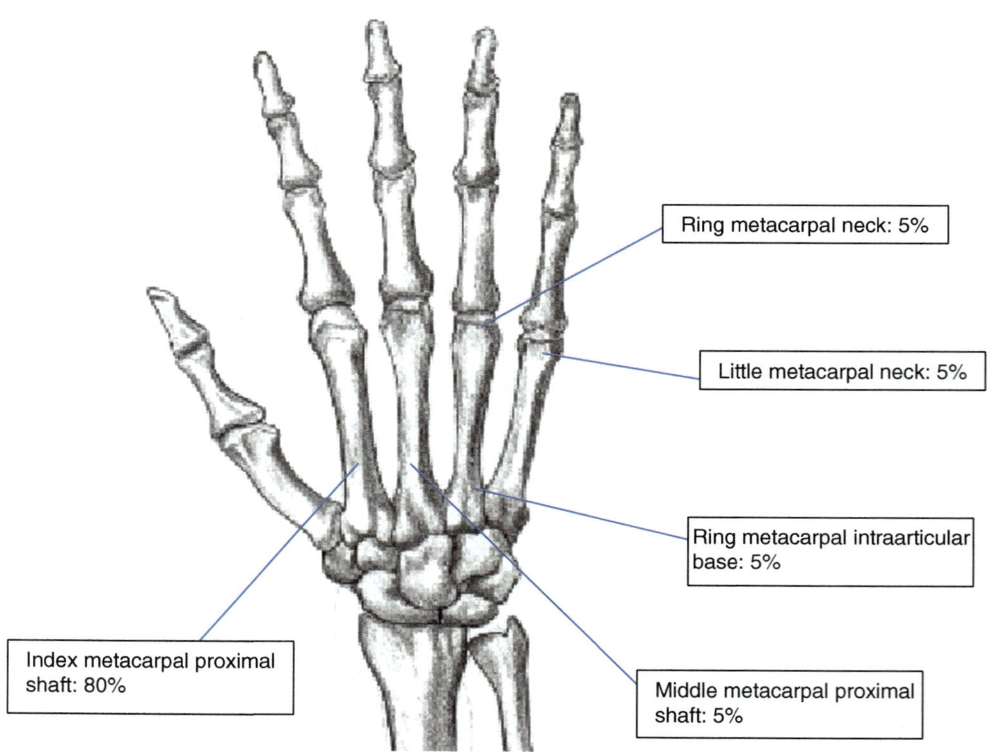

Fig. 23.1 Anatomical distribution of the incidence of reported stress fractures of the metacarpals

23.1.3 Diagnosis

Diagnosis is based on clinical suspicion and examination, and can be confirmed with further imaging.

23.1.3.1 History

The patient usually reports insidious onset of dorsal metacarpal pain. This often occurs at the point of striking the ball or gripping their sports equipment. There should be no history of acute precipitating trauma. Generally, symptoms progressively worsen, being provoked by incrementally less activity, until the patient is unable to continue playing or training. The presenting complaint is usually inability to play due to pain, which has often been present for several months. The patient should specifically be asked about recent increase in activity, training schedule, upcoming events, and any recent change in grip or equipment. Further questioning should focus on systemic symptoms include paraneoplastic symptoms, diet, and risk factors for metabolic bone disease including the female athlete triad.

23.1.3.2 Examination

The commonest finding is tenderness over the dorsal aspect of the metacarpal. This may be accompanied by a visible swelling or deformation of the finger. These injuries are commonly mistaken for carpometacarpal bossing. Grip strength may also be reduced.

23.1.3.3 Radiological Investigations

Plain radiographs are usually performed as a first line investigation. Plain radiographs may demonstrate a periosteal reaction, or a hairline crack, however these are normal in over 50% of cases [13]. The usefulness of plain radiographs centers around its role in excluding acute fractures.

Computed tomography (CT) can demonstrate cortical thickening [16] or reveal the fracture [17].

Magnetic resonance imaging (MRI) is the gold-standard investigation, and may demonstrate bone marrow oedema, a hairline crack, and local cortical thickening [18]. MRI can also distinguish between other important differentials including infection and neoplasia [7, 19].

Bone scintigraphy has also been performed and, if positive, will demonstrate increased tracer uptake at the site of the fracture [13]. However, the findings are non-specific and this imaging modality is unable to exclude other differential diagnoses [11].

23.1.4 Treatment

Reported treatment has been universally nonoperative. In all cases, cessation of aggravating activities was undertaken once the diagnosis was made. In most cases, cessation and rest was sufficient, however two authors treated their patients with hand immobilisation in a splint or cast [5, 10].

23.1.5 Complications

No complications have been reported in the literature. The most feared complication would be completion of the stress reaction to an acute fracture, which would require a longer period of immobilisation or surgical fixation. All patients were able to return to normal activities and to the same level of activity.

23.1.6 Rehabilitation

Median time for return to play from diagnosis was 8 weeks (range 4–16 weeks). For athletes who play racquet sports, grip modification is recommended: in the currently available literature four patients changed back from the Western to the Eastern grip [7, 9, 11, 13] as part of their rehabilitation. Three other patients modified their grip as part of their rehabilitation, however the authors of these reports do not specify which grip was utilised before or after the injury [5, 8, 13]. It would be reasonable to suggest a return to the grip which was used prior to the injury.

23.1.7 Preventative Measures

1. Clinicians should maintain a high index of suspicion for this injury in patients who play racquet sports. Immediate cessation of activity and investigation to facilitate early diagnosis and rehabilitation may reduce the recovery period. Consideration of changing racquet grip, usually from Western to Eastern grip, may prevent symptom recurrence.
2. As with all stress fractures, optimization of diet and general health should be undertaken to promote good bone health.

23.2 Stress Fractures of the Finger Phalanges

23.2.1 Epidemiology

Stress fractures of the finger phalanges represent a spectrum of injuries which almost invariably affect the physis in skeletally immature climbers. Previously published studies report a total of 72 cases, which occurred in 62 patients. Aside from a single case which occurred in a Ten-pin bowler,

Table 23.2 Summary of published reports of finger phalangeal stress fractures

Study	Number of cases	Sex	Age	Finger	Phalanx	Location	Side	Sport	Treatment	RTP (weeks)	Notes
Fakharzadeh [20]	1	M	28	Ring	P2	Shaft	Radial	10-pin bowling	Cessation	6	–
Hochholzer and Schöffl et al. [21]	24	23M 1F	14.5	Middle 7 Ring 17	P2	PIPJ	Dorsal	Rock climbing	Splint, physiotherapy, cessation	16–24	–
Chell et al. [22]	1	M	15	Middle; bilateral	P2	PIPJ	Dorsal	Rock climbing	Cessation	16	Bilateral
Bärtschi et al. [23]	21	12M 3F	13.7	Multiple	Multiple	PIPJ	Dorsal	Rock climbing	Cessation	–	
Sobel et al. [24]	1	M	15	–	P2	PIPJ	Dorsal	Rock climbing	Cessation	8	–
Kwon et al. [25]	1	F	11	Ring	P2	PIPJ	Dorsal	Rock climbing	Cessation and physiotherapy	4	–
Desaldeleer and Le Nen [26]	1	M	17	Middle	P2	PIPJ	Dorsal	Rock climbing	Physio and cessation	–	Chose to give up sport
Schöffl and Schöffl [27]	22	15M 3F	14.1	21 Middle, 1 unspecified	P2	PIPJ	Dorsal	Rock climbing	Physio and cessation	–	–

all cases occurred in Rock climbers. Data from currently-available literature is summarized in Table 23.2 [20–27].

The typical patient is an adolescent rock climber. Based on currently reported cases the average age at presentation is 16 years (range 11–28 years; standard deviation 5.5 years). 54 patients were male (87%). All reported cases to date have occurred in the middle and ring fingers, and all cases have occurred in the middle phalanx.

23.2.2 Classification

The single case which occurred in the Ten-Pin bowler occurred over the radial aspect of the ring finger middle phalangeal shaft. The remainder of cases represented intraarticular fractures of the proximal interphalangeal joint (PIPJ) (Fig. 23.2). These could be classified according to the Salter-Harris system, and all cases represented either a type II or type III fracture [28]. The fracture occurred over the dorsal aspect of the PIPJ in all cases.

23.2.3 Diagnosis

Diagnosis is based on clinical suspicion and examination, and is confirmed by radiological imaging.

23.2.3.1 History

The patient usually reports atraumatic dorsal PIPJ pain and swelling. As with metacarpal stress fractures, the patient should specifically be asked about recent increase in activity, training schedule, upcoming events, and any recent change in grip or training.

23.2.3.2 Examination

The commonest finding is tenderness over the dorsal aspect of the PIPJ. This is often accompanied by a visible swelling of the joint, along with a diminished range of motion. The patient may hold their finger with the PIPJ held in flexion, with inability to extend the joint due to pain. An important differential diagnosis is acute a2 pulley rupture, which is the most common finger injury in skeletally-mature competitive climbers [29]. However, this would typically present with volar pain, visible bowstringing, and a more acute history.

23.2.3.3 Radiological Investigations

Plain radiographs are performed as a first line investigation. Lateral plain radiography will usually demonstrate the dorsally displaced fragment clearly.

Ultrasound has been used to investigate phalangeal overuse injuries in climbers [30]. The typical finding is a PIPJ effusion, with malalignment of the metaphysis and epiphysis. Thickening of the volar plate and flexor tendons may also be present [30]. The use of ultrasound is limited by its small field of view, and its inability to detect subtle physeal abnormalities.

MRI has a wider field of view and is able to detect more subtle abnormalities, include bone oedema, physeal separation, and bone bridging [31].

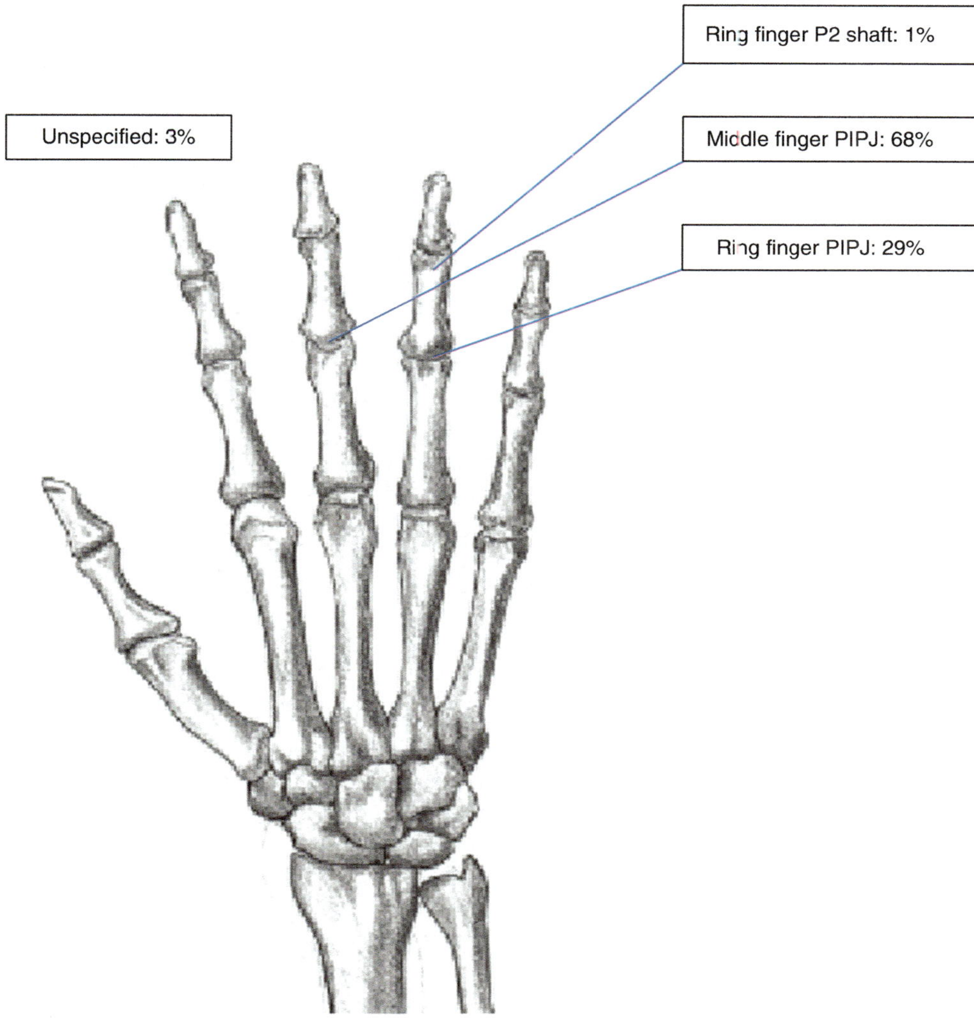

Fig. 23.2 Anatomical distribution of the incidence of reported stress fractures of the finger phalanges

23.2.4 Treatment

Treatment is universally nonoperative. Immediate cessation of precipitating activities is required, with physiotherapy to optimise hand function. In the vast majority of cases this has been sufficient, with 75% of patients able to return to climbing with conservative treatment [23]. There have been two cases of physeal separation with established nonunion, which required open epiphysiodesis after failure of conservative treatment [32].

23.2.5 Complications

Continuing to climb can result in premature malunion of the physis in adolescents, with deformity, or permanent articular surface incongruity resulting. There has been one reported case of PIPJ osteoarthritis as a result of this injury. Although 75% of athletes can expect to return to a similar level of activity, a significant proportion will not return to competitive climbing. This is either due to reduced function following the injury, or the patient electing not to return to climbing.

23.2.6 Rehabilitation

Complete cessation of activities, specifically with reduction in loading, is indicated. The patient should be counseled that, while the average time for rehabilitation is 24 weeks, it can take up to 1 year to regain full function following this condition.

23.2.7 Preventative Measures

The primary risk factors for this condition are adolescent age group, high-level competitive climbers, and routine finger strengthening exercises using a crimp grip or campus board. It is probably unrealistic to expect all competitive climbers to avoid this type of training, but discussion about the risks and benefits of this type of training should occur between the coach and athlete.

Clinical Pearls

- Always consider underlying metabolic abnormalities in any athlete presenting with an atraumatic fracture.
- Always question the athlete on recent changes in their training practices. Grip change, equipment change, or training intensity could all precipitate stress fractures.

Review

Questions

A 15-year-old female competitive tennis player presents to your clinic with a 6-month history of dorsal pain the radial border of her dominant hand. Examination reveals tenderness and swelling over the metacarpal shaft. She has recently increased her training intensity in preparation for forthcoming national championships in 3 weeks.

1. You suspect a metacarpal stress fracture. What is the most sensitive imaging modality to diagnose this?
2. Are there any other features, missing from the history, which must be considered in a patient presenting with this clinical picture?
3. How would you treat this injury?
4. How would you counsel the patient?

Answers

1. MRI is the most sensitive imaging modality. It can also rule out important differentials including neoplasia.
2. A low index of suspicion for neoplasia must be maintained in all patients with insidious and vague bony pain. A focused history asking about weight loss, night sweats, or other neoplastic symptoms should be obtained. Further questions relating to general bone health, such as diet and supplementation, are also valuable. Finally, asking if the patient had recently changed her equipment or racquet grip could provide a target for therapy.
3. The treatment for metacarpal stress fractures is non operative with rest followed by rehabilitation. If the patient has recently changed grip or equipment, changing back to their previous style may accelerate the healing process.
4. The patient can be counseled that these injuries generally heal well in a predictable pattern, and that, according to the literature, there is no reason to expect that they cannot return to sport in the fullness of time.

References

1. Iwamoto J, Takeda T. Stress fractures in athletes: review of 196 cases. J Orthop Sci. 2003;8(3):273–8.
2. Orava S, Puranen J, Ala-Ketola L. Stress fractures caused by physical exercise. Acta Orthop Scand. 1978;49(1):19–27.
3. Jowett AD, Brukner PD. Fifth metacarpal stress fracture in a female softball pitcher. Clin J Sport Med. 1997;7(3):220–1.
4. Rolison CJ, Smoot MK. Hand pain in a golfer. Sports Health. 2016;9(1):84–6.
5. Duarte ML, da Nóbrega RR, de Almeida Prado JL, Scoppetta LC. Metacarpal stress fracture in amateur tennis player—an uncommon fracture. Rev Bras Ortop. 2017;52(5):608–11.
6. Parsons EM, Goldblatt JP, Richmond JC. Metacarpal stress fracture in an intercollegiate rower: case report. Am J Sports Med. 2005;33(2):293–4.
7. Muramatsu K, Kuriyama R. Stress fracture at the base of second metacarpal in a soft tennis player. Clin J Sport Med. 2005;15(4):279–80.
8. Murakami Y. Stress fracture of the metacarpal in an adolescent tennis player. Am J Sports Med. 1988;16(4):419–20.
9. Waninger KN, Lombardo JA. Stress fracture of index metacarpal in an adolescent tennis player. Clin J Sport Med. 1995;5(1):63–6.
10. Busche MN, Knobloch K, Rosenthal H, Vogt PM. Stress fracture of the hamate body and fourth metacarpal base following military style push-ups: an unusual trauma mechanism. Knee Surg Sports Traumatol Arthrosc. 2008;16(12):1158.
11. Bespalchuk A, Okada K, Nishida J, Takahashi S, Shimada Y, Itoi E. Stress fracture of the second metacarpal bone. Skelet Radiol. 2004;33(9):537–40.
12. Fukuda K, Fujioka H, Fujita I, Uemoto H, Hiranaka T, Tsuji M, Kurosaka M. Stress fracture of the second metacarpal bone in a badminton player. Kobe J Med Sci. 2008;54(3):E159–62.
13. Balius R, Pedret C, Estruch A, Hernández G, Ruiz-Cotorro Á, Mota J. Stress fractures of the metacarpal bones in adolescent tennis players: a case series. Am J Sports Med. 2010;38(6): 1215–20.
14. Kollitz KM, Hammert WC, Vedder NB, Huang JI. Metacarpal fractures: treatment and complications. Hand. 2014;9(1):16–23.
15. Fullerton LR Jr, SNowdy HA. Femoral neck stress fractures. Am J Sports Med. 1988;18(4):365–77.
16. Boniotti V, Del EG, Fengoni E, Cerini R, Caudana R. Imaging of bone micro-injuries. Radiol Med. 2003;105(5–6):425–35.
17. Ostlie DK, Simons SM. Tarsal navicular stress fracture in a young athlete: case report with clinical, radiologic, and pathophysiologic correlations. The Journal of the American Board of Family Practice. 2001;14(5):381–5.
18. Umans HR, Kaye JJ. Longitudinal stress fractures of the tibia: diagnosis by magnetic resonance imaging. Skeletal radiology. 1996;25(4):319–24.
19. Howard RS, Conrad GR. Ice cream Scooper's hand. Report of an occupationally related stress fracture of the hand. Clin Nucl Med. 1992;17(9):721–3.
20. Fakharzadeh FF. Stress fracture of the finger in a bowler. J Hand Surg. 1989;14(2):241–3.
21. Hochholzer T, Schöffl VR. Epiphyseal fractures of the finger middle joints in young sport climbers. Wilderness Environ Med. 2005;16(3):139–42.

22. Chell J, Stevens K, Preston B, Davis TR. Bilateral fractures of the middle phalanx of the middle finger in an adolescent climber. Am J Sports Med. 1999;27(6):817–9.
23. Bärtschi N, Scheibler A, Schweizer A. Symptomatic epiphyseal sprains and stress fractures of the finger phalanges in adolescent sport climbers. Hand Surg Rehabil. 2019;38(4):251–6.
24. Sobel D, Constantin N, Or O. Climbing higher—common injuries in rock climbers. Harefuah. 2016;155(6):348–51.
25. Kwon SW, Hong SJ, Nho JH, Moon SI, Jung KJ. Physeal fracture in the wrist and hand due to stress injury in a child climber: a case report. Medicine. 2018;97(34)
26. Desaldeleer AS, Le Nen D. Bilateral fracture of the base of the middle phalanx in a climber: literature review and a case report. Orthop Traumatol Surg Res. 2016;102(3):409–11.
27. Schöffl I, Schöffl V. Epiphyseal stress fractures in the fingers of adolescents: biomechanics, pathomechanism, and risk factors. Eur J Sports Med. 2016;3(1)
28. Salter RB, Harris WR. Injuries involving the epiphyseal plate. JBJS. 1963;45(3):587–622.
29. Meyers RN, Potter MN, Hobbs S, Provance A. Finger stress fractures in youth elite rock climbers. Orthop J Sports Med. 2019;7(3_Suppl):2325967119S00065.
30. Garcia K, Jaramillo D, Rubesova E. Ultrasound evaluation of stress injuries and physiological adaptations in the fingers of adolescent competitive rock climbers. Pediatr Radiol. 2018;48(3):366–73.
31. Bayer T, Schöffl VR, Lenhart M, Herold T. Epiphyseal stress fractures of finger phalanges in adolescent climbing athletes: a 3.0-Tesla magnetic resonance imaging evaluation. Skelet Radiol. 2013;42(11):1521–5.
32. El-Sheikh Y, Lutter C, Schoeffl I, Schoeffl V, Flohe S. Surgical management of proximal interphalangeal joint repetitive stress epiphyseal fracture nonunion in elite sport climbers. J Hand Surg Am. 2018;43(6):572–e1.

Part VI

Stress Fractures in Sport: Lower Limb

Stress Fractures in Sport: Hip

24

Joshua D. Harris and Jessica T. Le

Learning Objectives

- To understand the patient presentation, including subjective history and objective physical examination, for patients with suspected stress-related bone injury around the hip.
- To understand the diagnostic imaging evaluation of patients with suspected stress fractures around the hip.
- To learn the classification of stress-related bone injuries around the hip.
- To accurately diagnose and treat patients with low- versus high-risk stress fracture.
- To understand the treatment outcomes of patients with stress-related bone injuries around the hip.

24.1 Femoral Neck Stress Fractures

24.1.1 Epidemiology

Stress fractures of the femoral neck are common injuries often related to overuse in athletes. These fractures account for approximately 5–11% of all stress fractures, making up about 50% of stress fractures of the femur [1–4]. Athletes who engage in sports with constant repetitive loading on the femur are at highest risk. This includes marathon runners, long-distance runners, basketball players, figure skaters and ballet dancers. Stress fractures of this type are also often seen in young military recruits.

Higher incidences of femoral neck stress fractures are reported in female athletes, often related to the female athlete triad of disordered eating, amenorrhea, and osteoporosis. RED-S (relative energy deficiency in sports) is a clinical syndrome that entails both significant health risks and performance problems, secondary to low energy availability. Low energy availability is the underlying theme of both RED-S and the Female Athlete Triad/Tetrad, and is the result of a simple imbalance between energy output (basal metabolism and sports/exercise/training) and input (caloric consumption) [5–7].

As opposed to the "Female Athlete Triad" (menstrual dysfunction, low bone mineral density, and low energy availability with or without eating disorder) and "Tetrad" (Triad plus endothelial dysfunction) syndromes, RED-S is applicable to both males and females. In women, low energy availability presents as menstrual irregularities: in men, this presents as low testosterone. These endocrinopathies are associated with decreased bone health and subsequent increased stress fracture risk [7]. Risk factors include female sex, smoking, alcohol use, low bone mineral density, sudden increase in training frequency and intensity, poor training, low baseline physical fitness, improper footwear, coxa vara alignment (femoral neck shaft angle <120°), and femoral acetabular impingement [1–14].

24.1.2 Classification

There are many systems used to classify stress fractures of the femoral neck, however one that is most clinically relevant is the Kaeding-Miller Classification [15]. This system utilizes both clinical and radiographic parameters for grading stress fracture severity. An advantage of this classification is its applicability to stress-related bone injuries of the femoral neck and shaft. The gradings of this classification system are:

- Grade I: Painless, asymptomatic. Stress response visible on imaging, without fracture line.
- Grade II: Symptomatic. Stress response visible on imaging, without fracture line.
- Grade III: Symptomatic. Non-displaced fracture line on imaging.

J. D. Harris (✉) · J. T. Le (✉)
Houston Methodist Orthopedics & Sports Medicine, Houston, TX, USA
e-mail: jle@houstonmethodist.org

G. A. J. Robertson, N. Maffulli (eds.), *Fractures in Sport*, https://doi.org/10.1007/978-3-030-72036-0_24

- Grade IV: Symptomatic. Displaced fracture line (>2 mm) on imaging.
- Grade V: Symptomatic. Non-union visible on imaging.

Another common classification is one described by Fullerton and Snowdy that is based on the anatomic location of the stress fracture on radiographic imaging. This classification has three types [16]:

- Type 1: tension-sided, nondisplaced;
- Type 2: compression-sided, nondisplaced;
- Type 3: displaced.

Provencher goes one step further adding an additional type to those mentioned by Fullerton & Snowdy: superior, incomplete tension-type [17].

The Blickenstaff and Morris classification also has three types that include [18]:

- Type 1: periosteal reaction or callus formation along the inferior femoral neck, without fracture line;
- Type 2: visible nondisplaced fracture line across the femoral neck or calcar;
- Type 3: complete displaced fracture.

Stress fractures of the femoral neck can also be classified simply as high risk or low risk based on their propensity to progress toward complete fractures, increasing the potential for further displacement, non-union, and avascular necrosis. High risk fractures are those that are tension-sided (superolateral), complete (from compression side to tension side), or displaced. Low risk fractures are those that are compression-sided (inferomedial) and/or non-displaced.

24.1.3 Diagnosis

A thorough history and physical examination is essential in the evaluation of athletes with stress fractures of the femoral neck. Patients with femoral neck stress fractures often present with the complaint of an insidious onset of pain, most commonly anteriorly, deep in the groin and hip. This pain may also be located in the anteromedial thigh or gluteal region, and sometimes radiates to the knee. History may reveal pain related to activity that is worse with weight-bearing and improves with rest. This pain often begins with the onset of weight-bearing, and continues to progress throughout training until it is over. The intensity of the pain will continue to increase as patients train through it, eventually limiting them from any further participation in activity. With continual stress to the fracture, the pain will begin to affect the patient in their regular daily activities, becoming more notable with rest. A "popping" or cracking" sensation may be reported with exercise, as the fracture completes or displaces [19]. Be sure to inquire about the patient's training regimen including information regarding activity frequency, duration, intensity, changes in form, or footwear. Patients often note a recent increase in various aspects of their training, such as to prepare for competition. Assess in detail the patient's dietary habits, caloric intake, and nutrition as well.

Physical exam findings for femoral neck stress fractures are often non-specific. Patients may have tenderness to palpation over the anterior aspect of the hip and in the inguinal area. Most consistently, pain is elicited at the extremes of hip range of motion, especially with internal rotation, which may mimic the physical examination findings of patients with Femoro- Acetabular Impingement (FAI) Syndrome [1]. Patients regularly present with an associated antalgic gait as well. All patients should undergo a thorough examination of the lower lumbar spine, pelvis, sacrum, lower extremities and contralateral hip, to ensure that other potential causes for the symptoms are not missed.

Plain radiographs are often the first imaging studies performed in the investigation of femoral neck stress fractures. An anteroposterior (AP) view of the pelvis and a cross-table lateral view are both indicated. If there is a high index of suspicion, then a supine AP pelvis is indicated, rather than a standing AP pelvis, due to the potential for fracture displacement. For this same reason, frog-leg laterals (or positional laterals, such as Dunn 45°, or Dunn 90°) are also contraindicated. Only about 15% of femoral neck stress fractures are seen on initial radiographs [10].

Magnetic resonance imaging (MRI) should be performed in all athletes with negative plain radiographs, if there is still a high suspicion of index of a femoral neck stress fracture. MRI is the preferred imaging study after plain radiographs, as it is more sensitive to detecting subtle changes in bone structure associated with the femoral neck stress fractures, such as changes in the periosteum and bone marrow edema [14]. Dual-energy X-ray absorptiometry (DEXA) should also be considered to assess the patient's bone mineral density (Fig. 24.1).

Laboratory analyses to assess stress-related bone injuries of the femur should include: comprehensive metabolic panel (especially for calcium), vitamin D, magnesium, phosphorus, endocrine and sex hormones, thyroid stimulating hormone (TSH), parathyroid hormone (PTH), estrogen, progesterone, gonadotropin releasing hormone (GnRH), follicle stimulating hormone (FSH), and luteinizing hormone (LH).

24.1.4 Treatment

Treatment of femoral neck stress fractures are dependent the location and stability of the fracture.

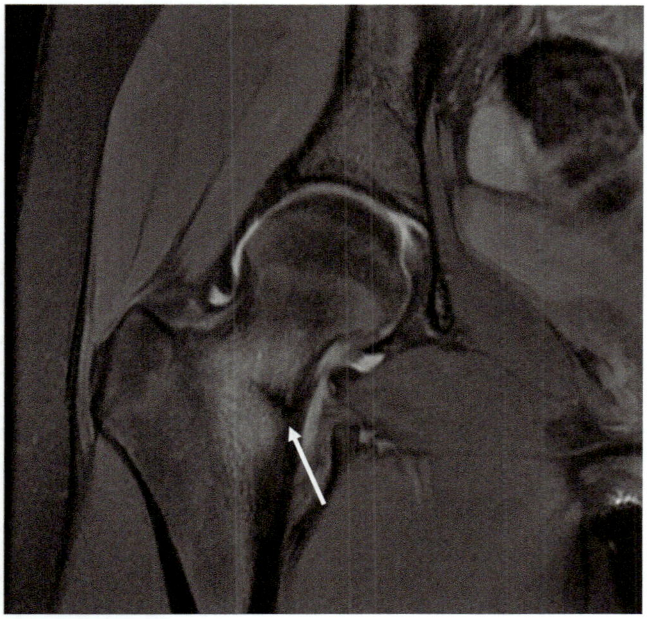

Fig. 24.1 15-Year-old female ballet dancer with a compression-sided femoral neck stress fracture. T2-weighted MRI

24.1.4.1 Non-Surgical Treatment

Compression-sided, non-displaced incomplete fractures of the femoral neck are treated non-surgically. This typically includes an initial 6 weeks of protective weight-bearing with crutch-assisted devices, after which they can slowly progress to full weight-bearing by 8–10 weeks post-diagnosis [1]. If after 6 weeks of protected weight-bearing, patients continue to have pain with axial loading, repeat imaging should be obtained. Any signs of non-union on plain films, such as persistent fracture lines with sclerotic ends, is an indication for surgical fixation.

24.1.4.2 Surgical Treatment

Indications for surgery in the presence of femoral neck stress fractures include:

- complete fractures, either tension-sided or compression-sided, with or without displacement;
- tension-sided incomplete fractures;
- displaced fractures;
- compression-sided incomplete fractures that have failed non-surgical treatment are also an indication for surgical fixation.

Compression-sided, non-displaced complete fractures should be treated with percutaneous cannulated hip screws or a sliding hip screw construct. Tension-sided, non-displaced complete fractures should be treated with a sliding hip screw construct [1]. All displaced fractures should undergo immediate anatomic reduction, followed by fixation with a sliding hip screw construct with or without a de-rotation screw, to limit rotation of the fracture (Table 24.1).

Table 24.1 Treatment of femoral neck stress fractures

Fracture type	Incomplete fracture	Complete fracture
Compression-sided	Conservative treatment, non-surgical	Surgical fixation – Cannulated screws – Sliding hip screw
Tension-sided	Surgical fixation – Sliding hip screw	Surgical fixation – Sliding hip screw
Displaced	–	Immediate reduction followed by surgical fixation – Sliding hip screw ± de-rotation screw

24.1.5 Complications

The rate of complications for femoral neck stress fractures is greatly dependent on the fracture type. Displaced fractures, which require surgical fixation, usually have a higher risk of developing complications.

Within the capsule surrounding the femoral neck lies the major blood supply to the femoral head—the lateral ascending vessels in the lateral synovial fold from the medial femoral circumflex artery. These vessels can be disrupted with displacement of femoral neck fractures increasing the risk for avascular necrosis (AVN) of the femoral head. Additionally, if the fracture disrupts the vessel(s) with subsequent hemarthrosis, the pressure in the joint can further compress these vessels, adding to the risk of AVN. The longer surgery is delayed in these patients, the higher the risk of AVN developing. Displaced femoral neck stress fractures should be taken to surgery as soon as possible, preferably within 12 h of displacement, if possible, to greatly reduce this risk.

As with other fractures, non-union, delayed union, and fixation failure are also potential complications. Non-union may appear as a persistent fracture line on plain radiographs with sclerotic ends. When fractures fail to reach bony union by 6 months after an injury, this is considered a delayed-union. Fixation failure often occurs due to either poor reduction or improper implant selection: taking the time to achieve appropriate anatomical reduction can help reduce this risk.

24.1.6 Rehabilitation

For patients undergoing non-surgical treatment, they may slowly progress from protective weight bearing at 6 weeks, to full weight bearing by 8–10 weeks post-diagnosis, as their pain allows. Following fixation of displaced fractures, it is recommended for patients to protect the reduction and fixation for a minimum of 6–8 weeks, by non-weight bearing with the use of crutch-assisted devices. They can then progress with 25% interval increases per week to full weight bearing by approximately 10–12 weeks [1, 19]. Once there is clear evidence of fracture union radiographically, and patients are pain free with normal daily activity, they may return to sports. This can be anywhere from 12–28 weeks post-injury [19].

24.1.7 Preventative Measures

When reviewing such patients, clinicians should assess patient nutrition at all visits, and ensure they have adequate caloric consumption for the intensity of their activities. Laboratory analyses (as above) should also be performed, if necessary. Patients should be educated on proper footwear to use for sports, and advised on appropriate progression in training regimens, to prevent them increasing their intensity too rapidly. Mental wellness screening is a vital adjunct to the management of patients with stress-related bone injuries, and this can be done with a variety of mental health practitioners, including psychiatry, psychology, and behavioural health.

24.2 Proximal Femur Stress Fractures

24.2.1 Epidemiology

Proximal femur stress fractures, more specifically in the subtrochanteric region, are generally found in a bimodal distribution, affecting both young active athletes and older adults on long-term bisphosphonate therapy. Athletes who engage in sports with constant repetitive loading on the femur are at highest risk. This includes marathon and ultramarathon runners, triathletes, military recruits, and ballet dancers.

Long-term bisphosphonate therapy (>5 years) in older adults has been shown to lead to impaired bone remodelling which subsequently results in the development of proximal femur stress fractures, with minimal to no trauma [20]. Higher incidences of proximal femur stress fractures are reported in female athletes, often related to the female athlete triad and RED-S.

24.2.2 Classification

The classification of risk in proximal femur fractures depends on patient demographics and location of the fracture. The Kaeding-Miller classification can be applied to this location (Table 24.2). Incomplete fractures on the medial cortex (calcar) of the femur are relatively low risk.

Table 24.2 Kaeding-Miller classification [15]

Grade	Radiographic findings	Pain
I	Stress response, without fracture line	–
II	Stress response, without fracture line	+
III	Fracture line, non-displaced	+
IV	Fracture line, displaced (>2 mm)	+
V	Non-union	+

Fractures of the lateral cortex are of moderate risk, due to the net tensile forces on the femur increasing the propensity for propagation and completion. Fractures in older adults on long-term bisphosphonate therapy, otherwise known as atypical femur fractures, are high risk. High risk fractures most commonly start on the lateral cortex, and due to the fragility of the bone, have a high propensity to propagate through to the medial cortex [21].

24.2.3 Diagnosis

A thorough history and physical examination is essential in the evaluation of athletes with potential stress fractures of the proximal femur. Patients with proximal femur stress fractures often complain of pain deep in the groin or the hip, much like with femoral neck stress fractures. Their pain is related to activity and worse with weight-bearing. While obtaining a full history, be sure to inquire about the patient's training habits and status, dietary habits, caloric intake, and nutrition.

Physical exam findings with proximal femur stress fractures are often non-specific. Patients may have tenderness to palpation over the anterior aspect of the hip and about the thigh. All patients should undergo a thorough examination of the lower lumbar spine, pelvis, sacrum, lower extremities and contralateral hip to ensure that other potential causes for the symptoms are not missed.

An anteroposterior (AP) view of the pelvis and a cross-table lateral view plain radiographs of the involved proximal femur should be obtained. With atypical femur stress fractures, localized periosteal or endosteal thickening of the lateral cortex or "beaking" is often noted. Fractures are often transverse or short oblique, and without comminution [21]. Films of the contralateral femur should always be obtained in patients on long-term bisphosphate therapy who are found to have a stress fracture. Up to 40% of patients with atypical femur fractures have bilateral involvement [22].

Magnetic resonance imaging (MRI) is the study of choice for delineating nondisplaced fractures or fractures that may not be initially apparent on plain radiographs. MRI is more sensitive to detecting subtle changes in bone structure, including bone marrow edema. Dual-energy X-ray absorptiometry (DEXA) should also be considered to assess patient bone density and help guide any preventative measures that should be taken for improving bone health and prevent future fractures.

Laboratory analyses to assess stress-related bone injuries of the femur should include: comprehensive metabolic panel (especially for calcium), vitamin D, magnesium, phosphorus, endocrine and sex hormones, thyroid stimulating hormone (TSH), parathyroid hormone (PTH), estrogen, progesterone, gonadotropin releasing hormone (GnRH), follicle stimulating hormone (FSH), and luteinizing hormone (LH).

24.2.4 Treatment

Treatment of proximal femur stress fractures is highly dependent on the patient, fracture stability, and location of the fracture. In young athletes, non-displaced stress fractures often do well with non-surgical treatment, consisting of protective weight-bearing with crutch-assisted devices, and gradual progression back to full-weight bearing over a period of 10–12 weeks. Older adults, who are found to have atypical proximal femur stress fractures, whether displaced or not, should be treated with an intramedullary nail. Prophylactic treatment of non-displaced fractures is important, due to the high incidence of future displacement in patients on bisphosphonate therapy.

24.2.5 Complications

Non-union and delayed union are both potential complications with proximal femur stress fractures. Atypical femur fractures have an increased risk of complication due the impaired bone remodelling that may result from bisphosphonate use. Non-union may appear as a persistent fracture line on plain radiographs with sclerotic ends. When fractures fail to reach bony union by 6 months after an injury, this is considered a delayed-union. Optimizing patient bone health with a thorough review of labs and medications will also help reduce the risk of complications.

24.2.6 Rehabilitation

For patients undergoing non-surgical treatment, they may slowly progress from protective weight bearing at 6 weeks, to full weight bearing as their pain allows by 10–12 weeks post-diagnosis. Following surgical treatment with intramedullary nail, with stabilization of the stress fracture, patients may weight bear as tolerated immediately after surgery.

24.2.7 Preventative Measures

When reviewing such patients, clinicians should assess patient nutrition at all visits, and ensure they have adequate caloric consumption for the intensity of their activities. Laboratory analyses (as above) should also be performed, if necessary. Patients should be educated on proper footwear to use for sports, and advised on appropriate progression in training regimens, to prevent them increasing their intensity too rapidly. Clinicians should always maintain a high index of suspicion for atypical stress fractures in patients on bisphosphonate therapy, presenting with hip and thigh pain.

24.3 Femoral Diaphyseal (Shaft) Stress Fractures

24.3.1 Epidemiology

Stress fractures of the femoral shaft most commonly occur in the proximal third of the femur. However, they can also occur in the mid-third or distal-third [23]. Femoral shaft stress fractures account for 3.5–7% of all athletic-related stress fractures [23–25]. Athletes who engage in activities with constant repetitive loading on the femur are at highest risk. This includes, but is not limited to, marathon and ultramarathon runners, triathletes, soccer players, gymnasts, and ballet dancers. Higher incidences of femoral shaft stress fractures are reported in female athletes, often related to the female athlete triad and RED-S. Risk factors include female sex, smoking, alcohol use, low bone mineral density, sudden increase in training frequency and intensity, poor training and improper footwear.

24.3.2 Classification

Femoral shaft stress fractures are generally classified as low risk fractures. These fractures tend to be on the medial (compression) side of the femur and have a low propensity for propagation and non-union [2]. The Kaeding-Miller classification is greatly applicable to stress-related bone injuries of the femoral shaft [15]. It includes both clinical and radiographic parameters for grading stress fracture severity. The gradings of this classification system are listed in Table 24.2.

24.3.3 Diagnosis

Assessing for femoral shaft stress fractures requires a high degree of suspicion. A detailed history, thorough physical exam, and imaging studies should be performed for confirmation. Up to 75% of these injuries may be missed on initial examination, if the diagnosis is not considered [24].

Patients with femoral shaft stress fractures often present with complaints of an insidious, vague, poorly localized thigh pain [23]. They may also have diffuse tenderness surrounding the thigh, without any history of trauma. Stress fractures of the femur generally have no effect on hip or knee range of motion. Pain is related to activity, worse with weight-bearing, and improves with rest. Initially, the pain may be thought to be from a muscle strain or tear. However, the intensity of pain will continue to increase, limiting patients from further participation in activity, affecting their regular daily activities, and becoming more notable with rest. Proximal femoral diaphyseal stress fractures are often also associated with an antalgic gait. Clinicians should inquire about the patient's training regimen (frequency, duration, intensity, changes in form, footwear, or running surface). Any recent sudden changes in training should lead to a strong suspicion for stress fracture. It is also important to inquire in detail about the patient's dietary habits, caloric intake, and nutrition.

Physical exam findings with femoral shaft stress fractures can often be non-specific. Patients may have tenderness about the thigh. Swelling is often absent due to the bulk of soft tissue surrounding the femur [25, 26]. A special test that is useful for helping to localize the stress fracture is the Fulcrum Test [23, 26, 27]. For this test, the patient is seated on the examination table with legs dangling off the edge. The examiner's arm is then used as a fulcrum under the thigh, and is moved distal to proximal along the thigh, as a gentle pressure is applied to the dorsal aspect of the knee with the opposite hand. At the point of fulcrum under the stress fracture, gentle pressure on the knee produces increased discomfort, which is described by the patient as a sharp pain and is usually accompanied by apprehension.

Plain radiographs are often performed first when evaluating for stress fractures of the femoral shaft. Anteroposterior (AP) and lateral views of the femur, hip, and knee should be included in the evaluation. When performed at the time of onset of symptoms, plain radiographs are only positive in about 30–70% of cases [23, 26].

Magnetic resonance imaging (MRI) can be performed if plain radiographs are negative and there is still a high suspicion for stress fracture. MRI is more sensitive in detecting early changes in bone structure, such as bone marrow edema.

Dual-energy X-ray absorptiometry (DEXA) should also be considered to assess patient bone mineral density. For every reduction of 1 standard deviation of femoral bone mineral density, patients are 2.6 times more likely to sustain a femoral shaft stress fracture [28] (Fig. 24.2a, b).

Laboratory analyses to assess stress-related bone injuries of the femur should include: comprehensive metabolic panel (especially for calcium), vitamin D, magnesium, phosphorus, endocrine and sex hormones, thyroid stimulating hormone (TSH), parathyroid hormone (PTH), estrogen, progesterone, gonadotropin releasing hormone (GnRH), follicle stimulating hormone (FSH), and luteinizing hormone (LH).

24.3.4 Treatment

Stress fractures of the femoral shaft are often managed successfully with non-surgical treatment, rarely requiring surgery. Non-displaced fractures of the femoral shaft, without evidence of complete cortical disruption, are best treated with protected weight-bearing and activity modification. Patients may initially get around with the assistance of gait assistive devices (e.g. crutches) to allow for pain-free ambulation for the first 6 weeks after diagnosis, then progressively discontinue their use as tolerated over the following 2–4 weeks.

Surgical fixation is warranted for completed or displaced fractures. It is also recommended as prophylactic treatment in patients with low bone density or over the age of 60. In such cases, where surgical fixation is indicated, an intramedullary nail should be used. With surgical fixation, patients may weight bear as tolerated immediately after surgery.

24.3.5 Complications

Non-union and delayed union are potential complications with femoral shaft stress fractures. Non-union may appear as a persistent fracture line on plain radiographs with sclerotic ends. When fractures fail to reach bony union by 6 months after an injury, this is considered a delayed-union. Optimizing patient bone health with a thorough review of laboratory analyses and medications will also help reduce the risk of complications.

24.3.6 Rehabilitation

Rehabilitation and return to exercise after femoral shaft stress fractures is guided by the patient's symptoms, and should be performed when the patient is pain-free with activity. Cross-training, with low-impact activities such as swimming or cycling, may be allowed early in the schedule, at the discretion of the provider, to maintain general conditioning. Patients may then gradually return to their sport after their injury, when they have no pain with weight-bearing during normal activity.

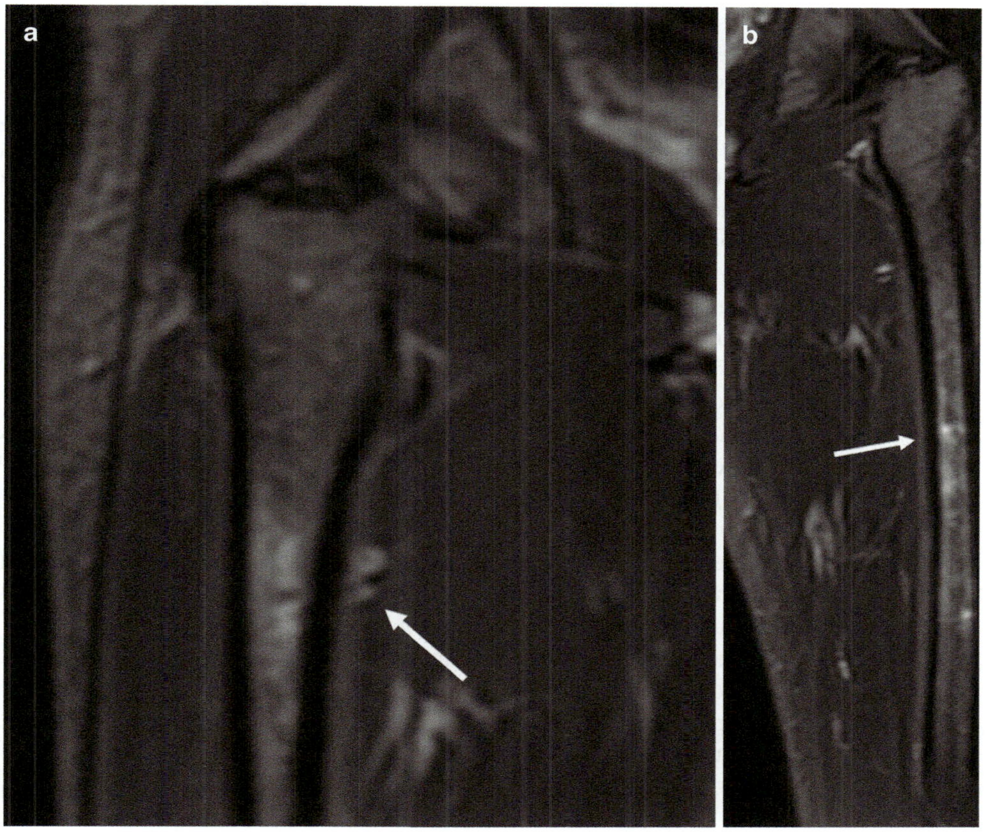

Fig. 24.2 (a) 40-Year-old female marathon runner found to have bilateral femoral shaft stress fractures. Proximal Femoral Shaft. T2-weighted MRI. (b) 40-Year-old female marathon runner found to have bilateral femoral shaft stress fractures. Mid-shaft Femur. T2-weighted MRI

24.3.7 Preventative Measures

When reviewing such patients, clinicians should assess patient nutrition at all visits, and ensure they have adequate caloric consumption for the intensity of their activities. Laboratory analyses (as above) should also be performed, if necessary. Patients should be educated on proper footwear to use for sports, and advised on appropriate progression in training regimens, to prevent them increasing their intensity too rapidly.

Clinical Pearls

- Vague, poorly localized pain to the hip and thigh in an athlete with negative plain radiographs does not exclude stress fractures from the diagnosis. A high index of suspicion for stress-related bone injury is required. Evaluate with more sensitive imaging such as MRI.
- High-risk stress fractures generally require surgical fixation, while low-risk stress fractures generally do well with non-surgical management.
- Stress fractures are frequently a multi-system problem, associated with relative energy deficiency in sports (RED-S): key areas to consider include bone health, menstrual function, growth and development, endocrine, metabolic, immunologic, gastrointestinal, cardiovascular, psychological, and hematologic systems.

Review

Questions

1. A 22-year-old female collegiate cross-country runner has deep anterior groin pain at the start of her senior season. She is running about 85 miles per week. Her body mass index is 16.9 kg/m^2. The pain occurs a few steps into each run, progressively gets worse with time and distance, and has recently caused her to stop runs before their scheduled end. She has no previous history of stress fracture. She states that her diet is "normal". The first meet of the season is in 4 days. The next appropriate step in management is:
   (a) Oral anti-inflammatory medications, continue running
   (b) Intra-articular corticosteroid hip injection, continue running
   (c) Physical therapy, continue running
   (d) Plain radiographs
   (e) Magnetic resonance imaging
2. A 44-year-old female recreational competitive marathon runner has vague mid-thigh pain with running. She is scheduled to run the Boston Marathon in two and a half months. She has recently joined a new running group,

started running in new carbon fiber plate shoes, with a goal time of a personal best below 3 h. She has had a fifth metatarsal stress fracture before in the past. Her body mass index is 17.5 kg/m^2. Her physical exam reveals no significant abnormalities. Plain radiographs of the hip and femur reveal no fracture. MRI revealed a stress response, without a fracture line, in the proximal third of the femoral shaft. The next appropriate step in management is:

(a) Increase calcium and Vitamin D intake, continue running and training
(b) Immediate femoral intramedullary nail, resume running in 1–2 weeks following surgery
(c) Immediate femoral dynamic compression plate, resume running in 1–2 weeks following surgery
(d) Non-surgical treatment, crutch-assisted protected weight-bearing for 6 weeks, withdraw from the marathon
(e) Non-surgical treatment, crutch-assisted protected weight-bearing for 6 weeks, resume training in 6–8 weeks and run the marathon
(f) Non-surgical treatment, change back to her previous running shoes, do not run in carbon fiber plate shoes, continue running but reduce mileage to 30 miles per week, run the marathon

Answers

1. (d)—Plain radiographs are often the first imaging studies performed in the investigation of stress fractures. Magnetic resonance imaging (MRI) should be performed if plain radiographs come back negative and there is still a high suspicion of fracture. MRI is more sensitive in detecting subtle changes in bone structure associated with stress fractures, such as changes in the periosteum and bone edema. It is not recommended for athletes to continue training if there is any suspicion of a stress fracture.
2. (d)—Non-displaced fractures of the femoral shaft without evidence of complete cortical disruption do well with protected weight-bearing and activity modification. It is recommended that this patient uses crutch-assisted weight-bearing for 6 weeks, then progressively discontinue their use as tolerated over 2–4 weeks. She may gradually return to running after she has no pain with weight-bearing during normal activity, however should take great caution in increasing the intensity too soon. She should withdraw from the upcoming marathon.

References

1. Harris JD, Chahal J. Femoral neck stress fractures. Oper Tech Sports Med. 2015;23(3):241–7.
2. Fredericson M, Jennings F, Beaulieu C, Matheson GO. Stress fractures in athletes. Top Magn Reson Imaging. 2006;17(5):309–25.
3. Behrens SB, Deren ME, Matson A, Fadale PD, Monchik KO. Stress fractures of the pelvis and legs in athletes: a review. Sports Health. 2013;5:165–74.
4. Carpintero P, Leon F, Zafra M, Serrano-Trenas JA, Román M. Stress fractures of the femoral neck and coxa vara. Arch Orthop Trauma Surg. 2003;123(6):273–7.
5. Civil R, Lamb A, Loosmore D, Ross L, Livingstone K, Strachan K, et al. Assessment of dietary intake, energy status, and factors associated with RED-S in vocational female ballet students. Front Nutr. 2018;5:136.
6. Keay N, Francis G, Hind K. Low energy availability assessed by a sport-specific questionnaire and clinical interview indicative of bone health, endocrine profile and cycling performance in competitive male cyclists. BMJ Open Sport Exerc Med. 2018;4(1):e000424.
7. Torstveit MK, Fahrenholtz IL, Lichtenstein MB, Stenqvist TB, Melin AK. Exercise dependence, eating disorder symptoms and biomarkers of Relative Energy Deficiency in Sports (RED-S) among male endurance athletes. BMJ Open Sport Exerc Med. 2019;5(1):e000439.
8. Egol KA, Koval KJ, Kummer F, Frankel VH. Stress fractures of the femoral neck. Clin Orthop Relat Res. 1998;348:72–8.
9. Devas MB. Stress fractures of the femoral neck. J Bone Joint Surg Br. 1965;47(4):728–38.
10. Maffulli N, Longo UG, Denaro V. Femoral neck stress fractures. Oper Tech Sports Med. 2009;17(2):90–3.
11. Joshi A, Kc BR, Shah BC, Chand P, Thapa BB, Kayastha N. Femoral neck stress fractures in military personnel. JNMA J Nepal Med Assoc. 2009;48(174):99–102.
12. Kupferer KR, Bush DM, Cornell JE, Lawrence VA, Alexander JL, Ramos RG, et al. Femoral neck stress fracture in Air Force basic trainees. Mil Med. 2014;179(1):56–61.
13. Neubauer T, Brand J, Lidder S, Krawany M. Stress fractures of the femoral neck in runners: a review. Res Sports Med. 2016;24(3):185–99.
14. Chalupa RL, Rivera JC, Tennent DJ, Johnson AE. Correlation between femoral neck shaft angle and surgical management in trainees with femoral neck stress fractures. US Army Med Dep J. 2016:1–5.
15. Kaeding CC, Miller TL. The comprehensive description of stress fractures: a new classification system. J Bone Joint Surg Am. 2013;95:1214–20.
16. Fullerton LR Jr, Snowdy HA. Femoral neck stress fractures. Am J Sports Med. 1988;16:365–77.
17. Provencher MT, Baldwin AJ, Gorman JD, Gould MT, Shin AY. Atypical tensile-sided femoral neck stress fractures: the value of magnetic resonance imaging. Am J Sports Med. 2004;32(6):1528–34.
18. Blickenstaff LD, Morris JM. Fatigue fracture of the femoral neck. J Bone Joint Surg Am. 1966;48(6):1031–47.
19. Robertson GA, Wood AM. Femoral neck stress fractures in sport: a current concepts review. Sports Med Int Open. 2017;1(2):E58–68.

20. Kwek EB, Goh SK, Koh JS, Png MA, Howe TS. An emerging pattern of subtrochanteric stress fractures: a long-term complication of alendronate therapy? Injury. 2008;39(2):224–31.
21. Phillips HK, Harrison SJ, Akrawi H, Sidhom SA. Retrospective review of patients with atypical bisphosphonate related proximal femoral fractures. Injury. 2017;48(6):1159–64.
22. Larsen MS, Schmal H. The enigma of atypical femoral fractures: a summary of current knowledge. EFORT Open Rev. 2018;3(9):494–500.
23. Ivkovic A, Bojanic I, Pecina M. Stress fractures of the femoral shaft in athletes: a new treatment algorithm. Br J Sports Med. 2006;40(6):518–20.
24. DeFranco MJ, Recht M, Schils J, Parker RD. Stress fractures of the femur in athletes. Clin Sports Med. 2006;25(1):89–103.
25. Kang L, Belcher D, Hulstyn M. Stress fractures of the femoral shaft in women's college lacrosse: a report of seven cases and a review of the literature. Br J Sports Med. 2005;39(12):902–6.
26. Matheson GO, Clement DB, McKenzie DC, Taunton JE, Lloyd-Smith DR, MacIntyre JG. Stress fractures in athletes: a study of 320 cases. Am J Sports Med. 1987;15 46–58.
27. Boden BP, Osbahr DC, Jimenez C. Low-risk stress fractures. Am J Sports Med. 2001;29(1):100–11.
28. Marshall D, Johnell O, Wedel H. Meta-analysis of how well measures of bone mineral density predict occurrence of osteoporotic fractures. Br Med J. 1996;312:1254–9.

Stress Fractures in Sport: Knee

25

Grace C. Plassche, Stephanie C. Petterson, and Kevin D. Plancher

Stress fractures are common injuries in the active population, with an incidence reaching 20% in athletes and military recruits [1]. The injury often results from repetitive impact stresses which exceed the remodeling capabilities of the bone itself. Two types of stress fractures are classically described: fatigue fractures and insufficiency fractures. Fatigue fractures, more common in younger and more active individuals, often result from a sudden increase in training intensity (e.g. increased weekly running mileage). In contrast, insufficiency fractures arise from an already weakened bone (e.g. osteopenia) undergoing normal stresses [1, 2]. Other predisposing factors include older age, rheumatoid arthritis, and various medications (e.g. corticosteroids) [3].

25.1 Distal Femur Stress Fractures

25.1.1 Epidemiology

The incidence of femoral stress fractures ranges from 2.8% to 33.3% [1, 2, 4]. These rates include femoral neck and shaft fractures as well as supracondylar, condylar, and subchondral stress fractures. Femoral neck stress fractures are the most common among these types, accounting for 50% of all femoral stress fractures and 3% of all stress fractures diagnosed in athletes (Fig. 25.1) [5, 6]. In comparison, the incidence and epidemiology of femoral shaft stress fractures are not well defined. Distal femoral stress fractures are more common across the active military, accounting for 51% of femoral stress fractures in this population [1, 7–10]. Niva et al. further classified specific incidence rates within military recruits; the most common stress fracture location was the condylar area (24%), followed by the subcondylar area (3%), and the distal shaft (0.5%) [10]. The true incidence rate of distal femur stress fractures is largely unknown in athletes given the variety of differential diagnoses related to knee pain, which results in underdiagnosis.

The prevalence of distal femur stress fractures is potentially associated with gender. The literature suggests a higher incidence of femoral stress fractures in female compared to male athletes (12.2% vs. 4.4%), a likely effect of the female athlete triad [2, 7, 9]. A combination of low energy availability (which can arise from an eating disorder), menstrual dysfunction (oligomenorrhea or amenorrhea), and low bone mineral density may predispose females to these injuries [1, 2, 4–10]. However, results are inconsistent [8].

25.1.2 Classification

Distal femur stress fractures are considered low-risk stress fractures. Displacement is unlikely, and these injuries occur on the compression side of the bone, thus resulting in a promising natural outcome once diagnosed [11]. As previously mentioned, in athletes and active military recruits, distal femur stress fractures are most commonly classified as fatigue fractures rather than insufficiency fractures. These are largely the result of an abrupt increase in training intensity [10, 12].

Stress fractures can be classified according to their radiographic appearance. While specific classification systems have been developed for femoral neck stress fractures (e.g. Naval Medical Center in San Diego Classification), there is no site-specific classification system for distal femur stress fractures [1, 13]. Several general stress fracture classification systems exist, though the accuracy of these systems is ques-

G. C. Plassche · S. C. Petterson
Orthopaedic Foundation, Stamford, CT, USA
e-mail: gplassche@ofals.org; spetterson@ofals.org

K. D. Plancher (✉)
Orthopaedic Foundation, Stamford, CT, USA

Department of Orthopaedic Surgery, Montefiore Medical Center/Albert Einstein College of Medicine, Bronx, NY, USA

Department of Orthopaedic Surgery, Weill Cornell Medical College, New York, NY, USA

Plancher Orthopaedics & Sports Medicine, New York, NY, USA
e-mail: kplancher@plancherortho.com

G. A. J. Robertson, N. Maffulli (eds.), *Fractures in Sport*, https://doi.org/10.1007/978-3-030-72036-0_25

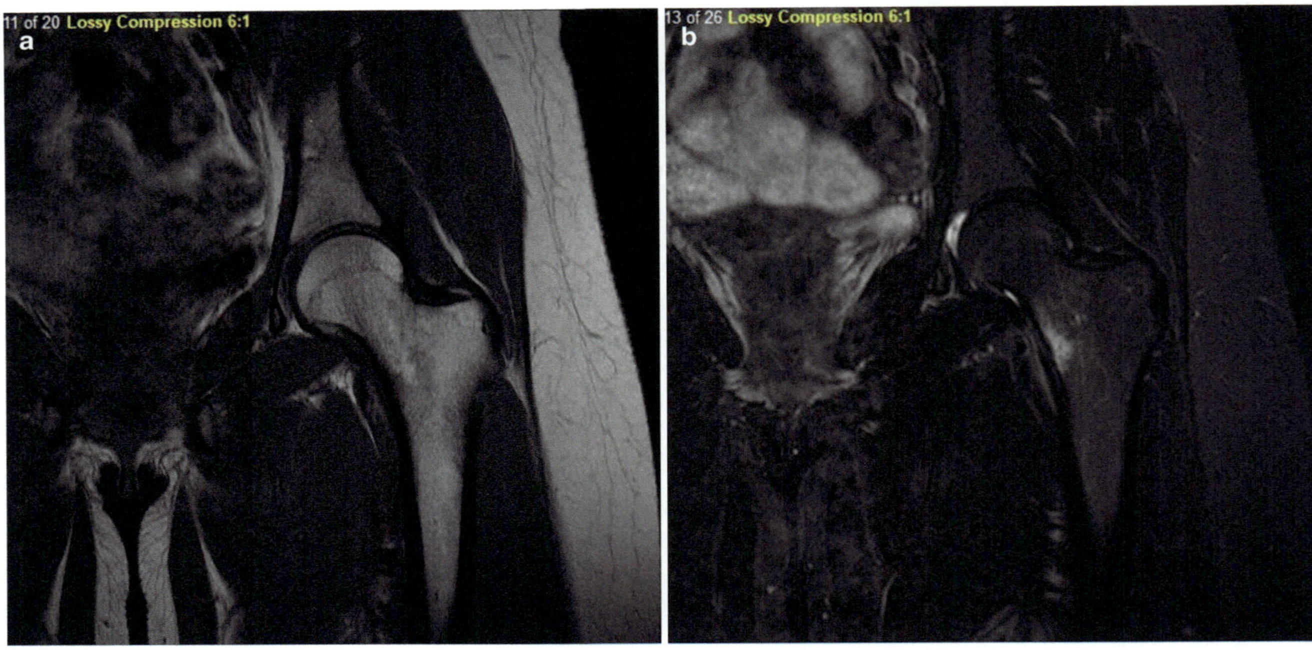

Fig. 25.1 19-year-old female with a left femoral neck stress fracture as seen on (**a**) T1-weighted MRI and (**b**) STIR MRI

Table 25.1 Classification System for Stress Fractures & Recommended Treatment

Grade	Radiograph Findings	MRI Findings	Recommended Treatment
1	Normal	Positive STIR image	3 weeks rest
2	Normal	Positive STIR, plus positive T2-weighted	3–6 weeks rest
3	Periosteal reaction	Positive T1- and T2-weighted, STIR without definite cortical break visualized	12–16 weeks rest
4	Injury or periosteal reaction	Positive injury line on T1- or T2-weighted scans	>16 weeks rest

tionable [13, 14]. One example combines both radiographic and magnetic resonance imaging (MRI) findings to guide physicians in their management (Table 25.1) [14, 15].

Although there is no universally accepted classification system for stress fractures, it is important to understand the implication of low risk versus high risk, fatigue versus insufficiency, and relevant grading with images [16]. These components must be factored into the treatment planning process upon diagnosis of a distal femur stress fracture.

25.1.3 Diagnosis

Misdiagnosis in initial evaluation occurs in up to 75% of all femoral stress fractures [1]. When stress fractures occur in the distal femur, their proximity to the knee joint can confound diagnosis, as several inflammatory, infectious, vascular, tumorous, and exertional pathologies of the soft tissue present with similar symptoms (Table 25.2) [10].

Table. 25.2 Differential Diagnoses for Distal Femur Stress Fractures

Femoral condyle avascular necrosis
Infection
Muscle strain
Knee arthritis (degenerative or inflammatory)
Patellofemoral pain syndrome
Plica syndrome
Neoplasm

25.1.3.1 History

Training history can raise suspicion for distal femur stress fractures and may aid in confirming the diagnosis when combined with physical examination and radiologic imaging (Table 25.3). Patients often report a sudden increase in training load over a very short period of time [1, 17]. Pain patterns can also aid in diagnosis. Patients with a distal femur stress fracture often report gradual onset of knee pain that worsens with activity and improves with rest. They may complain of an aching pain at night and, in the case of a condylar stress fracture, pain will be more focal at the knee, rather than a vague, diffuse pain along the thigh [17].

25.1.3.2 Physical Examination

Following a comprehensive review of the patient's history, a thorough physical examination is necessary to diagnose a distal femur stress fracture. With the primary focus on

Table 25.3 Risk Factors for Stress Fractures

Exercise Regimen • Prior levels of training • Abrupt increases in intensity/duration
Diet • Often lacking in vitamin D and calcium intake
Abnormal Metabolic Processes • Osteopenia, diabetes mellitus, Ricketts • More of a concern with insufficiency fractures
Menstrual Cycle Irregularities • Less of a concern with distal femur stress fractures

location of pain, a healthcare provider should begin with palpation. In contrast to deep femoral shaft stress fractures, distal supracondylar and condylar areas are subcutaneous, thus allowing for identification focal points of tenderness [1]. Swelling and erythema are often absent with these fractures [1, 18].

Passive and active knee range of motion will likely be painful or limited in flexion and extension. The Apley's Grind test, which uses compression and external rotation of the tibia against the knee joint, may be positive (i.e. produce pain), which may indicate concomitant meniscal pathology. Functional hop testing can also be used to reproduce repetitive inciting loads. The patient should be asked to hop on the affected leg in place to determine pain location. This test has proven confirmatory findings in nearly 70% of athletes with femoral stress fractures [1]. Specific to stress fractures of the supracondylar region, patients should also be observed for valgus or varus malalignment. Valgus limb alignment and the opposing forces of the medial collateral ligament and adductor muscles can cause stress fractures in the posteromedial cortex on the tension side of the femoral supracondylar region [10].

25.1.3.3 Imaging Investigations

Various modes of imaging are often necessary when diagnosing any type of stress fractures, as relevant symptoms can often be contributed to concomitant soft tissue conditions. Plain radiographs, the first imaging modality of choice, often appear normal until several weeks after the onset of pain [18]. Nondisplaced stress fractures of the distal femur are extremely difficult to identify on plain radiographs, and in the adolescent athletes they may present as a nondisplaced Salter-Harris fracture [1, 9]. These injuries occur at the relatively weak, cartilaginous growth plates at the distal end of the femur, often leading to inconclusive radiographic findings. For distal femur stress fractures, plain radiography may evidence radiolucency, cortical disruption, periosteal reaction, or early callus formation; however, the latter two are not present until at least 10 days after injury [10, 18]. Although these findings may indicate a distal femur stress fracture, a normal radiograph does not rule out the diagnosis.

Nuclear scintigraphy (i.e. technetium bone scans) may provide a helpful secondary imaging method in addition to radiographs. Radiotracer uptake is seen in areas of increased bony remodeling. Despite lacking specificity, bone scans are highly sensitive and can detect change in bone metabolic activity within first 72 hours of injury [1]. However, many conditions, such as osteogenic tumors, also cause increased bone cellular metabolic activity, potentially resulting in false positives as the radiotracer is taken up in these areas as well [1, 9]. Given the lack of specificity, bone scans cannot diagnose a stress fracture without additional reason for suspicion.

Magnetic resonance imaging (MRI) is considered the single most complete mode of imaging to diagnose stress fractures given the high specificity and the absence of radiation exposure compared to bone scans [11] and is the most commonly used mode of imaging for grading stress fractures [13]. MRI allows to visualize the surrounding soft tissue in conjunction with bony remodeling associated with stress fractures (Fig. 25.3). Additionally, fat bone marrow suppression can enhance early detection of endosteal bone marrow edema, specifically in insufficiency fractures of the femur [3, 16].

Ultrasound imaging can also be used to aid in the visualization of stress fractures with advantages of ease of use, accessibility in an outpatient setting, and the lack of radiation exposure [19].

25.1.4 Treatment and Rehabilitation

Nonoperative management is the first line of treatment for distal femur stress fractures given their low risk for displacement (Table 25.4) [1, 9]. Reduction in activity to avoid provocation of symptoms and allow for bone healing is vital. For the athlete, it is often important to maintain cardiovascular conditioning and strength during this period. Alternative low impact activities such as cycling, swimming, and elliptical training are recommended. Once callus formation is visualized on repeat imaging, approximately 6–8 weeks following diagnosis, a gradual return to impact activity can be implemented with return to normal activities by 8–12 weeks. Frequency, intensity, and duration of activities is closely monitored and progressed until pre-injury levels are reached to avoid any provocation of symptoms [9]. If non-operative management fails, internal fixation should be considered [1].

25.1.5 Complications

As the mode of treatment for distal femur stress fractures is often non-operative, complications are also rare. If vigorous activity is continued, the fracture may progress to displacement, malunion, or nonunion. Stress fractures of the femoral

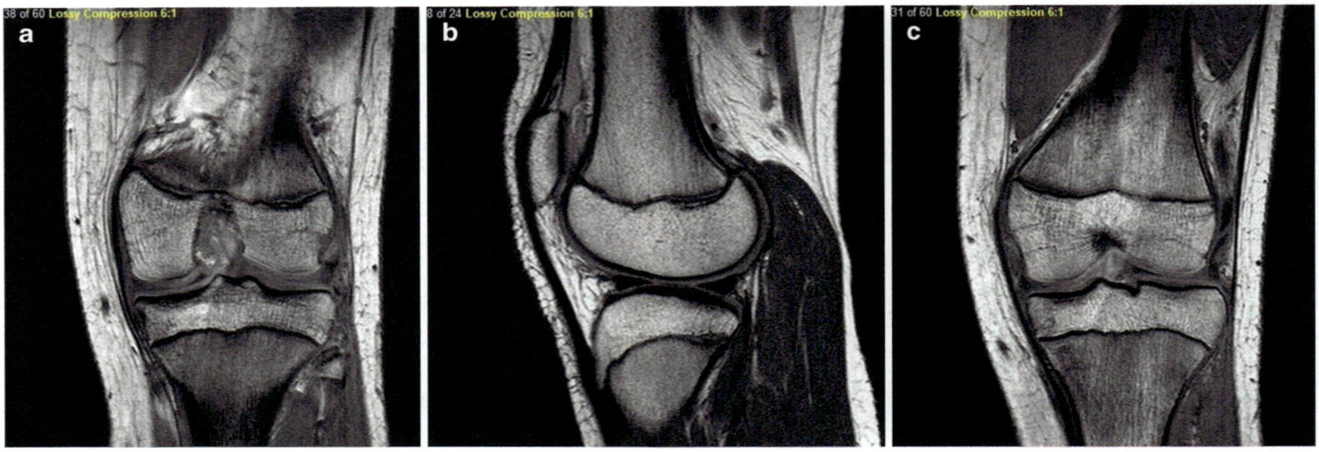

Fig. 25.3 13-year-old female athlete presenting with nondisplaced (**a**, **b**) posterior lateral distal femoral metaphysis stress fracture and (**c**) medial proximal tibial metaphysis stress fracture

Table 25.4 Non-Operative Treatment of Distal Femur Stress Fratures

Modify activity to pain free level
• 4–6 weeks depending on injury severity
Unloader braces to decrease stress on condylar stress fractures
• 6–8 weeks
Long leg cast immobilisation and crutches
• If fracture is greater than 50% the width of the bone
Resume low impact activities upon callus formation
• 6–8 weeks following diagnosis
Return to sports
• 8–12 weeks
• Must have no tenderness to palpation
Plain radiographs can be used to monitor healing
• Callus formation

condyles affect much of the surrounding tissue and cartilage; as a result, osteonecrosis and arthritic changes may arise if not given adequate time to heal [1]. If knee pain persists even with activity modification, alternative diagnoses should be considered to rule out any concomitant pathology.

25.1.6 Preventative Measures

Considering the rarity of distal femur stress fractures, specific preventative measures are not indicated. Therefore, athletes and their healthcare providers should focus on decreasing the relevant risk factors for all stress fractures. These include avoiding abrupt increases in training, allowing sufficient recovery time following large training loads, and ensuring proper nutrition with a diet rich in calcium and vitamin D. Despite variation in the thresholds designating vitamin D deficiency or insufficiency, recent studies agree on a recommended minimum vitamin D serum level of 40 ng/mL to safely prevent stress fractures in athletes. Vitamin D levels less than 20 ng/mL have been associated with a significantly higher risk of stress fractures when compared to athletes with levels greater than 40 ng/mL [20–22]. These serum levels can aid in guiding supplementation for athletes if a vitamin D deficiency or insufficiency is suspected. In a 2008 study of female military recruits, a regimen of 800 IU/day of vitamin D supplemented with 2000 mg of calcium resulted in a 20% lower incidence of stress fractures in comparison to a control group [23]. In the past decade, this dosage has become the accepted baseline level for prevention of stress fractures. In athletes, the vitamin D dosage increases to 2000–4000 IU/day, as these increased levels aid in recovery following eccentric exercises [21]. Furthermore, the higher range of these recommendations are often required for athletes who are experiencing low serum levels in combination with a lack of access to environmental sources of vitamin D, such as sunlight [22–24]. The ultimate goal of any supplementation is to maintain the athlete's vitamin D level above 40 ng/mL, and thus will be personalized to their specific needs.

Proper education, particularly in young female athletes is important. Education should be focused on the female athlete triad and warning signs that may indicate a trend towards insufficient bone mineral density, menstrual dysfunction, or insufficient energy intake [1]. Even when controlling for all of these variables, distal femur stress fractures can occur as a result of other factors such as alignment or specific training errors that are difficult to prevent. The mode of injury contributes to the injury's rarity, and further highlights the importance of diagnosing and treating distal femur stress fractures correctly.

25.2 Patella Stress Fractures

25.2.1 Epidemiology

Patella stress fractures are extremely rare, accounting for less than 1% of all stress fractures. First described by Devas in 1960, since then less than 40 case reports have been published on the topic [25–32]. When considering athletes specifically, the likelihood of a sports medicine healthcare provider diagnosing a patella stress fracture falls to 0.02% [25]. Of note, patients with cerebral palsy inordinately suffer from patella stress fractures. The characteristic crouched gait recruits a quadriceps muscle force that proves to be too large for the patella, thus causing a fatigue stress fracture from repetitive loads [25, 26]. Patients with cerebral palsy are also at risk for patellar insufficiency fractures; osteoporosis is not uncommon in these patients, as it often results from prolonged anti-seizure medication use [25].

The incidence of patella stress fractures is greater in male athletes and is almost always unilateral; only five bilateral cases have been detailed in the literature [28, 33–36]. Patella stress fractures may also be seen in athletes following an anterior cruciate ligament (ACL) reconstruction. These fractures are typically insufficiency fractures, as weakening occurs at the bone plug defect following harvest of a bone-patellar tendon-bone (BPTB) autograft [25, 37]. Furthermore, postoperative knee flexion contractures can increase stresses beyond the point the patella can withstand.

25.2.2 Classification

High-risk patella stress fractures are nearly always classified as fatigue fractures. Increased training intensity can result in repetitive tensile forces from the quadriceps muscle and patella tendon, with consequent overload on the patella [25]. The direction of the fracture, transverse versus longitudinal, is often dictated by the activity demand. Transverse patella stress fractures are more common in basketball and soccer players from sudden, forceful, compressive muscle contractions with repetitive jumping and loading [25]. Longitudinal patella stress fractures, on the other hand, are more common in long distance runners as a result of frequent repetitive, vertical stresses [25, 32]. Injury mechanism, fracture location, fracture pattern, and fracture progression can also help to classify these fractures (Table 25.5) [25, 28, 29, 31].

Radiographs and MRI findings can be used to grade patella stress fractures (Table 25.1) [15]. Patella stress fractures may present as nondisplaced or displaced and can then progress to a delayed union or nonunion [25, 29]. These classifications exist on a spectrum, and a fracture may progress from one stage to the next depending on when the fracture is diagnosed. Given this possibility, early diagnosis is of the utmost importance when managing patella stress fractures.

25.2.3 Diagnosis

The most common symptom of patella stress fractures is anterior knee pain. Therefore, there are numerous differential diagnoses that must be considered. It is important to be aware of these diagnoses to minimize the risk of misdiagnosis. These include (1) patellofemoral pain syndrome, (2) patellar tendinopathy, (3) osteochondritis dissecans, (4) bipartite patella, (5) and Sinding-Larsen-Johansson syndrome [25, 38]. Although these diagnoses may confound the identification of a patellar stress fracture, with the correct combination of history, physical examination, and imaging investigations the true cause of anterior knee pain should be elucidated.

25.2.3.1 History

In the case of a patella stress fracture, certain predisposing risk factors should be documented to induce substantial suspicion of the overuse injury in athletes [25, 32]. These include a history of BPTB ACL reconstruction and a tight iliotibial band or lateral retinaculum [25, 32]. The patient's pain profile is often described as anterior knee pain with increased activity and gradual worsening with continued activities. Any increase in intensity of sports that include

Table 25.5 Transverse Versus Longitudinal Patella Stress Fractures

	Transverse	Longitudinal
Underlying musculature	Excess loading of quadriceps and patellar tendons in early flexion	Tight lateral retinaculum or iliotibial band
Effect of musculature	Opposing forces on the patella cause vertical and posterior bending stress at fulcrum of patellofemoral reaction force	Patellofemoral joint reaction force is shifted to lateral side of patellar facet
Sport-specific cause	More common with sudden, intense muscle forces • Soccer, basketball	More common with lower forces at greater frequencies • Running
Specific location	Distal third of the patella • Start on anterior surface • Articulating point of patella moves from distal to proximal	Lateral side of the patella • Forces in the lateral facet of the posterior side translated to anterior surface

jumping or kicking may point to a transverse stress fracture, while increase of running frequency could be indicative of a longitudinal stress fracture [25]. Furthermore, the athlete may indicate a "pop" or "crack", which could suggest a displaced patella stress fracture [25]. Upon documenting the athlete's full history, including any failed prior treatment, physical examination must be thoroughly carried out.

25.2.3.2 Physical Examination

Tenderness to palpation of the distal third of the patella can be indicative of a transverse stress fracture. Alternatively, tenderness to palpation of the lateral border of the patella is characteristic of a longitudinal stress fracture. Nondisplaced patella stress fractures are not usually associated with swelling and inflammation. However, effusion may accompany a displaced patella stress fracture [25, 38]. Finally, ligamentous stability tests and gait analysis should be performed to fully understand the load patterns placed upon the patella.

25.2.3.3 Radiological Evaluation

Plain radiographs are the first choice of imaging modality. Transverse stress fractures are best visualized on lateral radiographs, while sunrise (skyline) view radiographs are best to view longitudinal stress fractures. The findings of interest are sclerotic edges surrounding the injury location. Anteroposterior radiographs can help distinguish between a patella stress fracture and a bipartite patella, as the differential characteristics of the bipartite patella's unfused zone and secondary ossification center will be visible. However, as radiographs have low sensitivity and specificity, they can often appear normal at the time of onset of symptoms, and alternative imaging modalities may be necessary. Although bone scintigraphy was used in early case studies of patella stress fractures, MRI is the optimal secondary imaging modality. STIR, T1-weighted, and T2-weighted images can be used to characterize patella stress fractures (Fig. 25.2). A high signal on STIR images and a low signal on T1-weighted images will indicate a grade three stress fracture [25, 38].

25.2.4 Management

With early diagnosis of a nondisplaced, transverse or longitudinal stress fracture, nonoperative management with activity modification and potential immobilisation of the affected leg can be enough to promote healing and return the athlete to low-impact activity within 3–6 weeks [25]. However, patella stress fractures are at high risk for displacement and nonunion; therefore, surgical treatment is often recommended. Small displaced fragments can be excised, but larger, displaced, transverse and longitudinal stress fractures should be internally fixed [25]. Transverse stress fractures of the distal third of the patella can be treated with either a tension band wire in a figure-8 pattern or cannulated screws inserted distal to proximal [25]. Longitudinal stress fractures do not require tension band wiring. Good results can be achieved with cannulated screws inserted from lateral to medial. A lateral retinacular release should also be considered if tight to avoid excessive lateral forces across the fracture site [2].

25.2.5 Complications

Delayed or missed diagnosis can lead to complications (Table 25.6) [25, 30, 31]. Continued tensile forces from the quadriceps and patella tendon will compress the patella against the underlying femur, which may result in worsening or completion of the stress fracture [29]. Other complications of nonoperative management include nonunion or

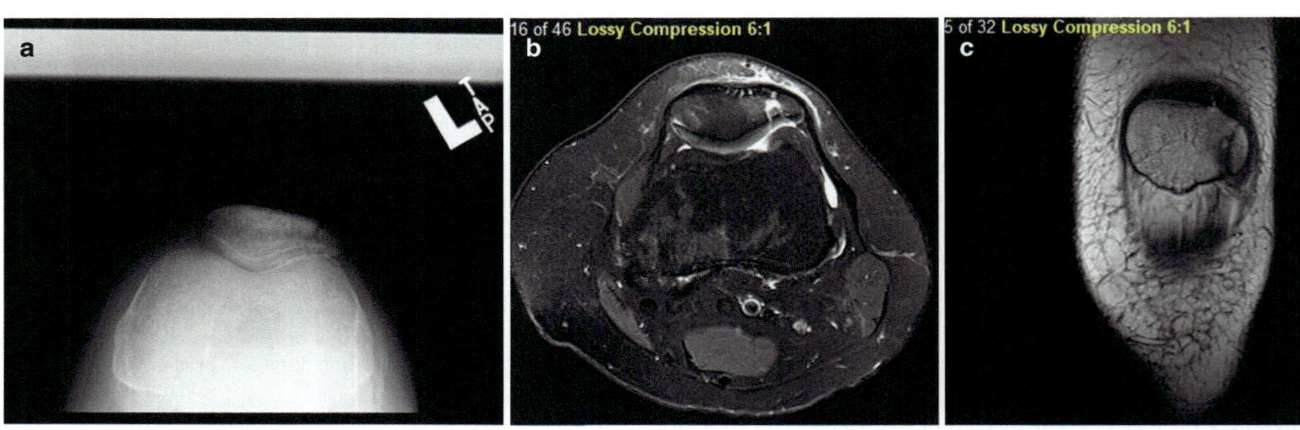

Fig. 25.2 25-year-old female with a nondisplaced left, lateral patella fracture as seen on (**a**) sunrise view radiographs, (**b**) axial, T2-weighted MRI, and (**c**) coronal, T1-weighted MRI sequences

osteonecrosis. While any surgical intervention is accompanied by potential complications, the consequences of missing the diagnosis are more severe.

25.2.6 Rehabilitation

The goal of nonoperative and postoperative management of patella stress fractures is to decrease load across patella to accelerate healing [27]. Activities such as running, jumping, kicking, and kneeling should be avoided. Postoperatively, protocols can help to guide the weight bearing status, range of motion, and therapeutic exercises throughout various stages of the rehabilitation process. Weightbearing is commonly allowed as tolerated by postoperative day one with a brace locked in extension to minimize the compressive forces across the patella stress fracture site. An adaptation of an example postoperative rehabilitation protocol is presented in Table 25.7 [39].

25.2.7 Preventative Measures

Patella stress fractures are rare in the general population, and even more so in the athlete. Therefore, preventative measures have not been widely published [25, 28, 29, 38]. The same general precautions outlined in Section 25.1.6 can be applied for prevention of patella stress fractures. Furthermore, an athlete can focus on minimizing the specific risk factors such as avoiding sudden increases in training and minimizing repetitive loads. The athlete should also be educated on gradual progression of intensity and duration of training [29].

25.3 Tibial Plateau Stress Fractures

25.3.1 Epidemiology

Posterior to the patella, articulating with the femoral condyles, the tibial plateau makes up the other half of the knee joint. Although tibial shaft overuse injuries are the most common in athletes, tibial plateau stress fractures are extremely rare. Furthermore, given the proximity to the stabilizing ligaments and menisci of the knee joint, it is often extremely difficult to correctly diagnose a tibial plateau stress fracture.

The prevalence of tibial plateau stress fractures is higher in active military personnel when compared to athletes [40]. Tibial plateau stress fractures account for up to 59% of all stress fractures in military recruits, with the majority occurring in the medial tibial plateau [40, 41]. The literature is inconclusive regarding whether females experience a greater risk, but these fractures are most commonly fatigue fractures [40–42]. A connection between running and tibial plateau stress fractures has been elucidated [42, 43]. While insufficiency fractures of the tibial plateau have been reported, they have not been reported in athletes [44–46]. Weakening can occur as a result of osteopenia, metabolic conditions, rheumatoid arthritis, and knee arthroplasty, all of which are more prevalent in the elderly, nonactive population [45, 46]. Given these trends, this section will focus on fatigue fractures of the

Table 25.6 Complications Based on Treatment Method

Nonoperative	Operative
A nondisplaced fracture can become displaced or complete	Internal fixation could result in more severe anterior knee pain
A displaced fracture could experience delayed union or nonunion	Hardware could become symptomatic or migrate
Osteonecrosis can occur with displacement	Osteonecrosis can occur with displacement and delayed treatment

Table 25.7 NYU Hospital for Joint Disease ORIF Patella Fracture Post-operative Rehabilitation Protocol

Phase	Specifications
I: 0–2 weeks	• **Knee immobilizer**: Worn at all times, converted to hinged knee brace at first postoperative visit • **Weightbearing**: As tolerated with knee locked in extension • **Range of motion**: 0–30° • **Therapeutic exercises**: Isometric quadriceps, hamstring, adductor, abductor strengthening, theraband exercises
II: 2–6 weeks	• **Knee brace**: Worn with weightbearing activities, locked in full extension, can be removed at night • **Weightbearing**: As tolerated with knee locked in extension • **Range of motion**: Add 15° of flexion per week, with a goal of 90° at week 6 • **Therapeutic exercises**: Isometric quadriceps, hamstring, adductor, abductor strengthening, theraband exercises, straight leg raises
III: 6–10 weeks	• **Knee brace**: Unlocked, worn with weightbearing activities • **Weightbearing**: Full • **Range of motion**: Progress to full ROM by week 10 • **Therapeutic exercises**: Isometric quadriceps, hamstring, adductor, abductor strengthening, theraband exercises, straight leg raises
IV: 10–12 weeks	• **Knee brace**: Discontinue • **Weightbearing**: Full • **Range of motion**: Full • **Therapeutic exercises**: Isometric quadriceps, hamstring, adductor, abductor strengthening, theraband exercises, straight leg raises, start stationary bicycle
V: 3–6 months	• **Return to full activities as tolerated**

tibial plateau which plague the active community, predominantly in training military recruits and runners.

25.3.2 Classification

The general mechanism of the fatigue stress fracture of the tibial plateau in athletes is repetitive stresses accumulating on a normal bone to a point that it cannot withstand. The next level of classification is high risk versus low risk, which considers the prognosis of the stress fracture. Although not directly commented upon, tibial plateau stress fractures, given their rarity, are not included amongst the high risk stress fractures, thus classifying them as low risk. Tibial plateau stress fractures in athletes and soldiers are generally self-limiting, unlikely to displace, and have a satisfactory natural progression when given time to heal [47]. The stress fracture pattern may be characterized as linear or stellate, which is most easily discerned with MRI [47].

The location of the stress fracture on the tibial plateau can be used to distinguish the injuries. Yukata et al. suggests additional stratification beyond medial and lateral [47]. The three classifications are anteromedial, posteromedial, and posterior type stress fractures, which can be discerned through pain pattern and imaging investigation [47]. The location of these stress fractures in athletes tend to correlate to the slope of the tibial plateau, indicating the value and necessity of physical examination and imaging investigation of the morphology of the tibia.

25.3.3 Diagnosis

There is an array of differential diagnoses related to the symptoms of an underlying tibial plateau stress fracture. Most often, lesions within the knee joint, meniscal injury, and pes anserinus bursitis are confounding conditions [48]. These are logical alternative diagnoses, as the menisci are in direct contact with the tibial plateau, and inflammation of the bursa in the knee joint will obscure pathologies of the plateau. These alternative causes can mask the actual injury, and therefore it is important for healthcare providers to be aware of them.

25.3.3.1 History

As tibial plateau stress fractures are more common in runners and military personnel, a history of activity associated with high impact loading of the lower extremities is generally expected. Furthermore, there is usually an onset of general knee joint pain related to an increase in intensity of training with no record of acute trauma. With the more common medial tibial plateau stress fracture, the pain will often emanate from the medial aspect of the proximal tibia and decrease with rest [47]. Of note, in comparison with other types of stress fractures, patients with tibial plateau injuries exhibit a shorter delay between onset of symptoms and seeking medical treatment for their pain [41, 49]. There are certain intrinsic and extrinsic risk factors which may predispose athletes to a wide variety of stress fractures, and it is therefore helpful to record their presence as they may eventually prove to be related to the mechanism of injury (Table 25.8) [42].

25.3.3.2 Physical Examination

A thorough physical examination is recommended to confirm the suspicion of a tibial plateau stress fracture, and should include the following [41]:

1. Palpation of knee—findings consistent with site of pain.
2. Knee range of motion—often not limited.
3. Ligamentous laxity—may be unequal between the injured and non-injured leg.
4. Joint effusion—likely not present.

Sports medicine healthcare providers should understand that these findings may be consistent with several different knee injuries, and therefore are not sufficient on their own to diagnose a tibial plateau stress fracture. Often physical examination will be unremarkable, but unique findings may point to an alternative diagnosis. For example, the presence of edema at the tendon insertion site can suggest pes anserine bursitis [41].

25.3.3.3 Imaging Investigations

The key to diagnosing tibial plateau stress fractures resides in imaging observation to help distinguish the condition from differential diagnoses. However, tibial plateau morphology and pathology are extremely difficult to detect using plain radiographs upon onset of symptoms [40, 47]. In fact, Yukata et al. reports that no fracture lines were present on

Table 25.8 Risk Factors with Examples Related to Tibial Plateau Stress Fractures

Intrinsic	Extrinsic
Anatomic factors • Varus or valgus alignment • Gait that causes more stress in the posterior aspect	Training errors • Change in training technique
Muscular fatigue • Muscles that are weakened and cannot dissipate load stress adequately	Training surface • Angle of surface can increase strain on tibial plateau
Physiologic factors • Menstrual disturbance in females	Shoe type • If shoe is not absorbing shock, muscles will be fatigued faster
Bone characteristics • Cancellous trabeculae handle load in plateau	Sport • Dance, Pilates, yoga, martial arts

plain radiographs in a cohort of patients with tibial plateau fatigue fractures within 2 weeks of symptom onset [47]. The vast majority of studies on tibial plateau stress fractures have highlighted MRI as the study of choice, as it is more specific than scintigraphy and more sensitive than computed tomography and radiographs [47]. Specifically, T2-weighted short tau inversion recovery (STIR) MR images suppress signals from blood and fat, allowing for more accurate visualization of edema of the cancellous bone and fracture lines of the tibial plateau [41, 42, 47]. Bone marrow edema is not a specific finding, and there must be the concomitant presence of a line of reduced signal intensity [41]. As mentioned previously, MRI can assist with determining the posterior slope of the tibia, along with related stresses, subsequently localizing the stress fracture as anteromedial, anteroposterior, or posterior.

25.3.4 Treatment and Rehabilitation

Given the low-risk nature of a tibial plateau stress fracture in athletes, there is no routine treatment plan reported in the literature. Therefore, modification of activity and rest are informed by the severity of pain and grade of injury. These methods prove successful in the majority of case studies with the primary evidence coming from a study by Engber et al. in, which no patient suffered a displacement of the stress fracture nor was there any recurrence of pain following adequate rest [49]. Limited studies suggest unique modes of treatment, such as ultrasound bone stimulation in combination with non-operative rehabilitation [42]. One study suggests resection, bone grafting, and internal fixation for the highly active patient does not want to limit their training [50]. However, this method of treatment for tibial plateau stress fractures is not widely commented, on and the indications for such treatment are unknown.

Recent literature has commented on a subchondroplasty as a potential treatment for knee stress fractures, specifically insufficiency fractures of the tibial plateau [51–53]. Upon confirmation of bone marrow lesions with T1 or T2 weighted MRI, minimally invasive surgery may be recommended and can be done in an outpatient setting [52]. In the procedure, calcium phosphate is injected into the trabeculae of the affected bone within the knee joint. The bone substitute material fills the defect and begins to crystallize, mimicking healthy cancellous bone and providing a scaffold for new endogenous bone to grow and replace the artificial scaffold [52]. In some patients with insufficiency fractures and concomitant osteoarthritis, subchondroplasty has resulted in relief of pain and improvement in function [53]. Based on these findings, this treatment may reduce pain, prevent progression of the injury, and return athletes suffering from tibial plateau stress fractures to sport faster [52]. However, there have only been a handful of case studies regarding the effectiveness of this management modality in athletes, and further investigation is needed [52]. Therefore, it is prudent to recommend activity limitation and rest until cessation of pain with daily activities. At this point, athletes may return gradually to activities such as running or marching, being cognizant of training that increases the stress load on the posterior tibia.

25.3.5 Complications

Tibial plateau stress fractures are rare and low risk, with a relatively minimal chance for complications. Issues may arise if diagnosis is delayed, as the stress fracture may be more severe and thus demand cessation of all activity rather than a simple modification of training regimen. Essentially, stress fractures operate along the rule that the earlier an injury is detected, the earlier an athlete will return to sport, pain free [43]. As a result, the most pressing complication with the general nonoperative management would be return of medial or lateral knee pain if adequate rest is not taken or if the correct alterations to training are not made.

25.3.6 Preventative Measures

Preventing a tibial plateau stress fracture is based upon the guidelines for preventing general stress fractures as outlined in Section 25.1.6. Avoiding intense increases in activities that stress the proximal tibia, sustaining adequate rest time within activity, and maintaining a healthy, nutrient rich diet are all simple steps an athlete can take to further minimize the chances of developing this rare stress fracture [40, 48]. Furthermore, preventing the abovementioned complications such as delayed return to sport will depend on whether the athlete seeks medical advice soon after the onset of medial knee pain.

25.4 Proximal Tibia Stress Fractures

25.4.1 Epidemiology

Separate from the transverse plane of the tibial plateau, the proximal tibia is the upper portion of the bone that widens to meet the femur in the knee joint. More specifically, the proximal tibia contains structures such as the tibial tuberosity on the anterior side, Gerdy's tubercle on the lateral aspect, the underlying formations of the medial and lateral tibial condyles, and the most proximal portion of the tibial diaphysis.

Overuse injuries in these structures contribute to the incidence of proximal tibia stress fractures in athletes, with the majority occurring in the posteromedial aspect [54]. The overall incidence of proximal tibial stress fractures in athletes is unknown; however, this specific injury inordinately affects distance runners [54]. Stress fractures in the proximal portion of the tibia are more common in adolescent athletes (Fig. 25.3) [54–56]. In skeletally immature athletes, a stress fracture incurred in the proximal tibia at a young age may become obscured. As the skeleton matures, athletes' tissue within the stress fracture may ossify, and result in a morphology that mimics overgrowth of the tibial tuberosity [57]. Proximal tibia stress fractures are rarer than their medial and distal counterparts, but case studies inform sports medicine healthcare providers on this overuse injury [48–50, 54–56].

25.4.2 Classification

Proximal tibial stress fractures can be categorized in a variety of ways, the first being the aforementioned fatigue classification, indicating that excessive stress loading causes the bone to fail. Furthermore, as proximal tibia stress fractures are nearly always in the posteromedial cortex, they are considered low risk stress fractures. These stress fractures are located in the compression side of the bone and are thus resistant to displacement and have predictable healing patterns [57]. The severity of a proximal tibia stress fracture can also be graded using a general classification system, such as the Arendt classification (Table 25.1) [15]. A more specific tibial grading system was published by Fredericson et al. and will be detailed in the forthcoming tibia diaphysis section [58].

25.4.3 Diagnosis

Several conditions can confound the diagnosis of a proximal tibia stress fracture. Many of them are also differential diagnoses of patella and tibial plateau stress fractures. This illustrates the difficulty of discerning these conditions given the proximity of the bones, ligaments, soft tissue, and tendons (Table 25.9) [56].

To correctly diagnose and manage a proximal tibia stress fracture, a thorough history and physical examination are necessary in concert with imaging investigations.

Table 25.9 Differential Diagnoses of Proximal Tibia Stress Fractures

Osgood-Schlatters disease in young athletes
Medial Plica syndrome
Patellar tendinopathy
Patellofemoral pain syndrome
Pes anserine bursitis
Bone tumor

25.4.3.1 History

In athletes complaining of proximal shin pain or knee pain, a relevant history is vital to raise the index of suspicion for a proximal tibia stress fracture. Several intrinsic and extrinsic risk factors can contribute to a proximal tibia stress fracture. The intrinsic risk factors to note are (1) Osgood-Schlatter Disease (specifically for stress fracture of the tibial tuberosity), (2) limb malalignment, (3) cavus deformity (high-arched foot), (4) hyperpronated foot, and (5) female athlete triad. Relevant extrinsic risk factors include (1) changes in running conditions, (2) uphill running which increases compressive forces, and (3) sudden increase in training intensity or load. Beyond these, the patient's pain history is important, as typically the athlete will experience pain upon this abrupt increase in activity [51, 56].

25.4.3.2 Physical Examination

Certain findings should be revealed on physical examination of athletes with a proximal tibia stress fracture [56]:

1. Focal point tenderness at site of fracture
2. Medial joint line tenderness
3. Tenderness with leverage motion
4. Tenderness with hop test
5. Joint effusion possible but not necessary

It is important to not only investigate these symptoms, but complete a thorough examination of both the injured and uninjured leg, as there may be discrepancies which could point towards the mechanism of injury and aid in future prevention. A comprehensive gait examination should evaluate faulty mechanics and implement targeted rehabilitation programs to address any muscular imbalances and improve movement patterns [56].

25.4.3.3 Imaging Investigations

The expected results of various imaging modes in the face of a proximal tibia stress fracture are summarized in Table 25.10 [51, 59]. Plain radiographs are the primary imaging method. Acute stress fractures will often be absent from radiographs around the time of onset of symptoms. However, a negative radiograph in the face of a compelling history and physical examination is not enough to rule out the overuse injury, but rather points to more extensive imaging. Extensive sclerosis at the onset of pain may point to a differential diagnosis, and findings of intercortical osteolysis are consistent with the differential diagnosis of a bone tumor [51, 59]. Bone scintigraphy has been used to diagnose proximal tibia stress fractures, but MR imaging is superior, allowing for visualization of the surrounding soft tissues and extent of bone marrow edema [55].

Table 25.10 Radiological Evidence of a Proximal Tibia Stress Fracture

Plain Radiographs	Magnetic Resonance Imaging
Sclerotic lines parallel to growth plates	Low intensity fracture lines surrounded by bone marrow edema
Interval radiographs may show periosteal bone formation and thickening of cortex	T1-weighted: edema will be lower intensity than normal bone marrow
If stress fracture is in cancellous bone will not be visible	T2-weighted fat suppressed: bone marrow edema will be high signal area with low signal fracture line

25.4.4 Treatment and Rehabilitation

Following a diagnosis of a proximal tibia stress fracture, conservative nonoperative management is the standard of care given the low risk of progression [54]. The first phase of management consists of activity modification and may include a brace for protective load bearing of the tibia to allow adequate healing time. The goal is for the patient to be asymptomatic while walking by 3–4 weeks following activity modification [56]. To maintain the athlete's level of cardiovascular conditioning, low impact training such as swimming or biking may be initiated 4–6 weeks after diagnosis [54]. If the athlete is pain free while weight-bearing, they may gradually return to impact activities between 6 weeks to 6 months after diagnosis. Ultimately, management and rehabilitation depend upon the athlete's pain status. Interval radiographs can be used to monitor the healing process of the stress fracture over the course of nonoperative treatment, as sclerotic lines should heal over time [54, 60]. If bone marrow edema is extensive or pain continues, complete cessation of running and immobilisation with a brace may be advised [54, 56].

25.4.5 Complications

Rest and activity modification protocols individualized to the athlete have proven successful in the treatment of proximal tibia stress fractures. There have been no cases reported in the literature of displacement, delayed union, or nonunion of proximal condylar tibia stress fractures [54]. Complications of persistent pain arise when nonoperative treatment is not aggressive enough. If activity modification does not include a period of complete cessation of running, it is possible that healing will be prolonged. This could lead to increased severity of bone marrow edema and conversion to non-weightbearing status on crutches, with immobilisation [56]. For active athletes, this complication can prove extremely inconvenient if the injury coincides with competition.

25.4.6 Preventative Measures

Modification of risk factors is the first step in preventing proximal tibia stress fractures. This includes strengthening the surrounding musculature to correct imbalances that may be placing inordinate stress on the tibia [57, 60]. A variety of intrinsic risk factors have been related to the foot, thus indicating that correct footwear or the use of insoles may aid in prevention [57]. For females, it is important to assess the possibility of the female athlete triad and determine the necessary steps to modify their condition. This may indicate an increase in caloric intake, addressing menstrual dysfunctions, or treating low bone density [14]. Assessment of running mechanics to identify and correct technique may help to prevent future recurrence. Furthermore, athletes should avoid abrupt increases in running distance or intensity and opt for progressive training programs which allow the necessary body adaptation [57].

25.5 Tibial Diaphysis Stress Fractures

25.5.1 Epidemiology

The final component of overuse injuries in the knee are stress fractures of the tibial diaphysis, the most common site of stress fracture among athletes and military recruits [43, 56]. Tibial diaphysis stress fractures account for 24–75% of all stress fractures in athletes [56, 61, 62]. Given their high incidence and prevalence, the mechanism of injury, diagnostic measures, and treatment protocol receive more attention in the literature compared to previously discussed stress fractures. As with the majority of athletic stress fractures, abnormal stresses affect a normal bone resulting in failure, otherwise known as a fatigue fracture. The tibia is the primary weight bearing bone in the lower leg and is responsible for 93% of load transmission [57]. Therefore, in the face of increased load magnitude or frequency, the tibia is disproportionately affected. Tibial diaphysis stress fractures have been reported in an extremely wide variety of sports including cross country, track and field, triathlons, soccer, basketball, ballet, American football, and skiing [56, 62]. There are two unique tibial diaphysis stress fractures: posteromedial stress fractures, which are more common in runners, and anterior stress fractures, which are more common in jumpers and ballet dancers [57].

25.5.2 Classification

The primary classification of any stress fracture is the risk level. In the case of tibial diaphysis stress fractures, there is potential for both low-risk and high-risk injuries. The most common site is the posteromedial cortex on the compression side of the tibia [56, 63]. Given the load pattern on the compression side of a long bone, these stress fractures are classified as low risk, indicating a reliable healing pattern with nonoperative treatment and a low rate of complications [57]. Posteromedial stress fractures may be transverse or longitudinal, though the former are more common [57]. The alternative tibial diaphysis stress fracture occurs in the anterior tibia, which, although rarer, is classified as a high risk stress fracture. The tension side of the bone presents decreased vascularization, and anterior tibia stress fractures are at an increased risk for propagation, displacement, delayed union, and non-union; they often must be treated operatively [56, 57, 63]. Tibial diaphysis stress fractures can be further categorized by severity. Fredericson et al. developed a tibial diaphysis specific classification system MRI which has been summarized in Table 25.11 [50]. These grades can aid with management and rehabilitation decisions.

Table 25.11 Adaptation of Fredericson et al. MRI Classification of Tibial Diaphysis Stress Fracture

Grade	MRI findings	Recommended treatment
1	Periosteal edema, no associated bone marrow abnormalities	2–3 weeks of rest followed by gradual return to running
2	Periosteal edema and bone marrow edema on T2-weighted images only	4–6 weeks of rest followed by gradual return to running
3	Periosteal edema and bone marrow edema on T1- and T2-weighted images	6–9 weeks of rest followed by non-impact training
4	Multiple or linear areas of intracortical signal abnormality and bone marrow edema on T1- and T2-weighted images	6 weeks of immobilisation in a cast, 6 weeks of non-impact training

25.5.3 Diagnosis

The differential diagnosis of pain in the tibial diaphysis is extensive, and includes tibial diaphysis stress fracture, medial tibial stress syndrome, posterior tibial tendinopathy, chronic exercise-induced compartment syndrome, bone tumors, and popliteal artery entrapment (Fig. 25.4) [56]. Correct diagnosis, especially of the high risk anterior tibia stress fracture, is vital.

25.5.3.1 History

An athlete's history should reveal the possible risk factors related to tibial diaphysis stress fractures. These include any rapid increase in intensity of training, change in running surface, change in sport, old worn running shoes, the presence of the female athlete triad, or metabolic deficiencies such as insufficient calcium or vitamin D [14]. A gradual onset of pain at the end of training sessions is indicative of a possible tibial diaphysis stress fracture. This pain will usually progress until it persists with walking and even resting [57]. An athlete's history of pain can aid in differentiating between tibial diaphysis stress fracture and medial tibial stress syndrome. If the athlete complains of worsening pain throughout a single training session to the point where they must halt activity, a tibial diaphysis stress fracture should be suspected. Alternatively, if the athlete complains of pain at the start of a training session that gradually lessens and eventually subsides with continued activity, medial tibial stress syndrome is more common [57].

25.5.3.2 Physical Examination

Physical examination of athletes with a suspected posteromedial or anterior tibia diaphysis stress fracture begin with palpation to the potential site of stress fracture. This should elicit pain and tenderness over a focal location of the tibia [57, 63]. In contrast, with shin splints, athletes will likely report more vague, diffuse pain that they are unable to localize [61–64]. Posteromedial tibial diaphysis stress fractures have occasional edema and palpable callus formation, while anterior stress fractures do not present with these symptoms given the avascularity of the site [57]. Other specific pain positive tests will include the tuning fork test and the single leg hop test [57]. With the former test, a vibrating tuning fork is placed on the site of pain, at which point the tenderness should be exacerbated. A similar result is derived from the single leg hop test; upon hopping on the affected leg, the patient should be able to more accurately localize their pain in the case of a tibial diaphysis stress fracture [57].

Beyond these tests, physicians should carry out a complete physical examination of both the affected and contralateral tibia in order to fully understand any deformities [63]. Examples of muscular and structural components that may affect the tibia are (1) a tight gastrocnemius-soleus complex which places large tensile stress on the anterior tibia thus affecting its convexity; (2) a pronated foot which will cause the athlete to lean slightly medially and place rotational torque on the tibia; (3) pes cavus, or a rigid, high arched foot, which cannot absorb load properly and therefore transmits excessive stress to the tibia; (4) pes planus, or an extremely

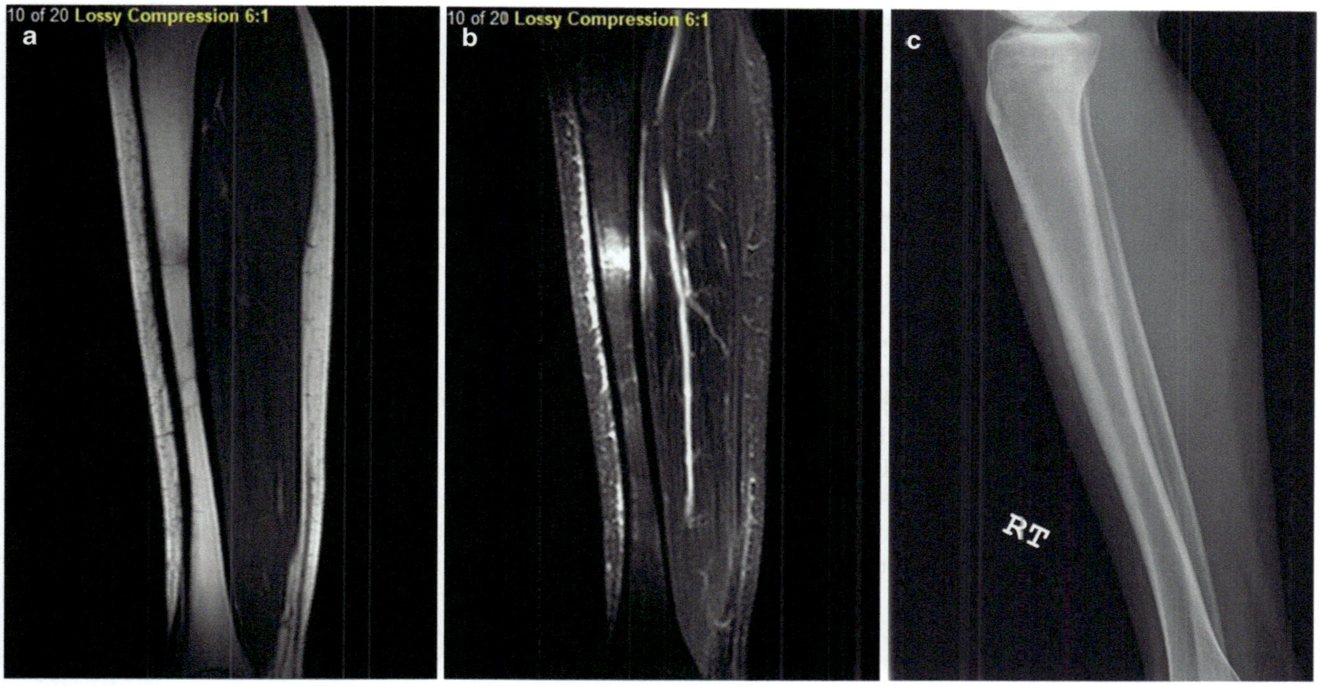

Fig. 25.4 16-year-old female athlete presenting with a differential diagnosis of right, medial tibial stress syndrome as seen on (**a**) sagittal T1-weighted MRI, (**b**) sagittal STIR MRI, and (**c**) plain radiographs

flat foot, which results in muscle fatigue that cannot support loads and; (5) a leg length discrepancy which can point to asymmetrical loading of one leg [57, 63]. Some physical examination findings should be absent to rule out various differential diagnoses. For example, chronic exertional compartment syndrome is uniquely characterized by swelling, numbness and tingling with activity, and diffuse leg pain [63]. Upon recording findings in the surrounding bony, soft tissue, tendon, and muscular structures, physicians may proceed to imaging investigations.

25.5.3.3 Imaging Investigations

Tibial diaphysis stress fractures may be visualized with a variety of imaging modalities, including plain radiographs, MRI, computed tomography, and bone scan. However, the first two have proven sufficient in most patients. Plain orthogonal radiographs should be pursued primarily for suspected posteromedial and anterior stress fractures [57]. With posteromedial diaphysis stress fractures, the expected result will be a sclerotic line in the middle third of the diaphysis; however, this finding may be absent [61]. Three weeks following the onset of symptoms, radiographs may show periosteal and cortical thickening, endosteal thickening, and callus formation [57].

This will also be the case for nondisplaced anterior stress fractures, but with the high-risk anterior injury there may be a radiographic "dreaded black line" if the injury has progressed [57, 61]. This is indicative of the prolonged healing and potential nonunion often associated with these stress fractures. This finding confirms the diagnosis of an anterior diaphysis stress fracture and physicians should proceed to treatment without delay, as the healing capacity will diminish as the fissure widens [57, 61, 63]. In the case of inconclusive or negative radiographs, MRI should be pursued. The Fredericson et al. classification system mentioned previously uses MRI to grade stress fractures by denoting the spectrum of periosteal edema and bone marrow edema [58]. T1-weighted and T2-weighted MRIs should be obtained in the axial, sagittal, and coronal plains in order to fully visualize the presence of these edemas and understand the surrounding tissue [57, 58, 61].

25.5.4 Management

The management of tibia diaphysis stress fractures is highly dependent upon whether the injury is a low risk posteromedial stress fracture or high risk anterior stress fracture.

25.5.4.1 Posteromedial Stress Fracture

These low risk stress fractures are treated nonoperatively beginning with rest and activity modification, potential immobilisation with a brace, and reduced weight bearing with crutches. Upon diagnosis, the athlete should cease all sports, specifically running, until they are asymptomatic while walking [56, 63]. In the meantime, non-impact training such as swimming may be employed to maintain fitness. Athletes may choose to use a walking boot or pneumatic brace to alleviate pain. The pneumatic brace unloads the tibia by compressing the lower leg, thus decreasing tibial bowing by redistributing forces from the surrounding musculature [56]. Once acute pain is alleviated, athletes may resume low impact exercises until pain is fully resolved, at which point they may follow a protocol to gradually return to impact [56]. The duration of these phases of treatment are often 4–8 weeks of initial activity modification to allow healing, and a total of 8–12 weeks until the athlete can fully return to sport [56, 63].

25.5.4.2 Anterior Stress Fracture

High risk stress fractures in the anterior tibia diaphysis often require operative treatment in the face of failed conservative management. Initially, athletes with nondisplaced anterior stress fractures will often undergo a prolonged period of rest and immobilisation at a minimum of 3–6 months [56, 63]. Upon subsequent imaging, if the fracture line widens or a "dreaded black line" is present on plain radiographs, surgical intervention is necessary [57]. There are several possible surgical techniques which physicians may opt for, including excision and bone grafting, open reduction with internal fixation, tibial reamed intra-medullary nailing, and compression plating [57]. The latter two methods have been shown to return more athletes to sport in a shorter amount of time [57]. Following surgery, the athlete should adhere to a rehabilitation program and return to play upon evidence of cortical bridging.

25.5.4.3 New Treatment Modalities

For competitive athletes at the college and professional level, the suggested activity restrictions can be detrimental to their athletic careers [65]. With athletes wanting to avoid the lengthy recovery period, new treatment modalities are being developed in order to accelerate return to sport. These include the use of bisphosphonates, pulsed ultrasound, and electrical stimulation [65]. These therapeutic options have limited evidence, and athletes should be informed of the risks involved prior to treatment. Furthermore, given the lack of robust evidence, there is no guarantee that such treatments will work for every athlete. Sports medicine healthcare providers should recommend the traditional protocol of rest prior to turning to these novel modalities. When they are employed, these therapeutic options should be used in combination with some type of activity modification. In the case of high-risk stress fractures that have progressed to displacement, surgery is necessary, and these treatment modalities should not be relied on.

25.5.4.4 Bisphosphonates

Bisphosphonates are used to suppress bone reabsorption by osteoclasts. They are commonly used to treat osteoporosis, but have been employed in an off-label use for the treatment of stress fractures [66]. In a study of five collegiate female athletes, the intravenous use of pamidronate accelerated return to sport and decreased pain [67]; athletes were able to play within 72 hours of the initial treatment. Bisphosphonates are thought to specifically aid in the treatment of remodeling-mediated stress fractures which are commonly seen in the tibia [66]. It is important to note the potential adverse side effects, which include nausea, fatigue, inflammatory reactions, arthralgias, and myalgias. However, the most important side effects of prolonged use of bisphosphonates are atypical fractures of the femur and aseptic necrosis of the mandible. The seriousness of the side effects of such drugs have prompted healthcare professionals to be extremely cautious in their use outside their string osteoporosis indications. The effectiveness of bisphosphonates in the treatment of stress fractures has not been confirmed, and healthcare providers should be prudent of the drawbacks. Further clinical studies are required to elucidate the potential of bisphosphonates in this setting.

25.5.4.5 Electrical Stimulation

Capacity coupled electric field (CCEF) stimulation, which uses calcium in the extracellular space, enhances the healing of traumatic fractures; electrical stimulation results in cellular stimulation and protein synthesis. Given the nature of stress fractures, CCEF stimulation may accelerate their healing in athletes [65]. Beck et al. found that severe stress fractures in athletes and military recruits responded well to a combination of CCEF stimulation and reduced weightbearing, indicated by a faster healing time [68]. Further research is needed in regards to how electrical stimulation accelerates the healing of stress fractures.

25.5.4.6 Low Intensity Pulsed Ultrasound

High frequency sound waves, as produced by ultrasound, have been found to stimulate healing through increased synthesis of extracellular matrix proteins. This method, much like electrical stimulation, has been found to aid in the treatment of acute fractures. For this reason, it is thought that ultrasound may reduce the time to osseous union, although the literature is mixed on this topic [48, 49, 59]. In a case study of an Olympic gymnast, low intensity pulsed ultrasound was used to treat a tibial stress fracture. The patient returned to activity within 3 weeks and went on to compete with minimal pain [69]. There is a lack of recent literature investigating the effectiveness of this treatment, but there is potential for ultrasound to result in accelerated healing of stress fractures [65].

25.5.5 Complications

With the new treatment modalities, if athletes return to play prior to adequate healing, there is a risk of progression. If a stress fracture becomes displaced or develops a delayed union or nonunion, surgical options must be explored. Thus, their time away from sport will ultimately be augmented and they may miss entire seasons of competition. Considering this, it is extremely important for athletes, along with their trainers and doctors, to exercise caution when utilizing new treatment modalities. The progression from rest and non-weightbearing to activity modification and low impact training prior to return to sports is detailed throughout this chapter and is the supported mode of treatment for nearly all stress fractures [11, 15, 57, 63]. As these new modalities lack reports in the literature, it is difficult to confirm their effectiveness in accelerating the healing process.

There are complications related to the traditional nonoperative and operative treatment of low risk and high risk stress fractures. With posteromedial stress fractures, even with conservative care there is a risk of a displacement if adequate activity modification is not achieved [62]. In this case, stress fractures require surgical treatment, and will be treated as previously described, likely with intra-medullary nailing [62]. The complications associated with high risk stress fractures are much more extensive. For example, if anterior stress fractures are treated conservatively, the fracture may complete and displace, at which point it is at risk for nonunion or delayed union [53, 63]. With operative treatment, issues may arise with the hardware used, as it may fail, or cause pain related to soft tissue damage [62]. Specific to athletes, the extensive time away from their sport associated with nonoperative treatment is often too large a burden for the in-season athlete. However, the surgical alternative poses its own significant risk to the athlete's ability to compete [63]. In the face of these obstacles, athletes may delay treatment, but this can result in a complete fracture which will ultimately increase the time away from sport drastically.

25.5.6 Rehabilitation

For conservative management, rehabilitation is often included in the protocol as activity modification, limited weightbearing with nonimpact alternative training, and gradual return to loading activities. Rehabilitation following surgical intervention includes a progressive weight-bearing program that commences within the first week after surgery. A physical therapist should be included in this program, guiding the athlete to full loading activities at 6–8 weeks postoperatively [57]. These rehabilitation programs should focus on stretching and strengthening the supporting structures such as the gastrocnemius-soleus complex, the iliotibial band, and the tibialis anterior as these will aid in the stabilization of loads transmitted to the tibia [70].

25.5.7 Preventative Measures

Preventing a tibial diaphysis stress fracture is based upon addressing the modifiable risk factors. Training regimens should be modified to avoid sudden increases in intensity [56, 63]. Addressing potential structural issues such as excessively high arched or flat feet, insoles and correct footwear may assist in alleviating the excessive loads [57]. Other abnormal biomechanics related to gait or leg length discrepancies should also be addressed to ensure that loads are evenly distributed upon initiation of high impact activities [63]. Maintaining proper nutrition and monitoring vitamin D levels recommended in Section 25.1.6 will further limit the athlete's risk of stress fractures. As detailed throughout this chapter, female athletes should be aware of the female athlete triad. Lack of sufficient energy intake, menstrual dysfunctions, or bone mineral density deficiencies may predispose these athletes to stress fractures and should be addressed [14].

25.6 Summary

Stress fractures of the knee are extremely variable in their incidence rates, classifications, and prognoses. Athletes most commonly experience fatigue fractures, a type of stress fracture caused by repetitive stresses on a bone which is incapable of remodeling at the necessary rate, thus leading to break down. Athletes may experience extreme setbacks from stress fractures depending on which bone is affected. Obtaining a detailed history of an athlete's training and pain, carrying out a thorough physical exam, and pursuing radiological investigations with plain radiographs and MRI is vital in the diagnose and treatment of each specific injury.

Stress fractures of the distal femur, tibial plateau, and proximal tibia are at low risk for displacement, and can usually be managed with activity modification and prevented with increased attention to training patterns and nutritional needs. In contrast, stress fractures of the patella and the tibia diaphysis, the most common stress fracture location in athletes, have the potential to progress to displacement which can lead to delayed union or nonunion. The operative treatments recommended for such stress fractures pose a heightened risk to an athlete's career by increasing the time away from competition. Given the limitations in traditional treatment options for stress fractures, new modalities have been experimented with to speed up an athlete's return to sport. However, such treatments are in their infancy, and the evidence for their efficacy and safety is limited. Thus, it is prudent for athletes to consider adhering to an activity modification and rehabilitation program to limit the risk for recurrence or displacement and return them to their sport.

Review

Questions

1. A collegiate female runner goes to her athletic trainer complaining of right knee and upper shin pain following an increase in her weekly mileage. She explains that she has been experiencing bouts of worsening pain throughout her training sessions and at times must stop running due to the intensity of her pain. In passing, the athlete mentions that her menstrual cycle has been irregular. When asked to point to the location of her pain, the athlete indicates a definitive location on her right, upper shin. She further indicates that there is no such pain in her left leg. At imaging, some edema is noted at the site of pain, and plain radiographs indicate periosteal thickening. After discussing her symptoms with her fellow teammates, the athlete is convinced she is suffering from "shin splints", a condition common in runners. What condition is this female athlete likely suffering from?
   A. Medial Tibial Stress Syndrome
   B. Anterior Tibial Diaphysis Stress Fracture
   C. Exertional Compartment Syndrome
   D. Bone Tumor
2. A professional male basketball player presents with acute anterior knee pain of the left knee. The pain arises during his competitive season, with his team averaging three games per week. The athlete's history consists of pain that has been increasing consistently with the increasing intensity of his team's schedule and a prior anterior cruciate ligament reconstruction. With physical exam, the athlete complains of increased pain with palpation to the knee, specifically towards the lower half.
   (a) What diagnosis should a sports medicine healthcare provider suspect with this athlete?
      A. Bipartite Patella
      B. Transverse Patella Stress Fracture
      C. Patellofemoral Pain Syndrome
      D. Longitudinal Patella Stress Fracture
   (b) Following this suspicion, which subsequent imaging modality should be pursued and used to visualize this specific injury?
      A. Anteroposterior View Radiographs
      B. Sunrise View Radiographs
      C. Lateral View Radiographs
      D. Rosenberg View Radiographs

Answers

1. This female collegiate runner is most likely suffering from an **(B) Anterior Tibial Diaphysis Stress Fracture**. There are several clues in the question that point to this diagnosis: (1) the athlete is a runner who just increased her mileage, indicating increased stress on her tibia through the repetitive loading associated with running; (2) the athlete mentions she has an irregular menstrual cycle, which could point to an underlying condition known as female athlete triad, a common predisposing factor for stress fractures in female athletes; (3) the athlete complains of increasing pain throughout training sessions, is able to point to a focal location of her pain, edema is present, and there are sclerotic lines on her radiographs. All of these characteristics help distinguish her condition from choice (A) Medial Tibial Stress Syndrome. This is the clinical name for "shin splints" which is the condition the athlete suspects she has due to conversations with teammates. This colloquial name is commonly used and is prevalent in the running world, but it can mask a tibial diaphysis stress fracture as it does in this case. It is extremely important to diagnose this athlete's anterior tibia diaphysis stress fracture as this injury is at a high risk for displacement and may require surgical intervention if the athlete does not take the necessary precautions.

2(a). In the case of the male professional basketball player, a sports medicine healthcare provider should suspect a **(B) Transverse Patella Stress Fracture**. The indications for this diagnosis are prevalent throughout the question and include (1) a prior ACL reconstruction which can weaken the patella at the tendon insertion site and render it more susceptible to injury; (2) the athlete has increased pain with palpation to the lower half of his knee and; (3) the athlete is a basketball player in the midst of an extremely intense season, thus indicating increased rates of abrupt muscle forces associated with common motions in basketball such as jumping. These final two clues aid in differentiating the athlete's patella stress fracture as transverse rather than longitudinal. Jumping and sudden increases in force are associated with transverse patella stress fractures which also are most common in the distal third of the sesamoid bone, thus explaining his focal location of pain.

2(b). Upon developing adequate suspicion of a transverse patella stress fracture, **(C) Lateral View Radiographs** should be used to visualize the injury. The other radiograph views can aid in the diagnosis of alternative injuries to the knee. For example, longitudinal patella stress fractures can be visualized with sunrise view radiographs and a bipartite patella can be differentiated using an anteroposterior radiograph which allows for visualization of the secondary ossification center. Although patella stress fractures are rare, they are at a high risk of displacement and must be properly diagnosed. There are several key findings which can indicate this injury, as detailed in this question.

References

1. Haro MS, Bruene JR, Weber K, Bach BR Jr. Stress fractures of the femur. In: Miller TL, Kaeding CC, editors. Stress fractures in athletes. Switzerland: Springer International; 2015. p. 111–24.
2. Rizzone KH, Ackerman KE, Roos KG, Dompier TP, Kerr ZY. The epidemiology of stress fractures in collegiate student-athletes, 2004-2005 through 2013–2014 academic years. J Athl Train. 2017;52(10):966–75.
3. Plett SK, Hackney LA, Heilmeier U, Nardo L, Yu A, Zhang CA, Link TM. Femoral condyle insufficiency fractures: associated clinical and morphological findings and impact on outcome. Skelet Radiol. 2015;44(12):1785–94.
4. Snyder RA, Koester MC, Dunn WR. Epidemiology of stress fractures. Clin Sports Med. 2006;25(1):37–52.
5. Robertson GA, Wood AM. Femoral neck stress fractures in sport: a current concepts review. Sports Med Int Open. 2017;1(2):E58–68.
6. Frassica FJ, Sponseller PD, Wilckens JH, editors. The 5-minute orthopaedic consult. 2nd ed. Philadelphia: Lippincott Williams & Wilkins; 2007. p. 424–5.
7. Waterman BR, Gun B, Bader JO, Orr JD, Belmont PJ Jr. Epidemiology of lower extremity stress fractures in the United States military. Mil Med. 2016;181:1308–13.
8. Mattila VM, Nica M, Kiuru M, Pihlajamaki H. Risk factors for bone stress injuries: a follow-up study of 102,515 person-years. Med Sci Sports Exerc. 2007;39(7):1061–6.
9. Ivkovic A, Bojanic I, Pecina M. Stress fractures of the femoral shaft in athletes: a new treatment method. Br J Sports Med. 2006;40(6):518–20.
10. Niva M. Fatigue bone stress injuries in the lower extremities in Finnish conscripts. 2006. Dissertation, University of Helsinki.
11. Kahanov L, Eberman L, Games K, Wasik M. Diagnosis, treatment, and rehabilitation of stress fractures in the lower extremity in runners. Open Access J Sports Med. 2014;6:87–95.
12. Matcuk GR, Mahanty SR, Skalski MR, Patel DB, White EA, Gottsegen CJ. Stress fractures: pathophysiology, clinical presentation, imaging features and treatment options. Emerg Radiol. 2016;23(4):365–75.
13. Miller T, Kaeding CC, Flanigan D. The classification systems of stress fractures: a systematic review. Phys Sportsmed. 2011;39(1):93–100.
14. Abbott A, Bird M, Brown SM, Wild E, Stewart G, Mulcahy MK. Part II: Presentation, diagnosis, classification, treatment and prevention of stress fractures in female athletes. The Physician and Sportsmedicine. 2019 [Epub ahead of print].
15. Arendt E, Agel J, Heikes C, Griffiths H. Stress injuries to bone in college athletes: a retrospective review of experience at a single institution. Am J Sports Med. 2003;31(6):959–68.
16. Warden SJ, Davis IS, Fredericson M. Management and prevention of bone stress injuries in long-distance runners. J Orthop Sports Phys Ther. 2014;44(10):749–65.
17. Knapik JJ, Reynolds K, Hoedebecke KL. Stress fractures: etiology, epidemiology, diagnosis, treatment and prevention. J Spec Oper Med. 2017;17(2):120–30.
18. Glorioso JE, Ross G, Leadbetter WB, Boden BP. Femoral supracondylar stress fractures: an unusual cause of knee pain. Phys Sportsmed. 2002;30(9):25–8.
19. Morrison E. Stress fracture of distal femur identified with musculoskeletal ultrasound after normal X-ray and magnetic resonance imaging. Ann Phys Rehabil Med. 2018;61:e164.
20. Sikora-Klak J, Narvy SJ, Yang J, Makhni E, Kharrazi FD, Mehran N. The effect of abnormal vitamin D levels in athletes. Perm J. 2018;22:17–216.
21. Moon AS, Boudreau S, Mussell E, He JK, Brabston EW, Ponce BA, Momaya AM. Current concepts in vitamin D and orthopaedic surgery. Orthop Traumatol Surg Res. 2019;105(2):375–82.
22. Shaker JL. Stress and insufficiency fractures. Clin Rev Bone Miner Metab. 2018;16(1):3–15.
23. Lappe J, Cullen D, Haynatzki G, Recker R, Ahlf R, Thompson K. Calcium and vitamin D supplementation decreases incidence of stress fractures in female navy recruits. J Bone Miner Res. 2008;23(5):741–9.
24. Dao D, Sodhi S, Tabasinejad R, Peterson D, Ayeni OR, Bhandari M, Farrokhyar F. Serum 25-hydroxyvitamin D levels and stress fractures in military personnel: a systematic review and meta-analysis. Am J Sports Med. 2014;43(8):2064–72.
25. Brown GA, Stringer MR, Arendt EA. Stress fractures of the patella. In: Miller TL, Kaeding CC, editors. Stress fractures in athletes. Switzerland: Springer International; 2015. p. 125–35.
26. Murphy KP. Cerebral palsy lifetime care – four musculoskeletal conditions. Dev Med Child Neurol. 2009;51(4):30–7.
27. Atsumi S, Arai Y, Kato K, Nishimura A, Nakazora S, Nakagawa S, Ikoma, Fujiwara H, Sudo A, Kubo T. Transverse stress fracture of the proximal patella: a case report. Medicine (Baltimore). 2016;95(6):e2649.
28. Baker S, Seales J, Newcomer S, Bruce J. A case report: bilateral patella stress fractures in a collegiate gymnast. J Orthop Case Rep. 2018;8(4):45–8.
29. Kizaki K, Yamashita F, Funakoshi N. Serial radiographs showing progression of a patellar stress fracture and beneficial surgical technique for a displaced patellar stress fracture. Knee Surg Relat Res. 2018;30(1):89–92.
30. Devas MB. Stress fractures of the patella. J Bone Joint Surg Br. 1960;42:71–4.
31. Orava S, Taimela S, Kvist M, Karpakka J, Hulkko A, Kujala U. Diagnosis and treatment of stress fracture of the patella in athletes. Knee Surg Sports Traumatol Arthrosc. 1996;4(4):206–11.
32. Keeley A, Bloomfield P, Cairns P, Molnar R. Iliotibial band release as an adjunct to the surgical management of patellar stress fracture in the athlete: a case report and review of the literature. Sports Med Arthrosc Rehabil Ther Technol. 2009;1(1):15.
33. Hanel DP, Burdge RE. Consecutive indirect patella fractures in an adolescent basketball player. A case report. Am J Sports Med. 1981;9(5):327–9.

34. Tibone JE, Lombardo SJ. Bilateral fractures of the inferior poles of the patellae in a basketball player. Am J Sports Med. 1981;9(4):215–6.
35. Hensal F, Nelson T, Pavlov H, Torg JS. Bilateral patellar fractures from indirect trauma. A case report. Clin Orthop Relat Res. 1983;178:207–9.
36. Careneiro M, Nery CA, Mestriner LA. Bilateral stress fracture of the patellae: a case report. Knee. 2006;13(2):164–6.
37. Morgan-Jones RL, Cross T, Caldwell B, Cross MJ. 'Silent' transverse patella fracture following anterior cruciate ligament reconstruction. Arthroscopy. 2001;19(9):997–9.
38. Patel DR, Villalobos A. Evaluation and management of knee pain in young athletes: overuse injuries of the knee. Transl Pediatr. 2017;6(3):190–8.
39. Post-operative rehabilitation protocol: patella fracture ORIF. NYU Hospital for Joint Diseases. https://www.sportssurgerynewyork.com/pdf/orif-patella-fracture-rehab-protocol.pdf. Accessed May 2020.
40. Harolds JA. Fatigue fractures of the medial tibial plateau. South Med J. 1981;74(5):578–81.
41. Niva MH, Kiuru MJ, Haataja R, Pihlajamäki HK. Bone stress injuries causing exercise-induced knee pain. Am J Sports Med. 2006;34(1):78–83.
42. Piccininni JJ, Berry DC. Diagnosis of a medial tibial stress fracture by ultrasound. Athl Today. 2007;12(2):16–20.
43. Brukner P, Bradshaw C, Bennell K. Managing common stress fractures: let risk level guide treatment. Phys Sportsmed. 1998;26(8):39–47.
44. Prasad Nm Murray JM, Kumar D, Davies SG. Insufficiency fracture of the tibial plateau: an often missed diagnosis. Acta Orthop Belg. 2006;72(5):587–91.
45. Chu EC, Bellin D. Insufficiency fracture of the tibial plateau: a disease of rare diagnosis. J Osteopor Phys Act. 2015;3(2)
46. Yokoyama M, Nakamura Y, Egusa M, Doi H, Onishi T, Hirano K, Doi M. Factors related to stress fracture after unicompartmental knee arthroplasty. Asia Pac J Sports Med Arthrosc Rehabil Technol. 2019;15:1–5.
47. Yukata K, Yamanaka I, Ueda Y, Nakai S, Ogasa H, Oishi Y, Hamawaki J. Medial tibial plateau morphology and stress fracture location: a magnetic resonance imaging study. World J Orthop. 2017;8(6):484–90.
48. Kiel J, Kaiser K. Stress reaction and fractures. Treasure Island, FL: StatPearls; 2019.
49. Engber WB. Stress fractures of the medial tibial plateau. J Bone Joint Surg Am. 1977;59:767–9.
50. Caroll JJ, Kelly SP, Foster JN, Mathis DA, Alderete JF. Bilateral proximal tibia stress fractures through persistent physes. Case Rep Orthop. 2018;2018:8181547.
51. Miller TL, Kaeding CC. Stress fractures. In: Rocha Piedade S, Imhoff A, Clatworthy M, Cohen M, Espregueira-Mendes J, editors. The sports medicine physician. Cham: Springer; 2019.
52. Farr J, Cohen S. Subchondroplasty as an emerging treatment option for sports-related subchondral stress fractures. Aspetar Sports Med J. 2016;10:284–91.
53. Abrams GD, Harris JD, Cole BJ. Subchondral bone treatment. In: Cole BJ, Harris JD, editors. Biologic knee reconstruction: a surgeon's guide. NJ: SLACK Incorporated; 2015.
54. Drabicki RR, Greer WJ, DeMeo PJ. Stress fractures around the knee. Clin Sports Med. 2006;25(1):105–15.
55. Posadzy M, Vanhoenacker F. Bilateral synchronous stress fracture of the tibia in a young female basketball player. J Belg Soc Radiol. 2016;100(1):61.
56. DeLee JC, Drez D Jr, Miller MD. DeLee and Drez's orthopaedic sports medicine: principles and practice. 3rd ed. Philadelphia: Saunders, Elsevier; 2010. p. 632–53.
57. Robertson GA, Wood AM. Lower limb stress fractures in sport: optimising their management and outcome. World J Orthop. 2017;8(3):242–55.
58. Fredericson M, Bergman AG, Hoffman KL, Dillingham MS. Tibial stress reaction in runners. Correlation of clinical symptoms and scintigraphy with a new magnetic resonance imaging grading system. Am J Sports Med. 1995;23(4):472–82.
59. Montgomery C, Couch C, Emory CL, Nicholas R. Giant cell tumor of bone: review of current literature, evaluation, and treatment options. J Knee Surg. 2019;32(4):331–6.
60. Daffner RH, Martinez S, Gehweiler JA Jr, Harrelson JM. Stress fractures of the proximal tibia in runners. Radiology. 1982;142:63–5.
61. Behrens SB, Deren ME, Matson A, Fadale PD, Monchik KO. Stress fractures of the pelvis and legs in athletes. Sports Health. 2013;5(2):165–74.
62. Robertson GAJ, Wood AM. Return to sports after stress fractures of the tibial diaphysis: a systematic review. Br Med Bull. 2015;114(1):95–111.
63. Harris JD, Varner KE. Stress fractures of the tibia. In: Miller TL, Kaeding CC, editors. Stress fractures in athletes. Switzerland: Springer International; 2015. p. 137–47.
64. Schilcher J, Bernhardsson M, Aspenberg P. Chronic anterior tibial stress fractures in athletes: no crack but intense remodeling. Scand J Med Sci Sports. 2019;29(10):1521–8.
65. Pereira H, Sousa D, d'Hooghe P, Gomes S, Oliveira JM, Reis RL, Espregueira-Mendes J, Ripoll PL, Hunt K. Return to play in stress fractures of the hip, thigh, knee, and leg. In: Musahl V, Karlsson J, Krutsch W, Mandelbaum B, Espregueira MJ, d'Hooghe P, editors. Return to play in football. Berlin, Heidelberg: Springer; 2018. p. 409–27.
66. Shima Y, Engebretsen L, Iwasa J, Kitaoka K, Tomita K. Use of bispohosphonates for the treatment of stress fractures in athletes. Knee Surg Sports Traumatol Arthrosc. 2009;17:542–50.
67. Stewart GW, Brunet ME, Manning MR, Davis FA. Treatment of stress fractures in athletes with intravenous pamidronate. Clin J Sport Med. 2005;15(2):92–4.
68. Beck BR, Matheson GO, Bergman G, Norling R, Fredericson M, Hoffman AR, Marcus R. Do capacitively coupled electric fields accelerate tibial stress fracture healing? A randomized controlled trial. Am J Sports Med. 2008;36(3):545–53.
69. Jensen JE. Stress fracture in the world class athlete: a case study. Med Sci Sports Exerc. 1998;30(6):783–7.
70. Kahanov L, Eberman LE, Games KE, Wasik M. Diagnosis, treatment, and rehabilitation of stress fractures in the lower extremity in runners. Open Access J Sports Med. 2015;6:87–95.

Stress Fractures in Sport: Ankle

26

Jensen K. Henry and Steve B. Behrens

Learning Objectives

- Recognize epidemiologic and clinical risk factors for stress fractures of the ankle.
- Understand the diagnostic and imaging principles of suspected ankle stress fractures.
- Identify high-risk and low-risk stress fractures.
- Apply appropriate nonoperative and operative treatment recommendations.

26.1 Introduction

Before the era of radiography, the first description of stress fractures was in 1855 by the military physician Breithaupt, who described the clinical condition of painful, swollen feet in Prussian soldiers [1]. Stress fractures were classically associated with military recruits for most of the nineteenth and early twentieth century. One century later, Devas and Sweetnam reported a series of 50 stress fractures of the fibula in their "athletes' clinic" [2]. Although stress fractures had been previously reported in the literature, the association with athletic participation had not been previously noted. Of the 49 athletes with stress fractures, 46 were competitive runners, and the majority were in the midst of their training season. Their report set the stage for greater awareness of the link between athletic participation and stress injury.

Participation in athletics has increased dramatically since then. This is largely in part due to Title IX of the 1972 Educational Amendments, which mandated equal access to school activities, including sports. As a result, an enormous shift of girls and women have transitioned off the sidelines and onto the playing field [3]. As a consequence, the number of high school girls participating in sports increased from under 300,000 in 1971 to nearly three million by the twenty-first century [3]. In the United States today, there are more than seven million high school athletes and 400,000 college athletes [3]. Beyond adolescence, more than half of adults exercise or play sports regularly each week [4]. Moreover, with the increased emphasis on exercise and physical ability in the media and pop culture, even older adults are regularly starting or continuing higher intensity exercise regimens. Road race participation increased by 300% from 1990 to 2013 [5], and, though adults aged 30–49 comprise the majority of marathoners, there has been a surge in nonagenarian participation [6].

Increased participation in athletics, combined with the fact that many individuals may be initiating training for the first time, all increases the likelihood of stress fracture. Therefore, physicians and orthopaedic surgeons must be aware of the presentation and workup for stress fractures, and be conversant with their management options, particularly when they should be referred to specialists. This chapter will focus on stress fractures of the ankle, specifically the distal tibia, medial malleolus, fibula, and talus.

26.2 Epidemiology

The rates of stress fractures may vary in the literature based on age, gender, sport/activity, and other predisposing factors. They are relatively rare in the general population, with reported rates of less than 0.5–1% [7]. Patients are typically young adults in their second or third decade of life [8–10]. Stress fractures are significantly more common in the elite athletic population, especially in running athletes. Track, cross country, volleyball, basketball, and gymnastics are the sports most commonly associated with ankle stress injuries [11]. In a survey of high school athletes, stress fractures were reported in 1.5% of the population, with a high rate in females (2.2%) than males (1.2%) [12]. Female sex conferred a 1.75 higher risk of stress fracture [12].

J. K. Henry (✉) · S. B. Behrens (✉)
Hospital for Special Surgery, Weill Cornell Medical College, New York, NY, USA
e-mail: henryj@hss.edu; behrenss@hss.edu

G. A. J. Robertson, N. Maffulli (eds.), *Fractures in Sport*, https://doi.org/10.1007/978-3-030-72036-0_26

Females, especially elite-level athletes, may be at increased risk to because of the female athlete triad of amenorrhea, inadequate caloric intake, and decreased bone density. In a study of National Collegiate Athletic Association (NCAA) athletes, more than a quarter had oligomenorrhea or amenorrhea, 6% met criteria for low bone mineral density, and 2% had a known eating disorder [13]. Moreover, nearly 1/3 of all female collegiate athletes met moderate- or high-risk criteria for future bone stress injuries [13].

In a survey of Japanese professional and recreational athletic injuries, the proportion of stress fracture was 1.91%, with a relatively similar rate between men and women [10]. Among all NCAA Division 1 athletes, 15% of female athletes had a history of stress fracture [14]. In a study of collegiate female competitive runners, the overall prevalence of stress fracture was 37% [15].

Injuries of the ankle constitute a significant proportion of lower extremity stress fractures: in competitive female runners, fractures at the distal tibia comprised 30%, with another 9% in the distal fibula [15]. Caucasians appear to have a higher likelihood of stress fractures, with rates of 39% versus 17% in African-Americans in one study [15]. Patients with lower extremity stress fractures in one location are also susceptible to stress injuries in other bones, especially the ankle—in patients with multiple stress fractures, 70% were in the tibia or fibula.

26.3 Etiology

26.3.1 Pathogenesis

Stress fractures differ from acute traumatic fractures in their pathogenesis. A list of contributing factors is shown in Table 26.1. Bone is a dynamic tissue, constantly remodeling through a balance of osteoclastic and osteoblastic activity. In fatigue stress fractures, submaximal stress is repeatedly applied to bone, which stimulates osteoclastic activity [15, 16]. In these periods of high intensity stress, new bone formation lags behind bone resorption [16, 17]. The hyperphysiologic loading to weakened bone predisposes it to microfracture, which can propagate and aggregate into stress fractures [16–18].

The period before the bone is structurally disrupted, but still has edema and changes as the cellular level, is considered to be a stress reaction (Fig. 26.1) [19]. Given the progression from stress reaction to fracture, fatigue injuries of bone can be considered along a spectrum. Comparatively, insufficiency stress fractures occur when normal stresses are applied to bone that is inherently weaker (i.e, osteoporosis) [15].

Table 26.1 Contributing factors to ankle stress fractures

Intrinsic factors	Extrinsic factors
Malalignment (tibia, ankle, foot)	Activity type
Cavovarus foot	Excessive activity/loading
Planovalgus foot	Rapid change in activity/ training regimen
Leg length discrepancy	
Tight Achilles tendon	Poor training conditions (i.e. hard surface)
Bone geometry	
Bone vascularity	Poor training mechanics
Tarsal coalition	Inadequate equipment/footwear
Prior surgery	
Estrogen or testosterone deficiency	
Obesity/overweight	

26.3.2 Mechanical

The most common reason for the bone resorptive imbalance seen in stress injuries is a change or increase in training. For example, in runners, initiation of a new exercise regimen, increase in distance, change to hard surfaces, and/or use of poorly supportive footwear may all increase the stress seen by the ankle bones. In Korean patients (both professional and recreational athletes) with stress fractures, more than 70% such fractures occurred after the athletes had increased their training by 100% [9]. The mean time from start of training to symptoms was 2.7 months, with a range of 1–6 months [9]. Extreme repetitive training may also increase fracture risk: in a study of ballet dancers, training for >5 hours per day increased the odds of stress fracture by more than sixfold [20]. Poor training choices—including inappropriate increases in the volume or pace of activity, or poor footwear and/or training surface—were cited in approximately one-fifth of ankle stress fractures [21].

Malalignment may also predispose to stress fracture at the ankle, and attention must be directed to varus/valgus alignment of the ankle and lower extremity. Various skeletal biomechanical factors have been associated with lower extremity stress fractures, including excessive external rotation at the hip, forefoot or subtalar varus, tibia varum, planovalgus or cavovarus foot, excessive foot pronation, increased hindfoot inversion, limited ankle dorsiflexion, and leg length discrepancy [22–24]. One study found a leg-length inequality in 83% of athletes with multiple (>1) stress fractures [24].

Among naval trainees, pes cavus and pes planus were both associated with twice as many stress fractures compared to feet with normal arches [23]. Moreover, in a study of athletes, forefoot varus and high arch were associated with recurrent stress fractures [24]. Finally, ankle stress fractures may occur in the postoperative setting. In a series of patients with prior ankle or hindfoot arthrodesis, 7% had subsequent stress fracture at the distal tibia, medial malleolus, or distal fibula [25].

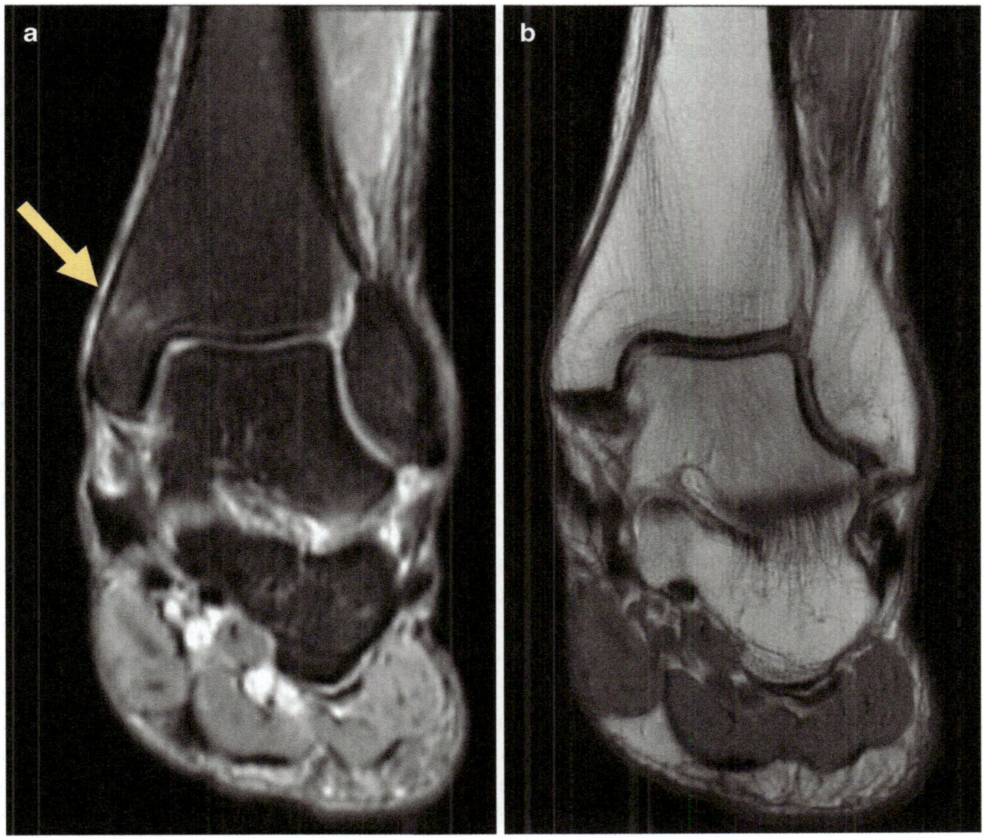

Fig. 26.1 Medial malleolar stress reaction. Coronal MRI images showing bony edema at the medial malleolus on the inversion recovery sequence (**a**), without cortical break on proton density sequence (**b**)

26.3.3 Biologic

The intrinsic nature of the bone, including its composition and vascular supply, may further predispose to fracture [16]. Sex-based and hormonal effects are imperative to consider as a contributing factor to stress reaction and fracture. The female athlete triad consists of amenorrhea, insufficient caloric intake (which may or may not manifest with an eating disorder), and osteoporosis. However, many athletes may have one or more of the conditions. Estrogen deficiency increases the rate of bone resorption and therefore decreases bone density, which predisposes to fracture [13, 16, 18].

Although the association between the female athlete triad and stress fracture has been well described, there is also growing awareness of the effect of endurance exercise on male athletes [18, 26]. Endurance training, such as in long-distance running, lowers testosterone levels in men, [27] potentially leading to increased osteoclastic activity and bone resorption [16]. In addition, while moderate-distance running and other athletic activities typically increase bone size and/or density, more extensive endurance running actually was actually associated with a decrease in bone mineral density in a study group of male runners [28].

26.4 Classification

Stress injuries of the bone are a continuum from stress reaction, which is characterized by bone marrow edema and periosteal reaction, to actual fracture [7]. In stress reaction, the bone has not been disrupted but does have an area of increased remodeling [16]. Stress fractures can also be characterized if they are high-risk or low-risk. Low-risk stress fractures, including those of the posteromedial tibia and fibula, have a favorable outcome with nonoperative management [7].

High-risk stress fractures include the anterior cortex of the tibia, the medial malleolus, and the talus. Characteristically these fractures have a higher chance of recurrence, progression to complete fracture, and non-union [7]. Often these injuries are subject to tensile—rather than compression—

forces, or have relative avascularity at the fracture site, which can predispose to poor healing [7]. In addition to high- and low- risk, stress fractures can also be categorized according to the extent of severity. Multiple scales have been developed based on imaging [29].

26.5 Diagnosis

26.5.1 History

As with any orthopaedic complaint, a thorough history should be obtained. Pain is a hallmark of stress fracture; further details about the quality, location, and duration should be elicited. Pain may be focal to the area or vague, difficult to localize, and/or radiating. In stress injuries, the onset is often insidious without an inciting injury or event. Symptoms may be chronic or subacute, although some patients may present acutely or with an acute worsening of their symptoms. Symptoms typically are present weeks to months prior to presentation or diagnosis; on average the period is 1–2 months [30].

Ameliorating and aggravating factors should also be identified. Classically in stress fractures, symptoms worsen with physical activity that loads the affected area and improve with rest or activity restriction. The physician or surgeon should investigate the patient's exercise/training regimen. Initiation of a new exercise program (for example, a patient who started training for a marathon) or escalation of training are hallmarks of the stress fracture diagnosis. The patient may report changes in the training surface (i.e., transition from a soft turf or field to a hard surface) [7]. Although stress fractures of the leg, ankle, and foot were traditionally linked to running, newer reports have shown stress injuries occurring in a wide variety of sports, including football, basketball, ballet, volleyball, rowing, and gymnastics [7, 8].

History from female patients should include age at menarche, any periods of amenorrhea, and contraceptive use. In a study of collegiate female runners, stress fractures occurred in nearly half of women with irregular menses compared to 29% of women with regular menses [15]. Moreover, oral contraceptive use may be associated with lower rates of stress fractures (one study reported a significant difference of 12% versus 29%) [15]. It is important to be cognizant of the female athlete triad, which increases fracture risk. In female college runners, 47% of women with menstrual irregularities also had disordered eating [15]. All patients, regardless of gender, should be asked about nutritional habits—including disordered eating—and vitamin/supplement use. Deficits in calcium and vitamin D are increasingly recognized as a risk factor for fracture [31].

26.5.2 Physical Examination

Although certain physical findings may be specific to the site of the stress fracture, all stress injuries of the ankle should be evaluated in a systematic manner. Visual inspection includes the identification of swelling, erythema, deformity, and/or callosities. Gait should be assessed, as many patients may present with an antalgic gait, or decreased time in stance phase on the affected side. Standing alignment of the feet and legs should be assessed for deformity, varus/valgus alignment, length discrepancy, and cavus or planovalgus position: all may predispose to stress fracture [32].

The site of concern should be examined for signs of inflammation including swelling or redness and palpated for tenderness. Neurovascular examination is normally negative. Muscle strength/bulk are usually unaffected. Provocative manuevers that reproduce the patient's pain should be assessed. Range of motion as well as Achilles or gastrocnemius contractures should be noted, as excessive stiffness or, conversely, ligamentous laxity, may lead to unequal forces across the joint—theoretically increasing fracture risk [32]. There are also descriptions of percussion tenderness or the "tuning fork test", in which a tuning fork is held to the bone at a distance from the involved site to see whether it reproduces the patient's symptoms [7, 9]. Anterior drawer and talar tilt tests should be performed to assess ligamentous stability. Ankle instability may be part of the differential diagnosis or even a contributing factor to stress fracture [33].

26.5.3 Imaging

Radiographs are the first imaging modality for nearly any clinical scenarios. Radiographs may show radiolucent lines or cortical disruption indicating fracture, periosteal reaction, or even early callus [7, 16]. However, negative radiographs do not exclude the diagnosis: in a study of 320 athletes with stress fractures, less than 10% had abnormal radiographs at the time of presentation [21]. Severity of the stress fracture is reflected in imaging findings—in low-grade stress fractures confirmed on bone scintigraphy, radiographs were positive in only 4% [34]. This number increased to 76% in higher-grade stress injuries [34].

Bone scan, or bone scintigraphy, was the traditional gold standard for advanced imaging evaluation of stress fracture (Fig. 26.2). Scintigraphy is highly sensitive and captures areas of increased tracer uptake at the stressed site. Techneitium-99 imaging is comprised of multiple phases which record perfusion as well as blood pooling [16]. While bone scanning is sensitive, it is not specific, and provides limited anatomic detail. It also requires clinical correlation, as infection, osteo-

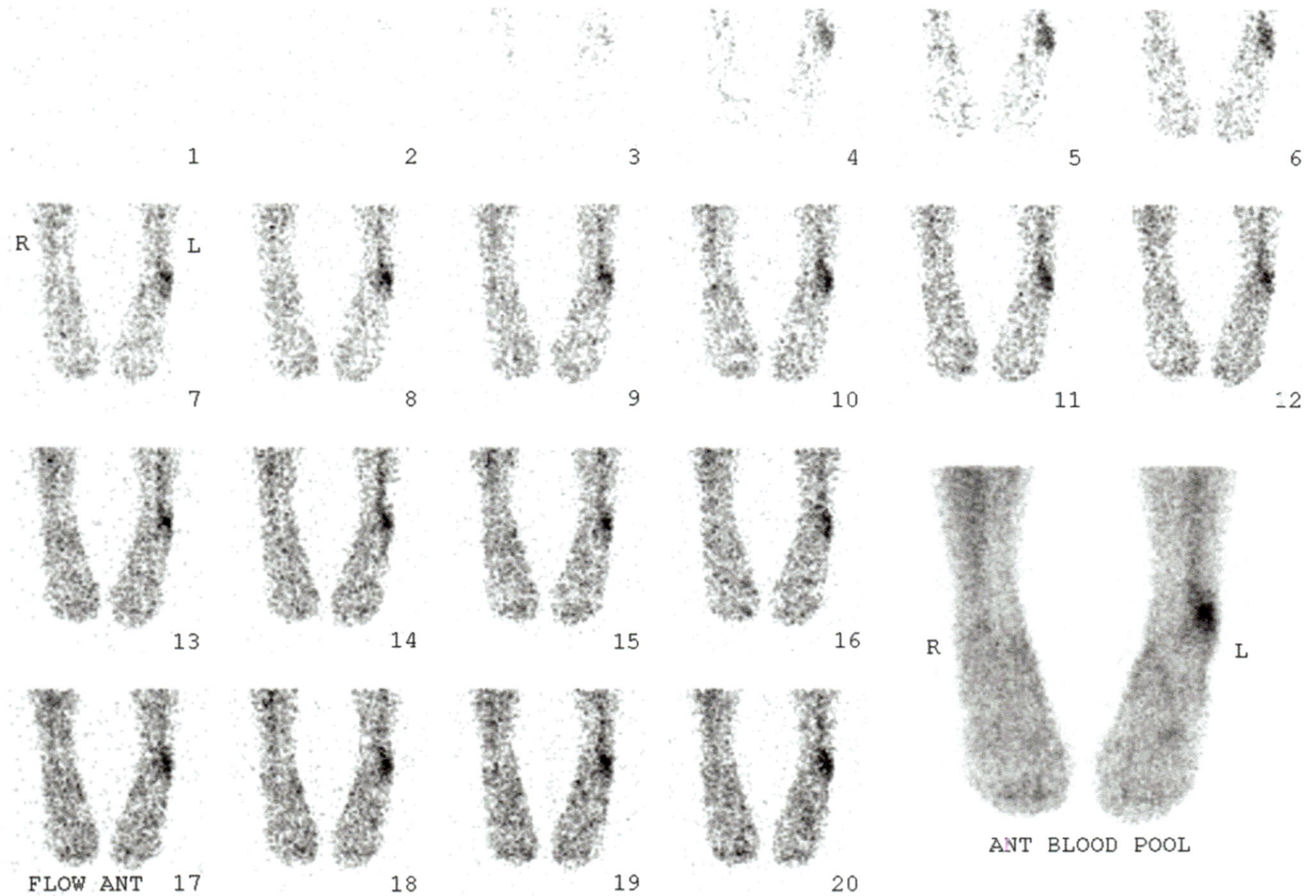

Fig. 26.2 Bone scan of a professional dancer with a fibular stress fracture

necrosis, and tumor can all resemble stress injury [19]. Moreover, activity intensity on imaging may linger for months after resolution of symptoms: therefore, it is not a useful modality to gauge healing or guide return to play [16].

Magnetic resonance imaging (MRI) has become the advanced imaging modality of choice for most cases. Specifically, MRI evaluation of stress injury should incorporate edema-sensitive sequences, such as short tau inversion recovery (STIR) or fat-suppressed T2 weighted images [19]. Contrast is not needed. At our institution, MRI protocols typically combine inversion recovery sequences, which are highly sensitive to edema, with proton density (fast spin echo), which provides anatomic detail, especially along joints. MRI has the same sensitivity and greater specificity than bone scan [19]. And because MRI can easily detect bone marrow edema, which is the hallmark of the stress response, it can help identify stress fracture weeks before any findings would be apparent on plain radiography [19]. In addition to being more specific than bone scan, MRI also provides information about the surrounding soft tissues, which may help in ruling a diagnosis in or out [19]. Severity of the stress fracture can be quantified based on MRI (Table 26.2).

Table 26.2 Radiologic grading of stress fractures

Grade	XR	Bone scan	MRI	Treatment
1	Normal	Increased activity, poorly defined	Edema on STIR sequence	3 weeks rest
2	Normal	Area of intensely increased activity, poorly defined	Edema on STIR and T2 sequences	3–6 weeks rest
3	Discrete line or periosteal reaction	Sharply defined area of uptake	Positive STIR and PD (or T1)	12–16 weeks rest
4	Definite fracture or periosteal reaction	Transcortical localized uptake	Positive STIR and PD (or T1) with fracture line	>16 weeks rest

Adapted from Arendt et al. [29]

Computed tomography (CT) is less sensitive than bone scan or MRI [19]. However, unlike MRI, bone scan, or plain radiographs, CT has the best ability to delineate cortical fracture lines [19]. Weight-bearing CT may provide additional information about bony alignment and mechanical predisposition to injury.

Table 26.3 Differential diagnosis for ankle stress fracture

Neoplastic
Solid tumor
Myeloma
Lymphoma
Leukemia
Osteoid osteoma
Ewing's sarcoma
Osteosarcoma
Metastasis
Pathologic fracture
Infectious
Osteomyelitis
Soft tissue infection
Bony or soft tissue injury
Tendinopathy
Plantar fasciitis
Exertional compartment syndrome
Nerve entrapment
Ligamentous injury or instability
Muscle strain
Acute trauma
Osteochondral defect
Peroneal tendon tear or subluxation/dislocation
Other
Metabolic disease
Tarsal coalition
Complex regional pain syndrome
Post-operative arthrodesis or fracture non-union

Ultrasound is not routinely used for diagnosis. However, given its highly user-dependent nature, certain centers may use it in limited or special circumstances. When used, ultrasonography of stress fractures demonstrates focal hyperechoic elevation of periosteum with bony irregularity and increased Doppler flow [35].

26.5.4 Differential Diagnosis

There is a wide differential diagnosis for stress fractures of the foot and ankle (Table 26.3). It is important to rule out nerve entrapment, infection, neoplasm, muscle strain, ligamentous injury, osteochondral injury, osteomalacia, and exertional compartment syndrome, among others [16, 19, 36].

While MRI can be used to differentiate stress fracture from most solid tumors, certain bone marrow diseases such as myeloma, lymphoma, leukemia, or early osteomyelitis may resemble stress fracture [19]. Bone marrow edema can also be seen in avascular necrosis, osteochondral defects, metabolic disease, tarsal coalition, tendinopathy, and plantar fasciitis [37]. A thorough history and physical examination are therefore critical.

26.6 Management

26.6.1 Initial Considerations

Hormonal, nutritional, and/or other medical abnormalities should be addressed to facilitate fracture healing. Vitamin D and calcium supplementation are often needed if the patient is deficient [31].

Female athletes with amenorrhea may require hormonal supplementation with estrogen, which helps to re-establish the normal menstrual state and improve bone mineral density [7]. Patients with stress fractures and caloric deficiencies or disordered eating should be referred to the appropriate specialists in nutrition or psychology to prevent potentially life-threatening effects of untreated eating disorders.

The diagnosis of a stress fracture should also prompt evaluation and any necessary modifications of unhealthy training practices. Athletes should be educated about proper footwear, safe surfaces for high endurance activity, cross-training to minimize repetitive stresses on the skeleton, and scheduled rest from sport. The physician or surgeon may need to emphasize the importance of these modifications to the coach, trainer, and family as well. Additional treatments may include physical therapy for generalized conditioning, performance mechanics, and strengthening. Finally, patients with poor running or fitness mechanics may benefit from gait analysis and retraining.

26.6.1.1 Low Risk

Low-risk stress fractures, such as the fibula, may be initially managed nonoperatively. This should include rest and cessation of activity for 2–6 weeks. After a period of rest, if the athlete has been pain-free, they may restart low impact activity (i.e. stationary bike, swimming). If they tolerate this without symptoms, they can gradually take on more progressive activities.

Weight-bearing status and immobilisation are based on the surgeon's clinical judgment. Although logically they would seem to decrease force on the tibia and facilitate healing, no studies have shown that they affect the stress fracture healing rate [7]. Low-risk stress fractures that are refractory to nonoperative management may be considered for surgical intervention. Often, changes in the radiographic appearance of these fractures—including lucency, cyst formation, and/or sclerosis—may prompt a more aggressive attitude. Some may advocate for early operative intervention in high-level athletes to decrease time to return to play.

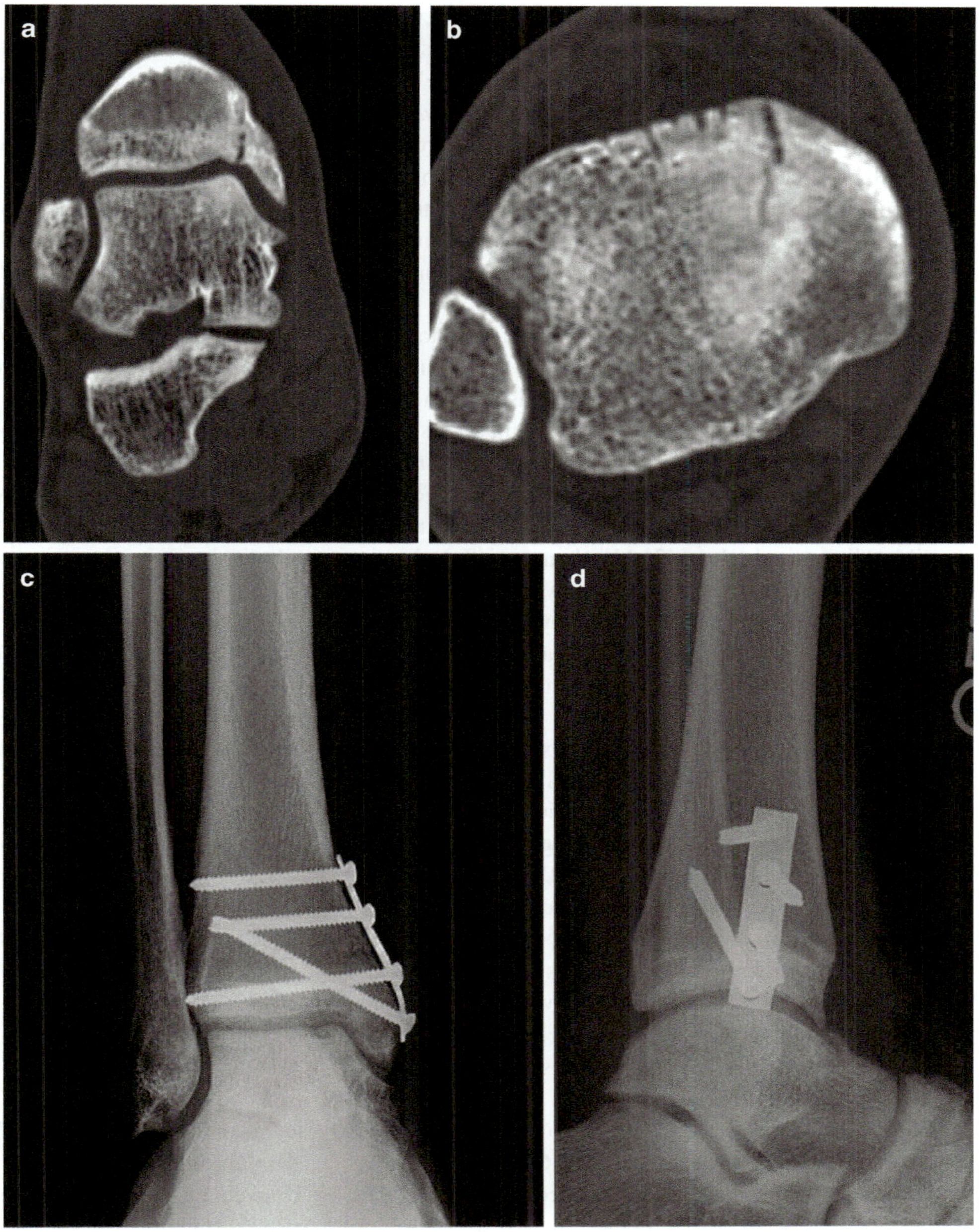

Fig. 26.3 Medial malleolar stress fracture in a professional athlete (**a**), treated with buttress plate fixation (**b**). The player was out for the season but was able to return to play at their previous level

26.6.1.2 High Risk

Some authors recommend treating high-risk stress fractures—like those of the medial malleolus and talus—similar to acute fractures due to the high risk of complications like progression to complete fracture or non-union [16]. If the fracture is displaced, surgical management with percutaneous internal fixation or open reduction and internal fixation (ORIF) is generally recommended. The majority of ankle stress fractures, though, even if high-risk, can be managed nonoperatively with immobilisation and limited weight-bearing.

However, if nonoperative treatment fails, or the patient is a high-demand athlete and there is concern for faster return-to-play, surgery is indicated (Fig. 26.3) [16]. Operative management is also indicated for fractures with radiographic findings indicative of impaired progression to healing or signs of non-healing, such sclerosis or cystic changes [16].

Novel management options include both operative and nonoperative methods to attempt to heal stress fractures. A pilot study found that teriparatide, a human recombinant parathyroid hormone typically used for osteoporosis treatment in postmenopausal women and men, improved bone density and bone biomarkers in premenopausal women with stress fractures [38]. Further research is needed to understand whether teriparatide reliably improves stress fracture healing.

There are limited reports of the use of extracorporeal shock wave therapy (ESWT) in stress fractures to stimulate healing in cases of delayed union or nonunion [39]. This has been described as an isolated management modality or as an adjuvant to operative management in high-risk stress fractures with delayed union, such as the medial malleolus [39]. Although this is a fairly new utility for ESWT, anecdotal reports are promising, citing faster improvement in symptoms and return to play [40]. Further evaluation is warranted.

Bone stimulators represent another possible nonoperative option for treatment of stress fractures [32]. Bone stimulators include electric/electromagnetic and ultrasound modalities [32]. Electric/electromagnetic bone stimulators stimulate intracellular calcium stores, which leads to increased calmodulin and ultimately cell proliferation [41]. Few studies have been published in human stress fractures, including the tibia, fibula, and talus [42, 43], demonstrating that coupled electric stimulation is safe and may even promote healing, though it is unclear whether they provide clinically relevant advantages [42, 43]. They may be considered in severe cases or elite-level athletes with high return-to-play needs.

Pulsed ultrasound bone stimulators exert multiple cellular effects, including collagen synthesis, cell proliferation, alterations in calcium levels, and stimulation of angiogenesis, and [44] have been successful in healing acute fractures and stress fractures in animal models [44, 45]. However, the literature regarding the efficacy of ultrasound bone stimulators in stress fractures in humans is limited [44].

Treatments with orthobiologic agents have been proposed in recent studies. Subchondroplasty, in which calcium phosphate is percutaneously injected into the injury site, has been utilized for osteochondral lesions but also stress fractures of the foot and ankle [46]. The data are too limited to draw conclusions, but this may be a novel way to provide a osteoconductive scaffold for bone remodeling [46].

The use of bone marrow aspirate concentrate (BMAC) has also been described as a method to heal stress fractures of the foot and ankle [47]. BMAC, which has applications throughout orthopaedics, may potentiate fracture healing via its hematopoietic and mesenchymal stem cell effects, as well as osteogenic effects via vascular endothelial growth factor (VEGF), transforming growth factor-beta (TGF-B), and platelet-derived growth factor (PDGF) [47].

26.7 Return to Play and Rehabilitation

Low-risk stress fractures usually benefit from a brief period of relative rest. However, the athlete generally can still bear weight or partial weight on the extremity. Importantly, individuals with low-risk stress fractures may still be allowed to participate to some form of physical activity. For elite athletes at high levels of activity, the decision to continue participation in the remainder of the season can be discussed [48]. For these patients, pain can be used as a guide for activity modification. The ultimate goal is to minimize the stress that caused the imbalance in resorption so that the body can rebuild bone at the necessary level [48].

For high-risk stress fractures, it is generally advised to completely rest from activity until thee fracture is healed. The goal of treatment of high-risk stress fractures is healing while minimizing the risk of delayed union, non-union, or propagation of the fracture [48]. Whether treated with immobilisation and limited weight bearing or surgery, the fracture must be healed before the patient returns to athletic activity.

For any of the ankle stress fractures, return to play should first start with low-impact activity such as stationary bicycle, elliptical training, stepping on the stepping machine, rowing or swimming. Return to running should only be initiated if the patient can tolerate lower impact activity without pain. A walk-jog program should be initiated first with gradual return to longer durations of running. The patient can gradually build up their tolerance to impact over a period of several weeks. Generalized conditioning and cross training should be recommended to minimize repeated stress and refracture. Treatment should be individualized to each patient, level of sport, timing in the season, and symptoms.

26.8 Preventative Measures

26.8.1 Vitamin D

Adequate vitamin D is essential to facilitate calcium absorption and the maintenance of normal calcium and phosphate levels in the body [31]. It is therefore critical for maintaining normal levels of bone formation and resorption. Low vitamin D levels have been associated with osteomalacia and higher risk of fracture [31, 49]. A study of female Navy recruits, who represent a higher-risk group due to their activity level, found that female recruits whose serum 25-hydroxyvitamin D levels were less than 20 ng/mL had double the risk of tibia and fibula stress fractures compared to recruits whose levels were greater than 40 ng/mL [49]. One strategy to prevent stress fracture, especially in high risk populations, may be vitamin D3 supplementation with 4000 IU daily in order to achieve levels of 40 ng/mL [49].

26.8.2 Surveillance

In female patients with stress fractures, surgeons should be keenly aware to look for amenorrhea and/or poor nutritional status to identify the female athlete triad. Any patient with the female athlete triad and stress fracture should undergo DEXA scan to diagnose and quantify osteoporosis. There are multiple studies detailing the incidence of recurrent stress fractures, or multiple stress fractures in different bones [24, 30]. The athlete and their coach, trainer, and family should be counselled about the importance of appropriate training conditions, progression of activity, and cross-training to minimize future injury.

26.9 Specific Anatomic Locations

26.9.1 Medial Malleolus

26.9.1.1 Overview/Epidemiology

Medial malleolus stress fractures are relatively uncommon but are considered high-risk injuries [16]. Medial malleolus stress fractures comprise approximately 0.6–4% of all stress fractures [8–10]. They are most common in patients participating in high-demand running and jumping sports, including track/cross-country, basketball, volleyball, fencing, and football [8, 10, 50]. In recreational and professional athletes, medial malleolus injuries represented approximately 16–17% of all stress fractures in basketball and volleyball players [10]. Another series of medial malleolar stress injuries reported a predominance of sprinting, hurdling, or running [51]..

As the ankle progresses repetitively through range of motion, the talus can impinge on the medial malleolus and cause stress fracture. The mechanism may be attributed to repetitive dorsiflexion and rotation, which reproduces the Lauge-Hansen supination-adduction injury pattern [52]. Anteromedial ankle impingement, in which the talar neck or anterior tibial osteophytes repeatedly impinge on the medial malleolus, have also been implicated [52, 53].

26.9.1.2 Diagnosis

History

Patients will usually report several weeks of pain or discomfort with running and jumping activities that should partially or completely resolve with rest [54]. They may or may not have an acute worsening event or injury that prompts the visit. The pain is usually centered over the medial malleolus but may be vague or difficult to localize early [51]. There is usually a lag of approximately 1–2 months between start of symptoms and presentation to the physician, but even with this delay, radiographs are often normal [51].

Physical Examination

Patients classically have tenderness over the medial malleolus and present with an ankle effusion [54]. Dorsiflexion may be limited as well [54].

Imaging

Radiographs show a vertically oriented fracture line extending from the junction where the tibial plafond meets the medial malleolus [54]. The fracture line may also extend obliquely from the tibial plafond-medial malleolus junction [54]. However, radiographic lucency may not always be present. In a case series of athletes, only 50% of patients with medial malleolus stress fractures had positive findings on radiographs [54]. In that case, advanced imaging is recommended (MRI or bone scan). Sclerotic changes along the fracture line, or cystic lobulated osteolytic changes, may be seen at the injury site [50].

26.9.1.3 Management

Nonoperative

In most cases, a trial of cast or boot immobilisation and non-weightbearing is appropriate [22]. In a limited series of six patients, Shelbourne et al. opted for nonoperative management for patients in whom radiographs were normal and there was only evidence on bone scan [54]. Patients were immobilized in braces for 6 weeks and refrained from training or other activity. Additional reports of medial malleolar stress fractures, even where the is a visible fracture line, have described success with nonoperative treatment [50]. Brief periods of immobilisation, potentially with casting, are recommended [50]. In a limited series of athletes with medial malleolar stress fractures, five of eight were management successfully with nonoperative treatment only [51]. The majority of these patients had positive findings on advanced imaging only, and there was a mean time of 4 months to healing from the time of diagnosis.

Operative

Indications for operative management of these high-risk stress fractures are debated, especially in elite or professional athletes. Failure of nonoperative management—i.e., recurrent or persistent symptoms despite adequate immobilisation and rest, or fracture propagation or displacement—is generally agreed upon as an indication for surgery [55]. Initial sclerosis or cystic change at the fracture site is another indication for operative treatment of medial malleolar stress fractures. Shelbourne et al. recommended operative fixation for patients with displacement or visible fracture lines on radiographs [54].

In a series of eight competitive athletes with medial malleolar stress fractures, only three were treated with surgery [51]. These fractures all demonstrated high-risk characteristics, including initial fracture displacement or persistent symptoms and delayed union [51]. Another group reported a medial malleolar stress fracture in an amenorrheic gymnast [56]. She was initially treated nonoperatively and progressed to normal activity over a 6-week period. However, with repeated competition, her symptoms recurred and the fracture had propagated. She subsequently underwent cancellous screw fixation [56]. Some surgeons advocate for early fixation of medial malleolar stress fractures in elite or professional athletes given both the high-risk nature of their sport as well as the necessity to return to play in a timely fashion.

Operative management generally should mimic the treatment for an acute traumatic medial malleolus fracture. Either open reduction or percutaneous fixation may be used. In open cases, a straight or curvilinear incision over the medial malleolus is utilized with care taken to protect the saphenous vein. Fixation is achieved with two 4.0 mm partially-threaded cancellous screws (Fig. 26.4) or anti-glide/buttress plating [55].

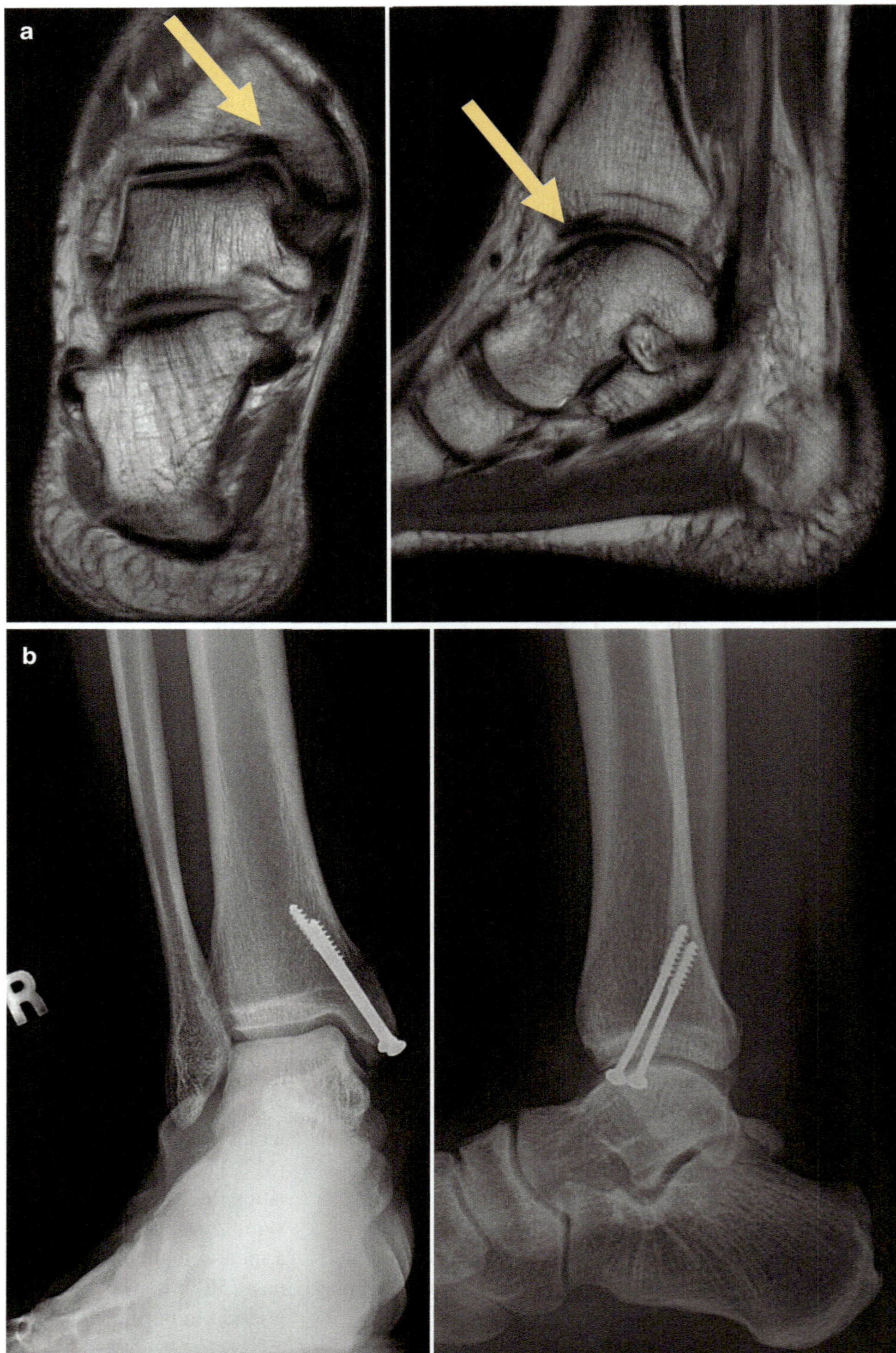

Fig. 26.4 Medial malleolar stress fracture seen on MRI (**a**, arrows) treated with screw fixation (**b**)

If there is fracture displacement and/or chronic sclerosis, bone graft can be used. Treatment of delayed union may include oblique drilling of the medial malleolus to stimulate healing [24]. Medial malleolus fractures are susceptible to high shear forces so surgeons should monitor closely for non-union.

The benefit of operative fixation is the ability to return to range of motion and weight bearing sooner. Patients are followed postoperatively with serial radiographs and typically demonstrate fracture union at 6–8 weeks, at which point they can start returning to activity. In a case of a football player treated operatively for a medial malleolar stress fracture, the patient was advanced to light running at 3 weeks postoperatively and was back to sport at 4 weeks, with complete union at 3 months [55]. In general, after the diagnosis is made and appropriate management is instituted, the average time to healing with normal radiographic appearance of bone is 5 months from the time of diagnosis (although certainly longer from the time of symptoms) [51]. Little has been studied on formal return to play statistics, but outcomes have been reported as good, with full return to pre-injury level of training at 6 months [51].

Special Considerations

Interestingly, one study reported a series of 5 elite athletes with medial malleolar stress fractures, all with an anteromedial bony spur on the tibia [53]. The authors believed that the stress fracture represented an end-stage presentation of anteromedial ankle impingement. They therefore treated patients surgically with internal fixation and arthroscopic debridement of the bony spur [53]. All patients achieved fracture union at 10 weeks and returned to their previous level of activity at final follow-up.

Another case report described a medial malleolar stress fracture in a baseball player which developed after multiple ankle sprains [33]. The authors believed this resulted from sustained varus force on the medial malleolus due to lateral ligament instability. The patient underwent fixation of the medial malleolus fracture with concomitant modified Brostrom procedure to address the lateral instability [33]. The patient had complete union and was gradually advanced to full activity at 3 months postoperatively. While there are limited data to support these proposed theories and treatment in all patients, certainly they may be beneficial in specific symptomatic athletes with characteristic findings on physical examination and imaging [53].

26.9.2 Distal Tibia

26.9.2.1 Overview/Epidemiology

Stress fractures of the tibia are common, with the distal tibia representing 25% of tibial stress fractures and just over 7% of all stress fractures [9, 24]. In a series of distal tibial stress fractures, 13 of 14 patients were runners, averaging 20–25 miles per week [57]. In addition to the typically susceptible high-impact running and jumping athletes, these injuries have been described in hockey players and gymnasts [58]. Distal tibia stress fractures may also occur in laborers who lift heavy loads or military recruits [59, 60]. There are rare reports of bilateral distal tibia stress fractures, so extensive loading with bilateral ankle pain should prompt further workup [58, 60].

26.9.2.2 Diagnosis

History

There is classically pain and swelling in the ankle or the supramalleolar region of the distal tibia.

Physical Examination

Patients usually have tenderness over the anterior ankle joint and may present with an antalgic gait [58]. Maximal dorsiflexion and plantarflexion may exacerbate anterior ankle pain as well [58].

Imaging

Distal tibia stress injuries typically occur in a transverse line that is parallel to the epiphysis and just proximal to the physeal scar [30, 58]. Although plain radiographs are often normal, radiographic features of stress fracture include cortical or periosteal thickening, a linear area of sclerosis, and/or focal areas of decreased cortical density (Fig. 26.5) [57].

26.9.2.3 Management

In the early setting, a brief period of immobilisation may be warranted. Rest from activity is the classic prescription, with resolution of symptoms over a 12-week period [58]. Supplementation with calcium or vitamin D may be recommended to minimize the risk of nonunion [61]. Surgery is reserved for those patients who fail nonoperative management, refractory cases, and elite or professional athletes with return-to-play considerations. There is a paucity in the literature describing operative treatment of distal tibia stress injuries.

26.9.3 Talus

26.9.3.1 Overview/Epidemiology

Stress fractures of the talus are also uncommon, but have been reported in running athletes as well as football players, gymnasts, ballet dancers, and pole vaulters [37, 62, 63]. Talar stress fractures have been described at the neck, body, and lateral process. The location often varies with the type of activity. In runners, the fracture or edema line is located in the neck, parallel to the talonavicular joint. In gymnasts, the stress injury extends from the body at an oblique angle to the talonavicular joint, and propagates into the posterior subtalar

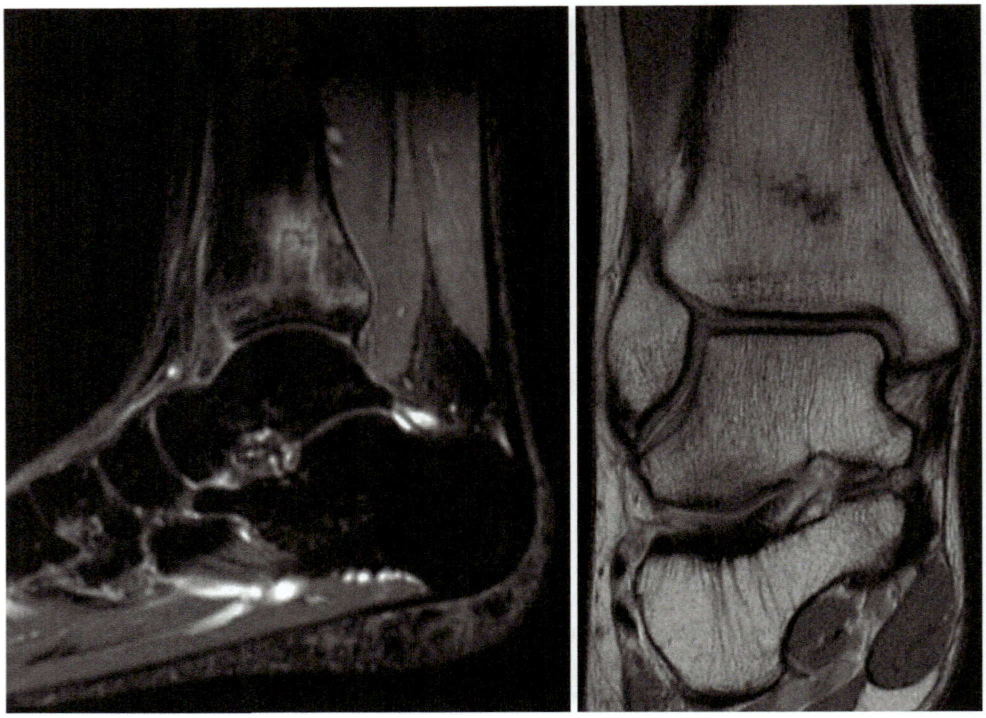

Fig. 26.5 MRI showing stress fracture of the distal tibia in a 25-year-old female runner with 3 weeks of ankle pain. The patient also had oligomenorrhea and disordered eating. She was treated nonoperatively with a CAM boot and rest from activity, as well as vitamin D and calcium supplementation

joint [63]. One purported mechanism is the impingement of the lateral process of the calcaneus on the posterolateral talus [62]. This occurs in athletes who are undergoing repeated plantarflexion and pronation [62].

26.9.3.2 Diagnosis

History

Talar stress fractures are typically seen in high-impact activities, especially those that require running or jumping. In a study of military trainees with ankle or foot stress injury, talus stress fractures represented the highest proportion at 15% [30]. Importantly, in this study, talar stress fractures were significantly more likely to occur simultaneously with other stress fractures, and clinicians should be aware that identification of stress fracture in one location does not preclude concomitant injuries [30].

Physical Examination

Patients may have lateral ankle or sinus tarsi pain that worsens with activity. The signs and symptoms of talar stress fracture may overlap with sinus tarsi syndrome; clinicians should have a high index of suspicion to work up potential stress fractures in these patients [62].

Imaging

Weight-bearing radiographs of the ankle should be obtained but are often negative [62]. Advanced imaging, such as CT or MRI, are therefore useful (Fig. 26.6). On MRI, the edema pattern is often perpendicular to the trabecular flow, parallel to the talonavicular joint [19]. Even prior to formal stress fracture, MRIs of professional ballet dancers showed patchy bone marrow edema in the talar neck or body, consistent with their tendency to perform extensive axial loading while in extreme plantar flexion (i.e., in the en-pointe and demi-pointe positions) [37]. This edema pattern may be reflect overuse prior to complete fracture.

26.9.3.3 Management

There are little data regarding long-term outcomes after treatment of talar stress fractures, and generally nonoperative management should be pursued first [62]. Four to six weeks of immobilisation in a cast or boot are recommended, with surgery reserved for fractures that are displaced or refractory to nonoperative treatment [63]. Because these injuries are relatively rare, there are little robust data regarding outcomes. Small series have demonstrated that symptom resolution occurs at approximately 4 months [63].

In a series of four athletes, only one was treated surgically [62]. However, even when the fractures had healed, the patients were either unable to return to their prior high level of activity or had persistent pain with activity [62]. In another series of gymnasts with talar body fractures, all three were able to return to activity at a high level [63]. Surgery is reserved for those patients who fail nonoperative management, refractory cases, and elite or professional athletes with return-to-play considerations.

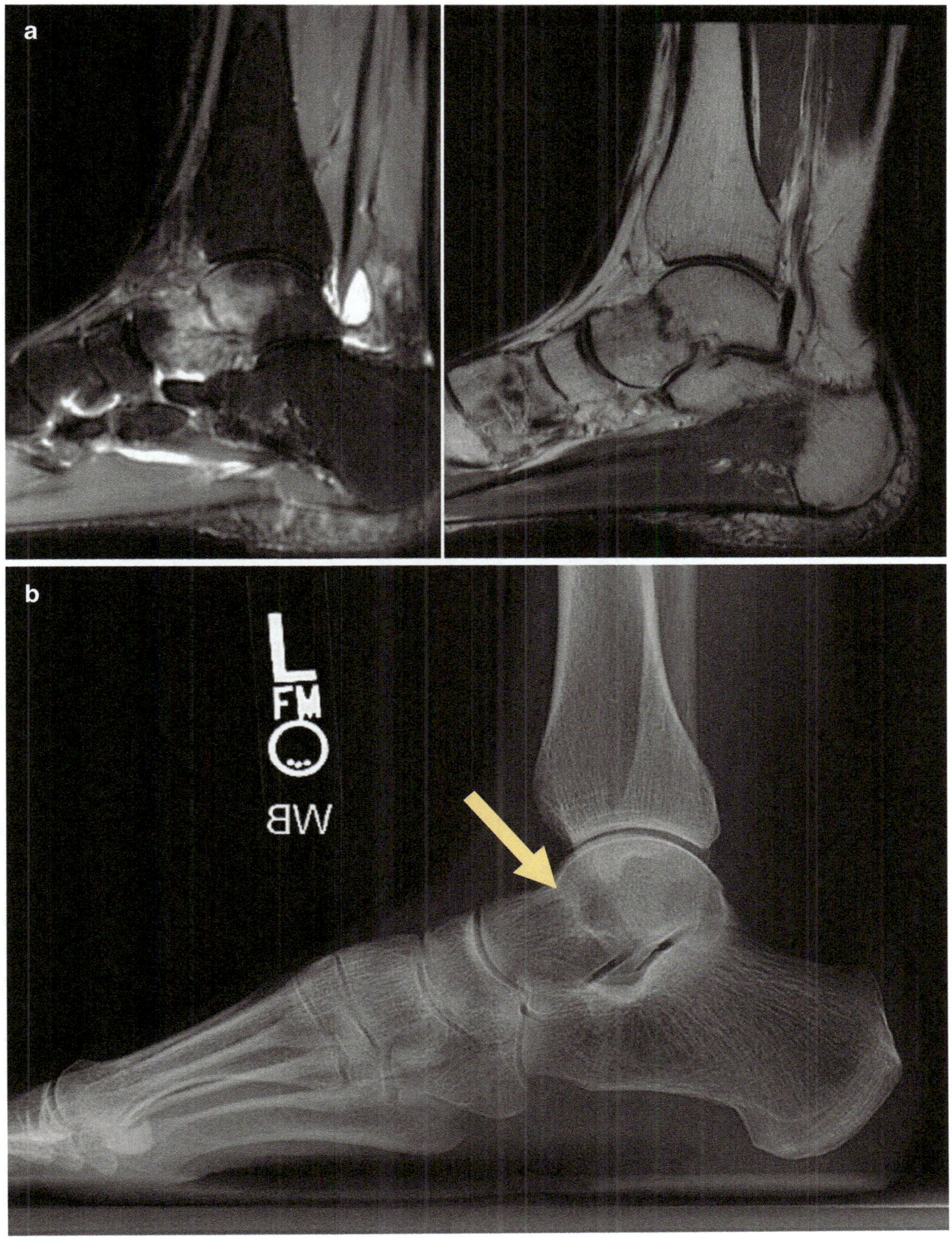

Fig. 26.6 Talar stress fracture in a female runner treated nonoperatively with a CAM boot and non-weightbearing. MRI at time of diagnosis demonstrated the fracture (**a**), and follow-up radiographs 3 weeks later (**b**) showed evidence of healing (arrow)

26.9.4 Fibula

26.9.4.1 Overview/Epidemiology

Fibula stress fractures are among the most common of ankle stress fractures, and are generally low-risk. They represent 3% of all athletic injuries [2]. Like most ankle stress fractures, they are typical in running athletes, especially those who train on hard surfaces [2, 36]. Among dancers, fibular stress fractures may arise from imbalance and/or fatigue when initiating a turn [64]. They may also occur in figure skaters, especially in the take-off leg, and hockey players [17, 65].

They commonly occur at the junction of cortical and cancellous bone in the distal fibula, just proximal to the inferior tibiofibular ligaments [36, 66]. Eversion of the foot strains the lateral fibula, leading to concentrated stress just below the interosseous ligament, may be the causative factor [66]. In dancers, fibular stress fractures are commonly located approximately 10 cm proximal to the tip of the lateral malleolus [64]. One theory purports that rhythmic contraction of the long toe flexors leads to micromotion of the fibula and ultimately stress injury [2, 36].

26.9.4.2 Diagnosis

History
Patients report days or weeks of insidious pain over the lateral portion of the ankle that worsens with activity and improves with rest.

Physical Examination
Tenderness and swelling directly at the fibula can easily be evidenced on physical examination. Patients will also have pain with compression across the tibiofibular joint distally. If the injury is subacute or chronic, callus may be palpable as the skin and soft tissue envelope is generally thinner over the distal fibula. Pain can be reproduced with ankle eversion or maximum ankle dorsiflexion [66].

Imaging
Initial radiographs may not show abnormalities, although by 6 weeks there is usually periosteal new bone visualized [2]. On plain radiographs, an oblique view with the extremity internally rotated shows the fibula in profile, and may be useful in detecting subtle changes [2]. Advanced imaging, such as MRI or bone scan, will show increased uptake or signal at the distal fibula (Fig. 26.7).

26.9.4.3 Management
Stress fractures of the distal fibula have an excellent prognosis when diagnosed and managed early. As these are low-risk injuries, even the presence of fracture lines on plain radiographs does not necessitate immediate surgical management or complete non-weightbearing. Patients should refrain from activity for 3–6 weeks. Immobilisation and limitations on weight bearing may vary with the patient and fracture. Generally, immobilisation with a CAM boot and rest suffice as initial treatment [17, 64].

Symptoms typically resolve by 4 months [66]. Despite successful outcomes with this treatment, it make take high-level athletes such as dancers up to a year to return to their pre-injury level of function and motion [64]. In figure skaters, return to activity occurs at approximately 3–7 months [65]. Without appropriate management, pain and disability may continue for 3–6 months or longer [2].

26.10 Summary

- Stress fractures of the ankle are common in athletes, especially in those who engage in high-impact and endurance-based exercise (classically, runners).
- The workup includes thorough history and physical examination, with attention to training regimen and potential endocrine or alignment abnormalities.
- Imaging should begin with plain radiographs, but usually includes MRI to visualize edema as well as fracture lines.
- Ankle stress fractures can be broadly categorized as low-risk, such as the fibula, or high-risk, such as the talus or medial malleolus. While both type of injuries can initially be managed nonoperatively with immobilisation and limited weight-bearing, high-risk stress fractures are more likely to result in delayed union, nonunion, or fracture propagation.
- Nonoperative management with immobilisation, refrain from activity, and limited weight-bearing is typically the first line of treatment.
- Surgery is reserved for cases that are refractory to nonoperative management, chronic cases with sclerosis and/or cystic changes, or potentially in elite athletes in whom prompt return to play is a priority.
- Novel treatments such as teriparatide, bone stimulators, shockwave therapy, and/or orthobiologic agents may play a future role in stress fracture treatment, but further research is warranted.
- Return to play starts with resumption of low-impact activity and eventual progression to higher-impact sports using pain and clinical/radiologic evidence of healing as a guide.
- The presence of a stress fracture should prompt clinicians to evaluate or refer patients to the appropriate specialist for potential disordered eating, menstrual irregularity, and/or endocrine or metabolic abnormality.
- Stress fractures should also direct clinicians to evaluate for abnormalities in limb biomechanics and/or training practices, which may necessitate modification to reduce the risk of future fractures.
- Generally, both low- and high-risk ankle stress fractures heal well with appropriate recognition and early treatment, and patients are able to resume their activities by 6–12 months after diagnosis.

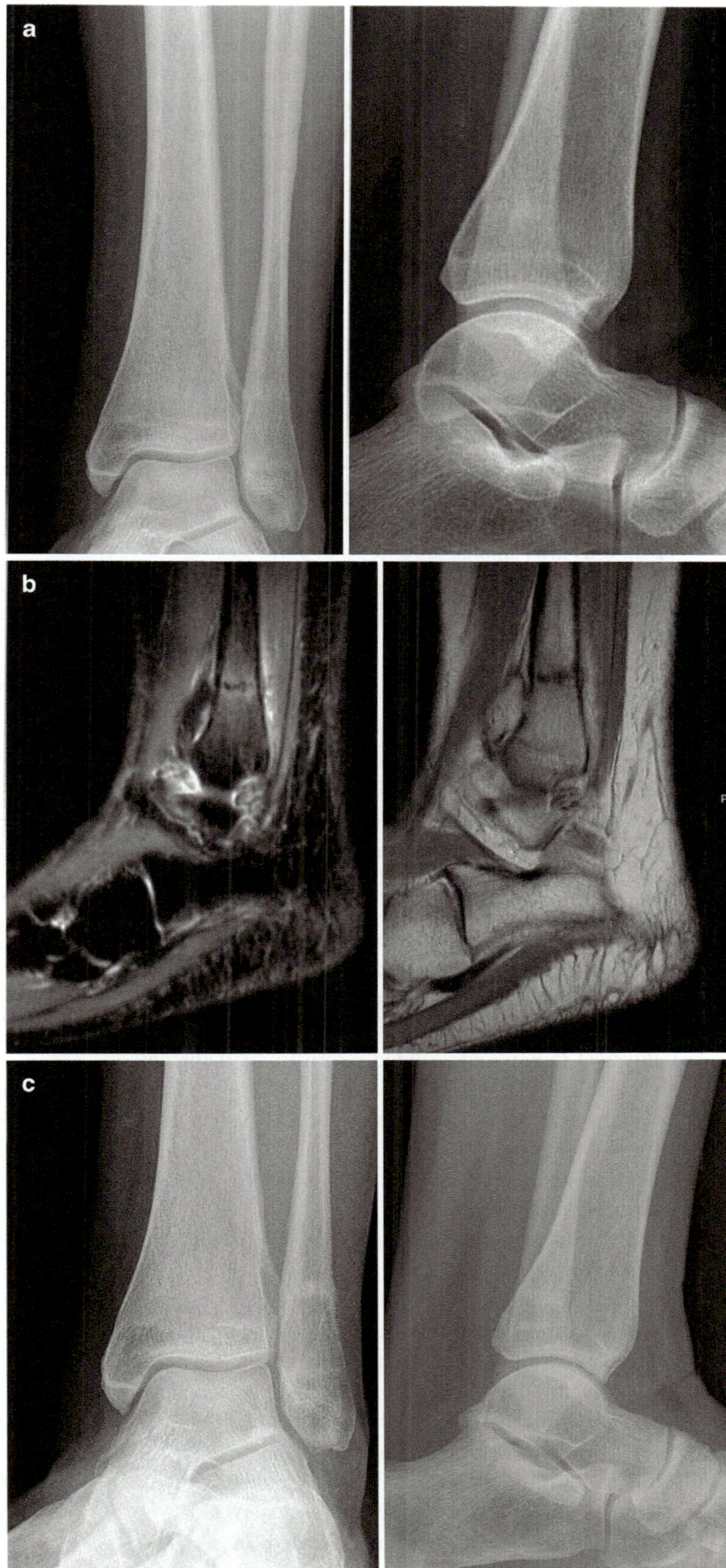

Fig. 26.7 Fibular stress fracture in a male patient, demonstrated at initial presentation on plain radiographs (**a**), MRI (**b**), and then with evidence of fracture healing 3 months later (**c**)

Clinical Pearls

- Ankle stress fractures can be broadly categorized as low-risk, such as the fibula, or high-risk, such as the talus or medial malleolus. While both type of injuries can initially be managed nonoperatively with immobilisation and limited weight-bearing, high-risk stress fractures are more likely to result in delayed union, nonunion, or fracture propagation.
- Nonoperative management with immobilisation, refrain from activity, and limited weight-bearing is typically the first line of management.
- Surgery is reserved for cases that are refractory to nonoperative management, chronic cases with sclerosis and/or cystic changes, or potentially in elite athletes in whom prompt return to play is a priority.
- Generally, both low- and high-risk ankle stress fractures heal well with appropriate recognition and early management, and patients are able to resume their activities by 6–12 months after diagnosis.

Review

Questions

1. A 23-year-old female recreational runner presents to your office with 4 weeks of lateral ankle pain. She is otherwise healthy and denies amenorrhea/oligomenorrhea and disordered eating. She has not seen any provider yet. Physical examination is notable for swelling and focal tenderness at the distal fibula. She is able to bear weight in the office. Plain radiographs of the ankle and foot show no abnormalities. An MRI is ordered and demonstrates increased signal in the distal fibula. What is the best initial treatment for this patient?
   (a) Physical therapy and guided return to sport therapy protocol
   (b) Weight-bearing as tolerated in a CAM walker boot for 4–6 weeks
   (c) Non-weight bearing in a cast for 6–8 weeks, with cessation of running
   (d) Open reduction internal fixation (ORIF) with plate and screw construct
2. A 19-year-old female competitive cross country athlete with a body mass index (BMI) of 16 kg/m^2 was referred by her athletic trainer for worsening medial ankle pain. It started in the middle of her season when she was increasing her daily mileage. She is otherwise healthy but does not have regular menstrual cycles, and she has a history of disordered eating in the past. MRI confirms medial malleolar stress fracture. What is the next best step?
   (a) Protected weight-bearing as tolerated in a CAM walker boot for 4–6 weeks
   (b) Open reduction internal fixation (ORIF) with either plate/screw construct or screws
   (c) Duel-energy X-ray absorptiometry
   (d) Vitamin D supplementation

Answers

1. b
2. c

References

1. Breithaupt J. Zur Pathologie des menschlichen Fusscess. Medizin Zeitung. 1855;24:169–77.
2. Devas MB, Sweetnam R. Stress fractures of the fibula; a review of fifty cases in athletes. J Bone Joint Surg Br. 1956;38-B:818–29.
3. Stevenson B. Title IX and the evolution of high school sports. Contemp Econ Policy. 2007;25:486–505.
4. Sharpe L. Gallup poll: Vermont no. 1 in frequent exercise, produce consumption. 2014.
5. Miller JA. The running bubble has popped. (You couldn't hear it in New York.) New York Times. 2017.
6. Hanson M, Iatsenko N, Luck P. Marathons 2014–2017. 2018.
7. Caesar BC, McCollum GA, Elliot R, Williams A, Calder JDF. Stress fractures of the tibia and medial malleolus. Foot Ankle Clin. 2013;18:339–55.
8. Brukner P, Bradshaw C, Khan KM, White S, Crossley K. Stress fractures: a review of 180 cases. Clin J Sport Med. 1996;6:85–9.
9. Ha KI, Hahn SH, Chung MY, Yang BK, Yi SR. A clinical study of stress fractures in sports activities. Orthopedics. 1991;14:1089–95.
10. Iwamoto J, Takeda T. Stress fractures in athletes: review of 196 cases. J Orthop Sci. 2003;8:273–8.
11. Rizzone KH, Ackerman KE, Roos KG, Dompier TP, Kerr ZY. The epidemiology of stress fractures in collegiate student-athletes, 2004–2005 through 2013–2014 academic years. J Athl Train. 2017;52:966–75.
12. Changstrom BG, Brou L, Khodaee M, Braund C, Comstock RD. Epidemiology of stress fracture injuries among us high school athletes, 2005–2006 through 2012–2013. Am J Sports Med. 2015;43:26–33.
13. Tenforde AS, Carlson JL, Chang A, Sainani KL, Shultz R, Kim JH, Cutti P, Golden NH, Fredericson M. Association of the female athlete triad risk assessment stratification to the development of bone stress injuries in collegiate athletes. Am J Sports Med. 2017;45:302–10.
14. Matheson GO, Anderson S, Robell K. Injuries and illnesses in the preparticipation evaluation data of 1693 college student-athletes. Am J Sports Med. 2015;43:1518–25.
15. Barrow GW, Saha S. Menstrual irregularity and stress fractures in collegiate female distance runners. Am J Sports Med. 1988;16:209–16.
16. Boden BP, Osbahr DC. High-risk stress fractures: evaluation and treatment. J Am Acad Orthop Surg. 2000;8:344–53.
17. Stanitski CL, McMaster JH, Scranton PE. On the nature of stress fractures. Am J Sports Med. 1978;6:391–6.
18. Voss LA, Fadale PD, Hulstyn MJ. Exercise-induced loss of bone density in athletes. J Am Acad Orthop Surg. 1998;6:349–57.
19. Datir AP. Stress-related bone injuries with emphasis on MRI. Clin Radiol. 2007;62:828–36.
20. Kadel NJ, Teitz CC, Kronmal RA. Stress fractures in ballet dancers. Am J Sports Med. 1992;20:445–9.

21. Matheson GO, Clement DB, Mckenzie DC, Taunton JE, Lloyd-Smith DR, Macintyre JG. Stress fractures in athletes: a study of 320 cases. Am J Sports Med. 1987;15:46–58.
22. Sherbondy PS, Sebastianelli WJ. Stress fractures of the medial malleolus and distal fibula. Clin Sports Med. 2006;25:129–37.
23. Kaufman KR, Brodine SK, Shaffer RA, Johnson CW, Cullison TR. The effect of foot structure and range of motion on musculoskeletal overuse injuries. Am J Sports Med. 1999;27:585–93.
24. Korpelainen R, Orava S, Karpakka J, Siira P, Hulkko A. Risk factors for recurrent stress fractures in athletes. Am J Sports Med. 2001;29:304–10.
25. Lidor C, Ferris LR, Hall R, Alexander IJ, Nunley JA. Stress fracture of the tibia after arthrodesis of the ankle or the hindfoot. J Bone Jointt Surg Am. 1997;79:558–64.
26. Hackney AC, Aggon E. Chronic low testosterone levels in endurance trained men: the exercise—hypogonadal male condition. J Biochem Physiol. 2018;1:1–4.
27. Wheeler GD, Wall SR, Belcastro AN, Cumming DC. Reduced serum testosterone and prolactin levels in male distance runners. JAMA. 1984;252:514–6.
28. MacDougall JD, Webber CE, Martin J, Ormerod S, Chesley A, Younglai EV, Gordon CL, Blimkie CJR. Relationship among running mileage, bone density, and serum testosterone in male runners. J Appl Physiol. 1992;73:1165–70.
29. Arendt EA, Griffiths HJ. The use of MR imaging in the assessment and clinical management of stress reactions of bone in high-performance athletes. Clin Sports Med. 1997;16:291–306.
30. Niva MH, Sormaala MJ, Kiuru MJ, Haataja R, Ahovuo JA, Pihlajamaki HK. Bone stress injuries of the ankle and foot: an 86-month magnetic resonance imaging-based study of physically active young adults. Am J Sports Med. 2007;35:643–9.
31. Holick MF. Vitamin D deficiency. N Engl J Med. 2007;357:266–81.
32. Mayer S, Joyner P, Almekinders L, Parekh S. Stress fractures of the foot and ankle in athletes. Sports Health. 2014;6:481–91.
33. Lee HS, Lee YK, Kim HS, Lee DW, Won SH, Jung KJ, Kim CH, Kim WJ. Medial malleolar stress fracture resulting from repetitive stress caused by lateral ankle instability: a case report. Medicine (Baltimore). 2019;98:1–5.
34. Zwas ST, Elkanovitch R, Frank G. Interpretation and classification of bone scintigraphic findings in stress fractures. J Nucl Med. 1987;28:452–7.
35. Amoako A, Abid A, Shadiack A, Monaco R. Ultrasound-diagnosed tibia stress fracture: a case report. Clin Med Insights Arthritis Musculoskelet Disord. 2017;10:0–2.
36. Boden BP, Osbahr DC, Jimenez C. Current concepts low-risk stress fractures. Am J Sports Med. 2001;29:100–11.
37. Elias I, Zoga AC, Raikin SM, Peterson JR, Besser MP, Morrison WB, Schweitzer ME. Bone stress injury of the ankle in professional ballet dancers seen on MRI. BMC Musculoskelet Disord. 2008;9:1–6.
38. Almirol EA, Chi LY, Khurana B, Hurwitz S, Bluman EM, Chiodo C, Matzkin E, Baima J, Leboff MS. Short-term effects of teriparatide versus placebo on bone biomarkers, structure, and fracture healing in women with lower-extremity stress fractures: a pilot study. J Clin Transl Endocrinol. 2016;5:7–14.
39. Taki M, Iwata O, Shiono M, Kimura M, Takagishi K. Extracorporeal shock wave therapy for resistant stress fracture in athletes: a report of 5 cases. Am J Sports Med. 2007;35:1188–92.
40. Leal C, D'Agostino C, Gomez Garcia S, Fernandez A. Current concepts of shockwave therapy in stress fractures. Int J Surg. 2015;24:195–200.
41. Brighton CT, Wang W, Seldes R, Zhang G, Pollack SR. Signal transduction in electrically stimulated bone cells. J Bone Jointt Surg Am. 2001;83:1514–23.
42. Benazzo F, Mosconi M, Beccarisi G, Galli U. Use of capacitive coupled electric fields in stress fractures in athletes. Clin Orthop Relat Res. 1995;(310):145–9.
43. Beck BR, Matheson GO, Bergman G, Norling T, Fredericson M, Hoffman AR, Marcus R. Do capacitively coupled electric fields accelerate tibial stress fracture healing?: a randomized controlled trial. Am J Sports Med. 2008;36:545–53.
44. Khan Y, Laurencin CT. Fracture repair with ultrasound: clinical and cell-based evaluation. J Bone Jointt Surg Am. 2008;90:138–44.
45. Li J, Waugh LJ, Hui SL, Burr DB, Warden SJ. Low-intensity pulsed ultrasound and nonsteroidal anti-inflammatory drugs have opposing effects during stress fracture repair. J Orthop Res. 2007;25:1559–67.
46. McWilliams GD, Yao L, Simonet LB, Haysbert CW, Giza E, Kreulen CD, Boutin RD. Subchondroplasty of the ankle and hindfoot for treatment of osteochoncral lesions and stress fractures: initial imaging experience. Foot Ankle Spec. 2019; https://doi.org/10.1177/1938640019863252.
47. Adams SB, Lewis JS, Gupta AK, Parekh SG, Miller SD, Schon LC. Cannulated screw delivery of bone marrow aspirate concentrate to a stress fracture nonunion: technique tip. Foot Ankle Int. 2013;34:740–4.
48. Diehl JJ, Best TM, Kaeding CC. Classification and return-to-play considerations for stress fractures. Clin Sports Med. 2006;25:17–28.
49. Burgi AA, Gorham ED, Garland CF, Mohr SB, Garland FC, Zeng K, Thompson K, Lappe JM. High serum 25-hydroxyvitamin D is associated with a low incidence of stress fractures. J Bone Miner Res. 2011;26:2371–7.
50. Okada K, Senma S, Abe E, Sato K, Minato S. Stress fractures of the medial malleolus: a case report. Foot Ankle Int. 1995;16:49–52.
51. Orava S, Karpakka J, Taimela S, Hulkko A, Permi J, Kujala U. Stress fracture of the medial malleolus. J Bone Joint Surg Am. 1995;77:362–5.
52. Mandell JC, Khurana B, Smith SE. Stress fractures of the foot and ankle: Part 2. Site-specific etiology, imaging, and treatment, and differential diagnosis. Skelet Radiol. 2017;46:1165–86.
53. Jowett AJL, Birks CL, Blackney MC. Medial malleolar stress fracture secondary to chronic ankle impingement. Foot Ankle Int. 2008;29:716–21.
54. Shelbourne KD, Fisher DA, Rettig AC, McCarroll JR. Stress fractures of the medial malleolus. Am J Sports Med. 1988;16:60–3.
55. Menge TJ, Looney CG. Medial malleolar stress fracture in an adolescent athlete. J Foot Ankle Surg. 2015;54:242–6.
56. Shabat S, Sampson KB, Mann G, Gepstein R, Eliakim A, Shenkman Z, Nyska M. Stress fractures of the medial malleolus – review of the literature and report of a 15-year-old elite gymnast. Foot Ankle Int. 2002;23:647–50.
57. Mulligan ME, Shanley DJ. Supramalleolar fatigue fractures of the tibia. Skelet Radiol. 1996;25:325–8.
58. O'Neill BJ, Ryan K, Burke NG, Moroney PJ. Bilateral distal tibial stress fractures in a healthy field-hockey goalkeeper. BMJ Case Rep. 2014; https://doi.org/10.1136/bcr-2014-205353.
59. Jensen A, Dahl S. Stress fracture of the distal tibia and fibula through heavy lifting. Am J Ind Med. 2005;47:181–3.
60. Sciberras N, Taylor C, Trimble K. Bilateral distal tibial stress fractures in a military recruit. BMJ Case Rep. 2012:2–4.
61. Van Demark RE, Allard B, Van Demark RE. Nonunion of a distal tibial stress fracture associated with vitamin D deficiency: a case report. S D Med. 2010;63:87–91. 93
62. Bradshaw C, Khan K, Brukner P. Stress fracture of the body of the talus in athletes demonstrated with computer tomography. Clin J Sport Med. 1996;6:48–51.
63. Rossi F, Dragoni S. Talar body fatigue stress fractures: three cases observed in elite female gymnasts. Skelet Radiol. 2005;34:389–94.
64. Goulart M, O'Malley MJ, Hodgkins CW, Charlton TP. Foot and ankle fractures in dancers. Clin Sports Med. 2008;27:295–304.
65. Pećina M, Bojanić I, Dubravcić S. Stress fractures in figure skaters. Am J Sports Med. 1997;18:277–9.
66. Richmond DA, Shafar J. A case of bilateral fatigue fracture of the fibula. Br Med J. 1955;1:264–5.

Stress Fractures in Sport: Foot

27

Amol Saxena, Robert Anderson, Richard T. Bouché, Magali Fournier, Brian Fullem, Ludger Gerdesmeyer, and Nicola Maffulli

Stress fractures of the foot can cause marked morbidity, especially in athletes, as they can be season and career ending [1–3]. The fact that one fourth of the bones of the body are located in the feet produces more "opportunity" for pathology. Stress fractures occur when bones are subjected to excessive and repetitive stresses, which, coupled with biomechanical and metabolic imbalances, accentuate the problem for the 56 weightbearing bones (including sesamoids of first MP) of this region. In general, if patients present with a stress fracture of this region, they should undergo a thorough metabolic assessment, particularly to exclude Vitamin D deficiency [1, 4, 5]. Approximately 83% of patients with stress fractures below the knee had a Vit D3 levels below 40 mg/dl, despite ranges up to 30 being considered normal in many countries [4].

The role of imaging in formulating a diagnosis of stress fracture in athletes is important. MRI imaging remains the most sensitive and specific study to diagnose stress fractures of the lower extremity, and is therefore considered the gold standard [5]. It is superior to nuclear scintigraphy which has high sensitivity but low specificity. Bone scan or SPECT may be more beneficial for athletes in season. Despite having low sensitivity (12–56%), plain radiographs are easy, cheap and readily available as first line modality. If positive, then no additional imaging study is necessary for diagnosis purposes. Ultrasonography is increasingly popular in diagnosing stress fractures and should be considered as a possible imaging option. Though not a first-line modality, it can adequately evaluate periosteum, adjacent tissue and focal interruptions of bone surface, and can be useful to follow the evolution of stress fractures healing. Ultrasonography does not expose patients to radiation, and is quick; however, it is operator-dependent [6].

27.1 Stress Injuries of Hallucal Sesamoids

27.1.1 Epidemiology

Injury to the hallucal sesamoids can result in a variety of pathologies; stress reaction/fracture (SRF) is one of the most common pathologies encountered, especially in a sports medicine setting. Diastasis of a bipartite sesamoid (DBS) parallels sesamoid SRF, and is managed similarly. SRF arises from overuse, and can vary from an asymptomatic stress reaction to a symptomatic stress reaction to a stress fracture, and ultimately to an overt fracture. DBS can result from an acute traumatic hyperextension injury of the hallux but more commonly to a non-traumatic overuse injury, resulting in pathologic stressing and eventual separation of the fibrous bridge of this bipartite bone. These injuries pose a significant clinical challenge, as the paucity of high-level research on such conditions makes the management of these injuries not necessarily evidence based. We will try and provide a practical overview of these two sesamoid stress injuries.

A. Saxena (✉)
Department of Sports Medicine, PAMF-Sutter, Palo Alto, CA, USA
e-mail: heysax@aol.com

R. Anderson
Titletown Sports Medicine and Orthopedics, Green Bay, WI, USA
e-mail: robert.anderson2@bellin.org

R. T. Bouché
The Sports Medicine Clinic, Brier, WA, USA

M. Fournier
Gundersen Health System, Lacrosse, WI, USA
e-mail: mfournie@gundersenhealth.org

B. Fullem
Elite Sports Podiatry, Dunedin, FL, USA

L. Gerdesmeyer
Department of Orthopedics, University of Schleswig-Holstein, Kiel, Germany

N. Maffulli
Department of Orthopedics and Trauma, University of Salerno, Salerno, Italy
e-mail: n.maffulli@qmul.ac.uk

G. A. J. Robertson, N. Maffulli (eds.), *Fractures in Sport*, https://doi.org/10.1007/978-3-030-72036-0_27

27.1.1.1 Diagnosis

Patients typically present with a gradual insidious onset of pain, swelling and reduced motion of the plantar first metatarsophalangeal joint (MTPJ), worse with activity (especially loading activities) and better with rest. Pain is reported to either one or both of the sesamoids, and varies from a "sharp stabbing pain" to an "intense dull aching." At times, proximal and/or distal radiation of the pain along the course of the plantar nerve can occur. As these problems become more chronic, pain can become intermittent, as patients avoid aggravating activities and attempt to compensate for their problem.

The pain is lower when walking flatfooted, and increased substantially with weight bearing during any toe-off manoeuvre. Patients do prefer the protection of a shoe, especially a shoe that offers a rigid rocker-sole design. Swelling is limited to the MTPJ (plantarly greater than dorsally), and occurs commonly in the acute/subacute setting with the foot least swollen early in the day, and becoming progressively more swollen as the day progresses. Chronic cases may exhibit minimal to no swelling, and, though pain may clinically improve, it will always be persistent especially during the toe-off phase of walking. Dysfunction of the first MTPJ will prevent patients from performing normal loading activities including running and jumping. If loading activities are pursued, patients typically will attempt to compensate by loading more on their heel, or rolling off the lateral aspect of their foot. Eventually, they may not be able to toe-off at all. These gait changes can result in symptoms affecting other areas of the foot and lower extremity.

27.1.1.2 Physical Examination and Classification

Evaluation of the sesamoids considers the vascular (e.g., perfusion), neurologic (e.g., sensation), dermatologic (e.g., skin lesions) and especially the musculoskeletal (MSK) system as it affects the foot. The MSK examination includes inspection, range of motion (ROM), muscle testing, palpation, and provocative testing. Patients should be evaluated statically while sitting and dynamically during standing and walking.

On inspection, the examiner assesses foot type, lower extremity alignment, deformities, asymmetries, presence of erythema, swelling and areas of callus formation. Patients typically have guarded ROM, especially hallux extension. Patients exhibit weakness of the flexion, especially in the flexor hallucis brevis (FHB) tendon on static and dynamic testing. On palpation, we recommend a systematic zonal approach to help differentiate the various pathologies that can present as plantar pain in the first MTPJ. There are three zones to consider: zone 1 (proximal to sesamoid zone), zone 2 (sesamoid zone), and zone 3 (distal to sesamoid zone). Commonly, structures other than sesamoids can be affected, and this zonal approach can help the examiner establish whether the sesamoids are directly involved. Zone 2 would be the "sesamoid zone", and with SRF and DBS there will be pain to palpation of potentially three areas of each sesamoid; therefore, six areas need to be palpated for full palpatory assessment of the sesamoids (Fig. 27.1).

After palpation, specific provocative testing can be performed; we suggest three static provocative tests and one dynamic provocative manoeuvre (with four stages). Static tests include: (1) maximum passive hallux extension test with palpation; (2) passive axial compression (PAC) test [1] and (3) first MTPJ ROM with concurrent sesamoid compression test [7]. In first test, maximum passive extension of hallux will lock the sesamoids against the metatarsal head; then, palpation can be performed. The second test also involves maximum dorsiflexion of hallux; the examiner's index finger is then used to palpate proximal to the involved sesamoid; the hallux is then passively plantarflexed with reproduction of pain with PF if test is positive. In the third test, each sesamoid is compressed against the metatarsal head while the first MTPJ is put through the whole range of motion. Dynamic provocative testing involves first assuming the tiptoe position (i.e. the demi-pointe or half-pointe position) on

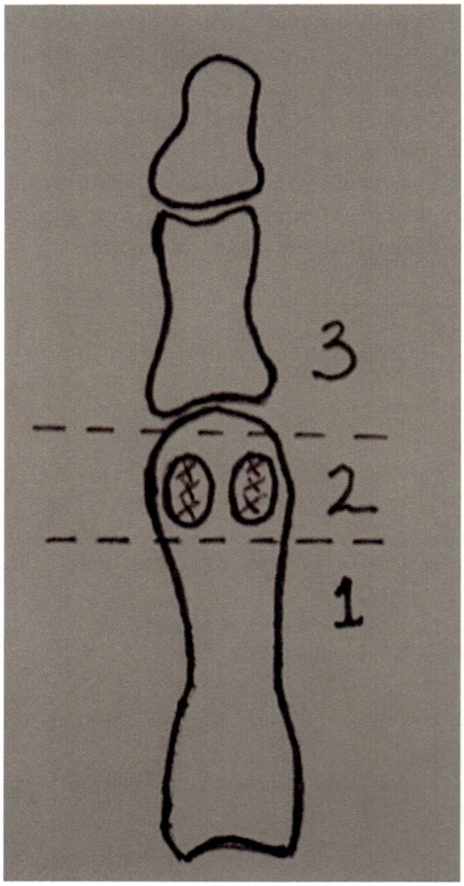

Fig. 27.1 Zone 1, 2 and 3 of sesamoid pathology

Table 27.1 Differential Diagnosis for Sesamoidopathy

Differential DX	
➢ Fracture	➢ DJD
➢ Diastasis	➢ Delayed/non union
➢ Contusion	➢ Rheumatic
➢ Capsule/PP tear	➢ "Frozen"
➢ AVN	➢ Plicae
➢ CD/OCD	➢ Infection/Osteo
➢ Sesamoiditis	➢ Neoplasm
➢ Neuritis	➢ Muscle/tendom

both feet concurrently. Then, with each foot separately, patients are asked to jump on both feet concurrently and then each hop on foot separately maintaining this tip-toe position through each challenge. In a positive test, pain is reproduced with any of these progressive manoeuvres. In the acute/sub-acute stage of injury, patients typically walk with an apropulsive antalgic gait favouring their medial forefoot. In the chronic state, patients may be able to walk reasonably well, but likely will have pain at toe-off.

27.1.1.3 Differential Diagnosis

A broad range of pathologies present with plantar pain and dysfunction of the first MTPJ . The problem could be related to specific sesamoid pathologies or other intraarticular and/or extra-articular pathologies of the first MTPJ (Table 27.1).

When referring to sesamoid pathologies, we suggest the term "sesamoidopathy", a general term indicating pathology affecting the hallucal sesamoids, though not specific for any one pathology. The commonly used term "sesamoiditis" should be reserved to inflammation of the sesamoids and periarticular soft tissue structures.

27.1.1.4 Diagnostic Tests

Based on history and physical examination, a differential diagnosis is established. The clinician can then proceed with a diagnostic work-up that should validate clinical suspicions. It is important of establishing a diagnosis before initiating treatment (especially on an athlete).

Following an algorithmic approach to diagnostic imaging when a sesamoidopathy is suspected, early in the evaluation weight-bearing (WB) radiographs are obtained, typically consisting of Dorsal-to-Plantar, Medial Oblique, Lateral Oblique, Lateral and Axial Sesamoid views. If radiographs are normal or equivocal, then a bone scan or SPECT bone scan can be considered: if positive, that would validate sesamoid bone involvement. A CT scan may then be indicated, focusing on the specific region of the positive bone scan and providing a high resolution three cardinal planes image of the pathologic area. If the bone scan is negative, a soft tissue problem (i.e., plantar plate tear) or avascular necrosis of the

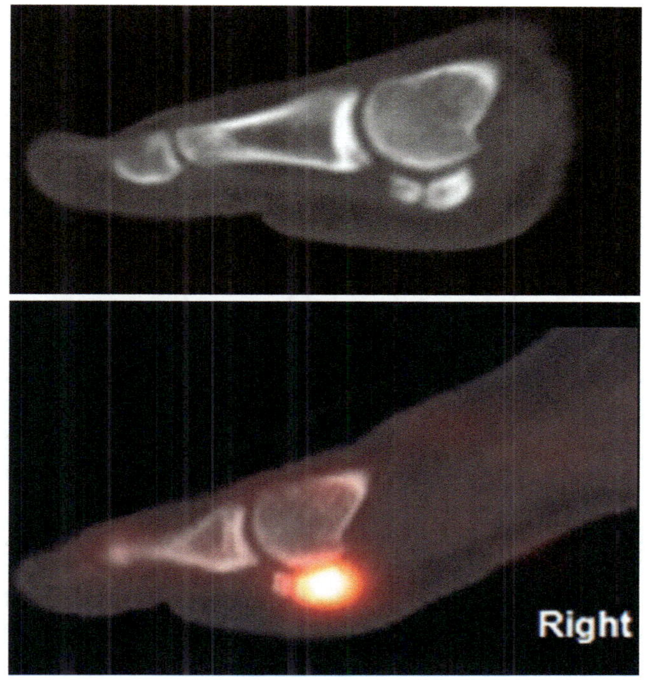

Fig. 27.2 SPECT scan showing sesamoid fracture

Table 27.2 Radiographic decision making for sesamoidopathy

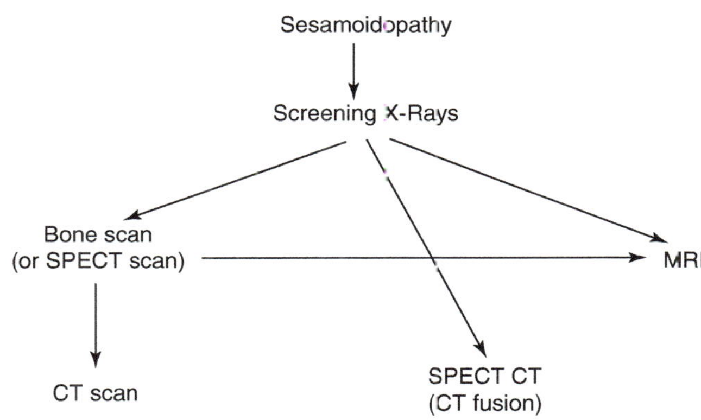

sesamoids is suspected, and then a magnetic resonance imaging (MRI) scan is indicated. Initially, if sesamoid bone involvement is highly suspected, a combination of bone scan and CT scan can be obtained together; this is called a SPECT CT or CT Fusion scan (Fig. 27.2 and Table 27.2).

Another helpful diagnostic tool is an injections of local anesthetic . This strategy is a good way to localize the problem to first MTPJ (intra-articular), outside the first MTPJ (extra-articular) or to hallucal sesamoid(s).

27.1.2 Treatment Options

27.1.2.1 Non-surgical Treatment

There are no high-level medical articles that describe and/or validate any conservative care modality for SRF and DBS injuries. Based on our experience, the following treatment protocol is suggested to prevent the onset of a "sick sesamoid." A "sick sesamoid." is a chronic, intractable sesamoidopathy which has failed all conservative treatments and is characterized by persistent pain and dysfunction. If accurate diagnosis is established early and appropriate aggressive conservative care initiated, then a sick sesamoid will be less likely.

For initial treatment of these two injuries, especially at the acute or subacute stage, patients should be NWB with crutches, roller-aid or crutchless walking device (i.e., iWalk-Free® Long Beach, CA USA or Freedom Leg® Edmonds, WA USA) for 4–6 weeks. The foot is maintained in a splint or hinged-boot allowing the foot and hallux to be positioned PF during the NWB period. This is followed by another 4 weeks in a walking boot.

Patients can be seen by a physiotherapist at 2–4 weeks to allow controlled first MTPJ range of motion avoiding extension of hallux to optimize healing potential. If SRF becomes chronic (i.e., delayed/non-union) and does not respond to conservative care, then bone stimulation and/or extracorporeal shockwave therapy (ESWT) can be effective. For DBS, if the initial conservative care pathway described above is ineffective, then ESWT can be considered; in sesamoid diastasis, bone stimulation has been singularly ineffective in our setting. If the initial aforementioned treatment is successful, then, once the patient is asymptomatic, rehabilitative and preventative measures are considered, including appropriate shoewear (with rigid-rocker sole), over-the- counter (OTC) or custom orthotics with the first metatarsal head "cut-out" to accommodate for the first MTPJ, avoiding barefoot walking, addressing potential predisposing factors and implementing a dynamic strengthening program. If patients do not respond to non-surgical treatment, then their problem is considered to have escalated to a "sick sesamoid", and surgery can be considered.

27.1.2.2 Surgical Treatment

Surgery for SRF non-union and chronically painful DBS is controversial, with minimal evidence-based medicine to guide our interventions. Many surgical options are available (Table 27.3).

Several procedures can be considered, but partial- [8, 9] and total sesamoidectomy [10–13] are the most predictable. The mechanical effects of sesamoidectomy have been studied assessing the effective tendon moment arm (ETMA) of the flexor hallucis brevis (FHB) and flexor hallucis longus (FHL) tendons after partial and total sesamoidectomy [14, 15]. Based on clinical presentation and imaging work-up, a decision can be made if a partial- or total sesamoidectomy should be considered. Surgery for these challenging problems can be highly successful if performed appropriately: the key to success of a partial or total sesamoidectomy is preservation of the flexor hallucis brevis (FHB) tendon slip(s) which contain the sesamoid(s) [16]. An ideal surgical approach would allow direct visualization of pathology, avoidance of neurovascular bundles and adequate exposure to assure ability to repair the FHB tendon and allow clean excision of the diseased sesamoid(s). The surgical approaches recommended for these procedures include a medial and plantar approach [17, 18]. The medial approach is through a longitudinal centrally placed incision equidistant between the dorsomedial and plantar medial neurovascular bundles (Fig. 27.3). The plantar approach is through a longitudinal centrally based incision immediately between the hallucal sesamoids (Fig. 27.4). The medial approach is considered when performing a partial tibial sesamoidectomy . The plantar approach is recommended when performing a total tibial, partial- or total fibular or total sesamoidectomy of both sesamoids (Fig. 27.5a–d). A plantar incision (vs. a medial incision) allows adequate exposure to repair the inter-sesamoidal

Table 27.3 Treatment options for sesamoidopathy

Surgical options	
• Total-excision	• MTPJ fusion
• Hemi-excision	• Lengthen PL
• Planing	• O or P-RIF
• Fenestration	• Autograft
• Relocation	• Implant
• Osteotomy	• Arthroscopy

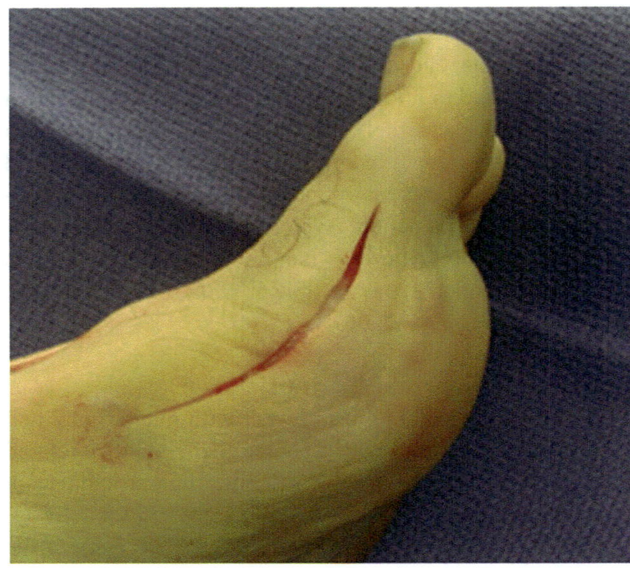

Fig. 27.3 Medial approach for tibial sesamoidectomy

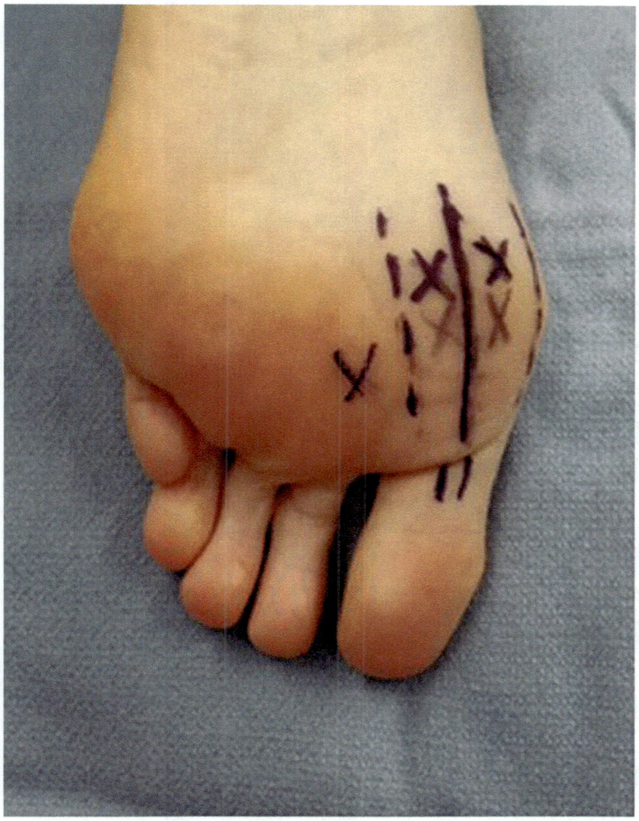

Fig. 27.4 Plantar approach for sesamoidectomy

ligament (ISL) to the medial FHB tendon slip. This ISL to FHB tendon repair prevents lateral migration of the fibular sesamoid and resultant bunion deformity which can happen if this repair is not performed. After tibial sesamoidectomy, there is a well reported significant incidence of hallux valgus deformity likely from weakening of the medial soft tissue structures and not repairing the ISL to the medial FHB [19].

A partial sesamoidectomy preserves part of an affected sesamoid if possible. This can be considered if clinical examination and imaging studies determined that there is a good, healthy portion of the sesamoid worth saving. It probably does not matter if the diseased portion of the sesamoid is distal or proximal, as surgical results are equally as good in the authors' experience. If a portion of the sesamoid can be preserved, patients should theoretically have less chance of developing functional deficits, and should rehabilitate faster. In the senior author's experience over the last 16 years, the author now prefers partial over total sesamoidectomy if patients meet the criteria for the partial excision, as these patients rehabilitate faster with minimal functional deficit.

Additional surgical procedures in addition to a sesamoid procedure may be needed depending on the clinical findings. For example, patients undergoing a tibial sesamoidectomy with a moderate to severe bunion deformity may need a concurrent structural bunion correction. If a mild bunion is present, a lateral capsulotomy/extensor hallucis brevis tendon release and adjunctive medial imbrication procedures can be considered (in lieu of a structural bunion correction). Medial imbrication procedures would include a medial capsulorraphy and/or an abductor hallucis tendon advancement.

On several occasions the senior author has performed a partial sesamoidectomy in an acute/subacute setting in patients with severe fracture and/or diastasis with significant separation between sesamoid segments and/or plantar plate injury. In this situation, early repair may be most efficient and predictable procedure for athletic patients who wish a timely return to pre-injury activities. This strategy can also avoid a long-term conservative management strategies that may be frustrating and uncertain for both patient and physician.

Post-operatively, patients with a partial tibial sesamoidectomy through a medial incision remain NWB for 2–3 weeks followed by 2–4 weeks in a walking boot. For all other procedures performed through a plantar approach patients are NWB for 4–6 weeks followed by 2–4 weeks in a walking boot. Patients begin a structured rehab program for all procedures at 2 weeks after the procedure under guidance of a physical therapist (PT). Controlled mobilization taking care to avoid hallux extension is recommended for the first 2 post-operative weeks.

Concerning return to athletic activities, it takes 4–6 months to return to pre-injury WB activities without limitations, though some patients can return sooner [20]. Anecdotally, partial (vs. total) sesamoidectomies and medial incisional procedures (vs. plantar incision procedures) allow return to sport earlier.

27.1.2.3 Complications

The biggest concern after sesamoid surgery in an athlete would be weakness of the sesamoid apparatus with resultant decreased push-off power and negative effect on performance, especially if the flexor apparatus is not repaired. Deviation of the hallux into varus or valgus can necessitate further surgery. "Cock-up toe" or hallux malleus can also occur, especially if the FHB and FHL are not repaired. Nerve entrapment and tendon adhesions are also potential complications. Arthritis of the inferior portion of the metatarsal head can occur in patients with chronic sesamoidopathy; this area should therefore be evaluated intra-operatively to advise the patients [8, 13, 20].

In summary, hallucal sesamoid problems pose a real challenge to the sports physician. Initial evaluation is critical to establish a diagnosis and plan appropriate treatment. Initial evaluation consists of comprehensive clinical examination followed by confirmatory diagnostic testing. Treatment options can be non-surgical or surgical depending on diagnosis. Appropriate early aggressive conservative care

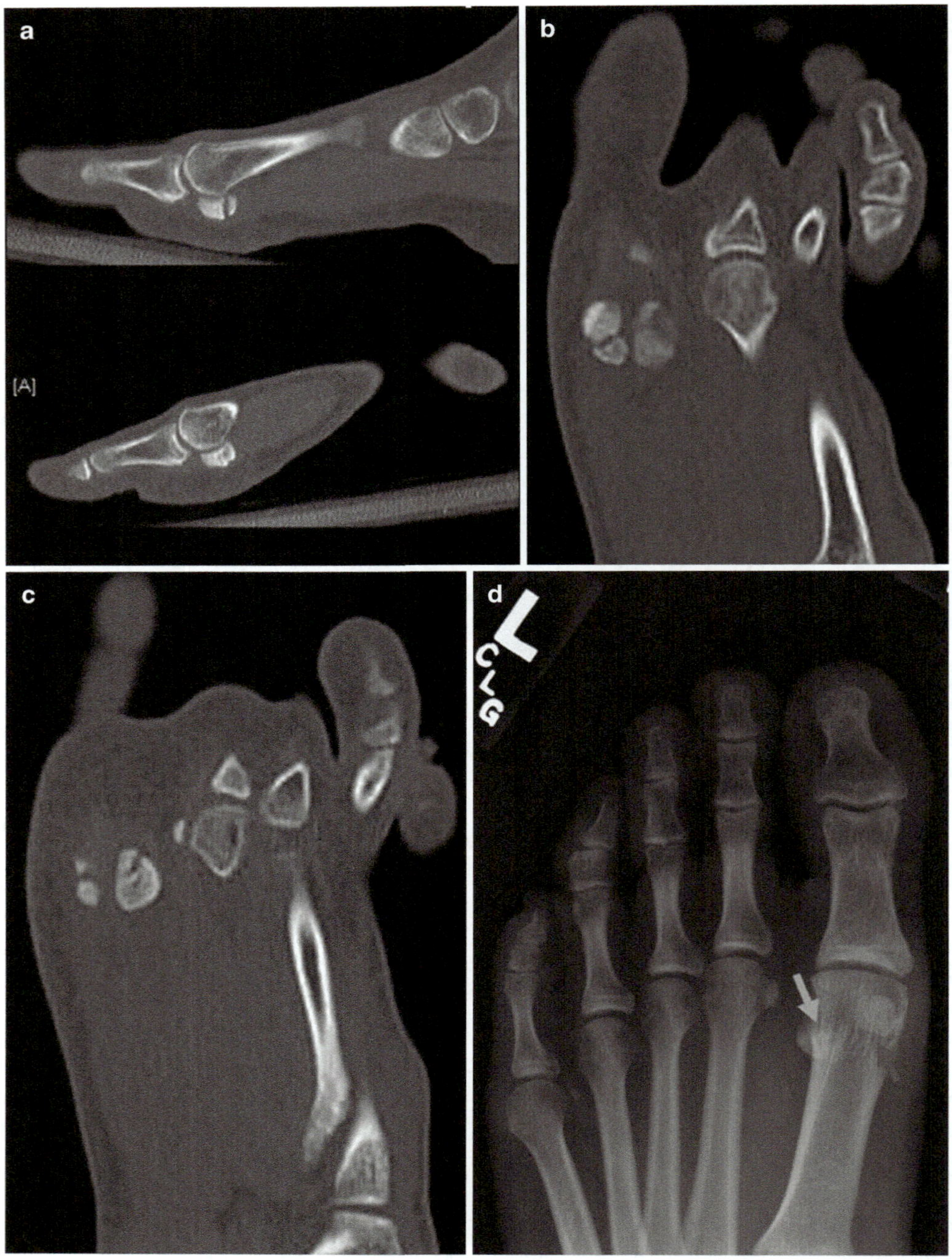

Fig. 27.5 (**a–d**) Patient with tibial and fibular sesamoid pathology

can be effective for SRF and DBS pathologies. If the sesamoid problem defies conservative care and results in a chronic "sick sesamoid" condition, then surgical options should be considered. There could be a role for early surgical intervention to allow patients to return to activities sooner and in a more predictable manner. Research is needed to assess best conservative care protocols and to document results of both partial and total sesamoidectomy procedures for SRF and DBS pathologies.

27.2 Central Lesser Metatarsal Stress Fractures

27.2.1 Epidemiology

The incidence of lesser metatarsal stress fractures has been reported to be 16% in the military population. They can be approximately 60% of all the lower extremity stress fractures in military trainees, especially the second and third metatarsals, and are more likely to occur early in training [21]. The percentage and incidence in the general population is harder to assess. The level of fracture and its healing potential dependent on location on the metatarsal [5, 22–26]. In general, mid- to distal metatarsal stress fractures heal faster than proximal metatarsal stress fractures [5, 22–24].

27.2.2 Classification

There are no accepted classification systems for stress fractures of the central metatarsals. The fracture is designated as occurring in the distal, central or proximal portion of the metatarsal. The proximal metatarsal region has been documented to be associated with delayed healing [5, 22, 25, 26].

27.2.3 Diagnosis (History/Physical Exam/ Radiological Investigations)

Patients with a stress fractures in this region report pain and swelling which worsen with activity. The provocative manoeuvre which would be to twist ("torque test") all three central metatarsals in sequence to ascertain which one is most painful (Fig. 27.6), though this may be equivocal. A thorough history should be obtained, particularly activity level, surface and shoe gear changes. Ballet dances going "en pointe", runners increasing mileage, swimmers initiating "dry-land" training, patients new to impact exercise regimens, all are common causes. Routine weight-bearing radiographs are taken, though actual confirmation of new callus formation may not occur for weeks [5]. When suspicion occurs for more proximal pathology, advanced imaging may be required. Radiologists claim that MRI is the best study to reveal stress fractures, but experienced sports clinicians often see these injuries can be missed even at MRI (Fig. 27.7a, b). "SPECT" is the preferred study when a critical judgement needs to be made, particularly with the "in-season" athlete (Fig. 27.8a–d).

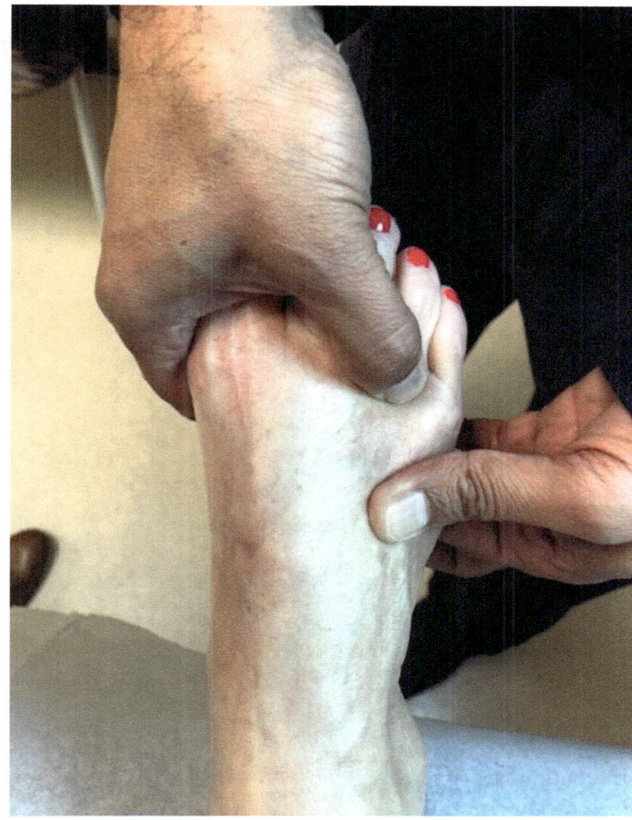

Fig. 27.6 "Torque test" performed to each metatarsal to determine which is painful

27.2.4 Treatment

For distal metatarsal stress fractures of the central rays, off-loading padding added to an insole is typically used (Fig. 27.9), along with a stiffer running shoe, but not necessarily a "post-operative" shoe. The shoe should off-load the affected metatarsal. "Metatarsal pads", though often used, are inferior to off-loading, and, in the senior author's experience, has actually caused this injury [27]. The usual time to return to sport is 4–8 weeks for distal metatarsal stress fractures. For mid-shaft stress fractures, in addition to the off-loading pad, a short "walker boot" is used. The usual time to return to sport is 6–12 weeks for these injuries. In proximal central metatarsals fractures, in addition to a boot, non-weightbearing is strongly advised. Proximal metatarsal stress fractures have a higher rate of delayed and non-union, similar to Jones fractures [5, 26]. If non-weightbearing is not maintained and the foot is not kept in neutral position, delayed healing is more likely [22]. If non-union is encountered, ORIF with autograft is recommended [22, 25, 26] (Fig. 27.10a–f). Post-operatively, patients are kept non-weightbearing at least 4 weeks or until confirmation of radiographic healing. The usual time to return to sport is 8–16 weeks. Use of shock absorptive insoles may help decrease the incidence of lower extremity stress fractures [28].

27.2.5 Complications

Central metatarsal stress fractures can incur malunion, delayed union and non-union. Malunion can lead to additional stress fractures, neuromas, capsulitis etc. Non-union can lead to arthrosis when the fracture extends into the joint such as with proximal metatarsal stress fractures. Mechanical off-loading and proper nutrition can decrease the potential of

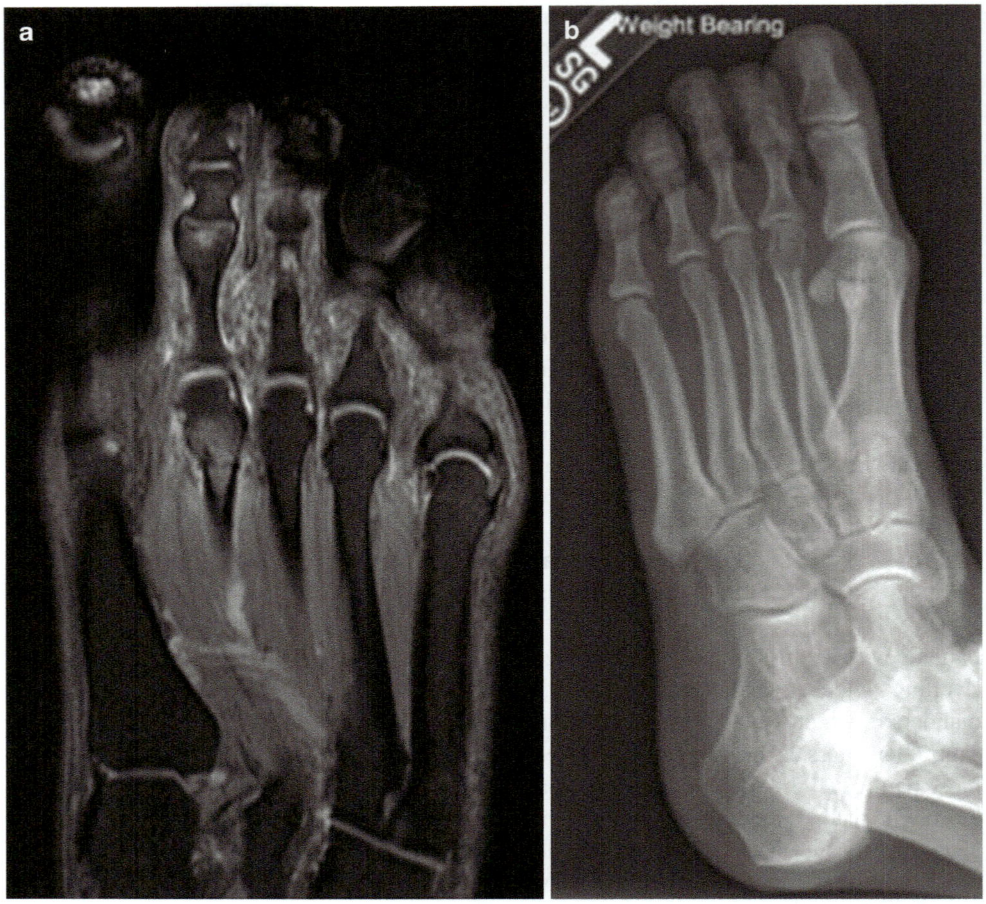

Fig. 27.7 (**a**) Second metatarsal stress fracture with initial MRI "negative" subsequent MRI showing second metatarsal neck stress fracture 3 weeks later. (**b**) X-ray showing malunion since the patient continued to run based on first MRI being "negative"

injury. Ascertaining the actual location of the injury helps guide treatment. Appropriate imaging is critical especially with in-season athletes.

27.3 Jones and Proximal Fifth Metatarsal Stress Fractures (Zone II and III)

27.3.1 Introduction

A fracture of the proximal aspect of the fifth metatarsal was initially described by Sir Robert Jones in 1902 after he sustained the injury himself while dancing [29]. Based on epidemiological studies of the general population and athletes, proximal fifth metatarsal fractures account for approximately 70% of metatarsal fractures, and are likely more common in subjects with cavovarus and lateral column overload [30, 31]. Fifth metatarsal fractures have been classified based on location of injury: tuberosity (zone I), metaphyseal-diaphyseal junction (zone II), or proximal diaphysis (zone III) [32]. Zone I fractures will not be discussed in this chapter. Zone II fractures are the classic Jones fracture: however, both these and zone III fractures are often treated in a similar fashion, despite a higher nonunion rate in the latter regardless of treatment [33]. In that light, the concern with an injury in zone II and II is the relatively high occurrence of delayed union, non-union and refracture, the result of poor blood supply in that region of the fifth metatarsal and stresses sustained with running activity [34, 35]. Anatomically, the vascular "water-shed" area is located at the metaphyseal-diaphyseal junction, as metaphyseal arteries enter the base and nutrient arteries enter the proximal shaft providing retrograde perfusion to the metaphyseal-diaphyseal junction [36]. A fracture at this site further compromises the intramedullary blood supply.

27.3.1.1 Epidemiology

Anatomy, morphology and osteology all play an intrinsic role in why Jones fractures occur [37]. Foot posture and bony malalignment may also predispose running athletes to fifth metatarsal fractures. Those with a supinated or underpronated posture have a significantly higher risk of an overuse injury [38]. A varus hindfoot leads to increased forces on the proximal fifth metatarsal which may lead to fracture [31]. This is also true for patients with metatarsus adductus or a skewfoot which result in lateral column overload [39]. In an

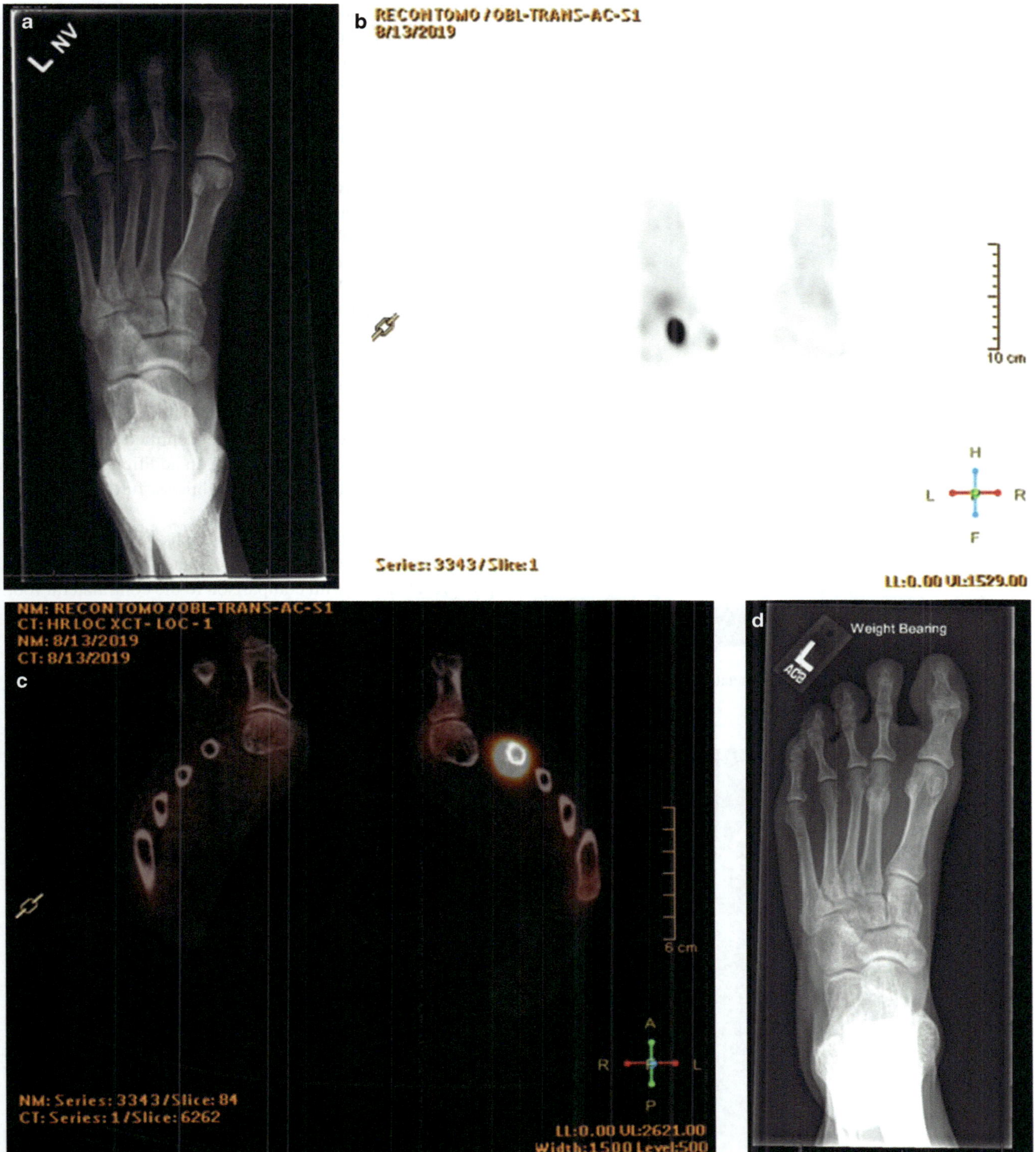

Fig. 27.8 (**a**) Negative X-ray of patient with positive "Torque test" of second Met. (**b**, **c**) Positive Bone scan and SPECT for second met shaft stress fracture. (**d**) Post-immobilisation with callus formation 3 weeks later

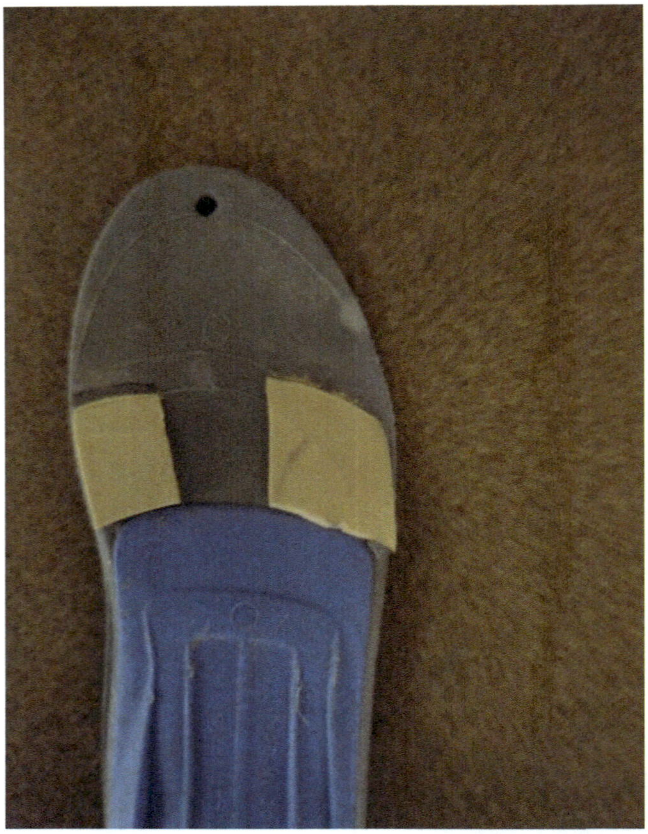

Fig. 27.9 Off-loading pad for second metatarsal stress fracture on the underside of an off-the-shelf insole

NFL study assessing foot sizing and shoe fitting, a remarkable number of players were wearing a shoe more narrow than the foot width itself. Ill fitting shoes have been speculated to allow the fifth metatarsal to "hang" over the lateral edge of the sole, thus increasing overload and pressures that may lead to stress induced changes [40, 41].

27.3.1.2 Diagnosis

Evaluation of a patient with lateral based foot pain should begin with a detailed history that includes the following questions: Was there an acute injury? Prior fracture? History of prior foot pain? What shoes/orthoses are being worn and has the individual been appropriately measured? Standing exam assesses for foot posture and any asymmetries, i.e. cavovarus, skew, metatarsus adductus. Sitting exam may determine swelling and tenderness along the fifth metatarsal and note swelling, which may be present with acute injuries [30, 31]. A plantar flexed first ray can be identified and a cause of cavus with lateral column overload. In addition, the Achilles tendon is assessed for excessive tightness, further adding to midfoot stresses.

Standard weight bearing radiographs of the foot in the anteroposterior, lateral and oblique plane should be obtained upon presentation, with comparison to the contralateral foot. Plain films alone may differentiate an acute fracture with a well-defined fracture line, compared to the presence of sclerosis or hypertrophy more consistent with a chronic situation or non-union. An MRI, or bone scan, can help determine the

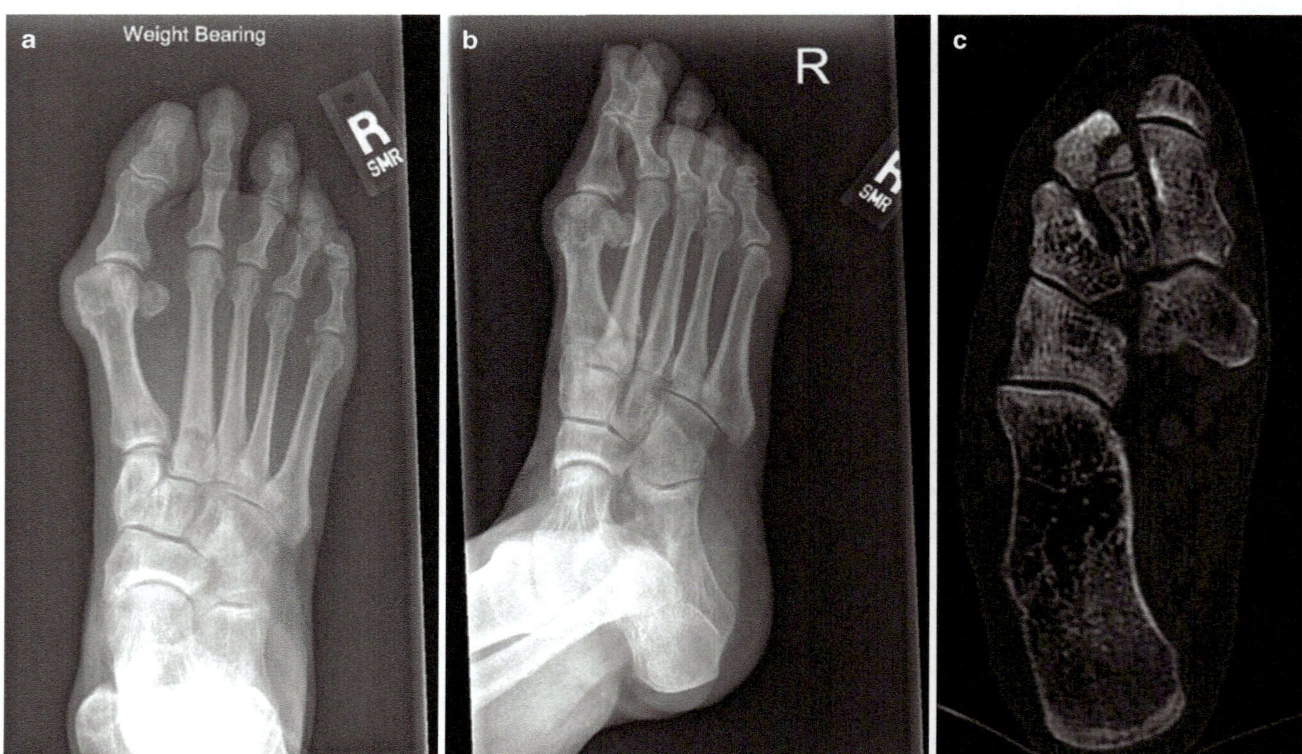

Fig. 27.10 (a–f) Pre-op X-rays, CT and post-op X-rays of a proximal second metatarsal, intra-articular fracture with delayed union treated with autograft

Fig. 27.10 (continued)

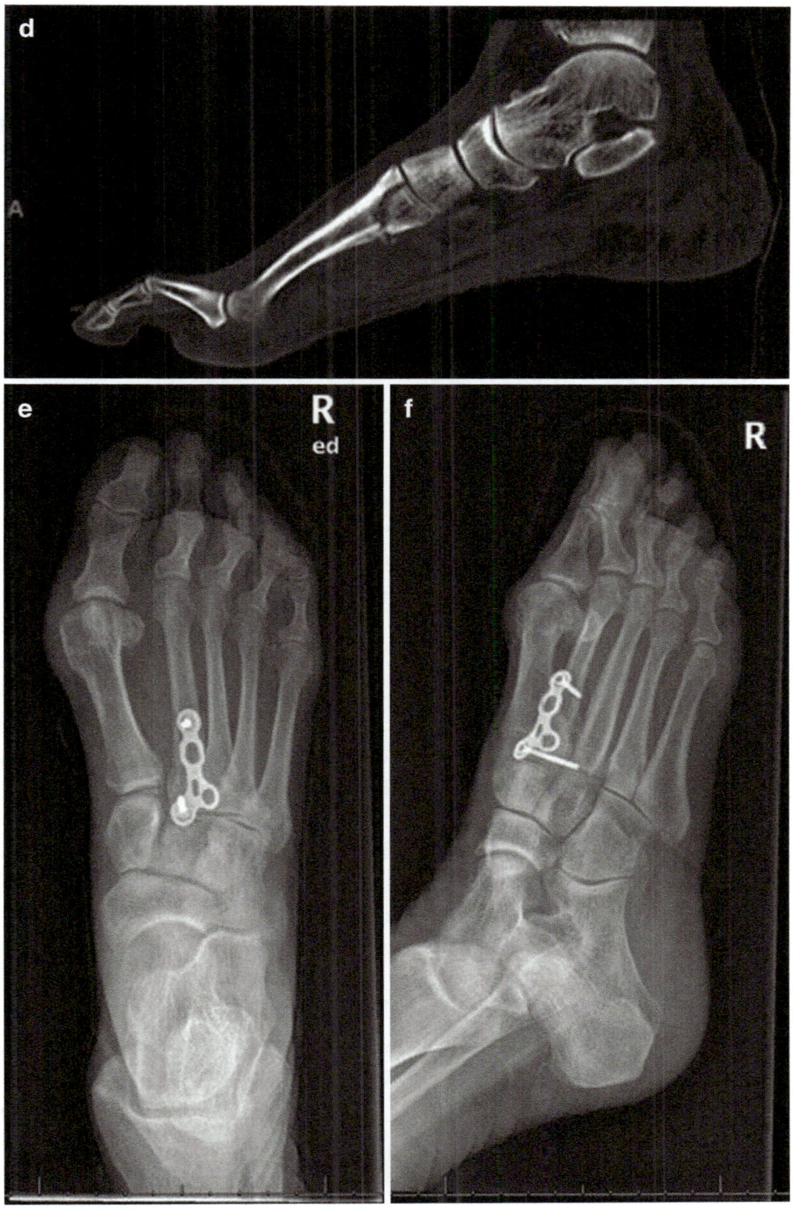

inflammatory activity (or acuteness) of the fracture. CT scans are useful to define the exact location and extent of the fracture (incomplete versus complete, occult presentations), but is more predominantly utilized post-operatively to assess bone healing.

27.3.1.3 Treatment

While nonoperative treatment with immobilisation and protected weight bearing can be attempted in all patients with a zone II/III fracture, the risk of delayed/non-union of up to 30% and refracture rates up to 50% is of concern to the elite or career athlete [34, 35, 41]. Therefore, immediate operative intervention is recommended in most athletes despite the inherent risks and costs. Operative treatment provides the potential for a quicker return to activity through a earlier rehabilitation program and is felt to reduce the incidence of non-union and refracture [42].

The gold standard for managing these Jones type fractures consists of axial/intramedullary screw fixation. A recent cadaveric study determined by digital measurement that the average intramedullary canal diameter is 6.475 ± 1.54 mm in the plantar to dorsal plane and 4.6 ± 0.85 mm in the medial to lateral plane. A 4.5 mm screw is the smallest diameter screw that can be efficaciously used for fifth metatarsal fractures [43]. Another radiographic study published evaluated 119 patients by CT scans, and determined the average coronal medullary canal diameter to be 5.0 mm at the isthmus and the length of the straight segment of the fifth metatarsal from proximal to distal to be 52 mm, approximately 68% of the metatarsal length. Based on this study, a screw greater than 4.5 mm is needed to obtain adequate purchase within the intramedullary canal while remaining shorter than 68% of the total length of the canal to prevent fracture displacement [44]. A variety of screws may be utilized for this axial fixation of the fifth metatarsal, and there are commercially available screws specific for this indication [45]. The senior author's preferes a solid partially threaded screw,. Newest generations of these screws include a chamfered head design to lessen the risk of cuboid impingement.

27.3.1.4 Surgical Technique

The patient is placed supine on the operative table with a bump under the ipsilateral hip, achieving about 30–45° of body angulation. To assist with lateral imaging, the foot itself is placed on blankets to elevate it above the level of the contralateral foot. A calf tourniquet or Esmarch bandage can be utilized to control blood loss. A fluoroscopy unit (mini C-arm) is placed at the foot of the bed to obtain appropriate orthogonal views. A guide wire is placed into the base of the fifth metatarsal under imaging guidance directed so that it is in line with the centre of the diaphyseal canal. Once achieved, an incision is made approximately 1 cm proximal and distal to the wire (Fig. 27.11). Blunt dissection through the subcutaneous tissues to the base of the fifth metatarsal will protect the peroneus brevis and the sural nerve, aided with the use of tissue protectors. The guide wire may be advanced to the fracture site but not further so as to avoid penetrating the diaphyseal cortex, a risk considering the natural curvature of the metatarsal distally (Figs. 27.12 and 27.13). A cannulated drill is advanced over the guide wire to the fracture site and then exchanged to a solid 3.2 mm drill that is then used "free-hand" into the midshaft intramedullary canal. This manoeuvre insures a straight line from entry to a point distal to the fracture while avoiding cortical perforation and the potential of creating a stress riser (Fig. 27.14). Sequential cannulated taps will determine the best diameter of screw to place, and are increased by 1 mm increments until the fifth metatarsal is adequately torqued (Fig. 27.15). This step also helps to determine the appropriate screw length, with the goal of having the screw threads extending just past the fracture site. To verify, the selected screw is placed adjacent to the metatarsal and assessed radiographically for length (Fig. 27.16a, b). Extending the screw too distal into the diaphysis may displace the fracture or create a lateral gap given the inherent curvature previously mentioned. In male adult athletes with a zone II fracture, the screw is typically 40–45 mm long and of 5.5 mm in diameter (Fig. 27.17a, b). Fluoroscopy should be used during screw insertion to confirm screw length, competency of diaphyseal cortices, and fracture site compression. If a gap is encountered after appropriate screw selection and insertion (typically plantar-lateral), a bone marrow aspirate concentrate mixed with a demineralized bone graft substitute or autogenous cancellous bone graft can be injected.

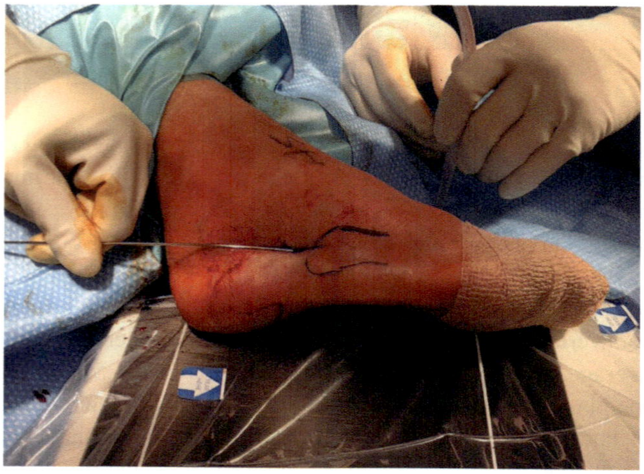

Fig. 27.11 incisional approach for Jones fracture

27.3.1.5 Postoperative Course

A splint is applied in the operating room and is removed after 1 week to allow for range of motion. Patients remain non-weight bearing for 2 weeks post-operatively and then transition to full weight bearing in a short walker boot. Walker boots significantly reduce contact pressure at the fifth metatarsal base with ambulation compared to post-operative shoe and running shoes [46]. In addition, orthotic devices can be placed into the boot for further protection. Cross training with non-impact activity is initiated early, and includes stationary bike and resisted muscle strengthening. Suspended pool running, and subsequent anti-gravity treadmill off loaded activity can be initiated when wounds have healed. Athletes are often advanced to a running shoe by 4–6 weeks if asymptomatic. As evidence for radiographic bony bridging may be significantly delayed, the authors allow advancement of activity when the patient is able to weight bear without pain, perform multiple single limb heel rise and hop. The gradual return to sport-specific training includes a shoe of appropriate width and modified with a full-length custom orthosis to provide shock absorption and arch support. Relief of pressure on the base of the fifth metatarsal is beneficial. A lateral flare or hindfoot post is used in athletes with a cavovarus foot [31]. The metatarsal may be further protected from excessive stresses during this time frame with either a clamshell orthosis or full-length turf toe plate. Most athletes return to play between 8 to 10 weeks post-operatively and

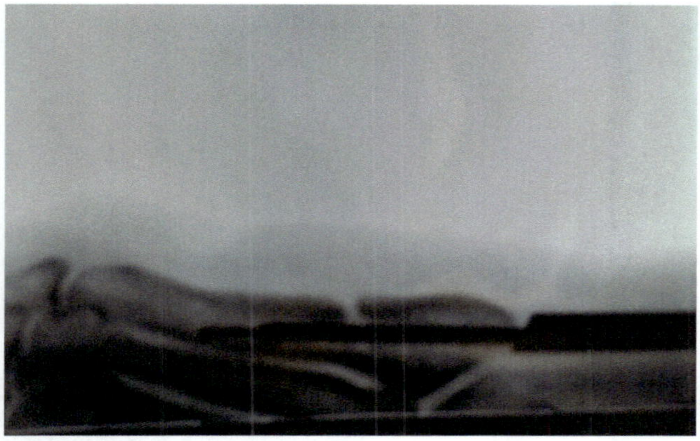

Fig. 27.12 Guide pin placement

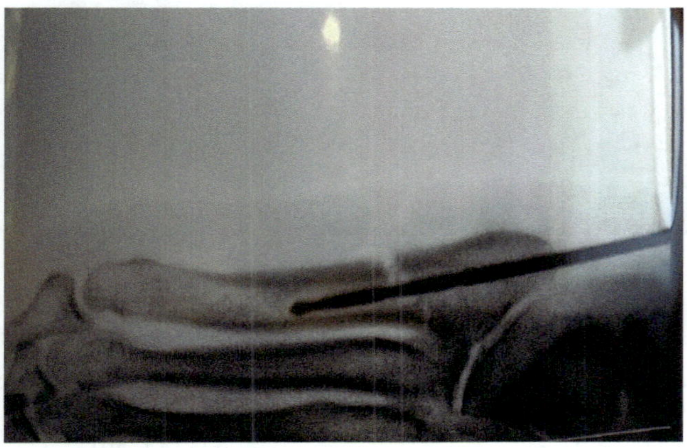

Fig. 27.13 Cannulated drill over guide pin

the use of this modified shoe wear is recommended for this first year, if not the duration of their sport career. Hardware is left in place indefinitely.

27.3.1.6 Complications

Revision surgery for symptomatic non-unions or refractures poses additional technical challenges. Open bone grafting is recommended, and some prefer to obtain the cancellous bone from the iliac crest in the running athlete. This is felt to obviate the risk of pain or fracture associated with harvesting in distal in the extremity. To fully manipulate and prepare the fracture site, hardware removal is performed through the previous insertion site. If the screw is broken, a broken screw removal set may be employed to remove the screw fragment. If unsuccessful, a cortical window may be created to remove a distal screw fragment. The non-union site is thoroughly debrided with currettes, ronguers and osteotomes, and drill bits are utilized to perforate all exposed bone surfaces. The intramedullary canal is cleared of sclerotic hypertrophic bone. Cancellous autograft from the calcaneus obtained is then placed abundantly in the refracture/non-union site before screw placement.

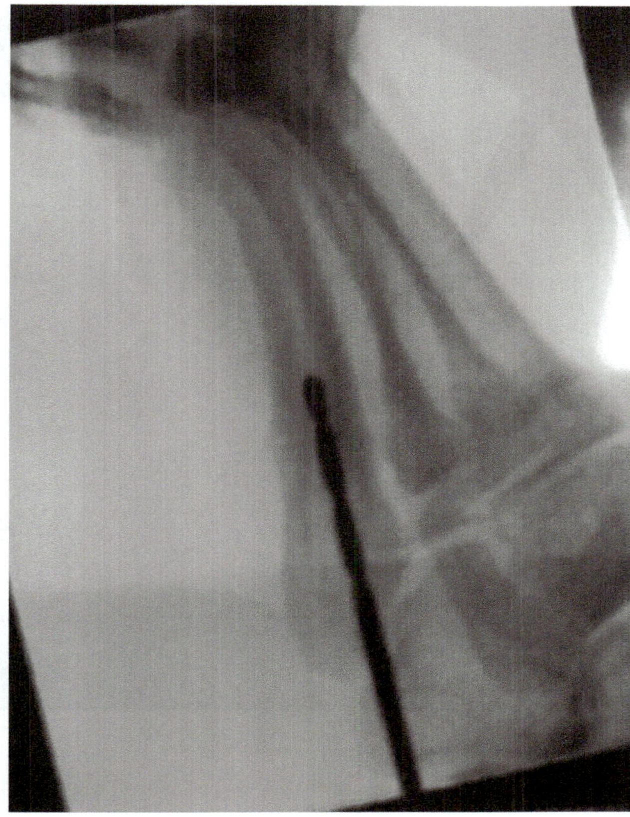

Fig. 27.14 Sequential drilling

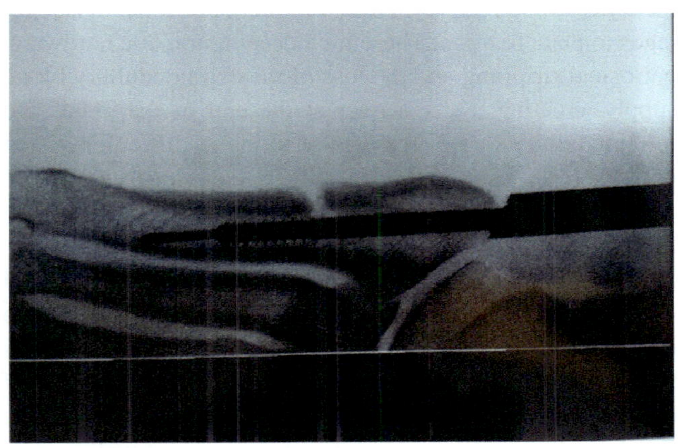

Fig. 27.15 Tap

There has been recent interest in plate fixation for zone II/III fractures [25, 45]. The use of a plate is particularly attractive in revision cases of non-union or refracture where open bone grafting is planned and direct access needed. Plate fixation is also helpful in instances of proximal bone loss or comminution. The plate can be placed on the tension side of the fracture, i.e. the plantar aspect of the metatarsal where is can be adequately covered with the adductor digiti mimini muscle and avoid shoe irritation. Biomechanical advantages

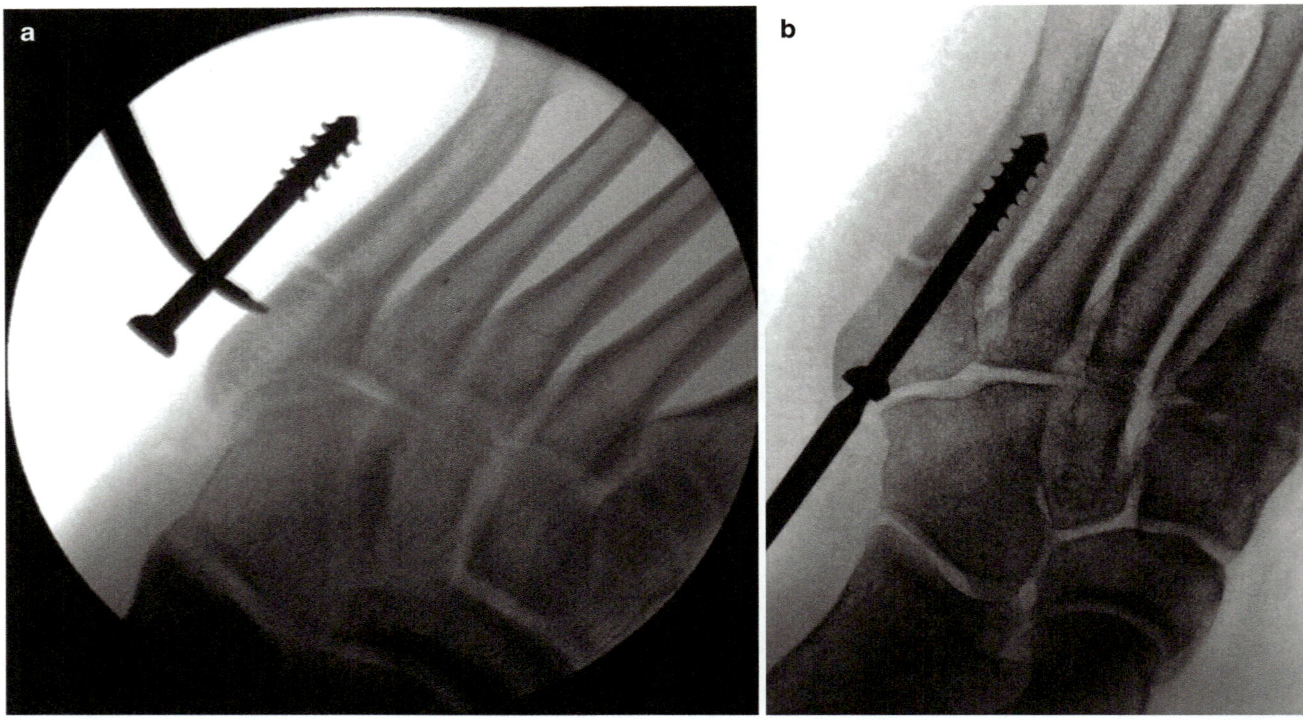

Fig. 27.16 (**a**, **b**) assessing screw length

of plate fixation have been described [46]. Advantages of plate fixation also include avoiding disruption of the intramedullary blood supply. However, there are some disadvantages to plate fixation. These include symptomatic hardware, periosteal stripping and the loss of the extramedullary blood supply, creating a stress riser at the end of the plate, and intramedullary screw breakage resulting in difficult revision options. In addition, this open technique obviously has a longer recovery than axial screw fixation and thus in-season implications in regard to return to sport.

Revision surgery for a non-union or refracture is followed by a slower, more conservative post-operative protocol than described previously for a primary situation. This includes non-weight bearing for 4–6 weeks, potentially longer if excessive bone is removed during screw retrieval. Patients are then advanced to weight bearing in a short walker boot for an additional 4–6 weeks. A running shoe with a protective orthosis is employed once the patient is asymptomatic and radiographic healing is present, often at 10–12 weeks. Patients are gradually advanced to running activity, first in a pool or on an anti-gravity treadmill. A CT is helpful to determine and confirm union, and is recommended prior to resuming court or field activity.

Adjuvant therapy is often utilized in the athletic population undergoing treatment of a Jones type fracture. Vitamin D and calcium levels should be obtained and monitored, with a low threshold for utilizing supplements in this situation: Vitamin D deficiency can occur in athletes and supplementation can decrease the rate of stress fractures [47–49].

Bone stimulators present another option during the recovery period. Bone stimulators improve healing of nonunions and delayed unions [50]. With regards to Jones fractures, all nine patients with delayed unions and non-unions achieved complete bony union with nonoperative management using a pulsed electromagnetic field [51]. More recently, a randomized clinical trial of patients with delayed unions or non-unions of the fifth metatarsal treated with intramedullary screw fixation with or without (control group) pulsed electromagnetic fields (PEMFS) showed that patients treated with PEMF achieved complete radiographic union 6 weeks sooner than controls. Furthermore, those treated with PEMF had significantly higher amounts of placental growth factor (a member of the VEGF subfamily) and higher levels of brain-derived neurotropic factor (BDNF). Both of these growth factors promote angiogenesis and vasculogenesis; therefore, increasing oxygenation and nutrient delivery to the fracture site may promote healing. BMP 5 and BMP 7 expression was also increased with PEMF, and BMPs can be used to optimise fracture union [52]. Extra-corporeal shockwave (ESWT) has been shown to be efficacious particularly for non-union. In one study, 0.35 mJ/mm^2 for 2000–4000 pulses was used to fractures of

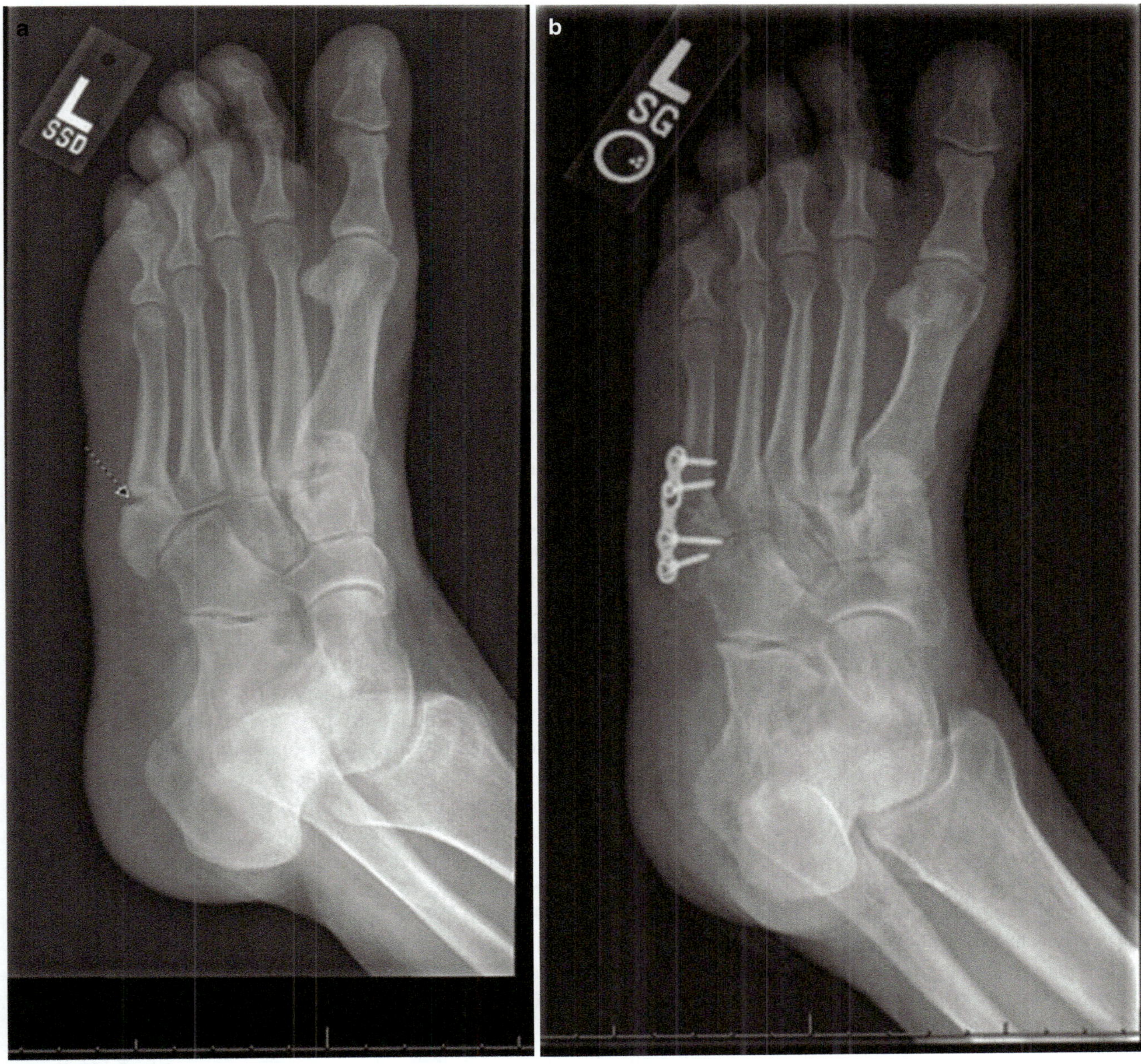

Fig. 27.17 Pre- and post-operative treatment of non-union with plate & dowel autograft

the fifth metatarsal base, though not all were "true" Jones fractures [53].

While no evidence for success has been reported, the off-label use of teriparatide, a recombinant human parathyroid hormone, may also be considered for revision situations. There have been rare incidences reported in humans, but patients need to be aware of the black box warning that this drug has been associated with an increased risk of osteosarcomas in laboratory rats.

27.3.1.7 Outcomes

The ultimate goal for managing zone II/III fifth metatarsal fractures is successful and sustained union and return to play to a pre-injury level of performance. A systematic review of 26 studies published in 2013 found that fractures treated non-operatively had a 76% union rate compared to a 96% union rate following operative treatment.Furthermore, delayed unions healed 44% with nonoperative care and 97% with operative treatment and non-unions had a 97% union rate with intramedullary screw fixation [41]. Another systematic review published in 2011 evaluated six studies of 330 patients, operative fixation with intramedullary screw fixation results in faster time to union, faster return to play with fewer complications compared to nonoperative management [54].

Another controversial issue concerns which is the ideal type of screw. The evidence comparing outcomes of different screw types varies. Our institution retrospectively compared the outcomes of treatment using indication specific screws to traditional screws in 47 patients. Both groups achieved a union rate greater than 95% with similar visual analog pain and satisfaction scores; however, the traditional screws had a significantly higher complication rate (four complications to none) [45]. Other authors report excellent results using headless compression screws for the treatment of Jones fractures with a 3.3% failure rate [55]. Biomechanical studies published in 2011 and 2012 compared traditional partially threaded screws to variable pitch screws [56, 57]. In simulated cadaveric Jones fracture models, the partially threaded screw generated more fracture site compression and less fracture site angulation; however, there was no difference in fracture stiffness [58]. Other studies have shown no difference in bending stiffness between variable pitch screws and partially threaded screws [59]. Another treatment option for fifth metatarsal fractures includes low profile hook plates. Using simulated cadaveric Jones fractures, Huh et al. compared intramedullary screws with the low profile plate. Biomechanically, the intramedullary screw resulted in greater bending stiffness, less fracture site angulation, and greater initial torsional stiffness compared to the hook plate [60].

While operative fixation of Zone II and Zone III fractures have a high union rate with fixation, nonunions and refractures still occur and in the range of 8–30% [59]. Managing these situations can be difficult given issues with retained hardware and bone loss. Bernstein et al. recently reported on their success with plate fixation. While a small sample size, they noted good success with plate fixation in elite athletes undergoing revision surgery [61]. Hunt et al. reported on the success of revision surgery utilizing screw exchange and biologics, the majority receiving autologous bone graft. A 100% union rate with return to preinjury competition level in 21 athletes at an average of 12.3 weeks was reported. One patient sustained a subsequent refracture following a traumatic injury that healed without further intervention [42]. Bigsby et al. reported on outcomes of 117 fifth metatarsal fractures, 55 of those being zone II and III injuries. Patients' Foot Function Index (FFI) scores improved from 22 at 1 month to 0 at 1 year. At 1 year, 28% of patients' with Zone I fractures and 33% with Zone III continued to report pain, but none of the Zone II patients reported any functional limitations but 10% of Zone III patients report functional limitations [62].

Athletes desiring to return to play following a fifth metatarsal fractures should have realistic expectations. In a recent retrospective study of professional athletes, 85% of basketball players were able to return to pre-injury level of function. In this study, 92% of the patients were treated operatively, 12% required reoperation and 19% had a recurrent injury [63]. National Football League (NFL) players are also at risk for sustaining a Jones fracture due to the repetitive strain placed on the fifth metatarsal. NFL players with Jones fractures treated with intramedullary screw fixation and iliac crest bone-marrow aspirate with demineralized bone matrix injected at the fracture site were retrospective reviewed. Post-operatively, the athletes underwent an aggressive rehabilitation program and 100% of athletes returned to play at an average of 8.7 weeks. Refracture occurred in 12% of athletes, and all returned to professional play after revision surgery [64].

27.3.1.8 Conclusion

In high-level athletes, nonoperative management of Zone II and Zone III fractures of the fifth metatarsal may prolong return to play because of the high rates of delayed union, refracture and nonunion. Therefore, we recommend minimally invasive primary operative fixation with a solid partial threaded intramedullary screw to obtain compression and provide inherent support. The screw threads should extend just distal to the fracture site with a typical screw length of 40 mm or greater. Furthermore, the screw size should be greater than 4.5 mm, ideally 5.0–6.5 mm in diameter [65]. It remains in question whether return to play should be delayed until complete radiographic union has been obtained to decrease the risk of refracture or nonunion [66]. Most importantly, it is felt necessary for the individual to be asymptomatic with activity and in appropriated sized shoes with protective modifications prior to return to sport [67].

27.4 Navicular Stress Fractures

27.4.1 Epidemiology

Navicular stress fractures were thought to be rare prior to advanced imaging beyond plain radiographs being available. Tarsal navicular stress fractures in humans were first described in 1970 [68]. The incidence of stress fractures of this bone is much higher in the athletic population compared to the general population, and appears to be common in track and field athletes, with an incidence in athletes of around 25% of the stress fractures in the lower extremity. In one study 32% of 180 stress fractures incurred in athletes were of the navicular; they also accounted for 73% of the track and field athletes stress fractures [69]. The healing potential for

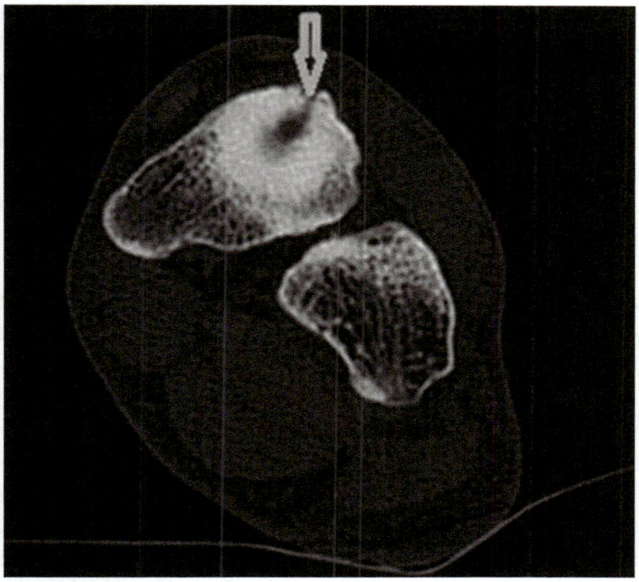

Fig. 27.18 Type I Navicular stress fracture (based on frontal plane image CT with <0.6 mm slices)

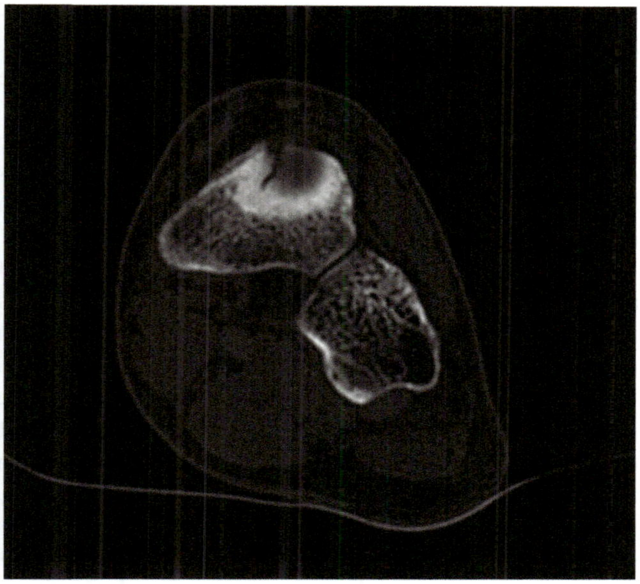

Fig. 27.19 Type II Navicular stress fracture

this injury is dependent on a timely diagnosis and the severity of the fracture. The closer the fracture is to being complete, the lower healing potential and increased probability that surgical management is required and arthrosis can occur regardless of treatment.

27.4.2 Classification

Saxena et al. proposed the only known classification of stress fractures of the navicular [70]. Type I fractures are only through the dorsal navicular cortex, (Fig. 27.18) Type II extend into the middle of the body of the bone, and Type III include penetration of a second cortex (Figs. 27.19 and 27.20). Modifiers help to further narrow down the prognosis of these injuries, "A" for avascular necrosis, "C" for cysts and "S" for sclerosis.

Saxena et al. [71] recently updated the classification to include stress reactions (Type 0.5) in which MRI shows signal change but CT confirms no actual fracture: (Table 27.4).

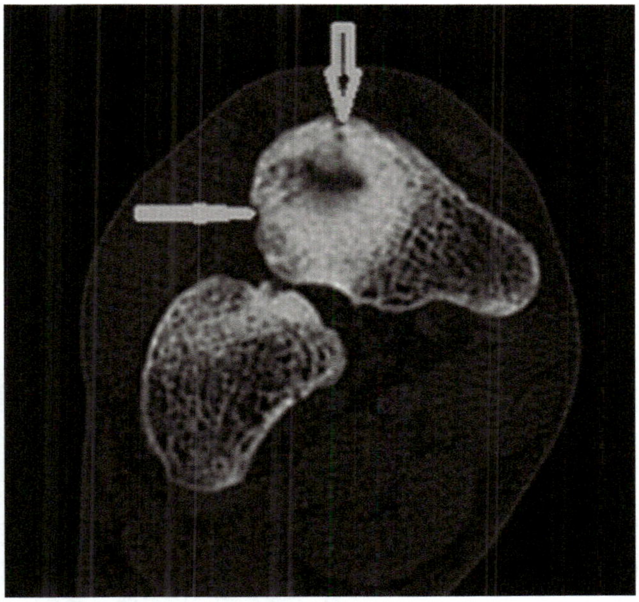

Fig. 27.20 Type III Navicular stress fracture

Table 27.4 Navicular stress fracture classification

Type	Description
0.5	Stress reaction: signal change on MRI noted, but stress fracture not imaged on CT
1	Dorsal cortical fracture on coronal image
2	Fracture extends into navicular body on coronal image
3	Complete propagation of fracture to second cortex (medial, lateral or plantar) on coronal image

Abbreviations: *CT* computed tomography, *MRI* magnetic resonance imaging
Adapted from Saxena et al. [71]

27.4.3 Diagnosis (History/Physical Exam/Radiological Investigations)

Clinicians must have a high index of suspicion to diagnose this stress fracture, as it presents differently than other stress injuries in lower extremity. Typically, the pain of a navicular stress fracture will be vague, the injury typically lacks any noticeable edema, and radiographs will typically not detect the presence of a bony injury. Patients will not usually recall a specific injury, and no foot type or activity has been specifically associated with this injury beyond impact activities.

Clinical examination can reveal pain dorsally over the highest dorsal point of the navicular, which is termed the "N" spot. Having the patient go into a crouched position or hop on their toes may also trigger the symptoms. Some patients claim medial ankle or arch pain, which can be confused with ankle impingement and plantar fasciitis.

Radiographs may detect the injury in advanced cases, but advanced imaging must be performed to properly assess this injury. MRI is often the initial advanced imaging ordered in many injuries and the injury can often be identified with the test. However, Computerized Tomography or "SPECT" are preferred as they provide better visualization of the extent of the injury. Patients in one of the largest studies were often mis-diagnosed using MRI, which was only 71% accurate, whereas CT was 100% accurate [71]. In that study, patients often were not correctly diagnosed until more than 8 months from symptom onset. Furthermore, since Saxena's classification is based on CT findings, we strongly recommend CT to confirm diagnosis, best treatment and healing potential.

27.4.4 Treatment

Early diagnosis and treatment are paramount for successful treatment of tarsal navicular stress fractures. Khan et al. reported on 86 navicular stress fractures, the largest series [72]. They found that 86% (19/22) of the patients treated initially with at least 6 weeks of non-weight bearing immobilisation returned to their sport compared to a return to sport of only 26% (9/34) who continued to bear weight on the injured foot. Fitch astutely pointed out that athletes will feel no pain in the area with relative rest within less than a week, but the symptoms will return with resumption of activity [73]. In a metaanalysis, Torg reported that the majority of failed conservative treatment of navicular stress fractures did not involve non-weight bearing immobilisation [74].

In a prospective study, Saxena and Fullem found an average return to activity for all treated navicular fractures of 4 months [75]. Type I fractures were treated with non-weight bearing and immobilisation: those athletes returned to activity in 3.8 months; Type II and III fractures underwent ORIF with an RTA of 3.7 and 4.0 months, respectively.

The gold standard of non-surgical treatment of a navicular stress fracture is 6–8 weeks of non-weight bearing immobilisation. For those who fail conservative treatment, surgical management should be considered, and in more severe stress fractures such as the Type III, which more closely resembles a complete fracture, it is advisable to immediately consider surgical management, especially if there was an initial delay in diagnosis and treatment. Athletic patients with Type II injuries should also be considered for ORIF, given the high incidence of delayed and non-union, re-fracture and arthrosis [71].

Surgical management through a dorsal approach with ORIF with a single screw placed from lateral can provide excellent results (Fig. 27.21a, b). The incision is typically made lateral to the neurovascular bundle. Care should be taken not to disrupt the vascular supply to the navicular in

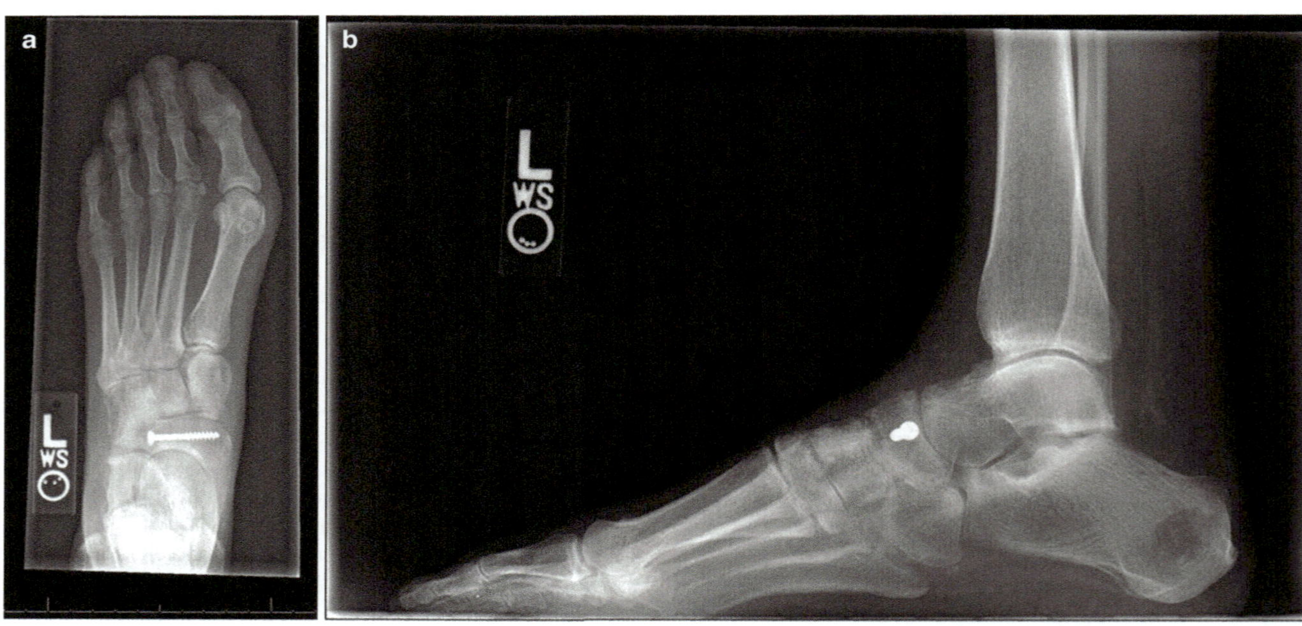

Fig. 27.21 (**a**, **b**) ORIF of navicular stress fracture

this region which comes from that lateral tarsal branch of the dorsalis pedis artery. In larger individuals and fractures, two screws may be required. Unlike Jones fractures which appear to have better outcome with solid screws, there is little data to show a distinct advantage over cannulated screws [57, 65, 76]. Curettage and drilling of fracture site with autogenous bone graft from the ipsilateral calcaneus will facilitate healing. Post-operatively, the patient should remain non-weight bearing in a short leg cast or boot 6 weeks, followed by another 2–6 weeks of weightbearing in a CAM boot until pain free. CT at 12 weeks, even in non-surgical cases, can confirm healing, especially in athletes trying to return to sport as soon as possible.

27.4.5 Complications

Navicular stress fractures can progress to a delayed, mal- or non-union, avascular necrosis, and degenerative arthrosis of the talo-navicular and or cuneo-navicular joints [71, 75]. On follow up of navicular stress fractures Saxena found that an osteochondral defect of the talo-navicular joint may develop following this injury, and an external fixation to produce arthrodiatasis following microfracture has been successfully performed on patients who develop this complication [71, 77].

27.4.6 Rehabilitation/Post-operative Care

Navicular stress fractures require a stricter conservative course than many other stress fractures in the lower limb. This injury involves a full loss of one or more seasons of sport, since the average time to return to sport is at least 4 months. Any exercise that even involves movements that will invert or evert the foot with the heel raised may place undue stress on the fracture and lead to failure. Not performing any relative exercise within the boot that involves the affected foot or leg can lead to significant atrophy and loss of proprioception, requiring physical therapy to restore function prior to returning to activity. Therefore, stationary biking for 20–30 min with the heel on the pedal with a cast or boot is encouraged to decreased atrophy when the patient is pain-free post-injury/surgery.

27.4.7 Preventative Measures

Since the exact etiology of this injury is unknown, there are not any known preventative measures beyond those already recommended for most fractures. These include replacing worn out shoe gear, monitoring calcium and Vitamin D intake and improving gluteal muscle activation ("CORE" strength).

27.4.8 Calcaneal Stress Fractures

27.4.8.1 Epidemiology

The calcaneus is composed predominantly of a thin cortex with a weaving cancellous bone made specifically to bear weight. This complex bone is especially subjected to high weight bearing forces during physical activities, with forces 110% and 250+% of body weight occurring during heel strike when walking and running, respectively [78].

Stress fractures of the calcaneus typically present as a nonspecific, vague exertional heel pain. It can be easily misdiagnosed as retrocalcaneal bursitis, Achilles tendinopathy, or plantar fasciitis, further delaying diagnosis and appropriate treatment. First described in 1939 in military recruits [79], it is the second most common foot stress fracture, after the second metatarsal [80]. It occurs in 21–28% of all lower extremity stress fractures, with a slightly higher incidence in females [5]. The posterior body of the calcaneus is injured most frequently (56%), followed by the anterior calcaneus (26%), then middle portion in 18% [3, 6, 80]. Calcaneal stress fractures are typically found in repetitive jumping, high impact sports and activities such as running. It is therefore hypothesised that the excessive pull of the Achilles tendon during activities produces excessive tension on the calcaneus. However, normal forces on abnormal bone can also lead to stress fractures, and therefore the quality of bone should always be evaluated.

27.4.8.2 Classification

There are no accepted classification methods for calcaneal stress fractures. Most often, these stress fractures occur in the posterior aspect of the calcaneus. Anecdotally, the fracture lines are perpendicular to the pull of the plantar fascia if there has been prior fasciitis. In cases of metabolic insufficiency, the fracture lines are parallel to the posterior subtalar joint (Figs. 27.22a–c and 27.23a, b). Stress fractures of the calcaneus can also occur in the region of the sustentaculum tali and anterior process (Fig. 27.24).

27.4.8.3 Diagnosis

Clinical evaluation can be deceiving, since their presentation is often non-specific. Patients report an insidious onset of increasing pain and tenderness over the calcaneus. The patient may lack specific physical findings such as edema, erythema or ecchymosis. Therefore, a high level of suspicion is necessary for a timely accurate diagnosis and proper treatment.

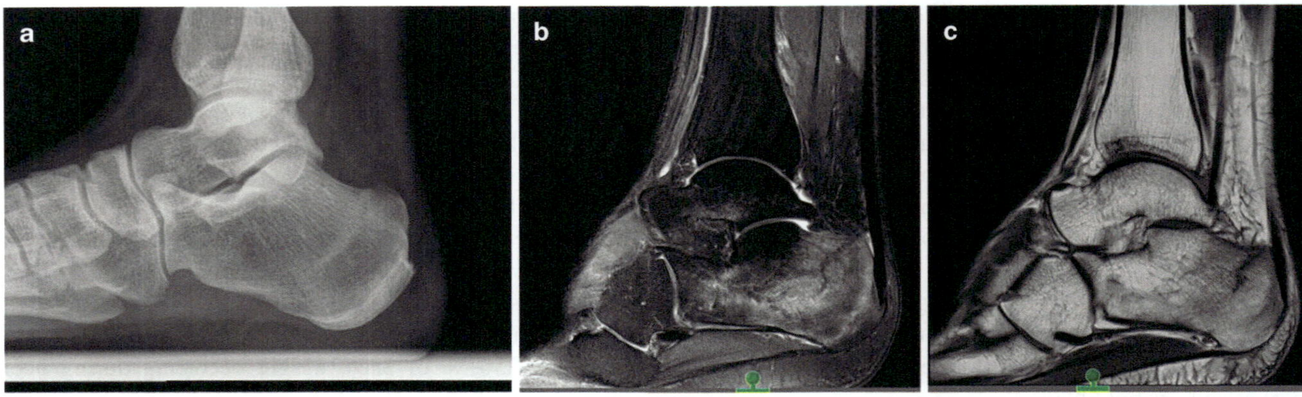

Fig. 27.22 (a) Calcaneal stress fracture X-ray. (b) T2 MRI showing calcaneal stress fracture. (c) T1 MRI showing calcaneal stress fracture

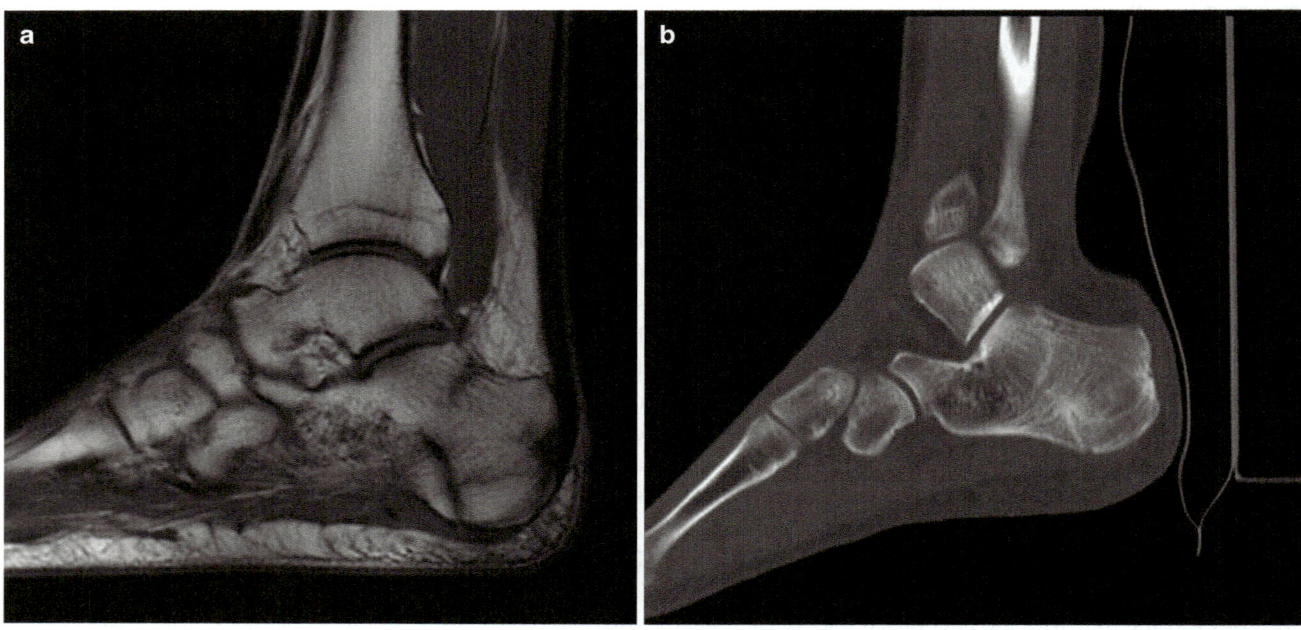

Fig. 27.23 (a) MRI of patient with calcaneal stress fracture; note fracture lines also perpendicular to plantar fascia, which is thickened. (b) CT of same patient after undergoing dry-needling for "plantar fasciitis" which created an inferior fracture

27.4.8.4 Treatment

When there is strong clinical suspicious of calcaneal stress fracture and initial radiographs are normal, appropriate treatment should begin immediately while awaiting confirmation with MRI imaging. Calcaneal stress fractures can be classified as being a low-risk fracture, which tends to heal well with activities modification, has a low risk of non-union, and does not require surgical intervention [79–81]. The treatment should be focused on the patient's symptoms by allowing weight bearing as tolerated in a protective cast boot, with or without a gait aid of choice to help with offloading of the foot. The causing sport and aggravating activities should be discontinued, but non-impact activities (such as bicycling and/or swimming) can be initiated to help maintain fitness. Activities should be modified for a period of 4–6 weeks, and it is recommended that the athlete be pain free and full weight bearing for a period of 2 weeks prior to resuming training [78].Typical return to sports is therefore 6–12 weeks after initiation of treatment. A sound return to activity plan should be followed and any reoccurrence of symptoms should be carefully monitored.

27.5 Other Less Common Stress Fractures of the Foot in Athletes

Stress fractures have been found in virtually all the bones of the foot. The etiology is often similar to the other more common stress fractures of the foot. MRIs and bone scans typically can reveal these. Other midfoot bones such as the

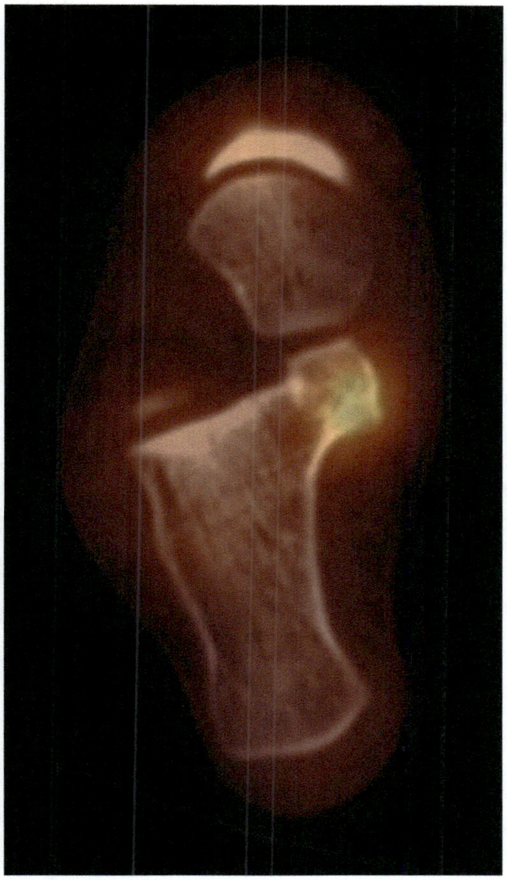

Fig. 27.24 Stress fracture of sustentaculum tali seen on SPECT

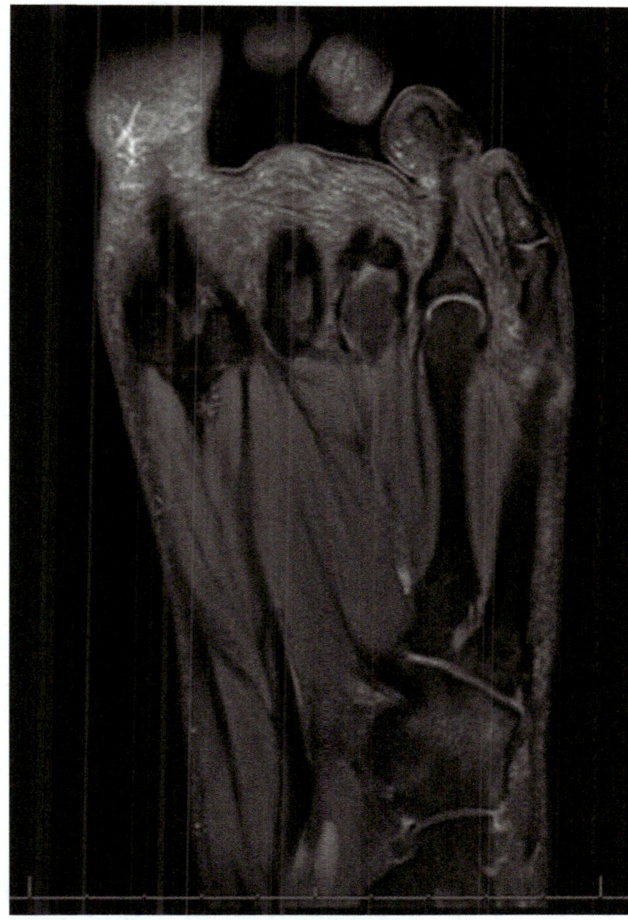

Fig. 27.25 MRI of cuboid stress fracture

cuneiforms and cuboid can incur stress fractures (Fig. 27.25). The treatment typically involves non-weightbearing for 2–3 weeks in a cast boot, and an additional 2–4 weeks in a boot until pain-free. In a study of over 900 extremity stress fractures in athletes, the talar body was involved in 0.3% of the cases, all teenage gymnasts [82]. The posterior talus has also been involved, and may require ORIF [83] (Fig. 27.26). Given the small number reported, it is difficult to determine best treat options, long-term prognosis and outcomes.

Stress fractures of the base of the proximal phalanges have been involved in dancers, gymnasts and other running/jumping athletes [84]. The treatment is symptomatic off-loading with a stiff shoe and, if needed, a cast boot and non-weightbearing. For intra-articular Salter-Harris III injuries of the phalangeal bases, ORIF is sometimes indicated [85]. Anecdotally, these may be misdiagnosed as plantar plate tears.

27.5.1 Rehabilitation of Stress Fractures

When patients require a boot, they can still exercise with their heel on the pedal, and run in the deep end of the pool. Gradual introduction of impact stress can be aided by using an anti-gravity treadmill (Fig. 27.27). Physical therapy using strengthening exercises are helpful to decrease atrophy and ensure equal range of motion of both limbs.

27.5.1.1 Preventative Measures and Future Treatment Options

Core strengthening, shock absorptive insoles, improving bone health and caloric intake and Vitamin D supplementation have all been shown to decrease stress fractures [4, 28] Interestingly, more experience and prior training does not appear to be protective in military recruits [23]. Evaluation of best treatment practices for "high-risk" stress fractures (sesamoid, Jones and other proximal metatarsal, and the navicular) are needed [86]. Non-invasive bone stimulators and particularly ESWT show favourable results [50, 51, 54]. Early use of ESWT and subsequent rehabilitation anti-gravity treadmills should be considered in athletes (Fig. 27.28a, b). More prospective studies are needed to determine best practices for stress fractures of the foot in athletes.

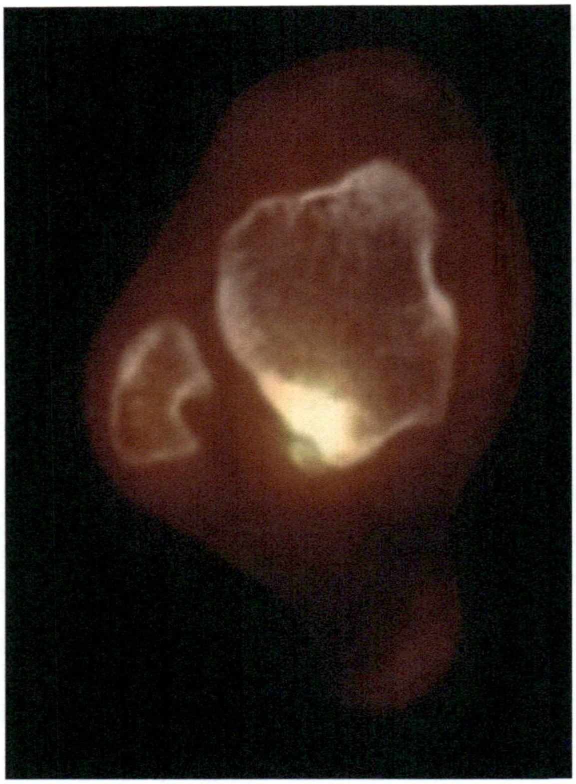

Fig. 27.26 SPECT showing stress fracture of posterior talus

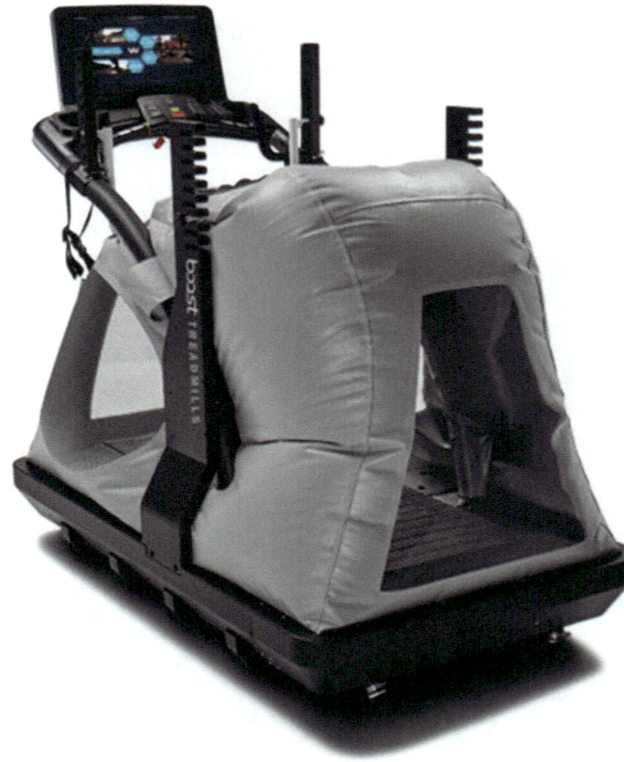

Fig. 27.27 Anti-gravity treadmill

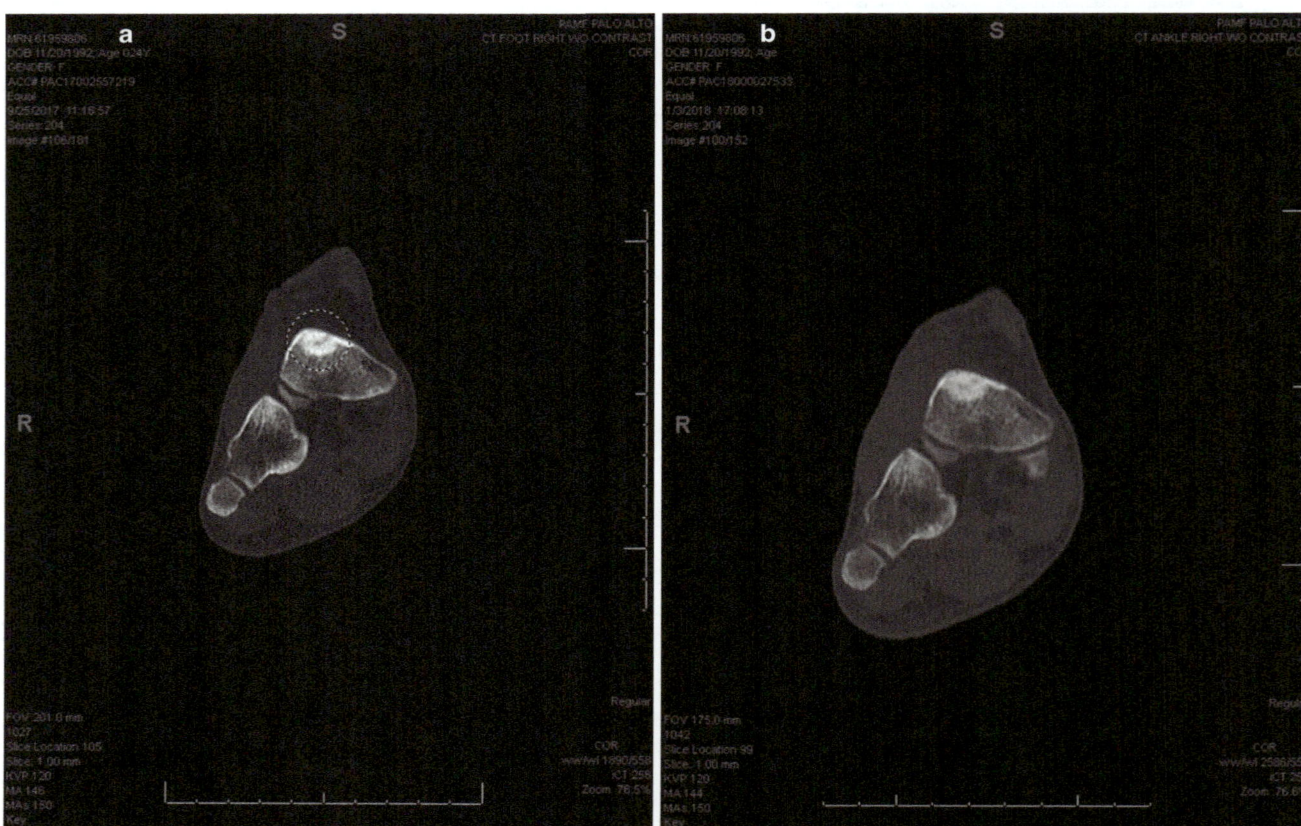

Fig. 27.28 (**a**) Olympian sprinter with Type I navicular stress fracture. (**b**) Same athlete 3 weeks after one treatment with focused ESWT, 6 weeks post-onset of symptoms, showing healed fracture

References

1. Khan M, Madden K, Burrus MT, Rogowski JP, Stotts J, Samani MJ, Sikka R, Bedi A. Epidemiology and impact on performance of lower extremity stress injuries in professional basketball players. Sports Health. 2018;10(2):169–74.
2. Sobrino FJ, Guillén P. Overuse injuries in professional ballet: influence of age and years of professional practice. Orthop J Sports Med. 2017;5(6):2325967117712704. https://doi.org/10.1177/2325967117712704.
3. Sandlin MI, Rosenbaum AJ, Taghavi CE, Charlton TP, O'Malley MJ. High-risk stress fractures in elite athletes. Instr Course Lect. 2017;66:281–92.
4. Miller JR, Dunn KW, Ciliberti LJ Jr, Patel RD, Swanson BA. Association of vitamin D with stress fractures: a retrospective cohort study. J Foot Ankle Surg. 2016;55(1):117–20. https://doi.org/10.1053/j.jfas.2015.08.002. Epub 2015 Sep 26.
5. Welck MJ, Hayes T, Pastides P, Khan W, Rudge B. Stress fractures of the foot and ankle. Injury. 2017;48(8):1722–6.
6. Wright AA, Hegedus EJ, Lenchik L, Kuhn KJ, Santiago L, Smoliga JM. Diagnostic accuracy of various imaging modalities for suspected lower extremity stress fractures. Am J Sports Med. 2016;44(1):255–63.
7. Allen MA, Cassillas MM. The passive axial compression (PAC) test: a new adjunctive provocative maneuver for the clinical diagnosis of hallucal sesamoiditis. Foot Ankle Int. 2001;22(4):345–6.
8. Biedert R, Hinterman B. Stress fractures of the medial great toe sesamoids in athletes. Foot Ankle Int. 2003;24(2):137–41.
9. Rodeo SA, Warren RF, O'Brien SJ, et al. Diastasis of bipartite sesamoids of the first metatarsophalangeal joint. Foot Ankle. 1993;14(8):425–34.
10. Shimozono Y, Hurley ET, Brown AJ, et al. Sesamoidectomy for hallux sesamoid disorders: a systematic review. J Foot Ankle Surg. 2018;57(6):1186–90.
11. Bichara DA, Henn F, Theodore GH. Sesamoidectomy for hallux sesamoid fractures. Foot Ankle Int. 2012;33(9):704–6.
12. Kane JM, Brodsky JW, Daoud Y. Radiographic results and return to activity after sesamoidectomy for fracture. Foot Ankle Int. 2017;38(10):1100–6.
13. Coetzee JC, Stone RM, Fritz JE, et al. Functional outcome of sesamoid excision in athletes. Orthop J Sports Med. 2016;4(Suppl 3)
14. Aper RL, Saltzman CL, Brown TD. The effect of hallux sesamoid resection on the effective moment of the flexor hallucis brevis. Foot Ankle Int. 1994;15(9):462–70.
15. Aper RL, Saltzman CL, Brown TD. The effect of hallux sesamoid excision on the flexor hallucis longus moment arm. Clin Orthop Relat Res. 1996;325:209–17.
16. Bouche RT. Letter to the editor. J Foot Ankle Surg. 1997;36:393–4.
17. Bouche RT, Heit E. Surgical approaches for hallucal sesamoid excision. J Foot Ankle Surg. 2002;41(3):192–6.
18. Ford SE, Adair CR, Cohen BE, Davis WH, Ellington JK, Jones CP, Anderson RB. Efficacy, outcomes, and alignment following isolated fibular sesamoidectomy via a plantar approach. Foot Ankle Int. 2019;40(12):1375–81. https://doi.org/10.1177/1071100719868734.
19. Nayfa TM, Sorto LA. The incidence of hallux abductus following tibial sesamoidectomy. J Am Pod Assoc. 1982;72(12):617–20.
20. Saxena A, Krisdakumtorn T. Return to activity after sesamoidectomy in athletically active individuals. Foot Ankle Int. 2003;24(5):415–9.
21. Dixon S, Nunns M, House C, Rice H, Mostazir M, Stiles V, Davey T, Fallowfield J, Allsopp A. Prospective study of biomechanical risk factors for second and third metatarsal stress fractures in military recruits. J Sci Med Sport. 2019;22(2):135–9.
22. Saxena A, Krisdakumtorn T, Erickson S. Proximal fourth metatarsal injuries in athletes: similarity to proximal fifth metatarsal injury. Foot Ankle Int. 2001;22(7):603–8.
23. Finestone A, Milgrom C, Wolf O, Petrov K, Evans R, Moran D. Epidemiology of metatarsal stress fractures versus tibial and femoral stress fractures during elite training. Foot Ankle Int. 2011;32(1):16–20.
24. Waterman BR, Gun B, Bader JO, Orr JD, Belmont PJ. Epidemiology of lower extremity stress fractures in the United States Military. Mil Med. 2016;181(10):1308–13.
25. Chuckpaiwong B, Cook C, Nunley JA. Stress fractures of the second metatarsal base occur in nondancers. Clin Orthop Relat Res. 2007;461:197–202.
26. Seidenstricker CL, Blahous EG, Bouché RT, Saxena A. Plate fixation with autogenous calcaneal dowel grafting proximal fourth and fifth metatarsal fractures: technique and case series. J Foot Ankle Surg. 2017;56(5):975–81.
27. Hähni M, Hirschmüller A, Baur H. The effect of foot orthoses with forefoot cushioning or metatarsal pad on forefoot peak plantar pressure in running. J Foot Ankle Res. 2016;9:44. eCollection 2016.
28. House C, Reece A, Roiz d SD. Shock-absorbing insoles reduce the incidence of lower limb overuse injuries sustained during Royal Marine training. Mil Med. 2013;178(6):683–9.
29. Jones RI. Fracture of the base of the fifth metatarsal bone by indirect violence. Ann Surg. 1902;35(6):697–700.2.
30. Petrisor BA, Ekrol I, Court-Brown C. The epidemiology of metatarsal fractures. Foot Ankle Int. 2006;27(3):172–4.
31. Raikin SM, Slenker N, Ratigan B. The association of a varus hindfoot and fracture of the fifth metatarsal metaphyseal-diaphyseal junction: the Jones fracture. Am J Sports Med. 2008;36(7):1367–72. https://doi.org/10.1177/0363546508314401.
32. Lawrence SJ, Botte MJ. Jones' fractures and related fractures of the proximal fifth metatarsal. Foot Ankle. 1993;14(6):358–65.
33. Chuckpaiwong B, Queen RM, Easley ME, Nunley JA. Distinguishing Jones and proximal diaphyseal fractures of the fifth metatarsal. Clin Orthop Relat Res. 2008;466(8):1966–70. https://doi.org/10.1007/s11999-008-0222-7.
34. Kavanaugh JH, Brower TD, Mann RV. The Jones fracture revisited. JBJS. 1978;60(6):776–82.
35. Fansa AM, Smyth NA, Murawski CD, Kennedy JG. The lateral dorsal cutaneous branch of the sural nerve: clinical importance of the surgical approach to proximal fifth metatarsal fracture fixation. Am J Sports Med. 2012;40(8):1895–8. https://doi.org/10.1177/0363546512448320.
36. Shereff MJ, Yang QM, Kummer FJ, Frey CC, Greenidge N. Vascular anatomy of the fifth metatarsal. Foot Ankle Int. 1991;11(6):350–3. https://doi.org/10.1177/107110079101100602.
37. Morris PM, Francois AG, Marcus RE, Farrow LD. The effect of peroneus brevis tendon anatomy on the stability of fractures at the fifth metatarsal base. Foot Ankle Int. 2015;36(5):579–84. https://doi.org/10.1177/1071100714565177.
38. Cain LE, Nicholson LL, Adams RD, Burns J. Foot morphology and foot/ankle injury in indoor football. J Sci Med Sport. 2007;10(5):311–9. Epub 2006 Sep 1.
39. Yoho RM, Carrington S, Dix B, Vardaxis V. The association of metatarsus adductus to the proximal fifth metatarsal Jones fracture. J Foot Ankle Surg. 2012;51(6):739–42. https://doi.org/10.1053/j.jfas.2012.08.008.
40. Crandall J. University of Virginia Biomechanics Lab and NFL Foot and Ankle Subcommittee.
41. Roche AJ, Calder JD. Treatment and return to sport following a Jones fracture of the fifth metatarsal: a systematic review. Knee Surg Sports Traumatol Arthrosc. 2013;21(6):1307–15. https://doi.org/10.1007/s00167-012-2138-8.
42. Hunt KJ, Anderson RB. Treatment of Jones fracture nonunions and refractures in elite athlete: outcomes of intramedullary screw fixa-

tion with bone grafting. Am J Sports Med. 2011;39(9):1948–54. https://doi.org/10.1177/0363546511408868.
43. Scott RT, Hyer CF, DeMill SL. Screw fixation diameter for fifth metatarsal jones fracture: a cadaveric study. J Foot Ankle Surg. 2015;54(2):227–9. https://doi.org/10.1053/j.jfas.2014.11.010.
44. Ochenjele G, Ho B, Switaj PJ, Fuchs D, Goyal N, Kadakia AR. Radiographic study of the fifth metatarsal for optimal intramedullary screw fixation of Jones fracture. Foot Ankle Int. 2015;36(3):293–301. https://doi.org/10.1177/1071100714553467.
45. Metzl J, Olson K, Davis WH, Jones C, Cohen B, Anderson R. A clinical and radiographic comparison of two hardware systems used to treat Jones fracture of the fifth metatarsal. Foot Ankle Int. 2013;34(7):956–61. https://doi.org/10.1177/1071100713483100.
46. Hunt KJ, Goeb Y, Esparza R, Malone M, Shultz R, Matheson G. Site-specific loading at the fifth metatarsal base in rehabilitative devices: implications for Jones fracture treatment. PM R. 2014;6(11):1022–9. https://doi.org/10.1016/j.pmrj.2014.05.011.
47. Constantini NW, Arieli R, Chodick G, Dubnov-Raz G. High prevalence of vitamin D insufficiency in athletes and dancers. Clin J Sport Med. 2010;20(5):368–71.
48. Lovell G. Vitamin D status of females in an elite gymnastics program. Clin J Sport Med. 2008;18(2):159–61.
49. Lappe J, Cullen D, Haynatzki G, Recker R, Ahlf R, Thompson K. Calcium and vitamin d supplementation decreases incidence of stress fractures in female navy recruits. J Bone Miner Res. 2008;23(5):741–9. https://doi.org/10.1359/jbmr.080102.
50. Bassett CA, Michell SN, Gaston SR. Pulsed electromagnetic field treatment in ununited fractures and failed arthrodesis. JAMA. 1982;247(5):623–8.
51. Holmes GB Jr. Treatment of delayed unions and nonunions of the proximal fifth metatarsal with pulsed electromagnetic fields. Foot Ankle Int. 1994;15(10):552–6.
52. Streit A, Watson BC, Granata JD, Philbin TM, Lin HN, O'Connor JP, Lin S. Effect on clinical outcome and growth factor synthesis with adjunctive use of pulsed electromagnetic fields for fifth metatarsal nonunion fracture: a double-blind randomized study. Foot Ankle Int. 2016; https://doi.org/10.1177/1071100716652621.
53. Smith TO, Clark A, Hing CB. Interventions for treating proximal fifth metatarsal fractures in adults: a meta-analysis of the current evidence-base. Foot Ankle Surg. 2011;17(4):300–7. https://doi.org/10.1016/j.fas.2010.12.005.
54. Schaden W, Mittermayr R, Haffner N, Smolen D, Gerdesmeyer L, Wang CJ. Extracorporeal shockwave therapy (ESWT)—first choice treatment of fracture non-unions? Int J Surg. 2015;24(Pt B):179–83. https://doi.org/10.1016/j.ijsu.2015.10.003. Epub 2015 Oct 9.
55. Murawski CD, Kennedy JG. Percutaneous internal fixation of proximal fifth metatarsal Jones fractures (zones II and III) with Charlotte Carolina screw and bone marrow aspirate concentrate: an outcome study in athletes. Am J Sports Med. 2011;39(6):1295–301. https://doi.org/10.1177/0363546510393306.
56. Horst F, Gilbert BJ, Glisson RR, Nunley JA. Torque resistance after fixation of Jones fractures with intramedullary screws. Foot Ankle Int. 2004;25(12):914–9. https://doi.org/10.1177/107110070402501212.
57. Sides SD, Fetter NL, Glisson R, Nunley JA. Bending stiffness and pull-out strength of tapered, variable pitch screws, and 6.5-mm cancellous screws in acute Jones fractures. Foot Ankle Int. 2006;27(10):821–5.
58. Nagao M, Saita Y, Kameda S, Seto H, Sadatsuki R, Takazawa Y, Yoshimura M, Aoba Y, Ikeda H, Kaneko K, Nozawa M, Kim SG. Headless compression screw fixation of jones fractures: an outcome study in Japanese athletes. Am J Sports Med. 2012;40(11):2578–82. https://doi.org/10.1177/0363546512459460.
59. OMalley M, DeSandis B, Allen A, Levitshy M, OMalley Q, Williams R. Operative treatment of fifth metatarsal Jones fractures (zones II and III) in the NBA. Foot Ankle Int. 2016;37(5):488–500. https://doi.org/10.1177/1071100715625290.
60. Huh J, Glisson RR, Matsumoto T, Easley ME. Biomechanical comparison of intramedullary screw versus low-profile plate fixation of a Jones fracture. Foot Ankle Int. 2016;37(4):411–8. https://doi.org/10.1177/1071100715619678.
61. Bernstein DT, Mitchell RJ, McCulloch PC, Harris JD, Varner KE. Treatment of proximal fifth metatarsal fractures and refractures with plantar plating in elite athletes. Foot Ankle Int. 2018;39(12):1410–5. https://doi.org/10.1177/1071100718791835.
62. Bigsby E, Halliday R, Middleton RG, Case R, Harries W. Functional outcome of fifth metatarsal fractures. Injury. 2014;45(12):2009–12. https://doi.org/10.1016/j.injury.2014.06.010.
63. Begly JP, Guss M, Ramme AJ, Karia R, Meislin RJ. Return to play and performance after Jones fracture in the National Basketball Association Athletes. Sports Health. 2016;8(4):342–6. https://doi.org/10.1177/1941738115621011.
64. Lareau CR, Hsu AR, Anderson RB. Return to play in National Football League players after operative Jones fracture treatment. Foot Ankle Int. 2016;37(1):8–16. https://doi.org/10.1177/1071100715603983.
65. Duplantier NL, Mitchell RJ, Zambrano S, Stone AC, Delgado DA, Lambert BS, Moreno MR, Harris JD, McCulloch PC, Lintner DM, Varner KE. Comparison of fifth metatarsal Jones fracture fixation methods. Am J Sports Med. 2018;46(5):1220–7. https://doi.org/10.1177/0363546517753376.
66. Quill GE. Fractures of the proximal fifth metatarsal. Orthop Clin North Am. 1995;26:353–61.
67. Jastifer J, Kent R, Crandall J, Sherwood C, Lessley D, McCullough K, Coughlin M, Anderson R. The athletic shoe in football: apparel or protective equipment? Sports Health. 2017;9(2):126–31. https://doi.org/10.1177/1941738117690717.
68. Towne LC, Blazina ME, Cozen LN. Fatigue fracture of the tarsal navicular. J Bone Joint Surg Am. 1970;52(2):376–8.
69. Brukner P, Bradshaw C, Khan KM, et al. Stress fractures: a review of 180 cases. Clin J Sport Med. 1996;6(2):85–9.
70. Saxena A, Fullem B, Hannaford D. Results of treatment of 22 navicular stress fractures and a new proposed radiographic classification system. J Foot Ankle Surg. 2000;39(2):96–103.
71. Saxena A, Behan SA, Valerio DL, Frosch DL. Navicular stress fracture outcomes in athletes: analysis of 62 injuries. J Foot Ankle Surg. 2017;56(5):943–8.
72. Khan KM, Fuller PJ, Brukner PD, Kearney C, Burry HC. Outcome of conservative and surgical management of navicular stress fracture in athletes. Am J Sports Med. 1992;20(6):657–66.
73. Fitch K, Blackwell J, Gilmour W. Operation for non-union of stress fracture of the tarsal navicular. J Bone Joint Surg Br. 1989;71-B(1):105–10.
74. Torg JS, Moyer J, Gaughan JP, Boden BP. Management of tarsal navicular stress fractures. Am J Sports Med. 2010;38(5):1048–53.
75. Saxena A, Fullem B. Navicular stress fractures: a prospective study on athletes. Foot Ankle Int. 2006;27:917–21.
76. Orr JD, Glisson RR, Nunley JA. Jones fracture fixation: a biomechanical comparison of partially threaded screws versus tapered variable pitch screws. Am J Sports Med. 2012;40(3):691–8. https://doi.org/10.1177/0363546511428870.
77. Saxena A, Fullem BW. A unique procedure for treatment of osteochondral lesions of the tarsal navicular: three cases in athletes. J Foot Ankle Surg. 2013;52(2):249–53.
78. Pegrum J, Dixit V, Padhiar N, Nugent I. The pathophysiology, diagnosis, and management of foot stress fractures. Phys Sportsmed. 2014;42(4):87–99.

79. Voormolen N, Cancete AN, Reijnierse M. Calcaneal stress fractures revisited. JBR-BTR. 2012;95(2):114–7.
80. Mandell JC, Khurana B, Smith SE. Stress fractures of the foot and ankle: Part 2. Site-specific etiology, imaging, and treatment, and differential diagnosis. Skelet Radiol. 2017;46:1165–18.
81. Bianchi S, Luong DH. Stress fractures of the calcaneus diagnosed by sonography. J Ultrasound Med. 2018;37:521–9.
82. Kubo M, Yasui Y, Miki S, Kawano H, Miyamoto W. Stress fractures of the posterior talus in a female long-distance runner treated by osteosynthesis with screw fixation via a two-portal hindfoot arthoscopy: a case report. BMC Musc. 2019;20:401–5.
83. Rossi F, Dragoni S. Talar body fatigue stress fractures: three cases observed in elite female gymnasts. Skelet Radiol. 2005;34(7):389–94. Epub 2005 May 12.
84. Munemoto M, Sugimoto K, Takakura Y. Stress fractures of the proximal phalanx of the great toe: a report of four cases. Foot Ankle Int. 2009;30(5):461–4. https://doi.org/10.3113/FAI.2009.0461.
85. Csonka A, Sikarinkul E, Gargyan I, Boa K, Varga E. Operative management of bilateral Salter-Harris type III fractures of the proximal phalanges of the great toes of a 10-year-old female ballet dancer: a case report. J Pediatr Orthop B. 2016;25(4):393–6. https://doi.org/10.1097/BPB.0000000000000284.
86. Kaiser P, Guss D, Digiovanni C. Stress fractures of the foot and ankle in the athlete. Foot Ankle Orthop. 2018;3(3). https://doi.org/10.1177/2473011418790078.

Part VII

Stress Fractures in Sport: Spine and Pelvis

Stress Fractures in Sport: Spine

28

Arash J. Sayari, James D. Baker, and Gregory D. Lopez

Learning Objectives

- Understand the mechanisms that lead to stress fractures in both the lumbar and cervical/thoracic spine.
- Recognize the clinical presentation of lumbar and cervical/thoracic stress fractures.
- Describe the various imaging modalities used to diagnose stress fractures of the spine.
- Develop a therapeutic and rehabilitation plan to treat spinal stress fractures.

28.1 Introduction

The spine is a mobile segment of the axial skeleton subjected to high weight bearing loads and motion-induced mechanical stresses. When these stressors compound over time, mechanical failure can lead to stress fractures, termed spondylolysis, or bony defects involving the pars interarticularis (pars). Functionally, the pars acts as the bony bridge, or isthmus, connecting the superior and inferior articulating facets of the vertebra. Historically, spondylolysis has been classified into five distinct types (Table 28.1) based on the etiology of the fracture: dysplastic (I), isthmic (II), degenerative (III), traumatic (IV), and pathologic (V) [1]. Stress fractures of the spine are classified as isthmic type II spondylolysis. Isthmic spondylolysis can be either unilateral or bilateral, and may begin initially as increased stress to the pars interarticularis. However, repeated mechanical insults to the pars can eventually progress to bony stress fracture. In extreme cases, spondylolisthesis one vertebrae relative to another can occur.

While fractures can occur anywhere along the spinal column, stress fractures are most common in the lumbar spine, particularly at L5 [2]. Uncommonly, avulsion-type stress fractures can also occur in the cervical and upper thoracic spine [3–5]. Regardless of location, repetitive mechanical stress appears to be a major factor in the development of spondylolysis. As such, young athletes are particularly at risk for developing spondylolysis. In fact, over 70% of cases of back pain in the young athlete occur due to spondylolysis [6]. Back pain usually is the presenting complaint [7], and may accompany a history of repetitive twisting, axial loading, and repeated back extension.

Prompt diagnosis and appropriate management of spondylolysis in the athlete is critical. Often, young athletes will attempt to self-treat injuries with extended periods of rest, and this can lead to delays in diagnosis [8]. A solid understanding of diagnostic factors, as well as treatment modalities, is essential for the clinician to accurately manage spondylolysis. The purpose of this chapter is to provide a concise discussion of the epidemiology, presentation, diagnostic workup, treatment, associated complications, and prevention strategies of stress fractures in the athlete. This chapter will include a discussion of the more common lumbar stress fractures, as well as less common stress fractures in the cervical and thoracic spine.

Table 28.1 Types of spondylolysis

Type	Classification	Pathophysiology
Type I	Dysplastic	Congenital
Type II[a]	Isthmic	Fracture of the pars interarticularis
Type III	Degenerative	Intervertebral disc degeneration causing instability
Type IV	Traumatic	Acute fracture, not involving pars
Type V	Pathological	Infection or tumor

[a]Type II subclassified into fatigue fracture (Type II-A), pars elongation due to healed stress fracture (Type II-B), and acute fracture (Type II-C)

A. J. Sayari (✉) · J. D. Baker · G. D. Lopez
Department of Orthopaedic Surgery, Rush University Medical Center, Chicago, IL, USA
e-mail: gregory.lopez@rushortho.com

G. A. J. Robertson, N. Maffulli (eds.), *Fractures in Sport*, https://doi.org/10.1007/978-3-030-72036-0_28

28.2 Lumbar Stress Fractures

28.2.1 Epidemiology

Epidemiological studies of spondylolysis in the lumbar spine are widely available, and have sought to establish a mechanism for the development of spondylosis. However, the exact cause is still up for debate. Several studies have found that the prevalence of spondylolysis is higher in males compared to women, and most studies have found a 2:1 male to female ratio [2, 9–12]. The reason men tend to have a higher prevalence of spondylolysis is unknown. Other studies have focused on the relationship between repetitive mechanical stress on the pars, and this appears to be the most widely accepted hypothesis. As humans have developed the ability to walk on two legs, the axial skeleton, and the lumbar spine in particular, have evolved to support increased loads. Therefore, spondylolysis may be an acquired condition as a result of bipedal ambulation. In fact, studies of both non-ambulatory patients and infants have demonstrated no incidence of pars defects or spondylolysis [13, 14].

The overall prevalence of lumbar spondylolysis appears to be 3–6% and is associated with increasing age [12, 15, 16]. In a 45-year longitudinal study, Beutler et al. examined a population of 500 six-year-old children and found the prevalence of spondylolysis to be 4.4% [12]. Over time, the prevalence increased to 6%. However, at 45-year follow-up, three unilateral defects resolved spontaneously, and the progression of bilateral defects tended to slow with time. A study by Sonne-Holm et al. followed 4001 subjects with lumbar spondylolysis, and similarly found an increase in prevalence of spondylolysis associated with advancing age [15]. However, another study found no significant increase in prevalence of spondylolysis in patients over 20 years old [17].

The risk of lumbar spondylolysis is much higher in athletes relative to the general population. Several studies have estimated the incidence of spondylolysis in athletes to be between 47–70% [18–20]. Young patients with underdeveloped spinal muscles, or dysplastic or hypoplastic facet joints, may not be equipped to handle motion-related shearing forces that occur in the lumbar spine [21]. Repetitive loading seen in athletes may further increase these shearing forces, resulting in fatigue and fracture of the pars. Repeated extension of the lumbar spine seen in certain dynamic sports also results in cyclic collision between the articular facet of the superior vertebrae with the facet of the inferior vertebrae, which can further increase the stress on the pars [22].

In addition, the type of sporting activity seems to play a role in the development of lumbar spondylolysis. In certain sports, the incidence of spondylolysis can be as high as 63% [23]. In an analysis of 590 elite athletes with evidence of spondylolysis, Rossi and Dragoni demonstrated that the implicated sports diving (40.35%), wrestling (25%), and weightlifting (22.32%) [19]. In their study of 3152 Spanish athletes, Soler and Calderon also found differences in rates of stress fracture across sports, implicating dynamic throwing, gymnastics, and rowing [24]. Other sports that have been found to be associated with spondylolysis include American football [25], rugby [26], swimming [27], and several others [19, 24].

28.2.2 Classification

Ninety-five percent of cases of lumbar spondylolysis occur at L5, and the incidence decreases at each subsequent cephalad level [28]. The lower lumbar levels, L5 in particular, bear the most dynamic and static stress associated with daily activities. Athletes place even more stress across their lower spine as a result of their sport's physical demands. For example, contact sports such as rugby and American football can place forces up to 8670 N across the lumbar spine [26]. Compressive forces combined with rotation or extension of the spine can also place particularly high levels of stress on the lower spine [29], and these movements are common in sports such as gymnastics, swimming, and diving. Other factors that increase the risk of spondylolysis at L5 include increased anterior tilt angle of the L5-S1 endplates and lumbar lordosis [30, 31]. These risk factors also result in poorer response to conservative treatment options [30, 31].

Spondylolysis can occur unilaterally or bilaterally. Often a unilateral stress fracture may progress to become bilateral, as the contralateral pars interarticularis can see 12.6-fold increases in stress following unilateral spondylolysis [32]. Unilateral stress fractures in athletes may be related to muscular asymmetry and differences in mechanical loading associated with throwing sports. Generally, unilateral spondylolysis is clinically benign, and more likely to respond to conservative treatment, whereas bilateral defects are less likely to achieve bony-union with conservative treatment and are associated with a higher risk of developing spondylolisthesis [12, 30, 33]. When an athlete initially presents with a unilateral spondylolysis but continues to experience persistent or worsening back pain, a bilateral spondylolysis should be suspected [32].

The severity of spondylolysis can be approximated using computerized tomography (CT). In 1995, Morita et al. proposed grading system based on CT findings, and divided spondylolysis in three categories: early, progressive, and terminal [33]. Early defects were characterized as minimal or hair-line fractures of the pars, progressive defects were grossly fractured, and terminal lesions were defined by sclerosis and pseudarthrosis. The grading of severity of the lesions is important, as clinical outcomes and expectations following treatment differ between the various classifications [30, 34].

28.2.3 Diagnosis

28.2.3.1 History and Physical Exam

Often, the presence of spondylolysis is an incidental finding in a young athlete. Findings of spondylolysis may have been picked up by imaging of the pelvis/abdomen. The athlete may present with no mechanical or neurological deficits, and not describe any traumatic event. They may endorse a history of paraspinal muscular fatigue and occasional back pain associated with overtraining. In such patients, a thorough work-up should be performed to rule out underlying spinal pathology.

When athletes with spondylolysis present, the most common complaint is low back pain [35]. The low back pain is localized to the midline, may involve the paramidline area where the facet joints are located, and may radiate to the buttock and upper thigh [35]. The pain is classically exacerbated by repetitive flexion and extension activities, and typically improves with rest. Radiculopathy, neurological symptoms, bladder dysfunction, and night pains are not typical, and may suggest another pathology.

Most patients will demonstrate a normal physical examination. Even in symptomatic patients, posture, gait, and strength is often normal. Patients can demonstrate hamstring or hip flexor tightness, both placing increased strain across the lower lumbar spine [36]. Direct inspection of the spine should be performed to look for signs of deformity, or hairy patches that suggest an underlying neurological condition such as spina bifida. Palpation of the lumbar spine, the paraspinal muscles, and sacroiliac joint should be performed, and may induce tenderness. Asking patients to "toe-walk" and "heel-walk" assesses gait, dorsiflexion and plantarflexion strength, and global balance. Neurological examination, as well as reflex testing, should be normal and not demonstrate any neurosensory deficits in myotomes or dermatomes. Special testing includes Adam's forward bend test to expose any underlying deformity, and the straight leg test to rule out radicular pain. The Stork test, or the one-legged hyperextension test, (Fig. 28.1) has been traditionally viewed as a pathognomonic diagnostic test for spondylolysis [37, 38]. The tests begins with the patient hyperextending one leg while flexing the contralateral leg at the hip and knee. The test is positive if the pain is reproduced in the extended leg. However, some researchers have questioned the diagnostic utility of this test. Masci et al. conducted a study to assess whether a positive hyperextension test was predictive of spondylolysis, and found that a positive test did not correlate with evidence of spondylolysis on single-photon emission computerized tomography or magnetic-resonance imaging, highlighting the insufficiency of physical examination alone in diagnosing spondylolysis [39].

28.2.3.2 Imaging Studies

Despite advancements in imaging modalities, plain radiography is the recommended first-line imaging method to evaluate symptomatic low back pain in young athletes. While anteroposterior (AP) and lateral views of the lumbar spine can be useful when evaluating adults, they may be insufficient in evaluating spondylolysis in the adolescent athlete [40, 41]. In cases of suspected spondylolysis, an oblique view, taken at roughly 45° from midline, provides the best view of the pars, highlighting the classic "Scotty-dog" appearance. Recently, however, the utility of oblique views has been challenged. Beck et al. compared the use of all three views (AP, lateral, and oblique) to only AP/lateral, and found no significant difference between the two approaches [41]. Furthermore, increased risks of additional radiation exposure may also negate the benefits of additional radiographic views, triggering the clinician to utilize alternative modalities in delineating spondylolysis.

Bone scintigraphy, or single-photon emission computerized tomography (SPECT), is a nuclear imaging test that identifies metabolic activity within the bone. SPECT is useful in distinguishing symptomatic pars defects with high metabolic activity from asymptomatic or chronic defects with less metabolic activity. Additionally, SPECT may be able to identify spondylolysis earlier than other imaging modalities such as CT or magnetic resonance imaging (MRI) [42]. However, this test lacks specificity, and additional imaging studies are needed to confirm, characterize, and distinguish spondylolysis from other spinal pathologies [43]. Limited resolution and added radiation exposure has called into question the utility of this imaging modality in spondylolysis and allowed for implementation of alternatives (Fig. 28.2).

CT similarly introduces ionizing radiation, and therefore CT (cut in 1 mm slices) is typically limited to the vertebral levels of interest, and offers excellent visualization of bony anatomy [44]. While useful for evaluating the extent and classification of spondylolysis, CT lacks the sensitivity of SPECT, and 20% of pars defects visualized with SPECT will not show up on CT [42]. Comparing CT to radiography, Fadell et al. demonstrated that CT outperformed 2-, 3-, and 4-view plain radiographs while maintaining a relatively low dose of radiation to the patient [45]. In their study, intergrader agreement was significantly higher in the CT group. These results suggest that CT may be the imaging modality of choice when evaluating an athlete with a high degree of suspicion for spondylolysis.

The applications of MRI have seen the greatest change in recent years. Specific to the adolescent athlete, MRI lends no ionizing radiation while allowing for evaluation of neurological and soft tissue structures, and can detect pars lesions earlier than CT [46]. Several studies have demonstrated the

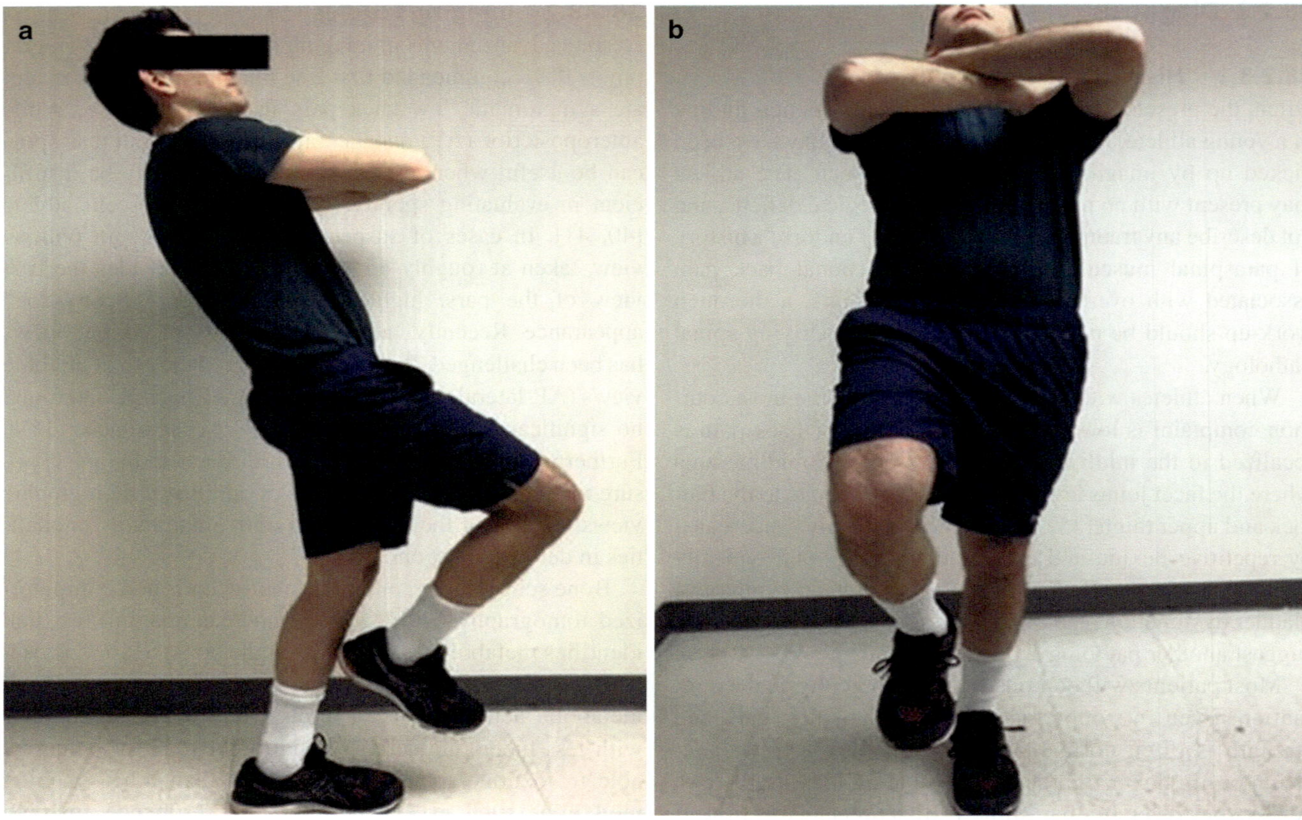

Fig. 28.1 Demonstration of the one-legged hyperextension test, or Stork test, as viewed from the side (**a**) and front (**b**). The patient is instructed to stand on one leg with the opposite leg flexed at the hip and the knee. Next the patient is asked to extend at the low back. The test is positive if the movement elicits pain on the weight-bearing side

utility of MRI in diagnosing spondylolysis [47, 48]. A recent systematic review by Tofte et al. assessed the utility of various imaging modalities in diagnosing spondylolysis, and the authors concluded that a majority of studies recommended using MRI as an early or first-line diagnostic tool [47]. Dhouib et al. performed a meta analysis to determine the sensitivity and specificity of MRI in diagnosing pars lesions [48]. They found MRI was able to identify 81% of pars lesions with 99% specificity. Furthermore, newer MRI protocols and techniques are being developed to expand its utility in the context of spondylolysis. In their cadaveric study, Finkenstaedt et al., developed an ultrashort time-to-echo MR protocol to identify simulated pars defects, and found this new protocol to be superior to traditional MR protocols at 3 T [49]. While still in its nascience, MRI will likely continue to be refined and developed in the future for use in diagnosing spondylolysis.

Given the breadth of imaging modalities available for diagnosis lumbar stress fractures, diagnostic algorithms have been proposed to streamline their use. Tofte et al. proposed one such system [47]. Briefly, in athletes with low back pain without neurological signs, 2-view plain radiography may be the first test ordered due to its cost effectiveness and low exposures to radiation relative to other options. If these results are inconclusive, decisions about follow-up imaging can be made based on the chronicity of the lesion. Acute lesions likely are better evaluated with MRI, as MRI may highlight bony edema and identify lesions earlier than CT. Additionally, MRI should be performed in athletes presenting with concurrent neurological signs or symptoms. Chronic lesions and those unresponsive to treatment benefit from CT evaluation of non-unions. The authors recommended against the routine use of SPECT, unless the use of CT or MRI is contraindicated.

28.2.4 Treatment

Treatment modalities in the adolescent athlete should be carefully considered based on clinical presentation, as outcomes following treatment will vary depending on the presenting features. Additional considerations include the patient's activity level, short and long term athletic goals, and preference for treatment. Many cases of spondylolysis will respond to conservative treatment. However, due to the variety of treatment options and relative lack of high-level

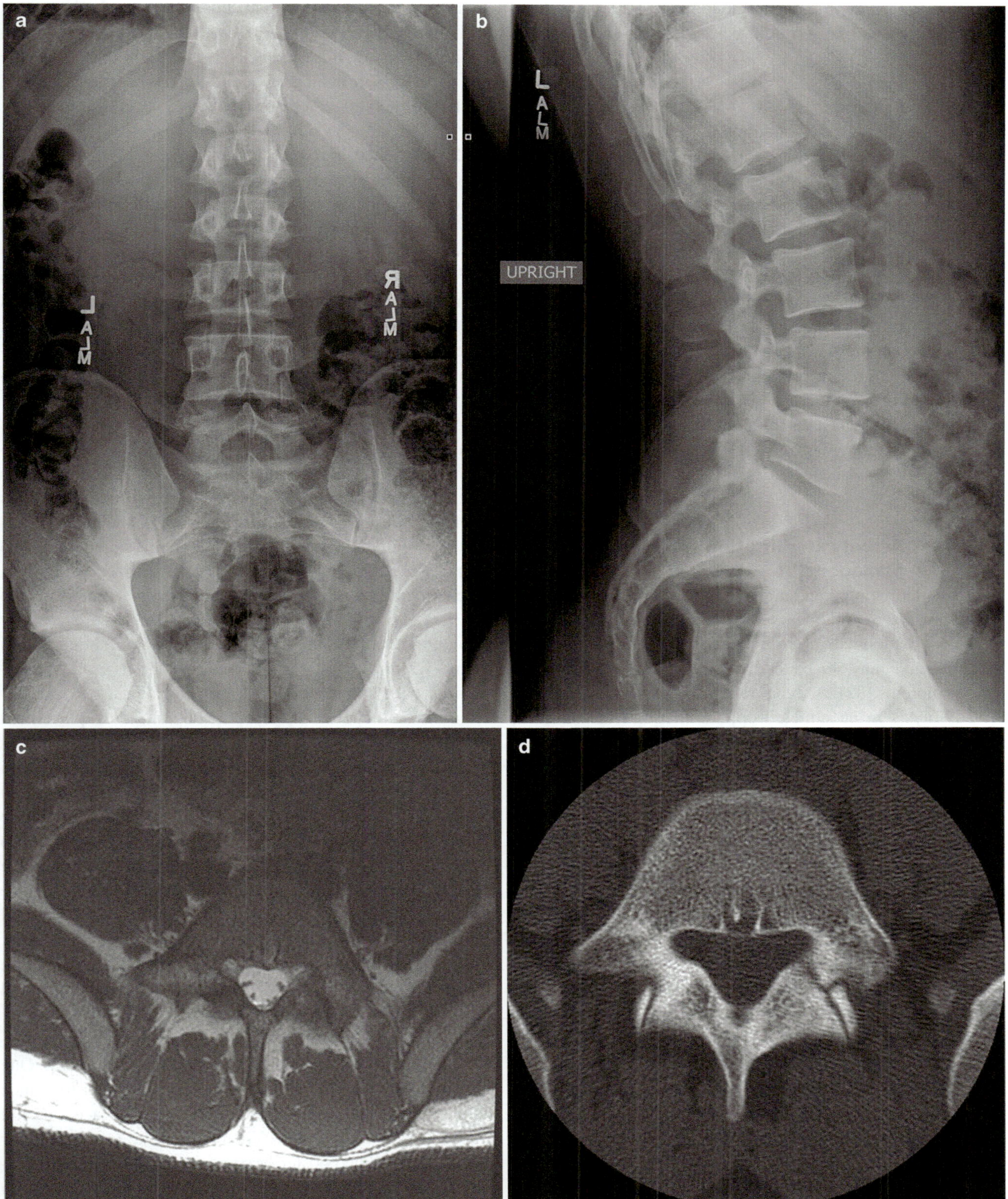

Fig. 28.2 (**a**) AP and (**b**) lateral radiographs of a 21-year-old elite-level baseball player with 1-month onset of back pain after batting. (**c**) Axial T2-weighted MRI and (**d**) axial CT further demonstrated an acute, left-sided unilateral L5 spondylolysis. He was successfully treated with rest and physical therapy

evidence regarding treatment guidelines in the literature, therapeutic plans likely should be defined on an individual basis.

28.2.4.1 Bracing

Overall, the literature surrounding lumbar orthosis devices is mixed [50, 51]. Some believe the use of a lumbosacral brace provides adequate stabilization of the low back and limits the motion of the pars. However, in a meta analysis, Klein et al. found that the use of lumbosacral braces did not significantly alter clinical outcomes compared to other treatment strategies [51]. Interestingly, the authors also noted that many lesions did not achieve bony arthrosis, despite satisfactory clinical outcomes, suggesting that bony fusion is not critical for a good outcome. The use of bracing as a treatment option can likely be left up to the patient and physician and demonstrates more utility in cases of acute stress reactions. While there is little evidence for clinical benefits associated with bracing, this strategy lends itself useful in cases of noncompliant athletes or those under pressure to return to play rapidly.

28.2.4.2 Activity Modification and Pain Management

Activity modification and management of symptomatic pain is a mainstay of treatment for spondylolysis, and patients who take 3 months off from their sport allow for healing potential and may do better than those who play through their symptoms [52]. A recent review by Panteliadis et al. on spondylolysis in an athlete population found that athletes who stopped sport returned to play at an average of 3.7 months, while those that were treated surgically required 8 months to return to play [6]. Currently, no clear guidelines for return to play exist, and patients should initially be treated conservatively with rest for around 3–4 months. Close monitoring should be implemented for evidence of deterioration, which may prompt more aggressive care. Once pain is adequately controlled, patients may begin to be reintroduced to their sport with conditioning protocols and incremental increases in activity to limit reinjury [43].

Techniques such as low-intensity pulsed ultrasound (LIPUS) have emerged to expand the realm of conservative treatment. A study by Arima et al. compared the use of LIPUS to conservative and bracing management strategies to treat progressive-grade spondylolysis, finding that the LIPUS cohort achieved bony union at significantly higher rates than the conventionally treated group [53]. In addition to promoting bony fusion, LIPUS may also enhance patient response to conservative treatments. Tsukada et al. performed a case-control study of 82 athletes with spondylolysis, and assessed the differences in conservative treatment with and without LIPUS [54]. They found that the 35 athletes treated with combined LIPUS and conservative treatment returned to sport significantly faster than those that were only treated with conservative measures (61 vs. 167 days, respectively). While promising, more evidence is necessary to evaluate the use of LIPUS in managing spondylolysis, particularly as it applies to specific athletic populations.

28.2.4.3 Surgical Management

Surgical management is considered in the subpopulation of patients in whom conservative management fails or spondylolysis deteriorates into a terminal-grade lesion, or when patients develop worsening pain symptoms or neurological compromise. Overall, 9–15% of symptomatic patients with spondylolysis will require surgery [55]. While some studies suggest that return to play is accelerated with surgery [56], others suggest that surgery may prolong return to play, highlighting the relevance of attempting 6–12 months of conservative management before surgery is considered [6].

A direct repair of pars defects is indicated in various clinical settings, including L1–L4 isolated cases of spondylolysis without disc involvement, cases of multiple stress fractures, and low-grade spondylolisthesis. In athletes, this approach preserves the motion segment of the spine, offering a more optimal clinical outcome in this population. The Buck procedure, developed in 1970, utilizes a 3.5 mm screw to apply a perpendicular compressive force across to the fracture [57]. This technique has been updated over time, and recent techniques have shown good bony fusion using 4.5 mm screws and cancellous bone graft supplemented with defect decortication [58] (Fig. 28.3). In athletes with osteopenia or dysplastic lamina, screw placement may be contraindicated, necessitating other options such as the Scott's technique, which involves placing two 2 mm holes in the bilateral transverse processes [59]. A 4 mm hole is then drilled into the spinous process and a 20-G wire is pulled through these holes in a figure-of-eight fashion to generate compression. More recently, minimally-invasive direct repair techniques have been proposed that have shown process to promote healing while sparing spinal musculature and preserving the native facet joint [60]. Other techniques have also been proposed, although the use of additional hardware may become symptomatic and require follow-up removal [61].

In more complex cases, such as those involving >30% slippage, stabilization techniques are preferred [62]. One area of controversy during stabilization is whether to reduce spondylolisthesis, as this could increase the surface area and improve fusion outcomes. When comparing *in situ* anterior fusion to combined posterior stabilization with anterior lumbar fusion, a study of 59 adolescent patients found that when posterior stabilization was coupled with anterior fusion, betters rates of fusion and shorter times to fusion were achieved [62]. Utilization of posterior instrumentation is therefore useful in cases of increased spondylolisthesis and minimizes

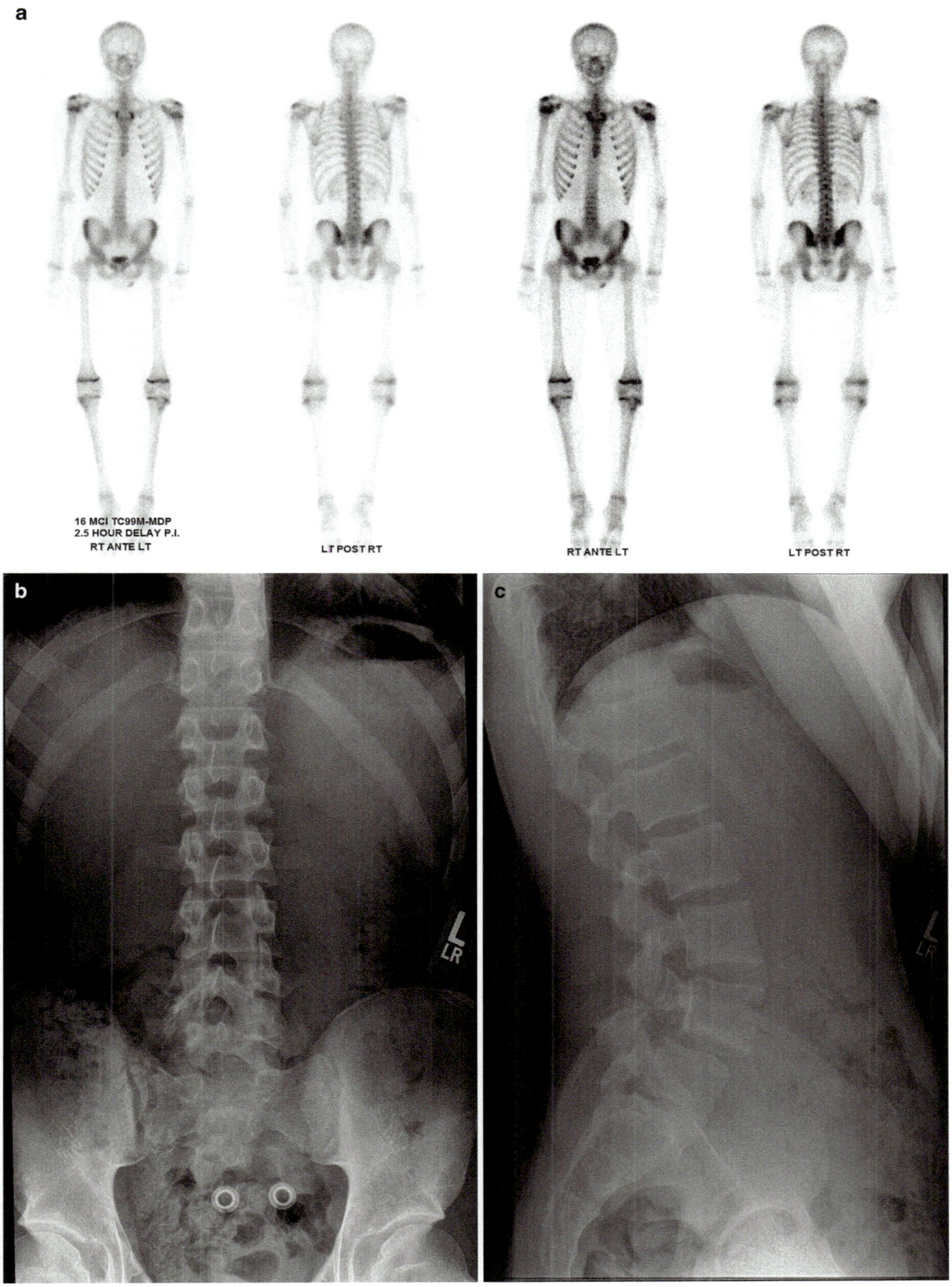

Fig. 28.3 (**a**) SPECT scan in an 18-year-old baseball player with 9 months of low back pain that failed rest, which suggested increased uptake in the lower lumbar spine. Follow-up (**b**) AP and (**c**) lateral radiographs demonstrated L4 spondylolysis, and L4–L5 grade I isthmic spondylolisthesis. Preoperative (**d**) Axial and (**e**) sagittal CT, and (**f**) axial T2-weighted MRI cuts demonstrated subacute bilateral pars defects without evidence of healing. Fibular strut and cancellous allografts were placed in bilateral pars defects followed by 4.0 × 40 mm partially threaded cannulated screws to compress across the fracture seen on postoperative (**g**) AP and (**h**) lateral radiographs

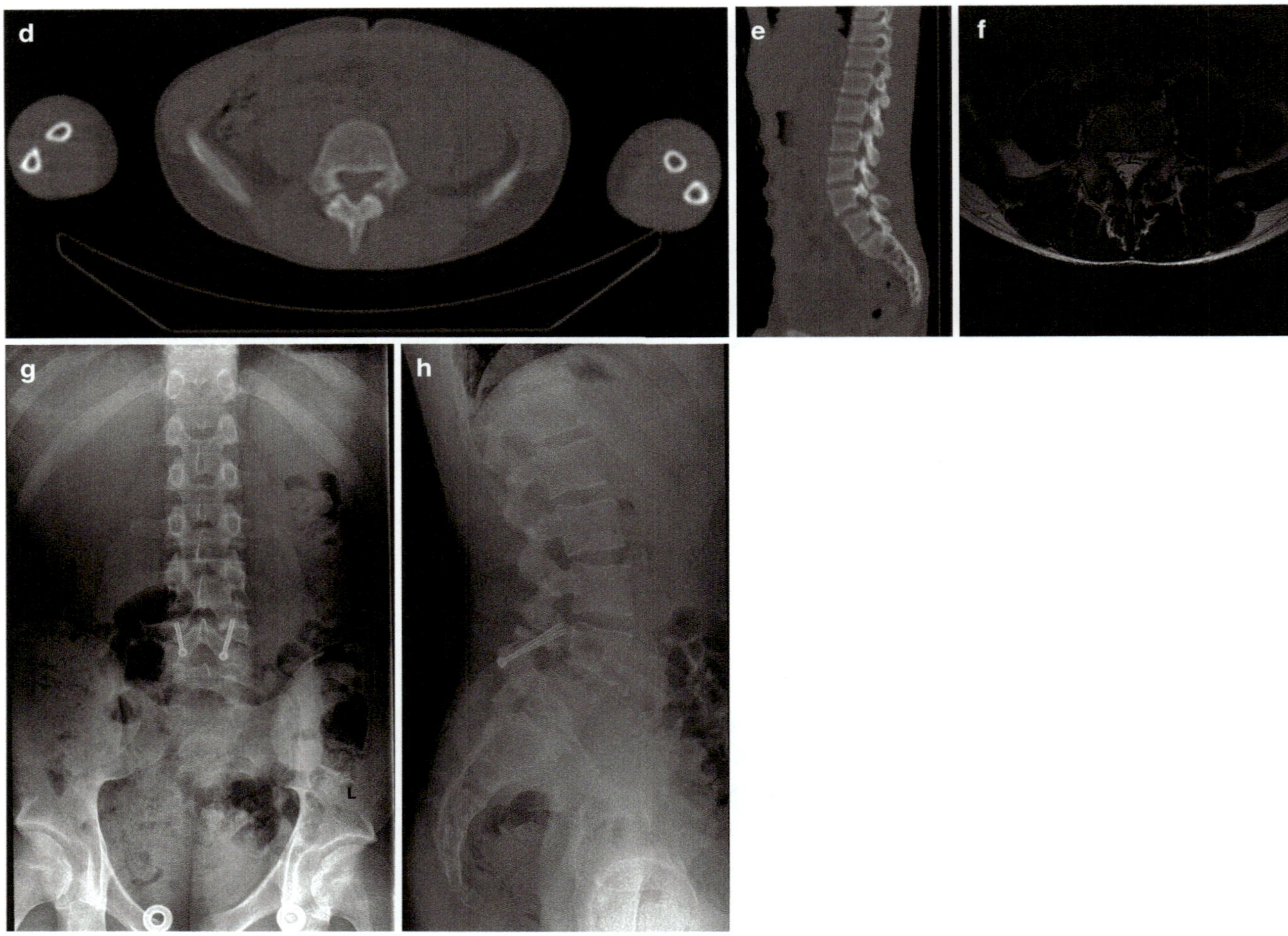

Fig. 28.3 (continued)

the risk of pseudarthrosis. However, in cases of high-grade spondylolisthesis, wedged vertebral bodies may be difficult to reduce and increase the risk of complications. Furthermore, attempts at reduction involve increased surgical exposures, blood loss, operative times, and risk of nerve stretch injury, leaving vertebral reduction as a topic of continued debate. The use of interbody devices may also increase the surface area during fusion, and may also be useful when reduction is challenging or not possible, as in cases where vertebral bodies are oriented more vertically and cannot be reached from an anterior approach (Fig. 28.4). Other technique options include placement of fibular dowels with a Bohlman technique through the sacrum and into the L5 vertebral body. This technique, though less utilized, has been shown to have a high success rate [63]. On the other hand, Gill-type laminectomies, foraminotomies, and isolated anterior approaches can be implemented in adult athletes, necessitating instrumentation to balance these destabilizing procedures (Fig. 28.5).

28.2.5 Complications

Though positive outcomes following management of spondylolysis can be expected, pseudarthrosis is the most common complication following surgical management. As decreases in contact surface area will likely increase the risk of non-union, pseudarthrosis is more likely following *in situ* fusions lacking partial reduction. However, this must be weighed against the risk of iatrogenic neurologic injury. Patients who develop pseudarthrosis must be monitored for progressive listhesis, deformity, neurologic compromise, or persistent back pain, which may necessitate revision. In such cases, circumferential instrumentation with or without decompression should be considered [64].

While rare, the risk for neurological injury is increased after attempted reduction of high-grade spondylolisthesis. Clinicians should monitor the patient for postoperative development of bladder, bowel, sexual dysfunction, or the development of an L5 radiculopathy. The rates of radicu-

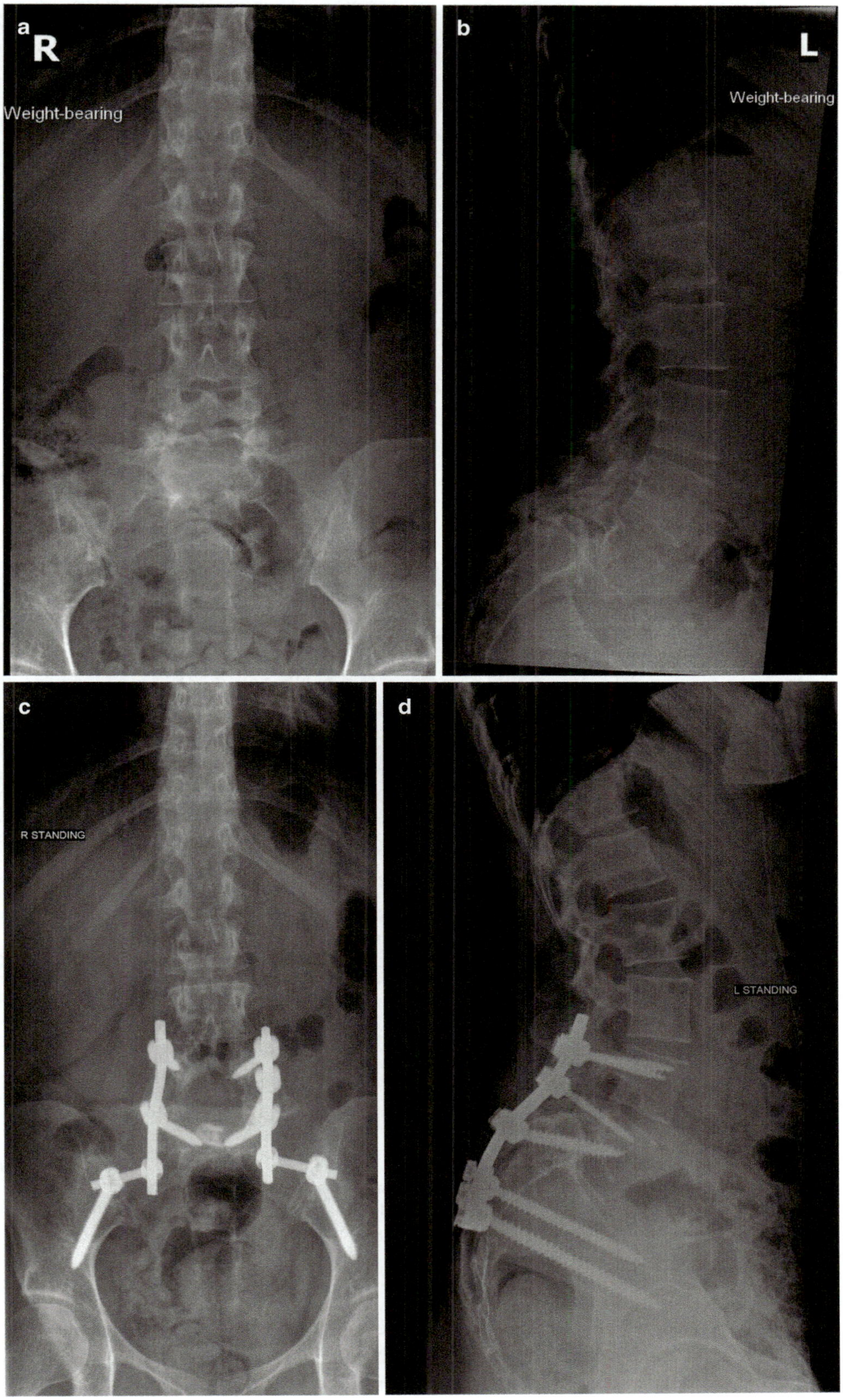

Fig. 28.4 (**a**) AP and (**b**) lateral radiographs of a 16-year-old elite gymnast, demonstrating bilateral L5 spondylolysis and Grade III spondylolisthesis. She was treated with an *in situ* L4-S1 decompression, sacral dome osteotomy, L5-S1 transforaminal lumbar interbody fusion, and posterior instrumentation L4-S1 utilizing both allograft and autograft as seen on postoperative (**c**) AP and (**d**) lateral radiographs. The patient healed uneventfully without complications

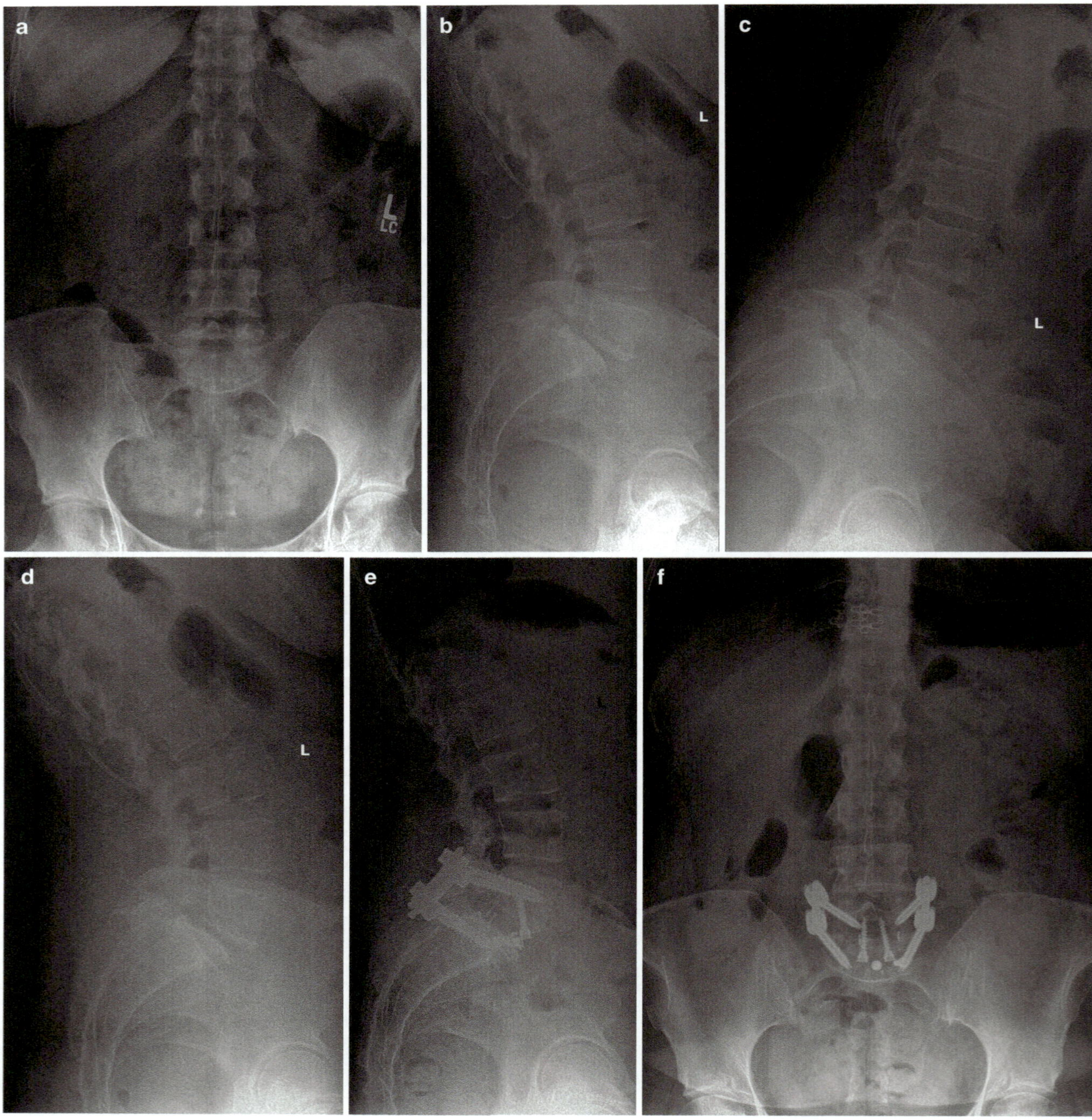

Fig. 28.5 (**a**) AP, (**b**) lateral, (**c**) flexion, and (**d**) extension radiographs of a 31-year-old prior athlete with chronic low back pain and an L5 radiculopathy. Imaging demonstrates bilateral L5-S1 grade II isthmic spondylolisthesis. Postoperative (**e**) AP and (**f**) lateral radiographs demonstrate how her neuroforaminal stenosis and spondylolisthesis was successfully treated with anterior lumbar interbody fusion (ALIF) and percutaneous posterior instrumentation

lopathy associated with motor dysfunction after surgery vary, with some studies reporting rates as high as 29%, though the same series reported improvement in symptoms by 3 months [65].

28.2.5.1 Outcomes

Outcomes following diagnosis of spondylolysis have been favorable, and patients can return to pre-injury levels of performance with or without bony union. A review of 40 athletes nearly a decade after diagnosis of spondylolysis demonstrated insufficient healing of bilateral defects, though healing potential may be improved with prompt diagnosis [66, 67]. Degenerative changes are often apparent following spondylolysis with spondylolisthesis, though rarely symptomatic or progressive following skeletal maturity [2]. Moreover, studies have found that return to sport in athletes is not associated progression of the slip [68]. Regardless, surveillance radiography is warranted biannually, or at least annually, until bony maturity is reached in adolescents with concurrent spondylolysis and spondylolisthesis, as those with progression, or persistence or worsening symptoms may require surgical intervention [69].

28.2.6 Rehabilitation

While no clear guidelines or specific rehabilitation protocols exist currently, the majority of rehabilitation in lumbar spondylolysis centers on a gradual return to play model. As such, the three-tiered approach developed by Radcliff et al. can likely be used as a treatment model [70]. In this approach, the patient is limited for the first 3 months to only aerobic activities that maintain a neutral orientation of the spine. If the patient continues to be pain-free and tolerant of increased activity, higher impact and sport-specific activities may be incorporated around 4–6 months. Finally, the patient may be cleared if strength is restored, range of motion is full, and the patient is completely pain-free with sports-related movements [70]. Generally, if the patient progresses well through rehabilitation, complete return to sport can be achieved roughly 5–7 months following initial diagnosis [71].

28.2.7 Preventative Measures

Prevention of any sporting injury includes maintaining a healthy and balanced diet combined with a physically active lifestyle. Many factors go into a solid preventative program for sport injuries, including training content, duration of the program, frequency, and compliance of the athlete to complete the program [72]. Athletes, family members, coaches, and physical trainers should all be aware of the risk factors and general preventative measures to reduce injury in young athletes [72]. Nau et al. proposed a series of exercises and activity modifications for athletes with spondylolysis [73]. Bodyweight strengthening exercises focusing on core stabilization and lower body strength are useful while implementing techniques that promote hip, pelvis, and lower extremity mobility and flexibility.

28.3 Cervical and Thoracic Stress Fractures

28.3.1 Epidemiology

Compared to lumbar spondylolysis, fewer studies have looked at stress fractures in the cervical and thoracic spine, most of which are isolated case reports. Termed "clay shoveler's fractures," these injuries are defined as isolated cervical or thoracic spinous process fractures stemming from twentieth century manual laborers who engaged in digging or shoveling heavy loads, though are now observed in athletes [4]. Asymmetric loading of the upper spine is believed to result in whip-like pulling forces from upper back muscles on the spinous processes of the lower cervical and upper thoracic levels, resulting in avulsion fractures [4]. Repetitive shear forces during golf swings can result in multi-level injuries [5], while other sports such as baseball, wrestling [74], paddling [75], American football [76], volleyball [77], powerlifting [78], and indoor rock-climbing [79].

The spinous processes of C7 and T1 are the most commonly affected vertebra, while multi-level injuries have been associated with increased trauma and can affect other levels of the lower cervical and upper thoracic spine [3, 4, 80, 81]. The increased incidence of fracture at C7 and T1 is related to the long and horizontally-oriented spinous processes at these two levels (Fig. 28.6). Such an orientation places greater perpendicular forces on the spinous processes during upper back muscle contraction. The insertion of the ligamentum nuchae, as well as the trapezius and rhomboid muscles, at C7 and T1 also increases pulling forces at these levels [4].

28.3.2 Diagnosis

28.3.2.1 History and Physical Exam

The clay-shoveler's fracture can occur as a result of acute trauma or repetitive pulling forces and muscular fatigue to the lower cervical and upper thoracic regions. Classically, patients will endorse an abrupt onset of severe "knife-like" upper back pain. The pain may be localized to between the shoulder blades. Additionally, a subset of patients may endorse an audible "pop" prior to the onset of symptoms.

Sensorineural evaluation should be intact in the upper and lower extremities. Upon inspection, the patient may demonstrate an antalgic posture, with slight neck flexion. The scapulae may be bilaterally elevated to limit motion through the upper spine. Upper extremity and neck range of motion will be limited secondary to pain, with often reproducible tenderness to palpation over the affected spinous processes as well as tight or spastic upper back musculature.

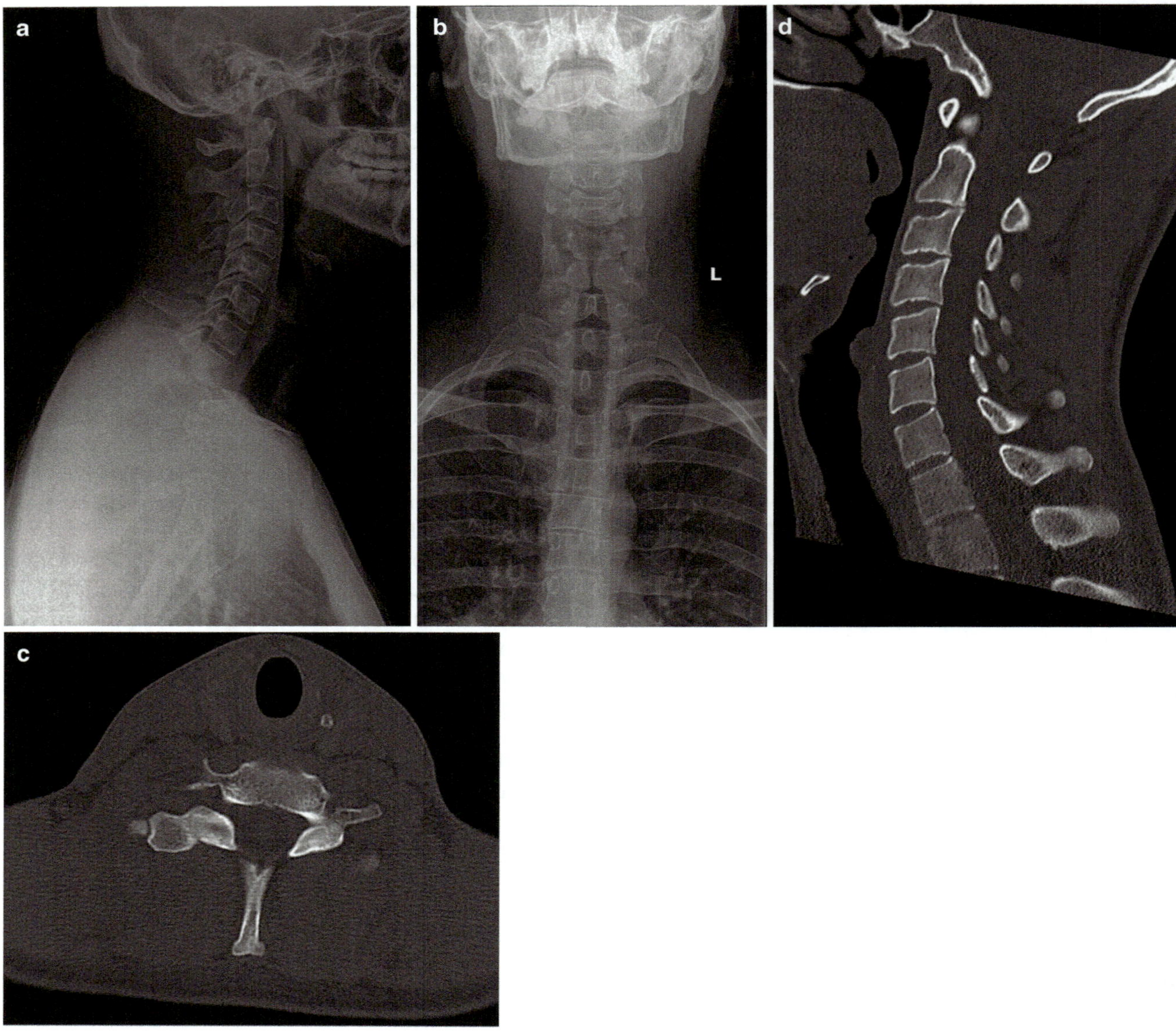

Fig. 28.6 (a) AP and (b) lateral images of a 26-year-old construction laborer with subacute neck pain that were initially interpreted as normal but demonstrate a subtle vertically-oriented fracture line of the T1 spinous process. This was redemonstrated on (c) axial and (d) sagittal CT cuts. He was successfully treated nonsurgically with rest and physical therapy

28.3.2.2 Imaging Studies

Initial AP and lateral radiographs of the cervical and thoracic spine are often sufficient in diagnosing stress injuries. One useful diagnostic clue visible on AP radiographs, the "double spinous sign," is the presence of a double shadow of the spinous process [82]. Importantly, the spinolaminar line should not be interrupted in a typical clay shoveler's fracture, which would suggest an unstable injury requiring further evaluation with CT or MRI may be necessary [80] (Fig. 28.5). When plain radiography is interpreted as normal despite increasing suspicion, follow-up imaging with CT and/or MRI is necessary [83].

28.3.3 Treatment

28.3.3.1 Bracing

Cervical bracing collars limit motion in the upper spine and specifically of the avulsed bony fragments, providing symptomatic relief, thereby limiting mobility may provide pain relief in the acute phase of treatment. Case reports have demonstrated a good patient response to cervical bracing for 3–4 weeks when applied to such stress injuries to the cervical and upper thoracic spine [5, 77, 80, 81]. Stress injuries to the mid- and lower-thoracic spine will not be addressed by cervical collars and requires thoracic-type bracing and may require a thorocolumbar orthosis. However, these injuries should be addressed on a case-by-case basis given the low incidence in the athletic population.

28.3.3.2 Activity Modification and Pain Management

Clay shoveler's fractures are generally viewed as stable fractures, and outcomes following conservative treatment are generally excellent [3, 77]. Therefore, rest and activity limitation is the first line approach to managing this type of fracture. Current management plans recommend an acute period of rest with analgesic therapies, followed by 4–6 weeks of activity modification [4]. Patients are typically able to return to activity once pain has been adequately managed. Physical therapy lends itself useful to maintain and optimize upper extremity strength and mobility. Furthermore, modalities for neck and posture control and modalities for pain management demonstrate further utility. However, physical therapy should be used cautiously as it may aggravate pain symptoms in select individuals [5].

28.3.3.3 Surgical Treatment

In cases of severe or persistent pain, surgical intervention is warranted [4]. Typically, surgery involves excision and removal of bony fragments. In a unique case report, a 38-year-old male presented with a C7 clay shoveler's fracture after playing a Wii video game [84]. He was treated conservatively with bracing and physical therapy for 3 months. However, his pain persisted and surgery was performed. Removal of the bone fragments completely resolved his pain. In a case series by Murphy and Hedequist, three athletes who were initially treated with rest and activity modification for a fracture at T1 continued to have persistent and debilitating pain after 10 months of treatment [85]. They were found to have non-union of the ossicle, and were treated with surgical removal of the loose fragments, followed by smoothing of the intact spinous process. This completely resolved their pain symptoms.

28.3.4 Complications and Rehabilitation

Overall, the outcomes following conservative treatment of cervical and thoracic stress fractures are excellent. Though rare, non-union is the most commonly-faced complication. Patients with chronic non-union may report chronic upper back pain and muscle weakness [4]. However, patients with a non-union may have positive outcomes, and therefore surgery should be reserved for those patients with persistent symptoms.

For most patients, a period of rest, with or without bracing, followed by activity modifications will likely result in symptom resolution. No explicit guidelines exist for managing the clay shoveler's fracture, although several case reports have detailed their management suggestions. In a case by Olivier et al., an amateur paddler with a fracture at T1 was initially treated with complete rest and analgesic medication 2 weeks. Between 2–4 weeks, the patient was allowed to begin cycling and running provided he was pain-free. At week 6, he was allowed to begin light swimming. By week 12, he was able to completely return to his normal sporting activities. In another case of a clay shoveler's in a rock climber, the patient was restricted from sport-specific activity for 4 months until his pain resolved [79]. With rest, pain management, and gradual reintroduction to activity, patients typically are able to return to full levels of activity anywhere from 3 weeks to 4 months [3, 74, 75, 79].

28.3.4.1 Preventative Measures

Prevention of cervical and thoracic stress fractures follows recommendations similar to those for the lumbar spine—maintaining a healthy lifestyle. Specific to the clay shoveler's fracture, athlete education regarding repetitive, strenuous movement involving the neck. There is no evidence to support restricting upper body exercises to prevent such injuries, though future investigations may shed light on specific preventative interventions and protocols to prevent stress injuries to the cervical and thoracic spine.

28.4 Summary

Athletes are often well-tuned to their bodies and are able to identify subtle changes in their physiology that alter their level of play. However, stress fractures of the spine may go undiagnosed as patients self-diagnose with muscular strains and rest, increasing the time to diagnosis. In cases of clinical suspicion, plain radiography is often able to diagnose fractures, though advanced imaging including CT and MRI should be implemented if symptoms persist or diagnosis. Bracing has demonstrated mixed results, though rest is most useful in the acute stage of treatment. Surgical intervention varies with the complexity of the case

Clinical Pearls

- Lumbar spondylolysis is a common stress injury in athletes, with an incidence between 47–70%.
- The development of lumbar stress fractures involves cyclical loading of the low back through a combination of flexion/extension, compression, and rotation.

- The treatment of lumbar spondylosis includes a combination of rest, pain management, activity modification, surgical repair if necessary, and a gradual return to play rehabilitation plan. Most athletes will completely recover in 5–7 months following the initial diagnosis.
- Clay shoveler's fracture is an uncommon upper spinal stress fracture that has been associated with several sports, including golf, paddling, rock climbing, volleyball, baseball, and American football.
- Patients will often report a "pop" and a knife-like plan in the upper spine following the avulsion fracture.
- Most patients will benefit from a brief period of bracing and pain management, followed by 4–6 weeks of activity modification before returning to their previous level of activity. In patients with persistent pain that does not improve with conservative management, surgical removal of loose bony fragments usually will resolve their pain.

Review

Questions

Multiple Choice

1. Lumbar spondylolysis involves injury to which anatomical structure:
   A. The vertebral body
   B. The nucleus pulposus
   C. Spinous process
   D. **Pars interarticularis**
2. Classification of spondylolysis is important due to all the following EXCEPT for:
   A. Unilateral lesions can progress to become bilateral lesions if not identified
   B. Early, progressive, and terminal lesions may require different treatment approaches and have different clinical outcomes
   C. **The upper levels of the lumbar spine are more commonly affected**
   D. Factors such as a steeper L5-S1 pelvic tilt and higher degree of lumbar lordosis can result in worse responses to conservative management
3. All the following are clinical exam findings associated with lumbar spondylolysis EXCEPT for:
   A. Midline low back pain that may radiate to the buttock
   B. **Radiculopathy**
   C. Pain worsens with low back extension
   D. Hamstring and/or hip flexor tightness
4. Treatment of clay shoveler's fracture may include all the following EXCEPT for:
   A. A brief period of cervical bracing
   B. Pain and symptom control
   C. **Immediate surgical management**
   D. A graduated return to sport

Answers

5. Briefly explain the pathogenesis of lumbar spondylolysis in athletes:
   ANSWER: Athletes, particularly those with underdeveloped paraspinal muscles and dysplastic facet joints, can place large amounts of strain on their low back when performing certain athletic movements. These movements include repeated extension and flexion of the low back that result in cyclic loading of the lower lumbar spine. In addition, a combination of compression and rotation in the low back can also place stress on the pars interarticularis. Eventually, repeated stress loading and paraspinal muscle fatigue may result in the formation of a stress fracture.
6. Describe the imaging workup of lumbar spondylolysis:
   ANSWER: The imaging workup begins with radiographs of the low back, and can include AP, lateral, and oblique views. If inconclusive, additional tests can be ordered based on the chronicity of the injury, If acute, MRI may be appropriate, as it may be able to diagnose stress fractures earlier than other modalities. Additionally, if the athlete presents with neurological signs, MRI may help identify nerve lesions. If chronic, CT can be used, as it offers better visualization of the bony anatomy. SPECT is also an option that can help diagnose early stress fractures, although it introduces radiation to the patient, and is generally reserved for patients whom MRI or CT is contraindicated.
7. What are the complications associated with surgical treatment of lumbar spondylolysis:
   ANSWER: The most common complication following surgical repair of lumbar spondylolysis is pseudarthrosis. However, non-union may not be necessary for a solid clinical outcome, and revision treatment should be decided on an individual basis. Other complications include progressive spondylolisthesis, neurological injury, and lumbar radiculopathy.
8. Why are C7 and T1 the most common sites for a clay shoveler's fracture?

ANSWER: The spinous processes of C7 and T1 are longer and more horizontally oriented than those at adjacent levels. Therefore, pulling from the upper spinal muscles exert a strong perpendicular force to these spinous processes that can result the avulsion fracture. In addition, the ligamentum nuchae, as well as the trapezius and rhomboid muscles, insert to the spine at these levels, resulting in stress during asymmetrical loading of the upper spine.

References

1. Wiltse LL, Newman PH, Macnab I. Classification of spondylolisis and spondylolisthesis. Clin Orthop Relat Res. 1976;(117):23–9.
2. Fredrickson BE, Baker D, McHolick WJ, Yuan HA, Lubicky JP. The natural history of spondylolysis and spondylolisthesis. J Bone Joint Surg Am. 1984;66:699–707.
3. Dellestable F, Gaucher A. Clay-shoveler's fracture. Stress fracture of the lower cervical and upper thoracic spinous processes. Rev Rhum Engl Ed. 1998;65:575–82.
4. Posthuma de Boer J, van Wulfften Palthe AFY, Stadhouder A, Bloemers FW. The clay Shoveler's fracture: a case report and review of the literature. J Emerg Med. 2016;51:292–7.
5. Kang D-H, Lee S-H. Multiple spinous process fractures of the thoracic vertebrae (Clay-Shoveler's fracture) in a beginning golfer: a case report. Spine. 2009;34:E534–7.
6. Panteliadis P, Nagra NS, Edwards KL, Behrbalk E, Boszczyk B. Athletic population with spondylolysis: review of outcomes following surgical repair or conservative management. Global Spine J. 2016;6:615–25.
7. Tallarico RA, Madom IA, Palumbo MA. Spondylolysis and spondylolisthesis in the athlete. Sports Med Arthrosc. 2008;16:32–8.
8. O'Brien CP, Williams C, Duffy G. Lumbar spine stress fracture in a young athlete. Phys Sportsmed. 1997;25:92–8.
9. Standaert CJ, Herring SA. Spondylolysis: a critical review. Br J Sports Med. 2000;34:415–22.
10. Ko S-B, Lee S-W. Prevalence of spondylolysis and its relationship with low back pain in selected population. Clin Orthop Surg. 2011;3:34–8.
11. Gregg CD, Dean S, Schneiders AG. Variables associated with active spondylolysis. Phys Ther Sport. 2009;10:121–4.
12. Beutler WJ, Fredrickson BE, Murtland A, Sweeney CA, Grant WD, Baker D. The natural history of spondylolysis and spondylolisthesis. Spine. 2003;28:1027–35.
13. Wiltse LL. 5 Etiology of spondylolisthesis. Clin Orthop Relat Res. 1957;10:48–60.
14. Rosenberg NJ, Bargar WL, Friedman B. The incidence of spondylolysis and spondylolisthesis in nonambulatory patients. Spine. 1981;6:35–8.
15. Sonne-Holm S, Jacobsen S, Rovsing HC, Monrad H, Gebuhr P. Lumbar spondylolysis: a life long dynamic condition? A cross sectional survey of 4.151 adults. Eur Spine J. 2007;16:821–8.
16. Amato M, Totty WG, Gilula LA. Spondylolysis of the lumbar spine: demonstration of defects and laminal fragmentation. Radiology. 1984;153:627–9.
17. Brooks BK, Southam SL, Mlady GW, Logan J, Rosett M. Lumbar spine spondylolysis in the adult population: using computed tomography to evaluate the possibility of adult onset lumbar spondylosis as a cause of back pain. Skelet Radiol. 2010;39:669–73.
18. Micheli LJ, Wood R. Back pain in young athletes. Significant differences from adults in causes and patterns. Arch Pediatr Adolesc Med. 1995;149:15–8.
19. Rossi F, Dragoni S. The prevalence of spondylolysis and spondylolisthesis in symptomatic elite athletes: radiographic findings. Radiography. 2001;7:37–42.
20. Berger RG, Doyle SM. Spondylolysis 2019 update. Curr Opin Pediatr. 2019;31:61–8.
21. Neumann DA. Kinesiology of the musculoskeletal system: foundations for rehabilitation. St. Louis: Mosby/Elsevier; 2010.
22. Sakai T, Sairyo K, Suzue N, Kosaka H, Yasui N. Incidence and etiology of lumbar spondylolysis: review of the literature. J Orthop Sci. 2010;15:281–8.
23. Rossi F. Spondylolysis, spondylolisthesis and sports. J Sports Med Phys Fitness. 1978;18:317–40.
24. Soler T, Calderón C. The prevalence of spondylolysis in the Spanish elite athlete. Am J Sports Med. 2000;28:57–62.
25. McCarroll JR, Miller JM, Ritter MA. Lumbar spondylolysis and spondylolisthesis in college football players. A prospective study. Am J Sports Med. 1986;14:404–6.
26. Castinel BH, Adam P, Prat C. A stress fracture of the lumbar spine in a professional rugby player. Br J Sports Med. 2007;41:337–8.
27. Nyska M, Constantini N, Calé-Benzoor M, Back Z, Kahn G, Mann G. Spondylolysis as a cause of low back pain in swimmers. Int J Sports Med. 2000;21:375–9.
28. Grogan JP, Hemminghytt S, Williams AL, Carrera GF, Haughton VM. Spondylolysis studied with computed tomography. Radiology. 1982;145:737–42.
29. Chosa E, Totoribe K, Tajima N. A biomechanical study of lumbar spondylolysis based on a three-dimensional finite element method. J Orthop Res. 2004;22:158–63.
30. Fujii K, Katoh S, Sairyo K, Ikata T, Yasui N. Union of defects in the pars interarticularis of the lumbar spine in children and adolescents. J Bone Joint Surg. 2004;86-B:225–31.
31. Bugg WG, Lewis M, Juette A, Cahir JG, Toms AP. Lumbar lordosis and pars interarticularis fractures: a case–control study. Skelet Radiol. 2012;41:817–22.
32. Sairyo K, Katoh S, Sasa T, Yasui N, Goel VK, Vadapalli S, Masuda A, Biyani A, Ebraheim N. Athletes with unilateral spondylolysis are at risk of stress fracture at the contralateral pedicle and pars interarticularis: a clinical and biomechanical study. Am J Sports Med. 2005;33:583–90.
33. Morita T, Ikata T, Katoh S, Miyake R. Lumbar spondylolysis in children and adolescents. J Bone Joint Surg. 1995;77-B:620–5.
34. Sairyo K, Katoh S, Takata Y, Terai T, Yasui N, Goel VK, Masuda A, Vadapalli S, Biyani A, Ebraheim N. MRI signal changes of the pedicle as an indicator for early diagnosis of spondylolysis in children and adolescents: a clinical and biomechanical study. Spine. 2006;31:206–11.
35. McCleary MD, Congeni JA. Current concepts in the diagnosis and treatment of spondylolysis in young athletes. Curr Sports Med Rep. 2007;6:62–6.
36. Purcell L, Micheli L. Low back pain in young athletes. Sports Health. 2009;1:212–22.
37. Anderson SJ. Assessment and management of the pediatric and adolescent patient with low back pain. Phys Med Rehabil Clin N Am. 1991;2:157–85.
38. Ciullo JV, Jackson DW. Pars interarticularis stress reaction, spondylolysis, and spondylolisthesis in gymnasts. Clin Sports Med. 1985;4:95–110.
39. Masci L, Pike J, Malara F, Phillips B, Bennell K, Brukner P. Use of the one-legged hyperextension test and magnetic resonance imaging in the diagnosis of active spondylolysis. Br J Sports Med. 2006;40:940–6; discussion 946.
40. Libson E, Bloom RA, Dinari G, Robin GC. Oblique lumbar spine radiographs: importance in young patients. Radiology. 1984;151:89–90.
41. Beck NA, Miller R, Baldwin K, Zhu X, Spiegel D, Drummond D, Sankar WN, Flynn JM. Do oblique views add value in the diagnosis of spondylolysis in adolescents? J Bone Joint Surg Am. 2013;95:e65–1.
42. Yang J, Servaes S, Edwards K, Zhuang H. Prevalence of stress reaction in the pars interarticularis in pediatric patients with new-onset lower back pain. Clin Nucl Med. 2013;38(2):110–4.
43. Standaert CJ, Herring SA. Expert opinion and controversies in sports and musculoskeletal medicine: the diagnosis and treatment of spondylolysis in adolescent athletes. Arch Phys Med Rehabil. 2007;88:537–40.
44. Miller R, Beck NA, Sampson NR, Zhu X, Flynn JM, Drummond D. Imaging modalities for low back pain in children: a review of

spondyloysis and undiagnosed mechanical back pain. J Pediatr Orthop. 2013;33:282–8.
45. Fadell MF, Gralla J, Bercha I, Stewart JR, Harned RK, Ingram JD, Miller AL, Strain JD, Weinman JP. CT outperforms radiographs at a comparable radiation dose in the assessment for spondylolysis. Pediatr Radiol. 2015;45:1026–30.
46. Campbell RSD, Grainger AJ, Hide IG, Papastefanou S, Greenough CG. Juvenile spondylolysis: a comparative analysis of CT, SPECT and MRI. Skelet Radiol. 2005;34:63–73.
47. Tofte JN, CarlLee TL, Holte AJ, Sitton SE, Weinstein SL. Imaging pediatric spondylolysis: a systematic review. Spine. 2017;42:777–82.
48. Dhouib A, Tabard-Fougere A, Hanquinet S, Dayer R. Diagnostic accuracy of MR imaging for direct visualization of lumbar pars defect in children and young adults: a systematic review and meta-analysis. Eur Spine J. 2018;27:1058–66.
49. Finkenstaedt T, Siriwanarangsun P, Achar S, Carl M, Finkenstaedt S, Abeydeera N, Chung CB, Bae WC. Ultrashort time-to-echo magnetic resonance imaging at 3 T for the detection of spondylolysis in cadaveric spines: comparison with CT. Investig Radiol. 2019;54:32–8.
50. Bouras T, Korovessis P. Management of spondylolysis and low-grade spondylolisthesis in fine athletes. A comprehensive review. Eur J Orthop Surg Traumatol. 2015;25(Suppl 1):S167–75.
51. Klein G, Mehlman CT, McCarty M. Nonoperative treatment of spondylolysis and grade I spondylolisthesis in children and young adults: a meta-analysis of observational studies. J Pediatr Orthop. 2009;29:146–56.
52. El Rassi G, Takemitsu M, Glutting J, Shah SA. Effect of sports modification on clinical outcome in children and adolescent athletes with symptomatic lumbar spondylolysis. Am J Phys Med Rehabil. 2013;92:1070–4.
53. Arima H, Suzuki Y, Togawa D, Mihara Y, Murata H, Matsuyama Y. Low-intensity pulsed ultrasound is effective for progressive-stage lumbar spondylolysis with MRI high-signal change. Eur Spine J. 2017;26:3122–8.
54. Tsukada M, Takiuchi T, Watanabe K. Low-intensity pulsed ultrasound for early-stage lumbar spondylolysis in young athletes. Clin J Sport Med. 2017; https://doi.org/10.1097/JSM.0000000000000531.
55. Syrmou E, Tsitsopoulos PP, Marinopoulos D, Tsonidis C, Anagnostopoulos I. Spondylolysis: a review and reappraisal. Hippokratia. 2010;14(1):17–21.
56. Eddy D, Congeni J, Loud K. A review of spine injuries and return to play. Clin J Sport Med. 2005;15(6):453–8.
57. Buck JE. Direct repair of the defect in spondylolisthesis. Preliminary report. J Bone Joint Surg Br. 1970;52:432–7.
58. Rajasekaran S, Subbiah M, Shetty A. Direct repair of lumbar spondylolysis by Buck's technique. Indian J Orthop. 2011;45:136.
59. Johnson GV, Thompson AG. The Scott wiring technique for direct repair of lumbar spondylolysis. J Bone Joint Surg Br. 1992;74:426–30.
60. Goldstein MJ, Bruffey J, Eastlack RK. New minimally invasive technique for direct pars interarticularis osteosynthesis using cortical screws and spinous-process modular link. Spine. 2016;41:E1421–4.
61. Cheung EV, Herman MJ, Cavalier R, Pizzutillo PD. Spondylolysis and spondylolisthesis in children and adolescents: II. Surgical management. J Am Acad Orthop Surg. 2006;14:488–98.
62. Muschik M, Zippel H, Perka C. Surgical management of severe spondylolisthesis in children and adolescents. Anterior fusion in situ versus anterior spondylodesis with posterior transpedicular instrumentation and reduction. Spine (Phila Pa 1976). 1997;22:2036–42; discussion 2043.
63. DeWald CJ, Vartabedian JE, Rodts MF, Hammerberg KW. Evaluation and management of high-grade spondylolisthesis in adults. Spine. 2005;30:S49–59.
64. Lenke LG, Bridwell KH, Bullis D, Betz RR, Baldus C, Schoenecker PL. Results of in situ fusion for isthmic spondylolisthesis. J Spinal Disord. 1992;5:433–42.
65. Schär RT, Sutter M, Mannion AF, Eggspühler A, Jeszenszky D, Fekete TF, Kleinstück F, Haschtmann D. Outcome of L5 radiculopathy after reduction and instrumented transforaminal lumbar interbody fusion of high-grade L5–S1 isthmic spondylolisthesis and the role of intraoperative neurophysiological monitoring. Eur Spine J. 2017;26:679–90.
66. Sys J, Michielsen J, Bracke P, Martens M, Verstreken J. Nonoperative treatment of active spondylolysis in elite athletes with normal X-ray findings: literature review and results of conservative treatment. Eur Spine J. 2001;10:498–504.
67. Miller SF, Congeni J, Swanson K. Long-term functional and anatomical follow-up of early detected spondylolysis in young athletes. Am J Sports Med. 2004;32:928–33.
68. Muschik M, Hähnel H, Robinson PN, Perka C, Muschik C. Competitive sports and the progression of spondylolisthesis. J Pediatr Orthop. 1996;16:364–9.
69. Tsirikos AI, Garrido EG. Spondylolysis and spondylolisthesis in children and adolescents. J Bone Joint Surg Br. 2010;92:751–9.
70. Radcliff KE, Kepler CK, Jakoi A, Sidhu GS, Rihn J, Vaccaro AR, Albert TJ, Hilibrand AS. Adjacent segment disease in the lumbar spine following different treatment interventions. Spine J. 2013;13:1339–49.
71. Standaert CJ. Spondylolysis in the adolescent athlete. Clin J Sport Med. 2002;12:119–22.
72. Frisch A, Croisier J-L, Urhausen A, Seil R, Theisen D. Injuries, risk factors and prevention initiatives in youth sport. Br Med Bull. 2009;92:95–121.
73. Nau E, Hanney WJ, Kolber MJ. Spinal conditioning for athletes with lumbar spondylolysis and spondylolisthesis. Strength Condit J. 2008;30:43–52.
74. Yamaguchi KT Jr, Myung KS, Alonso MA, Skaggs DL. Clay-shoveler's fracture equivalent in children. Spine. 2012;37:E1672–5.
75. Olivier EC, Muller E, Janse van Rensburg DC. Clay-shoveler fracture in a paddler: a case report. Clin J Sport Med. 2016;26:e69–70.
76. Nuber GW, Schafer MF. Clay shovelers' injuries. A report of two injuries sustained from football. Am J Sports Med. 1987;15:182–3.
77. Hetsroni I, Mann G, Dolev E, Morgenstern D, Nyska M. Clay shoveler's fracture in a volleyball player: revealing an unusual source of pain. Phys Sportsmed. 2005;33:38–42.
78. Herrick RT. Clay-shoveler's fracture in power-lifting. Am J Sports Med. 1981;9:29–30.
79. Kaloostian PE, Kim JE, Calabresi PA, Bydon A, Witham T. Clay-shoveler's fracture during indoor rock climbing. Orthopedics. 2013;36:e381–3.
80. Victor B, Feldman FA. An atypical clay shoveler's fracture: a case report. J Can Chiropr Assoc. 2001;45:213.
81. Umredkar A, Sura S, Mohindra S. Multiple contiguous isolated spinous process fracture (clay-shoveler's fracture) of the cervicodorsal spine. Neurol India. 2011;59:788–9.
82. Cancelmo JJ Jr. Clay shoveler's fracture. A helpful diagnostic sign. Am J Roentgenol Radium Therapy, Nucl Med. 1972;115:540–3.
83. Lin JT, Lee JL, Lee ST. Evaluation of occult cervical spine fractures on radiographs and CT. Emerg Radiol. 2003;10:128–34.
84. Brown CN, McKenna P. A Wii™-related clay-shoveler's fracture. ScientificWorldJournal. 2009;9:1190–1.
85. Murphy RF, Hedequist D. Excision of symptomatic spinous process nonunion in adolescent athletes. Am J Orthop (Belle Mead NJ). 2015;44:515–7.

Stress Fractures in Sport: Pelvis and Acetabulum

29

Emily K. Miller Olson, Emily Kraus, and Michael Fredericson

Learning Objectives

- Identify key aspects of the clinical presentation and examination that should encourage the examiner to obtain advanced imaging to rule out pelvic BSI.
- Describe the diagnostic findings on MRI associated with various grades of pelvic BSIs.
- Outline a basic treatment protocol for pelvic BSIs, including management of risk factors for recurrent BSI.
- List potential complications of misdiagnosed or untreated pelvic BSI and associated low energy availability.

29.1 Introduction

Although bone stress injuries (BSIs) of the pelvis and sacrum are relatively rare, comprising only 1–7% of all BSIs, they can be challenging to diagnose and manage [1–4]. These BSIs are considered medium-risk, meaning that they should be treated with caution even though they have a low likelihood of progressing to complete fracture or non-union [1, 3]. Unfortunately, pelvic BSIs are often missed since they are difficult to diagnose on plain radiographs, their presenting symptoms tend to be vague, and they are easily mistaken for other more common diagnoses. Given the risk for initial misdiagnosis, pelvic and sacral BSIs can progress to more severe grades by the time of diagnosis, leading to more prolonged recovery time and increased risk for progression to complete fracture.

The general pathophysiology of stress injuries is that repetitive stress leads osteoclastic activity to surpass the rate of osteoblastic new bone formation. This leads to temporary weakening of the bone, considered a stress reaction. As this continues, microfractures result and the bone responds by forming periosteal new bone for reinforcement. However, without activity modification, eventually a full cortical break eventually occurs [5, 6]., Athletes are particularly at risk for BSIs following a rapid change in training volume, such as during the transition from high school to collegiate athletics as a freshman, change in training surface or footwear, or generally running more than 32 km/week [5].

Compared to long bones, the pelvis, sacrum and spine bones have a much higher trabecular (cancellous) bone percentage [7]. Trabecular bone has a much higher surface area exposed to bone marrow and blood flow, leading to a higher turnover rate. Trabecular bone loss is prevented by estradiol in women. For women after menopause, bone loss tends to be much more rapid in trabecular bone due to the low levels of estrogen [8]. In men, 80% of estradiol is from aromatization of testosterone, so estradiol and androgen deficiencies are connected. Bioavailable estradiol has been more closely correlated with BMD than bioavailable testosterone. In men, as testosterone decreases or as testosterone aromatization decreases, BMD falls significantly [9]. As discussed previously, low energy availability can lead to hormonal dysregulation, especially of estrogen and testosterone, which, in turn, leads to bone loss. As hormones have a greater effect on trabecular bone, athletes with low energy availability may have increased trabecular bone loss. In fact, athletes who sustained BSIs in sites with a high trabecular bone percentage were more likely to exhibit disordered eating and oligomenorrhea or amenorrhea. These athletes had significantly lower bone mineral density at the lumbar spine, femoral neck, and the hip compared to those athletes who sustained BSIs at cortical bone sites such as the tibia [2]. Female NCAA athletes with moderate or high risk scores on the female athlete triad cumulative risk assessment [10] were 4.5-fold more likely to sustain bone stress injuries in trabecular rich sites than low risk athletes [11]. Male athletes with a history of BSI in trabecular rich sites had 4.6-fold increased risk for low BMD *Z*-scores for the lumbar spine and total body (less head) compared to athletes with BSIs in cortical rich sites only [9].

E. K. Miller Olson (✉) · E. Kraus · M. Fredericson
Physical Medicine and Rehabilitation, Stanford University, Stanford, CA, USA
e-mail: Emiller5@stanford.edu; ekraus@stanford.edu; mfred2@stanford.edu

G. A. J. Robertson, N. Maffulli (eds.), *Fractures in Sport*, https://doi.org/10.1007/978-3-030-72036-0_29

Table 29.1 MRI bone stress injury grading scale

Grade	Fredericson MRI description	Nattiv MRI description	Arendt MRI description
1	Periosteal edema noted on fat-suppressed T2 weighted images	Mild marrow edema or periosteal edema on fat-suppressed T2 weighted images	Marrow or periosteal edema present only on STIR images
2	Abnormal increased signal intensity within the marrow cavity or along the endosteal surface on fat-suppressed T2 weighted images	Moderate marrow edema or periosteal edema on fat-suppressed T2 weighted images	Marrow or periosteal edema present on both STIR and fat-suppressed T2 weighted images
3	Signal abnormalities seen on both T2 and T1 due to edema or hemorrhage related to accumulating microdamage and associated reparative response	Severe marrow edema or periosteal edema on both T2 and T1 weighted images without a fracture line	Marrow or periosteal edema present on STIR, T2 and T1 weighted images without a definite cortical break
4	Actual fracture line is present and seen on both T1 and T2	Actual fracture line is present and seen on either T1 or T2	Injury line on T1 or T2-weighted scans

Given the difficulty of diagnosing pelvic BSIs on plain radiographs, advanced imaging is necessary. The sensitivity of radiographs for any BSI is 10–35%, and even lower in the pelvis [5, 6]. For all BSIs, bone scintigraphy sensitivity reaches 93%, but its specificity is around 74%. CT is much less sensitive, but very specific, between 88–98%, and can be a good confirmatory test if clarification is needed regarding the extent of fracture. MRI is both very sensitive and specific, though there can still be some limitations especially in the very early period [5, 6]. The Fredericson, Nattiv and Arendt MRI grading scales are all very similar, and are based on a pattern of bone marrow and periosteal edema (see Table 29.1) [2, 5, 12]. These have been shown prospectively to be accurate and independent predictors of time to full return to sport [2]. While for all BSIs MRI grade correlates with prolonged return to sport, this difference is even more pronounced for BSIs in trabecular bone. Athletes with lower grade (Grades 1 and 2) trabecular BSIs (including pubic rami, sacrum, and femoral neck) took 17.1 ± 9.1 weeks to return to play, while those with higher grade (Grades 3 and 4) trabecular BSIs took 38.1 ± 6.4 weeks [2].

In this chapter, we discuss the epidemiology, presentation, diagnosis, and treatment of BSIs in the pubic rami, iliac wing, acetabular roof, and sacrum. Osteitis pubis is also included in this chapter since it is also a bone stress injury.

29.2 Common Bone Stress Injury Locations in the Pelvis and Acetabulum

29.2.1 Pubic Ramus or Ischium

29.2.1.1 Epidemiology and Mechanism

Despite being the most common location for pelvic BSIs [3], the overall incidence of pubic rami BSIs is relatively low. Over a five-year period, 32/211 NCAA track or cross-country athletes sustained 61 BSIs. Of those, only five were pelvic: three were sacral and two were in the pubic ramus. Pubic rami BSIs were 3% of the reported BSIs, and occurred in 0.9% of NCAA track and cross country athletes [2].

In the 1980s, Pavlov et al. [13] and Noakes et al. [14] published the two largest case series of pubic rami stress injuries, each with 12 runners. 20/24 ran more than 100 km/week and onset of symptoms occurred during or after more intense runs, either during competition or interval training. These BSIs all occurred in the inferior pubic ramus near the symphysis pubis. An additional case series in the military included three pubic rami BSIs in the same location [15]. This location is near the attachment of the adductor magnus muscle. A suggested mechanism is related to continuous and repetitive adductor magnus pulling on the bone insertion site, leading to bone absorption and localized osteoporosis, increasing risk for a BSI at that location. The vast majority of reported pubic rami BSIs occur in distance runners.

29.2.1.2 Presentation and Examination Findings

Patients often present with insidious onset pain that progressively got worse to the point of no longer being able to run, though some patients noted sudden onset pain without prior symptoms. 16/28 patients in various case reports reported insidious onset while 12 noted sudden onset [13–15]. The pain is most commonly located in the groin, but can present in the buttocks, posterior thigh, or low back. 10/15 athletes in two case series had pain in the groin, 4 had buttock pain and 2 had posterior thigh pain [13, 15].

On examination, all athletes had full painless range of motion. One study noted that 12/12 may be hypermobile based on the thumb to forearm test, and hypermobility could therefore be a predisposing factor [13]. In another study, 12/12 had a positive single leg standing sign, meaning they experienced significant pain when balancing on the affected leg or were unable to do so. Most patients will be unable to do a single leg hop due to pain. Additionally, 12/12 had severe tenderness to palpation at the inferior pubic ramus [14].

29.2.1.3 Diagnosis

Given the low incidence of pubic rami BSIs, these are commonly misdiagnosed initially. The differential is broad given patients can present with groin pain, buttock pain, or both. Some potential differential diagnoses include adductor, hip flexor, or hamstring muscle or tendon strain, discogenic low back pain, or intra-articular pathology like labral tear or femoral acetabular impingement. For this reason, diagnostic imaging is often targeted at ruling out other more common diagnoses. It has not been established whether physical examination tests like the single leg stance, single leg hop, or tenderness to palpation over the inferior pubic bone are specific to pubic rami BSIs. Therefore, diagnostic imaging confirmation is usually performed both to rule out other diagnoses and to evaluate for pubic rami BSIs.

As mentioned in the introduction, all pelvic BSIs are very difficult to diagnose on plain radiographs alone and are, therefore, historically underreported. Prior to the 1990s, all studies focused on radiographically diagnosed BSIs, since MRI was not in common use. Noakes et al. identified five pubic rami BSIs on radiographs, but an additional seven subjects with comparable clinical findings were included [14]. This gives an incidence of 5/1000 (0.5%) diagnosed radiographically or 12/1000 (1.2%) noted clinically. In a 2015 study on NCAA athletes, only 12/56 (21%) BSIs at any site were diagnosed on plain radiographs, including none of the five pelvic BSIs [2]. MRI of the pelvis should therefore be performed in athletes with severe groin or buttock pain preventing them from running and examination findings consistent with pubic rami BSI. By using the MRI grading scales defined in the introduction, a better prediction of the return to play timeline can be given. See Fig. 29.1.

29.2.1.4 Treatment and Rehabilitation

Rehabilitation following BSI typically follows a two-phase approach. The initial treatment, phase 1, for all pubic rami stress injuries is rest. Many authors recommend avoiding nonsteroidal anti-inflammatory medications during this phase since they may slow bone healing [3]. If athletes are unable to walk pain-free, a period of non-weight bearing using crutches or other assistive devices is recommended. Once they are able to walk pain-free, they can gradually wean from assistive devices and initiate non-impact aerobic exercise including swimming, aqua jogging, or anti-gravity treadmill running [3]. Most athletes are able to swim to maintain cardiovascular endurance, but cycling can be difficult as it may impose undue pressure over the inferior pubic ramus, and should therefore be avoided until the athlete is pain-free.

Rehabilitation during this period focuses on progressive resistance training, core and pelvic girdle stability, balance and proprioception training, and flexibility [3]. Strength training involves the whole body about 2–3 times per week, with load dependent on prior experience. More advanced athletes can use heavier loads for 10–25 repetitions, while athletes with little experience should limit themselves to lighter loads for 10–15 repetitions [3].

Phase 2 starts after the athlete is pain free with cross training and when focal point tenderness has resolved, usually about 6–8 weeks from the date of diagnosis. This initiates a return to running progression over 6–12 weeks dictated by pain recurrence. Initial running activity can start around 30–50% of the pre-injury level. Athletes then follow the 10% rule, increasing either mileage or intensity no more than 10% per week, although some athletes may be able to progress at a quicker rate, especially when recovering from a lower grade injury. If symptoms recur, mileage and intensity should decrease back to the prior level for an additional week before progression. During this return to run progression, athletes should be instructed to only run on flat surfaces, avoiding trails with lots of obstacles and preferably on a surface with some compliance, such as a rubber track instead of concrete. Full return to sport can follow completion of the running progression back to their pre-injury training level without pain [3]. Athletes with additional risk factors, such as low energy availability, may have a more prolonged return to sport from delays in bone healing.

As with any BSI, rehabilitation must occur in conjunction with identification of any risk factors. This includes screening for low energy availability and the female or male athlete triad. For any athletes found to have risk factors on this screening, more thorough work up should be performed, and these factors must be addressed as discussed in Chap. 1.1.4. One case report identified a BSI in the ischiopubic ramus in a patient with anorexia nervosa and excessive compulsive exercising. In this scenario, more aggressive treatment of the underlying eating disorder was required to adequately manage her BSI [16]. Additionally, other risk factors must be evaluated. If athletes increased training mileage abruptly or changed their shoes or running surface recently, these factors must be individually addressed through education. If a patient has repetitive BSIs without any notable risk factors, including more thorough screening for female or male athlete triad, a running evaluation prior to full return to sport may be beneficial to identify alterations in gait that may decrease risk for recurrent BSI.

29.2.1.5 Potential Complications

Potential complications of pubic rami BSIs include nonunion or progression to complete fracture. If the above regimen is followed, the risk of one of these complications is minimal. Pavlov et al. noted two athletes who continued running after diagnosis of BSI despite pain. Both athletes developed non-unions 13 and 27 months after initial diagnosis, which both healed with 4 months of rest [13]. Otherwise no complications were reported in 25/27 cases [13–15].

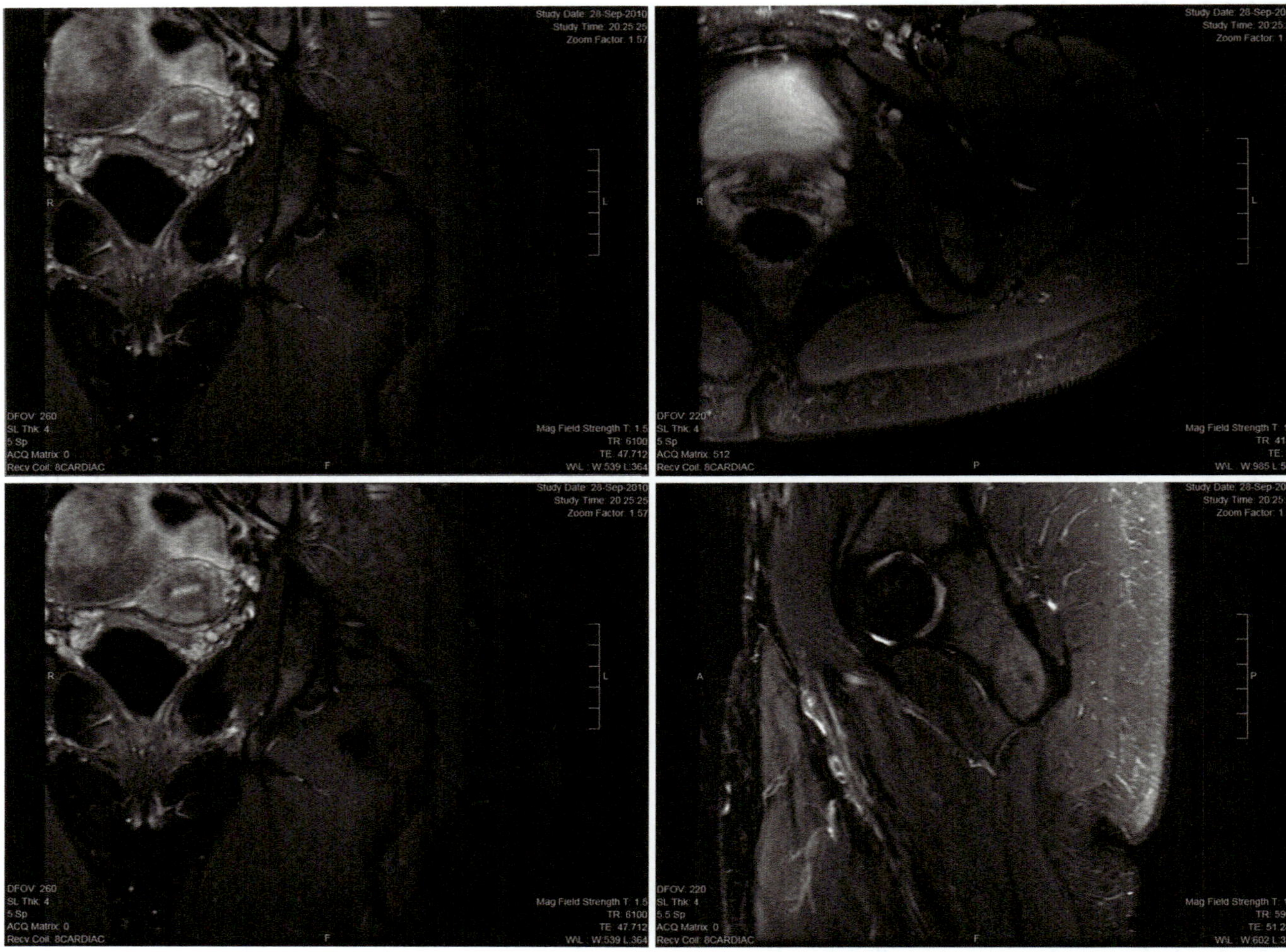

Fig. 29.1 Pubic rami bone stress injury in a 30 year old female distance runner with a history of prior femoral neck BSI who presented with progressive onset of left posteromedial thigh pain with tenderness to palpation of the left pubic ramus (coronal, axial, and sagittal T2)

29.2.2 Sacrum

29.2.2.1 Epidemiology and Mechanism

Sacral BSIs most commonly occur in the sacral ala, and are thought to be relatively rare, though more common than initially reported. Of all stress injuries, sacral BSIs are one of the least likely to be diagnosed on plain radiographs because of the obscuring bowel gas and soft tissues and attempts to shield reproductive organs [17, 18]., Additionally, there must be a 30–50% change in trabecular bone density before changes are evident on radiographs, meaning that all low-grade stress injuries would be missed [19]. As the pubic ramus, the sacrum has a high percentage of trabecular bone, and is much more strongly correlated to the Triad and low energy availability than other cortical BSIs such as the tibia or tarsal bones. For these reasons, sacral BSIs are likely under-reported, especially in long distance runners. Among 380 military recruits with unilateral hip pain, 31 were diagnosed with sacral BSIs on MRI after normal radiographs [20]. Among 312 children with sport-related low back pain for over 7 days, 1.6% were diagnosed with sacral BSIs. None of these were detected on plain radiographs, and all were located in the sacral ala. Of note, 33% of these children were diagnosed with lumbar BSIs, so these are much more common than sacral BSIs and should also be evaluated in sport-related low back pain [21].

In the sacrum, vertical body forces are dissipated from the spine and concentrated in the sacrum, potentially leading to sacral ala stress reactions with overuse, especially in the setting of leg length discrepancy [22]. Of note, sacral BSIs often occur in conjunction with other pelvic BSIs from abnormal shear stresses through the pelvic ring. In that military cohort, 12/31 had multiple pelvic BSIs including the femoral neck, ilium, inferior pubic ramus, and contralateral sacrum [20].

In addition to distance runners and military recruits, sacral BSIs are also seen in post-partum, potentially related to pregnancy- and lactation-related osteopenia. BMD decreases during the post-partum period following hormonal adaptation of calcium regulation during pregnancy and lactation, causing transient fragility of bones. These BSIs are particularly underdiagnosed given many more common reasons for low back pain post-partum. Therefore, patients need to be counseled on the risks of returning to run immediately post-partum and the need to restart a very gradual training program [23].

29.2.2.2 Presentation and Examination

Most commonly, athletes will present with unilateral pelvic pain localized to the sacroiliac joint area [5]. However, athletes may also present with vague, nonlocalized low back, buttock, or hip pain that is exacerbated by weight bearing [19]. The vast majority of reported cases have occurred in distance runners, including 23 collegiate cross country or distance track, 5 in a post-collegiate running club, and 4 recreational runners [19, 21, 22, 24]. However, there have been isolated reports in many other sports such as soccer and basketball [21]. Sacral BSIs are also commonly seen in military recruits, who are required to run or hike long distances while carrying a heavy load [20]. While outside of the military the vast majority (25/34) of reported cases are female [3, 19, 21, 25], within the military sacral BSIs are more evenly distributed, with 18 men and 13 women diagnosed with sacral BSI out of 380 patients with unilateral hip pain [20].

The most sensitive examination finding is tenderness to palpation of the unilateral sacrum and sacroiliac joint, which was seen in all reported cases [3, 19, 21, 25]. Additionally, all cases noted pain with single leg hopping on the affected side [3, 19, 25]. While multiple studies have mentioned that leg length discrepancy may be a risk factor for sacral BSIs, especially on the longer side, most reported cases do not include this exam finding [25].

29.2.2.3 Diagnosis

The differential diagnoses for low back pain in a young athlete include intervertebral disk pathology, sacroiliac joint dysfunction, sacroiliitis, spondylolysis, gluteal muscle strain, piriformis syndrome or strain, and high hamstring strain or tendinopathy [3, 25]. Since these other ailments are much more prevalent, sacral BSIs may not be on the list of initial differential diagnoses, leading to the risk of misdiagnosis. Particularly in distance runners presenting with unilateral pain and focal tenderness to palpation, the index of suspicion should remain high [22].

In reported cases, radiographs were negative in 48/52 sacral BSIs [3, 19, 21, 25]. MRI is considered the gold standard of diagnosis (see Fig. 29.2), but there are two reported cases when initial MRIs were negative approximately 1 week after onset of symptoms. Repeat MRIs approximately 4 weeks later, when athletes were unable to return to run, demonstrated sacral ala BSIs [22]. Sacral stress injuries can be graded using the MRI grading scales identified above, which can assist with predicting return to run (Table 29.1).

Since the sacrum is a very high trabecular bone site, it is commonly associated with low energy availability. Athletes should be screened for disordered eating, history of prior BSIs, and irregular menstruation. 13/17 female athletes in three case series had oligomenorrhea or amenorrhea [3, 19, 25]. Marx et al. reported a 3.3-fold increased risk for low BMD in female athletes with BSI in trabecular-rich locations, highlighting the need to screen athletes with sacral BSIs for low BMD. In published case reports, the lumbar BMD *T*-score and *Z*-score is often low, while that of the hip/femoral neck may be closer to normal [19].

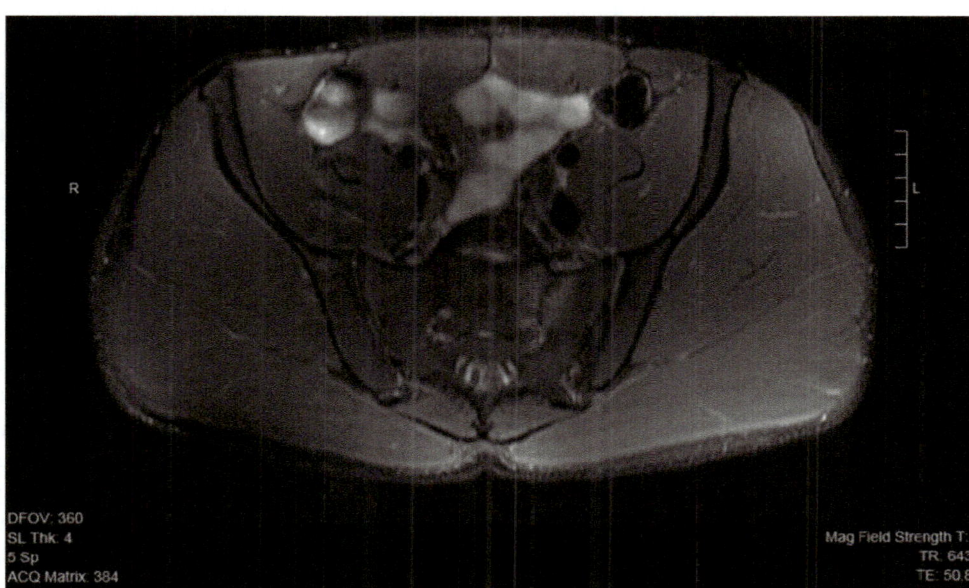

Fig. 29.2 Sacral bone stress injury in 21 year old male NCAA track athlete presenting with 12 days of gradually worsening left buttock pain with tenderness to palpation over the superior sacrum (axial T2)

29.2.2.4 Treatment, Rehabilitation, and Potential Complications

Treatment protocols following sacral BSIs are almost identical to those following pubic rami BSI. Phase 1 generally starts with a period of non-weight bearing on crutches for 1–2 weeks until the athlete is able to walk without pain. At that time, non-impact or limited impact cross training (swimming, aqua jogging, or cycling,) can start for approximately 6 weeks. This lasts at least 2 weeks after the athlete is pain free with all non-impact cross training activities. Phase two, a gradual return to run program over the next 3–6 months, can then be initiated, starting with an anti-gravity treadmill at approximately 60% and gradually progressing back to full weight-bearing. As an alternative to the anti-gravity treadmill, the elliptical machine is a reasonable option followed by a gradual walking and jogging progression. Both Phase one and two occur in conjunction with pelvic girdle and lower abdominal muscle strengthening programs to improve running biomechanics and decrease load [5, 19]. Overall, this is similar to that described for pubic rami stress injuries, though the time scale is slightly prolonged with a much more gradual return to run. One case series of eight female runners noted that it took 6 months for athletes to be entirely pain free with running, and 8 months to return to pre-injury activity level, though most other case series reported shorter times for return to sport [21]. There were no reported complications among the reviewed cases. However, as in other BSI, there is a theoretical risk of nonunion or progression with improper treatment.

29.2.3 Ileum

29.2.3.1 Epidemiology and Mechanism

BSIs of the ileum are even more rare than those of the sacrum or pubic rami. In fact, to our knowledge only eight case reports of ileum BSIs in athletes have been published [26–32], though adolescent apophyseal injuries were not included. Of these reported cases, only one was male and all were endurance runners. Many had one or more risk factors for the female or male athlete triad including low energy availability or oligomenorrhea [26, 27, 29, 31, 32]. At least three had a history of prior BSI [26, 31, 32]. Even more so than other pelvic BSIs, those in the ileum are very difficult to diagnose, and many athletes spend years with incorrect diagnoses.

One of the proposed mechanisms for iliac wing BSIs is thought to be related to the competing pulls of the iliacus muscle and the gluteal muscles while running. The competing muscle pulls of the gluteal and iliacus muscles or the sartorius muscle produce an increased stress response within the bone, increasing osteoclastic activity disproportionately, with localized weakening of the bone and microfractures [5, 29, 33].

29.2.3.2 Presentation and Examination

Most athletes present with poorly localized pain, often lasting for a prolonged period of time. At least five of the eight reported cases initially presented with pain for over 4 weeks [26, 29, 30, 32] usually located in the buttock, gluteal or sacral region, though lateral hip pain has also been described. Of note, several athletes mentioned a sensation of muscle tightness, either in the buttock or groin [26, 32], and potentially tenderness to palpation over the piriformis muscle [26, 32] in addition to tenderness over the iliac crest or sacroiliac joint [26, 27, 29, 32]. Athletes may present with physical exam findings that initially point towards alternative diagnoses, potentially delaying treatment [26, 27, 32].

29.2.3.3 Diagnosis and Classification

Like the sacrum, the ileum can be difficult to visualize on radiographs from obscuring bowel gas and soft tissues. All described cases used MRI for diagnosis, sometimes in conjunction with either screening bone scintigraphy or confirmatory CT. From the osteoporosis literature, there are three main types of iliac insufficiency fractures, which tend to follow the lines of attachment of the gluteal muscles. Type 1, supra-acetabular, has a fracture above and parallel to the acetabular roof. Type 2, oblique iliac, has a fracture extending diagonally across the iliac ala from the greater sciatic notch. Type 3, superomedial iliac, has a fracture adjacent to the sacroiliac joint with potential extension into the sacroiliac joint [33]. The majority of reported sport-related BSIs are type 3, superomedial [29–32]. However, there is one reported case of a BSI just superior to the ASIS and the attachment of the sartorius muscle [27]. These BSIs appear primarily as bone marrow edema within the ilium, with or without a distinct fracture line depending on the grade. See Fig. 29.3.

29.2.3.4 Treatment, Rehabilitation, and Potential Complications

Treatment follows the standard two-phase approach for all pelvic BSIs outlined under pubic rami BSIs. Many athletes will initially require a period of non-weight bearing on crutches because of pain while walking. This period typically lasts approximately 2 weeks, followed by approximately 4–6 weeks of decreased impact strengthening and cross training. Once pain-free with all rehab-related activities, the athlete can start phase two with a gradual return to run program over approximately 3 months [27, 29].

No complications were reported in the case reports. One athlete continued to run despite medical recommendations, but she was lost to follow up, and therefore it is unknown if she developed a non-union or fracture progression [29].

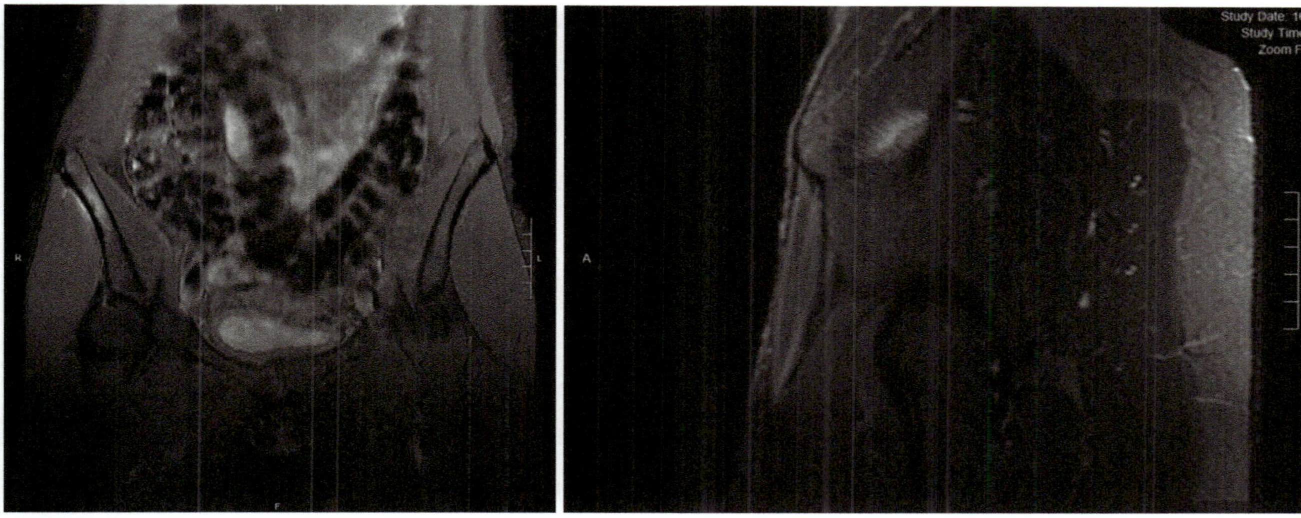

Fig. 29.3 Iliac wing bone stress injury in a 21 year old female NCAA track athlete presenting with a 3 week history of progressive low back pain with activity with tenderness to palpation of the right SI joint and sacrum (coronal and sagittal T2)

29.2.4 Acetabulum

29.2.4.1 Epidemiology and Mechanism

BSIs of the acetabulum are exceedingly rare. In a study of military recruits with unilateral hip pain, 12/178 (6.7%) had acetabular BSI [34]. When analyzed by gender, 10/167 (6.0%) men presenting with hip pain and 2/11 (18.2%) women presenting with hip pain were found to have acetabular BSIs. Almost all of these received a diagnosis of other BSIs of the hip and pelvis simultaneously, including the ispilateral inferior pubic rami BSIs, contralateral acetabulum, femoral neck and proximal femoral shaft [34]. In contrast to other pelvic BSIs, acetabular BSIs have not been reported in distance runners, but one has been found in a female gymnast with risk factors for female athlete triad [1], a male motocross athlete [35], and a male power lifter [36].

The nature of these cases suggest that acetabular BSIs may be related to higher impact activities as opposed to repetitive impact such as in distance running. The gymnast initially noted discomfort following a gainer full dismount from the balance beam [1], the weight lifter noted pain after attempting to deadlift 530 lb. during an amateur strongman competition [36], and the motocross athete, a sport that involves significant prolonged core musculature activation with ongoing impact, noted pain with both competition and practice [35]. The theoretical mechanism would be from repetitive high impact stress transmitted through the hip to the acetabular roof, leading to increased osteoclastic activity and subsequent weakening of the acetabulum making it susceptible to microfractures.

29.2.4.2 Presentation and Examination

Athletes may present with insidious onset groin pain or buttock pain which progressively worsens over time. On examination, patients may have tenderness to palpation given the bone's location lying deep within the muscular structures. Hip range of motion, especially hip flexion and internal or external rotation, may reproduce symptoms. Otherwise, full physical examination may be useful to exclude other diagnoses [1, 35, 36].

29.2.4.3 Diagnosis and Classification

The case studies of acetabular BSIs reported negative radiographs, but positive findings on bone scintigraphy and/or MRI. These BSIs were classified into two categories including acetabular roof and anterior column BSIs. In the first category, T2-weighted and STIR MRI imaging demonstrated increased marrow signal in the superior and lateral aspect of the acetabulum consistent with marrow edema. 5/7 of patients in this category had additional BSIs, including the ipsilateral inferior pubic ramus, the femoral neck, and the proximal femoral shaft. In the second category, T1-weighted and STIR MRI imaging demonstrated increased marrow signal with a vertical fracture line in the anterior column. 4/5 patients with anterior column BSIs had ipsilateral inferior pubic ramus BSI [34]. These BSIs can be classified in the same fashion full acetabular fractures, though the classification does not change treatment. The MRI grade of the BSI will affect timeline to recovery. See Fig. 29.4.

29.2.4.4 Treatment, Rehabilitation, and Complications

Treatment and rehabilitation following acetabular BSIs follows the same treatment algorithm described above starting with initial non-weight bearing, then cross training and strengthening, followed by gradual return to sport. The motocross athlete was able to return to full training at 4 months and competitions by 6 months. This is generally considered to be the typical timeline for healing of pelvic BSIs [35].

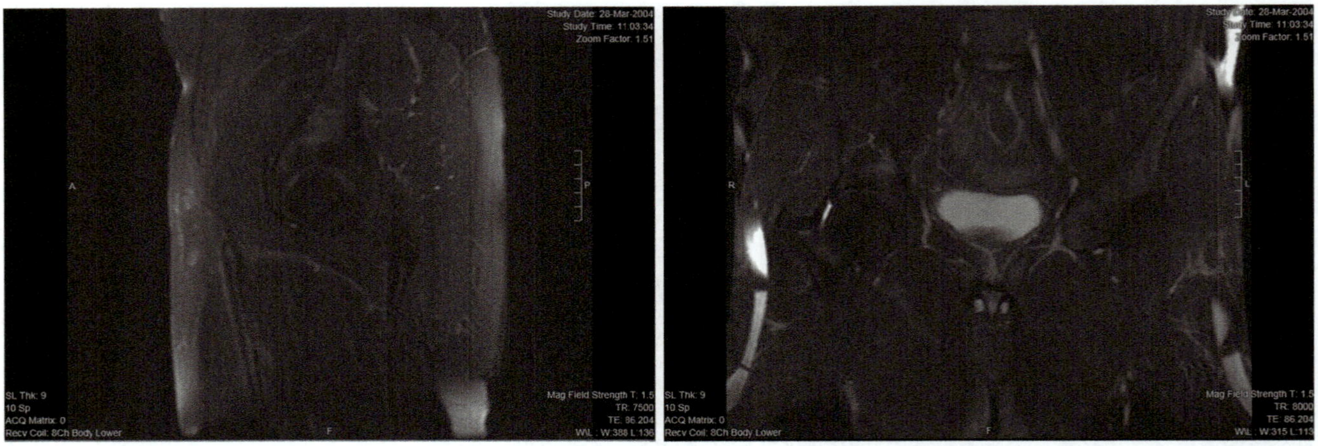

Fig. 29.4 Acetabular roof bone stress injury in a 20 year old male NCAA football player presenting with groin and buttock pain (sagittal and coronal T2)

Two of the three reported cases with acetabular BSIs experienced significant complications, including delayed healing and completion of fracture. The gymnast's bone healing was delayed because of her female athlete triad risk factors. Despite addressing her low energy availability with gradual weight gain (6.6 kg over several months), activity restrictions, and resumption of menses, she still had delayed healing at 16 weeks. She was prescribed supplemental teraparatide to assist with bone healing. She was asymptomatic by 27 weeks and gradually returned to gymnastics over the next 2 months, making her total recovery time approximately 8 months [1]. Non-unions or delayed healing are much more common if the athlete fails to follow weight bearing restrictions, or in the setting of low bone mineral density and/or low energy availability. Athletes with low energy availability benefit from a multidisciplinary team approach involving a sports dietician and, in some cases, an endocrinologist. The weight lifter, on the other hand, ignored his groin pain with activity for 3 months, ultimately leading to a complete fracture [36].

29.2.5 Osteitis Pubis

29.2.5.1 Epidemiology and Mechanism

Osteitis Pubis (OP) can be considered a bone stress injury of the symphysis pubis. It is often an overlapping condition with athletic pubalgia or sports hernia, and the literature has occasionally interchanged or combined these conditions [37]. The diagnosis can be difficult given the large number of potential sources of groin pain. For the purposes of this chapter, osteitis pubis refers to pubic BSI including edema of the pubic bones, pubic symphysis and adjacent structures in acute OP and other joint findings in chronic OP. Athletic pubalgia, with isolated microtearing of the rectus abdominis or adductor muscles, is considered a separate entity, though it may be a precursor to OP.

Groin pain in athletes occurs at a rate of 2–5%, and is much higher in field-based kicking sports such as soccer and rugby, though it is also common in ice hockey, fencing, and running [38]. Given the heterogeneity of diagnostic criteria in the literature, it is difficult to assess the exact incidence of OP, though it has been reported as high as 8% [37]. Of athletes presenting to clinic with chronic activity-related groin pain, up to 85% are diagnosed with OP [39]. Male soccer players are 10–18% of all athletes diagnosed with OP [37]. OP was thought to be much more common in men, with over 90% of reported cases in the literature being male prior to 2011 [40]. However, recently OP has been more commonly reported in women, potentially since more women are training at an elite level [41]. Of note, OP is particularly common following pregnancy or urological or gynecological procedures[xlii]. More women are returning to sports following pregnancy, and may be at increased risk for developing OP during this time frame.

The rectus abdominis tendon and the three adductor tendons stabilize the anterior pelvis through their attachment to the fibrocartilage plate of the symphysis pubis. The three adductor muscles work as antagonists, with the rectus elevating and the adductors depressing the anterior pelvis. The symphysis pubis acts as a fulcrum for force generated at the anterior pelvis. Injury or weakness in one of these muscle groups can increase the stress across the symphysis and alter biomechanics. In sports with multidirectional movements and/or kicking, the pubic symphysis is under continuous stress, thereby leading to stress in both the symphysis and the adjacent bones [42]. Femoro-acetabular impingement (FAI), especially Cam-type, may predispose athletes to the development of athletic pubalgia or OP since the decreased hip range of motion may lead to compensatory increased motion at the symphysis pubis and sacroiliac joint with resultant increased stress [43]. The prevalence of OP in patients with FAI can be as high as 43.48%, though a more recent study only found MRI evidence of OP in 1.8% (15/830) of patients undergoing arthroscopy for FAI [43].

29.2.5.2 Presentation and Examination

Athletes present with insidious onset of groin pain especially with kicking, running, jumping, cutting, or twisting. Pain may include the symphysis pubis, adductor muscles, lower abdominal muscles, perineal region, inguinal region, and scrotum and is exacerbated by eccentric loading [37]. Generally, the pain is described as deep and intense, and is often unilateral. It can also radiate into the perineum or scrotum [41]. Some athletes will note a clicking sensation at the symphysis pubis [44].

Many different examination techniques have been described, though most have not been validated [37]. Consistently, authors note tenderness to palpation of the symphysis pubis and adjacent pubic bones, though it is important to look for recreation of the athlete's typical pain. Classically, athletes present with an antalgic "waddling" gait [45] and may also have pain with active straight leg raise [46]. Weakness of the adductors or decreased hip range of motion due to FAI may be found on examination since these are potential predisposing factors [37]. While most of these tests are not validated, an increasing number of positive tests could raise your clinical suspicion for OP. The spring test, considered to be the most specific test, is performed by placing simultaneous downward pressure on both pubic rami. Pain at the pubic symphysis is considered a positive test [42, 45]. The lateral compression test is performed in the lateral decubitus position and downward pressure is placed on the superior iliac wing [45]. A positive test result is pain at the pubic symphysis. Verrall et al. described three pain provocation tests. The symphysis gap test or squeeze test is performed supine with hips and knees flexed to 90° with the examiners fist between their knees. The athlete then performs an isometric adductor contraction against the first. Pain in the groin and symphysis pubis is considered a positive test result. For the single adductor test, the athlete is supine with one leg at 0° of hip flexion and the other at 30°. They then have to resist abduction in the leg at 30°. Pain in either pubic bone or adductor region is a positive test. Finally, for the bilateral adductor test the athlete is supine and raises his/her legs to approximately 30° of hip flexion with slight abduction and internal rotation. The athlete then resists bilateral examiner abduction. Groin pain is considered a positive test [47].

29.2.5.3 Diagnosis and Classification

Unlike the other pelvic BSIs discussed above, OP does have findings noted on radiographs, though most of these findings present at later stages of the disease process. Bone scintigraphy will show tracer uptake in the pubic symphysis and parasymphyseal bone, but is non-specific [37]. As with other pelvic BSIs, MRI is now considered the gold standard. MRI in acute stages of OP demonstrates subchondral bone edema along the margins of the symphysis pubis, potentially with edema in the symphyseal joint or in surrounding muscles [41]. Bone marrow edema is the hallmark of the active phase of the disease, seen in 70–91% of patients, though it may disappear in the more chronic setting [39]. If the athlete has concomitant athletic pubalgia, they may have a superior cleft sign, from microtearing of the rectus abdominis or adductor longus attachment, or the secondary cleft sign from microtearing of the short adductor attachment [38]. Radiographs can become useful in the more chronic phases and demonstrate subchondral sclerosis, osteophytosis, bony irregularity, symphyseal lytic changes, symmetrical bone resorption with subsequent widening of the symphysis [37, 44]. MRI also demonstrates these same chronic findings. Of note, many of these findings have been identified in up to 76% of asymptomatic soccer players, and should only be interpreted in the setting of appropriate clinical suspicion [48]. The most specific findings for OP are seen on the flamingo views. These consist of two APs of the pelvis, one standing on both legs and the other standing on one leg. Greater than 7 mm of widening of the symphysis pubis or greater than 2 mm vertical displacement with the flamingo views are both considered specific for OP [44]. See Fig. 29.5.

A few classifications are available, though none have been externally validated by other groups. The initial proposed grading scale by Rodriguez et al. in 2001 was entirely based on clinical presentation. Stage 1 involved unilateral symptoms and inguinal pain in the adductor muscles that subsides after warm-up and recurs after training. Stage 2 consisted of bilateral inguinal pain that increases after training. Stage 3 included bilateral inguinal pain involving both the adductors and abdomen and the athlete is unable to continue sport participation. Stage 4 involved pain in the adductor and abdominal muscles referred to the pelvic girdle and lumbar spine with defecation, sneezing, or walking on uneven terrain that impairs the athlete's ability to perform activities of daily living. Based on this scale, stage 1 athletes were able to return to full play after 3.8 weeks, stage 2 after 6.7 weeks, stage 3 after 10 weeks, and stage 4 required surgery [49].

Two additional classifications based on MRI findings have been proposed, though one has not been found to correlate with clinical return to play or injury severity. The other, proposed by Gaudino et al., was based on a retrospective analysis of MRI findings which correlated to incomplete recovery after 18 months. For this scale, grade 1 requires bone marrow edema in the pubic bone with or without periarticular edema. Grade 2 also has bone marrow edema, but with both periarticular edema and edema in the muscles

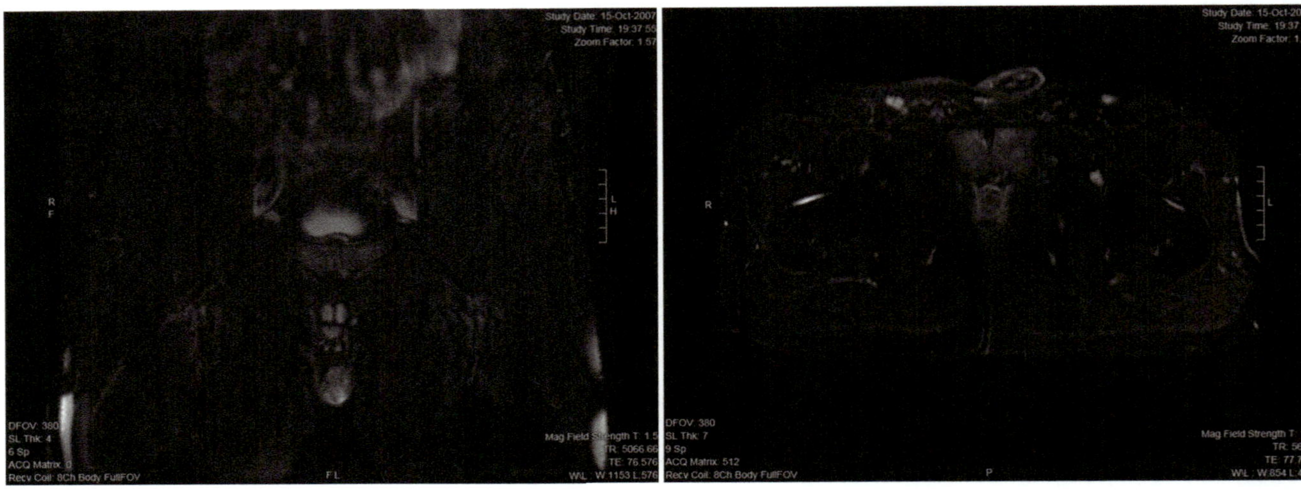

Fig. 29.5 Osteitis pubis with bone stress injury in a 26 year old recreational soccer player presenting with 3 months of gradual onset groin pain (coronal and axial T2)

around the symphyseal joint. Grade 3 has bone marrow edema, but with a highest mean normalized STIR signal greater than 3 and either periarticular edema or edema in the muscles around the symphyseal joint. Finally, grade 4 has bone marrow edema with a highest mean normalized STIR signal greater than 3 and both periarticular edema and edema in the muscles around the symphyseal joint. Based on their algorithm, 100% of those in grade 1 should make a full recovery with only conservative treatment, 50% in grade 2, 30% in grade 3, and 20% in grade 4 [41]. Since the degree of bone marrow edema may be prognostically important, diffusion weighted imaging is a key component of MRI evaluation [39]. While these grading scales may have some value, the lack of external validation of their findings leaves them with limited utility at this point.

29.2.5.4 Treatment, Rehabilitation, and Complications

The vast majority of athletes with OP will improve without surgery or injections. Choi et al. presented a comprehensive review in 2011. When analyzing six case series including 53 athletes treated with progressive rehabilitation (n = 52), NSAIDs (n = 36), and compression shorts (n = 11), the average return to play was 9.6 weeks with a range from 3 to 13 weeks. While the compression shorts mildly improved pain scores, there was no difference in their performance [40]. Generally, individualized progressive rehabilitation is the mainstay of treatment.

There have been several proposed rehabilitation protocols which move athletes through 3–5 stages of rehabilitation as they reach concrete markers. We have primarily based the protocol below on the one proposed by McAleer et al. (Fig. 29.6) [46]. Schöberl et al. in a level 1 randomized control trial found that the addition of shock wave therapy to a progressive rehabilitation model decreased the return to play time from approximately 102.6 days to 73.2 days. They also followed a control group, who had declined the progressive rehabilitation program, and noted that their return to play took over 8 months and many noted frequent recurrences of pain [50].

Various injections or non-surgical interventions have been investigated. One case series evaluated the use of prolotherapy in 24 athletes with 15 months of prior symptoms. Athletes received around three injections of a dextrose solution at eight sites, with 22 returning to sport in 9 weeks and two failing to respond [40]. Masala et al. in 2015 trialed pulse-dose radio frequency on 32 patients with refractory symptoms targeting the genital branches of the genitofemoral, ilioinguinal, iliohypogastric, and obturator nerves. Twenty-four had significant pain reduction after one treatment and an additional six had relief after a second treatment. There were no reported complications [37]. Recently, a single case report detailed the effects of needle tenotomy and platelet-rich plasma injection with return to play in 8 weeks [37]. Choi et al. reviewed multiple case series evaluating corticosteroid injections in patients with refractory symptoms. 17 of 29 were able to return to sport after 8 weeks without recurrence of pain, an additional five had some relief, but subsequent recurrent pain [40]. These findings suggest that, while various injections may be helpful to initiate recovery in athletes with refractory symptoms, they are not a replacement for progressive rehabilitation and should likely be done in conjunction.

In general, surgery is only considered after an athlete has already completed at least 3 months of a well-conducted rehabilitation protocol with no relief. Some authors

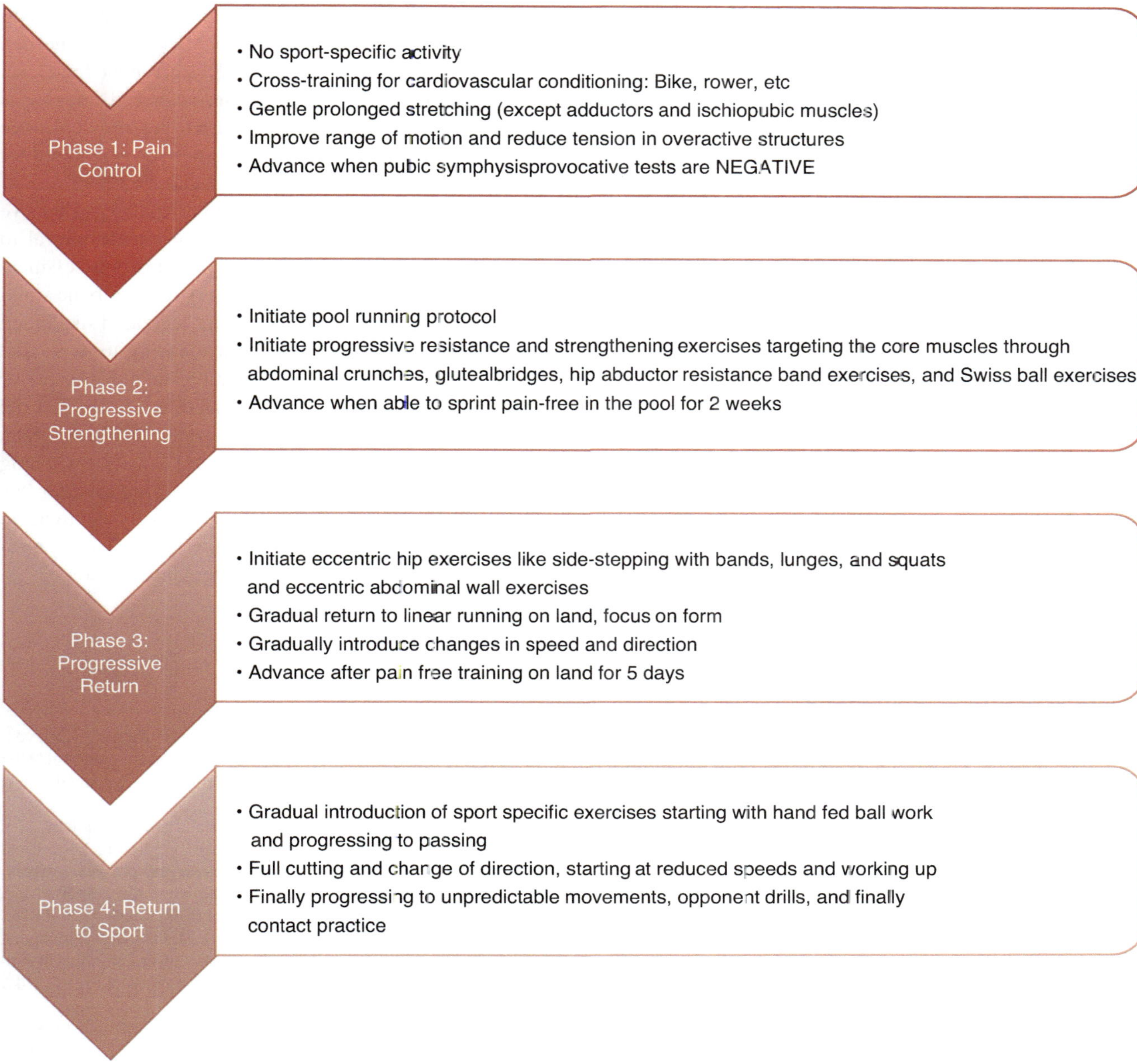
Phase 1: Pain Control
• No sport-specific activity
• Cross-training for cardiovascular conditioning: Bike, rower, etc
• Gentle prolonged stretching (except adductors and ischiopubic muscles)
• Improve range of motion and reduce tension in overactive structures
• Advance when pubic symphysisprovocative tests are NEGATIVE
Phase 2: Progressive Strengthening
• Initiate pool running protocol
• Initiate progressive resistance and strengthening exercises targeting the core muscles through abdominal crunches, glutealbridges, hip abductor resistance band exercises, and Swiss ball exercises
• Advance when able to sprint pain-free in the pool for 2 weeks
Phase 3: Progressive Return
• Initiate eccentric hip exercises like side-stepping with bands, lunges, and squats and eccentric abdominal wall exercises
• Gradual return to linear running on land, focus on form
• Gradually introduce changes in speed and direction
• Advance after pain free training on land for 5 days
Phase 4: Return to Sport
• Gradual introduction of sport specific exercises starting with hand fed ball work and progressing to passing
• Full cutting and change of direction, starting at reduced speeds and working up
• Finally progressing to unpredictable movements, opponent drills, and finally contact practice

Fig. 29.6 Progressive rehabilitation

report that surgical intervention is required for 5–10% of patients with OP. Many different surgical procedures have been proposed, including curettage of the symphysis pubis, arthrodesis of the symphysis with or without bone graft, and wedge resection, often with the associated release of adductor tendons or adductor enthesis repair. Most of the articles are retrospective case series, without clinical trials comparing various treatments. While time to return to play varies based on the surgical procedure, most report that most athletes are able to return to sport in 3–4 months without recurrence [37].

29.3 Conclusion

Pelvic BSIs are relatively rare, but can be difficult to diagnose. For all the above conditions, MRI is the gold standard of diagnosis and findings are often missed on plain radiographs. While severe complications are uncommon, rehabilitation for these BSIs tends to take longer than BSIs in other locations. With the right treatment algorithm including initial rest followed by gradual return to activity over months and management of contributing risk factors, pelvic BSIs will heal without surgical interventions or other complications.

Clinical Pearls

- Maintain a high index of suspicion for pelvic BSI in a repetitive stress athlete, especially distance runners, presenting with unilateral pelvic pain that is worse with activity with focal bony tenderness on examination.
- Prescribe a cautious treatment algorithm to patients with pelvic BSIs including initial activity modification, strengthening, and then gradual return to activity.

Review

Questions

1. A 21 year old female cross country runner presents to your clinic with left sided upper buttock pain with running that has been getting progressively worse over the last 2 weeks to the point that she is no longer able to run. She has focal tenderness to palpation over the left sacrum and sacroiliac joint. Initial radiographs are negative. What would be the best next step in management?
   (a) Advise the patient to avoid running for 2 weeks and then return to prior level of competition
   (b) MRI of the pelvis
   (c) Bone scintigraphy scan
   (d) DEXA scan
2. A 30 year old female ultra-marathon runner is seen in your clinic for a left sacral bone stress injury. She has a history of a right pubic rami bone stress injury 4 months ago and she returned to competition 2 months previously. Her BMI is 17.5. She is currently pain free with activities of daily living and is following a gradual return to activity protocol. What additional management is important in this case?
   (a) Referral to gynecology to assess for premature menopause
   (b) Bisphosphonate treatment for osteoporosis
   (c) Comprehensive treatment of likely female athlete triad with referral to sports nutritionist and bone mineral density assessment
   (d) Strongly encourage the athlete to quit running and start swimming since she is at high risk for recurrent bone stress injuries

Answers

1. The correct answer to this question is (b) MRI of the pelvis in order to evaluate for sacral bone stress injury (BSI). Sacral BSIs are notoriously difficult to diagnose on plain radiographs and MRI is the most sensitive and specific diagnostic test. While bone scintigraphy (c) is sensitive for BSI, it is very non-specific. DEXA scan (d) to assess bone mineral density can be helpful in the setting of BSI to evaluate for female athlete triad, MRI would be needed first to confirm the diagnosis. Finally, given the high level of suspicion for BSI in this case, advanced imaging is necessary prior to initiating a return to run protocol since a prolonged period of activity modification is required for full healing (a). See Sects. 29.2.2.3 and 29.2.2.4.
2. The correct answer to this question is (c) Comprehensive treatment of likely female athlete triad with referral to sports nutritionist and bone mineral density assessment given the low BMI (17.5) and history of prior bone stress injury. The most likely cause of her increased likelihood for BSI is low energy availability leading to decreased bone mineral density, not premature menopause (a) or premature osteoporosis (b). She needs treatment focused on the root issue, the low energy availability, rather than focusing only on the low bone mineral density. Switching to a sport such as swimming (d) will not improve her low bone mineral density since she will likely continue to struggle with low energy availability. The root issue must be targeted with a focused nutritional intervention.

References

1. Gende A, Thomsen TW, Marcussen B, Hettrich C. Delayed-union of acetabular stress fracture in female gymnast. Clin J Sport Med. 2019;30(5):e163–5. https://doi.org/10.1097/jsm.0000000000000739.
2. Nattiv A, Kennedy G, Barrack M, Abdelkerim A, Goolsby MA, Arends JC, Leanne L. Correlation of MRI grading of bone stress injuries with clinical risk factors and return to play: a 5-year prospective study in collegiate track and field athletes. Am J Sports Med. 2015;41(8):1930–41. https://doi.org/10.1177/0363546513490645.
3. Kahanov L, Eberman L, Games K, Wasik M. Diagnosis, treatment, and rehabilitation of stress fractures in the lower extremity in runners. Open Access J Sports Med. 2015;87 https://doi.org/10.2147/oajsm.s39512.
4. Behrens SB, Deren ME, Matson A, Fadale PD, Monchik KO. Stress fractures of the pelvis and legs in athletes: a review. Sports Health. 2013;5(2):165–74. https://doi.org/10.1177/1941738112467423.
5. Fredericson M, Jennings F, Beaulieu C, Matheson G. Stress fracture in athletes. Joint Bone Spine. 2018;85(3):307–10. https://doi.org/10.1016/j.jbspin.2017.04.013.
6. Bencardino JT, Stone TJ, Roberts CC, Appel M, Baccei SJ, Cassidy RC, et al. ACR Appropriateness Criteria® stress (fatigue/insufficiency) fracture, including sacrum, excluding other vertebrae. J Am Coll Radiol. 2017;14(5):S293–306. https://doi.org/10.1016/j.jacr.2017.02.035.
7. Dalstra M, Huiskes R, Odgaard A, van Erning L. Mechanical and textural properties of pelvic trabecular bone. J Biomech. 1993;26(4–5):523–35. https://doi.org/10.1016/0021-9290(93)90014-6.
8. Ott SM. Cortical or trabecular bone: what's the difference? Am J Nephrol. 2018;47(6):373–5. https://doi.org/10.1159/000489672.
9. Tenforde AS, Parziale AL, Popp KL, Ackerman KE. Low bone mineral density in male athletes is associated with bone stress injuries at anatomic sites with greater trabecular composition. Am J Sports Med. 2018;46(1):30–6. https://doi.org/10.1177/0363546517730584.
10. De Souza MJ, Nattiv A, Joy E, et al. 2014 female athlete triad coalition consensus statement on treatment and return to play of

the female athlete triad: 1st international conference held in san Francisco, California, May 2012 and 2nd international conference held in Indianapolis, Indiana, May 2013. Br J Sports Med. 2014;48(4):289.
11. Tenforde AS, Carlson JL, Chang A, Sainani KL, Shultz R, Kim JH, et al. Association of the female athlete triad risk assessment stratification to the development of bone stress injuries in collegiate athletes. Am J Sports Med. 2017;45(2):302–10. https://doi.org/10.1177/0363546516676262.
12. Arendt E, Agel J, Heikes C, Griffiths H. Stress injuries to bone in college athletes. A retrospective review of experience at a single institution. Am J Sports Med. 2003;31(6):959–68. https://doi.org/10.1177/03635465030310063601.
13. Pavlov H, Nelson T, Warren R, Torg J, Burstin A. Stress fractures of the pubic ramus. J Bone Joint Surg. 1982;64-A(7):1020–5.
14. Noakes TD, Smith JA, Lindenberg G, Wills CE. Pelvic stress fractures in long distance runners. Am J Sports Med. 1985;13(2):120–3. Retrieved from pm:3985259.
15. Lee SW, Lee CH. Fatigue stress fractures of the pubic ramus in the army: imaging features with radiographic, scintigraphic and MR imaging findings. Korean J Radiol. 2005;6(1):47–51. https://doi.org/10.3348/kjr.2005.6.1.47.
16. El Ghoch M, Bazzani P, Grave RD. Management of ischiopubic stress fracture in patients with anorexia nervosa and excessive compulsive exercising. BMJ Case Rep. 2014;2014:1–4. https://doi.org/10.1136/bcr-2014-206393.
17. Fredericson M, Salamancha L, Beaulieu C. Sacral stress fractures: tracking down nonspecific pain in distance runners. Phys Sportsmed. 2003;31(2):31–42. https://doi.org/10.3810/psm.2003.02.189.
18. Liong SY, Whitehouse RW. Lower extremity and pelvic stress fractures in athletes. Br J Radiol. 2012;85(1016):1148–56. https://doi.org/10.1259/bjr/78510315.
19. Johnson AW, Weiss CB, Stento K, Wheeler DL. Stress fractures of the sacrum. An atypical cause of low back pain in the female athlete. Am J Sports Med. 2001;29(4):498–508. https://doi.org/10.1177/03635465010290042001.
20. Ahovuo JA, Kiuru MJ, Visuri T. Fatigue stress fractures of the sacrum: diagnosis with MR imaging. Eur Radiol. 2004;14(3):500–5. https://doi.org/10.1007/s00330-003-1989-2.
21. Kaneko H, Murakami M, Nishizawa K. Prevalence and clinical features of sports-related lumbosacral stress injuries in the young. Arch Orthop Trauma Surg. 2017;137(5):685–91. https://doi.org/10.1007/s00402-017-2686-y.
22. Eller D, Katz D, Bergman A, Fredericson M, Beaulieu C. Sacral stress fractures in long-distance runners. Clin J Sport Med. 1997;7(3):222–5.
23. Yan CXB, Vautour L, Martin MH. Postpartum sacral insufficiency fractures. Skelet Radiol. 2016;45(3):413–7. https://doi.org/10.1007/s00256-015-2289-z.
24. Fredericson M, Moore W, Biswal S. Sacral stress fractures: magnetic resonance imaging not always definitive for early stage injuries – a report of 2 cases. Am J Sports Med. 2007;35(5):835–9. https://doi.org/10.1177/0363546506296519.
25. Harris CE, Vincent HK, Vincent KR. Sacral stress fractures: they see you, but are you seeing them? Curr Sports Med Rep. 2016;15(2):73. https://doi.org/10.1249/JSR.0000000000000245.
26. Tenforde AS, Watanabe LM, Moreno TJ, Fredericson M. Use of an antigravity treadmill for rehabilitation of a pelvic stress injury. PM R. 2012;4(8):629–31. https://doi.org/10.1016/j.pmrj.2012.02.003.
27. West AM, McInnis KC. Unusual iliac crest stress fracture in a marathoner: a case presentation. PM R. 2018;10(7):775–8. https://doi.org/10.1016/j.pmrj.2017.11.009.
28. Atlihan D, Quick D, Guanche CA. Stress fracture of the iliac bone in a young female runner. Orthopedics. 2003;26(7):729–30.
29. Vitale K, Smitaman E, Huang BK. Medial iliac stress fractures in athletes: report of two rare cases: review of literature and clinical recommendations. Skelet Radiol. 2019;48(7):1119–23. https://doi.org/10.1007/s00256-018-3117-z.
30. Battaglia M, Guaraldi F, Vannini F, Vanel D, Giannini S. Unusual supero-medial iliac fatigue stress fracture. Skelet Radiol. 2012;41(1):103–6.
31. Amorosa LF, Serota AC, Berman N, Lorich DG, Helfet DL. An isolated iliac wing stress fracture in a marathon runner. Am J Orthop. 2014;43(2):74–7.
32. Touhy J, Nattiv A. Iliac stress fracture in a male collegiate track athlete. Curr Sports Med Rep. 2008;7(5):252–4. https://doi.org/10.1249/JSR.0b013e3181873326.
33. Davies A, Bradley S. Iliac insufficiency fractures. Br J Radiol. 1991;64(760):305–9.
34. Williams TR, Puckett ML, Denison G, Shin AY, Gorman JD. Acetabular stress fractures in military endurance athletes and recruits: incidence and MRI and scintigraphic findings. Skelet Radiol. 2002;31(5):277–81. https://doi.org/10.1007/s00256-002-0485-0.
35. de Paiva Luciano A, Filho NF. Stress fracture in acetabular roof due to motocross: case report. Rev Bras Ortop. 2016;51(3):374–7. https://doi.org/10.1016/j.rboe.2016.03.004.
36. Karnes JM, Hagedorn JC, Hubbard DF. Catastrophic failure of an acetabular stress fracture in a healthy male power lifter. Am J Sports Med. 2015;43(10):2559–63. https://doi.org/10.1177/0363546515593953.
37. Giai Via A, Frizziero A, Finotti P, Oliva F, Randelli F, Maffulli N. Management of osteitis pubis in athletes: rehabilitation and return to training: a review of the most recent literature. Open Access J Sports Med. 2018;10:1–10. https://doi.org/10.2147/oajsm.s155077.
38. Byrne CA, Bowden DJ, Alkhayat A, Kavanagh EC, Eustace SJ. Sports-related groin pain secondary to symphysis pubis disorders: correlation between MRI findings and outcome after fluoroscopy-guided injection of steroid and local anesthetic. Am J Roentgenol. 2017;209(2):380–8. https://doi.org/10.2214/AJR.16.17578.
39. Erdem Toslak I, Cekic B, Turk A, Eraslan A, Parlak AE. Evaluation of diffusion-weighted MR imaging as a technique for detecting bone marrow edema in patients with osteitis pubis. Magn Reson Med Sci. 2017;16(4):317–24. https://doi.org/10.2463/mrms.mp.2016-0104.
40. Choi H, McCartney M, Best T. Symphysis in athletes: a systematic review. Br J Sports Med. 2011;45(1):57–64. https://doi.org/10.1136/bjsm.2008.050989.Treatment.
41. Gaudino F, Spira D, Bangert Y, Ott H, Beomonte Zobel B, Kauczor HU, Weber MA. Osteitis pubis in professional football players: MRI findings and correlation with clinical outcome. Eur J Radiol. 2017;94(April):46–52. https://doi.org/10.1016/j.ejrad.2017.07.009.
42. Mather RC, Ferrell MS. Athletic hip injuries. Orthop Knowl Update Sports Med. 2018;25(4):115–26. https://doi.org/10.5435/JAAOS-D-16-00171.
43. Krishnamoorthy VP, Kunze KN, Beck EC, Cancienne JM, O'Keefe LS, Ayeni OR, Nho SJ. Radiographic prevalence of symphysis pubis abnormalities and clinical outcomes in patients with femoroacetabular impingement syndrome. Am J Sports Med. 2019;47(6):1467–72. https://doi.org/10.1177/0363546519837203.
44. Miller C, Major N, Toth A. Pelvic stress injuries in the athlete: management and prevention. Sports Med. 2003;33(13):1003–12. https://doi.org/10.2165/00007256-200333130-00005.
45. Gomella P, Mufarrij P. Osteitis pubis: a rare cause of suprapubic pain. Rev Urol. 2017;19(3):156–63. https://doi.org/10.3909/riu0767.
46. McAleer SS, Lippie E, Norman D, Riepenhof H. Nonoperative management, rehabilitation, and functional and clinical progression of osteitis pubis/pubic bone stress in professional soccer players: a case series. J Orthop Sports Phys Ther. 2017;47(9):683–90. https://doi.org/10.2519/jospt.2017.7314.

47. Verrall GM, Slavotinek JP, Barnes PG, Fon GT. Description of pain provocation tests used for the diagnosis of sports-related chronic groin pain: relationship of tests to defined clinical (pain and tenderness) and MRI (pubic bone marrow oedema) criteria. Scand J Med Sci Sports. 2005;15(1):36–42. https://doi.org/10.1111/j.1600-0838.2004.00380.x.
48. Elattar O, Choi HR, Dills VD, Busconi B. Groin injuries (athletic pubalgia) and return to play. Sports Health. 2016;8(4):313–23. https://doi.org/10.1177/1941738116653711.
49. Rodriguez C, Miguel A, Lima H, Heinrichs K. Osteitis pubis syndrome in the professional soccer athlete: a case report. J Athl Train. 2001;36(4):437–40.
50. Schöberl M, Prantl L, Loose O, Zellner J, Angele P, Zeman F, et al. Non-surgical treatment of pubic overload and groin pain in amateur football players: a prospective double-blinded randomised controlled study. Knee Surg Sports Traumatol Arthrosc. 2017;25(6):1958–66. https://doi.org/10.1007/s00167-017-4423-z.

Correction to: Fractures in Sport

Greg A. J. Robertson and Nicola Maffulli

Correction to: **G. A. J. Robertson, N. Maffulli (eds.), Fractures in Sport, https://doi.org/10.1007/978-3-030-72036-0**

This book was inadvertently a spelling error in 2nd editor's surname. The correct name is Nicola Maffulli, this has been updated with this erratum.

The updated version of the book can be found at
https://doi.org/10.1007/978-3-030-72036-0

G. A. J. Robertson, N. Maffulli (eds.), *Fractures in Sport*, https://doi.org/10.1007/978-3-030-72036-0_3C

Index

G. A. J. Robertson, N. Maffulli (eds.), *Fractures in Sport*, https://doi.org/10.1007/978-3-030-72036-0

P

Q

R

GPSR Compliance

The European Union's (EU) General Product Safety Regulation (GPSR) is a set of rules that requires consumer products to be safe and our obligations to ensure this.

If you have any concerns about our products, you can contact us on ProductSafety@springernature.com

In case Publisher is established outside the EU, the EU authorized representative is:

Springer Nature Customer Service Center GmbH
Europaplatz 3
69115 Heidelberg, Germany

Batch number: 10731661

Printed by Printforce, the Netherlands